Basic Pharmacology for Nurses

Basic Pharmacology for Nurses

Bruce D. Clayton, B.S., Pharm.D., R.Ph.

Professor of Pharmacy Practice
College of Pharmacy
Butler University
Indianapolis, Indiana

Yvonne N. Stock, R.N., B.S.N., M.S.

Professor of Nursing
Health Occupations Department
Iowa Western Community College
Council Bluff, Iowa

TENTH EDITION

with 226 illustrations

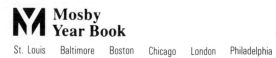
Mosby
Year Book

St. Louis   Baltimore   Boston   Chicago   London   Philadelphia   Sydney   Toronto

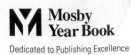

**Mosby
Year Book**

Dedicated to Publishing Excellence

Editor: Robin Carter
Project Manager: Allan S. Kleinberg
Designer: Susan Lane
Photographs: Renee Burgard

A NOTE TO THE READER

The authors and publisher have made every attempt to check dosages and nursing content for accuracy. Because the science of pharmacology is continually advancing, our knowledge base continues to expand. Therefore, we recommend that the reader always check product information for changes in dosage or administration before administering any medication. This is particularly important with new or rarely used drugs.

TENTH EDITION

Printed in the United States of America

Mosby−Year Book, Inc.
11830 Westline Industrial Drive
St. Louis, Missouri 63146

Library of Congress Cataloging in Publication Data

Clayton, Bruce D., 1947-
    Basic pharmacology for nurses / Bruce D. Clayton, Yvonne N. Stock.
  —10th ed.
     p.   cm.
    Includes bibliographical references and index.
    ISBN 0-8016-6431-4
    1. Pharmacology. 2. Nursing. I. Stock, Yvonne N. II. Title.
RM300.C5138 1993
615'.1—dc20   92-20875
                                                CIP

92 93 94 95 96 CL/VH 9 8 7 6 5 4 3 2 1

To **Francine**
for her unfailing support and encouragement
and to
Sarah *and* **Beth**
the lights of our lives

—BDC

To **Henry, Kyle,** *and* **Pamela**
who encouraged and supported me throughout this project
and to my mother
Vivian Washburn
who taught her children nothing was impossible
unless you made it thus

—YNS

Preface

The original purpose of this text, first published in 1957, was to motivate the learner to administer medication with concern for safety, precision, and attention to important physiologic factors. We have done our utmost to maintain these standards that have been synonymous with this book for the past 35 years. To accomplish this responsibility, we conducted extensive discussions and reviews with students, practitioners, and faculty at hospitals and schools of nursing concerning changes in goals, scope and depth of content, and educational format. We offer our gratitude and sincere appreciation for their assistance.

It became apparent very early in our discussions that the primary objectives of the book should not change. Students, practitioners, and faculty felt that it should remain a text to motivate the learner to administer and monitor medication with concern for safety, precision, and attention to important physiologic factors.

The information judged most valuable to our primary purpose is the correlation of pharmacological response to nursing actions (i.e., if a medication causes a certain side effect, how should the nurse respond?). A second major request was to place the role of pharmacology in perspective with the individual patient, the disease being treated, and the nursing process. Practitioners recognize that therapy is only as good as the patient's willingness to accept and follow a treatment regimen. We have therefore identified and correlated items of importance that the nurse must know to integrate patient education about medications into the patient's complete treatment plan.

Every chapter in this edition has been thoroughly reviewed, updated, and enhanced. At the beginning of each chapter is an *outline* of areas of nursing considerations and drug therapy emphasized, followed by *chapter goals*. Units within the chapter start with new *instructional objectives* and *key words* to guide the student in study of the unit. These instructional objectives are also part of the new *Instructor's Manual* that has been developed with this edition. A chapter has also been designed to describe the nursing process and its relationship to pharmacology. The chapter on nursing process includes the latest NANDA nursing diagnoses and incorporates the changes in wording of nursing diagnosis (i.e., a "potential" nursing diagnosis is now a "high risk" nursing diagnosis).

Unit I, Principles of Pharmacology, comprises two chapters. Chapter 1 provides introductory discussions of pharmacology, drug nomenclature, drug and patient information sources, and legal standards for both the United States and Canada. Chapter 2 is a foundational chapter on understanding drug actions, monitoring parameters, patient variables (e.g., pediatric and elderly patients), and drug interactions.

Unit II, Administration of Medications, has been redesigned to include photographs and illustrations to assist the student in learning the proper techniques of medication administration. Chapter 3 provides an extensive review of mathematics including examples of fractions, decimals, and conversions between the metric and avoirdupois systems of weights and measures to assist the student with dosage calculations. The *Instructor's Manual* has practice tests for students' use in perfecting these skills. Chapter 4 describes drug distribution systems, use of medication administration records (MARs), and medication profiles in the acute care and long-term care settings, the patient chart, the principles of nursing responsibilities and ethics, and the six Rights of Medication Administration. The text supports the sixth right—Documentation—by identifying the appropriate nursing actions needed to chart the details of drug administration, the therapeutic effectiveness of each medication administered, the patient teaching to be performed, and the degree of understanding of the medication regimen attained. Chapters 5 to 7 have comprehensive, illustrated sections on dosage forms, administration sites, and techniques of administration. Chapter 6 has been expanded to include information on administration of medications through peripheral, central, or vascular access devices. Procedures are also described for changing of IV dressings, and peripheral and central venous IV needles and catheters, and IV catheter care. The *Instructor's Manual* includes suggestions for the administration of practical exams to assess the student's understanding of dosage forms and principles of medication administration.

Chapter 8 discusses the relationship between the nursing process and pharmacology. This chapter stresses the need to collect, record, and analyze data obtained as part of the patient's drug history. Data collection must include information on the patient's drug history. Data collection must include information on the patient's health beliefs, existing health problems, desire and ability to learn and manage his or her own medication regimen, and prior compliance with prescribed treatment modalities. An extensive section on planning, with reference to the prescribed medications, provides the learner with a step-by-step guide to the important elements to be considered as part of the patient's care. The nursing intervention or implementation phase of the nursing process analyzes the dependent, interdependent, and independent nursing actions related to drug therapy. The section on evaluation of therapeutic outcomes guides the learner through the essential elements of patient education and the nurse's role in fostering patient responsibility for the maintenance of his or her well-being and the benefits to be derived from compliance to the prescribed treatment plan.

Unit III, Drugs Affecting Body Systems, and Unit IV, Other Pharmacologic Agents, have been undated with over 75 new drugs and expanded discussions on pain management, seizure disorders, control of emesis and hypertension. We have continued to expand our standardized format that emphasizes helping the nurse make knowledgeable assessments of the effects of drugs and patient teaching for nursing interventions.

The format in these units includes four sections. General Nursing Considerations for patients with particular diseases provides nurses with a brief, accurate synopsis of psychosocial, physiological, and nutritional assessment factors, health care measures, and patient teaching variables together with an overview of nursing responsibilities in relation to pathophysiology. This affords the practitioner a solid foundation upon which to base an evaluation of specific drug effects on individual patients. The Patient Education section compliments and fosters the expanded role of the nurse as a patient educator. Patient teaching variables can easily be extracted from this reference by the nurse for preparing teaching plans for patients based upon their specific medication regimen. Examples of written records that may be developed for patient use that will help the patient monitor therapy between follow-up visits have been included. Specific Drug Monographs provide a pronunciation guide, brand names available in the United States and Canada, actions and uses, side effects, availability, dosage and administration, and drug interactions. Finally, every aspect of the Nursing Intervention is considered, including side effects to expect, side effects to report, specific implementation considerations, and management of drug interactions. Examples and suggestions are offered for assessing and eliciting a

desired response in the patient (e.g., ways to detect ototoxicity, descriptions of palpitations, securing patient/family cooperation with I/O, and management of drug interactions). Moreover, the interventions are substantiated with sound, succinctly stated rationales that foster credibility and increased professional compliance.

The appendixes list common medical abbreviations, prescription abbreviations, mathematical conversions, temperature conversion tables, weight conversion tables, formulas for pediatric doses, sodium and potassium content of selected foods, nomograms for estimating body surface area, a table of normal values for commonly used laboratory tests for both standard and SI units, normal therapeutic ranges for plasma concentrations of drugs, and a template for developing a written record for patients to monitor their own therapy between visits. The Glossary is provided as a quick reference for defining many of the Key Words listed in chapter units and used throughout the text.

Finally, the *Instructor's Manual* has been completely updated to include information on the newly added drugs. Worksheets are revised and test questions have been added to cover the new content. Calculation problems have been integrated into the chapter tests to reinforce the importance of maintaining these skills.

This revised tenth edition reflects the nurse's responsibility to provide sound, knowledgeable care in the area of medication administration. We have tried to clarify content and reinforce learning throughout the text. We have also placed emphasis on assisting the patient to improve his or her health by providing appropriate physical care, emotional and social support, and information necessary for self-care. It is our hope that this revision will meet the needs of nurses for a book "to motivate the learner to administer medication with concern for safety, precision, and attention to important physiologic factors," and teaches and assists them to provide the best possible nursing care to their patients.

Bruce D Clayton

Yvonne N. Stock

Contents in Brief

APPENDIXES

Contents

8   The Nursing Process Applied to Pharmacology, 141

PRINCIPLES OF
PHARMACOLOGY

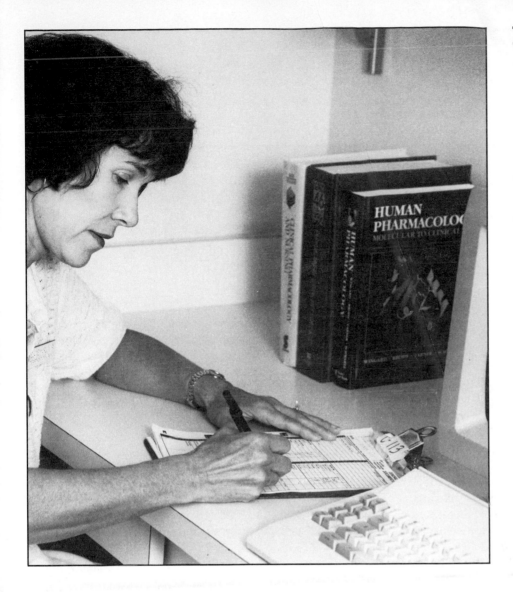

CHAPTER 1

Definitions, Names, Standards, and Informational Sources

CHAPTER GOALS

After completing this chapter, the student should be able to do the following:

1. Utilize nomenclature associated with the study of pharmacology.
2. Identify major sources of drug standards and drug information.
3. Describe the purpose of drug legislation and factors influencing the effectiveness of that legislation.

DEFINITIONS
OBJECTIVES

1. State the origin and definition of *pharmacology*.
2. Explain the meaning of *therapeutic methods*.

KEY WORD

pharmacology

Pharmacology

Pharmacology (Greek *pharmakon*, "drugs," and *logos*, "science") deals with the study of drugs and their actions on living organisms.

Therapeutic Methods

Diseases may be treated in several different ways. The approaches to therapy are called *therapeutic methods*. Most illnesses require a combination of therapeutic methods for successful treatment. The following are some examples of therapeutic methods:

• Drug therapy—treatment with drugs
• Diet therapy—treatment by diet, such as a low-salt diet for patients with cardiovascular disease
• Physiotherapy—treatment with natural physical forces such as water, light, and heat
• Psychological therapy—identification of stressors and methods to reduce or eliminate stress and/or the use of drugs

Drugs

Drugs (Dutch *droog*, "dry") are chemical substances that have an effect on living organisms. Therapeutic drugs, often called *medicines*, are those drugs used in the prevention or treatment of diseases. Up until a few decades ago, dried plants were the greatest source of medicines; thus the word *drug* was applied to them.

DRUG NAMES (UNITED STATES)
OBJECTIVES

1. Describe the process used to name drugs.
2. Differentiate among the *chemical, generic, official,* and *brand* names of medicines.

KEY WORDS

chemical name generic name
proprietary name official name
trademark   brand name

Many drugs have a variety of names. This may cause confusion to the patient, physician, and nurse, so care must be taken in obtaining the exact name and spelling for a particular drug. When administering the prescribed drug, the *exact* spelling on the drug package must correspond exactly to the spelling of the drug ordered.

Chemical Name

The chemical name is most meaningful to the chemist. By means of the chemical name, the chemist understands exactly the chemical constitution of the drug and the exact placing of its atoms or molecular groupings.

Generic Name (Nonproprietary Name)

Before a drug becomes official, it is given a generic name or common name. A generic name is simpler than the chemical name. It may be used in all countries, by any manufacturer. It is not capitalized.

Generic names are provided by the United States Adopted Names (USAN) Council, an organization sponsored by the United States Pharmacopeial Convention, the American Medical Association, and the American Pharmaceutical Association.

Official Name

The official name is the name under which the drug is listed by the United States Food and Drug Administration (FDA). The FDA is empowered by federal law to name drugs for human use in the United States.

Trademark or Brand Name

A trademark or brand name is followed by the symbol ®. This indicates that the name is registered and that its use is restricted to the owner of the drug, who is usually the manufacturer of the product. Some drug companies place their official drugs on the market under trade or proprietary names instead of official names. The trade names are deliberately made easier to pronounce, spell, and remember. The first letter of the trade name is capitalized.

> EXAMPLE: *Chemical name:* 4-dimethylamino-1, 4, 4a, 5, 5a, 6, 11, 12a-octahydro-3,6,10,12,12a-pentahydroxy-6-methyl-1,11,dioxo-2-naphthacenecarboxamide
> *Generic name:* tetracycline
> *Official name:* Tetracycline, USP
> *Brand names:* Achromycin, Panmycin, Tetracyn

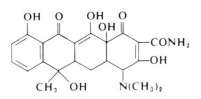

Figure 1-1 *Tetracycline, an antibiotic.*

DRUG NAMES (CANADA)
OBJECTIVES

1. Differentiate between the *official* and *proper* names of medicines.

Official Drug

The term *official drug* is used to mean any drug for which a standard is described either specifically in the *Food and Drug Regulations* or in any publication named in the *Food and Drugs Act* as satisfactory for officially describing the standards for drugs in Canada.

Proper Name

The proper name is the nonproprietary (generic) name used to describe an official drug in Canada.

SOURCES OF DRUG STANDARDS (UNITED STATES)
OBJECTIVE

1. List official sources of drug standards.

KEY WORD
USP/NF

Standardization is needed to ensure that drug products made by different manufacturers, or in different batches by the same manufacturer, will be uniformly pure and potent. Before 1820, many drugs were manufactured in different parts of the United States with varying degrees of purity. This problem was solved by the establishment of an authoritative book that set forth required standards of purity for drugs as well as methods to determine purity. It is called the *Pharmacopeia—National Formulary of the United States of America.*

The United States Pharmacopeia (USP), 22nd Revision, and the National Formulary (NF), 17th Revision

The USP and NF are now published as a single volume by the United States Pharmacopeial Convention, a nonprofit, nongovernmental corporation. The latest edition, published in 1990, represents the third time these two established reference books have been combined into one volume. This book is revised every 5 years. Supplements are published more frequently to keep it up to date.

The primary purpose of this volume is to provide standards for identity, quality, strength, and purity of substances used in the practice of health care. The standards set forth in the USP–NF have been adopted by the Food and Drug Administration as "official" standards for the manufacture and quality control of medicines produced in the United States.

USAN and the USP Dictionary of Drug Names

The USP dictionary is a compilation of more than 19,000 drug names. Each drug monograph contains the United States Adopted Name (USAN), a pronunciation guide, the molecular and graphic formula, chemical and brand name, manufacturer, and therapeutic category. It also contains the Chemical Abstracts Service registry numbers for drugs.

Manufacturers submit to the USAN Council a proposal for a name, in which they announce that a certain chemical compound has therapeutic potential and that they plan to investigate its use in human beings. The Council studies the chemical name, applies a series of nomenclature guidelines, and then selects the USAN (generic name). It is now customary for the Food and Drug Administration to accept the adopted generic name as the FDA "official name" for a chemical compound.

SOURCES OF DRUG STANDARDS (CANADA)
OBJECTIVE

1. List official sources of drug standards.

KEY WORDS
> *British Pharmacopoeia*
> *Pharmacopée Française*

The *Food and Drugs Act* recognizes the standards described by seven international authoritative books to be acceptable for Official Drugs in Canada. The acceptable publications are the *British Pharmacopoeia,* the *Pharmacopoeia of the United States of America,* the *Pharmacopoeia Internationalis,* the *Pharmacopée Française,* the *British Pharmaceutical Codex,* the *National Formulary (U.S.),* and the *Canadian Formulary.*

SOURCES OF DRUG INFORMATION (UNITED STATES)

OBJECTIVES

1. List and describe literature resources for researching prescription and nonprescription medications.
2. List and describe literature resources for researching drug interactions and drug incompatibilities.

KEY WORDS

> *American Drug Index*
> *American Hospital Formulary Service*
> *Drug Interaction Facts*
> *Facts and Comparisons*
> *Handbook on Injectable Drugs*
> *Handbook of Nonprescription Drugs*
> *Martindale*
> *PDR*

American Drug Index

The *American Drug Index* is edited annually by Norman F. Billups, Ph.D., and is published by J.B. Lippincott Company. It is an index of all drugs available in the United States.

Drugs in the *Index* are listed alphabetically by generic name and brand name. The generic name monographs indicate that the drug is recognized in the *United States Pharmacopeia—National Formulary* or *United States Adopted Names* and give the chemical name, use, and cross-references to brand names. Each brand name monograph lists the manufacturer, composition and strength, pharmaceutical forms available, package size, dosage, and use. Other features of this reference book include a list of common medical abbreviations; tables of weights, measures, and conversion factors; a glossary to aid in interpretation of the monographs; a labeler code index to identify drug products; and a list of manufacturers' addresses. The book is useful for quickly comparing brand names and generic names, and also for checking the availability of strengths and dosage forms.

American Hospital Formulary Service

The *American Hospital Formulary Service, Drug Information '92,* is a comprehensive reference book published annually by the American Society of Hospital Pharmacists in Bethesda, Maryland. It is updated with four supplements yearly. This volume contains monographs on virtually every single-drug entity available in the United States. The monographs emphasize rational therapeutic use of drugs. Each monograph is subdivided into sections on chemistry and statoxicity, drug interactions, dosage and administration, and available products. The index is cross-referenced by both generic and brand names.

The *American Hospital Formulary Service, Drug Information '92,* has been adopted as an official reference by the U.S. Public Health Service and the Veterans Administration. It has also been approved for use by the American Hospital Association, the Catholic Health Care Association of the United States, the National Association of Boards of Pharmacy, and the American Pharmaceutical Association and is included as a required or recommended standard reference in pharmacies in many states.

Drug Interaction Facts

Drug Interaction Facts is published by the Facts and Comparisons Division of J.B. Lippincott Company.

This three-ring, loose-leaf, 600-page book, first published in 1983, is currently the most comprehensive book available on the subject of drug interactions. The format is somewhat different from that of most other books: the index is in the front, and the book is not subdivided into chapters. Drugs are arranged alphabetically, and the book is then subdivided every 100 pages by a plastic tab sheet. Each page is a single monograph describing a drug interaction. Each monograph is subdivided into a table that lists the onset and severity of the drug interaction, expected outcomes, a statement on the expected effects, the proposed mechanism, and how to manage the interaction. A short discussion (with references) on the relevance of the interaction follows.

One of the most meaningful, although not obvious, benefits is the source of information used to develop *Drug Interaction Facts.* All the information reviewed is from the MEDIPHOR Group of the Stanford University School of Medicine. This internationally renowned group of physicians and pharmacists has the personnel, clinical experience, scientific background, library, and computer resources to collect, collate, review, and evaluate the scientific accuracy of descriptions of drug interactions from the world literature. Thus the book is an extremely reliable source of information. Subscribers receive an update supplement four times a year.

Facts and Comparisons

Facts and Comparisons is a large, loose-leaf compendium of over 2000 pages published by the Facts and Comparisons Division of J.B. Lippincott Company.

The book is divided into 12 chapters. At the beginning of each chapter is a detailed table of contents. All drugs within each chapter are subdivided by therapeutic classes. For each therapeutic class of drug, a monograph provides a brief description of drug action, pharmacokinetics, metabolism, uses, contraindications, warnings, precautions, adverse effects reported, treatment of overdosage, patient information in brief, and administration. The data base for the monographs is the most current FDA-approved package insert. The editors have reformatted the information and added additional information from the medical literature on investigational uses of the drugs.

At the end of each monograph are tables of all drugs in that therapeutic class. The tables are particularly valuable because they are designed to allow comparison of similar products, brand names, manufacturers, cost index, and available dosage forms.

The index is quite comprehensive and is updated both monthly and quarterly. Within each chapter, there is an excellent cross-referencing system as well, making it quite easy to gain information on drugs that may be categorized by more than one therapeutic class. Updated supplements for the entire book are provided monthly.

Handbook on Injectable Drugs

The *Handbook on Injectable Drugs*, the most comprehensive reference available on the topic of compatibility of injectable drugs, is written by Lawrence A. Trissel and published by the American Society of Hospital Pharmacists of Bethesda, Maryland. It is a collection of monographs on almost 300 injectable drugs. Each monograph is subdivided into sections on availability of concentrations, stability, pH, dosage and rate of administration, compatibility information, and other useful information about the drug.

Handbook of Non-Prescription Drugs

The *Handbook of Non-Prescription Drugs* is prepared and published by the American Pharmaceutical Association, Washington, D.C. It is the most comprehensive text available on medications that can be purchased over the counter in the United States.

Chapters are divided by therapeutic activity, such as antacid products, cold and allergy products, nutritional supplements, mineral and vitamin products, and feminine hygiene products. Each chapter provides a brief review of anatomy and physiology, evaluation of the symptoms being treated, suggested treatments with appropriate dosages, and a list of medications with their ingredients.

This book has three particular advantages for the health professional: (1) a list of questions to ask the patient to determine whether treatment should be recommended; (2) product selection guidelines for determining the most appropriate products; and (3) counseling to be conveyed to the patient on proper use of the recommended product.

Martindale—The Extra Pharmacopoeia

Martindale—The Extra Pharmacopoeia is a 1900 page volume edited by James E.F. Reynolds and published by The Pharmaceutical Press in London. It is one of the most comprehensive texts available for information on drugs in current use throughout the world. Part 1 contains extensive referenced monographs on the pharmacologic activity and side effects of about 4000 medicinal agents. Part 2 contains short monographs on another 800 agents that are considered either obsolete or too new for inclusion in Part 1. Part 3 gives the composition and manufacturers of more than 670 over-the-counter pharmaceutical products.

The index contains more than 62,000 entries. Medicinal agents are indexed by official names, chemical names, synonyms, and proprietary names.

Medical Letter

The *Medical Letter*, published by Drug and Therapeutic Information, Inc., New York, is a semi-monthly periodical newsletter. It contains brief comments on newly released drug products and related topics by an independent board of competent authorities. The board relies upon the knowledge of specialists in various fields for their experience with certain drugs. The primary purpose of the newsletter is to report new data on drug action and comparative clinical efficacy. The *Medical Letter* presents timely and critical summaries of data on new drugs during their early period of promotion. Such appraisals must, necessarily, be tentative.

Package Inserts

Before a new drug is marketed, the manufacturer develops a comprehensive but concise description of the drug, indications and precautions in clinical use, recommendations for dosage, known adverse reactions, contraindications, and other pharmacologic information relating to the drug. Federal law requires that this material be approved by the Food and Drug Administration before the product is released for marketing and that it be presented on an insert that accompanies each package of the product.

Physicians' Desk Reference (PDR)

The *PDR* is published annually by Medical Economics, Inc., of Oradell, New Jersey. It lists approximately

2500 therapeutic agents in seven sections. Each section uses a different page color for easy access.

Section 1 (white), Manufacturers' index

An alphabetic listing of each manufacturer, its addresses, emergency phone numbers, and a partial list of available products.

Section 2 (pink), Product name index

A comprehensive alphabetic listing of brand name products discussed in the Product Information section of the book.

Section 3 (blue), Product category index

Products are subdivided by therapeutic classes, such as analgesics, laxatives, oxytocics, and antibiotics.

Section 4 (yellow), Generic and chemical name index

Products are listed by their generic or chemical names, with references to the Product Information section.

Section 5, Product identification section

Each manufacturer has provided actual-size color pictures of their tablets and capsules, an invaluable aid in product identification.

Section 6 (white), Product information section

A reprint of the package insert for the major products of manufacturers, with information on action, uses, administration, dosages, contraindications, composition, and how each drug is supplied.

Section 7 (green), Diagnostic product information

An alphabetic listing by manufacturer of many diagnostic tests used in hospital and office practice.

SOURCES OF DRUG INFORMATION (CANADA)

OBJECTIVES

1. Describe the organization of the *Compendium of Pharmaceuticals and Specialties* and the information contained in each colored section.
2. Describe the organization of the *Canadian Self-Medication*.

Compendium of Pharmaceuticals and Specialties (CPS)

The *Compendium of Pharmaceuticals and Specialties* (CPS) is published annually by the Canadian Pharma-

ceutical Association. It provides a comprehensive list of the pharmaceutical products manufactured in Canada as well as other information of practical value to health professionals. The book is divided into six color-coded sections.

White pages

An alphabetic arrangement of manufacturer's brand information as well as numerous general monographs for common multi-source drugs; a few medical devices are described; a list of products discontinued since the previous edition is provided at the end of the section.

Blue pages

Tables and charts describing a wide range of information of interest to health professionals which otherwise would seldom be easily accessible, particularly in a single reference book; topics include the excipient content of selected pharmaceuticals, PVC plastic interactions with drugs, SI unit conversion factors, alcohol-free products, drugs banned in sports competition, a summary of Canadian regulations for narcotics and controlled drugs, the procedure to obtain on an emergency basis a drug not cleared for use in Canada, body surface area charts, treatment guidelines for sexually transmitted diseases and malaria prophylaxis, and the comparative content of vitamin products.

Product recognition section

Color photographs of drug products arranged according to the size and color shadings of individual dosage forms (tablets, capsules, liquids).

Pink pages

A "prescriber's guide" lists by brand name products available for numerous therapeutic use categories, as well as selected diagnostic or monitoring aids and medical devices.

Yellow pages

Names, addresses, and telephone numbers of the manufacturers and distributors of pharmaceutical products in Canada; also product markings for many of the manufacturers.

Green pages

An alphabetical cross-reference that lists drugs by both nonproprietary and brand names, also indicating whether the product was available in Canada at the time of publication.

Self-Medication

Self-Medication is published approximately every 4 years by the Canadian Pharmaceutical Association. It provides comprehensive information about the nonprescription drug products that are available in Canada.

Chapters are organized by therapeutic category, such as eye care, laxatives, sunscreens, common cold, and allergies. Each provides a review of the minor conditions suitable for self-medication. Treatment measures include both general and pharmacologic management suggestions and a review of the nonprescription drug alternatives available.

Appendixes include a table of chemicals with assorted pharmaceutical uses (e.g., alum, compound benzoin tincture) and a chart comparing multi-ingredient vitamin products. Brief product monographs supplied by manufacturers are listed in alphabetical order at the back of the text. Additional features include a therapeutic index, a manufacturer's index, and a "product ingredient index" that identifies the brands containing a specific substance in either single- or multiple-ingredient products.

SOURCES OF PATIENT INFORMATION

Objective

1. Cite literature resources for reviewing information to be given to the patient concerning prescribed medication.

KEY WORDS

Medication Guide for Patient Counseling
USP DI

Over the past two decades, it has become evident that health care providers must do a better job of informing patients of what they must do to assume responsibility for their own health care. The following books and reference materials are excellent sources of information for teaching patients how to use their medications properly.

Medication Guide for Patient Counseling

The *Medication Guide for Patient Counseling* is written by Dorothy L. Smith and published by Lea & Febiger of Philadelphia. This is an excellent resource book on the topic of patient counseling. It provides both a good discussion of how to counsel patients for health professionals and a comprehensive set of medication instructions for almost all of the medications available in the United States and Canada. The medication instructions have been translated from medical terminology into language that most patients can understand. Each of the drug monographs contains the important information (including administration techniques) that should be conveyed to the patient.

United States Pharmacopeia Dispensing Information

United States Pharmacopeia Dispensing Information (USP DI) is an annual publication written by the United States Pharmacopeial Convention, Inc.

USP DI is a two-volume set supplemented with bimonthly updates. The first volume includes dispensing information for health care providers arranged in alphabetically ordered monographs. Each monograph is subdivided into sections on the drug's use, mechanism of action, precautions, side effects, patient consultation information, general dosing information, and dosage forms available.

The second volume, *Advice for the Patient*, provides the layman's language for the patient consultation guidelines found in the first volume. The second volume is designed to be used at the discretion of the health care provider as an aid to counseling the patient if written information is to be given to the patient. The publisher permits all health care practitioners to reproduce the pages of advice for their patients receiving the prescribed drug. Generic and brand names are cross-referenced in the index of *Advice for the Patient.*

DRUG LEGISLATION (UNITED STATES)

Objectives

1. List legislative acts controlling drug use and abuse.
2. Differentiate among Schedule I, II, III, IV, and V medications, and describe nursing responsibilities associated with the administration of each type.

KEY WORDS

Federal Food, Drug, and Cosmetic Act
Controlled Substances Act
Scheduled Drugs

Drug legislation protects the consumer and patient. The need for such protection is great because manufacturers and advertising agents may make unfounded claims about the benefits of their products.

Federal Food, Drug, and Cosmetic Act, June 25, 1938 (Amended 1952, 1962)

The 1938 act authorizes the federal Food and Drug Administration of the Department of Health and Human Services to determine the safety of drugs before marketing and to assure that certain labeling specifications and standards in advertising are met in the marketing of products. Manufacturers are required to submit new drug applications to the FDA for review of safety studies before products can be released for sale.

The Durham-Humphrey Amendment in 1952 tightened control by restricting the refilling of prescriptions.

The Kefauver-Harris Drug Amendment in 1962 was brought about by the thalidomide tragedy. Thalidomide was an incompletely tested drug approved for use as a sedative-hypnotic during pregnancy. Infants exposed to thalidomide were born with serious birth defects. This amendment provides greater control and surveillance of the distribution and clinical testing of investigational drugs and requires that a product be proven both safe and effective before release for sale.

Harrison Narcotic Act, 1914

The Harrison Narcotic Act regulated the importation, manufacture, sale, and use of opium, cocaine, and all their compounds and derivatives. Its purpose was to limit the indiscriminate use of such drugs and to prevent the spread of the drug habit. The act was amended many times. However, it has been repealed and replaced by the Controlled Substances Act of 1970.

Controlled Substances Act, 1970

The Comprehensive Drug Abuse Prevention and Control Act was passed by Congress in 1970. This new statute, commonly referred to as the "Controlled Substances Act," repealed almost 50 other laws written since 1914 that relate to the control of drugs. The new composite law is designed to improve the administration and regulation of manufacturing, distributing, and dispensing of drugs found necessary to be controlled.

The Drug Enforcement Administration (DEA) was organized to enforce the Controlled Substances Act, to gather intelligence, and to train and conduct research in the area of dangerous drugs and drug abuse. The DEA is a bureau of the Department of Justice. The director of the DEA reports to the Attorney General of the United States.

The basic structure of the Controlled Substances Act consists of five classifications or "schedules" of controlled substances. The degree of control, the conditions of record keeping, the particular order forms required, and other regulations depend on these classifications. The five schedules, their criteria, and examples of drugs in each schedule are listed below:

Schedule I ℂ drugs

1. A high potential for abuse
2. No currently accepted medical use in the United States
3. A lack of accepted safety for use under medical supervision

   EXAMPLES: LSD, marijuana, peyote, STP, heroin, hashish

Schedule II ℂ drugs

1. A high potential for abuse
2. A currently accepted medical use in the United States

3. An abuse potential that may lead to severe psychologic or physical dependence

   EXAMPLES: secobarbital, pentobarbital, amphetamines, morphine, meperidine, methadone, Percodan

Schedule III ℂ drugs

1. A high potential for abuse, but less so than drugs in schedules I and II
2. A currently accepted medical use in the United States
3. An abuse potential that may lead to moderate or low physical dependence or high psychologic dependence

   EXAMPLES: Empirin with codeine, Doriden, Fiorinal, paregoric, Noludar, Tylenol with codeine

Schedule IV ℂ drugs

1. A low potential for abuse, compared with those in schedule III
2. A currently accepted medical use in the United States
3. An abuse potential that may lead to limited physical or psychologic dependence, compared with drugs in schedule III

   EXAMPLES: phenobarbital, Equanil, chloral hydrate, paraldehyde, Librium, Valium, Dalmane, Tranxene

Schedule V ℂ drugs

1. A low potential for abuse, compared with those in schedule IV
2. A currently accepted medical use in the United States
3. An abuse potential of limited physical or psychologic dependence liability, compared with drugs in schedule IV

   EXAMPLES: Lomotil, Robitussin A-C

The Attorney General, after public hearings, has authority to reschedule a drug, bring an unscheduled drug under control, or remove controls on scheduled drugs.

Every manufacturer, physician, dentist, pharmacy, and hospital that manufactures, prescribes, or dispenses any of the drugs listed in the five schedules must register biannually with the Drug Enforcement Administration.

A physician's prescription for substances named in this law must contain the physician's name, address, DEA registration number and signature, the patient's name and address, and the date of issue. The pharmacist cannot refill such prescriptions without the approval of the physician.

All controlled substances for ward stock must be ordered on special hospital forms that are used to help maintain inventory and dispersion control records of the schedule drugs. When a nurse administers a Schedule II drug, under a physician's order, the following information must be entered on the controlled substances record: name of the patient, date of administration, drug administered, and drug dosage.

Possession of Controlled Substances

Federal and state laws make the possession of controlled substances a crime, except in specifically exempted cases. The law makes no distinction between professional and practical nurses in regard to possession of controlled drugs. Nurses may give controlled substances only under the direction of a physician or dentist who has been licensed to prescribe or dispense these agents. Nurses may not have controlled substances in their possession unless they are giving them to a patient under a doctor's order, or the nurse is a patient for whom a doctor has prescribed schedule drugs, or the nurse is the official custodian of a limited supply of controlled substances on a ward or department of the hospital. Controlled substances ordered but not used for patients must be returned to the source from which they were obtained (the doctor or the pharmacy). Violation or failure to comply with the Controlled Substances Act is punishable by fine, imprisonment, or both.

DRUG LEGISLATION (CANADA)
OBJECTIVES

1. List legislative acts controlling drug use and abuse.
2. Differentiate between Schedule F and G, and describe nursing responsibilities with each.

Food and Drugs Act 1927; the Food and Drug Regulations 1953 and 1954, Revised 1979 and Periodic Amendments

The Food and Drugs Act and its Regulations empower the Department of National Health and Welfare of Canada to protect the public from foreseeable risks relating to the manufacture and sale of drugs. The administration of this legislation is carried out by the Health Protection Branch. It provides for a review of the safety and efficacy of drugs prior to their clearance for marketing in Canada as either prescription or nonprescription products. Also included in this legislation are requirements for good manufacturing practices, for adequate labeling, and for fair advertising.

Drugs requiring a prescription, except for narcotics, are listed on Schedule F or Schedule G of the Food and Drug Regulations.

Schedule F prescription drugs

Schedule F drugs may be prescribed only by qualified practitioners (physicians, dentists, or veterinarians) because they would normally be used most safely under supervision.

EXAMPLES: most antibiotics, antineoplastics, corticosteroids, cardiovascular drugs, antipsychotics

Schedule G controlled drugs

Schedule G drugs may be prescribed only by qualified practitioners. Because of a recognized abuse potential, these drugs are subject to additional requirements of record keeping for purchase, sale, or administration to a patient in a hospital.

EXAMPLES: amphetamines, barbiturates, diethylpropion, methaqualone, methylphenidate

The legitimate use of amphetamines in Canada is restricted to specific disorders such as narcolepsy or hyperkinetic disorders in children. It does not include obesity control.

Narcotic Control Act (1960-1961) and the Narcotic Control Regulations (Amended 1978)

The Narcotic Control Act and its Regulations establish the requirements for the control and sale of narcotic substances in Canada.

Generally, because of their abuse potential, narcotics are subject to more stringent requirements for inventory control than other prescription drugs.

EXAMPLES: meperidine (Demerol), morphine, propoxyphene (Darvon), codeine, oxycodone, hydrocodone

Recently, despite considerable controversy, special provision was made for the limited medical use of heroin in Canada for intractable pain.

The Narcotic Regulations also provide for the nonprescription sale of certain codeine preparations. The content must not exceed the equivalent of 8 mg codeine phosphate per solid dosage unit or 20 mg per 30 ml of a liquid and the preparation must also contain two additional nonnarcotic medicinal ingredients. These preparations may not be advertised or displayed and may be sold only by pharmacists. In hospitals, the pharmacy usually requires strict inventory control of these products as well as other narcotics.

EXAMPLES: Tylenol No. 1, Frosst "222," Benylin with codeine

Requirements for the legitimate administration of drugs to patients by nurses are generally similar in Canada and the United States. Individual hospital policy determines specific record-keeping requirements based upon federal and provincial laws. Violations of these laws would be expected to result in fines or imprisonment in addition to the loss of professional license.

Nonprescription Drugs

In Canada, the Health Protection Branch acknowledges two classes of nonprescription drugs. Provision is made in Division 10 of the Food and Drug Regulations for "proprietary medicines" that can be adequately labeled by manufacturers for direct use by consumers. Laws in each of the 10 provinces determine the actual conditions of distribution of nonprescription drugs. Proprietary medicines can generally be sold through any retail outlet, whereas other nonprescription drugs in some provinces may be sold only in pharmacies. In fact, a few provinces require the direct involvement of a pharmacist in the sale of certain nonprescription drugs. Most hospitals do not differentiate between prescription and nonprescription drugs, requiring physician's orders for both.

EFFECTIVENESS OF LEGISLATION OF DRUGS

The effectiveness of drug legislation depends on the interest and determination used to enforce these laws, the appropriation by government of adequate funds for enforcement, the vigor used by proper authorities in enforcement, the interest and cooperation of professional people and the public, and the education of the public concerning the dangers of unwise and indiscriminate use of drugs in general. Many organizations help in this education, including the National Coordinating Council on Patient Information and Education, the American Medical Association, the American Dental Association, the American Pharmaceutical Association, the American Society of Hospital Pharmacists, and local, state, and county health departments.

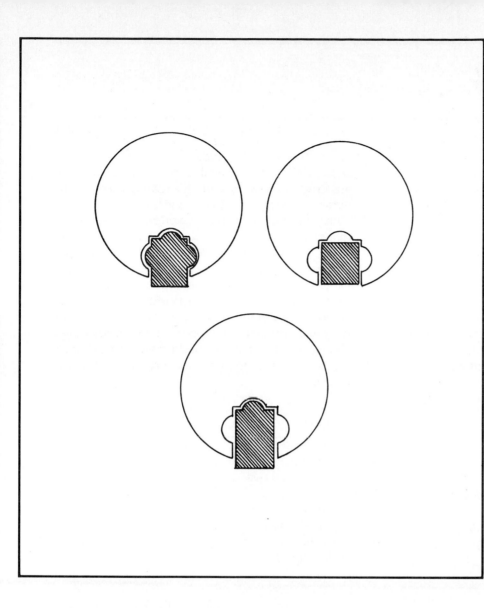

Principles of Drug Action and Drug Interactions

CHAPTER GOALS

After completing this chapter, the student should be able to do the following:

1. Utilize basic principles of drug action and interactions to make sound nursing judgments associated with medication therapy.
2. Correlate principles of drug interactions with information contained in drug monographs.

CHAPTER CONTENT:

Basic principles (p. 14)
Drug action (p. 17)

Variable factors influencing drug
action (p. 17)

Drug interactions (p. 19)

BASIC PRINCIPLES

OBJECTIVES

1. Identify five basic principles of drug action.
2. Explain nursing assessments necessary to evaluate potential problems associated with the absorption of medications.
3. Describe nursing interventions that can enhance drug absorption.
4. List three categories of drug administration, and state the routes of administration for each category.
5. Differentiate between general and selective types of drug distribution mechanisms.
6. Name the process that inactivates drugs.
7. Identify the meaning and significance to the nurse of the term *half-life* when used in relation to drug therapy.

KEY WORDS

receptors	enternal	excretion
antagonists	agonists	half-life
absorption	partial agonists	parenteral
metabolism	distribution	drug blood level
ADME	half-life	parenteral

How do drugs act in the body? A few key facts to remember are as follows:

1. Drugs do not create new responses, but alter existing physiological activity. Thus, drug response must be stated in relation to what the physiological activity was before the response to drug therapy (that is, an antihypertensive agent is successful if the blood pressure is lower during therapy than before therapy). Therefore, it is important to perform a thorough nursing assessment to identify the baseline data. Thereafter, regular assessments are performed by the nurse and compared to the baseline data by the physician, the nurse, and the pharmacist, in order to evaluate the effectiveness of the drug therapy.
2. Drugs interact with the body in several different ways. The most common way in which drugs act is by forming chemical bonds with specific sites called *receptors* within the body. Bonding occurs only if the drug and its receptor have similar shapes. The relationship between a drug and a receptor is like that between a key and a lock (see Figure 2-1, A).
3. Most drugs have several different atoms within the molecule that interlock into several locations on the receptor. The better the "fit" between the receptor and the drug, the better the response. The intensity

of a drug response is related not only to how well the drug molecule fits in the receptor but to the number of receptor sites occupied.

4. Drugs that interact with a receptor to stimulate a response are known as *agonists* (see Figure 2-1, B). Drugs that attach to a receptor but do not stimulate a response are called *antagonists* (see Figure 2-1, C). Drugs that interact with a receptor to stimulate a response, but inhibit other responses are called *partial agonists* (see Figure 2-1, D).
5. Once administered, all drugs go through four stages: absorption, distribution, metabolism, and excretion (ADME). Each drug has its own unique ADME characteristics.

Absorption

Absorption is the process by which a drug is made available to the body fluids for distribution. It is the way in which a drug is transferred from its site of entry into the body to the circulating fluids of the body, the blood and the lymphatic system. The rate at which this occurs depends on the route of administration, the blood flow through the tissue where the drug is administered, and the solubility of the drug. It is therefore important to administer oral drugs with an adequate amount of fluid; to give parenteral forms properly so that they are deposited in the correct tissue for enhanced absorption; and to reconstitute and dilute drugs only with the diluent recommended by the manufacturer in the package literature so that drug solubility is not impaired. Equally important are nursing assessments that imply poor absorption (for example, if insulin is administered subcutane-

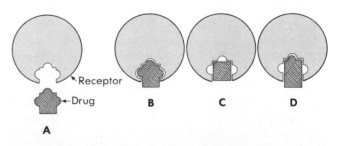

Figure 2-1 A, *Drugs act by forming a chemical bond with specific receptory sites, similar to a key and lock.* **B**, *The better the "fit," the better the response. Those with complete attachment and response are called* agonists. **C**, *Drugs that attach but do not elicit a response are called* antagonists. **D**, *Drugs that attach, elicit a small response, but also block other responses are called* partial agonists.

ously and a "lump" remains at the site of injection 2 to 3 hours later, absorption from that site may be impaired).

Drug administration is classified into three categories: the enteral, the parenteral, and the percutaneous routes. The *enteral* route is administration directly into the gastrointestinal tract by oral, rectal, or nasogastric routes. *Parenteral* routes of administration bypass the gastrointestinal tract by subcutaneous, intramuscular, or intravenous injection. Methods of *percutaneous* administration are inhalation or sublingual or topical administration. Absorption of topical drugs applied to the skin can be influenced by the drug concentration, length of contact time, size of affected area, thickness of skin surface, hydration of tissue and degree of skin disruption. Percutaneous absorption is greatly increased in newborns and young infants, who have thin, well-hydrated skin. Inhalation of drugs and their absorption can be influenced by depth of respirations and fineness of the droplet particles, available surface area of mucous membrane, contact time, hydration state, blood supply to the area, and concentration of the drug itself.

The rate of absorption by parenteral routes is partially dependent upon the rate of blood flow through the tissues. Circulatory insufficiency and respiratory distress may lead to hypoxia and further complicate this situation by resulting in vasoconstriction. (The nurse should therefore not give an injection where circulation is known to be impaired. Another site on the rotation schedule should be utilized.) Subcutaneous (SC) injections have the slowest absorption rate, especially if peripheral circulation is impaired. Intramuscular (IM) injections are more rapidly absorbed because of greater blood flow per unit weight of muscle. (Depositing the medication into the muscle belly is important. Nurses must carefully assess the individual patient for the correct length of needle to assure that this occurs.) Cooling an area of injection will slow the rate of absorption while heat or massage will hasten the rate of absorption. When administered intravenously (IV), the drug is dispersed throughout the body most rapidly. (Nurses must be thoroughly educated regarding the responsibilities and techniques associated with administering IV medications. Once the drug enters the bloodstream, it cannot be retrieved.)

Regardless of the route of administration, a drug must be dissolved in body fluids before it can be absorbed into body tissues. As an example, before a solid drug taken orally can be absorbed into the bloodstream for transport to the site of action, it must disintegrate and dissolve in the gastrointestinal fluids and be transported across the stomach or intestinal lining into the blood. The process of converting the drug into a soluble form can be partially controlled by the pharmaceutical dosage form used (that is, solution, suspension, capsule, and tablets with various coatings) or can be influenced by the time of administration in relation to the presence or absence of food in the stomach.

Distribution

The term *distribution* refers to the ways in which drugs are transported by the circulating body fluids to the sites of action (receptors), metabolism, and excretion. Drug distribution is both transport throughout the entire body by the blood and lymphatic systems, and transport from the circulating fluids into and out of the fluids that bathe the receptor sites. Organs having the most extensive blood supply, such as the heart, liver, kidneys, and brain, receive the distributing drug most rapidly. Areas with less extensive blood supply, such as the muscle, skin, and fat, receive the drug more slowly.

Once a drug has been dissolved and absorbed into the circulating blood, its distribution is determined by the chemical properties of the drug and how it is affected by the blood and tissues it contacts. Two of the factors that influence drug distribution are protein binding and lipid (fat) solubility. Most drugs are transported in combination with plasma proteins, especially albumin, which act as carriers for relatively insoluble drugs. Drugs bound to plasma proteins are pharmacologically inactive because the large size of the complex keeps them in the bloodstream and prevents them from reaching the sites of action, metabolism, and excretion. Only the free or unbound portion of a drug is able to diffuse into tissues, interact with receptors, and produce biologic effects (or be metabolized and excreted). The same proportion of bound and free drug is maintained in the blood at all times. Thus, as the free drug acts on receptor sites, the decrease in serum drug levels causes some of the bound drug to be released from protein to maintain the ratio between bound and free drug.

When a drug is circulating in the blood, a blood sample may be drawn and assayed to determine the amount of drug present. This is known as a *drug blood level*. It is quite important for certain drugs (e.g., anticonvulsants, aminoglycoside antibiotics) to be measured to make sure the drug is in the therapeutic range. If the blood level is low, either the dosage must be increased or the medicine must be administered more frequently. If the drug blood level is too high, the patient may develop toxicities; either the dosage must be reduced or the medicine administered less frequently. See Appendix I for therapeutic blood levels for selected medicines.

Once a drug leaves the bloodstream, it may become bound to tissues other than those with active receptor sites. The more lipid-soluble drugs have a high affinity for adipose tissue, which serves as a repository site for these agents. Because there is relatively low blood circulation to fat tissues, the more lipid-soluble drugs tend to stay in the body for much longer periods of time. An equilibrium is established between the repository site (lipid tissue) and circulation, so that as the amount of drug in the blood drops due to binding at the sites of biological activity, metabolism, or excretion, more drug is released from the lipid tissue. By contrast, if more drug is given, a new equilibrium will be established between the blood, activity sites, lipid tissue repository sites, and metabolic and excretory sites.

Distribution may be general or selective. Some drugs cannot pass certain types of cell membranes, such as the central nervous system (blood-brain barrier) or the placenta (placental barrier), while other types of drugs will very readily pass into these tissues. The distribution process is very important, because the amount of drug that actually gets to the receptor sites determines the extent of pharmacologic activity. If very little drug actually reaches and binds to the receptor sites, the response will be only minimal.

Metabolism

Metabolism, also called *biotransformation,* is the process by which the body inactivates drugs. The enzyme systems of the liver are the primary site of metabolism of drugs, but other tissues and organs metabolize certain drugs to a minor extent.

Excretion

Metabolites of drugs and, in some cases, the active drug itself, are eventually excreted from the body. The primary routes are through the gastrointestinal tract to the feces and through the renal tubules into the urine. Other routes of excretion include evaporation through the skin, exhalation from the lungs, and secretion into the saliva and mother's milk.

Since the kidneys are a major organ of drug excretion, it is appropriate for the nurse to review the chart for the results of the urinalysis and renal function tests. The patient with renal failure will often experience an increase in the action and duration of a drug if the dosage and frequency of administration are not adjusted to the patient's renal function.

Figure 2-2 is a schematic review of the absorption, distribution, metabolism, and excretion process of an oral medication. It is important to note how little of the active ingredient actually gets to the receptor sites for action.

Half-life

Elimination of drugs occurs by metabolism and excretion. A measure of the time required for elimination is the half-life. The *half-life* is defined as the amount of time required for 50% of the drug to be eliminated from the body. For example, if a patient were given 100 mg

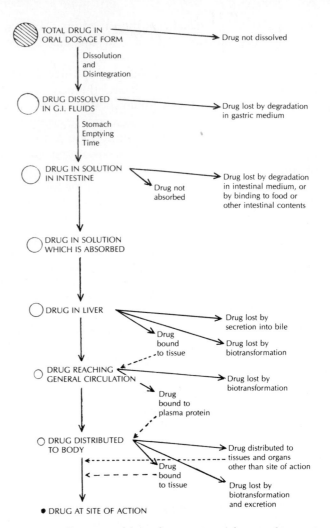

Figure 2-2 *Factors modifying the quantity of drug reaching a site of action after a single oral dose. (From Levine RR: Pharmacology, drug actions, and reactions, Boston, 1973, Little, Brown & Co.)*

of a drug that had a half-life of 12 hours, the following would be observed:

TIME (HR)	HALF-LIFE	DRUG REMAINING IN BODY
0	—	100 mg (100%)
12	1	50 mg (50%)
24	2	25 mg (25%)
36	3	12.5 mg (12.5%)
48	4	6.25 mg (6.25%)
60	5	3.12 mg (3.12%)

Note that as each 12 hours (one half-life) passes, the amount remaining is 50% of what was there 12 hours earlier. After six half-lives, more than 98% of the drug is eliminated from the body.

The half-life is determined by an individual's ability to metabolize and excrete a particular drug. Since most patients metabolize and excrete the same drug at about the same rate, the approximate half-lives of most drugs are now known. When the half-life of a drug is known, dosages and frequency of administration can be calculated. Drugs with a long half-life, such as digoxin at 36 hours, need to be administered only once daily, while drugs with a short half-life, such as aspirin at 5 hours, need to be administered every 4 to 6 hours to maintain therapeutic activity. In patients who have impaired hepatic or renal function, the half-life may become considerably longer due to the inability to metabolize or excrete the drug. An example is digoxin, with a half-life of about 36 hours in a patient with normal renal function, but a half-life of about 105 hours in a patient in complete renal failure. Monitoring diagnostic tests that measure renal or hepatic function is important. Whenever laboratory data reflect impairment of either function, the nurse should notify the physician.

DRUG ACTION
OBJECTIVE

1. Compare and contrast the following terms used in relationship to medications: desired action, side effects, adverse effects, allergic reactions, and idiosyncratic reactions.

KEY WORDS

desired action	allergic reaction
idiosyncratic reaction	carcinogenicity
adverse effects	teratogen

No drug has a single action. When a drug enters a patient and is absorbed and distributed, we usually see the *desired action*, the expected response. All drugs, however, have the potential to affect more than one body system at the same time, producing reactions known as *side effects* or *adverse effects*. Most of these side effects are predictable, and patients should be monitored for these side effects so that dosages can be adjusted to allow the maximum therapeutic benefit with a minimum of side effects. As described in Units 3 and 4 of this text, each drug has a series of *parameters* (therapeutic action to expect, side effects to expect, adverse effects to report, and probable drug interactions) that should be monitored by the nurse, physician, pharmacist, and patient in order to optimize therapy while reducing the possibility of serious adverse effects.

Two other types of drug action are much more unpredictable. These are idiosyncratic reactions and allergic reactions. An *idiosyncratic reaction* occurs when something unusual or abnormal happens when a drug is first administered. The patient usually shows an *overresponse* to the action of the drug. This type of reaction is usually due to a patient's inability to metabolize a drug due to a genetic deficiency of certain enzymes. Fortunately, this type of reaction is fairly rare.

Allergic reactions, also known as hypersensitivity reactions, occur in about 6% to 10% of patients taking medications. Allergic reactions occur in patients who have previously been exposed to a drug and have developed antibodies from their immune systems to it. Upon reexposure, the antibodies cause a reaction, most commonly seen as raised, irregular shaped patches on the skin with severe itching, known as *urticaria* or *hives*. Occasionally, a patient will have a severe, life-threatening reaction that causes respiratory distress and cardiovascular collapse, known as an *anaphylactic reaction*. This condition is a medical emergency and must be treated immediately. Fortunately, anaphylactic reactions occur much less frequently than the more mild urticarial reactions. If a patient has a mild reaction, it should be taken as a warning not to take the medication again. The patient is much more likely to have an anaphylactic reaction at the next exposure to the drug. Patients should receive information regarding the drug name and be told to tell health care professionals (such as nurses, physicians, pharmacists, and dentists) that they have had a reaction and must not receive the drug again. In addition, patients should wear an identification bracelet or necklace explaining the allergy.

Carcinogenicity is the ability of a drug to induce living cells to mutate and become cancerous. Many drugs have this potential, so all drugs are tested in several animal species prior to human investigation to help eliminate this potential.

A drug that induces birth defects is known as a *teratogen*. Organs of the body are particularly susceptible to malformation if exposed to a drug while being formed in the fetus. Since most organ systems are formed during the first trimester of pregnancy, the greatest potential for birth defects caused by drugs occurs during this trimester.

VARIABLE FACTORS INFLUENCING DRUG ACTION
OBJECTIVE

1. List factors that cause variations in absorption, metabolism, distribution, and excretion of drugs.

KEY WORDS

placebo
drug dependence
tolerance
cumulative effect

Many times we have heard patients complain, saying "That drug really knocked me out!" or "That drug didn't touch the pain!" The effects of drugs are unexpectedly potent in some patients, while other patients show little response to the same dose. In addition, some patients will react differently to the same dose of a drug administered at different times. Due to individual patient variation, exact responses to drug therapy are extremely difficult to predict. The following factors have been identified as contributors to a variable response to drugs:

1. Age

Infants and the very elderly tend to be the most sensitive to the response of drugs. There are important differences in the absorption, distribution, metabolism, and excretion of drugs in premature neonates, full-term newborns, and older children. Unfortunately, we do not know how clinically significant many of these differences are. There is no question, however, that we cannot assume that newborns are small versions of adults and that principles of drug administration can be applied to infants purely on the basis of size. Major differences that affect drug disposition in infants and children are a larger percentage of total body water and lower fat stores, variation in the content of circulating proteins in the blood, immature enzyme systems of the liver and lungs prolonging drug metabolism, and kidneys that function at only half the rate of young adult–aged kidneys.

The aging process brings about changes in body composition and organ function that can affect the elderly patient's response to drug therapy. Fat stores, lean body mass, percentage of total body water, cell solids, and bone are areas of change in body composition. Organ function is affected by changes in cell population, oxygen consumption, tissue blood flow, and functional efficiency. With advancing age, plasma concentrations of globulins rise, while that of albumin falls. The clinical importance of reduced serum albumin is that a greater unbound portion of highly protein-bound drugs is available for increased pharmacologic effects. Liver weight, the number of functioning hepatic cells, and hepatic blood flow decrease with increasing age. This results in a slower metabolism of drugs in the elderly. Decreasing renal function associated with aging is significant because many of the therapeutic agents used are eliminated by the kidneys. Renal function may be further impaired in the elderly secondary to dehydration, hypotension, heart failure, or other concurrent diseases. Other factors that place the elderly patient at greater risk for drug interactions or drug toxicity are chronic illnesses that require multiple drug therapy and a greater likelihood of malnourishment. All of these factors lead to accumulation of active drugs with the potential for serious adverse effects in these patients.

2. Body weight

In general, considerably overweight patients will require an increase in dosage to attain the same therapeutic response. Conversely, patients who are underweight (compared with the general population) tend to require lower doses for the same therapeutic response. Most pediatric doses are calculated by milligrams of drug per kilogram of body weight to adjust for rate of growth.

3. Metabolic rate

Patients with a higher metabolic rate tend to metabolize drugs more rapidly, thus requiring either larger doses or more frequent administration. The converse is true for those with lower metabolic rates. Chronic smoking enhances the metabolism of some drugs (e.g., theophylline), thus requiring higher doses to be given more often for a therapeutic effect.

4. Illness

Pathologic conditions may alter the rate of absorption, distribution, metabolism, and excretion. For example, patients in shock will have reduced peripheral vascular circulation and will absorb drugs injected intramuscularly or subcutaneously very slowly; vomiting patients may not be able to keep a medication in the stomach long enough for dissolution and absorption; diseases such as nephrotic syndrome or malnutrition may reduce the amount of serum proteins in the blood necessary for adequate distribution of drugs; patients with kidney failure must have significant reductions in the dosages of those medications that are excreted by the kidneys.

5. Psychological aspects

Attitudes and expectations play a major role in a patient's response to therapy and the willingness to take the therapy as prescribed. Patients with diseases that have relatively rapid consequences for ignoring therapy, such as insulin-dependent diabetes, have a fairly good rate of compliance. Patients with "silent" illnesses, such as hypertension, tend to be much less compliant with the treatment regimen.

Another psychological consideration is the "placebo effect." A *placebo* is a drug dosage form, such as a tablet or capsule, that has no pharmacologic activity, because the dosage form has no active ingredients. When taken, the patient may report a therapeutic response. This response can be beneficial in patients being treated for such illnesses as anxiety, because the patient tends to take fewer potentially habit-forming drugs.

6. Tolerance

Tolerance occurs when a person starts requiring higher doses to produce the same effects that lower doses once provided. An example is the person who is addicted to heroin. After a few weeks of use, larger doses will be required to provide the same "high." Tolerance can be due to psychological dependence, or the body may metabolize a particular drug more rapidly than before, causing the effects of the drug to wear off more rapidly.

7. Dependence

Drug dependence, also known as "addiction" or "habituation," is the inability of a person to control the ingestion of drugs. The dependence may be physical (in which the person develops withdrawal symptoms if the drug is withdrawn for a certain period of time) or psychological (in which the patient is emotionally attached to the drug). Drug dependence occurs most commonly with the use of schedule, or controlled, medications listed in Chapter 1 such as opiates and barbiturates.

8. Cumulative effect

A drug may accumulate in the body if the next doses are administered before previously administered doses have been metabolized or excreted. Excessive accumulation of a drug may result in drug toxicity. An example of drug accumulation is the excessive ingestion of alcoholic beverages. A person becomes "drunk" or "inebriated" when the rate of consumption exceeds the rate of metabolism and excretion of the alcohol.

DRUG INTERACTIONS
OBJECTIVES

1. State the mechanism by which drug interactions may occur.
2. Differentiate among the following terms used in relationship to medications: additive effect, synergistic effect, antagonistic effect, displacement, interference, and incompatibility.

KEY WORDS

additive effect   synergistic effect
antagonistic effect   displacement
interference   incompatibility

A *drug interaction* is said to occur when the action of one drug is altered by the action of another drug. Drug interactions are cited in two ways: (1) those agents that when combined *increase* the actions of one or both drugs; and (2) those agents that when combined *de-*crease the effectiveness of one or both of the drugs. Some drug interactions are beneficial, such as the use of caffeine, a central nervous system stimulant, with an antihistamine, a central nervous system depressant. The stimulatory effects of the caffeine counteract the drowsiness caused by the antihistamine without eliminating the antihistaminic effects.

The following terminology is used in describing drug interactions:

Additive effect—Two drugs, with similar actions, are taken for a doubled effect

EXAMPLE: propoxyphene + aspirin = added analgesic effect

Synergistic effect—The combined effect of two drugs is greater than the sum of the effect of each drug given alone

EXAMPLE: aspirin + codeine = much greater analgesic effect

Antagonistic effect—One drug interferes with the action of another

EXAMPLE: tetracycline + antacid = decreased absorption of the tetracycline

Displacement—The displacement of a drug by a second drug increases the activity of the first drug

EXAMPLE: warfarin + aspirin = increased anticoagulant effect

Interference—One drug inhibits the metabolism or excretion of a second drug, causing increased activity of the second drug

EXAMPLE: probenecid + spectinomycin = prolonged antibacterial activity from spectinomycin due to blocking renal excretion by probenecid

Incompatibility—One drug is chemically incompatible with another drug (causing deterioration) when the two drugs are mixed in the same syringe or solution; incompatible drugs should not be mixed together or administered together at the same site; signs of incompatibility are haziness, a precipitate, or a change in color of the solution when drugs are mixed

EXAMPLE: ampicillin + gentamicin = ampicillin inactivates gentamicin

ADMINISTRATION
OF MEDICATIONS

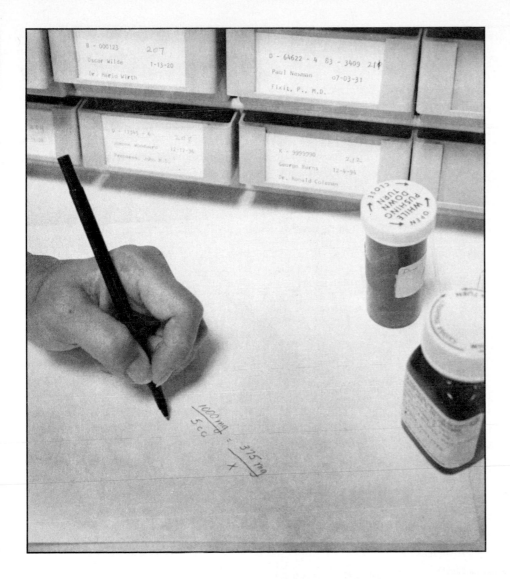

CHAPTER 3

A Review of Arithmetic

CHAPTER GOALS

After completing this chapter, the student should be able to do the following:

1. Learn to use formulas as a basis for performing calculations.
2. Apply basic mathematic principles to the calculation of problems associated with medication dosages.
3. Demonstrate proficiency in performing conversion problems related to medication administration using household, apothecary, and metric equivalents.
4. Convert temperature readings between the centigrade and Fahrenheit scales.

Although many hospitals are using the "unit dosage" system in dispensing drugs, it is still the nurse's responsibility to ascertain that the medication administered is exactly as prescribed by the physician. To give an accurate dosage, the nurse must have a working knowledge of basic mathematics. This review is offered so that individuals may determine areas in which improvement is needed.

ROMAN NUMERALS
OBJECTIVE

1. Read and write selected numerical values using Roman numerals.

Toward the end of the sixteenth century two systems of numbers emerged, Roman and Arabic. They are the basis for our communications in mathematics today, are used interchangeably, and are occasionally used by the physician in prescribing drugs. Roman numerals 1 through 100 are used frequently in medicine. Key symbols are

$$I = 1, V = 5, X = 10, L = 50,$$
$$C = 100, D = 500, M = 1000$$

Whenever a Roman numeral is repeated, or when a smaller numeral follows, the numerals are added.

EXAMPLES

I = 1,   II = 2,   III = 3,   VI = 6,
(1 + 0 = 1) (1 + 1 = 2) (1 + 1 + 1 = 3) (5 + 1 = 6)
VII = 7,   XI = 11,   XII = 12
(5 + 1 + 1 = 7) (10 + 1 = 11) (10 + 1 + 1 = 12)

Whenever a smaller Roman numeral appears before a larger Roman numeral, subtract the smaller numeral.

EXAMPLES

IV = 4,   IX = 9,   XC = 90
(5 − 1 = 4) (10 − 1 = 9) (100 − 10 = 90)

Whenever a smaller Roman numeral appears between two larger Roman numerals, subtract the smaller number from the numeral following it.

EXAMPLES

XIX = 19   XIV = 14
(10 + 10 − 1 = 19)   (10 + 5 − 1 = 14)
        XCIX = 99
    (100 − 10 + 10 − 1 = 99)

The most common Roman numerals associated with medication administration are s̈s̈ = ½, i = 1, ii = 2, iii = 3, iv = 4, v = 5, vi = 6, vii = 7, viis̈s̈ = 7½, viii = 8, ix = 9, x = 10 and xv = 15.

Express the following in Roman numerals:

3 _____   20 _____   101 _____
9 _____   18 _____   499 _____
10 _____   49 _____   1979 _____

Express the following in Arabic numerals:

iv _____   xxxix _____   xix _____
vi _____   ix _____   xv _____

FRACTIONS
OBJECTIVE

1. Demonstrate proficiency in calculating mathematical problems using the addition, subtraction, multiplication, and division of fractions.

KEY WORDS
numerator   denominator

Fractions are one or more of the separate parts of a substance, or less than a whole number or amount.

EXAMPLE: $1 - \dfrac{1}{2} = \dfrac{1}{2}$

Common Fractions

A common fraction is part of a whole number. The numerator (dividend) is the number above the line. The denominator (divisor) is the number below the line. The line separating the numerator and denominator tells us to divide.

Numerator (Names how many parts are used)
—————————————————————————
Denominator (Tabulates the pieces, or tells how
    many pieces the whole is divided into)

EXAMPLES
The denominator represents the number of parts or pieces the whole is divided into.

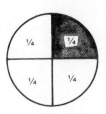

¼ means graphically that the whole circle is divided into four (4) parts; one (1) of the parts is being used.

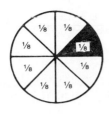

⅛ means graphically that the whole circle is divided into eight (8) parts; one (1) of the parts is being used.

From these two examples, ¼ and ⅛, you can see that the *larger* the *denominator* number, the *smaller* the *portion* is. (Each section in the ⅛ circle is smaller than each section in the ¼ circle.) This is an important concept to understand for persons who will calculate drug dosages. The drug ordered may be ¼ gr and the drug source available on the shelf ½ gr. Before proceeding to do any formal calculations you should first decide if the dose you need to give is smaller or larger than the drug source available on the shelf.

EXAMPLES
Visualize:

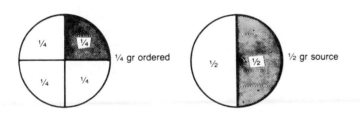

¼ gr ordered   ½ gr source

Decide: "Is what I need to administer to the patient a larger or smaller portion than the drug available on the shelf?"
Answer: ¼ is smaller; thus it would be less than one tablet.

Try a second example: ⅛ gr is ordered; the drug source on the shelf is ½ gr.

Visualize:

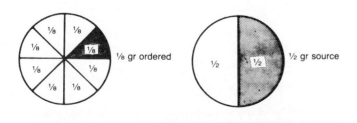

⅛ gr ordered   ½ gr source

Decide: "Is what I need to administer to the patient a larger or smaller portion than the drug available on the shelf?"
Answer: ⅛ is smaller than the drug source; thus it would be less than one tablet.

Types of Common Fractions

1. *Simple:* contains *one* numerator and *one* denominator: ¼, ½₀, ⅟₆₀, ⅟₁₀₀
2. *Complex:* may have a simple fraction in the numerator or denominator:

$$\frac{1}{2}\text{ over }4 = \frac{\frac{1}{2}}{4}$$

or
½ ÷ 4 =
½ ÷ ⁴⁄₁ =
½ × ¼ = ⅛

3. *Proper:* numerator is smaller than denominator: ⅛, ⅖, ⅟₁₀₀
4. *Improper:* numerator is larger than denominator: ⅓, ⁶⁄₄, ¹⁰⁰⁄₁₀
5. *Mixed number:* a whole number and a fraction: 4⅝, 6⅔, 1⁵⁄₁₀₀
6. *Decimal:* fractions written on the basis of a multiple of ten: 0.5 = ⁵⁄₁₀, 0.05 = ⁵⁄₁₀₀, 0.005 = ⁵⁄₁₀₀₀
7. *Equivalent:* fractions that have the same value: ⅓ and ²⁄₆

Working with Fractions

Reducing to lowest terms

Divide both the numerator and the denominator by a number that will divide into both evenly (a common denominator).

$$\text{EXAMPLE: } \frac{25}{125} \div \frac{25}{25} = \frac{1}{5}$$

Reduce the following:

$$\frac{5}{100} =$$

$$\frac{3}{21} =$$

$$\frac{6}{36} =$$

$$\frac{12}{44} =$$

$$\frac{2}{4} =$$

Finding the lowest common denominator of a series of fractions is not always easy. Here are some points to remember:

If the numerator and denominator are both even numbers, 2 will work as a common denominator, but may not be the smallest one.

If the numerator and denominator end with 0 or 5, 5 will work as a common denominator, but may not be the smallest one.

Check to see if the numerator divides evenly into the denominator; this will be the smallest term. When all else fails, use the prime number method to find the lowest common denominator. A prime number is a whole number, greater than 1, that can be divided only by itself and 1 (2, 3, 5, 7, 11, 19, 23, etc.).

Steps: (1) Write down all the denominators in a row, then proceed to divide each denominator by the lowest prime number, until you can no longer use that number, proceed to the next higher prime number and divide using it until it can no longer be used. Continue this procedure until all 1's are obtained. (2) Multiply all the prime numbers used to divide and you will have the lowest common denominator.

EXAMPLE

Fractions: $\dfrac{7}{16}$ $\dfrac{5}{9}$ $\dfrac{13}{30}$ $\dfrac{7}{22}$

Write down all denominators:

Prime numbers:

	16	9	30	22
2	8	9	15	11
2	4	9	15	11
2	2	9	15	11
2	1	9	15	11
3	1	3	5	11
3	1	1	5	11
5	1	1	1	11
11	1	1	1	1

2 is the smallest prime number. Keep dividing by this number until it no longer will divide into the denominators evenly. Proceed to next higher prime, reuse if possible. Go to next higher prime that will divide in evenly, continue until all 1's are obtained.

The lowest common denominator is

$$2 \times 2 \times 2 \times 2 \times 3 \times 3 \times 5 \times 11 = 7920$$

Addition

Adding common fractions

When denominators are the same figure, add the numerators.

EXAMPLE: $\dfrac{1}{4} + \dfrac{2}{4} + \dfrac{3}{4} = \dfrac{6}{4} = 1\dfrac{1}{2}$

Add the following:

$$\dfrac{2}{6} + \dfrac{3}{6} + \dfrac{4}{6} = \dfrac{9}{6} = 1\dfrac{1}{2}$$

$$\dfrac{1}{100} + \dfrac{3}{100} + \dfrac{5}{100} = \dfrac{9}{100}$$

When the denominators are unlike, change the fractions to equivalent fractions by finding the lowest common denominator.

EXAMPLE: $\dfrac{2}{5} + \dfrac{3}{10} + \dfrac{1}{2} = ?$

1. Determine the lowest common denominator. (Use 10 as the common denominator.)

2. Divide the denominator of the fraction being changed into the common denominator and multiply the product (answer) by the numerator.

$\dfrac{2}{5} = \dfrac{4}{10}$ [Divide 5 into 10 and multiply the answer (2) by 2]

$\dfrac{3}{10} = \dfrac{3}{10}$ [Divide 10 into 10 and multiply the answer (1) by 3]

$\dfrac{1}{2} = \dfrac{5}{10}$ [Divide 2 into 10 and multiply the answer (5) by 1]

$\dfrac{12}{10} = 1\dfrac{1}{5}$ [Add the numerators and place the total over the denominator (10); then convert the improper fraction to a mixed number and reduce to lowest terms.]

Add the following:

a. $\dfrac{2}{8} = \dfrac{}{64}$

$+ \dfrac{4}{64} = \dfrac{}{64}$

$+ \dfrac{5}{16} = \dfrac{}{64}$

$\dfrac{}{64}$ Answer: $\dfrac{5}{8}$

b. $\dfrac{3}{7} = \dfrac{}{28}$

$\dfrac{9}{14} = \dfrac{}{28}$

$+ \dfrac{1}{28} = \dfrac{}{28}$

$\dfrac{}{28}$ Answer: $1\dfrac{3}{28}$

Adding mixed numbers

Add the fractions first; then add the whole numbers.

EXAMPLE: $2\dfrac{3}{4} + 2\dfrac{1}{2} + 3\dfrac{3}{8} = ?$

1. Determine the lowest common denominator. (Use 8 as the common denominator.)

2. Divide the denominator of the fraction being changed into the common denominator and multiply the product (answer) by the numerator.

$2\dfrac{3}{4} = \dfrac{6}{8}$ [Divide 4 into 8 and multiply the answer (2) by 3]

$2\dfrac{1}{2} = \dfrac{4}{8}$ [Divide 2 into 8 and multiply the answer (4) by 1]

$+ 3\dfrac{3}{8} = \dfrac{3}{8}$ [Divide 8 into 8 and multiply the answer (1) by 3]

$\dfrac{13}{8}$ [Add the numerators and place the total over the denominator (8)]

[Convert the improper fraction

$7 + 1\dfrac{5}{8} = 8\dfrac{5}{8}$ $\left(\dfrac{13}{8}\right)$ to a mixed number $\left(1\dfrac{5}{8}\right)$

and add it to the whole numbers]

Add the following:

a. $+\dfrac{1}{4}$

$+\dfrac{3}{4}$

$\dfrac{}{\dfrac{}{4}}$ Answer: $\dfrac{4}{4}=1$

b. $\dfrac{1}{2}=\dfrac{}{6}$

$+\dfrac{1}{3}=\dfrac{}{6}$

$+\dfrac{1}{6}=\dfrac{}{6}$

$=\dfrac{}{6}$ Answer: $\dfrac{6}{6}=1$

c. $\dfrac{3}{5}=\dfrac{}{50}$

$+\dfrac{4}{50}=\dfrac{}{50}$ Answer: $\dfrac{34}{50}=\dfrac{17}{25}$

$=\dfrac{}{50}$ (Reduced to lowest term.)

Subtraction
Subtracting fractions
When the denominators are unlike, change the fractions to an equivalent fraction by finding the lowest common denominator.

EXAMPLE: $\dfrac{1}{4}-\dfrac{3}{16}=$

1. Determine the lowest common denominator. (Use 16 as the common denominator.)
2. Divide the denominator of the fraction being changed into the common denominator and multiply the product (answer) by the numerator.

$\dfrac{1}{4}=\dfrac{4}{16}$ [Divide 4 into 16 and multiply the answer (4) by 1]

$-\dfrac{3}{16}=\dfrac{3}{16}$ [Divide 16 into 16 and multiply the answer (1) by 3]

$\dfrac{1}{16}$ [Subtract the numerators and place the total over the denominator (16)]

Subtract the following:

a. $\dfrac{3}{8}$

$-\dfrac{2}{8}$

$\dfrac{}{8}$ Answer: $\dfrac{1}{8}$

b. $\dfrac{1}{100}=\dfrac{}{300}$

$-\dfrac{1}{150}=\dfrac{}{300}$

$\dfrac{}{300}$ Answer: $\dfrac{1}{300}$

Subtracting mixed numbers
Subtract the fractions first; then subtract the whole numbers.

EXAMPLE: $4\dfrac{1}{4}-1\dfrac{3}{4}=$?

$4\dfrac{1}{4}=3\dfrac{5}{4}$ [NOTE: You cannot subtract $\dfrac{3}{4}$ from $\dfrac{1}{4}$;

$-1\dfrac{3}{4}=1\dfrac{3}{4}$ therefore borrow 1 (which equals $\dfrac{4}{4}$) from

the whole numbers and add $\dfrac{4}{4}+\dfrac{1}{4}=\dfrac{5}{4}$.]

$2\dfrac{2}{4}=2\dfrac{1}{2}$ [Subtract the numerators, place answer over the denominator (4); reduce to lowest terms; subtract the whole numbers]

When the denominators are unlike, change the fractions to equivalent fractions by finding the lowest common denominator.

EXAMPLE: $2\dfrac{5}{8}-1\dfrac{1}{4}=$?

1. Determine the lowest common denominator. (Use 8 as the common denominator.)
2. Divide the denominator of the fraction being changed into the common denominator and multiply the product (answer) by the numerator.

$2\dfrac{5}{8}=2\dfrac{5}{8}$ [Divide 8 into 8 and multiply the answer (1) by 5]

$-1\dfrac{1}{4}=1\dfrac{2}{8}$ [Divide 4 into 8 and multiply the answer (2) by 1]

$1\dfrac{3}{8}$ [Subtract the numerators and place the total over the denominator (8); reduce to lowest terms; subtract the whole numbers.

Subtract the following:

a. $\dfrac{7}{8}=\dfrac{}{24}$

$-\dfrac{3}{6}=\dfrac{}{24}$

$\dfrac{}{24}$ Answer: $\dfrac{9}{24}=\dfrac{3}{8}$

b. $6\dfrac{7}{8}=\dfrac{}{16}$

$-3\dfrac{1}{16}=\dfrac{}{16}$

$\dfrac{}{16}$ Answer: $3\dfrac{13}{16}$

Multiplication
Multiplying a whole number by a fraction

EXAMPLE: $3\times\dfrac{5}{8}=$?

1. Place the whole number over 1. $\left(\frac{3}{1}\right)$
2. Multiply the numerators (top numbers) and multiply the denominators (bottom numbers).

$$\frac{3}{1} \times \frac{5}{8} = \frac{15}{8}$$

3. Change the improper fraction to a mixed number:

$$\frac{15}{8} = 1\frac{7}{8}$$

Multiply the following:

a. $2 \times \frac{3}{4} = ?$ Answer: $\frac{3}{2} = 1\frac{1}{2}$

b. $15 \times \frac{3}{5} = ?$ Answer: $\frac{9}{1} = 9$

Multiplying two fractions

EXAMPLE: $\frac{1}{4} \times \frac{2}{3} = ?$

1. Use cancellation to speed the process.

$$\frac{1}{\overset{}{\underset{2}{4}}} \times \frac{\overset{1}{2}}{3} =$$

2. Multiply the numerators (top numbers); multiply the denominators.

$$\frac{1}{2} \times \frac{1}{3} = \frac{1}{6}$$

Multiplying mixed numbers

EXAMPLE: $3\frac{1}{2} \times 2\frac{1}{5} = ?$

1. Change the mixed numbers (a whole number and a fraction) to an improper fraction (numerator is larger than denominator).

$3\frac{1}{2} \times 2\frac{1}{5} = ?$

$\frac{7}{2} \times \frac{11}{5} = ?$ (Multiply the denominator times the whole number and add the numerator.)

2. Multiply the numerators; multiply the denominators.

$$\frac{7}{2} \times \frac{11}{5} = \frac{77}{10}$$

3. Change the product (answer), an improper fraction, to a mixed number by dividing the denominator into the numerator; reduce to lowest terms.

$$\frac{7}{2} \times \frac{11}{5} = \frac{77}{10} = 7\frac{7}{10}$$

Multiply the following:

a. $1\frac{2}{3} \times \frac{3}{6} = ?$ Answer: $\frac{5}{6}$

b. $1\frac{7}{8} \times 1\frac{1}{4} = ?$ Answer: $\frac{75}{32} = 2\frac{11}{32}$

Division
Dividing fractions

EXAMPLE $4 \div \frac{1}{2} = ?$

1. Change the division sign to a multiplication sign.
2. Invert the divisor, the number after the division sign.
3. Reduce the fractions using cancellation.
4. Multiply the numerators and the denominators.

$$4 \div \frac{1}{2} = \frac{4}{1} \times \frac{2}{1} = \frac{8}{1} = 8$$

Dividing with a mixed number

1. Change the mixed number to an improper fraction.
2. Change the division sign to a multiplication sign.
3. Invert the divisor.
4. Reduce whenever possible

EXAMPLES

$$4\frac{1}{2} \div \frac{3}{4} = \frac{9}{2} \div \frac{3}{4} = \frac{\overset{3}{9}}{\underset{1}{2}} \times \frac{\overset{2}{4}}{\underset{1}{3}} = \frac{6}{1} \text{ or } 6$$

$$6\frac{1}{4} \div 1\frac{1}{4} = \frac{25}{4} \div \frac{5}{4} = \frac{\overset{5}{25}}{\underset{1}{4}} \times \frac{\overset{1}{4}}{\underset{1}{5}} = \frac{5}{1} \text{ or } 5$$

Fractions as decimals

Fractions can be changed to a decimal form by dividing the numerator by the denominator.

EXAMPLE: $\frac{1}{2} = 2\overline{)\overset{0.5}{1.0}}$

Change the following fractions to decimals:

a. $\frac{1}{100} = ?$ Answer: 0.01

b. $\frac{5}{8} = ?$ Answer: 0.625

c. $\frac{1}{2} = ?$ Answer: 0.5

Using cancellation to speed your work

1. Determine a number that will divide evenly into both a numerator and a denominator.

2. Continue the process of dividing both a numerator and denominator by the same number until all numbers are reduced to the lowest terms.
3. Complete the multiplication of the problem.

EXAMPLE: $\dfrac{\overset{1}{\cancel{5}}}{\cancel{6}} \times \dfrac{\overset{3}{\cancel{9}}}{\cancel{10}} = ?$

$\dfrac{1}{2} \times \dfrac{3}{2} = \dfrac{3}{4}$

4. Complete the division of the problem.

EXAMPLE: $\dfrac{6}{9} \div \dfrac{5}{8} = ?$

$\dfrac{2}{3} \times \dfrac{8}{5} = \dfrac{16}{15} = 1\dfrac{1}{15}$

(Change the division sign to a multiplication sign; invert the number after the division sign; reduce and complete the multiplication of the problem.)

DECIMAL FRACTIONS
OBJECTIVES

1. Demonstrate proficiency in calculating mathematical problems using the addition, subtraction, multiplication, and division of decimals.
2. Convert decimals to fractions and fractions to decimals.

When fractions are written in decimal form, the denominators are not written. The word *decimal* means "10."

When reading decimals, the numbers to the left of the decimal point are whole numbers. It helps to think of them as whole dollars.

EXAMPLES

        1. = one
       11. = eleven
      111. = one hundred eleven
     1111. = one thousand one hundred eleven

Numbers to the right of the decimal point are read as follows:

EXAMPLES

Decimal(s):	Fraction(s):
0.1 = one tenth	1/10
0.01 = one hundredth	1/100
0.465 = four hundred sixty-five thousandths	465/1000
0.0007 = seven ten thousandths	7/10000

Here is another way to view reading decimals:

ten thousands	thousands	hundreds	tens	one	DECIMAL POINT	tenths	hundredths	thousandths	ten thousandths
					.	1			
					.	2	2		
					.	1	1	2	
					.	0	1	1	2
				1	.				
			1	0	.				
		1	0	0	.				
	1	0	0	0	.				

| | Whole numbers | | | | | | Fractions | | |

. 1 equals one tenth (1/10)

. 2 2 equals twenty-two hundredths (22/100)

. 1 1 2 equals one hundred twelve thousandths (112/1000)

. 0 1 1 2 equals one hundred twelve ten thousandths (112/10000)

1 . equals number one

1 0 . equals number ten

1 0 0 . equals number one hundred

1 0 0 0 . equals number one thousand

On prescriptions another way of expressing the decimal is by using a slanted line.

EXAMPLES

1	mg = 0.001	g = 0/001	g
0.1	mg = 0.0001	g = 0/0001	g
30	mg = 0.030	g = 0/030	g
100	mg = 0.100	g = 0/100	g
1000	mg = 1.000	g = 1/0	g
250	mg = 0.250	g = 0/250	g

Multiplying Decimals

Multiplying whole numbers and decimals

1. Count as many places in the answer, starting from the right, as there are places in the decimal involved in the multiplication.
2. The multiplier is the bottom number with the × or multiplication sign before it.
3. The multiplicand is the top number.

EXAMPLES

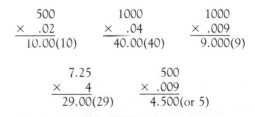

$$\begin{array}{r} 500 \\ \times\ .02 \\ \hline 10.00(10) \end{array} \qquad \begin{array}{r} 1000 \\ \times\ .04 \\ \hline 40.00(40) \end{array} \qquad \begin{array}{r} 1000 \\ \times\ .009 \\ \hline 9.000(9) \end{array}$$

$$\begin{array}{r} 7.25 \\ \times\ 4 \\ \hline 29.00(29) \end{array} \qquad \begin{array}{r} 500 \\ \times\ .009 \\ \hline 4.500(\text{or } 5) \end{array}$$

Rounding the answer

Note in the last example that the first number after the decimal point in the answer is 5. Instead of the answer remaining 4.5 it becomes the next whole number, 5.

This would be true if the answer were 4.5, 4.6, 4.7, 4.8, or 4.9. In each case the answer would become 5. If the answer were 4.1, 4.2, 4.3, or 4.4 the answer would remain 4.

When the first number after the decimal point is 5 or above, the answer becomes the next whole number. When the first number after the decimal point is less than 5, the answer becomes the whole number in the answer.

Multiply the following:

$$
\begin{array}{cccc}
1,200 & 575 & 515 & 510 \\
\times\ .009 & \times .02 & \times .02 & \times .04
\end{array}
$$

Multiplying a decimal by a decimal

1. Multiply the problem as if the numbers were both whole numbers.
2. Count decimal places in the answer, starting from the right, as many decimal places as there are in both of the numbers that were to be multiplied.

EXAMPLE:
$$
\begin{array}{r}
3.75 \\
\times\ .5 \\
\hline
1.875 = 2
\end{array}
$$

There are two decimal places in 3.75 and one decimal place in .5, making three decimal places. Count three decimal places from the right. Round off the answer to 2.

Multiplying numbers with zero

EXAMPLES

1. Multiply 223 by 40.
   a. Multiply 223 by 0. Write the answer, 0, in the unit column of the answer.
   b. Then multiply 223 by 4. Write this answer in front of the 0 in the product.

$$
\begin{array}{r}
223 \\
\times\ 40 \\
\hline
8920
\end{array}
$$

2. Multiply 124 by 304.
   a. First multiply 124 by 4. The answer is 496.
   b. Now multiply 124 by 0. Write the answer, 0, under the 9 in 496.
   c. Multiply 124 by 3. Write this answer in front of the 0 in the product.

$$
\begin{array}{r}
124 \\
\times\ 304 \\
\hline
496 \\
3720 \\
\hline
37696
\end{array}
$$

Dividing Decimals

1. If the divisor (number by which you divide) is a decimal, make it a whole number by moving the decimal point to the right of the last figure.

2. Move the decimal point in the dividend (the number dividend) as many places to the right as you moved the decimal point in the divisor.
3. Place the decimal point for the quotient (answer) directly above the new decimal point of the dividend.

EXAMPLES

$$
.25\overline{)10} = 25\overline{)1000.}^{\,40.} \qquad 0.3\overline{)99.3} = 3\overline{)993.}^{\,331.}
$$

$$
.4\overline{)1.68} = 4\overline{)16.8}^{\,4.2}
$$

Changing Decimals to Common Fractions

1. Remove the decimal point.
2. Place the appropriate denominator under the number.
3. Reduce to lowest terms.

EXAMPLES

$$
.2 = \frac{2}{10} = \frac{1}{5} \qquad .20 = \frac{20}{100} = \frac{1}{5}
$$

Change the following:

.3 = _____	.25 = _____
.4 = _____	.50 = _____
.5 = _____	.75 = _____
.05 = _____	.002 = _____

Changing Common Fractions to Decimal Fractions

Divide the numerator of the fraction by the denominator.

EXAMPLE: $\dfrac{1}{4}$ means $1 \div 4$ or $4\overline{)1.00}^{\,.25}$

Change the following:

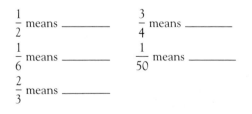

$\dfrac{1}{2}$ means _____ $\dfrac{3}{4}$ means _____

$\dfrac{1}{6}$ means _____ $\dfrac{1}{50}$ means _____

$\dfrac{2}{3}$ means _____

PERCENTS
OBJECTIVES

1. Demonstrate proficiency in calculating mathematical problems using percentages.
2. Convert percents to fractions, percents to decimals, decimal fractions to percents, and common fractions to percents.

Determining Percent One Number Is of Another

1. Divide the smaller number by the larger number.
2. Multiply the quotient by 100 and add the percent sign.

   EXAMPLE: A certain 1000 parts solution is 10 parts drug. What percent of the solution is drug?

$$\frac{.01}{1000)\overline{10.00}}$$
$$.01 \times 100 = 1. \text{ or } 1\%$$

Changing Percents to Fractions

1. Omit the percent sign to form the numerator.
2. Use 100 for the denominator.
3. Reduce the fraction.

   EXAMPLES: $5\% = \frac{5}{100} = \frac{1}{20}$ $75\% = \frac{75}{100} = \frac{3}{4}$

Change the following:

$25\% = \frac{25}{100} =$ $\qquad$ $2\% = \frac{2}{100} =$

$15\% = \frac{15}{100} =$ $\qquad$ $12\frac{1}{2}\% = \frac{12.5}{100} =$

$10\% = \frac{10}{100} =$ $\qquad$ $\frac{1}{4}\% = \frac{1/4}{100} =$

$20\% = \frac{20}{100} =$ $\qquad$ $150\% = \frac{150}{100} =$

$50\% = \frac{50}{100} =$ $\qquad$ $4\% = \frac{4}{100} =$

Changing Percents to Decimal Fractions

1. Omit the percent signs.
2. Insert a decimal point *two places to the left* of the last number, or express as hundredths, decimally.

   EXAMPLES: $5\% = .05$ $15\% = .15$

Change the following:

$4\% =$ $\qquad$ $25\% =$

$1\% =$ $\qquad$ $50\% =$

$2\% =$ $\qquad$ $10\% =$

Note in these examples that those numbers that were already hundredths, such as 10%, 15%, 25%, 50%, merely need to have the decimal point placed in front of the first number, since they are already expressed in hundredths; whereas 1%, 2%, 4%, 5% needed to have a zero placed in front of the number to express them as hundredths.

Change these percents to decimal fractions:

$12\frac{1}{2}\% =$ $\qquad$ $\frac{1}{4}\% =$

If the percent is a mixed number, it should have the fraction expressed as a decimal. Then change the percent to a decimal by moving the decimal point two places to the left.

EXAMPLES

$$12\frac{1}{2}\% = 12.5\% \text{ or } .125$$

$$\frac{1}{4}\% = 0.25\% \text{ or } .0025$$

Changing Common Fractions to Percents

1. Divide the numerator by the denominator.
2. Multiply the quotient by 100 and add the percent sign.

EXAMPLE: $\frac{1}{50} = 50)\overline{1.00}^{.02} = .02 \times 100 = 2\%$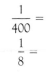

Change the following:

$$\frac{1}{400} =$$

$$\frac{1}{8} =$$

Changing Decimal Fractions to Percents

1. Move the decimal point two places to the right.
2. Omit the decimal point if a whole number results.
3. Add the percent signs. (This is the same as multiplying the decimal fraction by 100 and adding the percent sign.)

EXAMPLES: $.01 = 1.00 = 1\% \left(\text{or } \frac{1}{100} \right)$

Change the following:

$.05 =$

$.25 =$

$.15 =$

$.125 =$

$.0025 =$

Points to Remember in Reading Decimals

1. 1. is the whole number 1. When it is written 1.0, it is still one or 1.
2. The whole number is usually written like this: 1 or 2 or 3 or 4, and so on.
3. The whole number also can be written with the decimal point after the number: 1.0, 2.0, 3.0, 4.0.
4. Can you read this one? 0.1. This is one-tenth. There is one number after the decimal point.
5. Can you read this one? .1. This is also one-tenth. The zero in front of the decimal point does not change its value. One-tenth can be written, then, in two ways: 0.1 and .1.

6. Remember that in writing the number 1. or 1.0, the decimal point is after the number. This makes the number a whole number. It is read the whole number 1.

RATIOS
OBJECTIVE

1. Demonstrate proficiency in converting ratios to percentages and percentages to ratios, in simplifying ratios, and in use of the proportion method for solving problems.

A ratio expresses the relationship that one quantity bears to another.

EXAMPLES

1:5 means 1 part of a drug to 5 parts
of a solution.
1:100 means 1 part of a drug to 100 parts
of a solution.
1:500 means 1 part of a drug to 500 parts
of a solution.

A common fraction can be expressed as a ratio.

EXAMPLE: $\frac{1}{5}$ is the same as 1:5

The ratio of one amount to an amount expressed in terms of the same unit is the number of units in the first divided by the number of units in the second. The ratio of 2 ounces of a disinfectant to 10 ounces of water is 2 to 10 or 1 to 5 or ⅕. This ratio may be written ⅕ or 1:5.

The two numbers compared are referred to by using the term "ratio." The first term of a true ratio is always one, or 1. This is the simplest form of a ratio.

Changing Ratio to Percent

1. Make the first term of the ratio the numerator of the fraction whose denominator is the second term of the ratio.
2. Divide the numerator by the denominator.
3. Multiply by 100 and add the percent sign.

EXAMPLE: $5:1 = \frac{5}{1} \times 100 = 500\%$

Change the following:

1:5 =

Changing Percent to Ratio

1. Change the percent to a fraction and reduce the fraction to lowest terms.
2. The numerator of the fraction is the first term of the ratio, and the denominator is the second term of the ratio.

EXAMPLE: $\frac{1}{2}\% = \dfrac{\frac{1}{2}}{100} = \frac{1}{2} \div \frac{100}{1}$

$= \frac{1}{2} \times \frac{1}{100} = \frac{1}{200} = 1:200$

Change the following:

2% =
50% =
75% =

Simplifying Ratios

Ratios can be simplified as ratios or as fractions.

EXAMPLE: $25:100 = 1:4$ or $\dfrac{25}{100} = \dfrac{1}{4}$

Simplify the following:

4:12   =
5:10   =
10:5   =
75:100 =
¼:100   =
15:20   =
3:9   =

Proportions

A proportion shows how two *equal* ratios are related. This method is good because it is possible to prove that your answer is correct, and it is especially useful in solutions.

1. Three factors are known. The fourth *unknown* (what you are looking for) is represented by x.
2. The first and fourth terms of a proportion are called extremes. The second and third are the means. The product of the means equals the product of the extremes, or multiplying the first and fourth equals the second and third.

EXAMPLE

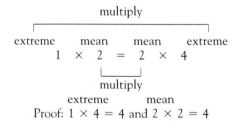

Proof: $1 \times 4 = 4$ and $2 \times 2 = 4$

If you did not know one number, you could solve for it as follows:

EXAMPLE

$$1:2 = 2:x$$
$$1x = 4$$
$$x = 4 \div 1 = 4$$
$$x = 4$$
Proof: $1 \times 4 = 4$ and $2 \times 2 = 4$

Solve the following:

a. $9 : x : : 5 : 300$ _____
b. $x : 60 : : 4 : 120$ _____
c. $5 : 3000 : : 15 : x$ _____
d. $0.7 : 70 : : : x : 1000$ _____
e. $\frac{1}{400} : : x : : 2 : 1600$ _____
f. $0.2 : 8 : : x : 20$ _____
g. $100,000 : 3 : : 1,000,000 : x$ _____
h. $\frac{1}{4} : x : : 20 : 400$ _____

NOTE: x is the unknown factor. It may be a mean or an extreme in any of the four positions in any problem.

SYSTEMS OF WEIGHTS AND MEASURES

OBJECTIVES

1. Memorize the basic equivalents of the household, apothecary, and metric systems.
2. Demonstrate proficiency in performing conversion of medication problems utilizing the household, apothecary, and metric systems.

KEY WORDS

household	apothecary
measurements	measurements
grains	minim
metric system	milliliter
centimeter	liter
milligram	gram
kilogram	

Three systems of measurement are used during the calculation, preparation, and administration of drugs: household, apothecary, and metric.

Household Measurements

Household measurements are the least accurate. However, they are often the way pharmacological agents are administered at home. The patient has grown up using this system of measurement and therefore understands it best. Household measurements include drops, teaspoons, tablespoons, teacups, cups, glasses, pints, quarts, and gallons. The first three measurements—drops, teaspoons, and tablespoons—would be used for medications, depending on the amount prescribed.

Common Household Equivalents

1 quart = 4 cups
1 pint = 2 cups
1 cup = 8 ounces
1 teacup = 6 ounces
1 tablespoon = 3 teaspoons
1 teaspoon = approximately 60 drops

Apothecary Measurements

The apothecary system of measurement is an ancient system; the word *apothecary* means "pharmacist" or "druggist." Physicians rarely order medicine using the apothecary system. The metric system is the preferred system of measurement because it is more accurate.

Apothecary weight

For weighing solids, the units of apothecary weight are, in increasing order of magnitude (smallest to largest), as follows:

20 grains (gr) = 1 scruple
3 scruples or 60 grains = 1 dram (ʒ)
(1 dram = 4 ml or 4 cc)
8 drams or 480 grains = 1 ounce (ʒ)
12 ounces = 1 pound (lb)

The grain was originally derived from the average weight of a grain of wheat. The symbol for grain is "gr." The dram (originally, drachma or drachm) was a Greek silver coin. The symbol for dram is ʒ. The ounce, whose symbol is ʒ, is $\frac{1}{12}$ of a troy pound. The pound is of Roman origin and signifies a balance. The symbol "lb" is the abbreviation for the Latin word *libra*, which means pound.

In apothecary weight, 12 ounces equal 1 pound (same weight as those of troy weight). In avoirdupois weight, 16 ounces equal 1 pound. Avoirdupois weight is used in weighing all articles *except* drugs, gold, silver, and precious stones.

Apothecary volume

For measuring fluids the units of apothecary volume are, from smallest to largest, as follows:

60 minims (♏) = 1 fluidram (f ʒ)
8 fluidrams or 480 minims = 1 fluidounce (f ʒ)
16 fluidounces = 1 pint (pt or O)
2 pints = 1 quart (qt)
4 quarts = 1 gallon (C)

The unit of fluid measure is a minim (see Figure 3-1). This is approximately the quantity of water that would weigh a grain. The symbol for minim is ♏. The symbol "O" is the abbreviation for the Latin word *octarius*. It means an eighth of a gallon and is the same as a pint. The symbol "C" is taken from the Latin word *congius*. It means a vessel or container that holds a gallon.

It might be of aid to visualize a dram as approximately equal to one teaspoonful in household measure.

The minim (♏) is the approximate equivalent of the drop, but it is not identical to the drop. Minims are not an accurate method of measuring medicines and, wherever possible, milliliters or cubic centimeters should be used.

Imperial system of volume

In Canada, the imperial system of volume measurement is used. The names of the units (that is, minims, fluid-

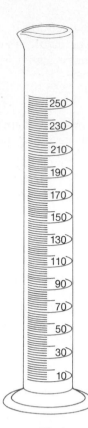

Figure 3-1 *Fluid measures.*

The International Metric Convention met in Paris in 1875, and as a result of this meeting the International Bureau of Weights and Measures was formed. The first task of the International Bureau of Weights and Measures was the preparation of an international standard meter bar and an international standard kilogram weight. Duplicates of these were made for all countries participating in the convention.

A measurement line was selected on the international standard meter bar. The distance between the two lines of measurement on the bar is the official unit of the metric system. The standards given to the United States are preserved at the National Institute of Standards and Technology, Gaithersburg, Maryland. There are 25.4 millimeters in 1 inch (2.5 centimeters).

The metric system uses the meter as the unit of length, the liter as the unit of volume, and the gram as the measurement of weight.

Units of Length (Meter)
1 millimeter = 0.001 meaning 1/1000
1 centimeter = 0.01 meaning 1/100
1 decimeter = 0.1 meaning 1/10
1 meter = 1 meter

Units of Volume (Liter)
1 milliliter = 0.001 meaning 1/1000
1 centiliter = 0.01 meaning 1/100
1 deciliter = 0.1 meaning 1/10
1 liter = 1 liter

Units of Weight (Gram)
1 microgram = 0.000001 meaning 1/1000000
1 milligram = 0.001 meaning 1/1000
1 centigram = 0.01 meaning 1/100
1 decigram = 0.1 meaning 1/10
1 gram = 1 gram

ounces, pints, quarts, gallons) are the same as those used in the apothecary system, but the volumes are somewhat different.

60 minims = 1 fluidram
8 fluidrams or 480 minims = 1 fluidounce
20 fluidounces = 1 pint
2 pints = 1 quart
4 quarts = 1 gallon

NOTE: In the imperial system, 20 fluidounces equals 1 pint; in the apothecary system, 16 fluidounces equals 1 pint.

Metric System

The metric system was invented by the French in the late eighteenth century. A committee of the Academy of Sciences, working under government authority, recommended a standard unit of linear measure. For a basis of measurement they chose a quarter of the earth's circumference measured across the poles. One ten-millionth of this distance was accepted as the standard unit of linear measure.

The committee calculated the distance from the equator to the North Pole from surveys that had been made along the meridian that passes through Paris. The distance divided by 10,000,000 was chosen as the unit of length, or the meter.

Metric standards were adopted in France in 1799.

Other prefixes

Deca means ten or 10 times as much. *Hecto* means one hundred or 100 times as much. *Kilo* means one thousand or 1000 times as much. These three prefixes can be combined with the words meter, gram, or liter.

EXAMPLES

1 decaliter = 10 liters
1 hectometer = 100 meters
1 kilogram = 1000 grams

Arabic numbers are used to write metric doses.

EXAMPLES: 500 milligrams, 5 grams, 15 milliliters

Prefixes added to the units (meter, liter, or gram) indicate smaller or larger units. All units are derived by dividing or multiplying by 10, 100, or 1000.

Common Metric Equivalents
1 milliliter (ml) = 1 cubic centimeter (cc)
1000 milliliters (ml) = 1 liter (L) = 1000 cubic centimeters (cc)
1000 milligrams (mg) = 1 gram (g)

1000 micrograms (mcg) = 1 milligram (mg)
1,000,000 micrograms (mcg) = 1 gram (g)
1000 grams (g) = 1 kilogram (Kg)

Differentiate between metric and apothecary weights. Mark each of the following M for metric or A for apothecary.

1. grain = _____
2. microgram = _____
3. milligram = _____
4. dram = _____
5. gram = _____

Differentiate between metric and apothecary volume. Mark each of the following M for metric or A for apothecary.

1. minim = _____
2. milliliter = _____
3. fluidram = _____
4. fluidounce = _____
5. liter = _____

Differentiate among metric weight, metric volume, apothecary weight, and apothecary volume. Mark each of the following MW for metric weight, MV for metric volume, AW for apothecary weight, or AV for apothecary volume.

1. minim = _____
2. microgram = _____
3. milliliter = _____
4. liter = _____
5. gram = _____

Conversion of Metric and Apothecary Units

The first step in calculating the drug dosage is to make sure that the drug ordered and the drug source on hand are *both* in the same *system of measurement* (preferably in the metric system) and in the *same unit of weight* (for example, both mg or both grams). See Table 3-1.

Converting grams (metric) to grains (apothecary) or milliliters (metric) to minims (apothecary)

(1 g = 15 grains; 1 ml = 15 ℥)
Multiply the number of grains (or milliliters) by 15.

EXAMPLES

1. Change 30 grams to grains.

$$30 \times 15 = 450 \text{ gr}$$

2. Change 1 gram to grains

$$\frac{1 \text{ g} \times 15 \text{ gr}}{\text{g}} = 15 \text{ gr}$$

Use ratio and proportion.

$$\frac{g}{1} : \frac{gr}{1} :: \frac{g}{15} : \frac{gr}{x}$$
$$x = 15$$
$$1 \text{ g} = \text{gr } 15$$

Change the following grams (metric) to grains (apothecary).

a. 15 g = _____ gr
b. 30 g = _____ gr
c. 1 g = _____ gr

Converting grains (apothecary) to grams (metric)

(1 gr. = 0.060 g)
Divide the number of grains by 15 (or multiply by 0.060).

EXAMPLES

1. Change 30 grains to grams.

$$30 \div 15 = 2g$$

2. Change 5 grains to grams.

$$\frac{0.060 \text{ g}}{\text{gr}} \times 5 \text{ gr} = 0.3 \text{ g}$$

Change grains (apothecary) to grams (metric).

a. 1 grain = _____ g
b. 5 grains = _____ g
c. 10 grains = _____ g
d. 15 grains = _____ g

In the following example, both the physician's order and the medication available are in the metric system. They are *not* both in the *same unit of weight* within the metric system.

EXAMPLE: The physician orders the patient to have 0.250 g of a drug. The label on the bottle of medicine says 250 mg, meaning that each capsule contains 250 mg of the drug.

To change the gram dose into milligrams multiply 0.250 by 1000 and move the decimal point three places to the right (a milligram is one thousandth of a gram), 0.250 g = 250 mg, so you would give one tablet of this drug.

TRY THIS ONE: The physician orders the patient to have 0.1 g of a drug. The label on the bottle states the strength of the drug is 100 mg/capsule.

To change the gram dose into milligrams, move the decimal point three places to the right: 0.1 g = 100 mg, exactly what the bottle label strength states.

Convert the following grams (g) to milligrams (mg):

0.2 g = _____ mg
0.250 g = _____ mg
0.125 g = _____ mg
0.0006 g = _____ mg
0.004 g = _____ mg

Table 3-1 *Metric Doses and Apothecary Equivalents*

LIQUID MEASURE		WEIGHT	
METRIC	APPROXIMATE APOTHECARY EQUIVALENTS	METRIC	APPROXIMATE APOTHECARY EQUIVALENTS
1000 ml[a]	**1 quart**	30 g	1 ounce
750 ml	1½ pints	15 g	4 drams
500 ml	**1 pint**	100 g	2½ drams
250 ml	8 fluidounces	7.5 g	2 drams
200 ml	7 fluidounces	6 g	90 grains
100 ml	3½ fluidounces	5 g	75 grains
50 ml	1⅓ fluidounces	3 g	45 grains
30 ml	**1 fluidounce**	2 g	30 grains (½ dram)
15 ml	4 fluidrams	1.5 g	22 grains
10 ml	2½ fluidrams	**1 g**	**15 grains**
8 ml	2 fluidrams	0.75 g	12 grains
5 ml	1¼ fluidrams	0.6 g	10 grains
4 ml	1 fluidram	**0.5 g**	**7½ grains**
3 ml	45 minims	0.4 g	6 grains
2 ml	30 minims	0.3 g	5 grains
1 ml	**15 or 16 minims**	0.25 g	4 grains
0.75 ml	12 minims	0.2 g	3 grains
0.6 ml	10 minims	0.15 g	2½ grains
0.5 ml	8 minims	0.12 g	2 grains
0.3 ml	5 minims	0.1 g	1½ grains
0.25 ml	4 minims	75 mg	1¼ grains
0.2 ml	3 minims	**60 mg**	**1 grain**
0.1 ml	1½ minims	50 mg	¾ grain
0.06 ml	**1 minim**	40 mg	⅔ grain
0.05 ml	¾ minim	30 mg	**½ grain**
0.03 ml	½ minim	25 mg	⅜ grain
		20 mg	⅓ grain
Metric	♣ *Imperial Equivalent*	**15 mg**	**¼ grain**
28.4 ml	1 fluidounce	12 mg	⅕ grain
568 ml	1 pint (20 fl oz)	10 mg	⅙ grain
1136 ml	1 quart	8 mg	⅛ grain
(1.136 L)	(40 fl oz)	6 mg	¹⁄₁₀ grain
4546 ml	1 gallon	5 mg	¹⁄₁₂ grain
(4.546 L)	(160 fl oz)	4 mg	¹⁄₁₅ grain
		3 mg	¹⁄₂₀ grain
		2 mg	¹⁄₃₀ grain
		1.5 mg	¹⁄₄₀ grain
		1.2 mg	¹⁄₅₀ grain
		1 mg	**¹⁄₆₀ grain**
		0.8 mg	¹⁄₈₀ grain
		0.6 mg	**¹⁄₁₀₀ grain**
		0.5 mg	¹⁄₁₂₀ grain
		0.4 mg	**¹⁄₁₅₀ grain**
		0.3 mg	**¹⁄₂₀₀ grain**
		0.25 mg	¹⁄₂₅₀ grain
		0.2 mg	¹⁄₃₀₀ grain
		0.15 mg	¹⁄₄₀₀ grain
		0.12 mg	¹⁄₅₀₀ grain
		0.1 mg	¹⁄₆₀₀ grain

Modified from United States Pharmacopeia XX. Equivalents in bold type should be memorized.
[a]A milliliter (ml) is approximately equivalent to a cubic centimeter (cc).

Converting milligrams (metric) to grams (metric)

(1000 mg = 1 g)
Divide by 1000 or move the decimal point of the milligrams three places to the left.

EXAMPLES: 200 mg = 0.2 g
0.6 mg = 0.0006 g

Convert the following milligrams to grams:

0.4 mg = _____ g
0.12 mg = _____ g
0.2 mg = _____ g
0.1 mg = _____ g
500 mg = _____ g
125 mg = _____ g
100 mg = _____ g
200 mg = _____ g
50 mg = _____ g
400 mg = _____ g

Can you take the gram dosages in these answers and convert them to milligrams?

Converting grains (apothecary) to milligrams (metric)

(1 gr = 60 mg)
Multiply the number of grains by 60.

EXAMPLE: Change gr to mg.
5 grains × 60 mg/gr = 300 mg

Solid dosage for oral administration

If the dosage on hand and dosage ordered are both in the same system (metric or apothecary) and in the same unit of weight, proceed to calculate the dosage using one of these methods.

EXAMPLE: Physician orders patient to have 1.0 g of Gantrisin. The Gantrisin bottle states that each tablet in the bottle contains 0.5 g.
PROBLEM: You do not have the 1.0 g as ordered. How many tablets will you give? (Both the amount ordered and the amount available are in the same system of measurement [metric] and the same unit of weight [grams].)

SOLUTION: You may use two methods.
Method 1:

1. $\dfrac{\text{Dosage desired}}{\text{Dosage on hand}} = \dfrac{1.0 \text{ g}}{0.5 \text{ g}} = 2$ You will give two 0.5 g capsules to give the 1.0 g ordered.

Method 2: (Proportional)
Metric dosage ordered: Drug form
Metric dosage available: Drug form

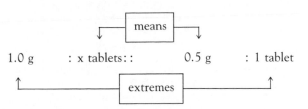

1.0 g   : x tablets ::   0.5 g   : 1 tablet

(means) = (extremes)
0.5x = 1.0
x = 2 tablets

Proof: Product of means: 2 (value of x) × 0.5 = 1.0
Product of extremes: 1.0 × 1 = 1.0

If the dosage on hand and dosage ordered are both in the same system of measurement (metric or apothecary) but they are *not* in the same unit of weight within the system, the units of weight must first be converted.

EXAMPLE: Physician orders: 1000 milligrams (metric) of ampicillin. On hand: 0.25 grams (metric) per tablet.
Rule: Converting Grams (metric) to Milligrams (metric) (1 g = 1000 mg)
Multiply the number of grams by 1000; move the decimal point of the grams three places to the right. 0.25 g = 250 mg

SOLUTION

1. $\dfrac{\text{Dosage desired}}{\text{Dosage on hand}} = \dfrac{1000}{250 \text{ mg}} = 4$ Give four 0.25 g tablets

2. $\dfrac{\text{mg}}{250} : \dfrac{\text{tablet}}{1} :: \dfrac{\text{mg}}{1000} : \dfrac{\text{tablet}}{x}$

$250x = 1000$
$x = \dfrac{1000}{250} = 4$ tablets

Proof: Product of means: 1 × 1000 = 1000
Product of extremes: 250 × 4 = (value of x) = 1000

Do the following conversions. (Make sure the amount ordered and source available are converted to the same system of measurement and unit of weight.)

1. Physician orders aspirin 600 mg. You have aspirin gr v per tablet. (metric and apothecary units)
2. Physician orders Gantrisin 0.25 g. You have Gantrisin 500 mg per tablet. (metric units, but different weight units)
3. Physician orders pentobarbital 200 mg. You have pentobarbital 1½ gr capsules. (metric and apothecary units)

Conversion problems

Some students understand problems in tablet dosage for oral administration if presented with their fractional equivalents as follows:

1. Physician orders patient to receive 2 g of a drug in oral tablet forms. The medicine bottle label states the strength on hand is 0.5 g. This means each tablet in the bottle is the strength 0.5 g.
How many tablets would be given to the patient? 1, 2, 3, 4, or 5? Answer: 4
What strength is ordered? 2 g

What strength is on the bottle label? 0.5 g
What is the fractional equivalent of 0.5 g? ½ g
How many ½ (0.5 g) tablets would equal 2 g? 4

$$2 \div \frac{1}{2} = \frac{2}{1} \times \frac{2}{1} = 4 \text{ tablets}$$

2. Physician orders patient to receive 0.2 mg of a drug in oral tablet form. The medicine bottle label states the strength on hand is 0.1 mg. This means each tablet in the bottle is the strength 0.1 mg.
   How many tablets would be given to the patient? 1, 2, 3, or 4? Answer: 2 tablets
   What strength is ordered? 0.2 mg
   What is the fractional equivalent of 0.2 mg? ²⁄₁₀
   What strength is on the bottle label (on hand)? 0.1 mg
   What is the fractional equivalent of 0.1 mg? ¹⁄₁₀
   How many ¹⁄₁₀ mg (0.1 mg) tablets would equal ²⁄₁₀ mg (0.2 mg)? 2

$$
\begin{array}{rl}
0.1 \text{ mg} = & \text{¹⁄₁₀ mg or 1 tablet} \\
+0.1 \text{ mg} = & \text{¹⁄₁₀ mg or 1 tablet} \\
\hline
0.2 \text{ mg} = & \text{²⁄₁₀ mg or 2 tablets}
\end{array}
$$

Dosage desired ÷ Dosage on hand =

$$or \ \frac{2}{10} \div \frac{1}{10} = \frac{2}{\cancel{10}} \times \frac{\cancel{10}}{1} = 2 \text{ tablets}$$

3. Physician orders patient to receive 0.5 mg of a drug in oral tablet form. The medicine bottle label states the strength on hand is 0.25 mg. This means each tablet in the bottle is the strength 0.25 mg.
   How many tablets would be given to the patient? 1, 2, 3, 4, or 5? Answer: 2 tablets
   What strength is ordered? 0.5 mg
   What fractional equivalent equals 0.5 mg? ½ mg
   What strength is on the bottle label? 0.25 mg
   What fractional equivalent equals the strength on hand? ¼ mg
   How many ¼ mg (0.25 mg) tablets would equal ½ mg (0.5 mg)? 2

$$
\begin{array}{rl}
0.25 \text{ mg} = & \text{¼ mg or 1 tablet} \\
+0.25 \text{ mg} = & \text{¼ mg or 1 tablet} \\
\hline
0.50 \text{ mg} = & \text{½ mg or 2 tablets}
\end{array}
$$

Dosage desired ÷ Dosage on hand =

$$or \ \frac{1}{2} \div \frac{1}{4} = \frac{1}{2} \times \frac{4}{1} = 2 \text{ tablets}$$

4. Physician orders patient to receive 0.25 mg of a drug in oral tablet form. The medicine bottle label states the strength on hand is 0.5 mg. This means that every tablet in the bottle is the strength 0.5 mg.
   How many tablets would be given? ½, 1, 1½, 2, 2½, 3, 4, or 5? Answer: ½ tablets
   What strength did the physician order? 0.25 mg

What is the fractional equivalent of the strength the physician ordered? ¼ mg
What strength is on the bottle label? 0.5 mg
What is the fractional equivalent of the strength on the bottle label (on hand)? ½ mg
Which is less: 0.5 mg (½ mg) or 0.25 mg (¼ mg)? Answer: 0.25 mg (¼ mg)
Was the amount ordered less than the strength on hand or more? Answer: Less

$$0.5 \text{ mg} = \frac{1}{2} \text{ mg or 1 tablet}$$
$$0.25 \text{ mg} = \frac{1}{4} \text{ mg or half as much or } \frac{1}{2} \text{ tablet}$$
$$or \ \frac{1}{4} \div \frac{1}{2} = \frac{1}{4} \times \frac{2}{1} = \frac{1}{2} \text{ tablet}$$

If the medication is also available in 0.25 mg tablets, request that size from the pharmacy. A tablet should be divided only when scored; even then the practice should be avoided.

Liquid dosage for oral administration

1. Physician orders 60 ml of a liquid medication. How many ounces will be given?
   To convert milliliters to ounces, divide milliliters by 30:

$$60 \text{ ml} \div 30 \ (30 \text{ ml} = 1 \text{ oz}) = 2 \text{ oz}$$

2. Physician orders 45 ml. How many ounces will be given?

$$45 \div 30 = 1\frac{1}{2} \text{ oz}$$

3. Physician orders 6 drams. How many milliliters (cubic centimeters) will you give?
   To convert drams to milliliters, multiply drams by 4:

$$4(4 \text{ ml} = 1 \text{ dram}) \times 6 = 24 \text{ ml (cc)}$$

Converting weight to kilograms (1 kg = 2.2 lb)

Many physicians request that the metric measure be used to record the body weight of the patient. Because the scales used in many hospitals are calibrated in pounds, the conversion from pounds to kilograms is required.

1. To convert weight in kilograms to pounds, multiply the kilogram weight by 2.2.

   EXAMPLE: 25 kg × 2.2 lb = 55 lb

Convert the following:

$$35 \text{ kg} = \underline{\hspace{2cm}} \text{ lb}$$
$$16 \text{ kg} = \underline{\hspace{2cm}} \text{ lb}$$
$$65 \text{ kg} = \underline{\hspace{2cm}} \text{ lb}$$

2. To convert weight in pounds to kilograms, divide the weight in pounds by 2.2.

EXAMPLE: 140 lb ÷ 2.2 kg = 63.6 kg

Convert the following:

125 lb = _____ kg
9 lb = _____ kg
180 lb = _____ kg

The weight of a liter of water at 40° C is 2.2 pounds.

FAHRENHEIT AND CENTIGRADE (CELSIUS) TEMPERATURES

OBJECTIVE

1. Demonstrate proficiency in performing conversions between the centigrade and Fahrenheit systems of temperature measurement.

KEY WORDS

centigrade   Celsius
Fahrenheit

It is necessary for the nurse to be familiar with both the centigrade and the Fahrenheit scale. Here are some of the main points about centigrade and Fahrenheit thermometers (Figure 3-2).

1. Centigrade and Fahrenheit thermometers look alike.

2. Both are made of the same-sized tube containing mercury.
3. The column of mercury in each thermometer rises to the same height when placed in a beaker of freezing water and to the same height in boiling water.
4. The centigrade and Fahrenheit thermometers differ from each other in the way they are graduated.
5. On the centigrade thermometer the point at which water freezes is marked "0."
6. On the Fahrenheit thermometer the point at which water freezes is marked "32."
7. The boiling point in centigrade is 100°.
8. The boiling point in Fahrenheit is 212°.
9. The space between the 0° point and the 100° point on the centigrade scale is divided into equal spaces or degrees.
10. The value of graduations (degrees) on the centigrade thermometer differs from the value of degrees on the Fahrenheit thermometer.
11. There are 180 spaces between the freezing and boiling points on the Fahrenheit thermometer.
12. In order to change readings on the centigrade thermometer to the Fahrenheit scale, the centigrade reading is multiplied by 180/100 or 9/5 and then added to 32.
13. To change Fahrenheit reading to centigrade scale, subtract 32 from the Fahrenheit reading and multiply by 5/9.

To understand why thermometer readings are interpreted in the way explained in Point 12 and to understand your conversion formula better, read Points 4 to 12 again several times.

Formula for Converting Fahrenheit Temperature to Centigrade Temperature

$$(\text{Fahrenheit} - 32) \times \frac{5}{9} = \text{centigrade}$$

$$(F - 32) \times \frac{5}{9} = C$$

EXAMPLE: Change 212° F to C.

$$(F - 32) \times \frac{5}{9} = C$$
$$212 - 32 = 180$$
$$180 \times \frac{5}{9} = \frac{900}{9} = 100° C$$

Convert the following Fahrenheit temperatures to centigrade:

98.6° F = _____ ° C
102.4° F = _____ ° C
95.2° F = _____ ° C

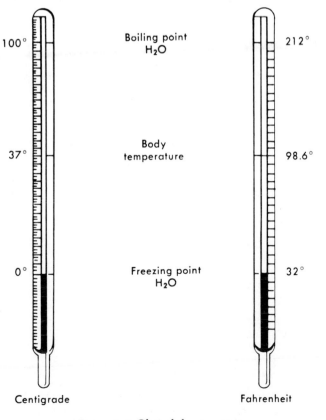

Figure 3-2 *Clinical thermometers.*

Formula for Converting Centigrade Temperature to Fahrenheit Temperature

$$\left(\text{Centigrade} \times \frac{9}{5}\right) + 32 = \text{Fahrenheit}$$

$$\left(C \times \frac{9}{5}\right) + 32 = F$$

EXAMPLE: Change 100° C to F.

$$\left(C \times \frac{9}{5}\right) + 32 = F$$

$$100 \times \frac{9}{5} = \frac{900}{5} = 180$$

$$180 + 32 = 212° F$$

Convert the following centigrade temperatures to Fahrenheit:

$$37° C = \underline{\hspace{1cm}} ° F$$
$$35° C = \underline{\hspace{1cm}} ° F$$
$$41° C = \underline{\hspace{1cm}} ° F$$

Try these problems in converting centigrade to Fahrenheit and Fahrenheit to centigrade.

1. The nurse takes the following temperatures with Fahrenheit clinical thermometers; patient A, 104° F; patient B, 99° F; patient C, 101° F. The physician asks what the centigrade temperature is for each patient. Work your problems to convert Fahrenheit temperatures to centigrade. Check your answers. (Answers: patient A, 40° C; patient B, 37.2° C; patient C, 38.3° C.)

2. The nurse takes the following temperatures with centigrade clinical thermometers: patient D, 37° C; patient E, 37.8° C; patient F, 38° C. The physician asks what the Fahrenheit temperature is for each patient. Work your problems to convert centigrade to Fahrenheit. Check your answers. (Answers: patient D, 98.6° F; patient E, 100° F; patient F, 100.4° F.)

Many hospitals today have conversion tables available on the wards. This saves time and possibility of error in doing problems. The nurse simply refers to the particular temperature on one scale and finds the conversion listed in a column beside it. However, try to remember the formula for each conversion.

Most larger hospitals currently use electronic thermometers which give centigrade readings or Fahrenheit readings.

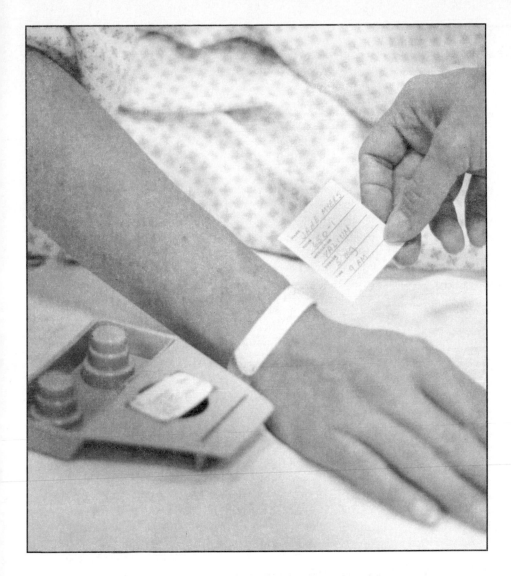

CHAPTER 4

Principles of Medication Administration

CHAPTER GOALS

After completing this chapter, the student should be able to do the following:

1. Cite ethical and legal considerations inherent in the administration of medications.
2. Identify and describe components of a patient's chart.
3. Describe drug distribution systems available for use.
4. Apply principles of drug distribution systems to experiences encountered in the practice setting.
5. State the six "rights" of drug administration and correlate these with the principles of medication administration in the practice setting.

Before medications are administered, it is important that the nurse understand the professional responsibilities associated with medication administration, drug orders, medication delivery systems, and the nursing process as it relates to drug therapy. Lack of knowledge of the nurse's overall responsibilities in the system will, at the least, result in delays in receiving and administering medications, but it may also result in serious administration errors. Either way, the patient loses and may suffer unnecessarily.

LEGAL AND ETHICAL CONSIDERATIONS
OBJECTIVES

1. Research the Nurse Practice Act in the state where practicing. Identify the limitations relating to medication administration placed on licensed practical nurses, registered nurses, and nurse clinicians.
2. Study the policies and procedures of the practice setting to identify specific regulations concerning medication administration by licensed practical nurses, registered nurses, and nurse clinicians.

KEY WORD

Nurse Practice Act

The practice of nursing under a professional license is a privilege, not a right. In accepting the privilege, the nurse must understand that this responsibility includes being held accountable for one's actions and judgments during the performance of professional duties. An understanding of the Nurse Practice Act and of the rules and regulations established by the state boards of nursing for the various levels of entry (that is, practical nurse, registered nurse, and nurse practitioner) is a solid foundation for beginning practice.

In addition to state rules and regulations, nurses must be familiar with the established policies and procedures of the employing health care agency. These policies must adhere to the minimum standards of the state board of nursing, but agency policies may be more stringent than those recognized by the state. Employment within the agency implies the willingness of the professional to adhere to established standards and to work within established guidelines to make necessary changes in the standards. Examples of policy statements relating to medication administration include the following: (1) educational requirements of professionals

authorized to administer medications (many health care facilities require that a written test be passed to attest to the necessary knowledge and skills of medication preparation, calculation, and administration prior to being granted approval to administer any medications); (2) approved lists of intravenous solutions and medications that the nurse can start or add to an existing infusion; (3) lists of restricted medications (such as antineoplastic agents, magnesium sulfate, allergy extracts, lidocaine, RhoGAM, Imferon, and heparin) that may be administered only by certain personnel.

Prior to the administration of any medication, the nurse must have (1) a current license to practice nursing, (2) a clear policy statement that authorizes the act, and (3) a medication order signed by a licensed physician or dentist. The nurse must understand the individual patient's diagnosis and presenting symptoms that correlate with the rationale for drug use. The nurse should also know why a medication is ordered, the expected actions, usual dosage, route of administration, minor side effects to expect, adverse effects to report, and contraindications of the use of a particular drug. If drugs are to be administered using the same syringe or at the same IV site, drug compatibility should be confirmed prior to administration. If unsure of any of these key medication points, the nurse must consult an authoritative resource or the hospital pharmacist *prior* to the administration of a medication. The nurse must be accurate in the calculation, preparation, and administration of medications. The nurse must assess the patient to be certain that both therapeutic and adverse effects associated with the medication regimen are reported. Nurses must be able to collect patient data at regularly scheduled intervals and to record observations in the patient's chart for evaluation of the effectiveness of the treatment. Claiming unfamiliarity with any of these nursing responsibilities, when an avoidable complication arises, is unacceptable; it is considered negligence of nursing responsibility.

Nurses must take an active role in the education of the patient and family in preparation for discharge from the health-care environment. (A person's health will improve only to the extent that the patient understands how to take care of himself or herself.) Specific teaching goals should be developed and implemented. Nursing observations and progress toward mastery of skills should be charted to verify the degree of understanding attained (see Health Teaching).

PATIENT CHARTS
OBJECTIVES

1. Identify the basic categories of information available in a patient's chart.
2. Study the patient charts at different practice settings to identify the various formats used to chart patient data.
3. Cite the information contained in a Kardex and describe the purpose of this file.

KEY WORDS

summary sheet	progress notes
graphic record	laboratory tests record
nurse's notes	Kardex records
consultation reports	narcotic inventory
history and physical	form
examination form	medication
physician's order form	administration record

The patient's chart is a major source of information that is necessary in patient assessment so that the nurse may make and implement plans for patient care. It is also the place for the nurse to provide a written record documenting nursing assessments performed, observations reported to the physician for further verification, basic nursing measures implemented (for example, daily bath and treatments), patient teaching performed, and observed responses to therapy.

This document serves as the communications link among all members of the health care team regarding the patient's status, care provided, and progress. It is a legal document that describes the patient's health, lists diagnostic and therapeutic procedures initiated, and describes the patient's response to these measures. The chart must be kept current as long as the patient is in the hospital. After the patient's discharge, it is stored in the medical records department until needed again. While in medical records, the chart may be used for research to compare responses to selected therapy in a sampling of patients with similar diagnoses.

Contents of Patient Charts

Although each hospital uses a somewhat different format, the basic patient chart consists of the following elements:

1. *Summary Sheet* This sheet gives the patient's name, address, date of birth, attending physician, sex, marital status, allergies, nearest relative, occupation and employer, insurance carrier and other payment arrangements, religious preference, date and time of admission to the hospital, previous hospital admissions, and admitting problem or diagnosis. The date and time of discharge will be added when appropriate.

2. *Physician's Order Form*—The physician orders all procedures and treatments on this form (Figure 4-1). These orders include general care (activity, diet, frequency of vital signs), laboratory tests to be completed, other diagnostic procedures (such as X-rays, ECG, CAT scans), and all medications and treatments (such as physical therapy, occupational therapy).

3. *Graphic Record*—This is a list of the vital signs, fluid intake and output, activity level, and other information used regularly for assessment of the patient's status (Figure 4-2, A and B).

4. *History and Physical Examination Form*—Upon admission to the hospital, the patient is interviewed by the physician and given a physical examination. The physician records the findings here and lists the problems to be corrected (the diagnoses).

5. *Progress Notes*—The physician uses this sheet to record frequent observations of the patient's health status. In some hospitals, other health professionals, such as pharmacists, dieticians, and physical therapists, may record observations and suggestions.

6. *Nurses' Notes* (Figure 4-3)—Here nurses record ongoing assessments of the patient's condition, responses to nursing interventions ordered by the physician (such as treatments or medications) or those initiated by the nurse (skin care or patient education); evaluations of the effectiveness of nursing interventions; procedures completed by other health professionals (such as wound cleaning by a physician or fitting for a prosthesis by a fitter); and other pertinent information, such as physician or family visits and the patient's responses after these visits. Entries may be made on the nurses' notes throughout a shift, but general guidelines include the following: (1) completing records immediately after making contacts with, and assessments of, the patient (that is, when first admitted or returning from a diagnostic procedure or therapy); (2) recording all p.r.n. medications immediately after administration, and the effectiveness of the medication; and (3) recording immediately before leaving the patient for extended periods of times, such as lunch or coffee breaks. In addition to accurately charting the observations in a clear, concise form, the nurse should report significant changes in a patient's status or assessments to the charge nurse. The charge nurse will then make a nursing judgment regarding notification of the attending physician.

7. *P.R.N. Medication Record*—Some clinical settings use a p.r.n. medication record rather than nurses' notes to record the date, time, p.r.n. medication

DOCTOR'S ORDER SHEET

Addressograph Here:

508-52-1917
Joseph Lorenzo
18 Bush Ave.
Hometown, U.S.A.

Martindale Hospital
Hometown, U.S.A.

Dr. M. Martin
Unit-6W, Rm. 622

PLEASE INDICATE ALLERGIES

None	Codeine	Penicillin	Sulfa	Aspirin	Others

Date	Time	Prob. No.	Physicians Orders	Doctor	Progress Record
1/6/93	3:00 pm	6	Erythromycin 250 mg, po Q 6 h × 8 days	M. Martin	

Figure 4-1 *Physician's order form and progress record.*

**Temperature Graph
and Vital Signs Record**

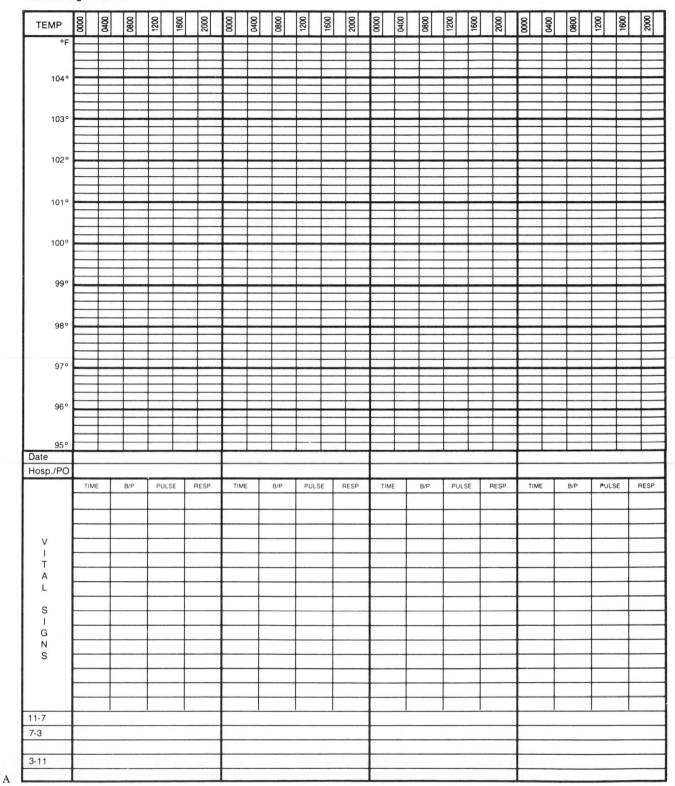

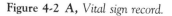

A

NS-22
Continued.

Figure 4-2 A, *Vital sign record.*

DATE							
HT-WT							
HYGIENE:							
Bedbath							
Partial							
Self							
Shower/tub							
Oral							
H.S.							
ACTIVITY:							
Bedrest							
BRP							
BRcBRP							
Dangle							
Chair/W.C.							
Amb							
Other							
Rails	7-3-11	7-3-11	7-3-11	7-3-11	7-3-11	7-3-11	7-3-11
DIET:	8-12-5	8-12-5	8-12-5	8-12-5	8-12-5	8-12-5	8-12-5
NPO							
Liquid							
Soft							
Regular							
Spec.							
HOLD							
OTHER:							

Intake	11-7	7-3	3-11	11-7	7-3	3-11	11-7	7-3	3-11	11-7	7-3	3-11	11-7	7-3	3-11	11-7	7-3	3-11	11-7	7-3	3-11
Oral																					
I.V. or Subq.																					
Blood																					
Other																					
Total 24 Hr. (cc.)																					
Output Urine																					
Total 24 Hr. (cc.) Urine																					
Emesis																					
Other																					
Total 24 Hr. (cc.)																					
Stool																					
Signature																					

B

Figure 4-2 B, *Patient care record.*

Time	Output	MEDS/TX/VS	

Figure 4-3 *Format of nurses' notes.*

administered and dose, reason for administering the p.r.n. medication, and patient's response to the drug given. (See Figure 4-4.)

8. *Laboratory Tests Record*—All laboratory test results are kept together in one section of the chart. Hospitals using computerized reports may list consecutive values of the same test once that test has been repeated several times (such as the electrolytes). Other hospitals may attach small report forms to a full sized backing sheet as each report returns from the laboratory. Since some medication dosages are based on daily blood studies, it is important to understand where to locate these data within the patient's chart. Figure 4-5 shows a daily series of prothrombin time (PT) results.

9. *Consultation Reports*—When other physicians (or other health professionals) are asked to consult on a patient, the specialist's summary of findings, diagnoses, and recommendations for treatment are recorded in this section.

10. *Other Diagnostic Reports*—Reports of surgery, EEG, ECG, pulmonary function tests, radioactive scans, and X-ray reports are usually recorded in this section.

11. *Medication Administration Record (MAR) or Medication Profile*—Today most medication administration records (MAR) or medication profiles are computer generated. This assures that the pharmacist and the nurse have identical medication profiles for the patient. Each clinical site arranges the MAR somewhat differently, but the following represents key components of the MAR.

The MAR lists all medications to be administered. The medications are usually grouped according to the following categories: Those *scheduled* on a regular basis (for example, every 6 hours or twice a day), *parenteral*, STAT, and *preoperative* orders. *P.r.n. medications* are usually listed at the bottom of the MAR.

The MAR provides a space for recording the time when the medication is administered and by whom it is given. Generally the nurse records and initials the time when the medication is given. The nurse also places his or her initials, name, and title in a designated place provided within the record for documentation.

MARs are kept in a notebook or clipboard file on the medication cart for the 24 hour period they are in use, then become a permanent part of the patient chart. In the acute-care setting, a new MAR is generated every 24 hours at the same time the unit dose cart is refilled. (See Figure 4-6.)

In the long-term care setting the MAR uses the same principles; however, it generally provides a space for medications to be recorded for up to 1 month. (See Figure 4-7.) The medication record also shows the name of the pharmacy dispensing the prescribed medications and the assigned prescription number. Medications prescribed for residents in the long-term care setting are required to be reviewed on a scheduled basis; therefore, the MAR identifies the reviewer and date. (See Figure 4-7.)

Additional forms included in a patient's chart depend upon the therapy prescribed. These may include separate medication administration reports; health teaching records; operative and anesthesiology records;

Last Name: _____　First Name: _____　Room & Bed No.: _____　Patient No.: _____　Physician: _____

PRN MEDICATION RECORD

DATE	TIME	MEDICATION	REASON	RESPONSE	NAME OF NURSE

Figure 4-4 *P. r. n. medication record.*

Martindale Hometown Hospital
Laboratory Summary Report

PATIENT NAME: Joseph Lorenzo   RM. 621-2   ADM: January 21
ID NO.   016-28-3978
DIAGNOSIS: Myocardial Infarction

PHYSICIAN: M. Martin, M.D.   TIME: 12:13 AM
    DATE: 1/28

	1/27	1/26	1/25	1/24	1/23	Normal
	07:00	07:00	07:00	07:00	07:00	Range
ProTime	19	18	24	18	16	11.0-13.0 sec
PTT	34	33	38	34	31	0-35 sec

Figure 4-5 *Laboratory test reports. Example of the prothrombin times for a patient receiving warfarin.*

recovery room records; physical, occupational, or speech therapy records; inhalation therapy reports; or a diabetic's daily record of insulin dosage and urine and blood sugar test results. Each page placed in the patient's chart will be imprinted with the patient's name, registration number, and unit or room number. Nurses often use data from all of these sections to formulate a plan of nursing care.

Kardex Records

The Kardex (Figure 4-8) is a large index-type card usually kept in a flip-file that contains pertinent information such as the patient's name, diagnosis, allergies, schedules of current medications with stop dates, treatments, and the nursing care plan. Since all ordered medications are listed in the Kardex, the nurse can assemble the medication cards (Figure 4-9) for all assigned patients and verify each medication card against the Kardex. When the unit dose system is used, all medications are still listed on the Kardex or the medication profile, but individual medication cards are not necessary. Although used primarily by nurses, the Kardex makes patient data quickly accessible to all members of the health team. The Kardex is often completed in pencil and updated by erasures. Since it is not a legal document, it is destroyed when the patient is discharged from the institution.

DRUG DISTRIBUTION SYSTEMS
OBJECTIVES

1. Cite the advantages and disadvantages of the ward stock system, the individual prescription order system, and the unit dose system of drug distribution.
2. Study the narcotic control system used at the assigned clinical practice setting and compare it to the requirements of the Controlled Substance Act, 1970.

KEY WORDS
    ward stock system
    individual prescription system
    narcotic control system
    unit dose system
    long-term care unit dose system

Before the administration of medications, it is important that the nurse understand the overall medication delivery system used at the employing health care agency. Although no two drug distribution systems function exactly alike, the following three general types are currently being used:

1. *Floor or Ward Stock System*—In this system, all but the most dangerous or rarely used medications are stocked at the nursing station in stock containers. This system has been used most often in very small hospitals and in hospitals where there are no charges directly to the patient for medications, such as in some government hospitals. Some advantages that may exist with the complete floor stock system are (1) ready availability of most drugs; (2) fewer inpatient prescription orders; and (3) minimal return of medications. The disadvantages of this type of system are (1) the increased potential for medication errors because of the large array of stock medications to choose

MARTINDALE HOMETOWN HOSPITAL

MEDICATION ADMINISTRATION RECORD

NAME	Joseph Lorenzo	RM-BD: 621-2
ID NO.	016-28-3978	AGE: 62
DIAGNOSIS	Myocardial Infarction	SEX: M
PHYSICIAN	M. Martin, M.D.	HT: 6' WT:

INIT	SIGNATURE	TITLE

SCHEDULED MEDICATIONS

DATES:	MEDICATION---STRENGTH---FORM---ROUTE	0030-0729	0730-1529	1530-0029
1/25	RANITIDINE (ZANTAC) ZANTAC 150 MG TABLET ORAL TWICE A DAY		0900	1800
1/25	DILTIAZEM HYDROCHLORIDE CARDIZEM 90 MG TABLET ORAL 4 TIMES DAILY		0900 1300	1800 2100
1/25	WARFARIN SODIUM COUMADIN 1 MG TABLET ORAL EVERY OTHER DAY	NOT GIVEN	TODAY	

IV AND PIGGYBACK ORDERS

DATES:	MEDICATION	0030-0729	0730-1529	1530-0029
1/25	CEFTAZIDIME (FORTAZ) 1 GM IV SODIUM CHLORIDE 0.9% 50 ML EVERY 8 HOURS INFUSE: 20 MIN	0200	1000	1800
1/25	GENTAMICIN PREMIX 80 MG IV ISO-OSMOTIC SOLN 100 ML BY IV PUMP EVERY 12 HOURS INFUSE: 30 MIN	0200	1400	
1/25	BY IV PUMP 1 IV DEXT-5/0.2 NACL 1000 ML RATE: 100 ML/HR			

PRN MEDICATIONS

DATES:	MEDICATION	0030-0729	0730-1529	1530-0029
1/25	ACETAMINOPHEN (TYLENOL) TYLENOL 650 MG (2X325) TABLET ORAL Q 4H AS NEEDED PRN			
1/25	MAGNESIUM HYDROXIDE MILK OF MAGNESIA 60 ML (CONC) ORAL CONC. ORAL AS NEEDED PRN			
1/25	ALBUTEROL PROVENTIL INHALER 90 MCG/INH AEROSOL INH AS NEEDED PRN SEE R.T. NOTES AT BEDSIDE			

AGE/SEX	HT WT DATE 1/25	ALLERGIES CODEINE
62/ M	6'0" 200 LBS	
ROOM-BD	NAME	
621 2	Joseph Lorenzo	

Figure 4-6 *Example of medication administration record (MAR). (Note: separation of scheduled orders, IVs, and p.r.n. medications.)*

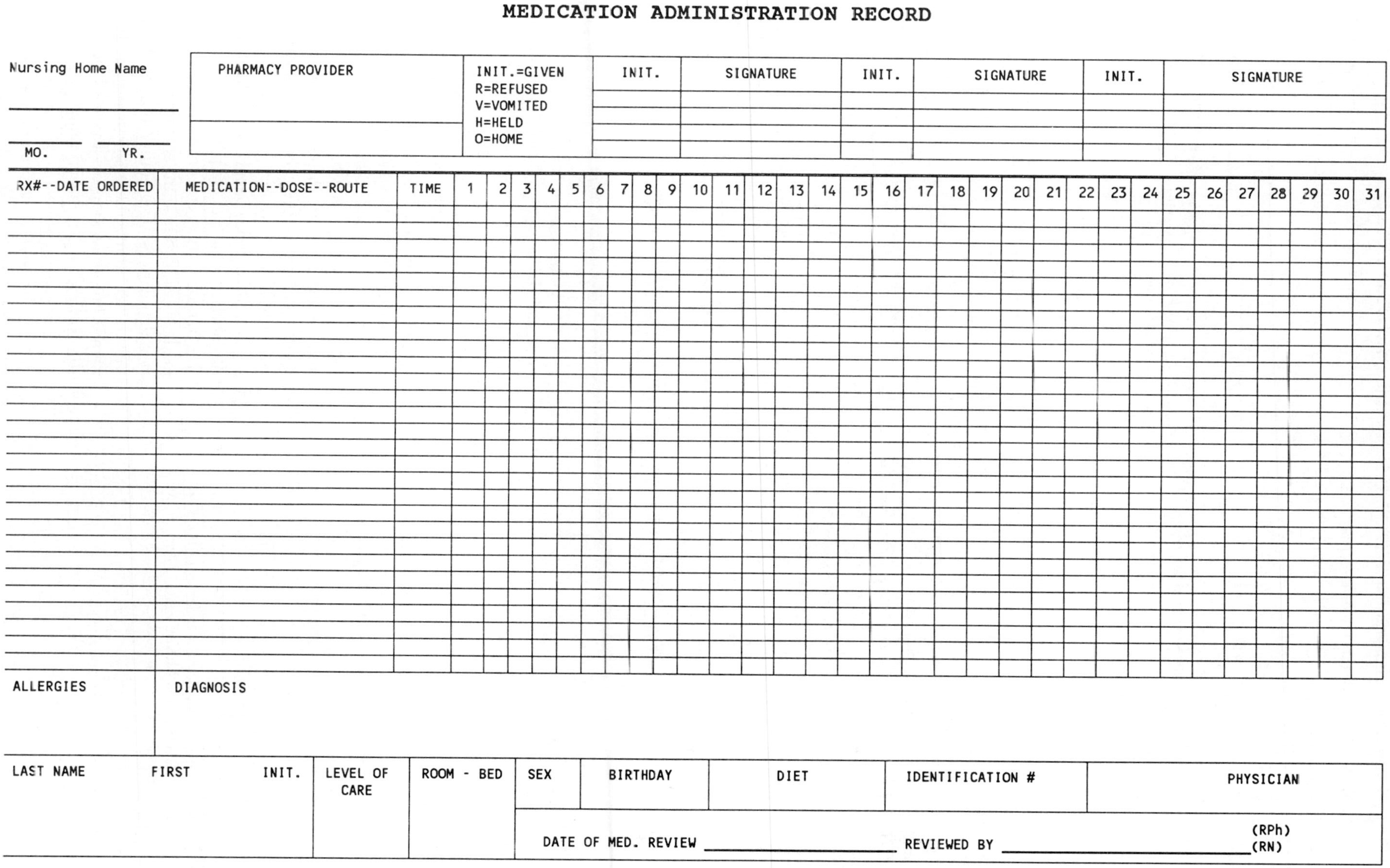

MEDICATION ADMINISTRATION RECORD

Nursing Home Name

MO. _____ YR. _____

PHARMACY PROVIDER

INIT.=GIVEN
R=REFUSED
V=VOMITED
H=HELD
O=HOME

RX#--DATE ORDERED | MEDICATION--DOSE--ROUTE | TIME

Days: 1 2 3 4 5 6 7 8 9 10 11 12 13 14 15 16 17 18 19 20 21 22 23 24 25 26 27 28 29 30 31

INIT. | SIGNATURE | INIT. | SIGNATURE | INIT. | SIGNATURE | INIT. | SIGNATURE

ALLERGIES

DIAGNOSIS

LAST NAME | FIRST | INIT. | LEVEL OF CARE | ROOM - BED | SEX | BIRTHDAY | DATE OF MED. REVIEW | DIET | IDENTIFICATION #

PHYSICIAN

REVIEWED BY _____

(RPh)
(RN)

Figure 4-7 *Example of medication administration record used in long-term care setting.*

JENNIE EDMUNDSON HOSPITAL

PATIENT ASSESSMENT/CARE PLAN

ALLERGIES _Penicillin_

REACTION _Hives on Trunk_   ALLERGY BAND APPLIED ☑

IN EMERGENCY CALL _Mary Doe (wife)_ (Home) 323-6421
(Name)   (Relationship)   (Phone)
John Jr. (son) (Home) 323-0644
(Name)   (Relationship)   (Phone)
(work) 536-1282

IV THERAPY _6/1 Heparin lock_
Rotate site 6/4 6/7 6/10 M.D.

CONSULTS/REFERRALS _Dr Krammer — cardiology_

O₂ THERAPY/IPPB _6/1 O₂ 2L N.C. Continuously_
6/5 O₂ PRN Chest pain   2L/N.C.

PHYSICAL THERAPY _____

SUPPORT SERVICES _____

TREATMENTS-OTHER _____

CURRENT MEDS BEING TAKEN _Lanoxin 0.125 mgm qd. Tenormin 50 mgm qd. Procardia 20 mgm qid, Transderm Nitro 5 -patch qid Persantine 25 mgm tid, N+G 1/150gr PRN chest pain Tylenol gr X PRN headache, minor discomforts_

OPERATIVE PROCEDURE _1/6/93 Cardiac catheterization Outcome: 2 Grafts blocked - severe coronary artery disease_

DIAGNOSIS _Angina CHF Hist MI 7/76 hypertension_

05-8/83

Physical Care: Bath _6/1 N.O. at bedside č Assistance if pain free_

Diet _6/1 2 gm Na; low cholesterol diet_

Fluid _As desires. Not to exceed 3000 cc/24 hr_

Help Needed _N/A_

Miscellaneous _B.P. basic Rhythm 6/1 S. tachy 120-130_

Daily Lab/Specimens

Activity/Limitations/Safety _6/1 Bedrest č BRP č pain_
Up as desires when pain free. Begin 1/6/93

Elimination _N.O. Note bowel activity daily. Allow to stand to void._

Not to SMOKE IN HOSP. D.O.
Smoker ✓ 1/2 pk/day   Dentures _upper only_
Non Smoker _____   Eye Glasses ✓
Hearing Aid _____   ② Other _#4 Telemetry_

I & O ✓   B.P. _q̄ 40_   T-P-R _q̄ 4°_   Weight _D.O. Daily at brkfst._
(N.O. Apical č Radial pulses q̄ 4 hr)

PATIENT CLASSIFICATION
KEY — 0-13 = I   14-18 = II   19 + = III

AMBUL	MEALS	BATH	Pr/Po OP	TRTMTS	TOT
1②3	1②3	1②3	2	3·1	PTS 14
BTH RM	MEDS	T&ES	UNCON'S	AGE	PT
②34	①o2	1 or ②	5	21	CAT 2

use pencil ONLY

PSYCHIATRIC PATIENT CLASSIFICATION
KEY — 0-15 = I   16-20 = II   21 + = III CONSTANT CARE

AMBUL	BATHRM	TRTMNTS	BEHAV'R	TOT PTS
123	1234	·1		
MEALS	MEDS	PR/PO-OP	531	
123	1 or 2	2	PHYS ACT	PAT CAT
BATHE	AGE	MENT ATT	531	
123	·1	531		

ADM DATE _1/6/93_

CHURCH/PARISH _St. Lukes_
RELIGION _Catholic_
90-540

NAME _Doe, John_   HOSP.# _43641_   AGE _58_   PHYSICIAN _Fitzgerald_   ROOM NO. _425_

Figure 4-8 *Example of a nursing care plan in a Kardex.*

Name: _Lorenzo, Joseph_

Room & bed: _621²_   Date started: _1/25/93_

Dr.: _Martin_

Noted by: _S. Over Rn_

Medication & route: _ERYTHROMYCIN 250 mg p.o. q. 6 hr._

Time: _12-6-12-6_

Figure 4-9 *Transcription of a medication order onto the Kardex or a medication card or ticket. (From McKenry LM, Salerno E: Mosby's pharmacology in nursing, ed 18, St Louis, 1992, Mosby–Year Book.)*

from and the lack of review by the pharmacist of each individual patient's medication order; (2) the increased danger of unnoticed drug deterioration, jeopardizing patient safety; (3) economic loss caused by misplaced or forgotten charges and misappropriation of medication by hospital personnel; (4) increased amounts of expired drugs to be discarded; (5) the need for larger stocks and frequent total drug inventories; and (6) storage problems on the nursing units in many hospitals.

2. *Individual Prescription Order System*—In this system, medications are dispensed from the pharmacy upon receipt of a prescription or a drug order for an individual patient. The pharmacist usually sends a 3- to 5-day supply of medication in a bottle labeled for a specific patient. Once received at the nurses' station, medications are placed in the medication cabinet in accordance with institutional practices. Generally, the medication containers are arranged alphabetically by the patient's name, but they may be arranged numerically by the patient's room or bed number.

This system provides (1) greater patient safety due to the review of prescription orders by both

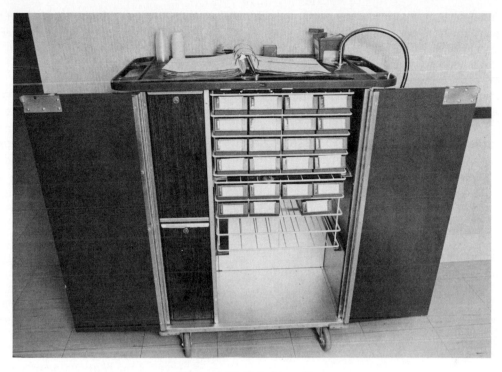

Figure 4-10 *Unit dose cabinet.*

the pharmacist and the nurse prior to administration; (2) less danger of drug deterioration and easier inventory control; (3) smaller total inventories; and (4) reduced revenue loss due to improved charging systems and less pilferage. While the dispensing of medication to individual patients is better than the floor stock system, the major disadvantages of this system are the very unwieldy and time-consuming procedures used to schedule, prepare, administer, control, and record the drug distribution and administration process.

3A. *Unit Dose System*—Unit dose drug distribution systems use single-unit packages of drugs, dispensed to fill each dosage requirement as it is ordered. Each package is labeled with generic and brand name, manufacturer, lot number, and expiration date. When dispensed by the pharmacy, the individual packages are placed in labeled drawers assigned to individual patients. The drawers are kept in a large "unit dose cabinet" (Fig. 4-10) that is kept at the nurses' station. Under most unit dose systems, the drawers are refilled by the pharmacist every 24 hours. In long-term care facilities, they are usually exchanged on 3- or 7-day schedules. The system was developed in the 1960s to overcome problems with inefficient use of nursing personnel, underutilization of pharmacists, excessively high rates of medication errors, poor drug control, waste of medications, and large inventories. The unit dose system is the safest and most economical method of drug distribution in

hospitals and long-term care facilities today. Advantages of the system include the following: (1) The time normally spent by nursing personnel in preparation of drugs for administration is drastically reduced. (2) The pharmacist has a profile of all medications of each patient, and is therefore able to analyze the prescribed medications for drug interactions or contraindications. This method increases the pharmacist's involvement and better utilizes his or her extensive drug knowledge. (3) No dosage calculations are necessary due to unit-of-use packaging, thus reducing errors. (4) The patient may double check drugs and dosages since each dose is individually packaged and labeled. (5) There is less waste and misappropriation since single units are dispensed. (6) Credit is given to the patient for unused medications, since each dose is individually packaged. (Under the individual prescription order system, returned bottles of unused medications were destroyed because of fear of contamination.)

An argument occasionally used by nurses against the unit or "single dose" system is that medications are prepared by someone else for the nurse to administer. Nurses have been taught: "Never administer anything you haven't prepared yourself." In principle, this is certainly true. A nurse should not administer any drug mixed and left unlabeled by another individual. However, for years nurses have administered medications that have been prepared and labeled by the pharmacist. The unit dose medication is prepared under rigid controls and is dispensed only after quality control procedures have been completed by pharmacists. Nurses should always continue to check medications prior to administration. If there is a discrepancy between the Kardex and the medication in the cart, the pharmacist and the original physician's order should be consulted.

At the time of administration, the nurse should check all aspects of the medication order as stated on the medication profile against the medication container removed from the patient's drawer for administration. The number of doses remaining in the drawer for the shift should also be checked. If the number of remaining doses is incorrect, check the medication order prior to continuing with the drug administration. Always consider the possibility that the drug has been discontinued, that someone else has given the dose, or that someone has omitted a dose or given the wrong patient the wrong medication. In the event that an error has been made, report it in accordance with hospital policies.

3B. *Unit Dose System in Long-Term Care Setting*—The unit dose medication system used in the long-term care system is an adaptation of that used in the acute care setting. The unit dose cart is designed with individual drawers to hold one resident's medication containers for 1 week. The drawer is labeled with the resident's name, room number, pharmacy name/telephone number, and the name of the facility. The pharmacist fills the medication container with the prescribed drug. Each container has enough compartments/cubicles to contain the prescribed number of doses of the drug for each day of the week. The individual compartments may be labeled with the days of the week. The medication cart has other compartments to store bottles of medication that cannot be placed in patient drawers. The cart has a storage area for medication cups, medicine crusher, drinking cups, straws, alcohol sponges, syringes, and other necessities for the preparation and administration of the medications prescribed. The entire cart has a locking system that should be locked at all times the medication cart is not in use or is unattended while medications are being dispensed.

The unit dose systems may use a color coding system to simplify finding the medication holder for a specific time of day, for example, purple = 6 AM, pink = 8 AM, yellow = noon, green = 2 PM or 4 PM, orange = early evening, red = p.r.n. Using this method to organize the medications allows the nurse or medication aide to remove all the pink holders to administer the prescribed 8 AM tablets or capsules. Each individual medication holder is also labeled with the resident's name, physician's name,

prescription number, generic/brand name of the drug, dose, frequency of drug order (for example, four times a day), and the actual time the drug within this holder is to be administered (for example, 8 AM).

At the time of administration, the nurse or medication aide checks all aspects of the medication order as stated on medication profile against the medication container that has been removed from one of the drawers. The number of doses remaining within the holder is checked against the days of the week that remain for the medication to be administered. If the resident refuses the medication, it must be charted on the record with the reason the medication was refused. In a long-term care setting, residents seldom wear identification bands; therefore, third-party identification of the resident must be relied upon until the nurse or medication aide is able to identify the residents. All medications administered should be charted as soon as given.

The medication aide has specific limitations on the types of medications he or she can administer; therefore, the nurse should be thoroughly familiar with the law/guidelines that exist in the state where functioning. The nurse is ultimately responsible for verifying the qualifications of the individual being supervised in the medication aide capacity and for the medications he or she is administering.

Narcotic Control Systems

As described in Chapter 1, laws regulating the use of controlled substances have been enacted and are rigidly enforced. Within hospitals, it is a standard policy that controlled substances are issued in single-unit packages and are kept in a separate, locked cabinet on each nursing unit. The key to the cabinet is controlled by the head nurse or a designated individual. When controlled substances are issued to a nursing unit, they are accompanied by an inventory sheet (Figure 4-11) that lists each type of controlled substance being supplied. This record is used to account for the disposition of each type of medication issued. At the time the controlled substance supply is dispensed to the nursing unit by the pharmacist, the nurse receiving the drug supply is responsible for counting and verifying the number and types of controlled substances received. The nurse then signs a record attesting to the accuracy and receipt of the controlled substances, and locks them in the controlled substances (narcotic) cabinet.

When a controlled substance is ordered for a particular patient, the nurse caring for the patient requests the key to the cabinet to obtain and prepare the medication for administration. At the time of removal from the cabinet, the inventory control record (Figure 4-11)

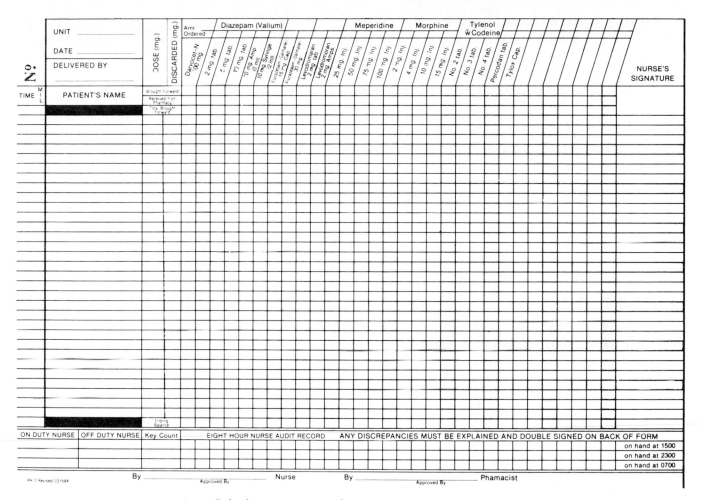

Figure 4-11 *Controlled-substances inventory form. (Courtesy of University Hospital, The University of Nebraska Medical Center; Copyright, Board of Regents of the University of Nebraska, Lincoln, Nebraska.)*

must be completed indicating time, patient's name, drug, dose, and the signature of the nurse responsible for checking out the controlled substance. If a portion of the medication is to be discarded due to a smaller prescribed dosage, two nurses must check the dosage, preparation, and the portion discarded. Both nurses must then co-sign the inventory control record to verify the transaction. The key is returned to the charge nurse after the dose is obtained and the paperwork is completed.

Prior to the administration of any controlled substance, the patient's chart should be checked to verify that the time interval since the last use of the drug has elapsed, as specified in the physician's orders. (See Chapter 8 for details of monitoring pain and the use of analgesics.) Immediately after the administration of a controlled substance, the chart should be completed by the nurse administering the medication. At appropriate intervals following the administration of a controlled substance, the degree and duration of effectiveness should be recorded in the nurse's notes.

At the end of each shift, the contents of the con-

trolled substances cabinet are counted (inventoried) by two nurses, one from the shift that is about to end and the other from the oncoming shift. Each individual container is counted and the remaining number of tablets, ampules and prefilled syringes is added to the amount used, according to the inventory control record. The amount of each drug remaining, plus the amount recorded as administered to individual patients, should equal the total number issued. During the counting procedure, packages of prefilled syringes that have not been opened are visually inspected to verify that the seal and the cellophane coverings are intact. Once the package seal is broken, closer scrutiny of the package is required. These observations should include tilting the package of prefilled syringes to observe the rate of air bubble movement inside the barrel, uniformity of color of the solutions in each of the barrels, and the similarity in fluid level in each of the barrels. The same medication in the same type of syringe should be the same color, travel within the barrel at the same rate, and all fluid levels should be similar. Discrepancies in the number of remaining doses are checked with nursing personnel on the unit to see if all narcotics used have been charted. If this does not reveal the source of the inaccuracy, each patient's chart is checked to be certain that all controlled substances recorded on the individual patient's charts for the shift coincide with the controlled substances inventory record. If the error still is not found, the pharmacy and the nursing service office should be contacted in accordance with the policy of the institution. In the event that the count appears to be accurate but tampering with the contents of the containers is suspected, a report should be made to the pharmacy and the nursing service office. When the controlled substances inventory is complete, the two nurses doing the counting sign the inventory control shift record to verify that the records and inventory are accurate at that time.

THE DRUG ORDER
OBJECTIVES

1. Define each of the four categories of medication orders used.
2. Describe the procedure used in the assigned clinical setting for taking, recording, transcribing, and verifying verbal medication orders.

KEY WORDS

stat orders	standing orders
renewal order	p.r.n. order
transcription	verification

Medications for patient use must be ordered by licensed physicians or dentists (or in some states by nurse practitioners and physician's assistants) acting within their areas of professional training. Placing an order for a medication or treatment is known as issuing a *prescription*. Initially it may be issued verbally or in written form. Prescriptions issued for nonhospitalized patients use a form similar to that shown in Figure 4-12, while prescriptions for hospitalized patients are written on the Physician's Order Form (see Figure 4-1). All prescriptions must contain the following elements: the patient's full name, date, drug name, route of administration, dosage, duration of the order, and signature of the prescriber. Additional information may be required for certain types of medications (for example, for intravenous administration, the concentration, dilution, and rate of flow should be specified in addition to the method— "IV push" or "continuous infusion").

Types of Medication Orders

Medication orders fall into four categories: the "stat" order, the single order, the standing order, and the p.r.n. order.

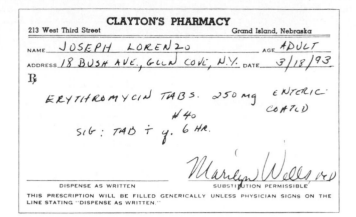

Figure 4-12 *A prescription showing patient name, patient address, date, drug and strength, number of tablets, directions for use, and the physician's signature.*

1. The *stat* order is generally used on an emergency basis. It means that the drug is to be administered as soon as possible, but only once. For example, if a patient is having a seizure, the physician may order "diazepam 10 mg IV stat," which is meant to be given immediately, and one time only.
2. The *single* order means administration at a certain time, but only one time. For example, a preoperative analgesic may be ordered "Demerol 100 mg IM to be given at the time the patient leaves the floor for surgery." Demerol would then be administered at that time, but once only.
3. The *standing* order indicates that a medication is to be given for a specified number of doses. For example, "TACE 72 mg q 12 h × 4 doses." A standing order may also indicate that a drug is to be administered until discontinued at a later date: For example, "Ampicillin 500 mg PO q 6 h."

   In the interest of patient safety, however, all accredited health agencies have policies that automatically cancel an order after a certain number of doses are administered or a certain number of days of therapy have passed (for example, prior to surgery, after 72 hours for narcotics, after one dose only for anticoagulants, after 7 days for antibiotics). A *renewal order* must be written and signed by the physician before the nurse can continue to administer the medication.
4. A *p.r.n.* order means "administer if needed." This order allows a nurse to judge when a medication should be administered based on the patient's need and when it can be safely administered.

Verbal orders

Health care agencies have policies regarding who may accept verbal orders and under what circumstances they should be accepted. The practice should be avoided whenever possible, but when a verbal order is accepted, the person who took the order is responsible for accurately entering it on the order sheet and signing it. The physician must co-sign and date the order, usually within 24 hours.

Nurse's Responsibilities Associated with the Drug Order

Verification of the drug order

Once a prescription has been written for a hospitalized patient, the nurse interprets it and makes a professional judgment on its acceptability. Judgments must be made regarding the type of drug, the therapeutic intent, the usual dose, and the mathematical and physical preparation of the dose. The nurse must also evaluate the method of administration in relation to the patient's physical condition, as well as any allergies and the patient's ability to tolerate the dosage form. If any part of an order is vague, the physician who wrote the order should be consulted for further clarification. Patient safety is of primary importance and the nurse assumes responsibility for verification and safety of the medication order. If, after gathering all possible information, it is concluded that it is inappropriate to administer the medication as ordered, the prescribing physician should be notified immediately. An explanation should be given why the order should not be executed. If the physician cannot be contacted or does not change the order, the nurse should notify the director of nurses and/or the nursing supervisor on duty. The reasons for refusal to administer the drug should be recorded in accordance with the policies of the employing institution.

Transcription of the order

Transcription of the prescriber's order is necessary to put it into action. After verification of an order, a nurse or another designated person transcribes the order from the physician's order sheet onto the Kardex or onto a medication administration record (MAR). (See Figure 4-9). These data may also be entered into a computer that produces a Kardex. When this process is delegated to a ward clerk or unit secretary, the nurse is still responsible for the verification of all aspects of the medication order. The nurse must sign the original medication order indicating that she received, interpreted, and verified the order. The nurse then sends a carbon copy of the original order to the pharmacy. A small supply is issued either in unit dose or in a container containing a multiday supply. The container is labeled with the date, patient's name, room number, and the drug name and strength/dose. When the supply arrives from the pharmacy it is stored in the medication room or in the patient's medication drawer of a medication cart.

In the long-term care setting, carbon copies of new medication orders are sent to the local pharmacy to be filled. If a stat dose is needed, or the medication must be started very soon, the pharmacy is notified via telephone and written verification of the medicine(s) ordered is also supplied to the pharmacy. Since the local pharmacy generates the medication administration record only on a monthly basis, new orders must be added to the current medication record by the nurse transcribing the order.

The nurse administers a drug by following the order on the medication administration record or drug profile according to the six rights of drug administration: right drug, right time, right dose, right patient, right route, right documentation.

THE SIX RIGHTS OF DRUG ADMINISTRATION

OBJECTIVES

1. Identify specific precautions needed to ensure that the RIGHT DRUG is prepared for the patient.
2. Memorize and recite standard abbreviations associated with the scheduling of medications.
3. Identify data found in the patient's chart that must be analyzed to determine if the patient has abnormal renal or hepatic function.
4. Describe specific safety precautions the nurse should institute to ensure that correct medication calculations are performed.
5. Review the policies and procedures of the practice setting to identify drugs of which dosages must be checked by two qualified persons.
6. Describe the methods that should be used to ensure that the correct patient receives the correct medication, by the correct route, in the correct amount, at the correct time.
7. Compare each safety measure described to ensure safe preparation and administration of medications with those procedures used at the clinical practice setting.
8. Identify appropriate nursing actions to document the administration and therapeutic effectiveness of each medication administered.

Right Drug

Many drugs have similar spellings and variable concentrations. *Before* the administration of the medication, it is imperative to compare the exact spelling and concentration of the prescribed drug with the medication card or drug profile and the medication container. Regardless of the drug distribution system used, the drug label should be read at least three times:

1. Before removing the drug from the shelf or unit dose cart

2. Before preparing or measuring the actual prescribed dose
3. Before replacing the drug on the shelf or before opening a unit dose container (just prior to administering the drug to the patient)

Right Time

When scheduling the administration time of a medication, factors such as timing abbreviations, standardized times, consistency of blood levels, absorption, diagnostic testing, and the use of p.r.n. medications must be considered.

1. *Standard Abbreviations*—The drug order specifies the frequency of drug administration. Standard abbreviations used as part of the drug order specify the times of administration (see Appendixes A and B). The nurse should also check institutional policy concerning administration of medications. Hospitals often have standardized interpretations for abbreviations (for example, "q 6 h" may mean 0600, 1200, 1800, and 2400; "q.i.d." may mean 0800, 1200, 1600 or 2000). The nurse must memorize and utilize standard abbreviations in interpreting, transcribing, and administering medications accurately.
2. *Standardized Administration Times*—For patient safety, certain medications are administered at specific times. This allows laboratory work or ECGs to be completed first, in order to determine the size of the next dose to be administered. For example, warfarin or digoxin would be administered at 1300, if ordered by the physician.
3. *Maintenance of Consistent Blood Levels*—The schedule for the administration of a drug should be planned to maintain consistent blood levels of the drug in order to maximize the therapeutic effectiveness.
4. *Maximum Drug Absorption*—The schedule for oral administration of drugs must be planned to prevent incompatibilities and maximize absorption. Certain drugs require administration on an empty stomach. Thus, they are given 1 hour before or 2 hours after meals. Other medications should be given with foods to enhance absorption or reduce irritations. Still other drugs are not given with dairy products or antacids. It is important to maintain the recommended schedule of administration for maximum therapeutic effectiveness.
5. *Diagnostic Testing*—Determine whether any diagnostic tests have been ordered for completion prior to initiating or continuing therapy. Before beginning antimicrobial therapy, assure that all culture specimens (such as blood, urine, or wound) have been collected. If a physician has ordered serum levels of the drug, coordinate the administration time of the medication with the time the phlebotomist is going to draw the blood sample. When completing the requisition for a serum level of a medication, always make a notation of the date and time that the drug was last administered. Timing is important; if tests are not conducted at the same time intervals in the same patient, the data gained are of little value.
6. *P.R.N. Medications*—*Before* the administration of any p.r.n. medication, the patient's chart should be checked to ensure that the drug has not been administered by someone else, or that the specified time interval has passed since the medication was last administered. When a p.r.n. medication is given, it should be charted immediately. Record the response to the medication.

Right Dose

Check the drug dosage ordered against the range specified in the reference books available at the nurses' station.

1. *Abnormal Hepatic or Renal Function*—Always consider the hepatic and renal function of the specific patient who will receive the drug. Depending on the rate of drug metabolism and route of excretion from the body, certain drugs require a reduction in dosage to prevent toxicity. Conversely, patients being dialyzed may require higher than normal doses. Whenever a dosage is outside the normal range for that drug, it should be verified *before* administration. Once verification has been obtained, a brief explanation should be recorded in the nurse's notes and on the Kardex (or drug profile) so that others administering the medication will have the information and the physician will not be repeatedly contacted with the same questions.

   The following laboratory tests are used to monitor liver function: aspartame aminotransferase (AST), alanine aminotransferase (ALT), gamma glutamyl transferase (GGT), alkaline phosphatase, and lactic dehydrogenase (LDH).

   The blood urea nitrogen (BUN), serum creatinine (Cr_s), and creatinine clearance (C_{cr}) are used to monitor renal function.
2. *Pediatric and Geriatric Patients*—Specific doses for some drugs are not yet firmly established for the elderly and for the pediatric patient. The nurse should question any order outside the normal range *before* administration. For pediatric patients, the most reliable method is by proportional amount of body surface area or body weight. (See Appendixes E and H.)
3. *Nausea and Vomiting*—If a patient is vomiting, oral medications should be withheld and the physician contacted for alternate medication orders, as the

parenteral or rectal route may be preferred. Investigate the onset of the nausea and vomiting. If it began after the start of the medication regimen, consideration should be given to rescheduling the oral medication. Administration with food usually decreases gastric irritation. Consult with a physician for changes in orders.

4. *Accurate Dose Forms*—Do not break a tablet unless it is scored. Consult with the pharmacy about other available dosage forms.
5. *Accurate Calculations*—Safety should always be maintained when calculating a drug dose. Whenever a dosage is questionable, or when fractional doses are calculated, check the dosage with another qualified individual. Most hospital policies require that certain medications (for example, insulin, heparin, IV digitalis preparations) be checked by two qualified nurses prior to administration.
6. *Correct Measuring Devices*—Accurate measurement of the volume of medication prescribed is essential. *Fractional doses require the use of a tuberculin syringe, while insulin is always measured in an insulin syringe that corresponds to the number of units in 1 ml (U-100 insulin is measured in a U-100 syringe).*

Right Patient

When using the medication card system, compare the name of the patient on the medication card with the patient's identification bracelet. With the unit dose system, compare the name on the drug profile with the individual's identification bracelet. When checking the bracelet under either system, always check for allergies, as well. Some institutional policies require that the individual be called by name as a means of identification. This practice must take into consideration the patient's mental alertness and orientation. It is much safer ALWAYS to check the identification bracelet.

1. *Pediatric Patients*—Never ask children their names as a means of positive identification. Children may change beds, try to avoid you, or seek attention by identifying themselves as someone else. Check identification bracelets EVERY TIME.
2. *Geriatric Patients*—It is a wise policy to check identification bracelets, in addition to confirming names verbally. In a long-term care setting, residents usually do not wear identification bracelets. In these instances, only a person who is familiar with the residents should administer medications.

Many errors may be avoided by carefully following the practices just presented. Make it a habit to check the identification bracelet EVERY TIME a medication is administered. The adverse effects of administration of the wrong medication to the wrong patient and the potential for a lawsuit can thus be avoided.

Right Route

The drug order should specify the route to be used for the administration of the medication. Never substitute one dosage form of medication for another unless the physician is specifically consulted and an order for the change is obtained. There can be a great variation in the absorption rate of the medication through various routes of administration. The intravenous route delivers the drug directly into the bloodstream. This route provides the fastest onset, but also the greatest danger of potential adverse effects such as tachycardia and hypotension. The intramuscular route provides the next fastest absorption rate, based upon availability of blood supply. This route can be quite painful, as is the case with many antibiotics. The subcutaneous route is next fastest, based on blood supply. In some instances the oral route may be as fast as the intramuscular route, depending on the medication being given, the dosage form (liquids are absorbed faster than tablets), and whether there is food in the stomach. The oral route is usually safe if the patient is conscious and able to swallow. The rectal route should be avoided, if possible, due to irritation of mucosal tissues and erratic absorption rates. In case of error, the oral and rectal routes have the advantage of recoverability for a short time after administration.

Right Drug Preparation and Administration

Maintain the highest standards of drug preparation and administration. Focus your entire attention on the calculation, preparation, and administration of the ordered medication. A drug reconstituted by a nurse should be clearly labeled with the patient's name, the dose or strength per unit of volume, the date and time the drug was reconstituted, the amount and type of diluent used, the expiration date and/or time, and the initials or name of the nurse who prepared it. Once reconstituted, the drug should be stored according to the manufacturer's recommendation.

- CHECK the label of the container for the drug name, concentration, and route of appropriate administration.
- CHECK the patient's chart, Kardex, medication administration record, or identification bracelet for allergies. If no information is found, ask the patient, prior to the administration of the medication, if he or she has any allergies.
- CHECK the patient's chart, Kardex or medication administration record for rotation schedules of injectable or topically applied medications.
- CHECK medications to be mixed in one syringe with a list approved by the hospital or the pharmacy for compatibility. Normally, all drugs mixed in a single syringe should be administered within 15 minutes after mixing. Immediately prior to administration, AL-

WAYS CHECK the contents of the syringe for clarity and the absence of any precipitate; if either is present, do not administer the contents of the syringe.

- CHECK the patient's identity EVERY TIME a medication is administered.
- DO approach the patient in a firm but kind manner that conveys the feeling that cooperation is expected.
- DO adjust the patient to the most appropriate position for the route of administration (for example, for oral medications, sit the patient upright to facilitate swallowing). Have appropriate fluids ready before administration.
- DO remain with the patient to be certain that all medications have been swallowed.
- DO use every opportunity to teach the patient and family about the drug being administered.
- DO give simple and honest answers or explanations to the patient regarding the medication and treatment plan.
- DO use a plastic container, medicine cup, medicine dropper, oral syringe, or nipple to administer oral medications to an infant or small child.
- DO reward the child who has been cooperative by giving praise; comfort and hold the uncooperative child after completing the medication administration.
- DO NOT prepare or administer a drug from a container that is not properly labeled or from a container where the label is not fully legible.
- DO NOT give any medication prepared by an individual other than the pharmacist. ALWAYS check the drug name, dosage, frequency, and route of administration against the order. Student nurses must know the practice limitations instituted by the hospital or school and which medications can be administered under what level of supervision.
- DO NOT return an unused portion or dose of medication to a stock supply bottle.
- DO NOT attempt to administer any drug orally to a comatose patient.
- DO NOT leave a medication at the patient's bedside to be taken "later"; remain with the individual until the drug is taken and swallowed. (NOTE: There are a few exceptions to this rule. One is that nitroglycerin may be left at the bedside for the patient's use. Secondly, in a long-term care setting certain patients are allowed to take their own medications. In both instances, a specific physician's order is required for *self-medication* and the nurse must still chart the medications taken and the therapeutic response achieved.)
- DO NOT dilute a liquid medication form unless there are specific written orders to do so.
- BEFORE DISCHARGE: (1) Explain the proper method of taking prescribed medications to the patient (for example, do not crush or chew enteric-coated tablets, or any capsules; sublingual medication is placed under the tongue and is not taken with water). (2) Stress the need for punctuality in the administration of medications, and what to do if a dosage is missed. (3) Teach the patient to store medications separately from other containers and personal hygiene items. (4) Provide the patient with written instructions reiterating the medication names, schedules, and how to obtain refills. Write the instructions in a language understood by the patient, and use LARGE, BOLD LETTERS when necessary. (5) Identify anticipated therapeutic response. (6) Instruct the patient, family member(s), or significant others on how to collect and record data for use by the physician to monitor the patient's response to drug and other treatment modalities. (7) Give the patient, or another responsible individual, a list of signs and symptoms that should be reported to the physician. (8) Stress measures that can be initiated to minimize or prevent anticipated side effects to the prescribed medication. It is important to do this to further encourage the patient to be compliant with the prescribed regimen.

Right Documentation

Documentation of nursing actions and patient observations has always been an important ethical responsibility, but now it is becoming a major medicolegal consideration as well. Indeed, it is becoming known as the sixth right. Always chart the following information: date and time of administration, name of medication, dosage, route, and site of administration. Documentation of drug action should be made in the regularly scheduled assessments for changes in the disease symptoms the patient is exhibiting. Promptly record and report adverse symptoms observed. Document health teaching performed and evaluate and record the degree of understanding exhibited by the patient.

- DO record when a drug is *not* administered and why.
- DO NOT record a medication until after it has been given.
- DO NOT record in the nurses' notes that an incident report has been completed when a medication error has occurred. However, data regarding clinical observations of the patient related to the occurrence should be charted to serve as a baseline for future comparisons.

Whenever a medication error does occur, an incident report is completed to describe the circumstances of the event. An incident report related to a medication error should include the following data: date, time the drug was ordered, drug name, dose, and route of administration. Information regarding the date, time, drug administered, and dose and route of administration should be given, and the therapeutic response or adverse clinical observations present should be noted. Finally, record the date, time, and physician notified of the error and any physician's orders given. Be FACTUAL; do not state opinions on the incident report.

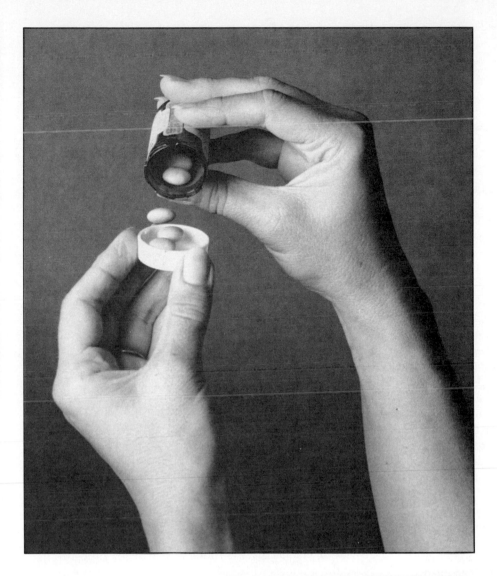

Preparation and Administration of Medications by the Enteral Route

Chapter Goals

After completing this chapter, the student should be able to do the following:

1. Give a detailed description of the dosage forms and procedures used to prepare and administer medications via the enteral route.

2. Differentiate between the techniques utilized to administer enteral medications using a "medication card" and a "unit dose" system of medication distribution.

3. Cite the specific methods used to document medication administration and therapeutic effectiveness of drugs administered via the enteral route.

4. Utilize the procedures and principles cited for the preparation and administration of medications via the enteral route in the practice setting.

The routes of drug administration can be classified into three categories: the enteral, the parenteral, and the percutaneous routes. The enteral route refers to those drugs administered directly into the gastrointestinal tract by oral, rectal, or nasogastric routes. The oral route is safe, most convenient, and relatively economical, and dosage forms are readily available for most medications. In the event of a medication error or intentional drug overdose, much of the drug can be retrieved for a reasonable time after administration. Disadvantages of the oral route are that it has the slowest and least dependable rate of absorption (and thus onset of action) of the commonly used routes of administration because of the frequent changes in the gastrointestinal environment produced by food, emotion, and physical activity. Another limitation on this route is that a few drugs, such as insulin and gentamicin, are destroyed by digestive fluids and must be administered parenterally for therapeutic activity. This route should not be used if the drug may harm or discolor the teeth or if the patient is vomiting, has gastric or intestinal suction, is likely to aspirate, or is unconscious and unable to swallow.

An alternative for those patients who cannot swallow or who have had oral surgery is the nasogastric route. The primary purpose of the nasogastric route is to bypass the mouth and pharynx. Advantages and disadvantages are quite similar to those of the oral route. The irritation caused by the tube in the nasal passage and throat must be weighed against the relative immobility associated with continuous intravenous infusions, expense, and the pain and irritation of multiple injections.

Administration via the rectal route has the advantages of bypassing the digestive enzymes and avoiding irritation of the mouth, esophagus, and stomach. It may also be a good alternative when nausea or vomiting is present. Absorption via this route varies depending on the drug product, the ability of the patient to retain the suppository or enema, and the presence of fecal material.

ADMINISTRATION OF ORAL MEDICATIONS
OBJECTIVES

1. Correctly define and identify oral dosage forms of medications.
2. Identify common receptacles used to administer oral medications.

KEY WORDS

capsules	lozenges
tablets	emulsions
suspensions	syrups
elixirs	soufflé cup
medicine cup	oral syringe

Dosage Forms

Capsules

Capsules are small, cylindrical gelatin containers (Figure 5-1) that hold dry powder or liquid medicinal agents. They are available in a variety of sizes and are a convenient way of administering drugs with an unpleasant odor or taste. They do not require coatings or additives to improve the taste. The color and shapes of capsules, as well as the manufacturer's symbols on the capsule surface, are means of identifying the product.

Timed-release capsules

Timed-release or sustained-release capsules (Figure 5-2) provide a gradual but continuous release of drug because the granules within the capsule dissolve at different rates. The advantage of this delivery system is that it reduces the number of doses administered per day. Trade names indicating that the drug is a timed-release product are Spansules, Gyrocaps, and Plateau Caps. The timed-release capsules should NOT be crushed or chewed or the contents emptied into food or liquids,

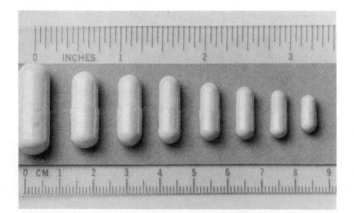

Figure 5-1 *Various sizes and numbers of gelatin capsules, actual size.*

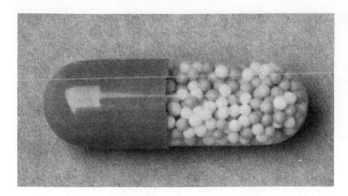

Figure 5-2 *Timed-release capsule.*

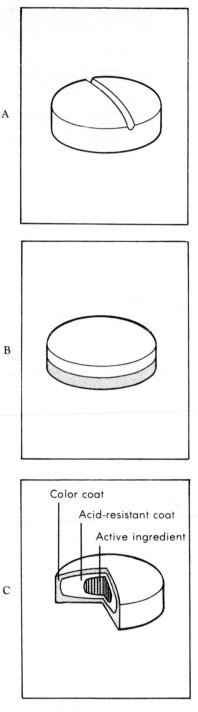

Figure 5-3 **A,** *Scored tablet.* **B,** *Layered tablet.* **C,** *Enteric coated tablet.*

because this may alter the absorption rate and could result in either drug overdose or subtherapeutic activity.

Lozenges

Lozenges are flat disks containing a medicinal agent in a suitably flavored base. The base may be a hard sugar candy or the combination of sugar with sufficient mucilage to give it form. Lozenges are held in the mouth to dissolve slowly, thus releasing the therapeutic ingredients.

Pills

Pills are an obsolete dosage form that are no longer manufactured due to the development of capsules and compressed tablets. Laypersons still use the term to refer to tablets and capsules.

Tablets

Tablets are dried, powdered drugs that have been compressed into small disks. In addition to the drug, tablets also contain one or more of the following ingredients: binders (adhesive substances that allow the tablet to stick together); disintegrators (substances that encourage dissolution in body fluids); lubricants (required for efficient manufacturing); and fillers (inert ingredients to make the tablet size convenient). Tablets are sometimes scored or grooved (Figure 5-3, A); the indentation may be used to divide the dosage. When possible, it is best to request the exact dosage prescribed rather than attempt to divide a tablet.

Tablets can be formed in layers (Figure 5-3, B). This method allows otherwise incompatible medications to be administered at the same time.

An enteric-coated tablet (Figure 5-3, C) has a special coating that resists dissolution in the acidic pH of the stomach but is dissolved in the alkaline pH of the intestines. Enteric-coated tablets are often used for administering medications that are destroyed in an acid pH. Enteric-coated tablets must NOT be crushed or chewed, or the active ingredients will be released prematurely and be destroyed in the stomach.

Elixirs

Elixirs are clear liquids made up of drugs dissolved in alcohol and water. Elixirs are used primarily when the drug will not dissolve in water alone. After the drug is dissolved in the elixir, flavoring agents are frequently

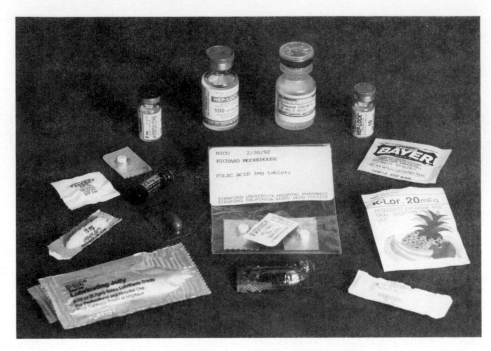

Figure 5-4 *Unit dose packages.*

added to improve taste. The alcohol content of elixirs is highly variable, depending on the solubility of the drug.

Emulsions

Emulsions are dispersions of small droplets of water in oil or oil in water. The dispersion is maintained by emulsifying agents such as sodium lauryl sulfate, gelatin, or acacia. Emulsions are used to mask bitter tastes or provide better solubility to certain drugs.

Suspensions

Suspensions are liquid dosage forms that contain solid, insoluble drug particles dispersed in a liquid base. All suspensions should be shaken well before administration to assure thorough mixing of the particles.

Syrups

Syrups contain medicinal agents dissolved in a concentrated solution of sugar, usually sucrose. Syrups are particularly effective for masking the bitter taste of a drug. Many preparations for pediatric patients are syrups, as children tend to like the flavored base.

Equipment

Unit dose or single dose

"Unit dose or single dose" packaging (Figure 5-4) provides a single dose of medication in one package, ready

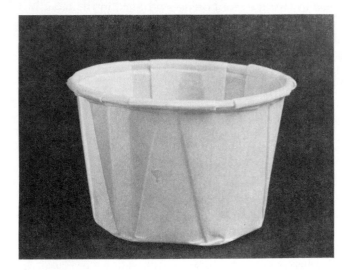

Figure 5-5 *Soufflé cup.*

for dispensing. The package is labeled with generic and brand names, manufacturer, lot number, and date of expiration. Depending on the distribution system, the patient's name may be added to the package by the pharmacy.

Soufflé cup

A small paper or plastic cup (Figure 5-5) may be used to transport solid medication forms, such as a capsule or tablet, to the patient to prevent contamination by handling. A tablet that must be crushed can be placed between two soufflé cups and then crushed with a pestle. This powdered form of the tablet can then be adminis-

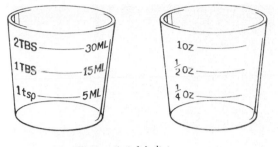

Figure 5-6 *Medicine cup.*

Table 5-1 *Commonly Used Measurement Equivalents*

HOUSEHOLD MEASUREMENT	APOTHECARY MEASUREMENT	METRIC MEASUREMENT
2 Tbsp	1 oz	30 ml
1 Tbsp	½ oz	15 ml
2 tsp	⅓ oz	10 ml
1 tsp	⅙ oz	5 ml

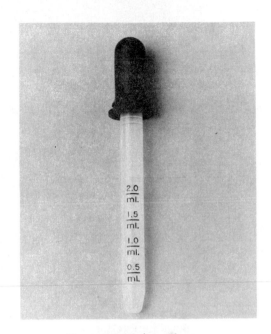

Figure 5-7 *Medicine dropper.*

tered in a solution if soluble, or it may be mixed with a small amount of food, such as applesauce.

Medicine cup

The medicine cup (Figure 5-6) is a glass or plastic container that has three scales (apothecary, metric, and household) for the measurement of liquid medications. The medicine cup should be carefully examined before pouring any medication to assure that the proper scale is being used for measurement (see Table 5-1). The medicine cup is inaccurate for the measurement of doses smaller than 1 teaspoonful, although it is reasonably accurate for larger volumes. A syringe comparable to the volume to be measured should be used for smaller volumes. For volumes less than 1 cc, a tuberculin syringe should be used.

Medicine dropper

The medicine dropper (Figure 5-7) may be used to administer eye drops, ear drops, and, occasionally, pediatric medications. There is great variation in the size of the drop formed, so it is quite important to use only the dropper supplied by the manufacturer for a specific liquid medication. Before drawing medication into a dropper, become familiar with the calibrations on the barrel. Once the medication is drawn into the barrel, the dropper should not be tipped upside down. The medication will run into the bulb, causing some loss of the medication. Medications should not be drawn into the dropper and then transferred to another container for administration because part of the medication will adhere to the second container, thus diminishing the dose delivered.

Teaspoons

Doses of most liquid medications are prescribed in terms using the teaspoon (Figure 5-8) as the unit of measure. However, there is great variation between the volumes measured by various teaspoons within the household. Within the hospital, 1 teaspoonful is converted to 5 ml (see Table 5-1) and is read on the metric scale of the medicine cup. For home use, an oral sy-

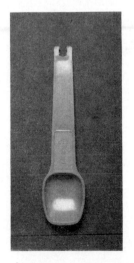

Figure 5-8 *Measuring teaspoon.*

ringe is recommended. If not available, a teaspoon used specifically for baking may be used as an accurate measuring device.

Oral syringes

Plastic oral syringes (Figure 5-9) may be used to measure liquid medications accurately. Various sizes are

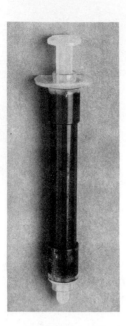

Figure 5-9 *Plastic oral syringe.*

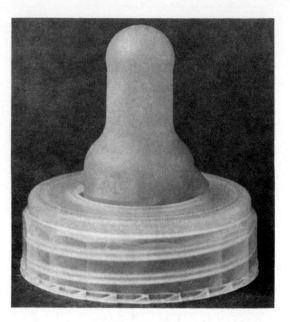

Figure 5-10 *Nipple.*

available to measure volumes from 0.1 ml to 15 ml. Note that a needle will not fit on the tip.

Nipples

An infant feeding nipple (Figure 5-10) with additional holes may be used for administering oral medications to infants. (See Techniques of Administration.)

ADMINISTRATION OF SOLID-FORM ORAL MEDICATIONS
OBJECTIVE

1. Describe general principles of administering solid forms of medications and the different techniques utilized with a "medication card" and "unit dose" distribution system.

Technique

Medication card system

Equipment:
  Medication tray
  Soufflé cup or medicine cup
  Medication cards

1. Wash hands.
2. Gather medication cards and verify against Kardex and/or physician's order for accuracy.
3. Gather remainder of equipment.
4. Read the entire medication card.
5. Obtain the medication prescribed from the cabinet.
6. COMPARE the label on the container against the medication card:

RIGHT PATIENT
RIGHT DRUG
RIGHT ROUTE OF ADMINISTRATION
RIGHT DOSAGE
RIGHT TIME OF ADMINISTRATION

7. Open lid of the bottle; pour correct number of capsules or tablets into the lid; return any extras to the container using the lid. (DO NOT touch the medication with your hands!)
8. Transfer correct number of tablets or capsules from the lid to a soufflé cup or medicine cup.
9. COMPARE the information on the medication card against the label on the stock bottle and the quantity of drug placed in the cup.
10. Replace lid of container.
11. RECHECK the 5 RIGHTS of the medication order.
12. Return the medication container to the shelf in the cabinet.
13. Place the patient's medication cup on the medication tray with the medication card (Figure 5-11).
14. Proceed to the patient's bedside when all medications are assembled for administration.
    —Check the patient's identification bracelet and verify against the medication card.
    —Explain what you are doing.
    —Check pertinent patient monitoring parameters (apical pulse, respiratory rate, etc.).
    —Hand medication to patient for placement in the mouth.

Unit dose system

Equipment:
  Medication cart   Medication profile

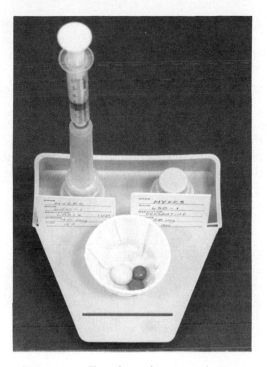

Figure 5-11 *Tray for medication card system.*

1. Wash hands.
2. Read the patient medication profile for drugs and times of administration.
3. Obtain the medication prescribed from the drawer that is assigned to the patient in the medication cart.
4. Check the label on the unit dose package against the patient medication profile.
   RIGHT PATIENT
   RIGHT DRUG
   RIGHT ROUTE OF ADMINISTRATION
   RIGHT DOSAGE
   RIGHT TIME OF ADMINISTRATION
5. Check the number of doses remaining in the drawer. (If the number of doses remaining is not consistent, investigate!)
6. Check the 5 RIGHTS of the medication order on the patient medication profile and unit dose package as removed from drawer.
7. Proceed to the bedside:
   —Check patient's identification bracelet and verify against the profile.
   —Explain carefully to the patient what you are doing.
   —Check pertinent patient monitoring parameters (apical pulse, respiratory rate, etc.).
8. Hand the medication to the patient and allow him or her to read the package label.
9. Retrieve the unit dose package and open it, placing the contents in the patient's hand for placement in the mouth.

General Principles of Solid-Form Medication Administration

1. Give the most important medication first.
2. Allow the patient to drink a small amount of water to moisten the mouth to make swallowing the medication easier.
3. Have the patient place the medication well back on the tongue. Offer appropriate assistance.
4. Give the patient liquid to swallow the medication. Encourage keeping the head forward while swallowing.
5. Drinking a full glass of fluid should be encouraged to ensure that the medication reaches the stomach and to dilute the drug to decrease the potential for irritation.
6. Always remain with the patient while the medication is taken. DO NOT leave the medication at the bedside unless an order exists to do so (medication such as nitroglycerin may be ordered for the bedside).
7. Discard the medication container (such as a soufflé cup or unit dose package).

Documentation

Provide the RIGHT DOCUMENTATION of medication administration and responses to drug therapy:

1. Chart the date, time, drug name, dosage, and route of administration.
2. Perform and record regular patient assessments for the evaluation of the therapeutic effectiveness (blood pressure, pulse, output, improvement or quality of cough and productivity, degree and duration of pain relief, etc.).
3. Chart and report any signs and symptoms of adverse drug effects.
4. Perform and validate essential patient education about the drug therapy and other essential aspects of intervention for the disease process affecting the individual.

ADMINISTRATION OF LIQUID-FORM ORAL MEDICATIONS
OBJECTIVE

1. Compare techniques used to administer liquid forms of oral medication utilizing "medication card" and "unit dose" system of distribution.

Technique

Medication card system

Equipment:
   Medication tray
   Plastic syringe or medicine cup
   Medication cards

1. Wash hands.
2. Gather medication cards and verify against Kardex and/or physician's order for accuracy.
3. Gather remainder of equipment.
4. Read the entire medication card.
5. Obtain the medication prescribed from the cabinet.
6. COMPARE the label on the container against the medication card:
   RIGHT PATIENT
   RIGHT DRUG
   RIGHT ROUTE OF ADMINISTRATION
   RIGHT DOSAGE
   RIGHT TIME OF ADMINISTRATION
7. Shake medication, if required.
8. Remove lid and place upside down on a flat surface to prevent contamination.
9. Proceed with one of the measuring techniques below:

Measuring with a medicine cup

—Hold the bottle of liquid so that the label is in the palm of the hand. This prevents the contents from smearing the label during pouring.
—Examine the medicine cup and locate the exact place to where the measured volume should be measured; place your fingernail at this level.
—While holding the medicine cup straight at eye level, pour the prescribed volume.
—Read the volume accurately at the level of the meniscus (Figure 5-12).
—COMPARE the information on the medication card against the label on the stock bottle and the quantity of drug placed in the cup.
—Replace lid on the container.
—RECHECK the 5 RIGHTS of the medication order.
—Return the medication container to the shelf of the cabinet.
—Place the patient's medication cup on the medication tray with the medication card (Figure 5-11).

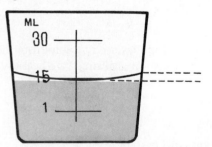

Figure 5-12 *Reading meniscus. The meniscus is caused by the surface tension of the solution against the walls of the container. The surface tension causes the formation of a concave or hollowed curvature on the surface of the solution. Read the level at the lowest point of the concaved curve.*

—Proceed to the patient's bedside when all medications are assembled for administration.

Measuring in an oral syringe (see Chapter 6 for reading calibrations of a syringe)

—Select a syringe in a size comparable to the volume to be measured.
—*Method 1*: With a large bore needle attached to the syringe, draw up the prescribed volume of medication. The needle is not necessary if the bottle opening is large enough to receive the syringe (Figure 5-13).
—*Method 2*: Using the cup and the method described above, pour the amount of medication needed into a medicine cup, then use a syringe to measure the prescribed volume (Figure 5-14).
—COMPARE the information on the medication card against the label on the stock bottle and the quantity of drug placed in the syringe.
—Replace the lid on the container.
—RECHECK the 5 RIGHTS of the medication order.

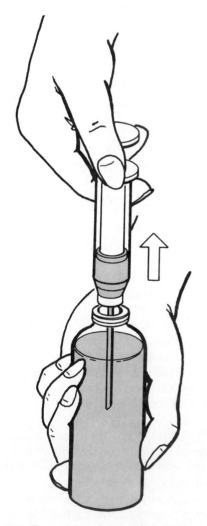

Figure 5-13 *Removing medication directly from a bottle.*

—Return the medication container to the shelf of the cabinet.

—Place the patient's medication syringe on the medication tray with the medication card directly under the syringe.

—Proceed to the patient's bedside when all medications are assembled for administration.

10. Check the patient's identification bracelet and verify against the medication card.
11. Explain what you are doing.
12. Check pertinent patient monitoring parameters (apical pulse, respiratory rate, etc.).
13. Hand medication cup to patient for placement of the contents in the mouth or administer via the oral syringe.

Unit dose system

Equipment:
   Medication cart
   Medication profile

1. Wash hands.
2. Read the patient medication profile for drugs and times of administration.
3. Obtain the medication prescribed from the drawer assigned to the patient in the medication cart.

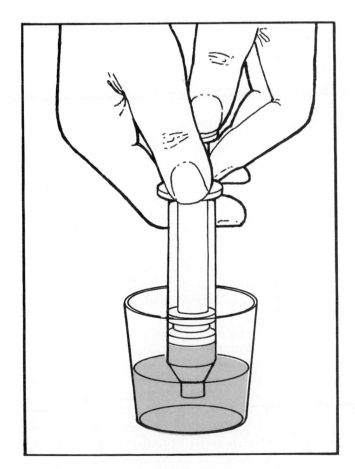

Figure 5-14 *Filling a syringe directly from a medicine cup.*

4. Check the label on the unit dose package against the patient medication profile:
   RIGHT PATIENT
   RIGHT DRUG
   RIGHT ROUTE OF ADMINISTRATION
   RIGHT DOSAGE
   RIGHT TIME OF ADMINISTRATION
5. Check the number of doses remaining in the drawer. (If the number of doses remaining is not consistent, investigate!)
6. Check the 5 RIGHTS of the medication order on the patient medication profile and unit dose package as removed from the drawer.
7. Proceed to the bedside:
   —Check patient's identification bracelet and verify against the profile.
   —Explain what you are doing.
   —Check pertinent patient monitoring parameters (apical pulse, respiratory rate, etc.).
8. Hand the unit dose medication to the patient and allow him or her to read the package label.
9. Retrieve the unit dose package and open it, placing the container in the patient's hand for placement of the contents in the patient's mouth.

General Principles of Liquid-Form Oral Medication Administration

For an adult or child

1. Give the most important medication first.
2. Never dilute a liquid medication unless specifically ordered to do so.
3. Always remain with the patient while the medication is taken. DO NOT leave the medication at the bedside unless an order exists to do so.

For an infant

1. Check the infant's identification bracelet and verify against the medication card or profile.
2. Be certain that the infant is alert.
3. Position the infant so that the head is slightly elevated (Figure 5-15).
4. Administration:
   Oral syringe or dropper

   —Place the syringe or dropper between the cheek and gums, halfway back into the mouth. This placement will lessen the chance that the infant will spit out the medication with tongue movements.

   —Slowly inject, allowing the infant to swallow medication. (Rapid administration may cause choking and aspiration!)
   Nipple

   —When the infant is awake (and preferably hungry), place the nipple in the infant's mouth.

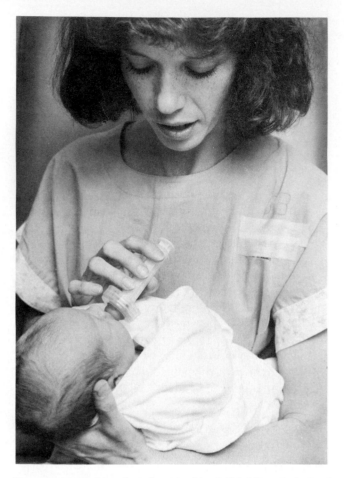

Figure 5-15 *Position the infant in a "football hold" with the head slightly elevated. Place the nipple in the infant's mouth. When the baby starts to suck, place the medication in the back of the nipple and allow the baby to suck.*

When the baby starts to suck, place the medication in the back of the nipple with a syringe or dropper and allow the baby to suck it in (Figure 5-15). (The size of the nipple holes may need to be enlarged for suspensions and syrups.) Follow with milk or formula, if necessary.

Documentation

Provide the RIGHT DOCUMENTATION of the medication administration and responses to drug therapy:

1. Chart the date, time, drug name, dosage, and route of administration.
2. Perform and record regular patient assessments for the evaluation of therapeutic effectiveness (blood pressure, pulse, output, improvement or quality of cough and productivity, degree and duration of pain relief, etc.).
3. Chart and report any signs and symptoms of adverse drug effects.
4. Perform and validate essential patient education about the drug therapy and other essential aspects of

intervention for the disease process affecting the individual.

ADMINISTRATION OF MEDICATIONS BY THE NASOGASTRIC TUBE
Objective

1. Cite the equipment needed, techniques utilized, and precautions necessary when administering medications via a nasogastric tube.

KEY WORD

nasogastric tube

Medications are administered via a nasogastric (NG) tube to patients who have impaired swallowing, are comatose, or have a disorder of the esophagus. Whenever possible, a liquid form of a drug should be used for NG administration. If it is necessary to use a tablet or capsule, the tablet should be crushed and the capsule pulled apart and the powder sprinkled in approximately 30 ml of water. (DO NOT crush enteric-coated tablets or timed-release capsules.)

Equipment

Glass of water
5 to 10 ml syringe (adult patient)
1 ml syringe (young child)
Stethoscope
Medication
Bulb syringe with catheter tip

Technique

Refer to the sections on the administration of solid-form or liquid-form oral medications for preparation of dosages.

1. Proceed to the patient's bedside when all medications are assembled for administration.
2. Check the patient's identification bracelet and verify against the medication card or drug profile.
3. Explain what you are going to do.
4. Sit the patient upright and check the location of the nasogastric tube before administering any liquid (Figure 5-16).
   —*Method 1*: Aspirate part of the stomach contents using the bulb syringe (Figure 5-16, A). Return of stomach contents confirms correct tube placement. If contents are not returned, use methods 2 and/or 3 to assess the location of the tube tip.
   —*Method 2*: Place a stethoscope over the stomach area; listen as 5 to 10 ml (adult) (0.5 up to 5 ml for child) of air are inserted (Figure 5-16, B). A gurgling sound should be heard if the na-

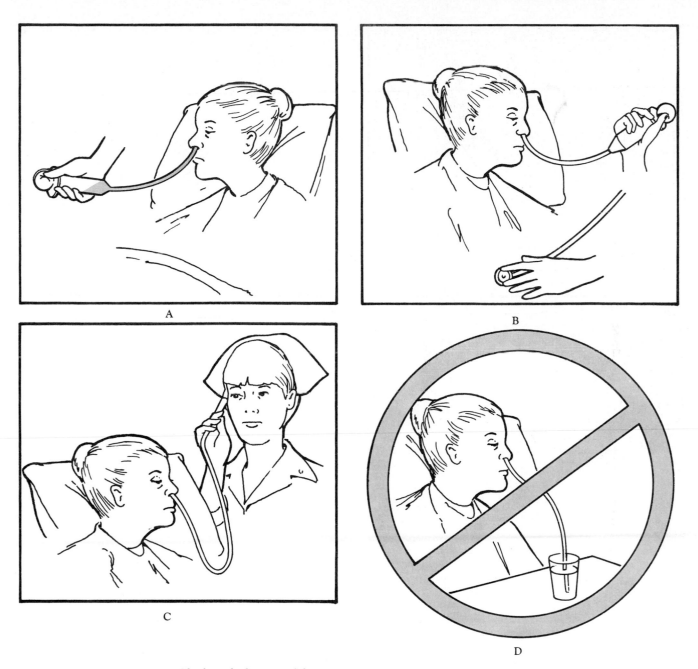

Figure 5-16 *Checking the location of the nasogastric tube.* **A,** *Aspiration of stomach contents.* **B,** *Place a stethoscope over the stomach area; listen for a "gurgling" sound as air is inserted.* **C,** *Listen for "crackling" sounds indicating placement of nasogastric tube in the lung.* **D,** *It is no longer recommended to place the end of the nasogastric tube in a glass of water. Although bubbling with respirations indicates placement of the tube in the lung, the patient may inadvertently inhale additional water from the glass into the lungs.*

sogastric tube is properly placed. Withdraw the amount of air inserted. (Although a bulb syringe is frequently used to insert the air, a syringe with an adapter may also be used for more accurate measurement.)

—*Method 3:* Place the unclamped NG tube next to the ear and listen for any crackling noise (Figure 5-16, C); if the crackling sounds are heard, the tube may be in the lung. Remove and reinsert.

5. Once the placement of the NG tube in the stomach is confirmed, do the following:

—Clamp the tubing and attach the bulb syringe; pour the medication into the syringe while the tubing is still clamped (Figure 5-17, A).

—Unclamp the tubing and allow the medication to run in by gravity (Figure 5-17, B); add the specified amount of water (at least 50 ml) (Figure 5-17, C) to flush the medication through the tube and into the stomach; clamp the tub-

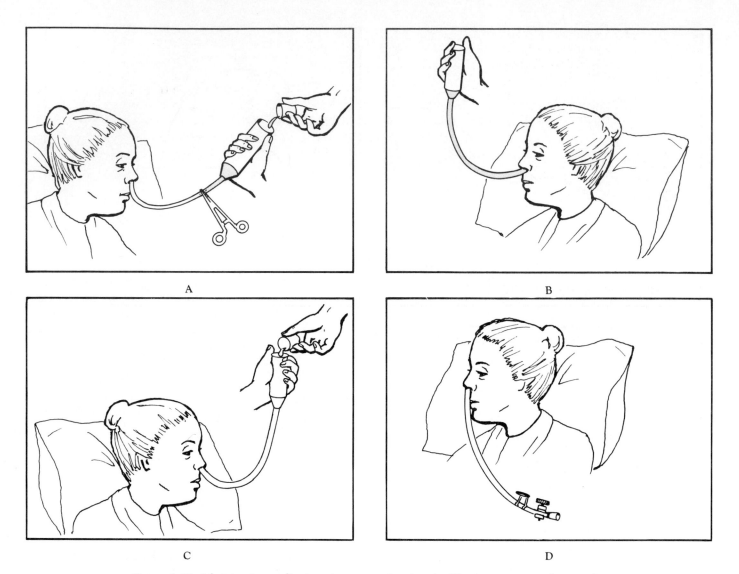

Figure 5-17 *Administering medication via nasogastric tube.* **A,** *Clamp nasogastric tube; attach a bulb syringe; and pour prescribed medication into syringe portion.* **B,** *Unclamp tubing and allow the medication to flow in by gravity.* **C,** *When medication is low in the syringe portion, pour in water to allow for thorough flushing of the medication from the tubing.* **D,** *Clamp tubing and secure end in place. Do not reattach to suction (if being used) for at least 30 minutes.*

ing as soon as the water has flowed through the bulb syringe (Figure 5-17, *D*).

—Clamp the tubing at the end of the medication administration. DO NOT attach to the suction source for at least 30 minutes, or the medication will be suctioned out.

—Give oral hygiene, if needed.

Documentation

Provide the RIGHT DOCUMENTATION of medication administration and responses to drug therapy:

1. Chart the date, time, drug name, dosage, and route of administration. Include all fluids administered on intake record.
2. Perform and record regular patient assessments for

the evaluation of the therapeutic effectiveness (blood pressure, pulse, output, improvement or quality of cough and productivity, degree and duration of pain relief, etc.).
3. Chart and report any signs and symptoms of adverse drug effects.
4. Perform and validate essential patient education about the drug therapy and other essential aspects of intervention for the disease process affecting the individual.

ADMINISTRATION OF RECTAL SUPPOSITORIES
OBJECTIVE

1. Cite the equipment needed and technique utilized to administer rectal suppositories.

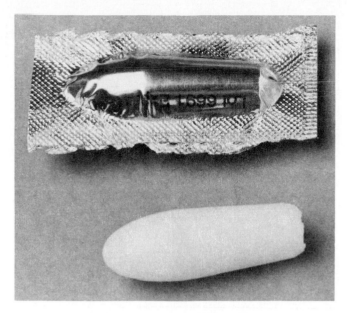

Figure 5-18 *Rectal suppositories.*

Dosage Form

Suppositories (Figure 5-18) are a solid form of medication designed for introduction into a body orifice. At body temperature, the substance dissolves and is absorbed by the mucous membranes. Suppositories should be stored in a cool place to prevent softening. If a suppository becomes soft and the package has not yet been opened, hold the foil-wrapped suppository under cold running water, or place in ice water for a short time until it hardens. Rectal suppositories should generally not be used for patients who have had recent prostatic or rectal surgery or recent rectal trauma.

Equipment

Finger cot or disposable glove
Water-soluble lubricant

Technique

1. Wash hands and assemble the necessary equipment and the prescribed rectal suppository.
2. COMPARE the label on the container against the medication card or drug profile:
    RIGHT PATIENT
    RIGHT DRUG
    RIGHT ROUTE OF ADMINISTRATION
    RIGHT DOSAGE
    RIGHT TIME OF ADMINISTRATION
3. Proceed to the patient's bedside.
4. Check the patient's identification bracelet and verify against the medication card or drug profile.
5. Explain what you are going to do.
6. Check pertinent patient monitoring parameters (time of last defecation, severity of nausea or vomiting, respiratory rate, etc.) as appropriate to the medication to be administered.
7. Whenever possible, have the patient defecate.
8. Provide for patient privacy; position and drape to avoid unnecessary exposure (Figure 5-19, A). Generally, the patient is placed on the left side (Sim's position).
9. Put on a disposable glove or finger cot (index finger for an adult; fourth finger for infants).
10. Ask the patient to bend the uppermost leg toward the waist.
11. Unwrap the suppository and apply a small amount of water-soluble lubricant to the tip of it. (If lubricant is not available, use plain water to moisten; DO NOT use Vaseline or mineral oil.) (Figure 5-19, B and C).
12. Place the tip of the suppository at the rectal entrance and ask the patient to take a deep breath and exhale through the mouth (many patients will have an involuntary rectal gripping when the suppository is pressed against the rectum). Gently insert the suppository (Figure 5-19, D) about an inch beyond the orifice past the internal sphincter.
13. Ask the patient to remain lying on the side for 15 to 20 minutes to allow melting and absorption of the medication.
14. In children, it is necessary to gently but firmly compress the buttocks and hold in place for the same time period to prevent expulsion.
15. Discard used materials and wash hands thoroughly.

Documentation

Provide the RIGHT DOCUMENTATION of medication administration and responses to drug therapy:

1. Chart the date, time, drug name, dosage, and route of administration.
2. Perform and record regular patient assessments for the evaluation of the therapeutic effectiveness (for example, when given as a laxative, chart color, amount, and consistency of stool; if given for pain relief, chart the degree and duration of pain relief; if given as an antiemetic, the degree and duration of relief of nausea and/or vomiting).
3. Chart and report any signs and symptoms of adverse drug effects.
4. Perform and validate essential patient education about the drug therapy and other essential aspects of intervention for the disease process affecting the individual.

ADMINISTRATION OF A DISPOSABLE ENEMA
OBJECTIVE

1. Cite the equipment needed and technique utilized to administer a disposable enema.

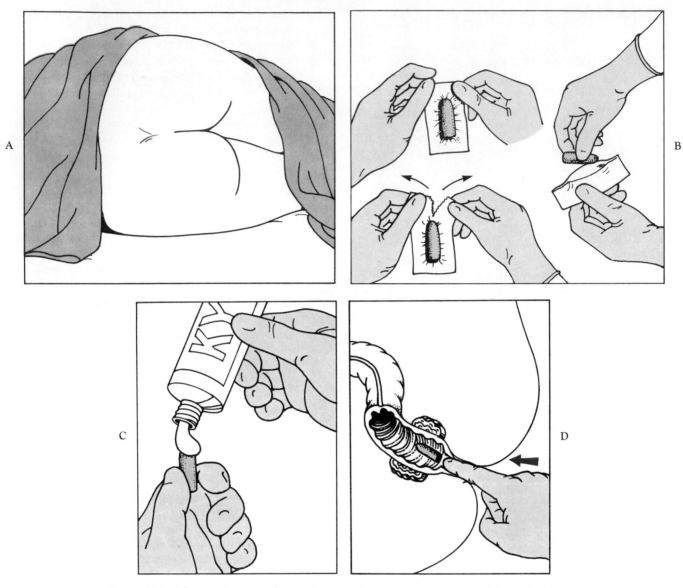

Figure 5-19 *Administering a rectal suppository.* **A,** *Position patient on side and drape.* **B,** *Unwrap suppository and remove from package.* **C,** *Apply water-soluble lubricant.* **D,** *Gently insert suppository about an inch past the internal sphincter.*

Dosage Form

A prepackaged, disposable-type enema solution of the type prescribed by the physician.

Equipment

Toilet tissue
Bedpan, if patient is not ambulatory
Water-soluble lubricant
Prescribed disposable enema kit
Gloves

Technique

1. Wash hands and assemble the necessary equipment and the prescribed rectal enema.

2. COMPARE the label on the container against the medication card or drug profile:
   RIGHT PATIENT
   RIGHT DRUG
   RIGHT ROUTE OF ADMINISTRATION
   RIGHT DOSAGE
   RIGHT TIME OF ADMINISTRATION
3. Proceed to the patient's bedside.
4. Check the patient's identification bracelet and verify against the medication card or drug profile.
5. Explain what you are going to do.
6. Check pertinent patient monitoring parameters (time of last defecation).
7. Provide for patient privacy; position patient on left side; drape to avoid unnecessary exposure (Figure 5-20, A).

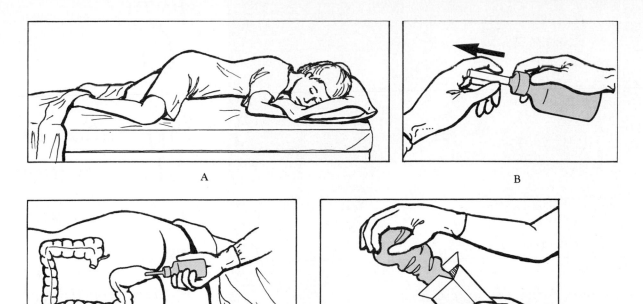

Figure 5-20 *Administering a disposable enema (Fleet enema). **A,** Place patient in a left lateral position, unless knee-chest position has been specified. **B,** Remove protective covering from rectal tube and lubricate tube. **C,** Insert lubricated rectal tube into rectum and dispense solution by compressing plastic container. **D,** Replace used container in original wrapping for disposal.*

8. Don gloves, remove protective covering from the rectal tube and lubricate (Figure 5-20, *B*).
9. Insert lubricated rectal tube into the rectum and insert solution by compressing plastic container (Figure 5-20, *C*).
10. Replace used container in its original container for disposal (Figure 5-20, *D*).
11. Encourage the patient to hold the solution for a short period of time (30 minutes) before defecating.
12. Assist the patient to a sitting position on the bedpan or to the bathroom, as orders permit.
13. Tell the patient NOT to flush the toilet until you return and can see the results of the enema. Instruct the patient regarding the location of the call light in case assistance is needed.
14. Wash hands thoroughly.

Documentation

Provide the RIGHT DOCUMENTATION of medication administration and responses to drug therapy:

1. Chart the date, time, drug name, dosage, and route of administration.
2. Perform and record regular patient assessments for the evaluation of the therapeutic effectiveness (color, amount, and consistency of stool).
3. Chart and report any signs and symptoms of adverse drug effects.
4. Perform and validate essential patient education about the drug therapy and other essential aspects of intervention for the disease process affecting the individual.

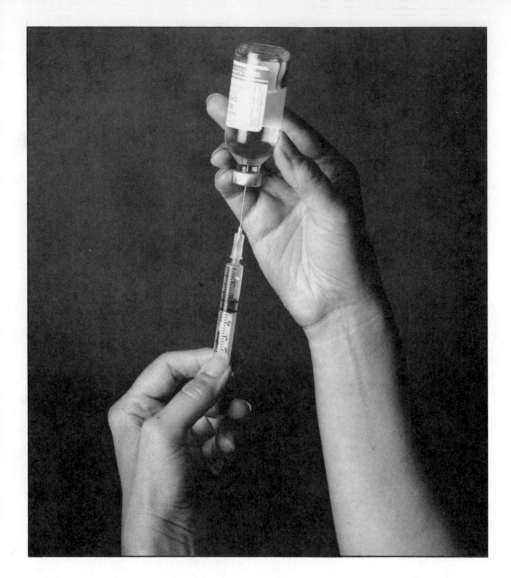

CHAPTER 6

Preparation and Administration of Medications by the Parenteral Route

CHAPTER GOALS

After completing this chapter, the student should be able to do the following:

1. Give a detailed description of the dosage forms and procedures used to prepare and administer medications via the parenteral route.

2. Accurately identify anatomic landmarks utilized in administering parenteral medications.

3. Cite the specific methods used to document medication administration and therapeutic effectiveness of drugs administered via the parenteral route.

4. Utilize the procedures and principles cited for the preparation and administration of intradermal, subcutaneous, intramuscular, and intravenous medications in the practice setting.

5. Cite the Centers for Disease Control recommendations for the prevention of HIV transmission.

The routes of drug administration may be classified into three categories: the enteral, the parenteral, and the percutaneous routes. The term *parenteral* means administration by any route other than the enteral, or gastrointestinal, tract. Technically, this definition could include topical or inhalation administration. However, as ordinarily used, *parenteral route* refers to intradermal, subcutaneous, intramuscular, or intravenous injections.

When drugs are given parenterally rather than orally, (1) the onset of drug action is generally more rapid but of shorter duration, (2) the dosage is often smaller, as drug potency tends not to be immediately altered by the stomach or liver, and (3) the cost of drug therapy is often greater. Drugs are administered by injection when it is important that all of the drug be absorbed as rapidly and completely as possible or at a steady, controlled rate, or when a patient is unable to take a medication orally because of nausea and vomiting.

Injection of drugs requires skill and special care because of the trauma at the site of needle puncture, the possibility of infection, the chance of allergic reaction, and because, once it is injected, the drug is irretrievable. Therefore, it is important that medications are prepared and administered carefully and accurately. Precautions must be taken to assure that (1) aseptic technique is used to avoid infection and (2) accurate drug dosage, proper rate of injection, and proper site of injection are used to avoid harm such as abscesses, necrosis, skin sloughing, nerve injuries, prolonged pain, or periosteitis. Thus, parenteral administration of drugs requires specialized knowledge and manual skill to ensure safety and therapeutic effectiveness.

EQUIPMENT USED IN PARENTERAL ADMINISTRATION
OBJECTIVES

1. Name the three parts of a syringe.
2. Read the calibrations of the minim and cubic centimeter or milliliter scale on different types of syringes.
3. Identify the sites where the volume of medication is read on a glass syringe and a plastic syringe.
4. Give examples of volumes of medications that can be measured in a tuberculin syringe, rather than a larger volume syringe.

5. State the advantages and disadvantages of using prefilled syringes.
6. Explain the system of measurement utilized to define the inside diameter of a syringe.
7. Identify the parts of a needle.
8. Explain how the gauge of a needle is determined.
9. Compare the usual volume of medication that can be administered at one site when giving a medication by intradermal, subcutaneous or intramuscular routes.
10. State the criteria used for the selection of the correct needle gauge and length.
11. Identify the parts of an intravenous administration set.
12. State where to find the number of drops per milliliter delivered by the drip chambers on intravenous administration sets purchased from different manufacturers.

KEY WORDS

barrel	plunger
minim scale	milliliter scale
insulin syringe	tuberculin syringe
prefilled syringes	butterfly needle
gauge	tip

Syringes

The syringe (Figure 6-1) has three parts:

—The *barrel* is the outer portion on which the calibrations for the measurement of the drug volume are located (Figure 6-2).
—The *plunger* is the inner, cylindrical portion that fits snugly into the barrel. This portion is used to draw up and eject the solution from the syringe.
—The *tip* is the portion that holds the needle. There are two types of tips, the plain tip and the LuerLok.

Syringes are made of glass or a hard plastic material. Each type has advantages and disadvantages.

Glass syringes

Advantages of the glass syringe include economy, easy-to-read calibrations, and availability in a wide range of sizes. In addition, they can be cleaned, packaged, sterilized, and reused. Disadvantages of the glass syringe are

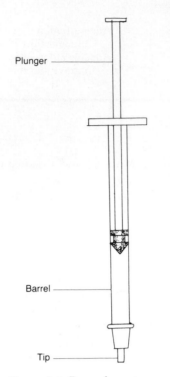

Figure 6-1 *Parts of a syringe.*

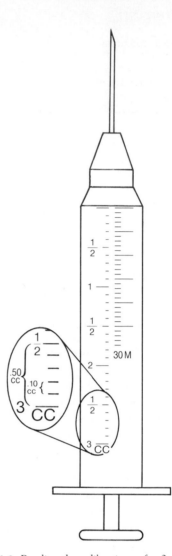

Figure 6-2 *Reading the calibrations of a 3 cc syringe.*

that it is easily breakable, time-consuming to clean and resterilize, and that the plunger may become loose with extended use, which causes medication to "creep" between the plunger and the barrel. This results in an inaccurate dose being administered to the patient.

Plastic syringes

Advantages of the plastic syringe include availability in a wide range of sizes, prepackaging with and without needles in a wide variety of gauges and needle lengths, disposability, and convenience. Disadvantages of the plastic syringe include expense, one-time use, and, in some instances, the unclear calibrations.

Syringe Calibration

The syringe is calibrated in *minims* (ɱ) and *milliliters* (ml) or *cubic centimeters* (cc) (Figure 6-2). The most commonly used syringes are 1, 3, and 5 cc syringes, but 10, 20, and 50 cc syringes are also available. (NOTE: Technically, millimeter is a measure of volume, while cubic centimeter is a three-dimensional measure of space. Even though it is technically inappropriate, many syringes are labeled in "cc" rather than "ml.")

Reading the Calibration of the Syringe

Minim scale (ɱ)

Using Figure 6-2 as a guide, note that 1 minim is indicated by *each* smaller line on the calibrated scale

marked (ɱ). Each of the longer lines on the scale equals 5 minims. Remember that 16 minims equals 1 ml or 1 cc. The use of the minim scale should be discouraged. The milliliter scale is more accurate and represents the units by which medications are routinely ordered. For volumes of 1 ml or less, use a 1 ml or "tuberculin" syringe.

Milliliter scale (ml)

Milliliters (or cubic centimeters) are read on the scale marked ml or cc (Figures 6-2 and 6-4). The shorter lines represent 0.1 cc. The longer lines on this scale each represent 0.5 cc (1 ml = 1 cc).

Insulin syringe

The insulin syringe has a scale specifically calibrated for the measurement of insulin. The most commonly used size is U-100, because insulin is now manufactured in this concentration.

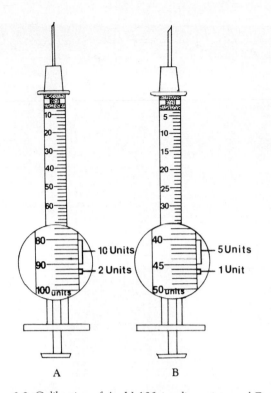

Figure 6-3 *Calibration of* **A,** *U-100 insulin syringe and* **B,** *low-dose insulin syringe.*

The U-100 syringe (Figure 6-3, A) holds 100 units of insulin per cc. On the scale, the shorter lines represent 2 units measured, while the longer lines measure 10 units of insulin. Low-dose insulin syringes (Figure 6-3, B) may be used for patients receiving 50 units or less of U-100 insulin. The shorter lines on the scale of the low-dose insulin syringe measure 1 unit, while the longer lines each represent 5 units.

Tuberculin syringe

The tuberculin syringe or "1 ml" syringe (Figure 6-4) was originally designed to administer tuberculin. Today it is used to measure small volumes of medication accurately. The volume should be measured on the cubic centimeter scale to achieve the greatest degree of accuracy. The syringe holds a total of 1 cc or 16 minims. On the minim scale, the longer lines represent 1 minim, while the shorter lines measure 0.5 ($^5/_{10}$ or $^1/_2$) minim; however, the use of the minim scale should be discouraged. On the cubic centimeter scale, each of the longest lines represents 0.1 ($^1/_{10}$) cc, the intermediate lines equal 0.05 ($^5/_{100}$) cc, and the shortest lines are 0.01 ($^1/_{100}$) cc.

The volumes within glass syringes are read at the point where the plunger is directly parallel with the calibration on the syringe (Figure 6-5). Volumes within disposable plastic syringes are read at the point where the rubber flange of the syringe plunger is parallel to the calibration scale of the barrel (Figure 6-6). Also

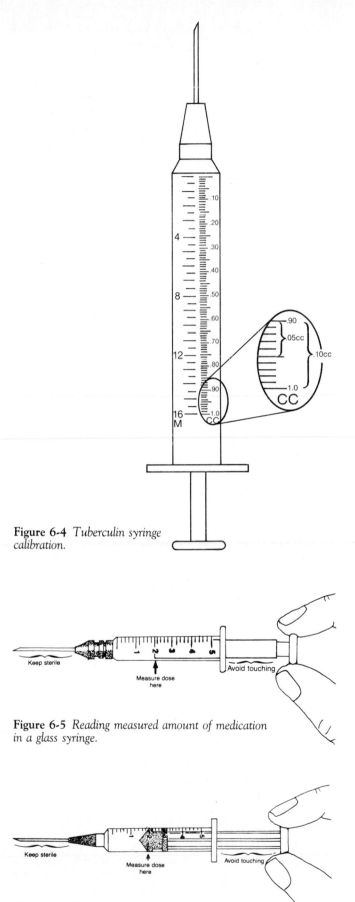

Figure 6-4 *Tuberculin syringe calibration.*

Figure 6-5 *Reading measured amount of medication in a glass syringe.*

Figure 6-6 *Reading measured amount of medication in a plastic syringe.*

note the area of the needle to keep sterile and the area on the syringe plunger to avoid touching.

Prefilled Syringes

Several manufacturers supply a premeasured amount of medication in a disposable cartridge-needle unit. These units are called by brand names such as Tubex and Carpuject. The cartridge contains the amount of drug for one standard dose of medication. The drug name, concentration, and volume are clearly printed on the cartridge. Certain brands of prefilled cartridges require a holder that corresponds to the type of cartridge being used (Figure 6-7, A,B, and C). Advantages of the prefilled syringe include the time saved in preparation of a standard amount of medication for one injection and the diminished chance of contamination between patient and hospital personnel, as the cartridge is in a sealed unit, which is used once and discarded. Disadvantages include additional expense, the need for different holders for different cartridges, and the limitation of the volume of a second medication that may be added to the cartridge.

Many hospital pharmacies "prefill" syringes for specific doses of medication for specific patients. The syringe is labeled with the drug name, dose, patient's name, room number, and date of preparation and expiration.

The Needle

Parts of the needle

The needle parts (Figure 6-8) are the hub, shaft, and beveled tip. The angle of the bevel can vary; the longer the bevel, the easier the needle penetration.

Needle gauge

The needle gauge is the diameter of the hole through the needle. The larger the number (which indicates the gauge), the smaller the hole. The gauge number is marked on the hub of the needle as well as on the outside of the disposable package. The proper needle gauge is usually selected based upon the viscosity (thickness) of the solution to be injected. A thicker solution requires a larger diameter; thus, a smaller gauge number is chosen (Figure 6-9). There are finer needles (for example, 28 and 29 gauge) for specialty use.

Needles for intravenous administration

All needles, if long enough, may be used to administer medications or fluids intravenously, but special equipment has been designed for this purpose.

The *butterfly*, *scalp*, and *wing-tipped* needles (Figure 6-10) are short, sharp-tipped needles designed to mini-

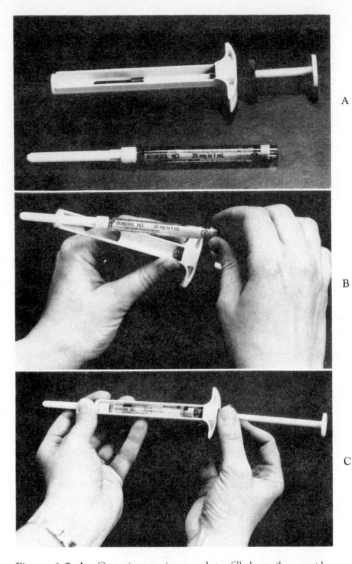

A

B

C

Figure 6-7 A, *Carpuject syringe and prefilled sterile cartridge with needle.* **B,** *Assembling the Carpuject.* **C,** *Cartridge slides into syringe barrel, turns, and locks at needle end. Plunger then screws into cartridge end.* (From Potter PA, Perry AG. Basic nursing: theory and practice, ed 2, 1991, St Louis, Mosby–Year Book.)

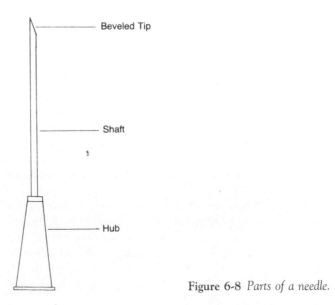

— Beveled Tip

— Shaft

— Hub

Figure 6-8 *Parts of a needle.*

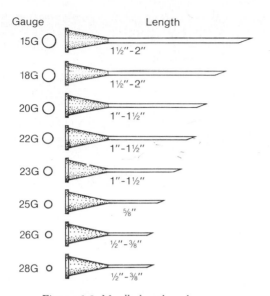

Gauge | Length

15G — 1½"–2"
18G — 1½"–2"
20G — 1"–1½"
22G — 1"–1½"
23G — 1"–1½"
25G — ⅝"
26G — ½"–⅜"
28G — ½"–⅜"

Figure 6-9 *Needle length and gauge.*

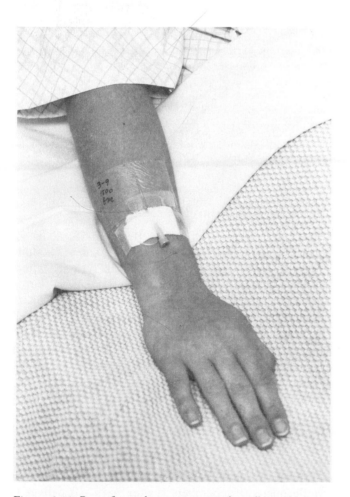

Figure 6-10 *Butterfly, scalp, or wing-tipped needle in place as a heparin lock. The tape should be labeled: Date, time, and initials of person inserting the heparin lock. Some practice settings also require the date and time the lock is to be changed on the label.*

mize tissue injury during insertion. The "winged" area can be pinched together to form a handle while the needle is being inserted, then laid flat against the skin to form a base for anchoring with tape. These needles come in gauges 17 to 27. A short plastic tubing with a plastic adapter at the end is attached to the needle. Butterfly needles are commonly used for venipuncture in infants and as "heparin locks" to allow patient mobility.

Plastic needles or *over-the-catheter* needles (Figure 6-11, A) are actually stainless steel needles coated with a teflonlike plastic. After penetrating the vein, the metal needle is removed, leaving the plastic catheter in place. This unit is used when intravenous therapy is expected to continue for several days or more. The rationale for use of the plastic catheter is that it does not have a sharp tip that may cause venous irritation and extravasation.

Intracatheters (Figure 6-11, B) use a large-bore needle for venipuncture. Then a 4- to 6-inch sterile, smaller-gauge plastic catheter is advanced through the needle into the vein. The needle is withdrawn and the skin forms a seal around the plastic catheter. The intravenous administration set is attached directly to the plastic catheter. This type of catheter is often used for hyperalimentation solutions and for IVs that will be running for a week or more.

Selection of the Syringe and Needle

The size of the syringe used is determined by the volume of medication to be administered, the degree of accuracy needed in measurement of the dose, and the type of medication to be administered.

Needle selection should be based upon the correct gauge for the viscosity of the solution, and the correct needle length for delivery of the medication to the correct site (subcutaneous, intramuscular, or intravenous). Table 6-1 may be used as a guideline to select the proper volume of syringe and length and gauge of needle for adult patients.

In small children and older infants, the usual maximum volume for intramuscular injection at one site is 1 ml. In small infants the muscle mass may only be able to tolerate 0.5 (⁵⁄₁₀ or ½) ml. For older children, the amount should be individualized; generally, the larger the muscle mass, the greater the similarity to the adult volume for one injection site. Pediatric intramuscular injections routinely use a 25 to 27 gauge needle 1 to 1½ inches long, depending on assessment of the depth of the muscle mass in the child. There are also 30 gauge, ½ inch needles available for pediatric use.

Clinical example: selection of needle length

Assess the depth of the patient's tissue for administration (muscle tissue for intramuscular administration,

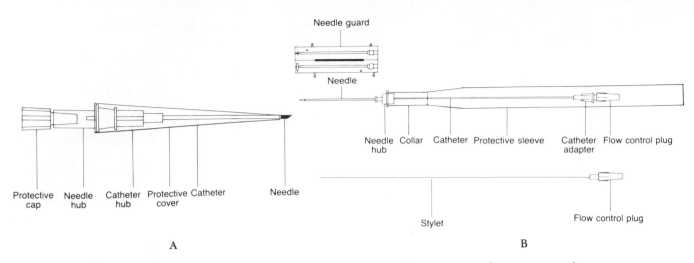

A

B

Figure 6-11 A, *Over-the-needle catheter. This unit is used when intravenous therapy is expected to continue several days.* **B,** *Intracatheters use a large-bore needle for venipuncture, then a 4- to 6-inch sterile, small-gauge plastic catheter is advanced through the needle into the vein. The needle is withdrawn and the skin forms a seal around the plastic catheter.*

Table 6-1 *Selection of Syringe and Needles*

ROUTE	VOLUME	GAUGE	LENGTH
Intradermal	0.01-0.1 ml	26-29 g	⅜-½ inch
Subcutaneous	0.5-2 ml	25-27 g	Individualize based on depth of appropriate tissue at site of injection†
Intramuscular	0.5-2 ml*	20-22 g	
Intravenous	1-2000 ml	20-22 g (solutions)	½-1¼ inch (butterfly)
		15-19 g (blood)	½-2 inch (regular needles)

*Divided doses are generally recommended for volumes that exceed 2-3 ml, particularly for medications that are irritating to the tissues.
†When judging the needle length, allow an extra ¼ -½-inch length to remain above the skin surface when the injection is administered. In the rare event of a needle breaking, this allows a length of needle to protrude above the skin to grasp for removal.

subcutaneous tissue for subcutaneous injection) and then choose a needle length to correspond with the findings.

> EXAMPLE: Compare the muscle depth of a 250-lb obese, sedentary female to the muscle depth of a 105-lb debilitated adult patient. The obese individual may require a 3- to 5-inch needle, the frail person a 1 to 1½ inch needle. A child may need a 1-inch needle (Figure 6-12).

Packaging of Syringes and Needles

Always inspect and verify the sterility of the syringe and needle to be used to prepare and administer a parenteral medication. Check cloth wrappers for holes, signs of moisture penetrating the wrapper, and the date of expiration. With prepackaged disposable items, check for continuity of the wrapper, loose lids or needle guards, and for any penetration of the paper or plastic container by the needle.

Intravenous administration sets

Intravenous administration sets (Figure 6-13, A, B, and C) are available with a variety of attachments (volume and size of drip chamber, "piggyback" portals, filters, drug administration chamber, clamps or rollers), but all sets have an insertion spike, a drip chamber, plastic tubing with a control clamp, a rubber injection portal, a needle adapter, and a protective cap over the needle adapter. The type of system used by a particular hospital is usually determined by the manufacturer of the physiologic solutions used by the institution. Each manufacturer makes adaptations to fit a specific type of glass or plastic large-volume solution container. A crucial point to remember about administration sets is that the drops delivered by drip chambers vary from different manufacturers. Macrodrip chambers (Figure 6-13, A and C) provide 10, 13, 15, or 20 drops per milliliter, while microdrip chambers (Figure 6-13, B) deliver 60 drops per milliliter of solution. It is essential to read the label of the box before opening it. The nurse must

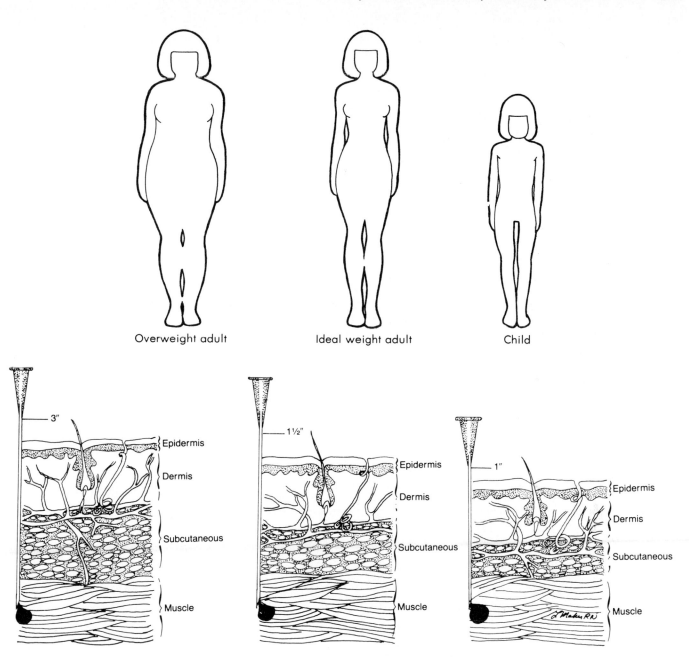

Overweight adult   Ideal weight adult   Child

Figure 6-12 *Clinical example: selection of needle length for intramuscular administration.*

know the number of drops per milliliter to calculate the flow rate for the intravenous solution.

PARENTERAL DOSAGE FORMS
OBJECTIVES

1. Differentiate among ampules, vials, and Mix-O-Vials.
2. Describe the different types of large-volume solution containers available.

KEY WORDS

ampules	vials
Mix-O-Vials	tandem setup
piggyback	IV rider
heparin lock	

All parenteral drug dosage forms are packaged so that the drug is sterile and ready for reconstitution (if needed) and administration.

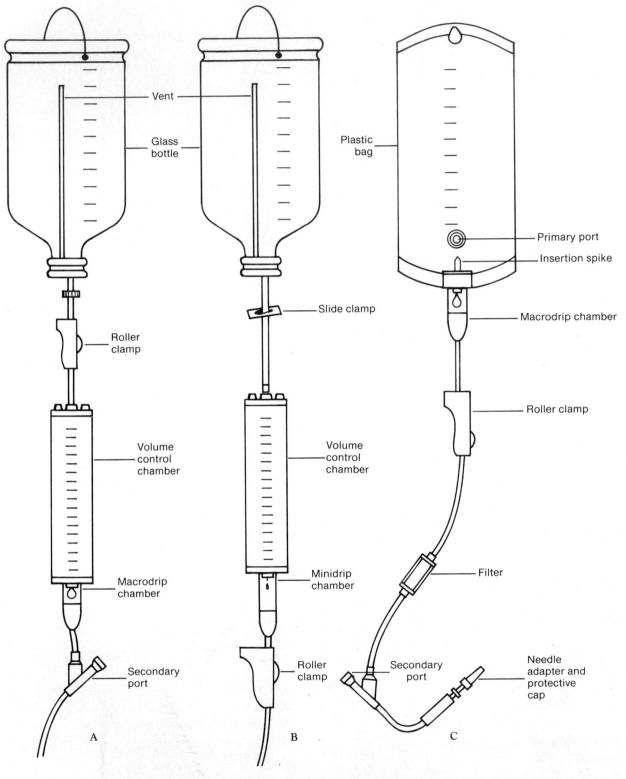

Figure 6-13 A-C, *Intravenous administration sets.*

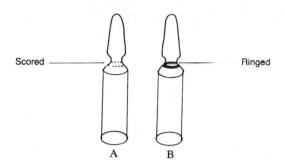

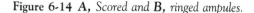

Figure 6-14 **A,** *Scored and* **B,** *ringed ampules.*

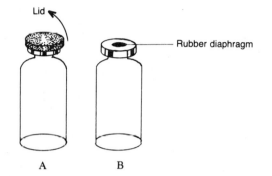

Figure 6-15 **A,** *Metal lid and* **B,** *rubber diaphragm vials.*

Ampules

Ampules are glass containers that usually contain a single dose of a medication. The container may be scored (Figure 6-14, A) or have a darkened ring around the neck (Figure 6-14, B). This marking is the location at which the ampule is broken open for withdrawing the medication.

Vials

Vials are glass containers that contain one or more doses of a sterile medication. The mouth of the vial is covered with a thick rubber diaphragm (Figure 6-15, B) through which a needle must be passed to remove the medication. Before use, the rubber diaphragm is sealed by a metal lid (Figure 6-15, A) to insure sterility. The medication in the vial may be in solution, or it may be a sterile powder to be reconstituted just prior to the time of administration.

Mix-O-Vials

Mix-O-Vials are glass containers with two compartments (Figure 6-16). The lower chamber contains the drug (solute) and the upper chamber contains a sterile diluent (solvent). Between the two areas is a rubber stopper. A single dose of medication is normally contained in the Mix-O-Vial. At the time of use, pressure

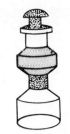

Figure 6-16 *Mix-O-Vial.*

Table 6-2 *Types of Intravenous Solutions**

SOLUTION	INGREDIENTS	ABBREVIATION
Electrolyte solutions	5% Dextrose in water	D5W
	10% Dextrose in water	D10W
	0.9% Sodium chloride (normal saline)	N.S.
	Ringer's lactate	R.L.
	5% Dextrose in 0.2% sodium chloride	D5/.2
	5% Dextrose in 0.45% sodium chloride	D5/.45
	5% Dextrose in Ringer's lactate	D5/LR
Nutrient solutions:		
Carbohydrate	Dextrose 5-25%	D5-25
Amino acids	Novamine	
	Travasol	
	Nephramine	
	Trophamine	
Lipids	Intralipid	
	Liposyn	
Blood volume expanders	Hetastarch	
	Dextran	
	Albumin	
	Plasma	
Alkalinizing solutions	Sodium bicarbonate	
	Tromethamine (THAM)	
	Lactate solutions	
Acidifying solutions	Ammonium chloride	

*A representative listing, not intended to be inclusive.

is applied on the top rubber diaphragm plunger. This forces the solvent and the rubber stopper to fall into the bottom chamber, dissolving the drug. A needle is then placed through the top plunger-diaphragm to withdraw the solution. (Change the needle after drug withdrawal, as puncturing the plunger-diaphragm may dull the needle bevel.)

Large-Volume Solution Containers

Intravenous solutions are available in both glass and plastic containers in a variety of types and concentrations (Table 6-2) and volumes ranging from 100 to 2,000 ml. Both the glass and plastic containers are vac-

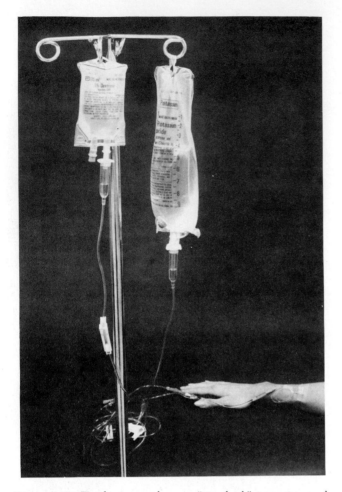

Figure 6-17 *Tandem, secondary, or "piggyback" intermittent administration setup. This illustrates a "piggyback" setup. Note that the smaller bottle is hung higher than the primary bottle.*

uum sealed. The glass bottles are sealed with a hard rubber stopper, then a metal disk, followed by a metal cap. Just before use, the metal cap and disk are removed, exposing the hard rubber stopper. The insertion spike of the IV administration set is pushed into a specifically marked area on the rubber stopper. Some brands also have another opening in the rubber stopper that serves as an air vent (Figure 6-13, A and B). As the solution runs out of the container, it is replaced with air. Other brands use a flexible plastic container (Figure 6-13, C). As the solution runs out of the bag, the flexible container collapses.

Plastic bags are somewhat different in that the entire bag and solution is sealed inside another plastic bag for removal just before administration. When the insertion spike is forced into the specifically marked portal, an internal seal is broken, allowing the solution to flow into the tubing.

Some drugs, such as antibiotics, are administered by intermittent infusion through an apparatus known as a *tandem setup, piggyback* (IVPB), or *IV rider* (Figure 6-17). They are given by a setup that is secondary to the primary IV infusion and that is hung in tandem and

connected to the primary setup. The secondary setup may consist of a drug infusion from a small volume of fluid in either a small bag or bottle (up to 250 ml) (Figure 6-17) or from a volume-control set (also known as a Volutrol, Pediatrol, or Buretrol) (see Figure 6-13, A and B). A volume-control set is made up of a calibrated chamber hung under the primary IV solution container that can provide the necessary 50 to 250 ml of diluent per dose of drug. Most intermittent diluted drug infusions are infused over 20 to 60 minutes.

PREPARATION OF PARENTERAL MEDICATION

OBJECTIVES

1. List the equipment needed for the preparation of parenteral medication.
2. Describe, practice, and perfect the preparation of medications using the various dosage forms for parenteral administration.
3. Describe, practice and perfect the technique of preparing two different drugs in one syringe, such as insulin or a preoperative medication.

Equipment

Drug in sterile, sealed container
Syringe of the correct volume
Needles of the correct gauge and length
Antiseptic swab
Special equipment based on the route of administration (such as heparin lock for insertion, IV administration set for starting intravenous infusion)

Technique

These are standard procedures for preparing all parenteral medications:

1. Wash hands *before* proceeding to prepare any medication or handling of sterile supplies. During the actual preparation of a parenteral medication, the primary rule is "sterile-to-sterile and unsterile-to-unsterile" when handling the syringe and needle.
2. Use the 5 RIGHTS of medication preparation and administration throughout the procedure:
   RIGHT PATIENT
   RIGHT DRUG
   RIGHT ROUTE OF ADMINISTRATION
   RIGHT DOSAGE (AMOUNT AND CONCENTRATION)
   RIGHT TIME OF ADMINISTRATION
3. Check the drug dosage form ordered against the source you are holding to prepare.
4. Check compatibility charts or contact the pharmacist before mixing two medications or adding medication to an intravenous solution.

5. Check medication calculations. When in doubt about a dose, check it with another qualified nurse. (Most hospital policies require that fractional doses of medications and doses of heparin and insulin be checked by two qualified personnel prior to administration.)
6. Be knowledgeable of the hospital policy regarding limitations on the types of medications to be administered by nursing personnel.
7. Prepare the drug in a clean, well-lighted area, using aseptic technique throughout the entire procedure.
8. Concentrate on this procedure; assure accuracy in preparation.

Guidelines for Preparing Medications

To prepare a medication from an ampule

1. Move all of the solution to the bottom of the ampule, flicking the side of the glass container with the fingers to displace the medication from the top portion of the ampule (Figure 6-18, A).
2. Cover the ampule neck area with a sterile gauze pledget or antiseptic swab while breaking the top off (Figure 6-18, B). Discard the swab and top.
3. Using an aspiration (filter) needle (Figure 6-18, C), withdraw the medication from the ampule (Figure 6-18, D and E).
4. Remove the aspiration needle from the ampule and point the needle vertically (Figure 6-18, F). Pull back on the plunger (this allows air to enter the syringe) (Figure 6-18, G) and replace the filter needle with a new sterile needle (Figure 6-18, H and I) of the appropriate gauge and length for administration.
5. Push the plunger slowly until the medication appears at the tip of the needle (Figure 6-18, J); or measure the amount of air to be included to allow total clearance of the medication from the needle when injected. (Never add air to a syringe that is to be used to administer an intravenous medication.)

Drugs in a *vial* may be in solution ready for administration (Figure 6-19) or may be in a powdered form for reconstitution prior to administration. To prepare medication from a vial:

Reconstitution of a sterile powder

1. Read the accompanying literature from the manufacturer and follow specific instructions for reconstituting the drug ordered. Add only the diluent specified by the manufacturer.
2. Cleanse the rubber diaphragm of the vial of diluent with an antiseptic swab (Figure 6-19, A).
3. Pull back on the plunger of the syringe to fill with an amount of air equal to the volume of solution to be withdrawn (Figure 6-19, B).
4. Insert the needle through the rubber diaphragm; inject air (Figure 6-19, C).

5. Withdraw the measured volume of diluent required to reconstitute the powdered drug (Figure 6-19, D and E). Remove the needle from the diaphragm of the diluent container.
6. Recheck the type and volume of diluent to be injected against the type and amount required.
7. Remove the needle and replace with a new, sterile needle (use principles illustrated in Figure 6-18, H, I, and J). Tap the vial containing the powdered drug to break up the caked powder (Figure 6-19, F). Wipe the rubber diaphragm of the vial of powdered drug with a new antiseptic swab (Figure 6-19, G).
8. Insert the needle in the diaphragm and inject the diluent into the powder (Figure 6-19, H).
9. Remove the syringe and needle from the rubber diaphragm.
10. MIX THOROUGHLY to ensure that the powder is entirely dissolved BEFORE withdrawing the dose (Figure 6-19, I).
11. Label the reconstituted medication:
    • Date, time of reconstitution
    • Volume and type of diluent added
    • Name of reconstituted drug
    • Concentration of reconstituted drug
    • Expiration date and time
    • Name of person reconstituting drug
    Store according to manufacturer's instructions.
12. Change the needle as described before. Attach a needle of the correct gauge and length to administer the medication to the patient.

Removal of a volume of liquid from a vial (Figure 6-19, A-E)

1. Calculate the volume of medication required for the prescribed dose of medication to be administered.
2. Cleanse the rubber diaphragm of the vial of diluent with an antiseptic pledget.
3. Pull back on the plunger of the syringe to fill with an amount of air equal to the volume of solution to be withdrawn.
4. Insert the needle through the rubber diaphragm; inject air.
5. Withdraw the volume of drug required to administer the prescribed dosage.
6. Recheck all aspects of the drug order.
7. Change the needle as described before. Attach a needle of the correct gauge and length to administer the medication to the patient.

Preparing a drug from a Mix-O-Vial

1. Check the drug order against the medication you have for administration.
2. To mix:
    —Tap the container in the hand a few times to break up the caked powder.

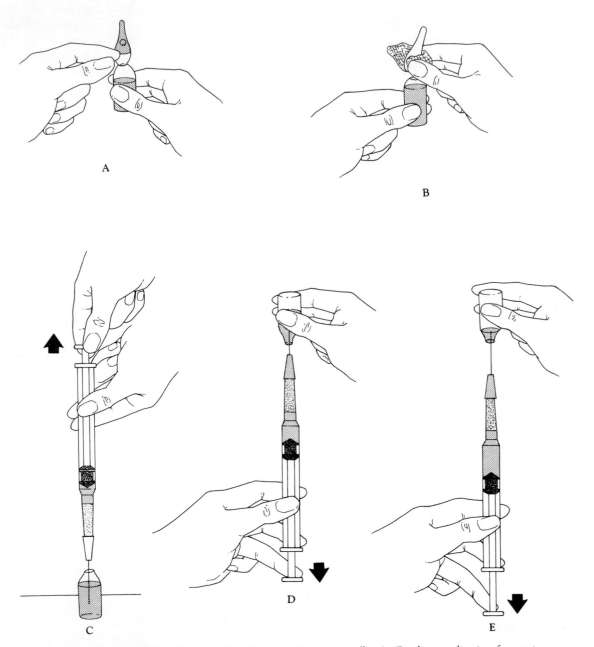

Figure 6-18 *Withdrawing from an ampule and changing needle.* **A,** *Displace medication from top portion of ampule.* **B,** *Cover ampule neck area with gauze sponge while breaking top off.* **C,** *Filter needle.* **D,** *Withdraw medication from ampule.* **E,** *Note that needle must be lowered to withdraw all solution from ampule.*

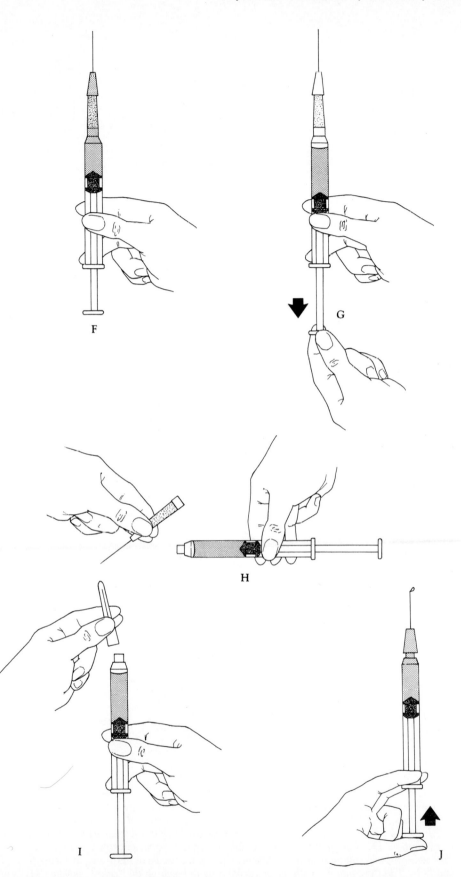

Figure 6-18, cont'd F, *Remove the filter needle from ampule and point needle vertically.* **G,** *Pull plunger downward to remove drug from needle.* **H,** *Remove filter needle.* **I,** *Replace filter needle with correct size needle for administering medication.* **J,** *Slowly push plunger until a drop of medication appears at needle tip. Recheck medication prepared against drug order.*

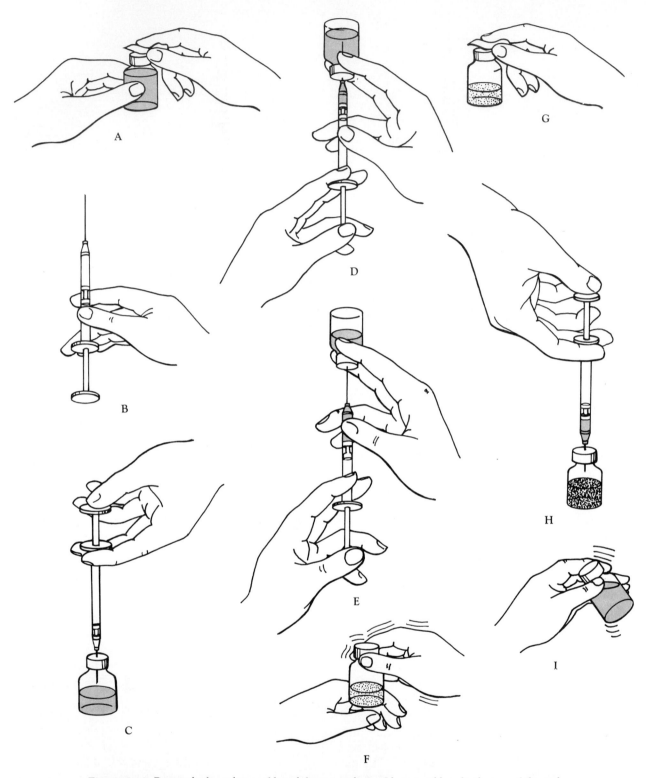

Figure 6-19 *Removal of a volume of liquid from a vial.* **A,** *Cleanse rubber diaphragm of the vial.* **B,** *Pull back on plunger of syringe to fill with an amount of air equal to the volume of solution to be withdrawn.* **C,** *Insert the needle through the rubber diaphragm; inject air with vial sitting in downward position.* **D,** *Withdraw the volume of diluent required to reconstitute the drug.* **E,** *Move needle downward to facilitate removal of diluent. Change the needle as illustrated in Figure 6-18, H, I, and J.* **F,** *Tap the container with the powdered drug to break up the "caked" powder.* **G,** *Wipe the rubber diaphragm of the vial of powdered drug with a new antiseptic swab.* **H,** *Insert the needle in the rubber diaphragm and inject the diluent into the powdered drug.* **I,** *Mix thoroughly to ensure the powdered drug is dissolved prior to withdrawing the prescribed dose.*

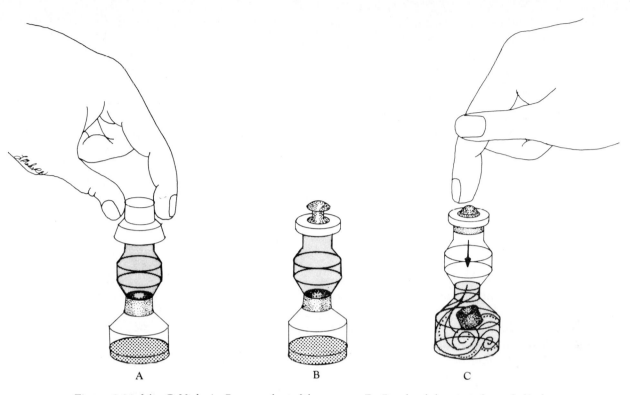

Figure 6-20 *Mix-O-Vial.* **A,** *Remove plastic lid protector.* **B,** *Powdered drug is in lower half; diluent is in upper half.* **C,** *Push firmly on the diaphragm-plunger. Downward pressure dislodges the divider between the two chambers.*

—Remove the plastic lid protector (Figure 6-20, A).

—Push firmly on the diaphragm-plunger. The downward pressure dislodges the divider between the two chambers (Figure 6-20, B and C).

—Mix thoroughly to ensure that the powder is COMPLETELY DISSOLVED before drawing up the medication for administration.

—Cleanse the rubber diaphragm and remove the drug in the same manner as described for removal of a volume of liquid from a vial (see Figure 6-19, A-E).

Preparing two medications in one syringe

Occasionally two medications may be drawn into the same syringe for a single injection. This is most commonly done when preparing a preoperative medication or when two types of insulin are ordered to be administered at the same time. Since mixing insulins is a routine procedure, it will be used to illustrate the technique (Figure 6-21).

1. Check the compatibility of the two drugs to be mixed before starting to prepare the medications.
2. Check the labels of the medications against the medication order.
3. Check
   Type: NPH, Regular, Lente, other
   Concentration: U-100 (U-100 = 100 units/ml)

Expiration Date: DO NOT use if outdated
Appearance: Clear, cloudy, precipitate present?
Temperature: Should be at room temperature

4. Philosophies: There are two philosophies concerning how insulins should be mixed. In one procedure, the volume of the shorter-acting insulin is drawn into the syringe first, followed by the longer-acting insulin. The rationale for this approach is that if a small amount of short-acting insulin is accidently displaced into the second (longer-acting insulin) bottle, the onset, peak, and duration of the longer-acting insulin will not be appreciably affected. If done in reverse order, the shorter-acting insulin would have its onset, peak, and duration affected due to the contamination by the longer-acting preparation.

   In the second procedure, the opposite is advocated. The rationale for this approach is that since the longer-acting insulin is cloudy, a change in clarity would be immediately visible if the longer-acting insulin contaminated the normally clear second (shorter-acting) insulin during preparation.

   We strongly recommend the use of the first procedure, but encourage you to check your institution's procedure manual for details.

5. Procedure:
   • Roll the bottle between the palms of the hands to thoroughly mix the contents. DO NOT SHAKE.
   • Check the insulin order and calculations of the

preparation with another qualified nurse, in accordance with hospital policy.
- Cleanse the top of BOTH vials with separate antiseptic swabs (Figure 6-21, A).
- Pull back the plunger on the syringe to an amount equal to the volume of the longer-acting insulin ordered (Figure 6-21, B).
- Insert the needle through the rubber seal of the longer-acting insulin bottle; inject air (Figure 6-21, C). (Do not inject air into the insulin solution because it may break up insulin particles.)
- Remove the needle and syringe. (Do not withdraw insulin at this time.)
- Pull back the plunger on the syringe to an amount equal to the volume of the shorter-acting insulin ordered (Figure 6-21, D).
- Insert the needle through the rubber seal of the second bottle; inject air (Figure 6-21, E). Invert the bottle and withdraw the volume of shorter-acting insulin ordered (Figure 6-21, F). NOTE: Check for bubbles in the insulin, flick the side of the syringe with the fingers to displace the bubbles, then recheck the amount in the syringe.
- Check the medication order against the label of the container and the amount in the syringe.
- Rewipe the lid of the longer-acting insulin container (Figure 6-21, G); recheck the drug order against this container; insert the needle of the syringe containing the shorter-acting insulin and withdraw the specified amount of longer-acting insulin (Figure 6-21, H). Be careful NOT to inject any of the first type of insulin already in the syringe into the vial.
- Remove the needle and syringe; recheck the drug order against the label on the insulin container and the amount in the syringe (Figure 6-21, I).
- Withdraw a small amount of air into the syringe and mix the two medications. Remove air carefully so that part of the medication is not displaced.
- Change needles and proceed to administer subcutaneously.

Preparing medications for use in the sterile field during an operative procedure

The following principles apply to the operating room:

1. All medications used during an operative procedure must remain sterile.
2. All medication containers (ampules, vials, "piggyback," and blood bags) used during the operative procedure should remain in the operating room until the entire procedure is completed. (In case a question arises, the container is available.)
3. Do not save an unused portion of medication for use in another operative procedure. Discard at the end of the operative procedure or send the patient's medication to the patient care unit with the patient, if appropriate (for example, antibiotic ointment for a patient having ophthalmic surgery).
4. Adhere to hospital policies concerning handling and storage of medications in the operating room.
5. ALWAYS tell the surgeon the name and dosage or concentration of the medication or solution being handed to him or her.
6. ALWAYS repeat the entire medication order back to the surgeon at the time the request is made to verify all aspects of the order. If in doubt, repeat again until accuracy is certain.

The following technique is used to prepare medications for use in the sterile operative field:

1. Prepare the drug prescribed according to the directions.
2. Always check the accuracy of the drug order against the medication being prepared at least three times during the preparation phase: (1) when first removed from the drug storage area; (2) immediately before removing the solution for use on the sterile field; (3) immediately after completing the transfer of the medication/solution to the sterile field. ALWAYS tell the surgeon the name and dose or concentration of the medication/solution when passing it to him or her for use.
3. The circulating (nonsterile) nurse retrieves the medication from storage, reconstitutes as needed, and turns the medication container so the scrubbed (sterile) nurse can read the label. It is best to read the label aloud to assure that both individuals are verifying the contents against the verbal order from the surgeon.

The following two methods may be used:
Method 1:

1. The circulating (nonsterile) nurse cleanses the top of the vial or breaks off the top of the ampule, as described above.
2. The scrubbed (sterile) person chooses a syringe of the correct volume for the medication to be withdrawn and attaches a large-bore needle to facilitate removal of the solution from the container.
3. The circulating (nonsterile) nurse holds the ampule or vial in such a way that the scrubbed (sterile) person can easily insert the sterile needle tip into the medication container (Figure 6-22, A).
4. The scrubbed person pulls back the plunger on the syringe until all the medication prescribed has been withdrawn from the container and from the needle used to withdraw the medication.
5. The needle is disconnected from the syringe and left in the vial or ampule (Figure 6-22, B).

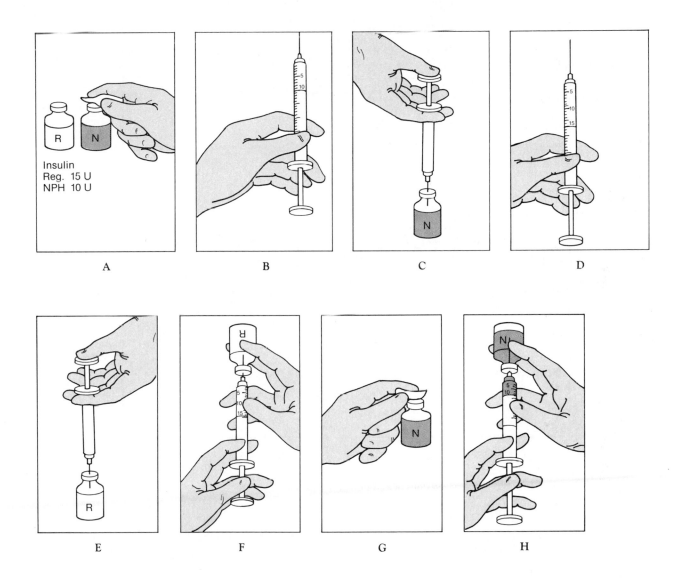

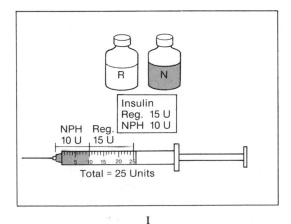

Figure 6-21 *Preparing two drugs in one syringe.* **A,** *Check insulin order; cleanse top of both vials with an antiseptic swab.* **B,** *Pull back on plunger to an amount equal to the volume of longer-acting insulin.* **C,** *Insert needle through the rubber diaphragm of the longer-acting insulin; inject air. Remove needle and syringe; do not remove insulin.* **D,** *Pull back the plunger on the syringe to a point equal to the volume of the shorter-acting insulin ordered.* **E,** *Insert needle through the rubber diaphragm; inject air.* **F,** *Invert the bottle and withdraw the volume of shorter-acting insulin ordered. Check amount withdrawn against amount ordered.* **G,** *Rewipe the lid of the longer-acting insulin.* **H,** *Insert needle; withdraw the specified amount of longer-acting insulin.* **I,** *Remove the needle and syringe; recheck the drug order against the labels on the insulin containers and the amount in the syringe. Pull plunger back slightly and proceed to mix two insulins (tilt syringe back and forth gently); change needle.*

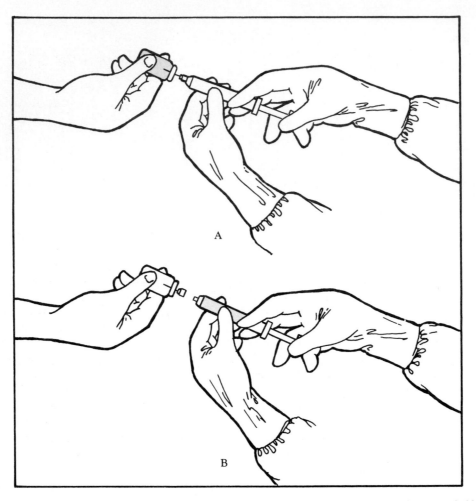

Figure 6-22 *Preparing a medication in the operating room.* **A,** *Circulating (unsterile) nurse holds vial to facilitate the "scrubbed" (sterile) person to insert the sterile needle tip into the medication container.* **B,** *The needle is disconnected from the syringe and left in the vial.*

6. The medication container is again shown to the scrubbed person and read aloud to verify all components of the drug prepared against the medication/solution requested.

Method 2:

1. The circulating (nonsterile) nurse removes the entire lid of the vial with a bottle opener, cleanses the rim of the vial, and pours the medication directly into a sterile medicine cup held by the scrubbed nurse.
2. The scrubbed person continues drug preparation on the sterile field in accordance with the intended use (such as irrigation or injection).

Regardless of the method used to transfer the medication to the sterile field, both the sterile scrubbed person and the nonsterile circulating nurse should know the location and exact disposition of each medication on the sterile field.

ADMINISTRATION OF MEDICATION BY THE INTRADERMAL ROUTE
OBJECTIVE

1. Identify the equipment needed and describe the technique used to administer a medication via the intradermal route.

KEY WORDS

wheal	erythema
papules	vesicles
intradermal	

Intradermal injections are made into the dermal layer of skin just below the epidermis (Figure 6-23). Small volumes, usually 0.1 ml, are injected to produce a wheal. The absorption from intradermal sites is slow, making it the route of choice for allergy sensitivity tests, desensitization injections, local anesthetics, and vaccinations.

Equipment

Medication to be injected

Tuberculin syringe with 26 gauge, ¼, ⅜, or ½ inch needle, OR a special needle and syringe for allergens

Metric ruler, if skin-testing procedure

Gloves

Antiseptic pledget

Sites

Intradermal injections may be made on any skin surface, but the site should be hairless and receive little friction from clothing. The upper chest, scapular areas of the back, and the inner aspect of the forearms are most commonly used (Figure 6-24, A and B).

Technique

The example of technique uses allergy sensitivity testing. CAUTION: Do not start any type of allergy testing unless emergency equipment is available in the immediate area in case of an anaphylactic response. Personnel should be familiar with the procedure to follow if an emergency does arise.

1. Check with the patient before starting the testing to be sure that he or she has not taken any antihistamines or anti-inflammatory agents (such as aspirin, ibuprofen, corticosteroids) for 24 to 48 hours preceding the tests. If the patient has taken antihistamines or anti-inflammatory agents, check with the physician before proceeding with the testing.
2. Cleanse the selected area thoroughly with an antiseptic pledget. Use circular motions starting at the planned site of injection, continuing outward in everwidening circular motions to the periphery. Allow the area to air-dry.
3. Prepare the designated solutions for injection using aseptic technique. Usual volumes to be injected range between 0.01 and 0.05 ml. A control injection of normal saline or diluent is also administered. Don gloves.
4. Insert the needle at a 15° angle with the needle bevel upward. The solution being injected is deposited in the space immediately below the skin; remove the needle quickly. A small *bleb* will appear on the surface of the skin as the solution enters the intradermal area (Figure 6-23). Be careful not to inject into the subcutaneous space and do not wipe the site with alcohol after injection.
5. Do NOT re-cap any needles that have been used. Dispose of used needles and syringes into a puncture-resistant container according to the policy of the employing institution.
6. Remove glove(s) and dispose of them according to agency policy. Thoroughly wash hands.

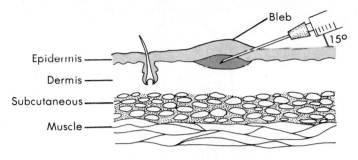

Figure 6-23 *Intradermal injection technique.*

7. Chart the times, agents, concentrations, and amounts injected (Figure 6-24, C). Make a diagram in the patient's chart numbering each location. Record what agent and concentration was injected at each site. (Subsequent "readings" of each area are then performed and charted on this record.)
8. Follow directions for the time of the "reading" of the skin testing being performed. Inspection of the injection sites should be performed in good light. Generally, a positive reaction (development of a wheal) to a dilute strength of suspected allergen is considered clinically significant. Measure the diameter in millimeters of erythema, and palpate and measure the size of any induration. Record this information in the patient's chart. No reaction should be noted at the control site.

The technique described above can easily be modified for desensitization injections and vaccinations.

Patient Teaching

Tell the patient the time, date, and place to return to have the test sites read. Tell the patient not to wash or scrub the area until the injections have been read.

If the patient develops an area of severe burning or itching, he or she should try not to scratch. Tell the patient to report immediately the development of any breathing difficulty, severe hives, or rashes. He or she should go to the nearest emergency room if unable to reach the physician who prescribed the skin tests.

Documentation

Provide the RIGHT DOCUMENTATION of the medication administration and responses to drug therapy.

1. Chart the date, time, drug name, dosage, and site of administration (Figure 6-24, C).
2. Perform a reading of each site after the application, as directed by the physician or the policy of the health care agency.
3. Chart and report any signs and symptoms of adverse drug effects.

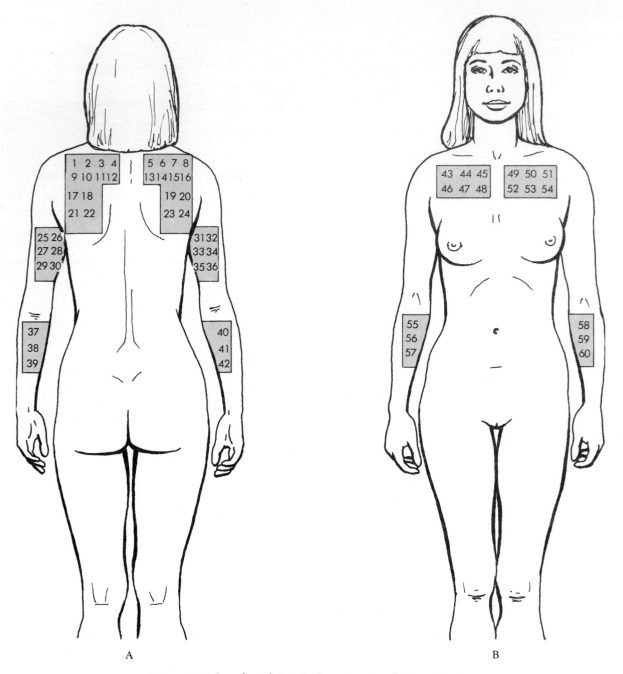

Figure 6-24 *Intradermal sites* **A,** *Posterior view.* **B,** *Anterior view.*

4. Perform and validate essential patient education about the drug therapy and other essential aspects of intervention for the disease process affecting the individual.

Commonly used readings of reactions and appropriate symbols are listed below.

+	(1+)	Redness of skin present (erythema)
++	(2+)	Redness and solid elevated lesions up to 5 mm in diameter (erythema and papules)

+++   (3+) Erythema, papules, and vesicles (blister-like areas 5 mm or less in diameter)

++++   (4+) Generalized fusing of blistered areas

Generally, a positive reaction to *delayed hypersensitivity* skin testing (to evaluate in vivo cell-mediated immunity) requires an *induration* of at least 5 mm in diameter.

Reading Chart for Intradermal Testing

Patient Name: _____
Identification Number: _____
Physician Name: _____

DATE:	TIME:	AGENT	CONCENTRATION	AMOUNT INJECTED	SITE NUMBER:*	Reading Time in Hours or minutes, i.e., 30 min. or 24, 48, or 72 hours		

* Refer to diagram of sites, Figure 6.24a,b.
  —Follow directions for the "reading" of the skin testing performed.
  —Inspect sites in a good light
  —Record reaction in upper half of box using the following guidelines, i.e.,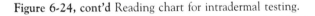
  +   (1⁺) Redness of skin present (erythema)
  + +   (2⁺) Redness and solid elevated lesion up to 5 mm in diameter (erythema and papules).
  + + +   (3⁺) Erythema, papules and vesicles (blister-like areas 5 mm or less in diameter).
  + + + + (4⁺) Generalized fusing of blisters.
  —Record measurement of induration (process of hardening) in mm. in lower half of box, i.e.,

Figure 6-24, cont'd Reading chart for intradermal testing.

ADMINISTRATION OF MEDICATION BY THE SUBCUTANEOUS ROUTE

OBJECTIVE

1. Identify the equipment needed and describe the technique used to administer a medication via the subcutaneous route.

KEY WORD

subcutaneous

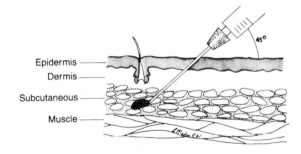

Figure 6-25 *Subcutaneous injection technique.*

Subcutaneous injections are made into the loose connective tissue between the dermis and muscle layer (Figure 6-25). Absorption is slower and drug action is generally longer with subcutaneous injections than with intramuscular or intravenous injections. If the circulation is adequate, the drug is completely absorbed from the tissue.

Many drugs cannot be administered by this route since no more than 2 ml can ordinarily be deposited at a subcutaneous site. The drugs must be quite soluble and potent enough to be effective in small volume, without causing significant tissue irritation. Drugs commonly injected into the subcutaneous tissue are heparin and insulin.

Equipment

Syringe size

Choose a syringe that corresponds to the volume of drug to be injected at one site. The usual amount injected subcutaneously at one site is 0.5 to 2 ml. Correlate syringe size with the size of the patient and the tissue mass.

Needle length

Assess each patient so that the needle length selected will deposit the medication into the subcutaneous tissue, not muscle tissue. Needle lengths of ⅜, ½, and ⅝ inch are routinely used. It is prudent to leave an extra ¼ inch of needle extending above the skin surface in case the needle breaks.

Needle gauge

Commonly used gauges for subcutaneous injections are 25 to 27 gauge.

Sites

Common sites used for the subcutaneous administration of medications include upper arms, anterior thighs, and abdomen (Figure 6-26, A and B). Less common areas are the buttocks and upper back or scapular region.

A plan for rotating injection sites should be developed for all patients who require repeated injections

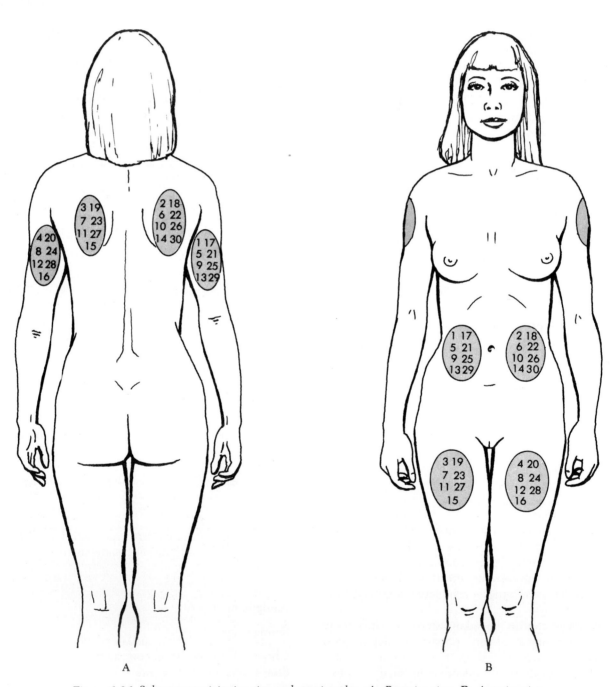

A   B

Figure 6-26 *Subcutaneous injection sites and rotation plan.* **A,** *Posterior view.* **B,** *Anterior view.*

(Figure 6-26, *A* and *B*). The anterior view (Figure 6-26, *B*) illustrates areas easily used for self-administration. The posterior view (Figure 6-26, *A*) illustrates less commonly used areas that may be used by other persons injecting the medication.

Technique

1. Prepare the medication as described before.
2. Check the accuracy of the drug order against the medication being prepared at least three times during the preparation phase: (1) when first removing the drug from the storage area; (2) immediately after preparation; and (3) immediately before administration.
3. Check your hospital policy regarding whether 1 to 2 minims of air are added to the syringe AFTER accurately measuring the prescribed volume of drug for administration (*Note:* The rationale for adding the air is that it will result in the needle being completely cleared of all medication at the time of injection. Conversely, if the volume of medication is completely drawn into the syringe before changing the needle, the drug volume ordered will still be administered as long as the same size needle is used for drawing up and injection. Thus, the needle should not need to be completely cleared of medication by air during administration. This issue can be critical when small volumes of potent drugs are administered to infants.)
4. Consult the master rotation schedule for the patient so that the drug is administered at the correct site.
5. Identify the patient prior to administration of the medication by checking the bracelet.
6. Explain what you are going to do.
7. Position the patient appropriately.
8. Expose the selected site and locate the landmarks. Don gloves.
9. Cleanse the skin surface with an antiseptic pledget starting at the injection site and working outward in a circular motion toward the periphery.
10. Let the area air-dry.
11. Consult the institution's policy regarding which of the following methods to use.

    Method 1:
    Grasp the skin area of the site selected, spread, hold firmly, and insert the needle quickly at a 45 degree angle; aspirate (DO NOT ASPIRATE FOR HEPARIN) and slowly inject the medication. If the aspiration draws blood, withdraw the needle and prepare an entirely new medication for administration (new syringe, needle, and drug).

    Method 2:
    Grasp the skin area of the site selected and cre-

ate a small roll or "bunch." Insert the needle quickly at a 90° angle, aspirate (DO NOT ASPIRATE FOR HEPARIN), and slowly inject the medication. If the aspiration draws blood, withdraw the needle and prepare an entirely new medication for administration (new syringe, needle, and drug).

12. As the needle is withdrawn, apply gentle pressure to the site with an antiseptic pledget.
13. Do NOT re-cap any needles that have been used. Dispose of used needles and syringes into a puncture-resistant container according to the policy of the employing institution.
14. Remove glove(s) and dispose of them according to agency policy. Thoroughly wash hands.
15. Provide emotional support for the patient.

Documentation

Provide the RIGHT DOCUMENTATION of the medication administration and response to drug therapy:

1. Chart the date, time, drug name, dosage, and route of administration.
2. Perform and record regular patient assessments for the evaluation of the therapeutic effectiveness (blood pressure, pulse, output, improvement or quality of cough and productivity, degree and duration of pain relief, etc.).
3. Chart and report any signs and symptoms of adverse drug effects.
4. Perform and validate essential patient education about the drug therapy and other essential aspects of intervention for the disease process affecting the individual.

ADMINISTRATION OF MEDICATION BY THE INTRAMUSCULAR ROUTE
OBJECTIVES

1. Identify the equipment needed and describe the technique used to administer medications in the vastus lateralis muscle, rectus femoris muscle, ventrogluteal area, dorsogluteal area, or the deltoid muscle.
2. For each anatomical site studied, describe the landmarks utilized to identify the site before administration of the medication.
3. Identify good sites for intramuscular administration of medication in an infant, a child, an adult, and an elderly person.

KEY WORDS

intramuscular	vastus lateralis
rectus femoris	ventrogluteal
dorsogluteal	deltoid
Z-track method	

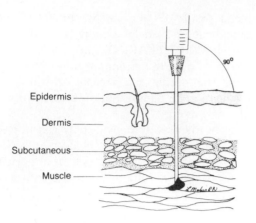

Figure 6-27 *Intramuscular injection technique.*

Intramuscular (IM) injections are made by penetrating a needle through the dermis and subcutaneous tissue into the muscle layer. The injection deposits the medication deep within the muscle mass (Figure 6-27). Absorption is more rapid than from subcutaneous injections because muscle tissue has a greater blood supply. Site selection is especially important with intramuscular injections because incorrect placement of the needle may cause damage to nerves or blood vessels. A large, healthy muscle free of infection or wounds should be used.

Equipment

Syringe size

Choose a syringe that corresponds to the volume of drug to be injected at one site. The usual amount injected intramuscularly at one site is 0.5 to 2 ml. In infants and children, the amount should not exceed 0.5 to 1 ml. Correlate syringe size with the size of the patient and the tissue mass. In adults, divided doses are generally recommended for amounts in excess of 3 ml; 1 ml may be injected in the deltoid area. Other factors that influence syringe size include the type of medication and site of administration, thickness of subcutaneous fatty tissue and the age of the individual.

Needle length

Assess each patient so that the needle length selected will deposit the medication into the muscular tissue (Figure 6-12). There is a significant difference among needle lengths appropriate for an obese patient, an infant, or an emaciated or debilitated patient. Needle lengths commonly used are 1 to 1½ inches long, although longer lengths may be required for an obese person. When estimating needle length, it is prudent to leave an extra ¼ inch of needle extending above the skin surface in case the needle breaks.

Needle gauge

Commonly used gauges for intramuscular injections are 20 to 22 gauge.

Sites

Common sites used for the intramuscular administration of medication include the following:

Vastus lateralis muscle

This muscle is located on the anterior lateral thigh away from nerves and blood vessels. The midportion is one handbreadth below the greater trochanter and one handbreadth above the knee (Figure 6-28, A and B). It is generally the preferred site for IM injections in infants since it has the largest muscle mass for that age group. The vastus lateralis muscle is also a good choice for an injection site in healthy, ambulatory adults (Figure 6-28, B). It will accommodate a large volume of medication and permits good drug absorption. In the elderly, debilitated, or nonambulatory adult, the muscle should be carefully assessed before injection as significantly less muscle mass may be present. If muscle mass is insufficient, an alternative site should be selected.

Rectus femoris muscle

The rectus femoris muscle lies just medial (Figure 6-29, A and B) to the vastus lateralis muscle, but does not cross the midline of the anterior thigh. The injection site is located in the same manner as the vastus lateralis muscle. It may be used in both children and adults when other sites are unavailable. A primary advantage to its use is that it may be used more easily by patients for self-administration. A disadvantage is that the medial border is quite close to the sciatic nerve and major blood vessels (Figure 6-29, A and B). If the muscle is not well developed, injections in this site may also cause considerable discomfort.

Gluteal area

The gluteal area is a commonly used site of injection because it is free of major nerves and blood vessels. *It must not be used in children under 3 years of age because the muscle is not yet well-developed from walking.* The area may be divided into two distinct injection sites: (1) the ventrogluteal area and (2) the dorsogluteal area.

Ventrogluteal area: This site is easily accessible when the patient is in a prone, supine, or side-lying position. It is located by placing the palm of the hand on the lateral portion of the greater trochanter, the index finger on the anterior superior iliac spine, and the middle finger extended to the iliac crest. The injection is made

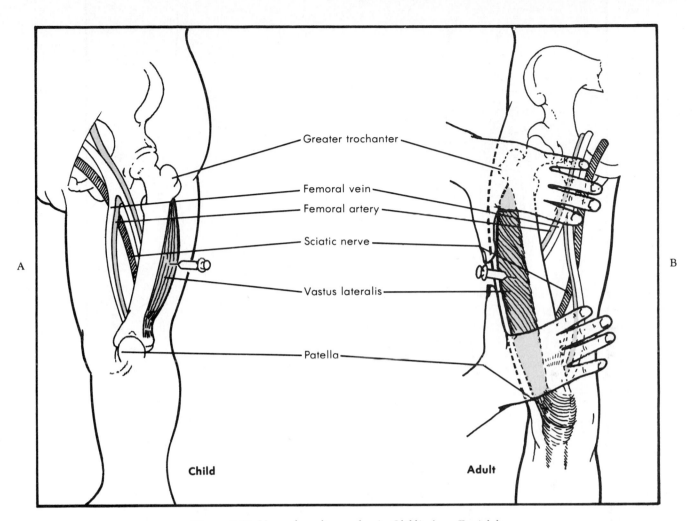

A

B

Greater trochanter

Femoral vein
Femoral artery

Sciatic nerve

Vastus lateralis

Patella

Child

Adult

Figure 6-28 *Vastus lateralis muscle.* **A,** *Child/infant.* **B,** *Adult.*

into the center of the "V" formed between the index and middle fingers with the needle directed slightly upward toward the crest of the ilium (Figure 6-30, A and B). Pain on injection can be minimized if the muscle is relaxed. The patient can aid in relaxation by pointing the toes inward while lying in a prone position (Figure 6-31) or by flexing the upper leg if lying on the side (Figure 6-32).

Dorsogluteal area: To use this injection site (Figure 6-33, A and B), the patient must be placed in a prone position on a flat table surface. The site is identified by drawing an imaginary line from the posterior superior iliac spine to the greater trochanter of the femur. The injection should be given at any point between the imaginary straight line and below the curve of the iliac crest (hipbone). The syringe should be held perpendicular to the flat table surface with the needle directed on a straight back-to-front course. Pain on injection can be minimized if the muscle is relaxed. The patient can

aid in relaxation by pointing the toes inward while lying in a prone position (Figure 6-31).

Deltoid muscle

The deltoid muscle is frequently used because of ease of access in the standing, sitting, or prone positions. However, it should be used in infants only when the volume to be injected is quite small, the drug is nonirritating, and the dose will be quickly absorbed. In adults, the volume should be limited to 2 cc or less and the substance must not cause irritation. Caution must also be exercised to avoid the clavicle, humerus, acromion, the brachial vein and artery, and the radial nerve. The injection site (Figure 6-34, A and B) of the deltoid muscle is located by drawing an imaginary line across the armpit at the level of the axilla and the lower edge of the acromion. The lateral borders of the rectangle are vertical lines parallel to the area one-third

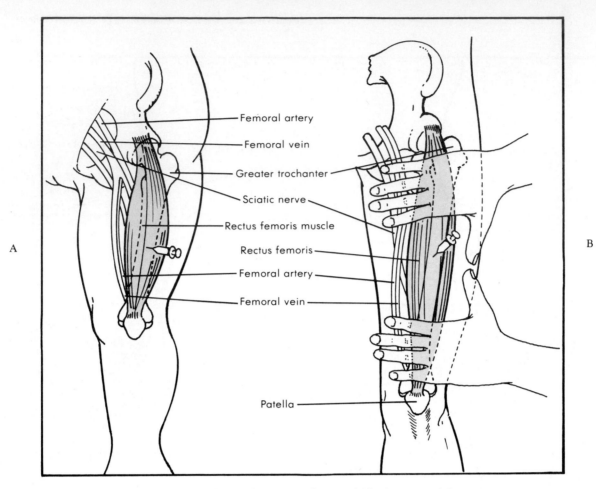

Figure 6-29 *Rectus femoris muscle.* **A,** *Child/infant.* **B,** *Adult.*

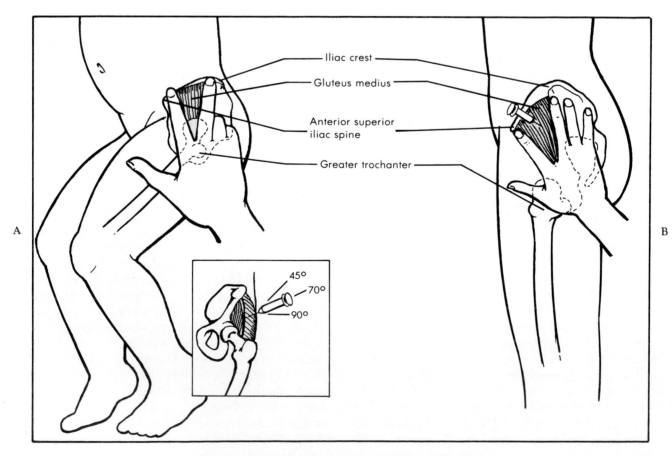

Figure 6-30 *Ventrogluteal site.* **A,** *Child/infant.* **B,** *Adult.*

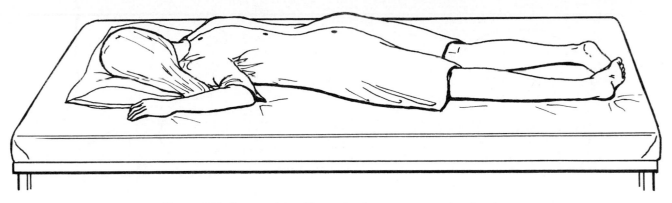

Figure 6-31 *Prone position. Toes pointed to promote muscle relaxation.*

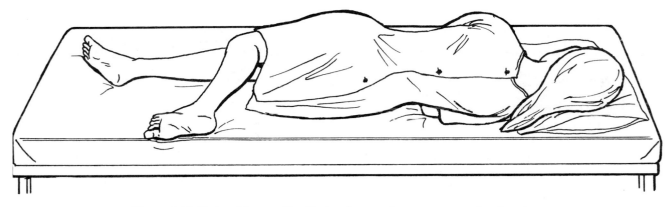

Figure 6-32 *Patient lying on side. Flexing the upper leg promotes muscle relaxation.*

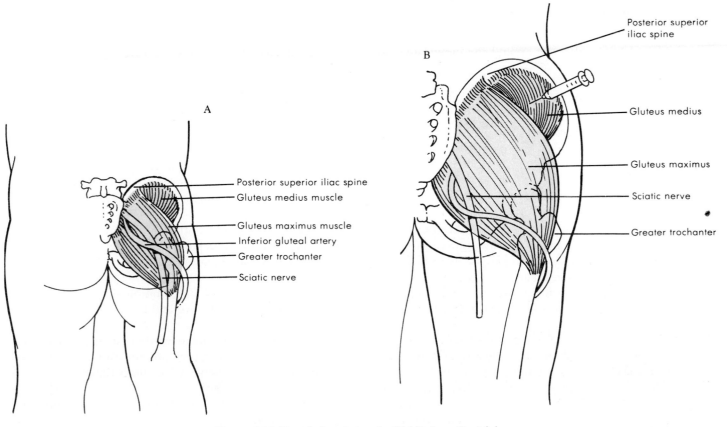

Figure 6-33 *Dorsal gluteal site.* **A,** *Child/infant.* **B,** *Adult.*

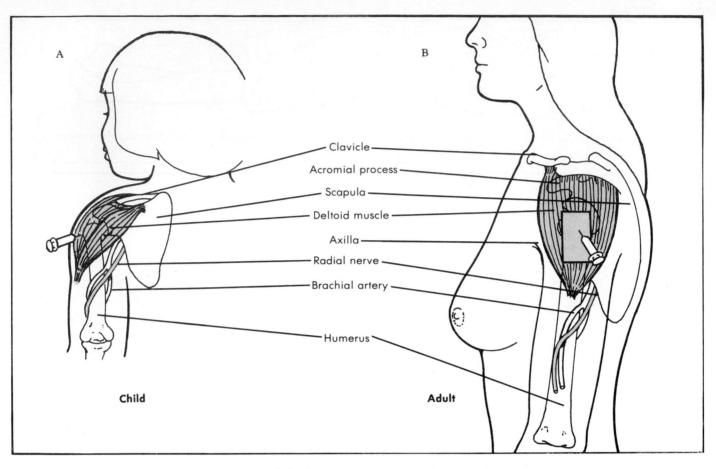

A

B

Clavicle

Acromial process

Scapula

Deltoid muscle

Axilla

Radial nerve

Brachial artery

Humerus

Child

Adult

Figure 6-34 *Deltoid muscle site.* **A,** *Child/infant.* **B,** *Adult.*

and two-thirds of the way around the outer lateral aspect of the arm.

Site Rotation

A master plan for site rotation should be developed and used for all patients requiring repeated injections (Figure 6-35, A and B).

Technique

1. Prepare the medication as described before.
2. Check the accuracy of the drug order against the medication being prepared at least three times during the preparation phase: (1) when first removing the drug from the storage area; (2) immediately after preparation; and (3) immediately before administration.
3. Check your hospital policy regarding whether 1 to 2 minims of air should be added to the syringe AFTER accurately measuring the prescribed volume of drug for administration. (NOTE: The rationale for adding the air is that it will result in the needle being completely cleared of all medication at the time of injection. Conversely, if the volume is completely drawn into the syringe before changing the needle, the drug volume ordered will still be administered as long as the same size needle is used for drawing up and injection. Thus, the needle should not need to be completely cleared of medication by air during administration. This issue can be critical when small volumes of potent drugs are administered repeatedly to infants.)
4. Consult the master rotation schedule for the patient so that the drug is administered at the correct site (Figure 6-35).
5. Identify the patient prior to administration of the medication by checking the bracelet.
6. Explain what you are going to do.
7. Position the patient appropriately (see Figures 6-31 and 6-32 for relaxation techniques).
8. Expose the selected site and locate the landmarks. Don gloves.
9. Cleanse the skin surface with an antiseptic pledget starting at the injection site and working outward in a circular motion toward the periphery.
10. Let the area air-dry.
11. Insert the needle at the correct angle and depth for the site being used.
12. Aspirate. If no blood returns, slowly inject the

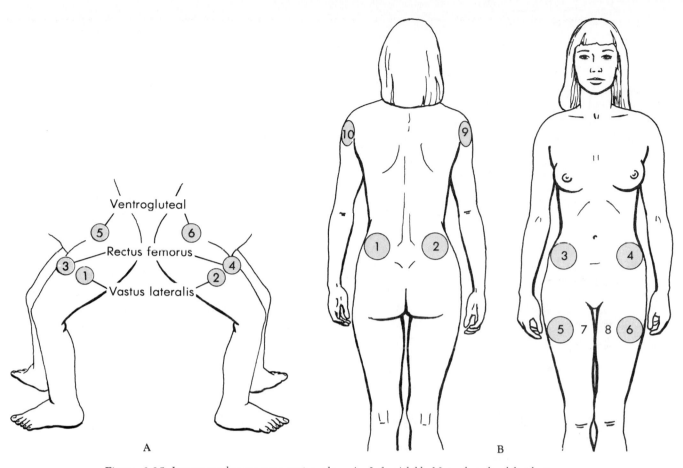

Figure 6-35 *Intramuscular master rotation plan.* **A,** *Infant/child. Note that the deltoid site may also be used in an infant or child; however, the volume of medication must be quite small and the drug nonirritating.* **B,** *Adult. In an adult, avoid the use of the rectus femoris (numbers 7 and 8) unless other sites are not available, due to the pain produced when this site is used and the location of the sciatic nerve, femoral artery, and vein. If used, be certain to insert the needle lateral to the midline.*

medication using gentle, steady pressure on the plunger. If blood does return, place an antiseptic pledget over the injection site as the needle is withdrawn. Start the procedure over with a new syringe, needle, and medication.

13. After removing the needle, apply gentle pressure to the site. Massage can increase the pain if the muscle mass is stressed by the amount of medication given.
14. Do NOT re-cap any needles that have been used. Dispose of used needles and syringes into a puncture-resistant container according to the policy of the employing institution.
15. Remove glove(s) and dispose of them according to agency policy. Thoroughly wash hands.
16. Apply a small bandage to the site.
17. Provide emotional support of the patient. Children should be given comfort during and after the injection. Sometimes letting a child hold your hand or say "ouch" helps. Praise the patient for assistance and cooperation.

The Z-track method

The use of a Z-track technique (Figure 6-36, A to D) may be appropriate for medications that are particularly irritating or that stain the tissue. Check the hospital policy concerning which personnel may administer by this method.

1. Expose the dorsogluteal site (Figure 6-36, A). Calculate and prepare the medication, and add 0.5 cc of air to ensure that the drug will clear the needle. Position the patient and cleanse the area for injection as previously described. Never inject into the arm or other exposed site. Don gloves.
2. Stretch the skin approximately 1 inch to one side (Figure 6-36, B).
3. Insert the needle. Choose a needle of sufficient length to ensure *deep* muscle penetration.
4. Aspirate and follow previous guidelines for use of the dorsogluteal site.
5. Gently inject the medication and wait approximately 10 seconds (Figure 6-36, C).

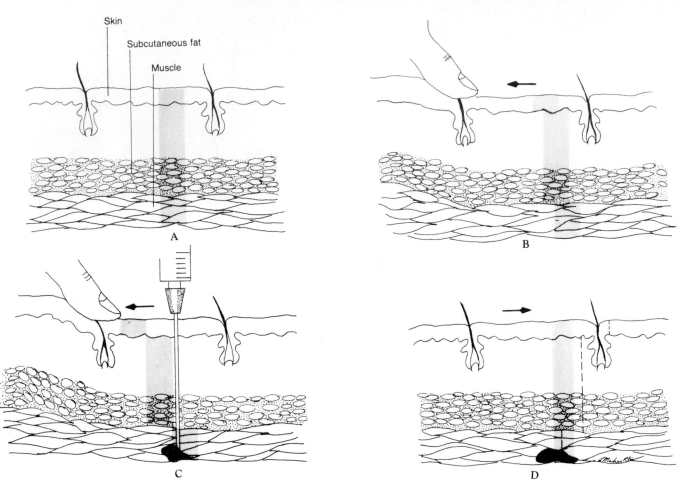

Figure 6-36 *Z-track method of intramuscular injection.* **A,** *Before starting Z tracking.* **B,** *Stretch skin slightly to one side, approximately one inch.* **C,** *Inject the medication; wait approximately 10 seconds.* **D,** *Remove needle and allow skin to return to normal position. Do not massage injection site.*

6. Remove the needle and allow the skin to return to the normal position (Figure 6-36, *D*).
7. DO NOT massage the injection site.
8. If further injections are to be made, alternate between dorsogluteal sites.
9. Do NOT re-cap any needles that have been used. Dispose of used needles and syringes into a puncture-resistant container according to the policy of the employing institution.
10. Remove glove(s) and dispose of them according to agency policy. Thoroughly wash hands.
11. Walking will help absorption. Vigorous exercise or pressure on the injection site (such as a tight girdle) should be temporarily avoided.

ADMINISTRATION OF MEDICATIONS BY THE INTRAVENOUS ROUTE
OBJECTIVES

1. Identify the dosage forms available, sites of administration, and general principles of administering medications via the intravenous route.

2. Describe the precautions needed to prevent the transmission of HIV that should be implemented for all patients requiring venipuncture.
3. Describe the correct techniques for administering medications by means of an established peripheral or central intravenous line, a vascular access device, a heparin lock, an intravenous bag, a bottle or volume-control device, or through a secondary piggyback set.
4. Describe the recommended guidelines and procedures for intravenous catheter care (including proper maintenance of patency of IV lines and implanted access device), IV line dressing changes, and for peripheral and central venous IV needle or catheter changes.
5. Discuss the proper baseline patient assessments needed to evaluate the intravenous therapy (such as phlebitis, extravasation, air in tubing).
6. Review the policies and procedures used at the practice setting to assure that persons performing venipunctures and intravenous therapy have the required proficiency.

KEY WORDS

intravenous   venipuncture
phlebitis   extravasation
pulmonary edema   embolism

Intravenous (IV) administration of medication places the drug directly into the bloodstream, bypassing all barriers to drug absorption. Large volumes of medications can be administered into the vein; there is usually less irritation; and the onset of action is the most rapid of all parenteral routes. Drugs may be given by direct injection with a needle and syringe, but more commonly drugs are given intermittently or by continuous infusion through an established peripheral or central venous line, or via an implantable venous access device also referred to as an "implantable subcutaneous port."

Intravenous drug administration is usually more comfortable for the patient, especially when several doses of medication must be administered daily. However, use of the intravenous route requires time and skill to establish and maintain an IV site; the patient tends to be less mobile; and there is an increased possibility of infection and severe adverse reactions from the drug.

Dosage Forms

Medications for intravenous administration are available in ampules, vials, and prefilled syringes. Be certain that the label specifically states that the medication is "for IV use."

Intravenous physiologic solutions come in a variety of volumes and concentrations in glass or plastic containers (Table 6-2).

Equipment

Gloves
Tourniquet
Administration set with appropriate needle, drip chamber, and filter
Medication
Physiologic solution ordered
Sterile dressing materials
Antiseptic solution
Syringe and needle (if by bolus)
Armboard
Tape
Standard IV pole or rod
Heparin lock, "piggyback," and additional solutions, as appropriate
(Additional supplies may be required to access, flush, change IV administration sets, in-line filters or dressings, depending on the type of peripheral, central, or implantable device being used.)

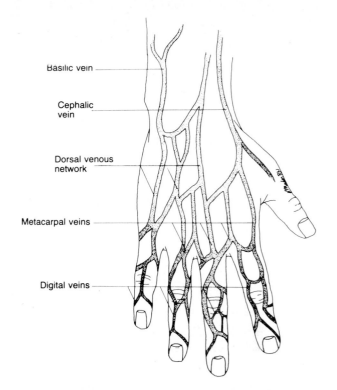

Figure 6-37 *Intravenous sites on the hand.*

Sites

Peripheral access

When selecting an intravenous site consider:

1. Length of time the IV will be required.
2. Condition and location of vein(s).
3. Purpose of infusion (for example, rehydration, delivery of nutritional needs (TPN), chemotherapy, antibiotics).
4. Patient status, cooperation, and patient preference for, and amount of self-care of, the injection site (if appropriate).

Peripheral intravenous devices include winged-tipped needle (Figure 6-10), over-the-needle catheter (Figure 6-11, A), and inside-the-needle catheter (Figure 6-11, B).

If a prolonged course of treatment is anticipated, start the first IV in the hand (Figure 6-37). The metacarpal veins, dorsal vein network, cephalic, and basilic vein are commonly used. To avoid irritation and leakage from a previous puncture site, the subsequent venipuncture sites should be made above the earlier site. Refer to Figure 6-38 for the veins of the forearm area that could be used for additional venipuncture sites.

- Avoid the use of vessels over bony prominences or joints unless absolutely necessary.
- In the elderly, the use of the veins in the hand area may be a poor choice due to the fragility of the skin and veins in this area.

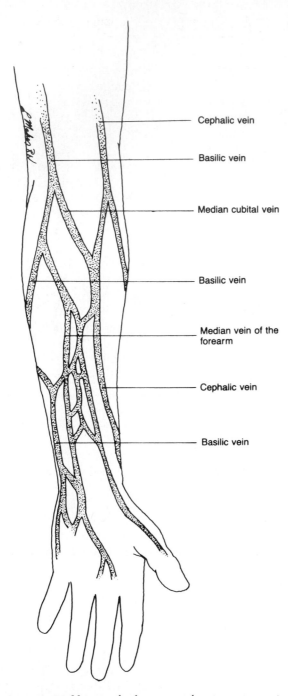

Figure 6-38 *Veins in the forearm used as intravenous sites.*

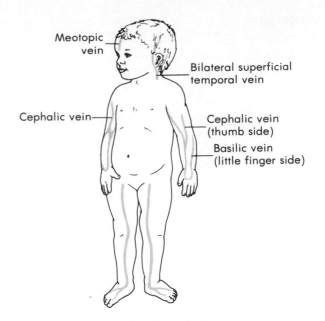

Figure 6-39 *Veins in infants and children used as intravenous sites.*

- Veins commonly used in infants and children for intravenous administration are on the back of the hand, dorsum of the foot, or the temporal region of the scalp (Figure 6-39).
- If possible, do not use the veins of the lower extremities because of the danger of developing thrombi and emboli.
- Do not use veins with varicosities or an extremity with impaired blood flow (for example, the affected side following a mastectomy and lymph node dissection).

- Whenever possible, initiate the IV in the nondominant arm.
- Do not initiate an IV in an arm with compromised lymphatic or venous flow.
- *Never start an IV in an artery!*

Central access

Central IV devices are used when:

1. The purpose of therapy dictates (for example, large volume, high concentration, or hypertonic solutions are to be infused).
2. Peripheral sites have been exhausted due to repeated use or condition of veins for access is poor.
3. Long-term or home therapy is required.
4. Emergency condition mandates adequate vascular access.

The central venous sites most commonly used for inside-the-needle catheters are the subclavian, jugular, or femoral veins (Figure 6-11). A physician can also elect to perform a venisection or "cutdown" to insert this type of catheter into the basilic or cephalic veins in the antecubital fossa.

Central sites commonly used for long-term silastic catheters (e.g., Hickman, Broviac, Groshong) are the jugular, subclavian, or cephalic veins. The distal end of the silastic catheter is positioned in the superior vena cava to allow maximal dilution of the IV fluid with blood. The proximal end of the catheter is tunneled in subcutaneous tissue that acts as a barrier to pathogens that may later attach to the catheter line and migrate to the vein causing an infection.

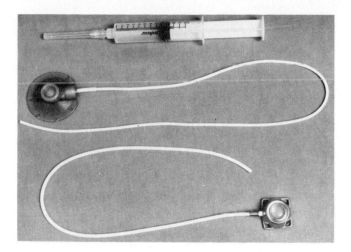

Figure 6-40 *Silicone venous catheters with infusion ports. (From Potter PA, Perry AG: Basic nursing: theory and practice, ed 2, 1991, St Louis, Mosby–Year Book.)*

Implantable vascular access devices

Vascular access devices, also known as implantable infusion ports (for example, Infus-A-Port, Port-A-Cath, Mediport, Chemoport) are used when long-term therapy is required and repeated accessing of the vein is required. Vascular access devices/ports (Figure 6-40) are implanted into a subcutaneous pocket in the chest area and are sutured in place. The distal end of the silicone catheter is threaded via the jugular, subclavian, or cephalic vein to the superior vena cava. The proximal end of the catheter is attached to the implanted port. The port itself contains a self-sealing silicone rubber septum specifically designed for repeated injections over an extended time period. A special noncoring Huber needle is used to penetrate the skin and the septum of the implanted device to minimize damage to the self-sealing septum.

General Principles of Intravenous Medication Administration

- Use appropriate barrier precautions (universal blood and body fluid precautions) to prevent the transmission of any infectious diseases, including HIV, as recommended by the Centers for Disease Control.
- Gloves should be worn throughout the venipuncture procedure. Care should be taken to wash the skin surface if the area is contaminated with blood.
- When the procedure is complete, remove the gloves and dispose of them in accordance with the policies of the practice setting. WASH hands thoroughly as soon as the gloves are removed. Care should be taken not to contaminate the IV tubing and rate regulator.
- Any used needles, syringes, venipuncture catheters, or vascular access devices should be placed in a punc-ture-resistant container in the immediate vicinity for disposal according to the policies of the practice setting.
- Never recap, bend, or break used needles because of the danger of inadvertently puncturing the skin.
- Be certain medications to be administered intravenously are thoroughly dissolved in the correct volume and type of solution. *Always* follow the manufacturer's recommendations.
- Most clinical practice sites now use transparent dressings over the IV insertion site that are changed in accordance with hospital policies, generally every 48 hours. Some clinical practice sites still use gauze dressings. When gauze is used, the four edges of the dressing should be sealed using tape. To prevent skin irritation, place tincture of benzoin on the skin directly under the edge of the gauze and allow it to dry before applying the dressing tape. Always check the specific policies of the employing institution as well as the physician's orders for frequency of dressing changes.
- At the time of the dressing change on any type of IV site, the area should be thoroughly inspected for any drainage, redness, tenderness, irritation, or swelling. The presence of any of these symptoms should be reported to the physician immediately. (Also take the patient's vital signs and report these at the same time.)
- Use in-line filters as recommended by the manufacturer of the drug to be delivered.
- DO NOT administer any drug or IV solution that is hazy or cloudy, or has foreign particles or a precipitate in it.
- DO NOT mix any other drugs with blood or blood products (such as albumin).
- DO NOT administer a drug in an IV solution if the compatibility is not known.
- Drugs must be entirely infused through the IV line before adding a second medication to the IV line.
- Once mixed, know the length of time an agent remains stable; all unused IV solutions should be returned to the pharmacy if not used within 24 hours.
- Check the hospital policy for the definition of "TKO" (to keep open). It is usually interpreted as "an infusion rate of 10 ml/hr" and should infuse less than 500 ml/24 hr.
- Shade IV solutions that contain drugs that should be protected from light (such as hyperalimentation solutions, nitrofurantoin, amphotericin B, nitroprusside).
- All intravenous solution bag/bottles should be changed every 24 hours (check hospital policy) to minimize the development of new infections. Label all intravenous solutions with the date and time initiated and the nurse's initials.
- Administration sets should be changed every 24 to 48 hours (check hospital policy). The sets must be la-

beled with the date and time initiated, the date to change the set, and the nurse's initials.

- Whenever a patient is receiving IV fluids, monitor intake and output accurately. Report declining hourly outputs and those of less than 30 to 40 ml/hour.
- Never "speed up" an IV flow rate to "catch up" when the volume to be infused has fallen behind. In certain cases, this could be dangerous. The physician should be consulted, particularly with patients who have cardiac, renal, or circulatory impairment.

Preparing an Intravenous Solution for Infusion

Dosage form

Check the physician's order for the specific IV solution ordered and for any medication to be added. If not already prepared by the pharmacy, check the accuracy of the drug order against the medication and/or solution being prepared at least three times during the preparation phase: (1) when first removing the drug/solution from the storage area, (2) immediately after preparation, and (3) immediately before administration. Check the expiration date on any additives and the primary solution.

Equipment

Administration set with appropriate drip chamber (microdrop or macrodrop), needle, IV catheter, and inline filter (if used)
Medications for intravenous delivery
Physiologic solution ordered
Antiseptic pads
IV Pole
Emesis basin

Technique

1. Assemble equipment and thoroughly wash hands.
2. Check the size and type of needle and/or catheter needed to access the vein selected for the IV or to access an implanted access device for the delivery of the IV solution or medication.
3. Check the physician's order against the physiologic solution chosen for administration.
4. Inspect the intravenous container for cloudiness, discoloration, or the presence of any precipitate.
5. Remove the plastic cover from the IV container and inspect the plastic IV bag to be certain it is intact; squeeze gently to detect any punctures. Inspect a glass container of IV solution for any cracks.
6. Choose the administration set appropriate for the type of solution ordered, the rate of delivery requested (microdrop vs. macrodrop), and for the type of IV container being used. Plastic bag IV

containers DO NOT require an air vent in the administration set. Glass containers for IV delivery must be vented or have an administration set with a vent in it. Remove the administration set from its container and inspect to ensure its sterility.

7. Move the roller or slide clamp to the upper portion of the IV line 6 to 8 inches from the drip chamber; close the clamp.
8. *Plastic IV bags:* Remove the tab from the spike receiver port; remove the tab from the administration set spike; insert the spike firmly into the bag port. Maintain sterility of port and spike throughout the process.

   Glass IV bottle: Peel back the metal tab and lift the protective metal disk from the container; remove the latex-type covering (if present) from the top of the rubber stopper. As the latex diaphragm is removed, a sudden noise should be heard as the vacuum within the glass container is released. If the noise is not heard, the contents of the IV container may not be sterile and should be discarded. Remove the tab from the administration set spike; insert the spike firmly into the port in the rubber stopper. Maintain sterility of the port and spike throughout the process.

   NOTE: When additive medications are ordered, they should be added to the large volume container before tubing is attached to help assure a uniform mixing of the medication and the physiologic solution. If medication is added to an existing IV solution, make sure adequate mixing takes place before the infusion is started again. (See technique used for adding a medication to an IV solution, p. 111.)
9. Hang the solution on an IV pole; squeeze the drip chamber and fill half way; prime the IV line by removing the protective tab from the distal end of the IV line; open the roller or slide clamp and allow the solution to run until all the air is removed from the line. Cover the end of the IV tubing with a sterile cap. Place an IV measuring device/tape strip on the plastic bag or glass IV container. Mark the container with the patient's name and date and time of preparation. If medication has been added, all details of the medication must be marked on the container: drug name, dose, rate of administration requested in physician's order, and the nurse's name who prepared IV.

   NOTE: It may be necessary to add in-line filters to the setup if recommended for the administration of the medication ordered.
10. The IV solution can now be taken to the bedside for attachment after a venipuncture is performed or for addition to an existing IV system. For safety, all aspects of the IV order should be checked again immediately before attaching the IV for infusion.

Always identify the patient by checking the bracelet before initiating any intravenous procedure.

Technique for adding medication to an existing IV solution

1. Prepare the medication as described previously.
2. Check the accuracy of the drug order against the medication and/or solution being prepared at least three times during the preparation phase: (1) when first removing the drug/solution from the storage area, (2) immediately after preparation, and (3) immediately before administration. Check the expiration date on the solution.
3. Determine that the drug being added to an existing IV line is compatible with the physiologic solution in the line by reviewing hospital policies or by consulting the pharmacist.
4. *Go to the bedside and identify the patient by checking the bracelet before initiating any intravenous procedure.*
5. Explain what you are going to do.
6. *Plastic IV container:* Clamp the IV tubing, wipe the injection port with an antiseptic pledget, then insert the needle a short distance and inject the prescribed medication into the IV bag; agitate the bag to thoroughly disperse the IV medication throughout the IV bag. (Use a short needle to prevent inadvertently puncturing the back of the container.) Add a label showing the type and amount of medication added, time and date added, and initials of the preparer.
   Glass IV container: Clamp the IV tubing, remove the protective cover from the air vent, remove needle from syringe and attach syringe to air vent port and insert the medication; replace the air vent cover; gently rotate the glass container to thoroughly disperse the IV medication throughout the bottle. Add a label containing the type and amount of medication added, the time and date added, and the initials of the preparer.
7. Before initiating IV therapy or administering IV medications, perform baseline assessments of the patient's current vital signs and state of hydration.

Venipuncture

Follow these steps in performing venipuncture.

1. Wash hands thoroughly.
2. Position the patient appropriately. Immobilize an infant or child for patient safety, if necessary.
3. Cut tape for stabilizing the IV needle or catheter before starting the procedure. Turn the ends of the tape back on itself to form a tab that will not adhere to a glove when the tape is to be applied or removed. The nurse must consider his or her gloves to be contaminated when they come in contact with

blood. If the gloves then contact the tape and dressing materials used at the venipuncture site, the outside of the dressings and tape are then potentially contaminated. Therefore, during the procedure the nurse must focus on allowing contamination only of the dominant gloved hand; the nondominant hand must be maintained as noncontaminated to handle the taping and stabilization of the needle or IV catheter. Once the needle or catheter is stabilized, the gloves can be removed; wash hands thoroughly and to apply the gauze or occlusive type of dressing materials according to the practice-setting policies.

4. Apply the tourniquet using a slip knot 2 to 6 inches above the site chosen (shaded area in Figure 6-41, A). Inspect the area to identify a vein of sufficient size to accommodate the needle and provide adequate anchorage. Palpate the vein to feel the depth and direction (Figure 6-41, B and C). To dilate the vein, it may be necessary to (1) place the extremity in a dependent position, (2) massage the vein against the direction of blood flow, (3) have the patient open and close the hand repeatedly, (4) lightly thump the vein with your fingertips, or (5) remove the tourniquet and apply a heating pad or warm, wet towels to the extremity for 15 to 20 minutes and then start the process all over.
5. Cleanse the skin surface with the antiseptic starting at the site of entry and working outward in a circular motion toward the periphery (Figure 6-41, D).
6. Let the area air-dry.
7. Put on gloves.
8. Provide tension on the skin surface to stretch the skin and stabilize the vein.

When using an *administration set* or a *needle and syringe:* (1) Hold the needle (bevel up) at an angle slightly less than 45° (Figure 6-41, E) and penetrate the skin surface approximately ½ inch below the intended entry site into the vein; decrease the angle to 15° (Figure 6-41, F) and slowly advance the needle along the course of the vein. (2) When blood flow is established, connect the tubing to the needle, release the tourniquet, cleanse the area to eliminate any blood that may have contacted the skin or IV tubing, remove gloves, and anchor the needle and tubing to the arm or hand with tape (Figure 6-42) and dressing as prescribed in the practice setting policy. (Because it is difficult to handle tape with gloves on, it is helpful to have a second person to anchor the needle and tubing and adjust the flow rate. The individual performing the venipuncture can then remove gloves and wash hands thoroughly.) (3) Adjust the rate of flow of the solution:

$$\frac{ml \text{ of solution} \times \text{number of drops/ml}}{\text{hours of administration} \times 60 \text{ minutes}} = \text{drops/minute}$$

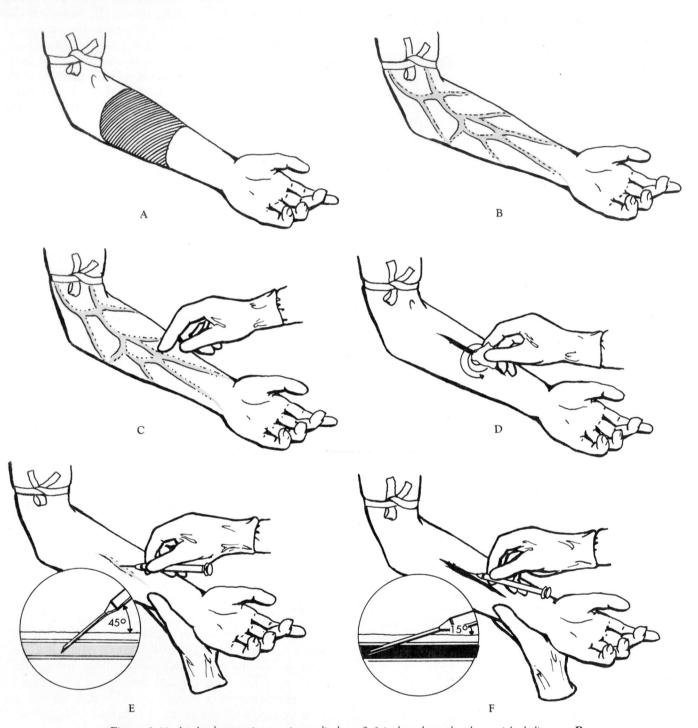

Figure 6-41 A, *Apply tourniquet using a slip knot 2-6 inches above the chosen (shaded) area.* **B,** *Allow veins to dilate.* **C,** *Palpate the vein to feel the depth and direction.* **D,** *Cleanse the skin surface with an antiseptic, starting at the anticipated site of entry, working outward in a circular motion to the periphery.* **E,** *Hold the needle (bevel up) at an angle slightly less than 45° to penetrate the skin surface.* **F,** *Decrease the angle to 15° and slowly advance the needle along the course of the vein.*

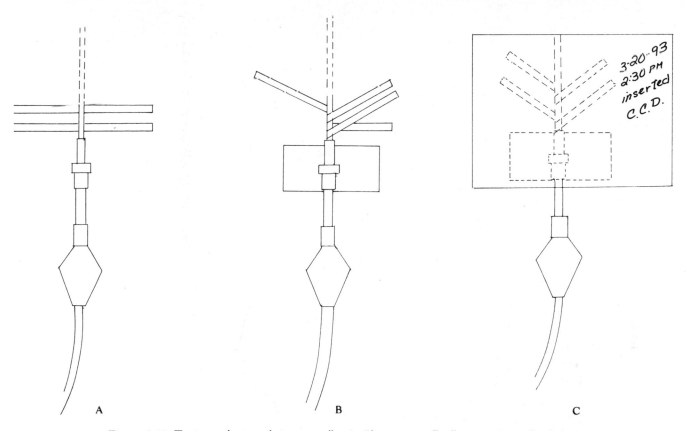

Figure 6-42 *Taping a plastic catheter or needle.* **A,** *Place two small adhesive strips under the needle or plastic catheter with the adhesive side up.* **B,** *Cross adhesive tapes one at a time to secure the plastic catheter or needle. The larger piece of tape is placed under the hub with adhesive side up. (It will adhere to larger tape to be applied later.)* **C,** *A larger piece of tape completes the stabilization of the plastic needle or catheter. Mark the date and time of insertion and the nurse's initials or signature. Note: There are several other methods for taping intravenous catheters or needles. Consult the procedure manual of the practice setting for the preferred method.*

(4) Regulate the flow by counting the drops for 15 seconds, multiply by 4, and adjust clamp on tubing for the appropriate rate.

When using a *plastic needle* (Figure 6-43): (1) Proceed as above until blood flow is established (Figure 6-42, A). (2) Remove the inner needle (Figure 6-43, B), connect the tubing to the plastic needle (Figure 6-43, C), release the tourniquet, cleanse the area to eliminate any blood that may have contacted the skin or IV tubing, remove gloves, and anchor the needle and tubing to the arm or hand with tape (Figure 6-42) and dressing as prescribed in the practice setting policy. (Because it is difficult to handle tape with gloves on, it is helpful to have a second person to anchor the needle and tubing, and adjust the flow rate. The individual performing the venipuncture can dispose of all soiled dressings or contaminated supplies according to the practice setting policy. Remove gloves and wash hands thoroughly.) (3) Adjust the rate of flow solution:

$$\frac{\text{ml of solution} \times \text{number of drops/ml}}{\text{hours of administration} \times 60 \text{ minutes}} = \text{drops/minute}$$

(4) Regulate the flow by counting the drops for 15 seconds, multiply by 4, and adjust clamp on tubing for the appropriate rate.

Regardless of the apparatus used, mark the tape with the date and time of insertion and the initials of the nurse who started it (Figure 6-42, C).

Many types of infusion pumps are available. The nurse should become familiar with the type used in his or her practice setting. Remember that the use of any type of equipment does not remove responsibility for visible monitoring of the rate of infusion and the infusion site at regularly scheduled intervals. Whenever an infusion pump is used, the danger of infiltration is increased.

Documentation

Provide the RIGHT DOCUMENTATION of the venipuncture, medication administration, and response to drug therapy:

1. Chart the date and time the venipuncture was performed.

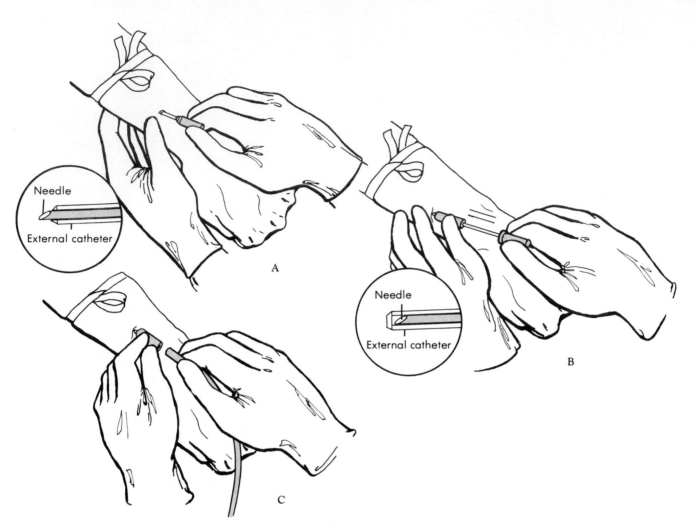

Needle

External catheter

A

Needle

External catheter

B

C

Figure 6-43 A, *"Over-the-catheter" type needle (see also Figure 6-11, A). When using a plastic needle, proceed as described in Figure 6-42, A-E, until blood flow is established.* **B,** *After the catheter has been advanced into the vein, remove the inner needle by withdrawing from the plastic needle.* **C,** *Connect the tubing to the plastic needle hub; release tourniquet.*

2. Chart the site used and the type and size of needle or catheter inserted.
3. Chart the type and amount of IV solution started or added to an existing line.
4. If a medication was added, chart the drug name and amount added, as well as the date and time of the addition.
5. Perform and record regular patient assessments for the evaluation of the therapeutic effectiveness (blood pressure, pulse, output, lung field sounds, degree and duration of pain relief, and so on).
6. Chart and report any signs and symptoms of adverse effects.
7. Perform and validate essential patient education about the drug therapy and other essential aspects of intervention for the disease process affecting the individual.

Administration of Medications into an Established IV Line

1. Prepare the medication as described before.
2. Identify the patient using the bracelet and explain what you are going to do.
3. Put on gloves. It is helpful to keep one gloved hand uncontaminated.
4. Swab the self-sealing portal of the injection site with an antiseptic sponge.
5. Using a short needle on the syringe, puncture the portal site. (The short needle reduces the possibility of penetrating the opposite wall of the portal.)
6. Draw back the plunger of the syringe until blood flow is seen in the tubing at the venipuncture site to establish that the line is open into the vein.
7. While pinching the IV tubing *above* the portal to stop flow (use the uncontaminated gloved hand) in-

ject the prescribed medication into the IV line at a rate recommended by the manufacturer.

8. When all the medication is administered, withdraw the needle from the portal, dispose of the syringe and needle in a puncture-resistant container using the contaminated gloved hand, and readjust the flow rate using the uncontaminated gloved hand. Cleanse the area of the skin and tubing contaminated by blood or fluid according to the policy of the practice setting. Remove gloves, and wash hands thoroughly. (Flushing the IV line is not recommended because the medication still in the line would be administered as a bolus. This is contrary to the manufacturer's safety recommendation. Sudden boluses of certain medications may also cause severe hypotension or other signs of toxicity.)

Administration of Medication by a Heparin Lock (see Figure 6-10)

1. Select a syringe several cc larger than that required by the volume of the drug. This allows room for aspiration of blood to assure placement of the needle and to allow blood to mix with the drug solution.
2. Prepare the medication as described before.
3. Identify the patient using the armband and explain what you are going to do.
4. Put on gloves.
5. Swab the self-sealing rubber diaphragm with an antiseptic sponge and hold the sides of the injection port with your free hand.
6. Using a short, small-gauge needle, puncture the rubber diaphragm and gently pull back on the plunger for blood return.
7. If blood return is established, inject the medication at the rate specified by the manufacturer.
8. Periodically pull back on the plunger to mix blood with the drug solution and to assure that the needle is in the vein.
9. After administration, withdraw the needle from the diaphragm and dispose of it in a puncture-resistant container.
10. Remove the syringe and insert another syringe containing (usually) 1 to 2 ml of normal saline to flush the remaining drug from the butterfly line.
11. Flush the lock with 1 ml of heparin (10 unit/ml to 100 unit/ml as directed by hospital policy). Maintain constant pressure on the plunger of the syringe while simultaneously withdrawing the needle from the diaphragm to prevent backflow of blood. *Always* verify heparin dosage with another qualified nurse.
12. Cleanse the site of any blood or fluids. Remove gloves and dispose of properly. Wash hands thoroughly.

The heparin in the lock should be replaced (1) when initially placed, (2) after administering medications, (3) after withdrawing blood samples, or (4) every 8 hours if medications are not administered more frequently.

Check the hospital policy to determine how long a heparin lock may remain in place before changing it. Monitor the lock venipuncture site as you would any other venipuncture site.

Adding a Medication to an Intravenous Bag, Bottle, or Volume Control

1. Prepare the medication as described before.
2. Identify the patient using the bracelet and explain what you are going to do.
3. Identify the injection port on the specific type of IV container or volume control set to be used; cleanse the portal with an antiseptic swab.
4. Clamp IV tubing.
5. Insert the sterile needle into the correct injection port and slowly add the prescribed medication to the intravenous solution. Always check to be certain the medication is being added to a compatible solution of sufficient volume to insure proper dilution of the medication as specified by the manufacturer.
6. For a volume-control apparatus, fill the volume chamber with the specified amount of intravenous solution; clamp the tubing between the intravenous bottle or bag and the volume control chamber.
7. Add the medication, as described before, via the cleansed injection port. Adjust the rate of flow solution:

$$\frac{\text{ml of solution} \times \text{number of drops/ml}}{\text{hours of administration} \times 60 \text{ minutes}} = \text{drops/minute}$$

8. Regulate the flow by counting the drops for 15 seconds, multiply by 4, and adjust clamp on tubing for the appropriate rate. *Note:* When IV medications are administered by a volume control apparatus, calculation of the rate of infusion to administer the drug over the proper time must include an allowance for the volume of the fluid in the IV tubing *and* the volume of medication.
9. Affix a label to the container. Indicate the medication name, dosage, date and time prepared, rate of infusion, length of infusion time, and the nurse's signature.

Adding a Medication with a Piggyback or Secondary Set

1. Prepare the medication as described before and add to an IV bag or bottle.

2. Identify the patient using the bracelet and explain what you are going to do.
3. Insert the administration set into the container, attach a short sterile needle, clear the line of air, and clamp the tubing.
4. Connect to the primary IV tubing in one of the following ways:

   Piggyback—Arrange the piggyback container so that it is elevated higher than the primary container (see Figure 6-17). Cleanse the secondary portal with an antiseptic swab and insert the needle, thereby connecting the piggyback tubing to the port of the tubing of the primary solution. Secure in place.

   Secondary set—Arrange both the primary and secondary containers at the same height and connect the secondary tubing to the port of the tubing of the primary solution in the same manner as described for piggybacks.

5. Always check specific orders for the infusion rate and sequence of solution or medication administration. Clamp the tubing of the primary solution if ordered to do so.
6. Affix a label to the container. Indicate the medication name, dosage, date and time prepared, rate of infusion, length of infusion time, and the nurse's signature.

Changing to the Next Container of IV Solution

1. Monitor the rate of infusion at least once per hour. When the container nears completion, notify the nurse responsible for adding the next container.
2. Slow the rate to keep the vein open if the level of solution in the container is low.
3. Using aseptic technique, clamp the tubing and quickly exchange the new container for the empty one. Fill the chamber at least half full; then unclamp.
4. Adjust the flow rate as previously described, and inspect the injection site.

Administering Medication by a Venous Access Device

Equipment

Two pair sterile gloves
Antiseptic pledgets
0.9% normal saline in vial
Sterile 10 ml syringe
18 to 22 gauge, ⅝ inch needle
Antiseptic solution or swabsticks
Huber point access needle
Extension tubing

1. Prepare the medication as described before and add to an IV bag or bottle, or leave in a sterile syringe.
2. Insert the administration set into the IV container, prime the IV line to remove all air, and cover the end of the IV line with a sterile cap.
3. Take all supplies and IV medication to the patient's bedside.
4. Identify the patient using the bracelet and explain what you are going to do.
5. Palpate the site where the venous access device is to be implanted.
6. Open the sterile gloves, using the package as a sterile field; drop the sterile syringe, Huber needle, and extension tubing on the sterile field.
7. Don sterile gloves and assemble the 10 ml syringe and 18 gauge needle; withdraw 10 ml normal saline from the vial (the hand touching the saline vial is CONTAMINATED); maintain sterility of the saline-filled syringe while dropping it onto the sterile field; remove and discard gloves.
8. Reglove; assemble saline syringe and extension tubing; prime the extension tubing line; clamp the tubing; attach to Huber needle.
9. Use the nondominant gloved hand to cleanse the site of the venous access device; cleanse from intended site of insertion outward in ever-widening circles. Repeat cleansing process two more times. Allow antiseptic to dry, then repeat cleansing process using isopropyl alcohol.
10. Using the sterile gloved hand, grasp the Huber needle by the winged flanges and insert the needle perpendicular to the patient's skin until the needle tip comes in contact with the bottom of the port.
11. Unclamp the extension tubing and withdraw the plunger of the saline syringe slightly until blood returns; inject normal saline to flush port of heparin; attach syringe with medication or IV infusion of medication using a piggyback container. Administer medication as prescribed by the bolus technique or provide support for the IV line that is attached to the Huber needle and tape it in place. Following completion of the administration of the medication, flush the line and refill the port with heparinized solution according to the practice setting policy. Maintain steady pressure on the plunger of the syringe as the needle is withdrawn from the access device to prevent the backflow of blood. Cleanse injection site with an antiseptic pledget following the removal of the Huber needle.
12. Dispose of used needles into a puncture resistant container. Dispose of used extension tubing and other supplies according to institution policy. Remove gloves and dispose according to policy. Wash hands thoroughly.
13. Document in the patient's record the medication administered and how well the procedure was tolerated.

Central Venous Catheter Care

Equipment

Clean gloves
Sterile gloves
Bag to discard old dressing
Antiseptic solution/swabsticks (for example, povidone-
   iodine, alcohol, chlorhexidine)
Dressing change kit or dressing supplies
Mask or cap
Antibiotic ointment

1. Assemble needed supplies; wash hands thoroughly; don clean gloves.
2. Explain procedure to the patient; position patient appropriately for access.
3. Remove old dressing; discard dressing and gloves used to remove the dressing into an impenetrable bag.
4. Inspect the catheter site thoroughly; report any signs of infection.
5. Open a sterile dressing tray and use this as a sterile field; put on a mask and don sterile gloves.
6. Clean the skin around the catheter site by starting at the catheter and wiping outward in ever-widening circles. Repeat this cleansing process three times using a new sterile antiseptic swab each time.
7. Cleanse the outside of the catheter with a new sterile antiseptic swab. Start at the insertion site and cleanse distally along the catheter.
8. Apply antiseptic ointment (for example, povidone iodine) to the catheter insertion site.
9. Apply the dressing (occlusive or gauze), being careful not to contaminate the outside of the dressing. Remove gloves and dispose of them. Cleanse the exposed portion of the catheter with alcohol; secure catheter. Wash hands thoroughly.
10. Label dressing with date and time changed and initials of nurse performing the procedure.
11. Document procedure in chart.

Discontinuing an Intravenous Infusion

You will need the following equipment to discontinue an IV infusion:

Tourniquet
Sterile sponges
Gloves
Dressing materials
Tape
Puncture-resistant container for needles, butterfly or other types of IV catheter

Perform the following technique:

1. Check the physician's orders. Verify that all intravenous solutions and medications have been completed.

2. Check the patient's identity using the bracelet before discontinuing the intravenous solutions.
3. Explain what you are going to do.
4. Adequately expose the intravenous site.
5. Clamp the intravenous tubing.
6. Loosen the tape at the venipuncture site while simultaneously stabilizing the needle to prevent venous damage. If the IV site is contaminated by blood or drainage, don gloves before handling the tape.
7. Review hospital policy regarding the placement of a tourniquet. (Some health care agencies state that a tourniquet should be applied prior to removal of the needle or intravenous catheter in case the tip breaks during removal. Other agencies state that the tourniquet should be loosely attached to the limb, but not tightened unless necessary.)
8. Put on gloves.
9. Using a gauze pad, gently apply pressure with the nondominant hand to the venipuncture site. Withdraw the needle, pulling out parallel to the skin surface. Inspect the tip of the needle or catheter to be sure it is intact. Release the tourniquet, if in place. Place the needle in the puncture-resistant container.
10. Cleanse the area if contaminated with any blood or fluid.
11. Continue to hold the IV site firmly until all bleeding ceases. If the venipuncture site was in the antecubital fossa, have the patient flex the elbow to hold the gauze in place.
12. Check for bleeding after 1 to 2 minutes. Remove gauze and discard with other contaminated dressings. Cleanse the area as appropriate.
13. Remove and discard gloves according to policy and wash hands thoroughly.
14. Apply a small dressing as stated by policy.
15. Provide patient comfort.

Provide the RIGHT DOCUMENTATION of termination of intravenous therapy.

1. Chart the date and time of termination.
2. Perform and record regular patient assessments (site data, size of site and color of skin at injection site).
3. Chart and report any signs of adverse effects (redness, warmth, swelling, and/or pain at the intravenous site).

Monitoring Intravenous Therapy

Prior to initiating therapy, perform baseline patient assessments to evaluate the patient's current status. Report at appropriate intervals throughout the course of treatment.

The patient and the intravenous site should be checked at least every hour for flow rate, infiltration (tenderness, redness, puffiness), and adverse effects. If the flow rate is falling behind schedule:

1. Check for mechanical obstruction of the tubing (closed clamp, kinking) or filter and either irrigate or change the tubing.
2. Check the drip chamber. If less than half full, squeeze it to fill more completely. (Do not over-fill.)
3. Check to make sure that the IV container is not empty. Also check to make sure the container is higher than 3 feet above the venipuncture site. The incorrect height may inadvertently occur if the patient is repositioned or the bed height is re-adjusted.
4. Check for tubing that has fallen below the veni-puncture site. If a significant amount has fallen, el-evate and carefully coil the tubing near the site of venipuncture.
5. Check to determine whether the bevel of the nee-dle is pushing against the wall of the vein. Do this by CAUTIOUSLY raising or lowering the angle of the needle slightly to see if flow is restored. If so, reposition slightly using a gauze pad in the most appropriate location.
6. Check the temperature of the solution being in-fused. Cold solutions can cause spasms in the vein.
7. Check to assure that a restraint or blood pressure cuff applied to the arm has not interfered with the flow.
8. If it appears that the syringe is clotted, DO NOT attempt to clear the needle by flushing with fluid. This will dislodge the clot and may cause a throm-boembolus. *Aspirate* the needle with a syringe to dislodge the clot.
9. Check medication administration record (MAR) or Kardex for IV medication and intravenous infu-sion orders for the patient(s) assigned. During shift report, identify the exact volume of intravenous solution and/or medication that has been infused on the previous shift and the volume remaining to be infused during the on-coming shift.
10. Immediately after receiving a report on your as-signed patients make rounds to perform a baseline assessment. Data that should be analyzed with ref-erence to IV therapy include:
    • Check that the ordered IV solution with or with-out medications is being administered to the cor-rect patient at the correct rate of infusion.
    • Check the total amount infused against the amount that should have infused. Is the volume of infused IV solution or IV medication "on tar-get," "ahead," or "behind?" Inspect the volume infused strips attached to the infusing solution bag or bottle.
    • Calculate the drip rate. If the IV tubing is run-ning by gravity, adjust it to the correct rate of in-fusion to deliver the milliliters per hour ordered. If an infusion pump is being used, check to be certain the drop sensor is positioned superior to fluid level in the drip chamber and inferior to port where the fluid drops from. Next be certain the infusion pump is set to deliver the prescribed volume (ml) per hour. Since there are several models of infusion pumps available, become thoroughly versed in the operation of this type of infusion pump being used in the practice setting. If in doubt about any facet of its operation, re-quest a service check on the equipment. In addi-tion to being knowledgeable about intravenous medications and solutions, the nurse must have expertise in the operation of the delivery systems used within the practice setting. Computerized equipment is only as good as the individual's op-erating knowledge of the infusion pump.
    • Check for in-line filters. If one is recommended for the medicine being infused, is it being used?
    • Check the date and time the infusing IV solution or IV medication was hung. Identify when the IV solution infusing, administration set and tub-ing, and the IV site needles, IV catheters, and/or dressing are to be changed in accordance with policies of the practice setting.
    • Check the date and time that procedures are or-dered to maintain the patency of the established IV lines. (Follow the practice-setting policies.) The patency of all IV lines used for the *intermit-tent* delivery of IV medications must be main-tained. The following are general guidelines:
      —Peripheral IV lines are usually flushed every 4 to 8 hours, or as stated in institution policy, using 1 to 2 ml of 10 or 100 units/ml hepa-rinized saline solution.
      —Central venous IV lines are usually flushed with 1 to 5 ml of 10 or 100 units/ml of hep-arinized saline solution; however, the intervals for flushing vary (once every 12 hours to one time per week). Always check specific policy of the institution where practicing.
      —Groshong catheters have a two-way valve that prevents backflow; therefore, these catheters do not require heparin. Groshong catheters are flushed with normal saline weekly or at an in-terval determined by institutional policy.
      —The amount of solution used to flush a Hick-man, Broviac, or Groshong catheter varies and must be sufficient to equal the volume required to fill the catheter lumen plus the volume of any extension tubing being utilized.
      —Implantable vascular access devices/ports (for example, Port-a-Cath, Mediport) require that the port be filled with sterile heparinized solu-tion, usually 100 units/ml, after each use. If not accessed regularly, flushes may only be per-

formed once each month or at an interval determined by the employing institution. REMEMBER THAT ONLY A HUBER NEEDLE IS USED TO ACCESS AN IMPLANTABLE VASCULAR ACCESS DEVICE/PORT.

—Whenever flushing a peripheral, central venous, or implantable vascular access device, the nurse should maintain positive pressure on the syringe barrel while simultaneously withdrawing the needle from the site. This will prevent backflow of blood and thus prevent occlusion.

—Prevent damage to any and all short- or long-term central venous catheters by only clamping the catheter with a padded hemostat or a smooth-edged clamp.

—Change the injection caps for lumen hubs on single or multiple lumen central venous catheter every 72 hours or as stated in the institutional policy.

- Check the IV tubing for any obstructions or air in the line. If running by gravity, be sure the tubing is not hanging below the level of the insertion site.
- Check the IV infusion site to validate that the IV is infusing properly into the arterial, peripheral, central venous, or implanted access device. Report and take immediate action if the infusion is infiltrated, improperly infusing, or if signs of infection exist.
- Finally, remain alert at all times for complications associated with IV therapy of any type (for example, phlebitis, infection, air in the tubing, circulatory overload, pulmonary edema, pyogenic reaction, pulmonary embolism, or drug reactions from the IV medications).
- Document all findings and procedures performed in association with IV therapy.

Phlebitis or infection

If signs of redness, warmth, swelling, and burning pain along the course of the vein are present, infection or phlebitis may be developing. Confirm the presence of these signs with the supervising nurse; then discontinue the IV. Insert a new IV using all new equipment at a different site. Many hospitals also require that the infection control nurse be notified, and that the site of phlebitis or infection be treated with hot or cold compresses. If purulent drainage is present, obtain a sample of the drainage for culture and sensitivity. If a fever and chills accompany these symptoms, a blood culture may also be indicated. Check practice setting policies about whether a physician's order is necessary to do this, or whether standing orders exist as part of the infection control procedures that mandate these actions.

Extravasation

Inspect the IV site at regular intervals for extravasation. Whenever a change in the limb's color, size, or skin integrity is observed, compare with the opposite limb. Apply a tourniquet *proximal* to the infusion site to constrict the flow. Continued flow with the tourniquet in place confirms infiltration. DO NOT rely on blood backflow into the tubing when the container is lowered. The venipuncture site could still be patent, but a laceration in the vessel may allow extravasation. Know the policies of your institution concerning the treatment of extravasation. Here are some general guidelines:

1. Stop the infusion.
2. Elevate the affected limb.
3. Remove the needle, as described above.
4. Apply heat to the site of extravasation to produce vasodilation and drug absorption.
5. Contact the physician for the possible use of antidotes to minimize tissue damage.

Air in tubing

If an air bubble is found in IV tubing, clamp the tubing immediately. Swab either the injection site in the rubber hub near the needle or the "piggyback" portal (whichever is closest to the air bubble) with an antiseptic sponge. Using sterile technique, insert a needle and syringe into the entry site below the air bubble and withdraw the air pocket.

If air has actually entered the patient via the IV tubing, turn the patient on the left side with the head in a dependent position. Administer oxygen and notify the physician immediately.

Circulatory overload and pulmonary edema

Signs of circulatory overload due to excessive volumes of fluid are engorged neck veins, dyspnea, reduced urine output, edema, bounding pulse, and shallow, rapid respirations. The signs of pulmonary edema are dyspnea, cough, anxiety, rales, rhonchi, and frothy sputum. When these symptoms develop, slow the IV immediately to a "keep open" rate. Place the patient in a sitting position, start oxygen, collect vital signs, and summon the physician immediately. Gather equipment for application of rotating tourniquets, but do not apply until an order is received.

Pyrogenic reaction

A pyrogenic reaction should be suspected if the patient develops sudden onset of chills, fever, headache, nausea, and vomiting. Check the patient's vital signs, stop the IV, and notify the physician of the findings immediately.

Save the unused portion of solution. Return it to the pharmacy or laboratory for testing as specified by hospital policy.

Pulmonary embolism

A pulmonary embolus may occur from foreign materials injected into the vein or from a blood clot that breaks loose. Emboli can be prevented by (1) using an in-line filter, (2) completely dissolving any medications added to a solution, (3) using proper diluents for reconstitution, (4) using IV solutions that are clear and have no visible signs of foreign matter or precipitate, and (5) avoiding the use of veins in the lower extremities.

Documentation

Provide the RIGHT DOCUMENTATION of the medication administration and responses to drug therapy:

1. Chart the date, time, drug name, dosage, and route of administration.
2. Perform and record regular patient assessments for the evaluation of the therapeutic effectiveness (blood pressure, pulse, intake and output, lung-field sounds, respiratory rate, pain at infusion site, etc.).
3. Chart and report any signs and symptoms of adverse drug effects.
4. Perform and validate essential patient education about the drug therapy, and other essential aspects of intervention for the disease process affecting the individual.
5. Chart dressing changes performed and cite any signs and symptoms of complications at the needle or central venous catheter site (for example, redness, tenderness, swelling, drainage).
6. Chart date and times that procedures are performed to maintain the patency of the IV needle, central venous catheter, or port (for example, heparinized flush or, for Groshong catheter, the saline flush).
7. Perform and validate essential patient education about the drug therapy, site or central venous catheter care, dressing care, or flushing of the IV system being used to administer medication. Always teach the patient (and/or significant others) signs and symptoms of complications that should be reported immediately to the physician. Depending on the type of IV delivery system being used to administer the medication, instruct persons being treated on an outpatient or home health setting when to return for the catheter to be changed and when to return for the next visit to the physician or clinic.

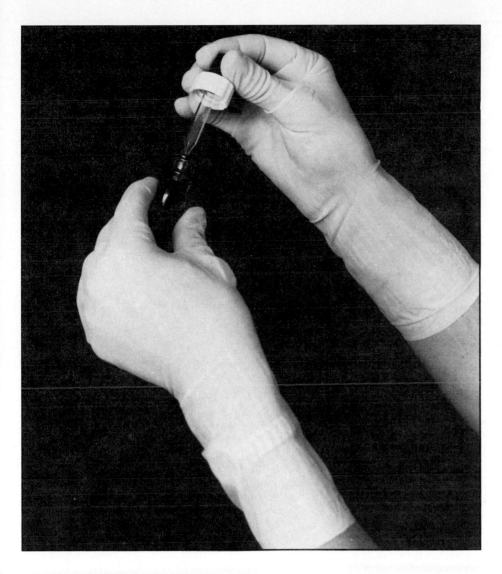

CHAPTER 7

Preparation and Administration of Medication by Percutaneous Routes

CHAPTER GOALS

After completing this chapter, the student should be able to do the following:

1. Give a detailed description of the dosage forms and procedures used to prepare and administer medications via the percutaneous routes.

2. Cite the specific methods used to document medication administration and therapeutic effectiveness of drugs administered via the percutaneous routes.

3. Utilize the procedures and principles cited for the preparation and administration of medications via the percutaneous routes at the practice setting.

4. Apply the Centers for Disease Control recommendations for prevention of HIV transmission.

5. Incorporate patient teaching as a part of the medication administration procedure.

6. Chart the health teaching performed.

ADMINISTRATION OF TOPICAL MEDICATIONS TO THE SKIN

Absorption of topical medications can be influenced by the drug concentration, the length of time the medication is in contact with the skin, the size of the affected area, the thickness of the skin, the hydration of tissues, and the degree of skin disruption.

Percutaneous administration refers to application of medications to the skin or mucous membranes for absorption. Methods of percutaneous administration include topical application of ointments, creams, powders, or lotions to the skin, instillation of solutions onto the mucous membranes of the mouth, eye, ear, nose, or vagina, and inhalation of aerosolized liquids or gases for absorption through the lungs. The primary advantage of the percutaneous route is that the action of the drug, in general, is localized to the site of application, which reduces the incidence of systemic side effects. Unfortunately, the medications are sometimes messy and difficult to apply. In addition they usually have a short duration of action and thus require more frequent reapplication.

ADMINISTRATION OF CREAMS, LOTIONS, AND OINTMENTS

OBJECTIVES

1. Describe the topical forms of medications used on the skin.
2. Cite the equipment needed and techniques utilized to apply each of the topical forms of medications to the skin surface.

KEY WORDS

creams
lotions
ointments

Dosage Forms

Creams

Creams are semisolid emulsions containing medicinal agents for external application. The cream base is generally nongreasy and can be removed with water. Many available over-the-counter creams are used as moisturizing agents.

Lotions

Lotions are usually aqueous preparations that contain suspended materials. They are commonly used as soothing agents to protect the skin and relieve rashes and itching. Some lotions have a cleansing action, whereas others have an astringent or drawing effect. To prevent increased circulation and itching, lotions should be gently but firmly patted on the skin, rather than rubbed in. Shake all lotions thoroughly immediately before application and use sparingly to avoid waste.

Ointments

Ointments are semisolid preparations of medicinal substances in an oily base such as lanolin or petrolatum. This type of preparation can be applied directly to the skin or mucous membrane and generally cannot be removed by water. The base helps keep the medicinal substance in prolonged contact with the skin.

Wet dressings

Solutions frequently used for wet dressings include potassium permanganate, silver nitrate, or Burow's solution. When used, these substances are added to plain water or physiologic saline at room temperature. If making the potassium permanganate from tablets, always strain the solution PRIOR to use. Potassium permanganate and silver nitrate *stain everything*. Use measure to prevent unnecessary staining.

Equipment

Prescribed cream, lotion, or ointment
2 × 2 gauze sponges
Cotton-tipped applicators
Tongue blade
Gloves

Sites

Skin surfaces affected by the disorder being treated.

Techniques

1. Wash hands and assemble the equipment.
2. Use the 5 RIGHTS of medication preparation and

administration throughout the procedure.
RIGHT PATIENT
RIGHT DRUG
RIGHT ROUTE OF ADMINISTRATION
RIGHT DOSAGE
RIGHT TIME OF ADMINISTRATION

3. Provide privacy for the patient and give a thorough explanation of what you are going to do.
4. Place the patient in a position so the surface where the topical materials are to be applied is exposed. Assess current status of symptoms. Provide for patient comfort before starting therapy.
5. Cleansing: Follow the specific orders of the physician for cleansing of the site of application. *Oil-based* products may be removed with cottonseed oil and gauze. *Coal tar* products may be removed with corn oil and gauze. *Water- or alcohol-based* products may be removed with soap and water or water alone.
6. Application: Use gloves during the application process. Many of the agents used may be absorbed through the skin of both the patient and the person applying the medication. *Lotions:* Shake well until a uniform appearance of the solution is obtained. *Ointments or creams:* Use a tongue blade to remove the desired amount from a wide-mouth container; squeeze the amount needed onto a tongue blade or cotton-tipped applicator from a tube-type container. Apply lotions firmly, but gently, by dabbing the surface. Apply ointments and creams with a gloved hand using firm but gentle strokes. Creams are gently rubbed into the area.
7. Dressings: Check specific orders regarding the type of dressing to be used. If a dressing is to be applied, spread the prescribed amount of ointment directly on the dressing material with a tongue blade; the impregnated dressing material can then be applied to the affected skin surface. Secure the dressing in place.
8. Wet dressings: Wring out wet dressings to prevent dripping. Always completely remove and reapply potassium permanganate or silver nitrate dressings to prevent excessive chemical irritation from buildup of residue at the site of application. Secure the dressing in place. A binder or Montgomery tapes may be needed for dressings requiring frequent changes.
9. Clean up the area and equipment used and make sure the patient is comfortable after the application procedure.
10. Wash hands.

Patient Teaching

1. If appropriate, teach the patient to apply the medication and dressings.
2. Teach personal hygiene measures appropriate to the underlying cause of the skin condition (for example, acne, contact dermatitis, infection).
3. When dressings are ordered, discuss materials readily available at home, such as clean, old muslin sheets or cloth diapers with no cotton filling. Or suggest the purchase of gauze and other necessary supplies.
4. Stress gentleness and moderation in the amount of medication to be applied.
5. Emphasize that the patient must avoid touching or scratching the affected area.
6. Tell the patient to wash hands before and after touching the affected area or applying the medication. Stress the prevention of spread of infection, when present.

Documentation

Provide the RIGHT DOCUMENTATION of the medication administration and responses to drug therapy.

1. Chart the date, time, drug name, dosage, and route of administration.
2. Perform and record regular patient assessments for the evaluation of the therapeutic effectiveness (change in size of affected area, reduced drainage, decreased itching, lowered temperature with an infection, etc.).
3. Chart and report any signs and symptoms of adverse drug effects as well as a narrative description of the area being treated.
4. Develop a written record for the patient to use in charting progress for evaluation of the effectiveness of the treatments being used. List the patient symptoms (such as rash on lower leg with redness and vesicles present; decubitus ulcer on the sacrum). List the data to be collected regarding the medication prescribed and the effectiveness (such as vesicles now crusted, weeping, or appear to be drying; redness in lower leg is lessening; area of decubitus is extending, remaining the same, or shrinking).
5. Perform and validate essential patient education about the drug therapy and other essential aspects of intervention for the disease process affecting the individual.

PATCH TESTING FOR ALLERGENS
OBJECTIVES

1. Describe the procedure used and purpose of performing patch testing.
2. Describe specific charting methods used with allergy testing.

KEY WORDS
patch testing
allergen
antibody
antigen

Patch testing is a method used to identify patient's sensitivity to contact materials (such as soaps, pollens, dyes, etc.). The suspected allergens (antigens) are placed in direct contact with the skin surface and covered with nonsensitizing, nonabsorbent tape. Unless marked irritation appears, the patch is usually left in place for 48 hours, then removed. The site is left open to air for 15 minutes, and then "read." A positive reaction is noted by the presence of redness and swelling, and indicates allergy to the specific antigen.

Intradermal tests may also be used to determine allergenicity to specific antigens. See Chapter 6 for further information on intradermal administration of allergens.

Equipment

Alcohol for cleansing the area
Solutions of suspected antigens
2 × 2 inch pieces of typewriter paper
1 × 1 inch gauze pads
Droppers
Mineral or olive oil
Water
Hypoallergenic tape
Record for charting data on substances applied and responses

Sites

The back, arms, or thighs are commonly used. (DO NOT use the face or areas receiving friction from clothing.) Selected areas are spaced every 2 to 3 inches apart. The type of allergen applied and the site of application are documented on the patient's chart (Figure 7-1). Hair is shaved from sites to ensure that the antigen is kept in close contact with the skin surface, thereby preventing a false-negative reaction.

Technique

CAUTION: DO NOT start any type of allergy testing unless emergency equipment is available in the immediate area in case of an anaphylactic response. Personnel should be familiar with the procedure to follow if an emergency does arise.

1. Check with the patient before starting the testing to be sure that he or she has not taken any antihistamines or anti-inflammatory agents (such as aspirin, ibuprofen, corticosteroids) for 24 to 48 hours preceding the tests. If the patient has taken an antihistamine or anti-inflammatory agent, check with the physician before proceeding with the testing.
2. Wash hands and assemble the equipment.
3. Use the 5 RIGHTS of medication preparation and administration throughout the procedure.

RIGHT PATIENT
RIGHT DRUG
RIGHT ROUTE OF ADMINISTRATION
RIGHT DOSAGE
RIGHT TIME OF ADMINISTRATION

4. Provide privacy for the patient and give a thorough explanation of what you are going to do.
5. Place the patient in a position so the surface where the test materials are to be applied is horizontal. Provide patient comfort before starting testing.
6. Cleanse the selected area thoroughly using an alcohol pledget. Use circular motions starting at the planned site of injection and continuing outward in ever-widening circular motions to the periphery. Allow the area to air-dry.
7. Prepare the designated solutions using aseptic technique.
8. Follow specific directions of the employing health-care agency for the application of liquid and solid forms of suspected allergens. Generally, a dropper is used to apply suspected liquid contact-type materials; solid materials are applied directly to the skin surface and then moistened with mineral or olive oil.
9. After application, each area used should be covered first with a 1 × 1 gauze followed by a 2 × 2 piece of typewriter paper; secure with hypoallergenic tape. (If the patient is known to be allergic to all types of tape, then consider the use of a binder.)

or

Designated amounts of standardized-strength chemical solutions are arranged in metal receptacles that are backed with hypoallergenic adhesive. These are applied to the selected site. It is important to identify the contents of each receptacle correctly.

or

Patches impregnated with designated antigens are available for direct application to the prepared site(s).

10. Chart the times, agents, concentrations, and amounts applied. Make a diagram in the patient's chart numbering each location. Record what agent and concentration was placed at each site. Subsequent readings of each area are then performed and charted on this record.
11. Follow directions for the time of the reading of the skin testing being performed. Inspection of the testing sites should be performed in good light. Generally, a positive reaction (development of a wheal) to a dilute strength of suspected allergen is considered clinically significant. Measure the diameter of erythema in millimeters and palpate and measure the size of any induration. Record this information in the patient's chart. No reaction should be noted at the control site.

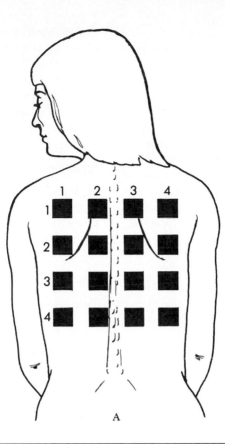

A

DATE:	TIME:	AGENT	CONCENTRATION	AMOUNT INJECTED	SITE NUMBER:*	Reading Time in Hours or minutes i.e. 30 min. or 24, 48, 72 hours		

Patient Name: _____

Identification Number: _____

Physician Name: _____

* Refer to diagram of sites, Figure 6.24a,b.
—Follow directions for the "reading" of the skin testing performed.
—Inspect sites in a good light
—Record reaction in upper half of box using the following guidelines, i.e.,
    +   (1⁺) Redness of skin present (erythema)
    + +   (2⁺) Redness and solid elevated lesion up to 5 mm in diameter (erythema and papules).
    + + +   (3⁺) Erythema, papules and vesicles (blister-like areas 5 mm or less in diameter).
    + + + + (4⁺) Generalized fusing of blisters.
—Record measurement of induration (process of hardening) in mm. in lower half of box, i.e.,

B

Figure 7-1 *Patch test for contact dermatitis.* **A,** *Patch testing sites.* **B,** *Reading chart, patch testing.*

Patient Teaching

1. Tell the patient the time, date, and place of the return visit to have the test sites read.
2. Tell the patient not to take a bath or shower until the patches are read and removed. Explain the need to avoid activities that could cause excessive perspiration.
3. If the patient develops an area of severe burning or itching, lift the patch and gently wash the area. Tell the patient to report immediately the development of any breathing difficulty, severe hives, or rashes. The patient should be told to go to the nearest emergency room if unable to reach the physician who prescribed the skin tests.

Documentation

Provide the RIGHT DOCUMENTATION of the medication administration and responses to drug therapy.

1. Chart the date, time, drug name, dosage, and site of administration (Figure 7-1).
2. Read each site 24-48-72 hours after the application, as directed by the physician or policy of the health care agency. Additional readings may be required up to 5 days after application.
3. Chart and report any signs and symptoms of adverse drug effects.
4. Perform and validate essential patient education about the testing and other essential aspects of intervention for the disease process affecting the individual.

Commonly used readings of reactions and appropriate symbols are listed below.

+	(1+)	Redness of skin present (erythema)
++	(2+)	Redness and solid elevated lesions up to 5 mm in diameter (erythema and papules)
+++	(3+)	Erythema, papules, and vesicles (blisterlike areas 5 mm or less in diameter)
++++	(4+)	Generalized fusing of blistered areas

ADMINISTRATION OF NITROGLYCERIN OINTMENT

OBJECTIVES

1. Identify the equipment needed, sites used, techniques utilized, and patient education required when nitroglycerin ointment is prescribed.
2. Describe specific documentation methods utilized to record the therapeutic effectiveness of nitroglycerin ointment therapy.

Dosage Form

Nitroglycerin ointment (Nitro-Bid, Nitrol) provides relief of anginal pain for several hours longer than sublingual preparations. When properly applied, nitroglycerin ointment is particularly effective against nocturnal attacks of anginal pain. Specific instructions for nitroglycerin ointment are reviewed in this text because it is the only ointment currently available for which dosage is critical to the success of use. (See Chapter 11, "Drugs Affecting the Cardiovascular System.")

Equipment

Nitroglycerin ointment
Applicator paper
Clear plastic wrap
Nonallergenic adhesive tape

Sites

Any area without hair may be used. Most people prefer the chest, flank, or upper arm areas (Figure 7-2). (Do NOT shave an area to apply the ointment; shaving may cause skin irritation.)

Techniques

1. Wash hands and assemble the equipment.
2. Use the 5 RIGHTS of medication preparation and administration throughout the procedure.
   RIGHT PATIENT
   RIGHT DRUG
   RIGHT ROUTE OF ADMINISTRATION

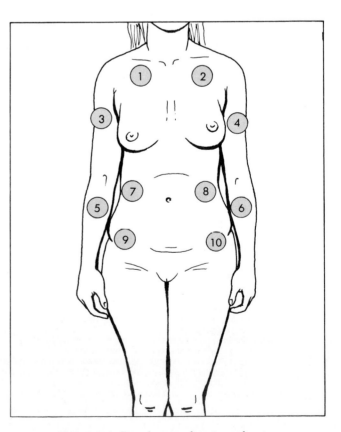

Figure 7-2 *Sites for nitroglycerin application.*

RIGHT DOSAGE
RIGHT TIME OF ADMINISTRATION

3. Provide privacy for the patient and give a thorough explanation of what you are going to do.

4. Place the patient in a position so the surface where the topical materials are to be applied is exposed. Provide patient comfort before starting therapy. *Note:* When reapplying ointment, remove plastic wrap, remove dose-measuring applicator paper from prior dose and cleanse the area of remaining ointment on the skin surface. Select a new site for application of the medication then proceed with steps 5 through 9 below.

5. Lay the dose-measuring applicator paper with the print side DOWN on the site (Figure 7-3, A). (The ointment will smear the print.)

6. Squeeze a ribbon of ointment of the proper length onto the applicator paper.

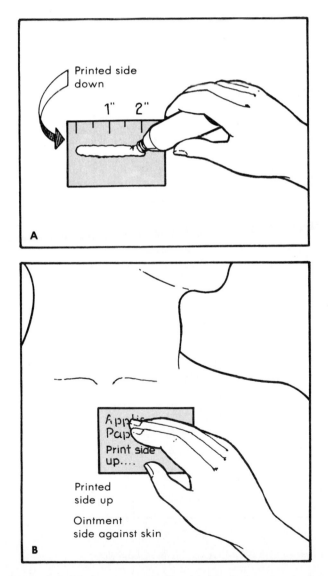

Figure 7-3 *Administering nitroglycerin topical ointment.* **A,** *Lay applicator paper print side down, and measure ribbon of ointment.* **B,** *Apply applicator to skin site, ointment side down. Spread in a uniform layer under applicator; leave paper in place.*

7. Place the measuring applicator on the skin surface at the site chosen on the rotation schedule, ointment side DOWN. Spread in a thin, uniform layer under the applicator. DO NOT RUB IN. Leave the paper in place. NOTE: Use of the applicator paper allows you to measure the prescribed dose and prevents absorption through the fingertips as you apply the medication (Figure 7-3, B).

8. Cover the area where the paper is placed with plastic wrap and tape it in place.

9. Wash hands after applying the ointment.

Patient Teaching

1. Guide the patient in learning how to apply the ointment.

2. Tell the patient that the medication may discolor clothing. Use of clear plastic wrap protects clothing.

3. When the dose is regulated properly, the ointment may be used every 3 to 4 hours and at bedtime.

4. Tell the patient to wash hands after application to remove any nitroglycerin that came in contact with the fingers.

5. When terminating the use of this topical ointment, the dose and frequency of application should be gradually reduced over a 4- to 6-week period. Tell the patient to contact the physician if he or she feels that the dosage needs to be adjusted. Encourage the patient not to discontinue the medication abruptly. (See Chapter 11, "Drugs Affecting the Cardiovascular System," for further information.)

Documentation

Provide the RIGHT DOCUMENTATION of the medication administration and responses to drug therapy.

1. Chart the date, time, drug name, dosage, site, and route of administration.

2. Perform and record regular patient assessment for the evaluation of therapeutic effectiveness (blood pressure, pulse, output, degree and duration of pain relief, etc.).

3. Chart and report any signs and symptoms of adverse drug effects.

4. Perform and validate essential patient education about the drug therapy and other essential aspects of intervention for the disease process affecting the individual.

ADMINISTRATION OF TRANSDERMAL DRUG DELIVERY SYSTEMS
OBJECTIVES

1. Identify the equipment needed, sites used, techniques utilized, and patient education required when transdermal medication systems are prescribed.

2. Describe specific documentation methods utilized to

record the therapeutic effectiveness of medications administered using a transdermal delivery system.

KEY WORD
transdermal disks

Dosage Form

The transdermal patch provides controlled release of a prescribed medication (e.g., nitroglycerin, clonidine, estrogen, nicotine, scopolamine) through a semipermeable membrane for 24 hours when applied to intact skin. The dosage released depends upon the surface area of the disk in contact with the skin surface and the individual drug. See specific monographs for onset and duration of action of drugs using this delivery system.

Equipment

Transdermal disk
Shaving equipment as appropriate for the site and skin condition

Sites

Any area without hair may be used. Most people prefer the chest, flank, or upper arm areas. Develop a rotation schedule for use (Figure 7-2).

Techniques

1. Wash hands and assemble the equipment.
2. Use the 5 RIGHTS of medication preparation and administration throughout the procedure.
   RIGHT PATIENT
   RIGHT DRUG
   RIGHT ROUTE OF ADMINISTRATION
   RIGHT DOSAGE
   RIGHT TIME OF ADMINISTRATION
3. Provide for patient privacy and give a thorough explanation of what is to be done.
4. Place the patient in a position so the surface where the topical materials are to be applied is exposed. Provide for patient comfort. NOTE: When reapplying a transdermal disk, remove the old disk and cleanse thoroughly. Select a new site for application.

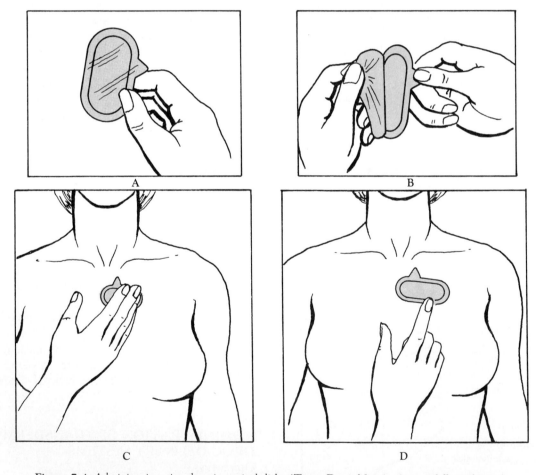

Figure 7-4 *Administering nitroglycerin topical disks (Trans-Derm Nitro).* **A,** *carefully pick up the system lengthwise, with the tab up.* **B,** *Remove clear plastic backing from system at the tab. Do not touch inside of exposed system.* **C,** *Place the exposed adhesive side of the system on the chosen skin site; press firmly with the palm of the hand.* **D,** *Circle the outside edge of the system with one or two fingers. (Courtesy of CIBA Pharmaceutical Co., Summit, N.J.)*

5. Apply the small adhesive topical disk. Figure 7-4, *A-D* illustrates nitroglycerin being applied to one of the sites recommended by the rotation schedule. The frequency of application will depend on the specific medication being applied in the transdermal disk and the duration of action of the prescribed medication. Nitroglycerin is applied once daily whereas clonidine is applied once every 7 days.
6. Wash hands after application.

Patient Teaching

1. Guide the patient in learning how and when to apply the disks. NOTE: Trans-Derm Nitro and Nitrodur may be worn while showering; Nitrodisc should be replaced after bathing or showering. Scopolamine, used for motion sickness, must be applied at least four hours prior to travel. Clonidine transdermal systems are applied once every 7 days.
2. If a disk becomes partially dislodged, the recommendations of the product should be followed. Nitroglycerin disks are removed and a new one is applied. Clonidine transdermal disks, on the other hand, come with a protective adhesive overlay to be applied over the patch to ensure skin contact of the transdermal system should the disk become loosened.
3. Patients receiving nitroglycerin transdermally may require sublingual nitroglycerin for anginal attacks, especially while the dosage is being adjusted.

Documentation

Provide the RIGHT DOCUMENTATION of the medication administration and the responses to drug therapy.

1. Chart the date, time, drug name, dosage, and route of administration.
2. Perform and record regular patient assessments for the evaluation of therapeutic effectiveness (blood pressure, pulse, degree and duration of pain relief, etc.).
3. Chart and report any signs and symptoms of adverse drug effects.
4. Perform and validate essential patient education about the drug therapy and other essential aspects of intervention for the disease process affecting the individual.

ADMINISTRATION OF TOPICAL POWDERS
OBJECTIVE

1. Describe the dosage form, sites utilized, and techniques employed to administer medications in topical powder form.

Dosage Form

Powders are finely ground particles of medication contained in a talc base. They generally produce a cooling, drying, or protective effect where applied.

Equipment

Prescribed powder

Site

To the skin surface of the body, as prescribed.

Technique

1. Wash hands.
2. Use the 5 RIGHTS of medication preparation and administration throughout the procedure.
   RIGHT PATIENT
   RIGHT DRUG
   RIGHT ROUTE OF ADMINISTRATION
   RIGHT DOSAGE
   RIGHT TIME OF ADMINISTRATION
3. Provide privacy for the patient and give a thorough explanation of what you are going to do.
4. Place the patient in a position so the surface where the topical materials are to be applied is exposed. Provide patient comfort before starting therapy.
5. Wash and thoroughly dry the affected area before applying the powder.
6. Apply powder by gently shaking the container. This distributes the powder evenly over the area. Gently smooth over the area for even coverage.

Patient Teaching

Tell the patient to clean and reapply powder to external surface as directed by the physician. The patient should avoid inhaling the powder during application.

Documentation

Provide the RIGHT DOCUMENTATION of the medication administration and the responses to drug therapy.

1. Chart the date, time, drug name, dosage, site, and route of administration.
2. Perform and record regular patient assessments for the evaluation of therapeutic effectiveness.
3. Chart and report any signs and symptoms of adverse drug effects.
4. Perform and validate essential patient education about the drug therapy and other essential aspects of intervention for the disease process affecting the individual.

ADMINISTRATION OF MEDICATIONS TO MUCOUS MEMBRANES

OBJECTIVES

1. Describe the dosage forms, sites, equipment used, and techniques for administration of medications to the mucous membranes.
2. Identify the dosage forms safe for administration to the eye.
3. Describe patient education necessary for patients requiring ophthalmic medications.
4. Compare the techniques utilized to administer ear drops in a child under 3 years of age and in patients over 3 years old.
5. Describe the purpose, precautions necessary, and patient education required for persons requiring medications by inhalation.
6. Describe the dosage forms available for vaginal administration of medications.
7. Identify the equipment needed, site, and specific techniques required to administer vaginal medications or douches.
8. State the rationale and procedure used for cleansing vaginal applicators or douche tips following use.
9. Develop a plan for patient education of persons taking medications via the percutaneous routes.

KEY WORDS

buccal	aerosols
ophthalmic	metered dose inhalers
otic	nebulae

Drugs are well absorbed across mucosal surfaces, and it is easy to obtain therapeutic effects. However, mucous membranes are highly selective in absorptive activity and differ in sensitivity. In general, aqueous solutions are quickly absorbed from mucous membranes, whereas oily liquids are not. Drugs in suppository form can be used for local effects on the mucous membranes of the vagina, urethra, or rectum. A drug may be inhaled and absorbed through the mucous membranes of the nose and lungs. It may be dissolved and absorbed by the mucous membranes of the mouth, or applied to the eyes or ears for local action. Or it may be painted, swabbed, or irrigated on a mucosal surface.

Administration of sublingual and buccal tablets

Dosage Forms

Sublingual tablets are designed to be placed under the tongue for dissolution and absorption through the vast network of blood vessels in this area. Buccal tablets are designed to be held in the buccal cavity (between the cheek and molar teeth) for absorption from the blood vessels of the cheek. The primary advantage of these routes of administration is the rapid absorption and onset of action since the drug passes directly into systemic circulation with no immediate pass through the liver, where extensive metabolism usually takes place. Contrary to most other forms of administration to mucous membranes, the action from these dosage forms is usually systemic, rather than localized to the mouth.

Equipment

Prescribed medication. NOTE: The medications available to be administered by this route are forms of nitroglycerin. Once the self-administration technique is taught, the patient should carry the medication or keep it readily available at bedside for use as needed.

Site

Sublingual area (under tongue) (Figure 7-5, A) or buccal pouch (between molar teeth and cheek) (Figure 7-5, B).

Technique

For administration by the nurse

Refer to Chapter 5, "Administration of Solid-Form Oral Medications," for correct technique with either the medication card system or the unit dose system.

1. Wash hands and assemble the equipment.

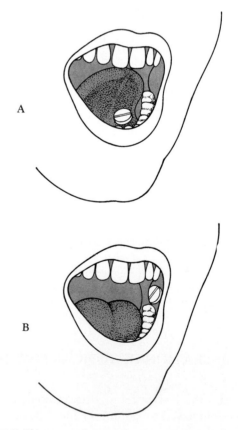

Figure 7-5 *Placing medication in the mouth.* **A,** *Under the tongue (sublingual).* **B,** *In the buccal pouch.*

2. Use the 5 RIGHTS of medication preparation and administration throughout the procedure.
   RIGHT PATIENT
   RIGHT DRUG
   RIGHT ROUTE OF ADMINISTRATION
   RIGHT DOSAGE
   RIGHT TIME OF ADMINISTRATION
3. Provide privacy for the patient and give a thorough explanation of what you are going to do.
4. Put on a glove and place the medication under the tongue (sublingual) (Figure 7-5, A) or between the upper molar teeth and the cheek (buccal) (Figure 7-5, B). The tablet is meant to dissolve in these locations. Do not administer with water. Encourage the patient to allow the drug to dissolve where placed.
5. Remove glove and dispose according to policy.
6. Wash hands thoroughly.

Teaching self-administration

Explain the exact placement of the medication and the dosage and frequency of taking the medication. The patient should be told what side effects to expect, what adverse effects to report, where to carry the medication, how to store the medication, and how to refill the prescription when needed. (See Chapter 11, "Drugs Affecting the Cardiovascular System," Nitroglycerin.)

Documentation

Provide the RIGHT DOCUMENTATION of the medication administration and responses to drug therapy.

1. Chart the date, time, drug name, dosage, site, and route of administration.
2. Perform and record regular patient assessments for the evaluation of therapeutic effectiveness (blood pressure, pulse, degree and duration of pain relief, number of doses taken, etc.).
3. Chart and report any signs and symptoms of adverse drug effects.
4. Perform and validate essential patient education about the drug therapy and other essential aspects of intervention for the disease process affecting the individual.

NOTE: When the patient is self-administering a medication, the nurse is still responsible for all aspects of the charting and monitoring parameters to document the drug therapy and response achieved.

Administration of eye drops and ointment

Dosage Form

Medications for use in the eye should be labeled OPHTHALMIC. If not labeled as such, do not administer to the eye. Ocular solutions are sterile, easily administered, and usually do not interfere with vision when instilled. Allow eye medication to warm to room temperature before administration.

Ocular ointments do cause alterations in visual acuity. However, they have a longer duration of action than solutions.

Always use a separate bottle or tube of eye medication for each patient. (See Chapter 18, "Drugs Affecting the Eye.")

Equipment

Gloves
Eye drops or ointment prescribed (check strength carefully)
Dropper (use only the dropper supplied by the manufacturer)
Paper tissues and/or sterile cotton balls
Sterile eye dressing (pad), as appropriate
Normal saline solution, if needed for cleaning off exudate

Site

Eye(s). O.D. = right eye, O.S. = left eye, O.U. = both eyes.

Techniques

1. Wash hands and assemble *ophthalmic* medication.
2. Use the 5 RIGHTS of medication preparation and administration throughout the procedure.
   RIGHT PATIENT
   RIGHT DRUG
   RIGHT ROUTE OF ADMINISTRATION
   RIGHT DOSAGE
   RIGHT TIME OF ADMINISTRATION
3. Provide privacy for the patient and give a thorough explanation of what you are going to do.
4. Position the patient so that the back of the head is firmly supported on a pillow and the face is directed toward the ceiling. With children, restraints may be necessary if the child is too young to cooperate voluntarily. Always ensure patient safety.
5. Check to be certain that you have the correct medication according to the 5 RIGHTS. Put on gloves. Inspect the affected eye to determine the current status. As appropriate, remove exudate from the eyelid and eyelashes using sterile saline solution. Always use a separate cotton ball for each wiping motion. Start at the inner canthus and wipe outward.
6. Expose the lower conjunctival sac by applying gentle traction to the lower lid at the bony rim of the orbit.
7. Approach the eye from below with the medication dropper or tube of ointment. (Never touch the eye

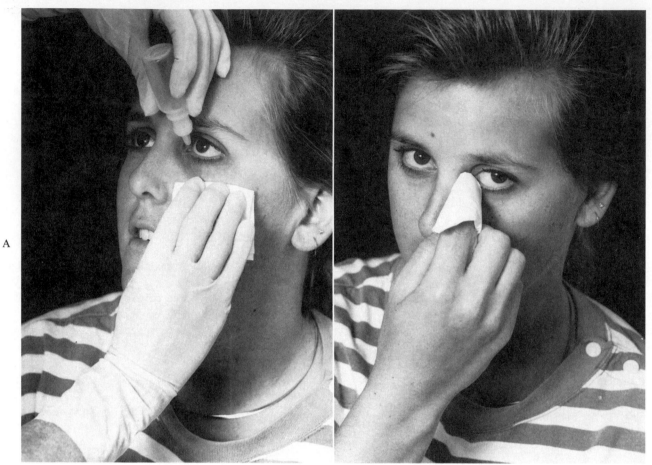

Figure 7-6 *Administering ophthalmic drops.* **A,** *Have the patient look upward; apply gentle traction to lower lid to expose conjunctival sac. Instill drops into sac.* **B,** *Using a tissue, apply gentle pressure to the inner corner of eyelid on bone for 1 to 2 minutes.*

dropper or ointment tip against the eye or face.)
Drops (Figure 7-6):

- Have the patient look upward over your head.
- Drop the specified number of drops into the conjunctival sac. Never drop directly onto the eyeball.
- After instilling the drops, apply gentle pressure, using a cotton ball, to the inner corner of the eyelid on the bone for approximately 1 to 2 minutes. This prevents the medication from entering the canal where it would be absorbed in the vascular mucosa of the nose and produce systemic effects. It also ensures an adequate concentration of medication in the eye.
- When more than one type of eye drop is ordered for the same eye, wait 1 to 5 minutes between instillation of the different medications. Use only the dropper provided by the manufacturer. Apply a sterile dressing as ordered.

Ointment:

- Gently squeeze the ointment in a strip fashion into the conjunctival sac (Figure 7-7). Do not allow the tip to touch the patient.
- Tell the patient to close the eye(s) gently and move the eyes with the lid shut, as if looking around the room, to spread the medication. Apply a sterile dressing as ordered.

8. At conclusion of either procedure remove the gloves and discard according to the policy of the practice setting.
9. Wash hands thoroughly.

Patient Teaching

1. Guide the patient in learning how to apply his or her own ophthalmic medication.
2. Tell the patient to wipe the eye(s) gently from the nose outward to prevent contamination between the eyes and possible spread of infection, and to use a separate tissue to wipe each eye.
3. Have the patient wash hands frequently and avoid touching the eye or immediate areas surrounding it,

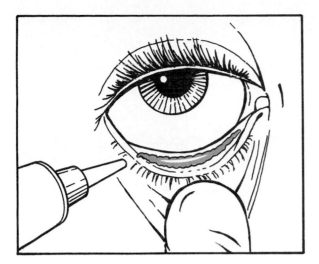

Figure 7-7 *Administering ophthalmic ointment. To instill the ointment, gently pull the lower lid down as patient looks upward. Squeeze ophthalmic ointment into lower sac. Avoid touching tube to eyelid.*

especially when an infection is present. Dispose of tissues in a manner that prevents spread of an infection.

4. Stress punctuality in administration of eye medications, especially when used for treating infections or increased intraocular pressure.
5. Tell the patient to discard eye medications that have changed color, become cloudy, or contain particles. (If the patient's visual acuity is reduced, someone else should check clarity.)
6. The patient must not use over-the-counter eye washes without first consulting the physician managing the eye disorder.
7. Emphasize the need for careful follow-up of any eye disorder until the physician releases the patient from further care.

Documentation

Provide the RIGHT DOCUMENTATION of the medication administration and responses to drug therapy:

1. Chart the date, time, drug name, dosage, site, and route of administration.
2. Perform and record regular patient assessments for the evaluation of therapeutic effectiveness (redness, discomfort, visual activity, changes in infection or inflammatory reaction, degree and duration of pain relief, etc.).
3. Chart and report any signs and symptoms of adverse drug effects.
4. Perform and validate essential patient education about the drug therapy and other essential aspects of intervention for the disease process affecting the individual.

Administration of ear drops

Dosage Form

Ear drops are a solution containing a medication which is used for the treatment of localized infection of inflammation of the ear. Medications for use in the ear should be labeled OTIC. If not labeled as such, do not administer to the ear. Ear drops should be warmed to room temperature before use, and separate bottles of ear drops should be used for each patient.

Equipment

Gloves
Otic solution prescribed
Dropper provided by the manufacturer

Site

Ear(s)

Techniques

1. Review the policy of the practice setting and follow guidelines regarding whether gloves are to be worn during instillation of ear medications.
2. Wash hands and assemble the equipment.
3. Use the 5 RIGHTS of medication preparation and administration throughout the procedure.
   RIGHT PATIENT
   RIGHT DRUG
   RIGHT ROUTE OF ADMINISTRATION
   RIGHT DOSAGE
   RIGHT TIME OF ADMINISTRATION
4. Provide privacy for the patient and give a thorough explanation of what you are going to do.
5. Place the patient in a position so the affected ear is directed upward; don gloves (according to policy).
6. Assess the ear canal for wax accumulation. If wax is present, get an order to irrigate the canal before instilling the ear drops.
7. Allow the medication to warm to room temperature, shake well, and draw up into the dropper.
8. Administration: *Children under 3 years of age:* Restrain the child, turn the head to the appropriate side, and gently pull the earlobe *downward* and *back* (Figure 7-8, A). Instill the prescribed number of drops into the canal. Do not allow the dropper tip to touch any part of the ear. *Children over 3 years of age and adults:* Enlist cooperation, or restrain as necessary, turn the head to the appropriate side, and gently pull the earlobe *upward* and *back* (Figure 7-8, B) to straighten the external auditory canal. Instill the prescribed number of drops into the canal. Do not allow the dropper tip to touch any part of the ear.
9. Have the patient remain on the side for a few min-

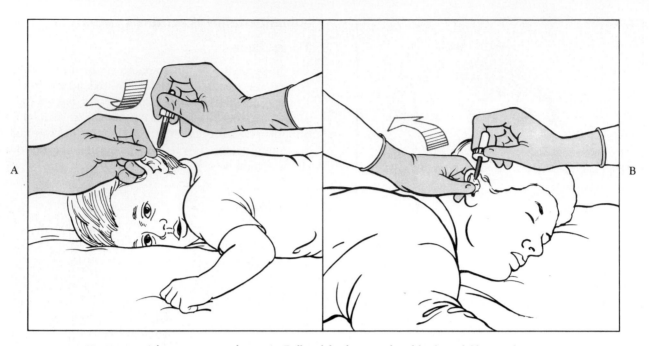

Figure 7-8 *Administering ear drops.* **A,** *Pull earlobe downward and back in children under 3 years of age.* **B,** *Pull earlobe upward and back in patients over 3 years of age.*

utes following instillation; insert a cotton plug *loosely* if ordered.

10. Repeat the procedure if ear drops are ordered for both ears.
11. Remove gloves and dispose according to policy.

Patient Teaching

1. Explain the importance of administering the medication as prescribed.
2. Teach self-administration or administration to another person as appropriate.

Documentation

Provide the RIGHT DOCUMENTATION of the medication administration and the responses to drug therapy:

1. Chart the date, time, drug name, dosage, site, and route of administration.
2. Perform and record regular patient assessments for the evaluation of therapeutic effectiveness (redness, pressure, degree, and duration of pain relief, color and amount of drainage, etc.).
3. Chart and report any signs and symptoms of adverse drug effects.
4. Perform and validate essential patient education about the drug therapy and other essential aspects of intervention for the disease process affecting the individual.

Administration of nose drops

Nasal solutions are used to treat temporary disorders affecting the nasal mucous membrane. Always use the dropper provided by the manufacturer and provide each patient with a separate bottle of nose drops.

Equipment

Gloves
Nose drops prescribed
Dropper supplied by the manufacturer
Tissue to blow the nose

Site

Nostril(s)

Techniques

1. Review the practice setting policy and follow guidelines regarding whether gloves are to be used during the instillation of nose drops to prevent possible contact with body fluid secretions.
2. Wash hands and assemble the equipment.
3. Use the 5 RIGHTS of medication preparation and administration throughout the procedure.
   RIGHT PATIENT
   RIGHT DRUG
   RIGHT ROUTE OF ADMINISTRATION
   RIGHT DOSAGE
   RIGHT TIME OF ADMINISTRATION

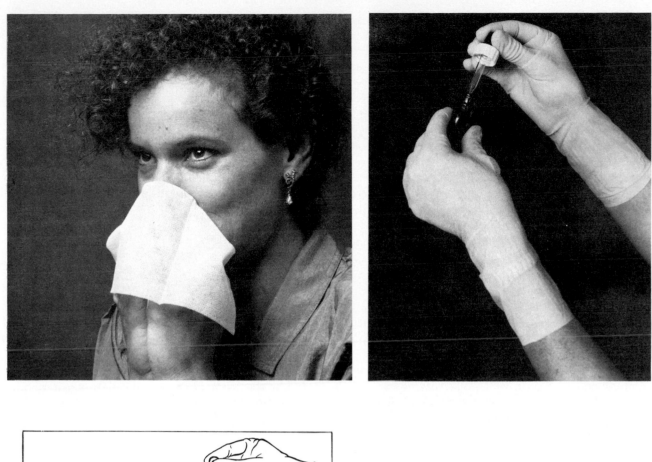

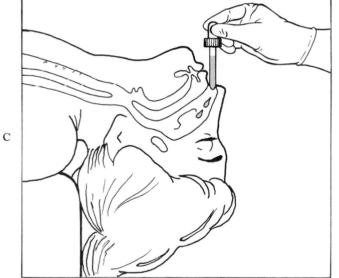

Figure 7-9 *Administering nose drops.* **A,** *Gently blow nose.* **B,** *Open medication and draw up to calibration on dropper.* **C,** *Instill medication. Have patient remain in position for 2 to 3 minutes. Repeat on other side if necessary.*

4. Provide privacy for the patient and give a thorough explanation of what you are going to do.
5. Administration (Figure 7-9):
   Adults and older children
   • Instruct the patient to blow the nose gently.
   • Have the patient lie down and hang the head backward over the edge of the bed.
   • Draw the medication into the dropper. Hold the dropper just above the nostril and instill the medication.

• After a brief time, have the patient turn the head to the other side and repeat the administration process in the second nostril, if needed.
• Have the patient remain in this position for 2 to 3 minutes to allow the drops to remain in contact with the nasal mucosa.
   Infants and young children
• Position the infant or small child with the head over the edge of the bed or pillow. Or, use the "football" hold to immobilize the infant.

- Administer nose drops in the same manner as for the adult.
- For the child who is cooperative, offer praise. Provide appropriate comforting and personal contact for all children or infants.
6. Have paper tissues available for use if absolutely necessary to blow the nose.

Patient Teaching

Guide the patient in learning self-administration of nose drops if necessary. Tell the patient that overuse of the nose drops can cause a "rebound effect," which causes the symptoms to become worse. If symptoms have not resolved after a week of nasal drop therapy, the physician should be consulted again.

Documentation

Provide the RIGHT DOCUMENTATION of the medication administration and responses to drug therapy:

1. Chart the date, time, drug name, dosage, site, and route of administration.
2. Perform and record regular patient assessments for the evaluation of the therapeutic effectiveness (nasal congestion, degree and duration of relief achieved, improvement in overall status, etc.).
3. Chart and report any signs and symptoms of adverse drug effects.
4. Perform and validate essential patient education about the drug therapy and other essential aspects of intervention for the disease process affecting the individual.

Administration of nasal spray

The mucous membranes of the nose absorb aqueous solutions very well. When applied as a spray, the small droplets of solution containing medication coat the membrane and are rapidly absorbed. The advantage of spray over drops is less waste of medication, since some of the drops often run down the back of the throat before absorption can take place. As with drops, each patient should have a personal container of spray.

Equipment

Gloves
Nasal spray prescribed
Paper tissues to blow the nose

Site

Nostril(s)

Techniques

1. Review the policy of the practice setting and follow guidelines regarding whether gloves are to be used during the instillation of nasal sprays.
2. Wash hands and assemble the equipment.
3. Use the 5 RIGHTS of medication preparation and administration throughout the procedure.
   RIGHT PATIENT
   RIGHT DRUG
   RIGHT ROUTE OF ADMINISTRATION
   RIGHT DOSAGE
   RIGHT TIME OF ADMINISTRATION
4. Provide privacy for the patient and give a thorough explanation of what you are going to do.
5. Instruct the patient to gently blow the nose (Figure 7-10, A-C).
6. Sit the patient upright.
7. Block one nostril.
8. Holding the spray bottle upright, shake the bottle.
9. Immediately after shaking, insert the tip into the nostril. Ask the patient to inhale through the open

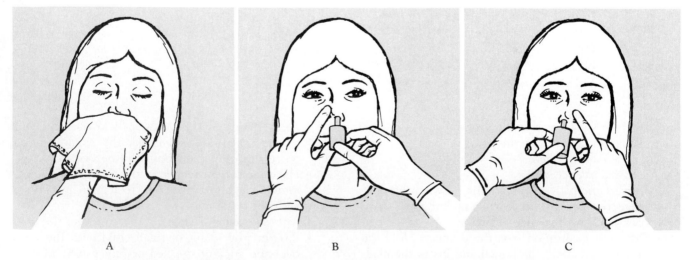

A   B   C

Figure 7-10 *Administering nasal spray.* **A,** *Gently blow nose.* **B,** *Block one nostril; shake bottle, insert tip into nostril and squeeze a puff of spray while inhaling through the open nostril.*

nostril and squeeze a puff of spray into the nostril at the same time.

10. Have paper tissues available for use if absolutely necessary to blow the nose.

Patient Teaching

Guide the patient in learning self-administration of nose drops if necessary. Tell the patient that overuse of nasal spray can cause a "rebound effect," which causes the symptoms to become worse. If symptoms have not resolved after a week of nasal spray therapy, the physician should be consulted again.

Documentation

Provide the RIGHT DOCUMENTATION of the medication administration and responses to drug therapy:

1. Chart the date, time, drug name, dosage, site, and route of administration.
2. Perform and record regular patient assessments for the evaluation of therapeutic effectiveness (nasal congestion, degree and duration of relief achieved, improvement in overall status, etc.).
3. Chart and report any signs and symptoms of adverse drug effects.
4. Perform and validate essential patient education about the drug therapy and other essential aspects of intervention for the patient's disease process.

Administration of medications by inhalation

The respiratory mucosa may be medicated by means of inhalation of sprays (nebulae) or aerosols. Nebulae are sprayed into the throat by a nebulizer. Aerosols use a flow of air or oxygen under pressure to disperse the drug throughout the respiratory tract. Oily preparations should not be applied to the respiratory mucosa, as the oil droplets may be carried to the lung and cause lipid pneumonia (see also Chapter 12, "Drugs Affecting the Respiratory System"). Although saliva as a body fluid has not been implicated in the transmission of the HIV at the time of this writing, the practice setting policy manual should reflect current standards of "universal precautions" for all patients and health care personnel. Follow these procedures faithfully to prevent the transmission of this disease.

Equipment

Gloves
Liquid aerosol or spray forms of medications

Site

Respiratory tract

Techniques

1. Wash hands and assemble the equipment.
2. Use the 5 RIGHTS of medication preparation and administration throughout the procedure.
   RIGHT PATIENT
   RIGHT DRUG
   RIGHT ROUTE OF ADMINISTRATION
   RIGHT DOSAGE
   RIGHT TIME OF ADMINISTRATION
3. Provide privacy for the patient and give a thorough explanation of what you are going to do.
4. Place the patient in a sitting position. This allows maximum lung expansion. Don gloves (according to policy).
5. Prepare the medication according to the prescribed directions and fill the nebulizer with diluent. (This may be done before sitting the patient up if time is a factor to the patient's well-being.)
6. Direct the patient to exhale through pursed lips.
7. Put the nebulizer mouthpiece in the mouth: DO NOT seal the lips completely.
8. Activate the inhalation equipment while simultaneously having the patient inhale and breathe to full capacity.
9. Direct the patient to exhale *slowly* through pursed lips.
10. WAIT approximately 1 minute and repeat the sequence according to the physician's directions, or until all of the medication in the nebulizer is used.
11. Clean the equipment according to the manufacturer's directions.
12. Assist the patient to a comfortable position.
13. Remove gloves and wash hands.

Patient Teaching

1. As appropriate to the circumstances, teach the patient or significant others to operate the nebulizer to be used at home.
2. Explain the operation and cleansing of the equipment.
3. Have the patient or significant others administer the treatment using the equipment and medications prescribed for at-home use before discharge.
4. Stress the need to perform the procedure exactly as prescribed and to report any difficulties experienced after discharge for physician evaluation.

Documentation

Provide the RIGHT DOCUMENTATION of the medication administration and responses to drug therapy:

1. Chart the date, time, drug name, dosage, and route of administration.
2. Perform and record regular patient assessments for the evaluation of therapeutic effectiveness (blood

pressure, pulse, improvement or quality of breathing, cough, and productivity, degree and duration of pain relief, ability to operate the nebulizer, activity and exercise restrictions, etc.).
3. Chart and report any signs and symptoms of adverse drug effects.
4. Perform and validate essential patient education about the drug therapy and other essential aspects of intervention for the disease process affecting the individual.

Administration of medications by metered dose inhalers

Dosage Forms

Bronchodilators and corticosteroids may be administered by inhalation through the mouth using an aerosolized, pressurized metered dose inhaler (MDI). The primary advantage of the aerosolized inhalers is that the medication is applied directly to the site of action, the bronchial smooth muscle. Smaller doses are used, with rapid absorption and onset of action. The valve of the pressurized container also helps assure that the same dose of medication is administered with each inhalation.

Approximately 25% of patients do not use the MDIs properly, and therefore do not receive the maximal benefit of the medication. Devices known as "extenders" or "spacers" have been designed for patients who cannot coordinate the release of the medication with inhalation. The extender devices can be adapted to most pressurized canisters of the MDIs. These devices "trap" the aerosolized medication in a chamber that the patient inhales through within a few seconds after releasing the medication into the chamber.

Equipment

Gloves
Prescribed medication packaged in a metered dose inhaler

Site

Respiratory tract

Technique

1. Wash hands and assemble the equipment.
2. Use the 5 RIGHTS of medication preparation and administration throughout the procedure.
   RIGHT PATIENT
   RIGHT DRUG
   RIGHT ROUTE OF ADMINISTRATION
   RIGHT DOSAGE
   RIGHT TIME OF ADMINISTRATION
3. Provide privacy for the patient and give a thorough explanation of what you are going to do; don gloves.

4. (The following principles apply to all metered dose inhalers. Read and adapt the technique to directions provided by the manufacturer for a specific inhaler, and extender if needed.)
   - If the medication is a suspension, shake the canister. This disperses and mixes the active bronchodilator and propellant together.
   - Open the mouth and place the canister outlet 2-4 inches in front of the mouth, or use an "extender." This space allows the propellant to evaporate and prevents large particles from settling in the mouth.
   - Activate the metered dose inhaler and have patient inhale deeply over 10 seconds to ensure that airways are open and that the drug is dispersed as deeply as possible.
   - Have patient hold breath, then exhale slowly to permit the drug to settle into pulmonary tissue.
   - If prescribed, repeat in 2-3 minutes. Using small doses with 2-3 inhalations enhances deposition of the drug in the smaller, peripheral airways for longer therapeutic effect.
   - Cleanse the apparatus according to the manufacturer's recommendations; remove gloves and dispose of according to hospital policy.
   - The patient should not wait until the canister is empty before having the prescription refilled. The last few doses in a canister are often subtherapeutic due to an imbalance in the remaining amounts of medication and propellant.

Patient Teaching

Explain the procedure and allow the patient to demonstrate the technique. Teaching aids of MDIs without active ingredients are available from the pharmacy department to encourage patients to practice the technique prior to medication administration. In addition to technique, the patient should be told what side effects to expect, what adverse effects to report, how to carry the medication, how to store it, and how to have it refilled when needed. (See Chapter 12, "Drugs Affecting the Respiratory System.")

Documentation

Provide the RIGHT DOCUMENTATION of the medication administration and responses to drug therapy:

1. Chart the date, time, drug name, dosage, site and route of administration.
2. Perform and record regular patient assessments for the evaluation of therapeutic effectiveness (blood pressure, pulse, improvement or quality of breathing, cough and productivity, degree and duration of pain relief, ability to operate the metered dose inhaler, activity and exercise restrictions; etc.).
3. Chart and report any signs and symptoms of adverse drug effects.

4. Perform and validate essential patient education about the drug therapy and other essential aspects of intervention for the disease process affecting the individual.

Administration of vaginal medications

Women with gynecologic disorders may require the administration of a medication intravaginally, usually for localized action. Vaginal medications may be creams, jellies, tablets, foams, suppositories, or irrigations (douches). The creams, jellies, tablets, and foams are inserted using special applicators provided by the manufacturer, while suppositories are usually inserted with a gloved index finger. (See Administration of a Vaginal Douche, p. 140.)

Equipment

Prescribed medication
Vaginal applicator
Perineal pad
Water-soluble lubricant (for suppository)
Gloves
Paper towel

Site

Vagina

Techniques

1. Wash hands and assemble the equipment.
2. Use the 5 RIGHTS of medication preparation and administration throughout the procedure.
   RIGHT PATIENT
   RIGHT DRUG
   RIGHT ROUTE OF ADMINISTRATION
   RIGHT DOSAGE
   RIGHT TIME OF ADMINISTRATION
3. Provide privacy for the patient and give a thorough explanation of what you are going to do. Have the patient void to ensure that the bladder is empty. Don gloves.
4. Fill the applicator with the prescribed tablet, jelly, cream, or foam.
5. Place the patient in the lithotomy position and elevate the hips with a pillow. Drape the patient to prevent unnecessary exposure.
6. Administration. *For creams, foams, and jellies:* With the gloved, nondominant hand, spread the labia to expose the vagina. Assess the status of presenting symptoms (such as color of discharge, volume, odor, level of discomfort). Gently insert the vaginal applicator as far as possible into the vagina and push the plunger to deposit the medication (Figure 7-11). Remove the applicator and wrap it in a pa-

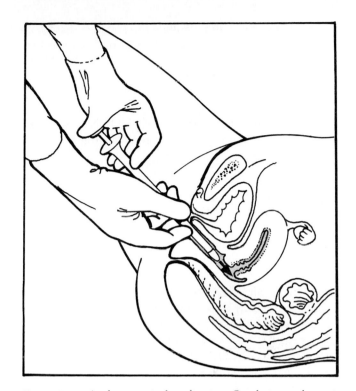

Figure 7-11 *Applying vaginal medication. Gently insert the vaginal applicator as far as possible into the vagina and push plunger to deposit the medication.*

per towel for cleaning later. *For suppositories:* Unwrap a vaginal suppository that has warmed to room temperature and lubricate with a water-soluble lubricant. Lubricate the gloved, dominant index finger. With the gloved, nondominant hand, spread the labia to expose the vagina. Insert the suppository (rounded end first) as far into the vagina as possible with the dominant index finger.
7. Remove glove by turning inside out; place on paper towel for later disposal.
8. Apply a perineal pad to prevent drainage onto the patient's clothing or bed.
9. Instruct the patient to remain in a supine position with hips elevated for 5 to 10 minutes to allow melting and spreading of the medication.
10. Dispose of all waste and wash your hands.

Patient Teaching

1. Guide the patient in learning how to administer the medication correctly.
2. The applicator should be washed in warm soapy water after *each* use.
3. Review personal hygiene measures such as wiping from the front to the back after voiding or defecating.
4. Tell the patient not to douche and to abstain from sexual intercourse after inserting the medication.
5. With most types of infection, both the male and fe-

male partners require treatment. Partners should abstain from sexual intercourse until both partners are cured to prevent reinfections.

Documentation

Provide the RIGHT DOCUMENTATION of the medication administration and responses to drug therapy:

1. Chart the date, time, drug name, dosage, and route of administration.
2. Perform and record regular patient assessments for the evaluation of the therapeutic effectiveness (type of discharge present, irritation of labia, discomfort, degree and duration of pain relief, etc.).
3. Chart and report any signs and symptoms of adverse drug effects.
4. Perform and validate essential patient education about the drug therapy and other essential aspects of intervention for the disease process affecting the individual.

ADMINISTRATION OF A VAGINAL DOUCHE

Douches (irrigants) are used for washing the vagina. This procedure is not necessary for normal female hygiene, but may be required if a vaginal infection and discharge are present. It should also be noted that douches are not effective methods of birth control.

Equipment

IV pole
Gloves
Water-soluble lubricant
Douche bag with tubing and nozzle
Douche solution

Site

Vagina

Techniques

1. Wash hands and assemble the equipment.
2. Use the 5 RIGHTS of medication preparation and administration throughout the procedure.
   RIGHT PATIENT
   RIGHT DRUG
   RIGHT ROUTE OF ADMINISTRATION
   RIGHT DOSAGE
   RIGHT TIME OF ADMINISTRATION
3. Provide privacy for the patient and give a thorough explanation of what you are going to do.
4. Ask the patient to void prior to the procedure.
5. If teaching this procedure to a patient for home use, the patient would customarily recline in a bathtub. Depending on the patient's condition in the hospital, this too could occur. However, it may

be necessary to place the patient on a bedpan and drape for privacy.
6. Hang the douche bag on an IV pole, about 12 inches above the vagina; don gloves; apply water-soluble lubricant to plastic vaginal tip.
7. Cleanse the vulva by allowing a small amount of solution to flow over the vulva and between the labia.
8. Gently insert the nozzle, directing the tip backward and downward 2 to 3 inches.
9. Hold the labia together to facilitate filling the vagina with solution. Rotate nozzle periodically to help irrigate all parts of the vagina.
10. Intermittently release the labia allowing the solution to flow out.
11. When all the solution has been used, remove the nozzle. Have the patient sit up and lean forward to thoroughly empty the vagina.
12. Pat the external area dry.
13. Clean all equipment with warm soapy water after *every* use; rinse with clear water and allow to dry.
14. Thoroughly clean and disinfect the bathtub, if used. Remove gloves and dispose of according to hospital policy.
15. Wash hands.

Patient Teaching

1. Guide the patient in learning how to correctly administer the douche.
2. Explain that the bag and tubing should be washed in warm soapy water after each use so as not to become a source of reinfection.
3. Review personal hygiene measures such as wiping from the front to the back after voiding or defecating.
4. Explain that douching is not recommended during pregnancy.
5. With most types of infection, both the male and female partners require treatment. Partners should abstain from sexual intercourse until both partners are cured to prevent reinfections.

Documentation

Provide the RIGHT DOCUMENTATION of the medication administration and responses to drug therapy:

1. Chart the date, time, drug name, dosage, and route of administration.
2. Perform and record regular patient assessments for the evaluation of therapeutic effectiveness (type of discharge present, irritation of labia, discomfort, degree and duration of pain relief, etc.).
3. Chart and report any signs and symptoms of adverse drug effects.
4. Perform and validate essential patient education about the drug therapy and other essential aspects of intervention for patient's disease process.

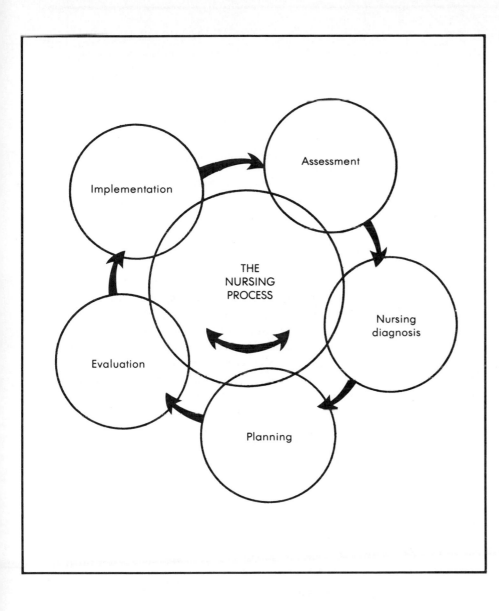

The Nursing Process Applied to Pharmacology

CHAPTER GOALS

After completing this chapter, the student should be able to do the following:

1. Describe the concept of the "nursing process."
2. Use the nursing process to gather and analyze data in order to detect potential problems that may be encountered during the course of the patient's treatment.
3. Describe the nursing responsibilities associated with drug administration.
4. Develop a teaching plan; implement and document actual teaching performed relative to drug therapy and monitoring of the therapeutic regimen.

THE NURSING PROCESS

OBJECTIVES

1. Identify the purpose for using the nursing process methodology.
2. State the five steps in the nursing process and describe in terms of a problem-solving method used in nursing practice.

KEY WORD

nursing process

The practice of nursing is an "art and science" that uses a systematic approach to identify and solve the potential problems individuals may experience as they strive to maintain basic human function along the wellness–illness continuum. The focus of all nursing care is to help individuals maximize their potential for maintaining the highest possible level of independence in meeting self-care needs. Conceptual frameworks of the basis of nursing practice such as Henderson's Complementary-Supplement Model (1980), Roger's Life Process Theory (1979, 1980), Roy's Adaptation Model (1976), and the Canadian Nurses' Association Testing Service (1980) are examples of models used today.

The nursing process is the foundation for the clinical practice of nursing. It provides the framework for consistent nursing actions, using a problem-solving approach rather than an intuitional approach. It provides a systematic method of working with patients to identify potential patient problems, particularly those related to drug therapy, and helps determine what actions must be taken to correct the problems. When implemented properly, it also provides a method to evaluate the outcomes of the therapy delivered. In addition to quality of care, the nursing process provides a scientific, transferable method for health-care planners to assign nursing staff to patients and to determine and justify the cost of providing nursing care in this age of soaring health-care expense.

Some nursing education programs and health-care facilities use a five-step model that includes assessment, nursing diagnosis, planning, implementation, and evaluation. Other programs prefer a four-step model, in which analysis of data (nursing diagnosis in the five-step model) is the final part of the assessment phase, followed by the planning, implementation, and evaluation phases (Table 8-1). The five-step model is used here for purposes of discussion. Regardless of the model used, it is not the number of steps but the quality of nursing care provided and documented by the process that counts.

Nurses should examine the nurses' practice act in the state where they practice to identify the educational and experiential qualifications necessary to perform physical assessment and developing nursing diagnoses. Formulation of nursing diagnoses requires a broad knowledge base to make the discriminating judgments needed to identify the individual patient's care needs. All members of the health care team need to contribute data regarding the patient's care needs and response to the prescribed treatment regimen.

Just as bodily functions are constantly undergoing adjustments to maintain homeostasis in the internal and external environment, so is the nursing process an ongoing, cyclic process that must respond to the changing requirements of the patient. The nurse must continually interact with people in a variety of settings to creatively and cooperatively establish and execute nursing functions to meet the holistic care needs of patients (Figure 8-1).

Assessment

OBJECTIVES

1. Describe the components of the assessment process.
2. Compare current methods used to collect, organize, and analyze information about the health care needs of patients and their significant others.

KEY WORD

assessment

Assessment is an ongoing process that starts with the admission of the patient and is completed at the time of dismissal. It is the problem-identifying phase of the nursing process. The initial assessment must be performed by registered nurses who have the necessary assessment skills to perform the physical examination and the knowledge base to analyze the data assembled and to identify patient problems based on defining characteristics (signs, symptoms, clinical evidence). Further, the nurse should identify risk factors that make an individual or group of persons more vulnerable to develop certain problems in response to a disease process or to the prescribed therapeutic interventions when used (for example, side effects to drugs that may require modification of the regimen).

Table 8-1 *Principles of the Nursing Process*

ASSESSMENT	PLANNING	INTERVENTION	EVALUATION
Collect all relevant data associated with the individual patient's diagnosis to detect potential problems needing intervention. Primary data sources Secondary data sources Tertiary data sources Based on the data collected, formulate a statement of the behaviors or problems of concern and the cause. This is referred to as an "actual" nursing diagnosis when the defining characteristics are present; as a "high-risk" nursing diagnosis when there is a likelihood of the diagnosis developing or being prevented; or as a "possible" nursing diagnosis* when more data are required to substantiate or refute the problem. (Check hospital policies for the level of nursing required for this function.)	Prioritize the problems identified from the assessment data, with the most severe or life-threatening first. Other problems are arranged in descending order of importance. (Maslow's hierarchy is frequently used as a basis for prioritizing; other approaches may be equally valid.) Develop short- and long-term patient goals in measurable statements to describe the behavior to be observed. Identify the monitoring parameters to be used to detect possible complications of the disease process or treatments being used. Plan nursing approaches to correlate with each identified long-term goal. More than one short-term goal may be required to actually lead to the broader, more encompassing long-term goals.	Perform the nursing intervention planned to achieve the individualized short- and long-term goals. Monitor the patient's response to treatments, and monitor for complications related to existing pathophysiology. Provide for patient safety. Perform ongoing assessments on a continuum. Document care given and additional findings on the chart.	Evaluation is an ongoing process that occurs at every phase of the nursing process. Review and analyze the data regarding the patient and modify the care plan so that goals of care (usually, returning the patient to the highest level of functioning) are attained. Unrealistic goals may require revision or discontinuation. Follow a systematic approach to recording progress, depending on the setting and charting methods used. Document goal attainment, partial attainment, or failure to achieve goals. Continue the nursing process, initiate referral to a community-based health agency, or execute discharge procedures as ordered by the physician.

*Nursing Diagnosis: As not all patient problems are amenable to resolution by nursing actions, those complications associated with the medical diagnosis or from treatment-related complications are placed in a category known as *collaborative problems* that the nurse monitors.

During the assessment phase, the nurse collects a comprehensive information base about the patient from the physical exam, the nursing history, the medication history, and professional observation. Formats commonly used for data collection, organization, and analysis are the "head-to-toe" assessment, "body systems" assessment, or Gordon's Functional Health Patterns Model. Both the "head-to-toe" and "body systems" approaches focus on physiology and thereby limit the nurse's knowledge of sociocultural, psychological, spiritual, and developmental factors affecting the individual's needs. (See box, p. 144, Gordon's Functional Health Patterns Model.)

Nursing Diagnosis

OBJECTIVES

1. Define "nursing diagnosis" and discuss the wording used in formulating nursing diagnosis statements.
2. Define a "collaborative problem."
3. Differentiate between a "nursing diagnosis" and a "medical diagnosis."
4. Differentiate between problems that require formu-

lation of a nursing diagnosis and those categorized as collaborative problems, which may not require nursing diagnosis statements.

KEY WORDS

nursing diagnosis	collaborative problem
medical diagnosis	actual problem
high-risk problem	possible problem

Nursing diagnosis is the second phase of the five-step nursing process. The Ninth Conference (1990) of the North American Nursing Diagnosis Association (NANDA) approved the following official definition of nursing diagnosis:

> Nursing diagnosis is a clinical judgment about individual, family or community response to actual or potential health problems/life processes. Nursing diagnosis provides the basis for selection of nursing intervention to achieve outcomes for which the nurse is accountable.

Using his or her knowledge and skill (in anatomy, physiology, nutrition, psychology, pharmacology, mi-

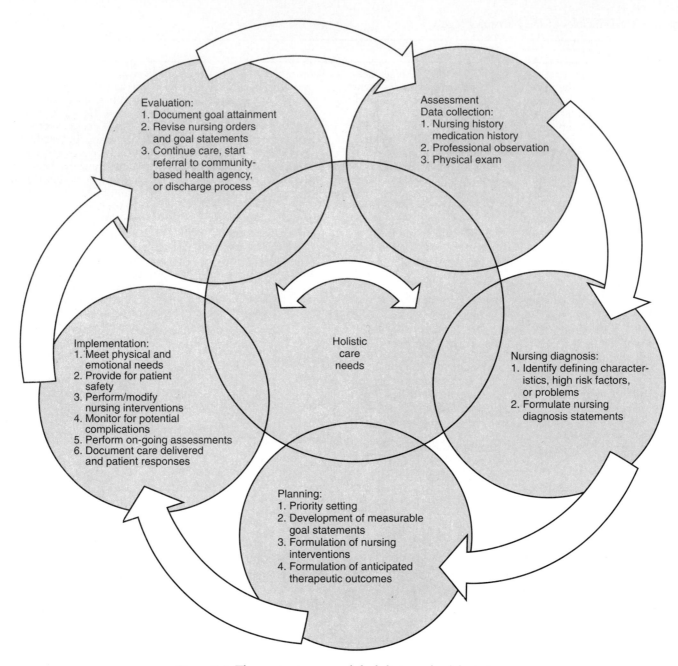

Figure 8-1 *The nursing process and the holistic needs of the patient.*

Gordon's functional health patterns model

1. Health perception–health management pattern
2. Nutritional–metabolic pattern
3. Activity–exercise pattern
4. Sleep–rest pattern
5. Cognitive–perceptual pattern
6. Self-perception pattern
7. Role–relationship pattern
8. Sexuality–reproduction pattern
9. Coping–stress tolerance pattern
10. Value–belief pattern

crobiology, nursing practice skills, and communication techniques), the nurse analyzes the data collected to identify whether certain major and minor *defining characteristics* (signs, symptoms, and clinical evidence) that may be present relate to a particular patient problem. If so, the nurse may conclude that certain actual problems are present. These patient-related problems are referred to as "nursing diagnosis."

It should be noted that not all patient problems identified during an assessment are treated by the nurse alone. Many of the identified problems require a multidisciplinary approach. When the nurse cannot legally

Differentiating Nursing Diagnoses from Other Client Problems

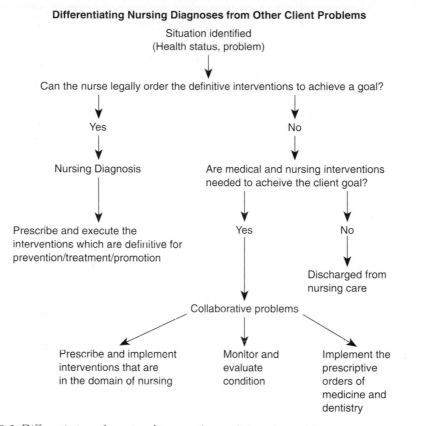

Figure 8-2 *Differentiation of nursing diagnoses from collaborative problems. (From Carpenito LJ: Nursing diagnosis application to clinical practice, 4th ed, Philadelphia, 1992, JB Lippincott, p. 40. © 1992 Lynda Juall Carpenito.)*

order the definitive interventions required under the presenting circumstances, a collaborative problem exists (Figure 8-2).

As nursing care has gained recognition as a cognitive process in planning patient care, several national conferences have been held to identify the diagnostic terms that describe areas of potential health problems that nurses should anticipate and may treat. As of 1990, the NANDA has recognized the approved listing of nursing diagnoses (see box, p. 146).

There is a difference between a medical diagnosis and a nursing diagnosis. A medical diagnosis is a statement of the patient's alterations in structure and function and results in a diagnosis of a disease or disorder that impairs normal physiologic function. A nursing diagnosis usually refers to the patient's ability to function in activities of daily living in relation to the impairment induced by the medical diagnosis; it identifies the individual's or group's response to the illness. A medical diagnosis also tends to remain unchanged throughout the illness, whereas nursing diagnoses may vary depending upon the patient's state of recovery. Concepts that help distinguish a nursing diagnosis from a medical diagnosis include the following:

1. Conditions described by nursing diagnoses can be accurately identified by nursing assessment methods.

2. Nursing treatments, or methods of risk factor reduction, can resolve the condition described by a nursing diagnosis.
3. Because the necessary treatment to resolve nursing diagnoses are within the scope of nursing practice, nurses assume accountability for outcomes.
4. Nursing assumes responsibility for the research required to clearly identify the defining characteristics and etiological factors and to improve methods of treatment and treatment outcomes for conditions described by nursing diagnoses (Gordon, 1987, p. 15).

The wording of an "actual" nursing diagnosis takes the form of a three-part statement. These statements consist of: (1) a diagnostic label (from the NANDA-approved list), (2) the contributing factors (cause if known or stated as etiology unknown), and (3) the defining characteristics (signs and symptoms). As of January 1992, problems previously referred to as "potential" problems are referred to as "high-risk" nursing diagnoses.

The high-risk statements consist of the diagnostic label (from the NANDA-approved list) and the risk factors that make the individual or group more susceptible to the development of the problem. Validation of a high risk diagnosis is the presence of the risk factors

NANDA-approved nursing diagnoses

Activity intolerance
Altered family processes
Altered growth and development
Altered health maintenance
Altered nutrition: less than body requirements
Altered nutrition: more than body requirements
Altered nutrition: potential for more than body requirements
Altered oral mucous membrane
Altered parenting
Altered patterns of urinary elimination
Altered protection†
Altered role performance
Altered sexuality patterns
Altered thought processes
Altered (specify type) tissue perfusion (cerebral, cardiopulmonary, renal, gastrointestinal, peripheral)
Anticipatory grieving
Anxiety
Bathing/hygiene self-care deficit
Body-image disturbance
Bowel incontinence
Chronic low self-esteem*
Chronic pain
Colonic constipation*
Constipation
Decisional conflict (specify)*
Decreased cardiac output
Defensive coping*
Diarrhea
Dressing/grooming self-care deficit
Dysfunctional grieving
Dysreflexia*
Effective breastfeeding†
Family coping: potential for growth
Fatigue*
Fear
Feeding self-care deficit
Fluid volume deficit (1)
Fluid volume deficit (2)
Fluid volume excess
Functional incontinence
Health-seeking behaviors (specify) or desire for high-level wellness (specify)*
Hopelessness
Hyperthermia
Hypothermia
Impaired adjustment
Impaired gas exchange
Impaired home maintenance management
Impaired physical mobility

Impaired skin integrity
Impaired social interaction
Impaired swallowing
Impaired tissue integrity
Impaired verbal communication
Ineffective airway clearance
Ineffective breastfeeding
Ineffective breathing pattern
Ineffective denial*
Ineffective family coping: compromised
Ineffective family coping: disabled
Ineffective individual coping
Ineffective thermoregulation
Knowledge deficit (specify)
Noncompliance (specify)
Pain
Parental role conflict*
Perceived constipation*
Personal identity disturbance
Post-trauma response
Potential activity intolerance
Potential altered body temperature
Potential fluid volume deficit
Potential for aspiration*
Potential for disuse syndrome*
Potential for infection
Potential for injury
Potential for poisoning
Potential for suffocating
Potential for trauma
Potential for violence: self-directed or directed at others
Potential impaired skin integrity
Powerlessness
Rape-trauma syndrome
Rape-trauma syndrome: compound reaction
Rape-trauma syndrome: silent reaction
Reflex incontinence
Self-esteem disturbance*
Sensory/perceptual alterations (specify) (auditory, gustatory, kinesthetic, olfactory, tactile, visual)
Sexual dysfunction
Situational low self-esteem*
Sleep pattern disturbance
Social isolation
Spiritual distress (distress of the human spirit)
Stress incontinence
Toileting self-care deficit
Total incontinence
Unilateral neglect
Urge incontinence
Urinary retention

*Diagnosis accepted in 1988.
†Diagnosis accepted in 1990.

that would contribute to the individual/group developing the stated problem. "Possible" nursing diagnosis identifies a problem that may occur, but the assembled data are insufficient to confirm it.

Further discussion of the philosophy and clinical use of nursing diagnoses, the specifics regarding the wording of "actual," "high-risk," and "possible" nursing diagnoses, and the new categories of "wellness" nursing diagnoses and "syndrome" nursing diagnoses can be found in other primary texts and reference works, especially those developed solely for the purpose of explaining nursing diagnosis.

Collaborative Problems

Not all patient problems identified by the nurse can be resolved by nursing actions. The nurse is, however, responsible for *monitoring* the patient on a continuum for potential complications that are associated with the medical diagnosis, diagnostic procedures, or treatments prescribed. To differentiate between a problem requiring a nursing diagnosis and a collaborative problem, the nurse must judge whether he or she can order the definitive interventions to prevent or treat the problem to maintain the health status of the patient (Carpenito, 1985, 1987, 1990). See Figure 8-2 for an illustration of this decision-making process.

Planning

OBJECTIVES

1. Identify the steps included in the planning of nursing care.
2. Explain the process of prioritizing individual patient needs utilizing Maslow's hierarchy of needs.
3. Formulate measurable goal statements for a patient for whom you are actively caring in the clinical practice setting.
4. State the behavioral responses around which goal statements revolve when the discharge of a patient is planned.
5. Identify the purposes and uses of a "patient care plan."
6. Differentiate between nursing interventions and therapeutic outcomes.

KEY WORDS

priority setting	measurable goal
nursing interventions	statements
anticipated therapeutic	nursing actions
outcomes	

Once the patient has been assessed and problems have been diagnosed, plans should be formulated to meet the patient's needs. Planning usually encompasses four phases: (1) priority setting, (2) development of measurable goal statements, (3) formulation of nursing interventions, and (4) formulation of anticipated therapeutic outcomes that can be used to evaluate the patient's status. The written document that evolves from this planning process is called the *nursing care plan*. When completed, it is placed in the patient's Kardex or chart, where it serves as a communication system for all health care providers. Because care needs are constantly changing, the care plan and priorities will also need to be evaluated and modified on a continuing basis to meet the patient's needs.

Maslow's hierarchy of needs	
HIGH	Self-Actualization Needs
	Esteem Needs
	Social Needs
	Safety Needs
LOW	Physiologic Needs

Priority Setting

After the nursing diagnoses and collaborative problems have been identified, they must be prioritized. Maslow's hierarchy of needs (see box above) is a model frequently used to establish priorities. Using Maslow's hierarchy, priority is given to those needs that directly affect the maintenance of homeostasis. Generally, physiologic needs such as oxygenation, temperature maintenance, or nutritional and fluid requirements would take precedence over psychologic needs. The box on p. 148 lists the priority ranking of Maslow's subcategories of human needs.

Measurable Goal Statements

After priorities of needs have been set, goals must be established and statements written. Goals are usually divided into short-term, intermediate, and long-term plans. The statements start with an action word (verb), followed by the behavior(s) to be performed by the patient or family, with a specific time allocated for attainment.

All goal statements must take into consideration the patient's individual needs, ability to learn (cognitive, psychomotor, and affective domains), and a realistic level of health rehabilitation based on the underlying disease pathology and on situational, environmental, and maturational factors (Carpenito, 1987).

When goals are being established, it is important to include the patient and appropriate significant others in decision-making, as the patient and his or her support persons will be responsible for the accomplishment of the goals. Involvement of the patient is essential to promote cooperation and compliance with the therapeutic regimen and a sense of control over the disease process and course of treatment. The goals established should be *patient goals*, not nursing goals for the patient.

The planning process may be scheduled with all significant persons present at one or more meetings. It is important to establish an openness that conveys a willingness to consider each person's input into the final plan. The strengths and weaknesses of each participant in the final care plan must be analyzed, and the goal statements must be realistic for the group to achieve.

Priority ranking of Maslow's subcategories of human needs

Physiologic needs

Oxygen, circulation
Water-salt balance
Food balance
Acid-base balance
Waste elimination
Normal temperature
Sleep, rest, relaxation
Activity, exercise
Energy
Comfort
Stimulation
Cleanliness
Sexuality

Safety needs

Protection from physical harm
Protection from psychologic threat
Freedom from pain
Stability
Dependence
Predictable, orderly world

Belonging needs

Love and affection
Acceptance
Warm, communicating relationship
Approval from others
Unity with loved ones
Group companionship

Self-esteem needs

Recognition
Dignity
Appreciation from others
Importance, influence
Reputation of good character
Attention
Status
Dominance over others

Self-actualization needs

Personal growth and maturity
Awareness of potential
Increased learning
Full development of potential
Improved values
Religious, philosophical satisfaction
Increased creativity
Increased reality perception and problem-solving abilities
Less rigid conventionality
Less of the familiar, more of the novel
Greater satisfaction in beauty
Increased pleasantness
Less of the simple, more of the complex

From Campbell C: *Nursing diagnosis and intervention in nursing practice,* New York, 1978; © John Wiley & Sons.

Most goal statements revolve around the patient's need to do the following:

1. Reduce or resolve the symptoms (usually the chief complaint) of the disease that caused the person to seek medical attention
2. Understand the disease process and its effect on lifestyle and activities of daily living
3. Gain knowledge and skills associated with the treatment procedures so as to attain the highest level of function possible (nutrition, comfort measures, medication regimen, physical therapy)
4. Understand reasonable expectations of the therapy, including signs and symptoms of improvement versus complications requiring physician consultation
5. Identify monitoring parameters that should be maintained on a written record that reflects the response to the prescribed therapy
6. Establish a schedule for follow-up evaluation

The beginning practitioner should consult a text on nursing diagnosis for further information on the correct wording of measurable goal statements associated with nursing diagnosis and collaborative problems.

Nursing Actions or Nursing Interventions

Nursing action or *intervention statements* list in a concise form exactly what the nurse will do to achieve each goal statement developed for each nursing diagnosis. A nursing action is a statement that describes nursing interventions applicable to any patient (for example, "promote adequate respiratory ventilation"). *Nursing orders* describe how specific actions will be implemented for an individual patient.

Example: (date): cough, turn, deep breath: 0800, 1000, 1200, 1600, 1800, 2000, 2200

(date): Educate patient re: abdominal breathing, splinting the abdomen and purselip breathing, assuming correct position to facilitate breathing.

(date): Auscultate breath sounds 0800, 1200, 1600, 2000

(date): Increase fluid intake to at least 2000 ml/24 hr:

0700–1500: 1000 ml
1500–2300: 800 ml
2300–0700: 200 ml

(date): Assess respiratory depth and rate at 0800, 1200, 1600, 2000, 2400

Anticipated Therapeutic Outcome Statements

Measurable *anticipated therapeutic outcome statements* are also developed to document the effectiveness of the care delivered. In the above example, the patient will do the following:

1. Improve in the ability to perform coughing technique
2. Maintain an adequate fluid intake as evidenced by achieving a mutually set goal of 2000 ml within 24 hours
3. Attain a respiratory rate between 18 to 24 per minute
4. Perform activities of daily living without feeling fatigued

Nursing Intervention or Implementation

OBJECTIVE

1. Compare the types of nursing functions classified as dependent, interdependent, and independent and give examples of each.

KEY WORDS

nursing actions   nursing interventions
dependent actions   independent actions
interdependent actions

Nursing intervention or *implementation* is the actual process of carrying out the established plan of care. Nursing care is directed at meeting the physical and emotional needs of the patient, at providing for patient safety, at monitoring for potential complications, and at performing ongoing assessments as a part of the continual process of data collection and evaluation to identify changes in the patient's care needs. Nursing actions are suggested by the etiologies of the problems identified in the nursing diagnoses and are used to implement plans. They may include activities such as counseling, teaching, providing comfort measures, coordinating, referring, using communication skills, and carrying out a physician's orders. Documentation of all care given, including patient education and the patient's apparent response, should be done regularly, both to assist in evaluation and reassessment and to make other health professionals aware of the patient's changing needs.

Nursing Actions

Within the nursing process, there are three types of nursing actions: (1) dependent, (2) interdependent, and (3) independent. *Dependent* actions are those performed by the nurse based on the physician's orders (such as the administration of prescribed medications and/or treatments). It is important to note that, even though this is a dependent function, the nurse is still responsible for exercising professional judgment in carrying out the orders. *Interdependent* nursing actions are those actions the nurse implements cooperatively with

other members of the health team for restoration or promotion of health maintenance. This allows nurses to coordinate their interventions with those of other health professionals to maximize knowledge and skills from various disciplines for the well-being of the patient. *Independent* nursing actions are those actions not prescribed by a physician that a nurse can provide by virtue of the education and licensure he or she has attained. These actions are usually written in the nursing care plan and originate from the nursing diagnosis.

Evaluating and Recording Therapeutic Outcomes

OBJECTIVE

1. Describe the evaluatory process used to establish whether patient behaviors are consistent with the identified short-term, intermediate, or long-term goals.

The final step of the nursing process is evaluation of the expected outcomes of the patient's behavior. All care is evaluated against the established nursing diagnoses (goal statements), planned nursing actions, and anticipated therapeutic outcomes. In order for the evaluation process to be successful, the participants (patient, family, nurse) must be willing to receive the feedback. Therefore, plans for evaluation must involve the patient and family from the beginning.

Although the evaluation phase is the last step in the nursing process, it is not an end in itself. Evaluation recognizes successful completion of previously established goals, but it also provides a means for input of new, significant data indicating the development of additional problems or a lack of therapeutic responsiveness that may require additional nursing diagnoses and/or collaboration with the physician or other professionals on the health care team as plans for therapy are revised.

RELATING THE NURSING PROCESS TO PHARMACOLOGY
Assessment

OBJECTIVES

1. State the information that should be obtained as a part of a medication history.
2. Identify primary, secondary, and tertiary sources of information used to build a patient information base.

Assessment is an ongoing process that starts with the admission of the patient and is completed at the time of discharge. In relating the nursing process to the nursing functions associated with medications, assessment includes taking a drug history, for three reasons: to evaluate the patient's need for medication; to obtain his or her current and past use of over-the-counter medication, prescription medication, and street drugs; and to identify problems related to drug therapy. Nurses will also want to identify risk factors such as allergy to certain medications (for example, penicillins) or the presence of other diseases (such as hypertension) that may limit the use of certain types of drugs (as with sympathomimetic agents).

The nurse draws upon three sources to build the medication-related information base. Whenever the patient is able to provide reliable information, he or she should be utilized as the *primary* source of information. Subjective and objective data serve as the baseline for the formulation of drug-related nursing diagnoses. Subjective data are information provided by the patient (such as "Whenever I take this medicine I feel sick to my stomach"). Objective data are gained from observations that the nurse makes using physiologic parameters (such as "Skin pale, cold and moist"; "temperature 99.2° F orally"). Other objective information needed will be the patient's height and weight, which may be needed to select dosages of medications and later as a monitoring parameter for drug therapy.

In some cases it is necessary to obtain information from *secondary* sources (for example, relatives, significant others, medical records, laboratory reports, nursing notes, or other health professionals). Secondary sources of information are subject to interpretation by someone other than the patient. Data collected from secondary sources should be analyzed using other portions of the data base to validate the conclusions reached.

Tertiary sources of information, such as a literature search, provide a "textbook picture" of the characteristics of a disease, nursing interventions, diagnostic tests used, pharmacological treatment prescribed, diets, physical therapy, and other factors pertinent to the patient's care requirements. (When utilizing these sources, the student should be aware that the patient has individual needs and that the plan of care must be adapted to the patient's identified needs.)

Assessment related to drug therapy continues on an ongoing basis through the hospitalization. Examples of ongoing assessment activities include visiting with the patient, the need for p.r.n. medication, monitoring vital signs, and observation for therapeutic effects, side effects to expect, side effects to report, and potential drug interactions.

In preparation for the patient's eventual discharge and need for education about new health-related responsibilities, the assessment process should include collection of data related to the patient's health beliefs, existing health problems, prior compliance with prescribed regimens, readiness for learning both emotionally and experientially, and ability to learn and execute the skills required for self-care.

Nursing Diagnoses

OBJECTIVES

1. Define "problem."
2. Describe the process that is used to identify factors that could result in patient problems when medications are prescribed.
3. Review the content of several drug monographs to identify information that may result in patient problems from the medication therapy.

To deal effectively with identified problems (diagnoses), the nurse must recognize the etiology and contributing factors.

> The etiological and contributing factors are those clinical and personal situations that can cause the problem or influence its development. . . . Situations can be pathophysiological, treatment related, situational, or maturational. (Carpenito, 1987)

When identifying problems related to medication therapy, the nurse should review the drug monographs given later in this text for each prescribed drug. Several nursing diagnoses can be formulated based on the patient's drug therapy. The most commonly observed are those associated with drug *treatment* of a disease or the *side effects* from drug therapy, but nursing diagnoses can also originate from pathophysiology caused by drug interactions.

> EXAMPLE: Drugs prescribed for Parkinson's Disease are administered to provide relief of symptoms (muscle tremors, slowness of movement, muscle weakness with rigidity, and alterations in posture and equilibrium). An actual nursing diagnosis of "Mobility, impaired physical: related to neuromuscular impairment (Parkinson's Disease)" would be formulated based on the defining characteristics established for this nursing diagnosis. Evaluation of the therapeutic outcomes from the prescribed medications would be based on the degree of improvement noted in the symptoms present.
>
> A second nursing diagnosis would be "Injury, high risk for: related to amantadine side effects (confusion, disorientation, dizziness, light-headedness)."
>
> In this example, the drug amantadine, prescribed to *treat* the symptoms of the disease, is also the basis of the first nursing diagnosis. The second nursing diagnosis is a collaborative problem that requires the nurse to *monitor* the development of these side effects. In other words, a patient with Parkinson's Disease is at risk of developing the defining characteristics needed to have this occur. When the defining characteristics are observed, notification of the physician is required, and the nurse would need to intervene to provide for the patient's safety.

Two nursing diagnoses that apply to all types of medications prescribed are as follows:

1. Knowledge deficit (actual, high risk, or possible),

related to: the medication regimen (patient education).

2. Noncompliance (actual, high risk, or possible) related to: the patient's value system, cognitive ability, cultural factors, or economic resources.

Planning

OBJECTIVES

1. Identify steps used to plan nursing care in relation to a medication regimen prescribed for a patient.
2. Describe an acceptable method of organizing, implementing, and evaluating the patient education delivered.
3. Practice developing short- and long-term patient education objectives and have them critiqued by the instructor.

KEY WORD

therapeutic intent

Planning, with reference to the prescribed medications, must include the following steps:

1. Identification of the *therapeutic intent* for each prescribed medication. (Why was the drug prescribed? What symptoms should be relieved?)
2. Review of the drug monograph in this text to identify the *side effects to expect* (symptoms that can be alleviated or prevented by actions of the nurse or patient will require immediate planning for patient education).
3. Review of the drug monograph in this text to identify the *side effects to report* (a collaborative problem in which the nurse has a responsibility to *monitor* the patient for adverse effects of drug therapy and report suspected adverse effects to the physician).
4. Identification of the *recommended dosage* and *route of administration* (compare the recommended dosage with the dosage ordered; confirm that the route of administration is correct and that the dosage form ordered can be tolerated by the patient).
5. Scheduling of the administration of the medication based on the physician's orders and the policies of the health care facility (medications prescribed must be reviewed for drug-drug interactions and drug-food interactions; laboratory tests may also need to be scheduled if serum levels of the drug have been ordered).
6. Teaching the patient to keep written records of his or her responses to the prescribed medications (see the template in Appendix K).
7. Additional education as needed on techniques of self-administration (such as injection, topical patches, instillation of drops).

8. Information as needed on proper storage, how to refill a medication, or how to fill out an insurance claim for reimbursement.

Priority ranking in preparation for health education may encompass several factors: (1) the patient's concerns and priorities; (2) the urgency or time available for the learning to take place; (3) a sequence that allows the patient to move from the simple to the more complex concepts; and (4) a review of the overall needs of the individual. The content taught to the patient should be well planned in advance and delivered in increments that the patient is capable of mastering. The complete teaching plan should be in the Kardex or on the patient's chart.

EXAMPLE: Mr. Jones will be able to state the:

1. Drug name
2. Dosage
3. Route and administration times
4. Anticipated therapeutic response
5. Side effects to expect
6. Side effects to report
7. What to do if a dosage is missed
8. When, how, or if to refill the medication

for each prescribed medication by *(date)* and will show retention of this information by repeating it on *date*.

To attain this goal, the patient's ability to name all these factors would need to be checked at the initial time of exposure and on subsequent meetings to validate retention. Once the goals have been formulated, they should not be considered final but should be reevaluated as needed throughout the course of treatment.

Nursing Intervention or Implementation

OBJECTIVE

1. Differentiate among dependent, interdependent, and independent nursing actions and give an example of each.

Nursing actions applied to pharmacology may be categorized as dependent, interdependent, or independent.

Dependent Nursing Actions

The physician admits the patient, states the admitting diagnosis, and orders diagnostic procedures and medications for the immediate well-being of the patient. The physician reviews data on a continuing basis to determine the risks and benefits of maintaining or modifying the medication orders. Maintenance or modification of the medication orders is the physician's responsibility; however, the data collected and recorded by the nurse on the patient's chart are essential for evaluation of the effectiveness of the medications prescribed.

Interdependent Nursing Actions

The nurse will perform baseline and subsequent assessments that will be valuable in establishing therapeutic goals, duration of therapy, detection of drug toxicity, and frequency of reevaluation.

The nurse should approach any problems related to the medication prescribed collaboratively with appropriate members of the health care team. Whenever the nurse is in doubt about medication calculations, monitoring for therapeutic efficacy and side effects, or the establishment of nursing interventions or patient education, another qualified professional should be consulted.

The pharmacist reviews all aspects of the drug order, then prepares the medications and sends them to the unit for storage in a medication room or a unit dose medication cart. If any portion of the drug order or the rationale for therapy is unclear, the nurse and pharmacist may consult with each other and/or the physician for clarification.

The frequency of medication administration is defined by the physician in the original order. The nurse and pharmacist establish the schedule of the medication based on the standardized administration times used at the practice setting. The nurse, and occasionally the pharmacist, also coordinates the schedule of the medication administration and the collection of blood samples with the laboratory phlebotomist to monitor drug serum levels.

The nurse completes laboratory test requisitions based upon the physician's orders to monitor drug therapy, establish dosages, and/or identify the most effective medication for pathogenic microorganisms.

As soon as laboratory/diagnostic test results are available, the nurse and pharmacist review them to identify values that could have a bearing on drug therapy. The results of the tests are conveyed to the physician. The nurse should also have current assessment data available for collaborative discussion of signs and symptoms that may relate to the medications prescribed, dosage, therapeutic efficacy, or adverse effects.

Patient education (including discharge medications) requires that an established plan be developed, written in the patient's medical record, implemented, documented, and reinforced by all persons delivering care to the patient (see box, p. 153).

Independent Nursing Actions

The nurse visits with the patient, performing the nursing history, which includes a medication history. The history of current and past medications—including prescription, over-the-counter, and street drugs—is reviewed to identify treatment-related problems.

The nurse verifies the drug order and assumes responsibility for correct transcription of the drug order to the nurse's Kardex, medication administration record (MAR), or computer. As part of this process, the nurse makes professional judgments concerning the class of drug, therapeutic intent, usual dosage, and the patient's ability to tolerate the drug dosage form ordered. If all aspects of the verification and transcription procedure are considered to be correct, the carbon copy of the original order is sent to the pharmacy.

The nurse formulates appropriate nursing diagnoses and actions to monitor for therapeutic effects and side effects of medications. (The nurse may need to review drug monographs to formulate the diagnoses and goal statements.) Criteria for therapeutic responses should describe the improvement expected in symptoms of the disease for which the medication was prescribed.

The nurse prepares the prescribed medications using procedures to insure patient safety. As part of this process, nursing professional judgments required include the following:

1. Selection of the correct supplies (needle gauge, length, type of syringe) for administration of the medications.
2. Verification of all aspects of the medication order before preparing the medication; the order should be verified again immediately following preparation and again prior to actual patient administration (patients should always be identified immediately prior to administration of the medication, each time a medication is to be administered).
3. Collection of appropriate data to serve as a baseline for later assessments of therapeutic effectiveness and/or to detect adverse effects of drugs.
4. Administration of the medication by the correct route at the correct site (selection and rotation of sites for medication should be based on established practices for rotation of sites and on principles of drug absorption, which in turn may be affected by the presence of pathophysiology, such as poor tissue perfusion).
5. Documentation in the chart of all aspects of medication administration; subsequent assessments should be documented to identify the drug efficacy, the development of expected side effects, or any adverse effects.
6. Implementation of nursing actions to minimize expected side effects and to identify side effects to be reported promptly.
7. Education of patients as appropriate for the medications prescribed, in addition to other facets of the therapeutic regimen; when noncompliance is identified, the nurse should attempt to ascertain the patient's reasons for not following the regimen and collaboratively discuss approaches to the problems viewed by the patient as hindrances to following the prescribed regimen.

Sample teaching plan for a patient with diabetes mellitus taking one type of insulin[*]

Understanding of health condition
- Assess the patient's and family's understanding of diabetes mellitus.
- Clarify the meaning of the disease in terms the patient is able to understand.
- Establish learning goals through mutual discussion. Arrange to teach most important data first. Set dates for teaching of content after discussion with patient.

Food and fluids
- Arrange for the patient, family members, and significant others to attend nutrition lectures and demonstrations on food preparation.
- Reinforce knowledge of exchange lists (or other dietary method) by tactful questioning and by giving the patient a chance to practice food selections for daily meals from menus provided.
- Explain management of the diabetic diet during illness (that is, nausea and vomiting, need for increase in fluid) and when to contact the physician.
- Stress interrelationship of food and onset, peak, and duration of the prescribed insulin.

Monitoring tests
- Demonstrate the collection and testing of blood glucose samples and, as appropriate, urine testing.
- Validate understanding by having the patient collect, test, and record results of the testing for the remainder of the hospitalization.
- Stress performing serum glucose testing and urine tests (e.g., ketones) before meals and at bedtime.
- Explain the importance of regular follow-up laboratory studies (that is, fasting plasma glucose testing or postprandial, glycosylated hemoglobin) to monitor the patient's degree of control.

Medications and treatments
- Teach the name, dose, route of administration, desired action, storage, and refilling of the type of insulin prescribed.
- Explain the principles of insulin action, onset, peak, and duration (see Index).
- Demonstrate preparation and administration of the prescribed dose of insulin.
- Teach site location and rotation schedule for self-administration of insulin.
- Give specific instructions on reading the syringe to be used at home (glass or disposable plastic).
- Teach sterilization of glass syringe and needle, and storage and assembly, if necessary. Teach how to obtain disposable syringes.
- Cite usual times for "reactions," signs and symptoms of hypoglycemia or hyperglycemia, and management of each complication.
- Validate the patient's understanding of the side effects to expect and those that require reporting.
- Teach and validate family members' and significant others' understanding of the signs and symptoms of hypoglycemia and hyperglycemia and management of each complication.
- Teach general approach to management of illnesses (e.g., if nausea and vomiting or fever occur—actions required; stress glucose monitoring before meals and at hour of sleep; and need to call physician).

Personal hygiene
Discuss the management of personal hygiene measures of great importance to the patient with diabetes mellitus:
- Regular foot care.
- Meticulous oral hygiene and dental care.
- Care of cuts, scratches, minor and major injuries.
- Stress management and needed alterations in insulin dosage; reporting to physician for guidance and discussion.

Activities
- Assist the patient to develop a detailed time schedule for usual activities of daily living. Incorporate diabetic care needs into the schedule.
- Encourage maintenance of all usual activities of daily living; discuss anticipated problems and possible interventions.
- Correlate personal care needs not only in the home environment, but also in the work setting as appropriate. (Consider involvement of the industrial nurse if available in the work setting.)
- Discuss effects of an increase or decrease in activity level on the management of the diabetes mellitus.

Home or follow-up care
- Arrange for outpatient or physician follow-up appointments and for scheduling ordered laboratory tests.
- Tell the individual to seek assistance from the physician or from the nearest emergency room service for problems that may develop.
- Arrange appropriate referral to community health agencies if needed.
- Complete a Diabetic Alert card or other means of alerting people to the individual's needs (such as an identification necklace or bracelet).

Special equipment and instructional material
- Develop a list of equipment and supplies to be purchased; have a family member purchase and bring to the hospital for use during teaching sessions (urine testing and blood glucose monitoring supplies, syringes, needles and sterilizing equipment, alcohol, cotton balls, etc.).
- Show audiovisual materials available on insulin preparation, storage, administration on serum glucose and urine testing, etc.
- Develop a written record (Chapter 16) and assist the patient to maintain data during hospitalization.

Other
- Teach measures to make travel easier.
- Tell the patient of the American Diabetes Association and material available through this resource.

[*]Each item listed needs to be assessed for the individual's current knowledge base and level of understanding throughout the course of teaching. The process is reassessed and the teaching continued until the patient masters all facets of self-care needs. With the advent of shorter hospitalizations, inpatient and outpatient teaching may be necessary. Referral to community-based health care agencies may be necessary. Discharge charting and referral should carefully document those facets of the teaching plan mastered and those to be taught. The physician should be notified of deficits in learning ability and/or mastery of needed elements in the teaching plan.

Evaluating Therapeutic Outcomes

OBJECTIVE

1. Describe the procedure for evaluating the therapeutic outcomes obtained from prescribed therapy.

Evaluation associated with drug therapy is an ongoing process that assesses response to the medications prescribed, observation for signs and symptoms of recurring illness or the development of adverse effects of the medication, determination of the patient's ability to receive patient education and self-administer medications, and the potential for compliance. Table 8-2 illustrates an overview of the application of the nursing process to the nursing responsibilities associated with drug therapy.

PATIENT EDUCATION ASSOCIATED WITH MEDICATION THERAPY

OBJECTIVES

1. Describe essential elements of patient education in relation to the prescribed medications.
2. Describe the nurse's role in fostering patient responsibility for the maintenance of well-being and for compliance with the therapeutic regimen.
3. Identify the types of information that should be discussed with the patient and/or significant others in order to establish reasonable expectations for the prescribed therapy.
4. Discuss specific techniques used in the practice setting to document the patient education performed and degree of achievement attained.

Over the past 2 decades, health teaching has evolved from an abstract form of intervention that occurred only if a specific need existed at discharge (and if the physician approved of providing the information to the patient), to the current state of formalized development of learning objectives to direct the individual toward attainment of goals based on the needs of the patient. Today, health teaching is an important nursing responsibility that carries with it legal implications for failure to provide and document education.

The content taught to the patient should be thoroughly planned in advance and delivered in increments that the patient is capable of mastering. The complete teaching plan should be in the Kardex or on the patient's chart. Each segment should be expressed in measurable behavioral terms. Once the goals have been formulated, they should not be considered final but should be reevaluated throughout the course of treatment and modified if necessary. All teaching should be documented in the nurse's notes or on the health teaching record, along with observations that verify the patient's degree of understanding or proficiency of skill mastered. As mastery of an item is attained, it should be checked off on the Kardex or health teaching form in the patient's chart.

Assessing the patient's readiness for learning is crucial to success. When anxiety is high, the ability to focus on details is reduced. The nurse should anticipate periods during the hospitalization when teaching can be more effectively implemented. Some teaching is most successful when done spontaneously, such as when the patient asks direct questions regarding progress toward discharge. The nurse also must learn to anticipate inopportune times to initiate teaching, such as during times of withdrawal after learning of a diagnosis with a poor prognosis. With reduced hospital stays, the ability to time patient education ideally and to perform actual teaching is a challenge. It is imperative that the nurse document those aspects of the health teaching that have been mastered and, of equal importance, document what has not been accomplished and request referral to an appropriate agency for follow-up teaching and assistance.

During the process of patient education, the nurse should address the areas of communication and responsibility, expectations of therapy, changes in expectation, and changes in therapy through cooperative goal setting.

Communication and Responsibility

Nurses tend to think that patients will do what is suggested simply because they have been told it is beneficial. In the hospital, the nurse and other health team members reinforce the basic therapeutic regimen; at dismissal, however, the patient leaves the controlled environment and is free to choose to follow the prescribed treatment or to alter it as he or she deems appropriate based on personal values and beliefs. In order for learning to take place, the patient must perceive the information as relevant. Whenever possible, start with simple, attainable teaching goals to build the patient's confidence. It is important to correlate the teaching with the patient's perspective on the illness and ability to control the signs and symptoms or course of the disease process.

Expectations of Therapy

Before dismissal, discuss reasonable responses to the planned therapy. The patient should know what signs and symptoms can be expected to be altered by the prescribed medications. The precautions necessary when taking a medication need to be explained by the nurse and understood by the patient (for example, caution in operating power equipment or a motor vehicle or in avoiding direct sunlight, or the need for follow-up laboratory studies).

Text continued on p. 159.

Table 8-2 *The Nursing Process Applied to the Patient's Pharmacologic Needs*

ASSESSMENT	PLANNING	INTERVENTION	EVALUATION
Data collection			
Collect data on patient symptoms; disease process as based on the history and physical, patient, and/or family information; nursing assessments and interview	Identify and prioritize: • Patient problems • Baseline assessment data to be monitored to evaluate the patient's symptoms • Anticipated drug side effects and those to report	Perform the identified baseline patient assessments on a regularly scheduled basis (such as blood pressure, pulse, respirations, pain level [frequency, duration, activity associated with onset], leg pain)	Analyze data collected on a continuum; chart and report *changes* of significance in the baseline data and/or patient's status; report escalating of symptoms or ineffective response to drug therapy
Drug history: ask questions in a simple, direct manner to elicit information regarding drugs currently being taken, or those taken during the preceding year; ask about over-the-counter drugs used on a regular or casual basis	Plan to monitor patients total drug needs; develop goals to deal with any drug interactions, incompatibilities, or diagnostic tests potentially affected by drugs being administered	Perform drug preparation, scheduling, and administration to coincide with specific patient needs or problems	Analyze data collected on a continuum
Ask about any prior drug "allergies" and specifics of the "reaction" and treatment used	Plan to monitor patients at risk for the development of an allergic reaction	Implement monitoring parameters	Analyze observed symptoms for potential drug reaction or interactions
Age and disease process present	Plan modifications in dosage, administration technique, and observations based on the individual's age and physiologic status that may indicate a problem with drug absorption, distribution, metabolism, or excretion; confirm drug dosages BEFORE administering any drug in question	Implement the proper administration of confirmed drug dosages	As therapy continues, analyze the patient's weight, mental status, and disease processes that may be indicative of a problem with drug absorption, distribution, metabolism, or excretion; report abnormal laboratory values or *changes* in the patient's baseline assessment data
Body weight	Plan to weigh the patient daily or as needed	Perform the procedure of weighing the patient at the same time, in the same weight clothing, on the same scale at the intervals ordered	Report weight gains or losses (this is of particular importance with some types of drugs such as digitalis glycosides, corticosteroids, thyroid medications, and chemotherapy)
Metabolic rate	Plan nursing intervention to correlate with diseases that alter metabolic rate (such as hyperthyroidism, hypothyroidism, congestive heart failure)	Institute nursing measures directed at nutritional status, activity/exercise needs, environmental alterations needed	Analyze effectiveness of approaches utilized; observe closely for an increase or decrease in therapeutic effect
Monitoring parameters			
Laboratory data (See Appendix for normal values): review data to determine potential problems in the absorption, distribution, metabolism and elimination of the prescribed drug	Follow hospital policies for ordering and assisting with laboratory/diagnostic test; always check for drugs that may interact with scheduled laboratory tests		
Hepatic function	AST, ALT, alkaline phosphatase, LDH, GGT	Complete appropriate forms to order the tests; assist in drawing of blood samples and in providing patient support during procedure	As soon as results are received on the unit, report any diagnostic value outside the normal range to the physician

Continued.

Table 8-2 *The Nursing Process Applied to the Patient's Pharmacologic Needs—cont'd*

ASSESSMENT	PLANNING	INTERVENTION	EVALUATION
Monitoring parameters—cont'd			
Renal function	Serum creatinine, creatinine clearance, BUN (Blood Urea Nitrogen), Urinalysis	Same as above Same as above Collect urine sample by clean catch or, if ordered, by catheterization Check for drugs being given and record on urinalysis slip Send urine samples to laboratory promptly after collection. Be certain it is refrigerated/iced as appropriate. Always record the exact start date/time and end date/time on laboratory slip for 12 hr/24 hr urine collection (e.g., urine creatinine)	Elevated serum creatinine levels generally indicate renal disease Elevated BUN levels occur in renal disease, dehydration, a high protein diet, or a catabolic state Depressed BUN levels are found in severe hepatic damage, overhydration, and malnutrition Urinalysis: Always report RBCs, casts, crystals, proteinurea, glycosuria, high or low pH, or specific gravity outside the normal range (1.001-1.017)
In addition to the above tests, the following tests may be used to monitor disease and drug therapy: Infectious disease Assessment for site/source of the infection	Culture and sensitivity (C&S)	Collect specimen properly to maintain sterility of the culture tip so that the source examined is the only surface touched. Label appropriately; take to lab immediately	Report results of a culture and sensitivity promptly; particularly important are results that indicate that the drug being administered is not effective against the organism cultured
Complete blood count	Plan intervention based on the organism, the site of the infection, fever, hematuria, and drainage	Implement nursing measures to deal effectively with the patient's needs—fever, pain, drainage, and degree of precautions appropriate to the organism	Elevated WBCs, bands, segs, lymphocytes need to be reported to the physician Analyze subsequent CBC reports for significant changes; continue performing baseline assessments to detect degree of responsiveness to therapy
Monitoring of drug levels			
Routinely monitored: digitalis glycosides, theophylline, aminoglycosides, lithium, lidocaine, phenytoin, procainamide, quinidine, vancomycin (see Appendix I)	Plan to requisition the laboratory tests ordered by the physician to monitor serum blood levels at the scheduled times; ensure that the patient will be available at the required times	Record drug name, dosage, and times and route of administration on requisition	Therapeutic doses of certain drugs can be established through a combination of monitoring of serum levels and patient assessments of essential data Example: aminophylline—The patient's age and disease factors modify the dosage needs; therefore patients with cardiac, pulmonary, or renal dysfunction may require serum concentration as a guide to dosage.

Table 8-2 *The Nursing Process Applied to the Patient's Pharmacologic Needs—cont'd*

ASSESSMENT	PLANNING	INTERVENTION	EVALUATION
Monitoring of drug levels—cont'd			
			The current clinical status of the patient is always important; therefore, regular assessments specifically planned to detect therapeutic and toxic activity are imperative to effective patient management
			Check specific drug monographs for other drugs that may alter laboratory results; report results promptly for the physician's evaluation
Other laboratory tests	Prothrombin time (PT) (for warfarin) Partial thromboplastin time (PTT) (for heparin)	Requisition the prescribed laboratory test so that the drug dosage can be ordered by the physician; perform nursing assessments associated with anticoagulant therapy and the disease process specifically being treated	Be certain the correct date and patient data are relayed to the physician when seeking or confirming the anticoagulant drug order; always double check the date, time, and specific dosage of the anticoagulant drug order; anticoagulants should be checked with a second qualified nurse at the time of preparation and administration
	Blood glucose and urine glucose	Withhold daily insulin until blood sugar sample is drawn; test urine or blood for glucose as ordered or ac and hs	Correlate the results of the laboratory reports to the patient's status and degree of response to drug therapy; carefully evaluate patient symptoms for hyper- and hypoglycemia. Report laboratory data and patient status changes to the physician
	Glycosylated hemoglobin	Measures average blood glucose control for past 120 days. No food or fluid restrictions.	
	Fructosamine	Measures average blood glucose control for previous 1 to 3 weeks.	
Nursing research of prescribed drugs			
Drug action Consult "General Nursing Considerations" in specific drug monographs to correlate drug action and monitoring parameters to the patient's presenting symptoms and disease process	Develop goal statements for monitoring presence or absence of response Plan the administration schedule to correlate with known information about time of administration in relation to food, tests, and planned sleep Plan interventions to minimize or alleviate drug-related complications (side effects)	Assess the patient for baseline data before administering the drug; perform subsequent assessments at regular intervals to collect data to evaluate therapeutic response to the drug Administer the prescribed drug: RIGHT patient RIGHT drug RIGHT dose RIGHT route RIGHT time RIGHT documentation	Document all assessments by carefully recording all pertinent observations in the patient's chart Analyze the collected data and compare to the baseline data gathered before initiation of drug therapy; report significant changes in the patient's status

Continued.

Table 8-2 *The Nursing Process Applied to the Patient's Pharmacologic Needs—cont'd*

ASSESSMENT	PLANNING	INTERVENTION	EVALUATION
Nursing research of prescribed drugs—cont'd			
Side effects to expect	Consult specific drug monographs for side effects to expect; plan assessments to detect and intervention to manage these as they occur	Monitor the patient for development of expected side effects; implement measures designed to effectively manage or minimize effects; assist patient to understand and cope with specific symptoms as developed	Once expected side effects develop, it is important to evaluate the nursing measures designed to minimize or reduce the effects; report lack of responsiveness; modify intervention appropriately; analyze the patient's level of tolerance of the side effects
	Plan specific teaching that incorporates side effects to expect	Teach which side effects to expect and how to alleviate discomfort	Document specific teaching performed and the degree of understanding observed through direct questioning and return demonstrations
		Encourage the patient to discuss relevant symptoms with the physician and to adhere to the medication prescribed; suggest discussion of symptoms and encourage cooperative planning for modifications in the medications taken; discourage discontinuance or self-adjusted dosages	Analyze verbal and nonverbal behaviors observed to detect patient response to suggestion of cooperative goal-setting between the physician and patient
Side effects to report	Plan nursing assessments and intervention for side effects that are serious and require reporting	Perform regularly scheduled nursing assessments to detect any side effects from drug therapy that should be reported	Analyze data collected on a continuum; report deviations appropriately
	Develop a specific teaching plan that incorporates teaching of side effects to report	Perform health teaching of the observations the patient should make and the findings that require reporting	Carefully evaluate the patient's attitude toward compliance with drug therapy and intent to report problems for discussion and needed modifications
	Plan teaching of necessary monitoring parameters (blood pressure, pulse, respirations, daily weights, etc.)	Teach and repeat at appropriate intervals to achieve patient/family mastery	Evaluate the degree of accuracy attained by the patient or family members; refer to social services or community agencies if assistance is needed at time of discharge
Patient understanding of drug therapy	Plan teaching of drug name, dosage, route of administration, and exact time schedule; record overall teaching plan on the Kardex or chart	Throughout the hospitalization, discuss medication information and how it will benefit the course of treatment; seek cooperation and understanding of the following points so that medication compliance may be enhanced:	Document teaching and understanding achieved; try role-playing a situation or, when appropriate during hospitalization, have the patient describe what needs to be done
	Plan teaching of medications taken on a p.r.n. basis (such as nitroglycerin) and establish goals to evaluate understanding of frequency and dose, repeating of dose, lack of response	1. Name 2. Dosage 3. Route and administration times 4. Anticipated therapeutic response 5. Side effects to expect 6. Side effects to report	Document the individual's understanding of the directions given; try role-playing a situation or, when appropriate during hospitalization, have the patient describe what needs to be done
	Plan teaching of any self-administration techniques (oral, inhalation, injection, rectal, etc.)	7. What to do if a dosage is missed 8. When, how, or if to refill the medication prescription	Validate the patient/significant other's understanding by return demonstration; document teaching of administration techniques and degree of understanding in nurse's notes

Table 8-2 *The Nursing Process Applied to the Patient's Pharmacologic Needs—cont'd*

ASSESSMENT	PLANNING	INTERVENTION	EVALUATION
Nursing research of prescribed drugs—cont'd			
Patient understanding of drug therapy—cont'd		Teach name of drug being taken, symptoms that can be relieved by the p.r.n. drug, when to take it, amount to take, what to do if not effective Teach administration techniques to be used at home; give simple written instructions to follow at home	
Patient understanding of entire treatment plan	Develop goal statements for teaching the individual's care that will assist the patient in gaining knowledge of *all* aspects of self-care for the disease process present (nutritional status, activity or exercise modifications, psychological, medication, physical therapy, etc.) Incorporate assessments to determine the individual's readiness and capability to learn, degree of understanding, and tolerance for needed alterations	Implement planned nursing measures appropriate to the specific disease process affecting the individual Incorporate teaching techniques (visual aids, demonstrations and return demonstrations, role playing, etc.)	Analyze the patient's response to *each* component of the entire treatment plan Throughout the course of teaching, evaluate the degree of understanding exhibited by having the patient perform appropriate activities (for example, choose the therapeutic diet from the hospital menu) Evaluate the tolerance exhibited to restrictions and modifications implemented, or to drug side effects expected and present; document all facets of health teaching performed, degree of understanding attained, or intolerances observed or experienced

Changes in Expectations

Assess changes in expectations as therapy progresses and the patient gains understanding and skill in the management of the diagnosis. The expectations about therapy of patients with acute illnesses may vary widely from those of patients with chronic illnesses.

Changes in Therapy through Cooperative Goal Setting

An attitude of shared input into the goals can encourage the patient into therapeutic alliance. Therefore, the patient should be taught to help monitor the parameters used to evaluate therapy. It is imperative that the nurse nurture a cooperative environment that encourages the patient to (1) keep records of the essential data needed to evaluate the prescribed therapy and (2) contact the physician for advice rather than altering the medication dosages or schedule or discontinuing the medication entirely. For each major class of drugs in this book, written records are provided to help the nurse identify essential data that the patient needs to

understand and record on a regular basis to assist the physician in monitoring therapy. (See the template in Appendix K; also box on p. 153 for a sample teaching plan for a patient with diabetes mellitus receiving one type of insulin.) In the event that the patient, family, or significant others do not understand all aspects of the continuing therapy prescribed, they may be referred to a community-based agency for the achievement of long-term health care requirements.

At Dismissal

A summary statement of the patient's unmet needs must be written and placed in the medical chart. The physician should be consulted concerning the possibility of a referral to a community-based agency for continued monitoring and/or treatment. The nurse's dismissal notes must identify the nursing diagnoses that are unmet and potential collaborative problems that require continued monitoring and intervention. All counseling information should be carefully written out in a manner that the patient can read and understand.

DRUGS AFFECTING BODY SYSTEMS

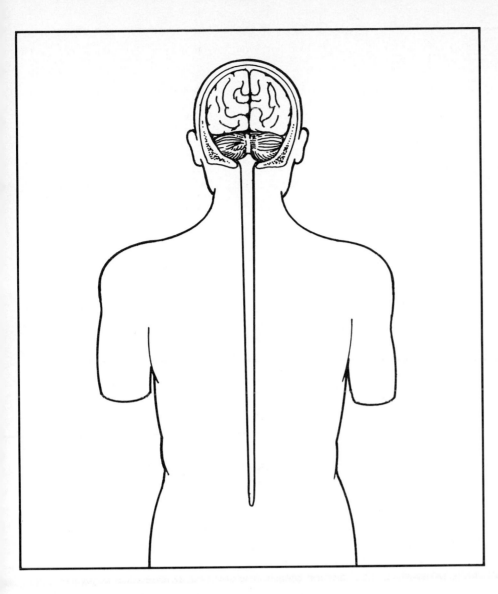

Drugs Affecting the Central Nervous System

CHAPTER GOALS

After completing this chapter, the student should be able to do the following:

1. Explain the major action (effects) of drugs used to treat disorders of the central nervous system.

2. Identify baseline data the nurse should collect on a continuous basis for comparison and evaluation of drug effectiveness.

3. Identify important nursing assessments and interventions associated with the drug therapy and treatment of diseases associated with the central nervous system.

4. Identify essential components in planning patient education that will enhance compliance with the treatment regimen.

THE CENTRAL NERVOUS SYSTEM

All human functions, from the most complex (abstract reasoning and creative thought) to the most basic (heart rate and respiration), require coordination to perform as a whole. The main coordinator of these functions is the central nervous system.

The central nervous system consists of the brain, the spinal cord, and many nerve cells called neurons. External-world information, such as sound, sight, smell, touch, and taste, and internal-world information, such as oxygen or carbon dioxide blood levels, body temperature, and muscle tension, are integrated. Instructions are relayed to the appropriate cells or tissues to produce the necessary actions and environmental adjustments. Information concerning these actions and adjustments is again relayed to the central nervous system. This feedback permits continuous adjustment in the instructions sent to various tissues for efficient control of body function.

Drugs act to decrease or increase the activity of nerve centers and conducting pathways. Many stimulants and depressants for the brain, the spinal cord, or specific centers of each have been developed, and the effects of such drugs can be predicted accurately. This chapter is subdivided into sections in which drugs are described based on their primary use.

SLEEP AND SLEEP DISTURBANCE
OBJECTIVES

1. Differentiate between the terms *sedative* and *hypnotic*; initial, intermittent, and terminal insomnia; and between *rebound sleep* and *paradoxical sleep*.
2. Identify alterations found in the sleep pattern when hypnotics are discontinued.

3. Cite nursing interventions that can be implemented as an alternative to administering a sedative-hypnotic.
4. Compare the effects of barbiturates and benzodiazepines on the central nervous system.
5. Explain the major benefits of administering benzodiazepines rather than barbiturates.
6. Identify laboratory tests that should be monitored when benzodiazepines or barbiturates are administered over an extended period of time.
7. Develop measurable short- and long-term objectives for patient education whenever a sedative or hypnotic is prescribed.

KEY WORDS

sedative   blood dyscrasias
hypnotic   delirium
insomnia   paradoxical sleep
rebound sleep

Sleep is a state of unconsciousness from which a patient can be aroused by appropriate stimulus. It is a naturally occurring phenomenon that occupies about one-third of an adult's life. It is a different state of unconsciousness from that produced by deep anesthesia or coma.

The constitution of optimal or sound sleep is a characteristic of each individual patient, but adequate sleep is important. Natural sleep is a rhythmic progression through four stages that provide physical and mental rest. Stages I and II are light sleep periods that allow easy arousal. Stage III is a transition from the lighter to deeper state of sleep, stage IV. Each stage is characterized by a specific set of brainwave activities. Stage IV sleep is called *deep sleep* and is dreamless, very restful, and associated with a 10% to 30% decrease in blood pressure, respiratory rate, and basal metabolic rate.

In a normal night of sleep, a person will rhythmically cycle through the four stages of sleep. About every 90 minutes or so, a patient will develop a sleep pattern called *paradoxical sleep*, or *REM sleep*. It is superimposed on stages I and II of sleep. This type of sleep represents up to 20% of sleep time and is characterized by rapid eye movements (REM), dreaming, increased heart rate, irregular breathing, secretion of stomach acids, and some muscular activity. REM sleep appears to be an important time for our subconscious minds to release anxiety and tension and reestablish a psychic equilibrium. The elderly take longer to move through the relaxation stages of non-REM sleep. There is an increased frequency and duration of awakenings. It is not necessarily true that the elderly require more sleep. In fact, they often sleep less but take frequent naps throughout the day. Consequently, the geriatric patient may have difficulty sleeping through the night.

Insomnia is the most common sleep disorder known. It is defined as the inability to sleep. Insomnia is not a disease but a symptom of physical or mental stress. It is usually mild and lasts for only a few nights. Common causes are changes in lifestyle or environment (such as hospitalization), pain, illness, excess consumption of products containing caffeine, eating large or "rich" meals shortly before bedtime, or anxiety. *Initial* insomnia is the inability to fall asleep when desired, *intermittent* insomnia is the inability to stay asleep, and *terminal* insomnia is characterized by early awakening with the inability to fall asleep again.

Measures that may be taken to alleviate or avoid insomnia include eliminating environmental and human noises and providing the patient with such comforts as back rubs, better ventilation, clean linens, a bedpan or urinal if needed, a change of position, extra pillows, an extra blanket, light nourishment (such as warm milk, hot chocolate, one or two crackers), and reassurance (listening to the patient's concerns).

If these measures are not successful, a sedative-hypnotic may be prescribed. A hypnotic is a drug that produces sleep. A sedative quiets the patient and gives a feeling of relaxation and rest, not necessarily accompanied by sleep. Hypnotics and sedatives are not always different drugs; their effects may depend on the dose and the condition of the patient. A small dose of a drug may act as a sedative, whereas a larger dose of the same drug may act as a hypnotic and produce sleep.

A good hypnotic should provide the following action within a short period: a restful natural sleep, a duration of action that will allow the patient to awaken at the usual time, a natural awakening with no "hangover" effects, and no danger of habit formation. Unfortunately, the ideal hypnotic is not available. The most frequently used sedative-hypnotics do increase total sleeping time, especially in stages II and IV; however, they also decrease the number of REM periods and the total time in REM sleep. When REM sleep is decreased, there is a strong tendency to "make it up." Compensatory, or *rebound*, REM sleep seems to occur even when hypnotics are used for only 3 or 4 days. After chronic administration of sedative-hypnotic agents, REM rebound may be severe, accompanied by restlessness and vivid nightmares. Depending on the frequency of hypnotic administration, normal sleep patterns may not be restored for weeks. It is suspected that the effects of REM rebound may enhance chronic use of—and dependence on—these agents to avoid the unpleasant consequences of rebound.

The sedative-hypnotics may be classified into three groups: the barbiturates, the benzodiazepines, and the miscellaneous agents (see Tables 9-1, 9-2, and 9-3).

General Nursing Considerations for Patients with Sleep Disturbance

Nurses can control many of the factors that cause sleep disturbances in the hospital setting. Therefore all efforts should be made to facilitate sleep within this new and strange environment prior to the administration of a hypnotic agent. This is a nursing challenge to be met by implementing nursing measures that will alleviate anxiety and provide for basic comfort needs. Persons with respiratory disorders and those who snore heavily may have low respiratory reserve and should not receive hypnotics because of the potential for causing respiratory depression.

Sedative-hypnotics may also be prescribed as a preanesthetic medication. If so, the primary purpose is to produce a restful sleep and thereby reduce anxiety in preparation for the planned surgical intervention.

Patient Concerns: Nursing Intervention/Rationale

Insomnia. Assess the patient's usual pattern of sleep and obtain information on the pattern of sleep disruption (such as difficulty in falling asleep, inability to sleep the entire night, or awakening in the early morning hours unable to return to a restful sleep).

Ask the patient about the amount of sleep (hours) he or she considers normal and how insomnia is managed at home. If the patient is taking medications, determine the drug, dose, and frequency of administration.

Anxiety level. Assess the patient's exhibited degree of anxiety. Is it really a sedative-hypnotic the patient needs, or is it someone to *listen* and intervene therapeutically?

Patients with persistent insomnia should be carefully monitored for the number of "naps" taken during the daytime. Investigate the type of activities performed immediately prior to retiring for sleep. A quiet "unwinding" time may be helpful. For children, try a bedtime story that is pleasant and soothing, not one that will cause anxiety or fear. Playing soft music may also promote relaxation.

Environmental control. Provide for adequate ventilation, subdued lighting, correct room temperature, and control of traffic in and out of the patient's room.

Organize nursing activities so that the patient is disturbed as infrequently as possible while maintaining safe nursing care.

Provide for the patient's well-being and personal safety. Leave a night light on, place the call light within reach, and, if appropriate, put the bed in the *low* position with the side rails up. Playing soft music may also promote relaxation. *Do not* allow a patient who has been medicated to smoke in bed.

Nutritional needs. Help the patient avoid products containing caffeine, such as coffee, tea, soft drinks, and chocolate. Limit the total daily intake of these items and give warm milk and crackers as a bedtime snack. Protein foods and dairy products contain an amino acid that synthesizes serotonin, a neurotransmitter that is found to increase sleep time and decrease the time required to fall asleep.

Exercise. Daytime exercise and being outside in the fresh air may also promote sleep.

Routine orders. Many physicians order a sedative-hypnotic on a p.r.n. basis. Do not offer it unless the patient is having difficulty sleeping and other measures to meet his or her comfort and psychological needs have failed to produce the desired effect. Never leave a medication at the bedside "in case" it is needed later.

p.r.n. If giving p.r.n. medications, assess the record for the effectiveness of the therapy. It is sometimes necessary to repeat a medication if an order exists to do so. This is up to the nurse's discretion based on the evaluation of a particular patient's needs.

A paradoxical response may occur if the patient is showing increasing signs of excitement, restlessness, euphoria, or confusion. In such cases, it would be harmful to repeat the medication.

Reassess the underlying cause of sleeplessness. Is it really pain control that is needed? If so, repeating the order for a hypnotic will not meet the patient's needs.

When a medication is administered, carefully assess the patient at regular intervals for therapeutic and adverse effects.

Personal comfort. Position the patient for maximum comfort, provide a back rub, encourage the patient to empty his or her bladder, and be certain that bedding is clean and dry. Take time to meet patients' individual needs and calm their fears. Foster a trusting relationship.

Patient Education Associated with Sedative-Hypnotic Therapy

Communication and responsibility. Encourage open communication with the patient concerning frustra-

tions and anger as attempts are made to adjust to the diagnosis and need for treatment. The patient must be guided to insight into the disorder if he or she is to assume responsibility for the continuation of treatment. Keep emphasizing those things the patient can do to alter the progression of the disease, including maintenance of good general health through adequate rest, activity, and proper nutrition.

Nutrition. Teach appropriate nutrition information concerning the basic four food groups, adequate intake of fluids, and use of vitamins. Communicate the information at the educational level of the patient.

Caffeine consumption should be reduced or discontinued. Introduce the patient to decaffeinated products that can be substituted for previously used foods containing caffeine.

For insomnia, suggest warm milk about 30 minutes before the patient attempts to sleep.

Environmental control. Encourage the patient to provide for insomnia relief by attempting to sleep in the proper environment—a quiet, darkened room free from distractions.

Activity and exercise. Plan daily activities so that the patient obtains sufficient exercise and is tired enough to sleep. Also plan a quiet "unwinding" time prior to retiring for the night.

Stress management. Some stressors that create insomnia may be within the work environment; therefore involvement of the industrial nurse, along with a thorough exploration of work factors, may be appropriate.

Teach the patient relaxation techniques and personal comfort measures, such as a warm bath, to relieve stress.

Referral for mastery of biofeedback or other techniques to reduce stress levels may be necessary.

Stress produced within the dynamics of the family may require professional counseling.

Encourage the patient to express *feelings* openly with regard to stress and insomnia. The adjustment to this situation involves working through great personal fears, frustrations, hostilities, and resentments.

Try to identify the coping mechanisms the person uses in response to stress and identify methods of channeling these toward positive realistic goals and alternatives to the use of medication.

Expectations of therapy. Discuss the expectations of therapy and the degree of relief from previous symptoms that caused the need for medications. Has the sleep pattern improved; muscle pain been decreased; seizures been controlled; anxiety been decreased?

If a substance-abuse problem exists, denial and manipulation may be major problems. See a mental health text for appropriate nursing intervention.

Changes in expectations. Assess changes in expectations as therapy progresses and the patient gains understanding and skill in the management of the diagnosis.

Patient Education and Monitoring of Therapeutic Outcomes for Patients Receiving Sleeping Pills

Medications	Color	To be taken

Name _____

Physician _____

Physician's phone _____

Next appt.* _____

	Parameters	Day of discharge							Comments
Time:	Arising								
	Bedtime								
	Last cup of coffee								
Sleep pattern	Took ___ hr. or min. to get to sleep.								
	Awaken during night; takes ___ hr. or min. to get back to sleep.								
	Slept all night								
	Couldn't sleep								
	Went right to sleep								
Dreams	Dreamed all night								
	No. of dreams								
	Did not dream								
Feelings the next morning?	Very tired when I woke up.								
	Awoke refreshed.								
Exercise	No desire to exercise								
	Usual routine, including work.								
	Unable to work								
Stress level No time to relax — Time to relax 10 5 1									
Medication	Took (#) sleeping pills								

*Please bring this record with you to your next appointment.
Use the back of this sheet for additional information.

Figure 9-1 *Patient education and monitoring of therapeutic outcomes for patients receiving sleeping pills.*

Changes in therapy through cooperative goal setting. Work mutually with the patient to encourage adherence to the treatment as prescribed. When the patient feels that a change should be made in a treatment plan, encourage discussion with the physician.

Written record. Enlist the patient's aid in developing and maintaining a written record of monitoring parameters (such as extent of insomnia, frequency; see Figure 9-1) and response to prescribed therapies for discussion with the physician. The patient should be encouraged to bring this record on follow-up visits.

Fostering compliance. Discuss medication information and how it will benefit the course of treatment. Seek cooperation and understanding of the following points so that medication compliance may be enhanced:

1. Name.
2. Dosage: Lowest dose for the shortest time possible.
3. Route and administration times: Do not leave medication at bedside; the patient may forget and repeat the dose too frequently.
4. Anticipated therapeutic response: When sedative-hypnotics are prescribed, the degree of response the patient anticipates should be discussed; all attempts should be made to substitute changes in daily activities, control of the environment, or assistance with underlying problems for the use of this medication.
5. Side effects to expect: Sedation, lethargy, and "morning hangover" or grogginess.
6. Side effects to report: Excessive drowsiness, slurred speech, tremors, alteration in mental alertness and the ability to use sound judgement, motor incoordination, mental depression, hives, rash, pruritus, fever.
7. What to do if a dosage is missed: Ignore it and substitute alternative methods of relaxation whenever possible.
8. When, how, or if to refill the medication: Try to avoid refills of sedative-hypnotic agents.

Difficulty in comprehension. If it is evident that the patient or the patient's family is not understanding all aspects of continuing therapy being prescribed (such as administration and monitoring of medications, exercises, diets, follow-up appointments), consider use of social service or visiting nurse agencies.

Associated teaching. Always inform the physician or dentist of any prescription or over-the-counter medication being taken.

Over-the-counter medications should not be taken without discussion first with the physician or pharmacist.

Always report side effects of rash, itching, or hives immediately. Nausea, vomiting, or diarrhea should also be reported for the physician's evaluation if it is a new symptom.

Keep all medications out of the reach of children.

If pregnancy is suspected, consult an obstetrician as soon as possible about continuation of medication therapy.

At discharge. Items to be sent home with the patient should include the following:

1. Written instructions for the item's use.
2. Labels in a level of language and size of print appropriate for the patient.
3. If needed, identification cards or bracelets.
4. A list of additional supplies to be purchased after discharge.
5. A schedule for follow-up appointments.

Drug Therapy for Sleep Disturbance

Barbiturates

The first barbiturate was placed on the market as a sedative-hypnotic in 1903. It became so successful that chemists identified some 2500 barbiturate compounds, of which more than 50 were distributed commercially. Barbiturates became such a mainstay of therapy that fewer than a dozen other sedative-hypnotic agents were successfully marketed through 1960. The release of the first benzodiazepine (chlordiazepoxide) in 1961 started the decline in the use of barbiturates. However, several barbiturate compounds are still prescribed today (see Table 9-1).

Barbiturates can reversibly depress the activity of all excitable tissues. The central nervous system is particularly sensitive, but the degrees of depression (ranging from mild sedation to deep coma and death) depend on the dosage, route of administration, tolerance from previous use, degree of excitability of the central nervous system at the time of administration, and condition of the patient. Usual hypnotic doses produce mild respiratory depression similar to that of natural sleep; with large doses, the rate, depth, and volume of respiration are markedly diminished.

Barbiturates are classified according to their duration of action: ultrashort-, short-, intermediate-, and long-acting. Since the duration of action depends on the dose and the rate of metabolism of the barbiturate, it is important to use the duration-of-action information as a guideline only.

Barbiturate-induced sleep varies from normal sleep in that there is decreased REM time. With chronic administration of hypnotic doses, the amount of REM sleep gradually returns to normal as tolerance develops to the REM suppressant effect. When barbiturate therapy is discontinued, a rebound increase in REM sleep occurs in spite of the tolerance. Irregularities in REM sleep cycles may take weeks to dissipate fully.

Barbiturates are used primarily for their sedative and hypnotic effects. Long-acting barbiturates (that is, phenobarbital, metharbital) are also used for their anticonvulsant activity. The ultrashort-acting agents (metho-

Table 9-1 *Barbiturates*

GENERIC NAME	BRAND NAME	AVAILABILITY	ADULT ORAL DOSE	COMMENTS
Amobarbital	Amytal, ✚Isobec	Tablets: 30, 50, 100 mg Capsules: 65, 200 mg	Sedation: 30-50 mg 2-3 times daily Hypnosis: 100-200 mg 30 minutes before bedtime	Intermediate-acting; Schedule II Used primarily as a daytime sedative and bedtime hypnotic; may also be used as a sedative prior to anesthesia or during labor Also available for rectal, IM, and IV use
Aprobarbital	Alurate	Elixir: 40 mg/5 ml	Sedation: 40 mg 3 times daily Hypnosis: 40-160 mg prior to bedtime	Intermediate-acting; Schedule III Used primarily as a daytime sedative and bedtime hypnotic Elixir contains 20% alcohol
Butabarbital	Butisol, Butatran, Butalan, ✚Neo-Barb	Tablets: 15, 30, 50, 100 mg Capsules: 15, 30 mg Elixir: 30, 33.3 mg/5 ml	Sedation: 15-30 mg 3-4 times daily Hypnosis: 50-100 mg at bedtime	Intermediate-acting; Schedule III Used primarily as a daytime sedative and bedtime hypnotic Elixir contains 7% alcohol
Mephobarbital	Mebaral	Tablets: 32, 50, 100, mg	Sedation: 32-100 mg 3-4 times daily Anticonvulsant: 400-600 mg daily	Long-acting; Schedule IV Used primarily as an anticonvulsant; may also be used as a daytime sedative
Metharbital	Gemonil	Tablets: 100 mg	Anticonvulsant: up to 600-800 mg daily	Long-acting; Schedule III Used as an anticonvulsant, usually in combination with other anticonvulsant agents
Pentobarbital	Nembutal, ✚Pentogen	Capsules: 50, 100 mg Elixir: 18.2 mg/5 ml	Sedation: 30 mg 3-4 times daily Hypnosis: 100 mg at bedtime	Short-acting; Schedule II Used primarily as a daytime sedative and bedtime hypnotic; may also be used as a preanesthetic sedative Elixir contains 18% alcohol Also available for IM and IV use
Phenobarbital	Luminal, Solfoton, Barbita, ✚Gardenal	Tablets: 8, 16, 30, 32, 65, 100 mg Capsules: 16 mg Elixir: 15, 20 mg/5 ml	Sedation: 8-30 mg 2-3 times daily Hypnosis: 100-320 mg Anticonvulsant: 50-100 mg 2-3 times daily	Long-acting; Schedule IV Used most commonly now as an anticonvulsant; may also be used as a daytime sedative, preanesthetic, or hypnotic agent Also available for IM and IV use Elixir contains 13.5% alcohol
Secobarbital	Seconal	Tablets: 100 mg Capsules: 100 mg	Hypnosis: 100-200 mg at bedtime	Short-acting; Schedule II Used primarily as a daytime sedative or bedtime hypnotic Therapy is not recommended for longer than 14 days Also available for IM and IV use

✚Available in Canada only.

hexital, thiopental) may be administered intravenously as general anesthetics.

Side effects. The habitual use of barbiturates may result in physical dependence. Rapid discontinuance of barbiturates after long-term use of high dosages may result in symptoms similar to alcohol withdrawal. These may vary from weakness and anxiety to delirium and grand mal seizures. Treatment consists of cautious and gradual withdrawal of barbiturates over a 2- to 4-week period.

General adverse effects of barbiturates include drowsiness, lethargy, headache, muscle or joint pain, and mental depression. Barbiturate "hangover" frequently occurs after administration of hypnotic doses of the long-acting barbiturates. Patients may display a dulled affect, subtle distortion of mood, and impaired coordination.

Elderly patients and those in severe pain may respond paradoxically to barbiturates with excitement, euphoria, restlessness, and confusion.

Hypersensitivity reactions to barbiturates are infrequent but may be serious. Barbiturate therapy should be discontinued immediately if the patient develops symptoms of hypersensitivity.

Rarely, barbiturates may induce blood dyscrasias.

Availability. See Table 9-1.

Dosage and administration. See Table 9-1.

• Nursing Interventions: Monitoring barbiturate therapy

See also General Nursing Considerations for Patients with Sleep Disturbance (p. 165).

Side effects to expect

"HANGOVER," SEDATION, LETHARGY. Patients may complain of "morning hangover," blurred vision, and transient hypotension on arising.

Explain to the patient the need for arising first to a sitting position, equilibrating, and then standing. Assistance with ambulation may be required.

If hangover becomes troublesome, there should be a reduction in the dosage, a change in the medication, or both.

People working around machinery, driving a car, pouring and giving medicines, or performing other duties in which they must remain mentally alert should not take these medications while working.

Side effects to report

EXCESSIVE USE OR ABUSE. Assist the patient to recognize the abuse problem.

Identify underlying needs and plan for more appropriate management of those needs.

Discuss the case with the physician and make plans to cooperatively approach gradual withdrawal of the medications being abused.

Provide for emotional support of the individual; display an accepting attitude—be kind but firm.

PARADOXICAL RESPONSE. Provide supportive physical care and safety during these responses.

Assess the level of excitement and deal calmly with the individual. During periods of excitement, protect people from harm and provide for physical channeling of energy (for example, walk with them).

Seek change in the medication order.

HYPERSENSITIVITY. Report symptoms of hives, pruritus, rash, high fever, or inflammation of mucous membranes for evaluation by the physician. Withhold further barbiturate administration until physician's approval has been granted.

BLOOD DYSCRASIAS. Routine laboratory studies (RBC, WBC, and differential counts) should be scheduled. Stress the importance of patient's returning for this laboratory work.

Monitor for the development of sore throat, fever, purpura, jaundice, or excessive and progressive weakness.

Drug interactions

DRUGS THAT INCREASE TOXIC EFFECTS. Antihistamines, alcohol, analgesics, anesthetics, tranquilizers, valproic acid, chloramphenicol, monoamine oxidase inhibitors, and other sedative-hypnotics: Monitor the patient for excessive sedation and reduce the dosage of the barbiturate if necessary.

PHENYTOIN. The effects of barbiturates on phenytoin are variable. Serum levels may be ordered, and a change in phenytoin dosage may be required. Observe patients for increased seizure activity and for signs of phenytoin toxicity: nystagmus, sedation, and lethargy.

BARBITURATES DECREASE THE EFFECTS OF:

Warfarin. Monitor the prothrombin time and increase the dosage of warfarin if necessary.

Digitoxin. Monitor the digitoxin serum levels for signs of increased congestive heart failure: dyspnea, orthopnea, edema. The dosage of digitoxin may need to be increased.

Estrogens. This drug interaction may be critical in patients receiving oral contraceptives containing estrogen. If patients develop spotting and breakthrough bleeding, a change in oral contraceptives and the use of alternative forms of contraception should be considered.

Corticosteroids, propranolol, doxycycline, antidepressants, quinidine, and chlorpromazine. The patient should be monitored for signs of increased activity of the illness for which the medication was prescribed. Dosage increases may be necessary or the barbiturate may have to be discontinued.

Benzodiazepines

Benzodiazepines, as a class of compounds, have been extremely successful products from a marketing and safety standpoint. A major advantage over the barbiturate and nonbarbiturate sedative-hypnotics is the wide safety margin between therapeutic and lethal dosages. Intentional and unintentional overdoses of several hundred times the normal therapeutic doses are well tolerated and are not fatal.

Over 2000 benzodiazepine derivatives have been identified, and over 100 have been tested for sedative-hypnotic or other activity. While there are many similarities among the benzodiazepines, they are difficult to characterize as a class. This is so because certain benzodiazepines are effective anticonvulsants (p. 205), others serve as antianxiety agents (p. 187), while still others are used as sedative-hypnotics (below). It is thought that they are all similar in mechanisms of action as CNS depressants but that individual derivatives act more selectively at specific sites, thus allowing for a variety of uses.

Six benzodiazepine derivatives are used as sedative-hypnotics (see Table 9-2). When benzodiazepine ther-

Table 9-2 *Benzodiazepines Used for Sedation-Hypnosis*

GENERIC NAME	BRAND NAME	AVAILABILITY	ADULT ORAL DOSAGE	COMMENTS
Estrazolam	ProSom	Tablets: 1, 2 mg	Hypnosis: 1-2 mg at bedtime	Intermediate-acting; Schedule IV Used for insomnia Tapering therapy recommended to reduce rebound insomnia Minimal "morning hangover"
Flurazepam	Dalmane, ✚Novoflupam	Capsules: 15, 30 mg	Hypnosis: 15-30 mg at bedtime	Long-acting; Schedule IV Used for short-term treatment of insomnia, up to 4 weeks Morning hangover may be significant Rebound insomnia and REM sleep occur less frequently
Lorazepam	Ativan, ✚Novolorazepam	Tablets: 0.5, 1, 2 mg Inj: 2 mg and 4 mg/ml in 1, 10 ml vials; 4 mg prefilled syringes	Hypnosis: 2-4 mg at bedtime	Used primarily for insomnia, but may also be used for preoperative anxiety IM, IV administration also available
Midazolam	Versed	Inj: 1, 5 mg/ml in 1, 2, 5, 10 ml vials; 2 ml prefilled syringes	Preop: IM—0.07-0.08 mg/kg 1 hr prior to surgery Induction of Anesthesia; IV—0.2-0.3 mg/kg Endoscopy: IV—0.1-0.15 mg/kg	Short-acting; Schedule IV Onset: IM—15 minutes IV—3-5 minutes Duration: IM—30-60 minutes IV—2-6 hours Causes amnesia in most patients Lower doses in patients over age 55
Quazepam	Doral	Tablets: 7.5, 15 mg	Hypnosis: 7.5–15 mg at bedtime	Long-acting; Schedule IV Used for insomnia Tapering therapy recommended to reduce rebound insomnia "Morning hangover" may be significant
Temazepam	Restoril	Capsules: 15, 30 mg	Hypnosis: 15-30 mg at bedtime	Intermediate-acting; Schedule IV Used for insomnia Minimal if any "morning hangover" Rebound insomnia may occur
Triazolam	Halcion	Tablets: 0.125, 0.25 mg	Hypnosis: 0.25-0.5 mg at bedtime	Short-acting; Schedule IV Used for insomnia, but tends to lose effectiveness within 2 weeks Tapering therapy is recommended to reduce rebound insomnia Rapid onset of action No "morning hangover"

✚ Available in Canada only.

apy is started, patients feel a sense of deep or refreshing sleep. Benzodiazepine-induced sleep varies, however, from normal sleep in that there is less REM sleep. With chronic administration, the amount of REM sleep gradually increases as tolerance develops to the REM suppressant effects. When benzodiazepines are discontinued, a rebound increase in REM sleep occurs in spite of the tolerance. During the rebound period, the number of dreams stays about the same, but many of the dreams are reported to be bizarre in nature. After chronic use of most benzodiazepines, there is also a rebound in insomnia. Consequently it is important to use these agents only for short courses of therapy.

Midazolam (Table 9-2) is the first of a new series of short-acting, parenterally administered benzodiazepine CNS depressants. It is used intramuscularly as a preoperative sedative and intravenously for conscious sedation prior to short diagnostic procedures or for induction of general anesthesia. It has a more rapid onset of action then diazepam and a much shorter duration. It also produces a greater degree of amnesia than diazepam, again making it beneficial for short diagnostic and operative procedures. Because the amnesic effect may persist for several hours after the administration of midazolam, it is suggested that outpatients who are treated with the drug should be given postoperative instructions in writing.

Side effects. The more common side effects of benzodiazepines are extensions of their pharmacologic properties. Drowsiness, fatigue, lethargy, and "morning hangover" are relatively common.

The habitual use of benzodiazepines may result in physical and psychological dependence. Rapid discontinuance of benzodiazepines after long-term use may result in symptoms similar to alcohol withdrawal. These may vary from weakness and anxiety to delirium and grand mal seizures. The symptoms may not appear for several days after discontinuation. Treatment consists of gradual withdrawal of benzodiazepines over a 2- to 4-week period.

Benzodiazepines should be administered with caution to patients with a history of blood dyscrasias or hepatic damage.

Availability. See Table 9-2.

Dosage and administration. See Table 9-2.

• Nursing Interventions: Monitoring benzodiazepine therapy

See also General Nursing Considerations for Patients with Sleep Disturbance (p. 165).

Side effects to expect

"HANGOVER," SEDATION, LETHARGY. Patients may complain of "morning hangover," blurred vision, and transient hypotension on arising.

Explain to the patient the need for arising first to a sitting position, equilibrating, and then standing. Assistance with ambulation may be required.

If hangover becomes troublesome, there should be a reduction in the dosage or a change in the medication or both.

Persons who are working around machinery, driving a car, pouring and giving medicines, or performing other duties in which they must remain mentally alert should not take these medications while working.

Side effects to report

EXCESSIVE USE OR ABUSE. Assist the patient to recognize the abuse problem.

Identify underlying needs and plan for more appropriate management of those needs.

Discuss the case with the physician and make plans to cooperatively approach gradual withdrawal of the medications being abused.

Provide for emotional support of the individual; display an accepting attitude—be kind but firm.

BLOOD DYSCRASIAS. Routine laboratory studies (RBC, WBC, and differential counts) should be scheduled. Stress the patient's returning for these tests.

Monitor for the development of a sore throat, fever, purpura, jaundice, or excessive and progressive weakness.

HEPATOTOXICITY. The symptoms of hepatotoxicity are anorexia, nausea, vomiting, jaundice, hepatomegaly, splenomegaly, and abnormal liver function tests (elevated bilirubin, AST, ALT, GGT, alkaline phosphatase, prothrombin time).

Drug interactions

DRUGS THAT INCREASE TOXIC EFFECTS. Antihistamines, alcohol, analgesics, anesthetics, tranquilizers, narcotics, cimetidine, and other sedative-hypnotics.

SMOKING. Smoking enhances the metabolism of the benzodiazepines. Larger doses may be necessary to maintain sedative effects in patients who smoke.

Miscellaneous sedative-hypnotic agents

The nonbarbiturate, nonbenzodiazepine sedative-hypnotics are listed in Table 9-3. All have somewhat variable effects on REM sleep, development of tolerance, and rebound REM sleep and insomnia. Because of the safety factor, the use of these agents is diminishing in favor of the benzodiazepines.

Side effects. The habitual use of these sedative-hypnotic agents may result in physical dependence. Rapid discontinuance after long-term use may result in symptoms similar to alcohol withdrawal. These may vary from weakness and anxiety to delirium and grand mal seizures. Treatment consists of gradual withdrawal over a 2- to 4-week period.

General adverse effects include drowsiness, lethargy, headache, muscle or joint pain, and mental depression. "Morning hangover" frequently occurs after administration of hypnotic doses. Patients may display dulled affect, subtle distortion of mood, and impaired coordination. Some patients experience transient restlessness and anxiety before falling asleep.

Table 9-3 *Miscellaneous Sedative-Hypnotic Agents*

GENERIC NAME	BRAND NAME	AVAILABILITY	ADULT ORAL DOSE	COMMENTS
Acetylcarbromal	Paxarel	Tablets: 250 mg	Sedation: 250-500 mg 2-3 times daily	Short-acting Metabolized to bromide, prolonged use may result in bromide toxicity; discontinue use if dizziness, impaired thought and memory, incoordination (bromism) develop Rarely used today because of availability of safer and more effective sedatives
Chloral hydrate	Noctec, Aquachloral, ♣Novochlorhydrate	Capsules: 250, 500 mg Syrup: 250, 500 mg/5 ml Suppositories: 325, 500, 650 mg	Sedation: 250 mg 3 times daily after meals Hypnosis: 500 mg to 1 g 15-30 minutes before bedtime	The original "Mickey Finn"; Schedule IV Used primarily as a bedtime hypnotic, but also is used as a preoperative sedative because it does not depress respirations or cough reflex May cause nausea; administer with full glass of water; do not chew capsules See Drug Interactions
Ethchlorvynol	Placidyl	Capsules: 200, 500, 750 mg	Hypnosis: —Usual dose 500 mg at bedtime —100-200 mg may be administered if patient wakes up after 500-750 mg	Short-acting; Schedule IV Used for short-term insomnia Therapy is not recommended beyond 1 week
Ethinamate	Valmid	Capsules: 500 mg	Hypnosis: 500 mg to 1 g 20 minutes before bedtime	Short-acting; Schedule IV Used for short-term insomnia; loses effectiveness after about 7 days
Glutethimide	Doriden	Tablets: 250, 500 mg	Hypnosis: 250-500 mg at bedtime	Short-acting; Schedule III Used for short-term insomnia; not recommended for use beyond 3-7 days See Drug Interactions
Methyprylon	Noludar	Tablets: 200 mg Capsules: 300 mg	Hypnosis: 200-400 mg 15-30 minutes before bedtime	Intermediate-acting; Schedule III Used for short-term insomnia; requires 45 minutes for sleep but lasts 5-8 hours
Paraldehyde	Paral	Liquid: 30 ml (for oral or rectal use)	Sedation: 4-8 ml	Bitter-tasting, unpleasant odor; administer in milk or iced fruit juice to mask taste and odor Dispense only in a glass container; do not use a plastic spoon or container Used predominantly as a sedative in treating delirium tremens This agent imparts a strong, foul odor to the breath for up to 24 hours after administration; the patient is often unaware of the foul smell Schedule IV

♣Available in Canada only.

Elderly patients and those in severe pain may respond paradoxically with excitement, euphoria, restlessness, and confusion.

Hypersensitivity reactions are infrequent but may be serious. Therapy should be discontinued immediately if the patient develops symptoms of hypersensitivity.

Availability. See Table 9-3.

Dosage and administration. See Table 9-3.

- **Nursing Interventions: Monitoring sedative-hypnotic therapy**

See also General Nursing Considerations for Patients with Sleep Disturbance (p. 165).

Side effects to expect

"HANGOVER," SEDATION, LETHARGY. Patients may complain of "morning hangover," blurred vision, and transient hypotension on arising.

Explain to the patient the need for arising first to a sitting position, equilibrating, and then standing. Assistance with ambulation may be required.

If hangover becomes troublesome, there should be a reduction in the dosage or a change in medication or both.

Persons who are working around machinery, driving a car, pouring and giving medicines, or performing other duties in which they must remain mentally alert should not take these medications while working.

RESTLESSNESS, ANXIETY. These side effects are usually mild and do not warrant discontinuation of the medication. Encourage the patient to try to relax and let the sedative effect take over.

Safety measures such as maintenance of bed rest, side rails, and observation should be used during this period.

Implementation

PARALDEHYDE. Dilute oral form in milk or iced fruit juice to mask taste and odor.

Dispense only in glass container; do not use a plastic spoon or container.

Drug interactions

CNS DEPRESSANTS. CNS depressants, including sleeping aids, analgesics, anesthetics, narcotics, tranquilizers, and alcohol, will increase the sedative effects of the sedative-hypnotics.

WARFARIN. Glutethimide and ethchlorvynol may diminish the anticoagulant effects of warfarin. Monitor the prothrombin time and increase the dosage of warfarin if necessary.

Chloral hydrate may enhance the anticoagulant effects of warfarin. Observe for the development of petechiae, ecchymoses, nosebleeds, bleeding gums, dark tarry stools, and bright red or "coffee-ground" emesis. Monitor the prothrombin time and reduce the dosage of warfarin if necessary.

DISULFIRAM. Disulfiram may prolong the activity of paraldehyde. Monitor the patient for excessive sedation.

CLINITEST. Chloral hydrate may produce false-positive Clinitest results. Use Clinistix or Tes-tape to measure urine glucose.

PARKINSON'S DISEASE
OBJECTIVES

1. Prepare a list of signs and symptoms of Parkinson's disease and accurately define the vocabulary utilized for the pharmacological agents prescribed and the disease state.
2. Name the neurotransmitter that is found in excess and the neurotransmitter that is deficient in persons with parkinsonism.
3. Describe reasonable expectations of medications prescribed for treatment of Parkinson's disease.
4. Identify the period of time necessary for a therapeutic response to be observable when drugs used to treat parkinsonism are initiated.
5. List symptoms that can be attributed to the cholinergic activity of pharmacological agents.
6. Name the action of bromocriptine mesylate, carbidopa, and levodopa on neurotransmitters involved in Parkinson's disease.
7. Cite the specific symptoms that should show improvement when anticholinergic agents are administered to the patient with Parkinson's disease.
8. Develop measurable short- and long-term objectives for patient education for persons with Parkinson's disease.
9. Describe specific adaptations in patient education needed for a patient recently diagnosed with Parkinson's disease as opposed to the needs of a patient under long-term treatment who requires a medication adjustment.

KEY WORDS

Parkinson's disease	neurotransmitter
propulsive movements	dyskinesia
livido reticularis	cholinergic crisis
anticholinergic agents	anticholinergic activity

Parkinson's disease, or paralysis agitans, is a chronic disorder of the central nervous system. An estimated 200,000 to 400,000 patients in the United States are afflicted by this disorder, and an estimated 40,000 new cases are diagnosed annually. Characteristic symptoms are muscle tremors, slowness of movement, muscle weakness with rigidity, and alterations in posture and equilibrium. The cause of Parkinson's disease is unknown, but it is thought to reflect an imbalance in neurotransmitters within the brain. There is a relative excess of acetylcholine (causes excitation) and an absolute deficiency of dopamine in the basal ganglia. Parkinsonian symptoms may also be associated with the use of higher doses of antipsychotic agents such as the phenothiazines. The phenothiazines act by inhibition of dopamine, leaving an excess of acetylcholine in the basal ganglia. The treatment of these drug-induced symptoms may require therapy with anticholinergic agents, some of the same agents used in the treatment of Parkinson's disease.

Treatment of parkinsonism remains palliative rather than curative. Goals are to provide maximal relief of symptoms and to maintain some independence of movement and activity. Drug therapy includes the use of anticholinergic agents to inhibit the relative excess in cholinergic activity and levodopa, carbidopa, bromocriptine, pergolide, selegiline, or amantadine to enhance dopaminergic activity.

General Nursing Considerations for Patients with Parkinson's Disease

Parkinson's disease affects the entire family. The disease frequently occurs during middle adult years when the high expenses of educating a family or of planning and saving for retirement are at a peak.

The patient and family need assistance to learn the medical regimen aimed at controlling the symptoms and maintaining the patient at an optimal level of participation in the activities of daily living. The drug therapy presents the potential for many side effects that all involved parties must understand.

Nurses can have a major influence in the positive use of coping mechanisms as the patient and family express varying degrees of anxiety, frustration, hostility, conflict, and fear. The primary goal of nursing intervention should be to keep the patient socially interactive and participatory in daily activities. This can be accomplished through the use of physical therapy, adherence to the drug regimen, and management of the course of treatment.

Patient Concerns: Nursing Intervention/Rationale

Characteristics of Parkinsonism

Stages of Parkinson's disease. Parkinson's disease has five stages, based on the degree of disability exhibited by the patient:

Stage 1: involvement of one limb; mild disease
Stage 2: involvement of two limbs
Stage 3: significant gait alterations and moderate generalized disability
Stage 4: Akinesia (abnormal state of motor and psychic hypoactivity or muscle paralysis), rigidity, and severe disability
Stage 5: unable to perform all activities of daily living

Facial appearance. The patient typically appears expressionless, as if wearing a mask; eyes are wide open and fixed in position. Some patients have almost total eyelid closure.

Tremors. Tremors are often observed in the hands and may involve the jaw, lips, and tongue. A "pill rolling" motion in the fingers and thumbs is a characteristic movement. Tremors are usually reduced with voluntary movement. Emotional stress and fatigue may increase the frequency of tremors.

Assess the degree of tremor involvement and specific limitations in activities being affected by the tremors.

Salivation. As a result of excessive cholinergic activity, patients salivate excessively. As the disease progresses, patients may be unable to swallow all secretions and will frequently drool. If pharyngeal muscles are involved, the patient will have difficulty chewing and swallowing.

Dyskinesia. Dyskinesia is the impairment of the individual's ability to perform voluntary movements. This symptom commonly starts in one arm or hand. It is usually most noticeable because the patient ceases to swing the arm on the affected side while walking.

As the dyskinesia progresses, movement, especially in small muscle groups, becomes slow and jerky. This motion is often referred to as "cogwheel rigidity." Muscle soreness, fatigue, and pain are associated with the prolonged muscle contractibility. The patient develops a shuffling gait, and once-automatic movements such as getting out of a chair or walking require a concentrated effort to be accomplished.

Along with the shuffling gait, the head and spine flex forward and the shoulders become rounded and stooped.

As mobility deteriorates, steps quicken and become shorter. Propulsive, uncontrolled movement forward or backward is evident. Patient safety becomes a primary consideration.

Emotional lability. The disease does *not* affect the intellectual capacity of the patient. The chronic nature of the disease and physical impairment produce mood swings and serious depression. Patients commonly display a delayed reaction time. The individual should be observed for the development of signs of dementia, which may be associated with the disease, may be a result of medications, or may be a new medical diagnosis.

Patient assessment. Assess the patient's degree of alertness and orientation to name, place, and time prior to initiating therapy. Also assess the quality, rate, volume, and flow of speech.

Evaluate the patient's strengths and resources available to assist in working with the disease.

Activity and exercise. Assess the individual's current level of exercise and compare it to daily life prior to diagnosis.

Stress. Take a detailed history of how the patient has controlled physical and mental stress in the past.

Family resources. Determine what family resources are available and the closeness of the family during daily as well as stress-producing events.

Strive to develop a trusting relationship by listening and providing support for patient and family concerns.

Patient Education Associated with Therapy for Parkinson's Disease

Communication and responsibility. Encourage open communication with the patient concerning frustrations and anger as attempts are made to adjust to the diagnosis and need for treatment. The patient must be guided to insight into the disorder if he or she is to assume responsibility for the continuation of the treatment. Keep emphasizing those things the patient can do to alter the progression of the disease, including the factors listed below.

Posture. The minimization of deformities is imperative to the long-term well-being of the patient. Erect posture and joint mobility through active and passive exercise must be maintained.

Head and neck. Perform prescribed exercises to maintain head and neck strength, mobility, and erectness. Encourage the patient to lie on a firm mattress without a pillow. Exercises should include a regimen to maintain the strength of facial muscles and for the tongue to facilitate speech clarity and the ability to swallow.

Gait training. Prescribed gait training is essential if the patient is to delay the onset of shuffling and propulsion of the gait.

Nutrition. As the disease progresses, dietary modification will be necessary.

Adequate fluid intake to maintain hydration and foods to promote bulk and stool softness should be used to minimize constipation.

Vitamins should not be given unless recommended by the physician. Pyridoxine (B$_6$) will reduce the therapeutic effect of levodopa.

The type and consistency of foods given must be tailored to current individual symptoms. In advanced disease, many patients have difficulty swallowing and may aspirate food or water. Because of fatigue and difficulty in eating, assistance appropriate to the degree of impairment should be given. Do not rush the individual when he or she is eating; cut foods in bite-sized pieces. Plan six smaller meals rather than three large meals.

The patient should be weighed weekly with periodic evaluation of the trend in body weight.

Self-reliance. Encourage patients to perform as many activities of daily living as they are able to do. Do not "take over"; encourage self-maintenance. Provide for socialization and activities such as hobbies.

Stress management. The avoidance of stress and the need for relaxation are essential; symptoms such as tremors are enhanced by anxiety.

Depression and mood alterations are secondary to disease progression (for example, lack of ability to participate in sex, immobility, incontinence) and may be expected.

Expectations of therapy. Discuss the expectations of therapy. With medications such as levodopa, several weeks of therapy may be required before any degree of improvement in symptoms may be noted.

Generally, patients expect an increase in joint mobility and relief from rigidity and tremor activity. When excessive salivation and drooling are present, relief from these symptoms is desired.

Because of the many side effects from these drugs, individualized teaching of the patient and family is imperative.

Cooperatively, set realistic goals. Family members and the patient need assistance in the establishment and continued refinement of goals as the symptoms of disease improve or worsen.

Changes in expectations. Assess changes in expectations as therapy progresses and the patient gains understanding and skill in the management of the diagnosis.

Changes in therapy through cooperative goal setting. Work mutually with the patient to encourage adherence to the treatment prescribed. When the patient feels that a change should be made in a treatment plan encourage discussion first with the physician.

Written record. Enlist the patient's aid in developing and maintaining a written record (Figure 9-2) of monitoring parameters (such as degree of tremor relief, stability, changes in mobility and rigidity, sedation, constipation, drowsiness, mental alertness or deviations) and response to prescribed therapies for discussion with the physician. Patients should be encouraged to bring this record with them on follow-up visits.

Fostering compliance. Throughout the hospitalization, discuss medication information and how it will benefit the course of treatment. Seek cooperation and understanding of the following points so that medication compliance may be increased.

1. Name.
2. Dosage.
3. Route and administration times: Sudden withdrawal of medication may precipitate a parkinsonian crisis characterized by anxiety, sweating, and tachycardia and an exacerbation of tremors, rigidity, and dyskinesia; administer medication after meals to prevent gastric irritation.
4. Anticipated therapeutic response: Improved gait, posture, speech, mobility, and ability to perform activities of daily living; decreased salivation and sweating may be observed with anticholinergic agents.
5. Side effects to expect: Nausea, vomiting, and anorexia can be reduced by administering medications after meals or with food; orthostatic hypotension may be manifested by dizziness and weakness, particularly during initiation of therapy or therapy changes; confusion, disorientation, mental depres-

Patient Education and Monitoring of Therapeutic Outcomes for Patients Receiving Antiparkinson Agents

Medications	Color	To be taken

Name _____

Physician _____

Physician's phone _____

Next appt.* _____

Parameters		Day of discharge								Comments
Weight										
Blood pressure										
Pulse										
Tremor relief or pain relief Little relief — Moderate relief — Good relief 10 — 5 — 1										
Mobility and rigidity — gait training, working or not? No improvement — Less rigidity 10 — 5 — 1										
Control of secretions? Worse — Improved — No problem 10 — 5 — 1										
Alertness and orientation to time, person, and place (T.P.P.). Poor — Good 10 — 5 — 1										
Exercise: Note present level of activity: Walking, getting out, performing range of motion (R.O.M.) exercises.										
Bowel and bladder	Constipated = C Normal = N (Check one)	C___ N___	C___ N___	C___ N___	C___ N___	C___ N___	C___ N___	C___ N___		
	Difficulty urinating = D									
	Occasional problem urinating									
Dietary needs	No problem eating or drinking.									
	Drinks (_#_) glasses fluid per day.									
	Needs frequent small meals.									
	Needs a lot of time to eat.									
Socialization Withdrawn — Active, involved 10 — 5 — 1										

*Please bring this record with you to your next appointment.
Use the back of this sheet for additional information.

Figure 9-2 *Patient education and monitoring of therapeutic outcomes for patients receiving antiparkinson agents.*

sion, insomnia, and hallucinations require careful assessment; with anticholinergic agents, constipation is to be anticipated; careful dietary management aimed at adequate fluid intake and sufficient bulk is important; dryness in the mouth may be relieved by sucking on hard candy or ice chips, or by chewing gum.

6. Side effects to report: Changes in mental clarity, tachycardia, palpitations, apparent deterioration of clinical status; dosage adjustments may be required.

7. What to do if a dosage is missed, and when, how, or if to refill the medication: Sudden withdrawal of medications may produce a parkinsonian crisis; keep an adequate supply of medications available.

Difficulty in comprehension. If it is evident that the patient or family does not understand all aspects of continuing therapy being prescribed (that is, administration and monitoring of medications, exercises, diets, follow-up appointments), consider use of social service or visiting nurse agencies.

Associated teaching. Always inform the physician or dentist of any prescription or over-the-counter medication being taken.

Over-the-counter medications should not be taken without first discussing with the physician or pharmacist; this includes vitamin preparations.

Always report side effects of rash, itching, or hives immediately. Nausea, vomiting, or diarrhea should also be reported for the physician's evaluation if it is a new symptom.

Take all of the medication as prescribed for the full course of treatment. Do not discontinue use when feeling improved; do not save for future use or give medicine to another individual. Sudden discontinuation of certain medications may produce harmful effects.

Keep all medications out of the reach of children.

If pregnancy is suspected, consult an obstetrician as soon as possible about continuation of medication therapy.

At discharge. Items to be sent home with the patient should include the following:

1. Written instructions for the item's use.
2. Labels in a level of language and size of print appropriate for the patient.
3. If needed, identification cards or bracelets.
4. A list of additional supplies to be purchased after discharge (such as eating aids, walker).
5. A schedule for follow-up appointments.

Drug Therapy for Parkinson's Disease

amantadine hydrochloride (ah-man′tah-deen)

Symmetrel (sim′eh-trel)

Amantadine is a compound developed originally to treat viral infections. It was administered to a patient with parkinsonism who also had the Asian flu. During the course of therapy for the flu, the patient showed definite improvement in the parkinsonian symptoms. The exact mechanism of action is unknown but appears to be unrelated to the drug's antiviral activity. Amantidine seems to slow the destruction of dopamine, thus making the small amount present more effective. It may also aid in the release of dopamine from its storage sites. Unfortunately, about half the patients who benefit from amantadine therapy will begin to notice a reduction in benefit after 2 or 3 months. An increase in dosage or temporary discontinuation followed by a reinitiation of therapy several weeks later may restore the therapeutic benefits.

Side effects. Most of the adverse effects of amantadine therapy are dose-related and reversible. Common side effects include confusion, disorientation, mental depression, dizziness and light-headedness, nervousness, insomnia, and gastrointestinal complaints manifested by nausea, anorexia, abdominal discomfort, and constipation.

A dermatologic condition known as livido reticularis is frequently observed in conjunction with amantadine therapy. It is characterized by diffuse, rose-colored mottling of the skin, often accompanied by pedal edema, predominantly in the extremities. It is more noticeable when the patient is standing or exposed to cold. It is reversible within 2 to 6 weeks after discontinuation of amantadine but generally does not require discontinuation of therapy.

Amantadine should be used with caution in patients with a history of seizure activity, liver disease, uncontrolled psychosis, or congestive heart failure. Amantadine may cause an exacerbation of these disorders.

Availability

PO—100 mg capsules, 50 mg/5 ml syrup.

Dosage and administration

Adult

PO—Initially, 100 mg 2 times daily. Maximum daily dose is 400 mg.

- **Nursing Interventions: Monitoring amantadine therapy**

See also General Nursing Considerations for Patients with Parkinson's Disease (p. 175).

Side effects to expect

CONFUSION, DISORIENTATION, MENTAL DEPRESSION. Perform a baseline assessment of the patient's degree of alertness and orientation to name, place, and time *prior* to initiating therapy. Make regularly scheduled subsequent evaluations of mental status and compare findings. Report development of alterations.

DIZZINESS, LIGHT-HEADEDNESS, ANOREXIA, NAUSEA, ABDOMINAL DISCOMFORT. These side effects are usually mild and tend to resolve with continued therapy. Encourage the patient not to discontinue therapy without first consulting the physician. Provide for patient safety during periods of dizziness or light-headedness.

LIVIDO RETICULARIS (SKIN MOTTLING). These side effects are usually mild and tend to resolve with continued therapy. Symptoms are enhanced by exposure to the cold or by prolonged standing. Encourage the patient not to discontinue therapy without first consulting the physician.

Side effects to report
LIVER DISEASE. The symptoms of liver disease are anorexia, nausea, vomiting, jaundice, hepatomegaly, splenomegaly, and abnormal liver function tests (elevated bilirubin, AST, ALT, GGT, alkaline phosphatase, prothrombin time).

SEIZURE DISORDERS, PSYCHOSIS. Provide for patient safety during episodes of dizziness; report symptoms for further evaluation.

DYSPNEA EDEMA. If amantadine is used with patients who have a history of congestive heart failure, assess lung sounds, additional edema, and weight gain on a regular basis.

Implementation
ADMINISTRATION SCHEDULE. Because of the possibility of insomnia, plan the last dose to be administered in the afternoon, not at bedtime.

Drug interactions
ANTICHOLINERGIC AGENTS (TRIHEXYPHENIDYL BENZTROPINE, PROCYLIDINE, DIPHENHYDRAMINE). Amantadine may exacerbate the side effects of anticholinergic agents that may also be used to control the symptoms of parkinsonism. Confusion and hallucinations may gradually develop. The dosage of amantadine and/or the anticholinergic agent should be reduced.

bromocriptine mesylate (bro-mo′krip-teen)

Parlodel (par-lo′del)

Bromocriptine stimulates dopamine receptors in the basal ganglia of the brain. Since parkinsonian patients are deficient of dopamine in this neurologic center, there is marked improvement in the symptoms of the disease with bromocriptine therapy. Bromocriptine appears to be nearly as effective as levodopa in treating parkinsonism and is occasionally useful with patients who are no longer benefiting from levodopa therapy.

Side effects. Side effects with bromocriptine therapy are very common, particularly when the dosage is greater than 15 to 20 mg daily. They can be minimized by starting with low dosages, then increasing dosages gradually to effective levels, and by administering medication in the evening with food. If severe side effects do appear, they can also be minimized by reducing the dosage for a few days, then increasing the dosage more gradually. Side effects based on organ system are as follows:

Gastrointestinal. Nausea, vomiting, anorexia, abdominal cramps, and constipation on long-term use are very common.

Neurologic. Involuntary movements, headache, migraine, dizziness, light-headedness, and sedation have been reported. Patients taking doses greater than 100 mg daily have a higher incidence of delusions, confusion, hallucinations, and a painful burning of the skin, usually of the feet and hands, accompanied by a mottled redness of the affected areas.

Cardiovascular. Orthostatic hypotension is very common, particularly with higher dosages.

Other side effects. Dryness of the mouth, double vision, nasal congestion, and metallic taste may also occur.

Availability
PO—2.5 mg tablets and 5 mg capsules.

Dosage and administration
Adult
PO—Initially, 1.25 mg 2 times daily with meals. Increase the dosage by 2.5 mg/day every 2 to 4 weeks. The dosage must be adjusted according to the patient's response and tolerance. Dosages in the 50 to 100 mg daily range are not uncommon for maximal therapeutic benefit.

• Nursing Interventions: Monitoring bromocriptine therapy

See also General Nursing Considerations for Patients with Parkinson's Disease (p. 175).

Side effects to expect
GASTROINTESTINAL EFFECTS. Most of these effects may be minimized by temporary reduction in dosage, administration with food, and use of stool softeners for constipation.

Side effects to report
NEUROLOGIC. As described above, neurologic effects often occur with higher dosages.

Perform a baseline assessment of the patient's degree of alertness and orientation to name, place, and time *prior* to initiating therapy. Make regularly scheduled subsequent evaluations of mental status and compare findings. Report development of alterations.

Provide for patient safety, be emotionally supportive, and assure the patient that these adverse effects dissipate within 2 to 3 weeks of discontinuing therapy.

ORTHOSTATIC HYPOTENSION. Monitor the blood pressure daily in both the supine and standing positions.

Anticipate the development of postural hypotension and take measures to prevent an occurrence. Teach the patient to rise slowly from a supine or sitting position; encourage the patient to sit or lie down if feeling "faint."

Implementation
PO. Dosage must be adjusted according to the patient's response and tolerance.

Side effects can be minimized by starting with small doses, then increasing the dosage gradually, and by administering medication with food in the evening.

Drug interactions
LEVODOPA. Bromocriptine and levodopa have additive neurological effects.

This interaction may be advantageous because it often allows a reduction in dosage of the levodopa.

ANTIHYPERTENSIVE AGENTS. Dosage adjustment of the antihypertensive agent is frequently necessary because of excessive orthostatic hypotension.

carbidopa (kar'be-do-pah), levodopa

Sinemet (sin'eh-met)

Sinemet is a combination of carbidopa and levodopa used for treating the symptoms of Parkinson's disease. Carbidopa is an enzyme inhibitor that reduces the metabolism of levodopa, allowing a greater portion of the administered levodopa to reach the desired receptor sites in the basal ganglia. Carbidopa reduces the dose of levodopa required by approximately 75%. When administered with levodopa, carbidopa increases both plasma levels and the plasma half-life of levodopa. Patients with irregular, "on and off" responses to levodopa do not show benefit from Sinemet.

Side effects. Carbidopa has no effect when used alone; it must be used in combination with levodopa. The side effects seen with combined therapy are actually an enhancement of the effects of levodopa because the carbidopa is allowing more levodopa to reach the brain. See Levodopa.

Availability
PO—Sinemet is a combination product containing both carbidopa and levodopa. The combination product is available in ratios of 10/100, 25/100, and 25/250 mg of carbidopa/levodopa respectively. There is also a sustained release product, Sinemet CR, which contains 50 mg/200 mg of carbidopa/levodopa.

Dosage and administration
Adult. PO—Patients not currently receiving levodopa: Initially, Sinemet 10/100 or 25/100 3 times daily, increasing by 1 tablet every other day until a dosage of 6 tablets daily is attained. As therapy progresses and patients show indications of needing more levodopa, substitute Sinemet 25/250, 1 tablet 3 to 4 times daily. Increase by 1 tablet every other day to a maximum of 8 tablets daily.

Drug interactions. Sinemet may be used to treat parkinsonism in conjunction with amantadine or anticholinergic agents. The dosages of all medications may need to be reduced due to combined therapy. See also Levodopa below.

• Nursing Interventions: Monitoring carbidopa therapy

See also General Nursing Considerations for Patients with Parkinson's Disease (p. 175). See also Levodopa following.

levodopa (le-vo-do'pah),

Larodopa (lar-oh-do'pah), Dopar (do'par)

As stated in the introductory remarks on Parkinson's disease, the symptoms of parkinsonism are thought to result from an absolute deficiency of dopamine and a relative excess of acetylcholine. Dopamine itself, when administered orally, does not enter the brain. Levodopa does cross into the brain, is metabolized to dopamine, and replaces the dopamine deficiency in the basal ganglia.

About 75% of patients with parkinsonism respond favorably to levodopa therapy, but after a few years the response diminishes, becomes more uneven, and is accompanied by many more side effects. This loss of therapeutic effect reflects the progression of the underlying disease process.

Side effects. Levodopa causes many side effects but most are dose-related and reversible. Side effects vary greatly, depending on the stage of the disease.

Side effects based on organ system are as follows:

- *Gastrointestinal.* Nausea, vomiting, and anorexia are frequently reported at the initiation of therapy.
- *Cardiovascular.* Orthostatic hypotension and arrhythmias such as sinus tachycardia and premature ventricular contractions occur.
- *Central nervous system.* Abnormal involuntary movements occur in half the patients taking levodopa for more than 6 months. These movements are observed as chewing motions, bobbing of the head and neck, facial grimacing, active tongue movements, and rocking movements of the trunk.
- *Psychiatric.* Levodopa may cause nightmares, restlessness, anxiety, insomnia, depression, dementia, loss of memory, and hallucinations. Reduction in dosage may control these symptoms.
- *Ophthalmic.* All patients should be screened for the presence of closed-angle glaucoma. Levodopa may precipitate an acute attack of angle-closure glaucoma. Patients with open-angle glaucoma can safely use levodopa in conjunction with mitotic therapy.
- *Secretions.* Sweat and urine may be darkened. Patients should be counselled that this is a harmless effect.

Levodopa therapy may cause the following abnormalities in laboratory tests:

- False-positive tests for urinary ketones are reported with Ketostix and Labstix. Acetest tablets are generally not affected.
- False-negative tests for urine glucose are reported with Tes-tape and Clinistix. A false-positive "trace" reading with Clinitest may also occur.
- The urine may turn red to black on exposure to air or alkaline substances (bowl cleaners). Patients should be told not to be alarmed.

Availability
PO—100, 250, and 500 mg tablets and capsules.
Dosage and administration
Adult
PO—Initially, 0.5 to 1 g daily in divided doses, administered with food. Do not exceed 8 g per day. Therapy for at least 6 months may be necessary to determine full therapeutic benefits.

• **Nursing Interventions: Monitoring levodopa therapy**

See also General Nursing Considerations for Patients with Parkinson's Disease (p. 175).

Side effects to expect

NAUSEA, VOMITING, ANOREXIA. These effects can be reduced by slowly increasing the dose, dividing the total daily dose into 4 to 6 doses, and administering the medication with food or antacids.

ORTHOSTATIC HYPOTENSION. Although generally mild, levodopa may cause some degree of orthostatic hypotension manifested by dizziness and weakness, particularly when therapy is being initiated. Tolerance usually develops after a few weeks of therapy.

Monitor the blood pressure daily in both the supine and standing positions.

Anticipate the development of postural hypotension and take measures to prevent an occurrence. Teach patients to rise slowly from a supine or sitting position; encourage them to sit or lie down if feeling "faint."

Side effects to report

CHEWING MOTIONS, BOBBING, FACIAL GRIMACING, ROCKING MOVEMENTS. These involuntary movements occur in about half the patients taking levodopa more than 6 months. A reduction in dosage may be beneficial.

NIGHTMARES, DEPRESSION, CONFUSION, HALLUCINATIONS. Perform a baseline assessment of the patient's degree of alertness and orientation to name, place, and time *prior* to initiating therapy. Make regularly scheduled subsequent evaluations of mental status and compare findings. Report development of alterations.

Provide for patient safety during these episodes.

Reduction in the daily dosage may control these adverse effects.

TACHYCARDIA, PALPITATIONS. Take the pulse at regularly scheduled intervals. Report for further evaluation.

Implementation

GLAUCOMA. All patients should be screened for the presence of angle-closure glaucoma *prior* to the initiation of therapy.

Patients with open-angle glaucoma can safely use levodopa.

PO. Administer medication with food or milk to reduce gastric irritation.

Drug interactions

PHENELZINE, ISOCARBOXAZID. These agents unpredictably exaggerate the effects of levodopa. They should be discontinued at least 14 days before the administration of levodopa.

ISONIAZID. Use with caution in conjunction with levodopa. Discontinue isoniazid if patients taking levodopa develop hypertension, flushing, palpitations, and tremor.

PYRIDOXINE. Pyridoxine (vitamin B_6) in oral doses of 5 to 10 mg reverses the toxic and therapeutic effects of levodopa. Normal diets contain less than 1 mg of pyridoxine, so dietary restrictions are not necessary. The ingredients of multiple vitamins should be considered, however.

There is a pyridoxine-free multiple vitamin (Larobec) made specifically for patients taking levodopa.

DIAZEPAM, CHLORDIAZEPOXIDE, PAPAVERINE, PHENYLBUTAZONE, CLONIDINE, PHENYTOIN. These agents appear to cause a deterioration in the therapeutic effects of levodopa. Use with caution in patients with parkinsonism and discontinue if the patient's clinical status deteriorates.

PHENOTHIAZINES, RESERPINE, HALOPERIDOL, METHYLDOPA. A side effect associated with these agents is a parkinson-like syndrome. Since this will nullify the therapeutic effects of levodopa, do not use concurrently.

EPHEDRINE, EPINEPHRINE, ISOPROTERENOL, AMPHETAMINES. Levodopa may increase the therapeutic and toxic effects of these agents. Monitor for tachycardia, arrhythmias, and hypertension. Reduce the dose of these agents if necessary.

ANTIHYPERTENSIVE AGENTS. Dosage adjustment of the antihypertensive agent is frequently necessary because of excessive orthostatic hypotension.

KETOSTIX, LABSTIX. This drug may produce false-positive urine ketone results with these products. Use Acetest tablets.

CLINITEST. This drug may produce a false-positive "trace" of urinary glucose.

TES-TAPE, CLINISTIX. This drug may produce false-negative urine glucose results with these products.

BOWL CLEANERS. The metabolites of this drug will react with toilet-bowl cleaners to turn the urine a red to black color. This may also occur if the urine is exposed to air for long periods of time. Inform the patient that there is no cause for alarm.

pergolide mesylate (per-goh′lyd)

Permax (per′maks)

Pergolide is a potent dopamine receptor stimulant. It is thought to exert its therapeutic effect in patients with Parkinson's disease by directly stimulating postsynaptic dopamine receptors in the nigrostriatal system. Pergolide is used in combination with levodopa/carbidopa in the management of Parkinson's disease.

Side effects. Side effects with pergolide are fairly common. About 25% of those patients receiving pergolide must discontinue therapy due to side effects. Adverse effects can be minimized by starting with low dosages, then increasing dosages gradually. Side effects based on organs systems are as follows:

• *Neurologic.* Most commonly reported are dyskinesias, hallucinations, somnolence, and insomnia.
• *Cardiovascular.* About 10% of patients receiving pergolide in combination with carbidopa/levodopa report orthostatic hypotension and dizziness. Patients are also more prone to develop atrial arrhythmias and sinus tachycardia.

- *Gastrointestinal.* Nausea, constipation, diarrhea, upset stomach. Many other adverse effects have been reported, but occur with a frequency of less than 1%.

Availability

PO—0.05, 0.25, and 1 mg tablets.

Dosage and administration

Adult

PO—Initiate with a daily dose of 0.05 mg for the first 2 days. Gradually increase the dosage by 0.1 or 0.15 mg/day every third day over the 12 days of therapy. The dosage may then be increased by 0.25 mg/day every third day until an optimal dose is achieved. Pergolide is usually administered in divided doses 3 times daily. During dosage titration, the dosage of concurrent carbidopa/levodopa should be cautiously decreased. The usual total daily dose of pergolide is 3 mg.

- **Nursing Interventions: Monitoring pergolide therapy**

See also General Nursing Considerations for Patients with Parkinson's Disease (p. 175).

Side effects to expect

GASTROINTESTINAL EFFECTS. Most of these effects may be minimized by temporary reduction in dosage, administration with food, and use of stool softeners for constipation.

Side effects to report

NEUROLOGIC. About 14% of patients develop hallucinations. Perform a baseline assessment of the patient's degree of alertness and orientation to name, place, and time *prior* to initiating therapy. Make regularly scheduled subsequent evaluations of mental status and compare findings. Report development of alterations.

Provide for patient safety, be emotionally supportive, and assure the patient that these adverse effects usually dissipate as tolerance to the adverse effects develops over the next few weeks.

ORTHOSTATIC HYPOTENSION. Monitor the blood pressure daily in both the supine and standing positions.

Anticipate the development of postural hypotension and take measures to prevent an occurrence. Teach the patient to rise slowly from a supine or sitting position; encourage the patient to sit or lie down if feeling "faint."

Implementation

PO. Dosage must be adjusted according to the patient's response and tolerance.

Side effects can be minimized by starting with small doses, then increasing the dosage gradually.

Drug interactions

LEVODOPA. Pergolide and levodopa have additive neurological effects. This interaction may be beneficial because it often allows a reduction in dosage of the levodopa.

DOPAMINE ANTAGONISTS. (e.g., phenothiazines, butyrophenones, thioxanthenes, metoclopramide). As dopamine antagonists, these agents will diminish the effectiveness of pergolide, a dopaminergic agonist.

ANTIHYPERTENSIVE AGENTS. Dosage adjustment of the antihypertensive agent is frequently necessary because of excessive orthostatic hypotension.

selegiline (sel-edg'il-een)

Eldepryl (el-deh-pril')

Levodopa/carbidopa are the current drugs of choice for the treatment of Parkinson's disease. Unfortunately, these agents lose effectiveness (on-off phenomenon) and develop more adverse effects (dyskinesias) over time. It is often necessary to add other dopamine receptor agonists such as bromocriptine and pergolide to improve the patient response and tolerance. Selegiline has been found to have similar adjunctive activity to levodopa/carbidopa in the treatment of Parkinson's disease. The mechanism of antiparkinsonian action of selegiline is unknown. It is known to be a potent monoamine oxidase-type B inhibitor, but this does not explain all of its actions. The combination of selegiline and levodopa/carbidopa improves memory and motor speed and may increase life expectancy by interfering with the degeneration of striated dopaminergic neurons.

Side effects. Selegiline causes relatively few adverse effects. It may increase the adverse dopaminergic effects of levodopa such as chorea, confusion, or hallucinations, but these can be controlled by reducing the dose of levodopa. Other reported side effects include transient nausea, orthostatic hypotension, agitation, confusion, and insomnia.

Availability

PO—5 mg tablets.

Dosage and administration

Adult

PO—5 mg at breakfast and lunch. Do not exceed 10 mg daily. After 2 to 3 days of treatment, the dose of levodopa/carbidopa should start being titrated downward. Levodopa/carbidopa dosages may be able to be reduced by 10 to 30%.

- **Nursing Interventions: Monitoring selegiline therapy**

See also General Nursing Considerations for Patients with Parkinson's Disease (p. 175).

Side effects to expect

GASTROINTESTINAL EFFECTS. Most of these effects may be minimized by temporary reduction in dosage, administration with food, and use of stool softeners for constipation.

Side effects to report

NEUROLOGIC. Selegiline may increase the adverse dopaminergic effects of levodopa, such as chorea, confusion, and hallucinations. Perform a baseline assessment of the patient's degree of alertness and orientation to name, place, and time *prior* to initiating therapy. Make regularly scheduled subsequent evaluations of mental status and compare findings. Report development of alterations.

Provide for patient safety, be emotionally supportive and assure the patient that these adverse effects usually dissipate as tolerance to the adverse effects develops over the next few weeks.

ORTHOSTATIC HYPOTENSION. Monitor the blood pressure daily in both the supine and standing positions.

Anticipate the development of postural hypotension and take measures to prevent an occurrence. Teach the patient to rise slowly from a supine or sitting position; encourage the patient to sit or lie down if feeling "faint."

Implementation

PO. Dosage must be adjusted according to the patient's response and tolerance.

Drug interactions

LEVODOPA. Selegiline and levodopa have additive neurological effects. This interaction may be beneficial because it often allows a reduction in dosage of the levodopa.

MEPERIDINE. Fatal drug interactions have been reported between monoamine oxidase inhibitors and meperidine. Whereas this interaction has not been reported with selegiline, it is recommended that the two agents not be given concurrently.

ANTIHYPERTENSIVE AGENTS. Dosage adjustment of the antihypertensive agent is frequently necessary because of excessive orthostatic hypotension.

Anticholinergic agents

It is hypothesized that parkinsonism is induced by the imbalance of neurotransmitters in the basal ganglia of the brain. The primary imbalance appears to be a deficiency of dopamine, with a relative excess of the cholinergic neurotransmitter acetylcholine. Anticholinergic agents are thus used to reduce hyperstimulation caused by excessive acetylcholine. The anticholinergic agents reduce the severity of the rigidity, sweating, drooling, depression, and tremor that characterize parkinsonism. Anticholinergic agents may be useful for patients with minimal symptoms, for those unable to tolerate the side effects of levodopa, and for those who have not benefited from levodopa therapy. Combination therapy with levodopa and anticholinergic agents is also successful in controlling symptoms of the disease more completely in about half the patients already stabilized on levodopa therapy.

Side effects. Most side effects observed with anticholinergic agents are direct extensions of their pharmacologic properties. Frequently seen adverse effects that usually dissipate with therapy are dryness and soreness of the mouth and tongue, blurring of vision, dizziness, mild nausea, and nervousness.

Psychiatric disturbances such as mental confusion, delusions, euphoria, paranoia, loss of memory, and hallucinations may be indications of overdosage.

Other side effects include constipation; urinary hesitancy or retention; tachycardia; palpitations; and mild, transient hypotension.

All patients should be screened for the presence of closed-angle glaucoma. Anticholinergic agents may precipitate an acute attack of angle-closure glaucoma. Patients with open-angle glaucoma can safely use anticholinergic agents in conjunction with mitotic therapy.

Availability. See Table 9-4.

Dosage and administration

Adult

PO—See Table 9-4.

• Nursing Interventions: Monitoring anticholinergic agent therapy

See also General Nursing Considerations for Patients with Parkinson's Disease (p. 175).

Side effects to expect

BLURRED VISION, CONSTIPATION, URINARY RETENTION, DRYNESS OF MUCOSA OF THE MOUTH, THROAT, AND NOSE. These symptoms are the anticholinergic effects produced by these agents. Patients taking these medications should be monitored for the development of these side effects.

Dryness of the mucosa may be relieved by sucking hard candy or ice chips, or by chewing gum.

If patients develop urinary hesitancy, assess for distension of the bladder. Report to the physician for further evaluation.

Give stool softeners as prescribed. Encourage adequate fluid intake and foods to provide sufficient bulk.

Caution the patient that blurred vision may occur and make appropriate suggestions for personal safety of the individual.

Side effects to report

NIGHTMARES, DEPRESSION, CONFUSION, HALLUCINATIONS. Perform a baseline assessment of the patient's degree of alertness and orientation to name, place, and time *prior* to initiating therapy. Make regularly scheduled subsequent evaluations of mental status and compare findings. Report development of alterations.

Provide for patient safety during these episodes.

Reduction in the daily dosage may control these adverse effects.

ORTHOSTATIC HYPOTENSION. Although the instance is infrequent and generally mild, all anticholinergic agents may cause some degree of orthostatic hypotension manifested by dizziness and weakness, particularly when therapy is being initiated.

Monitor the blood pressure daily in both the supine and standing positions.

Anticipate the development of postural hypotension and take measures to prevent an occurrence. Teach the patient to rise slowly from a supine or sitting position; encourage the patient to sit or lie down if feeling "faint."

Table 9-4 *Agents with Anticholinergic Properties Used to Treat Parkinsonism*

GENERIC NAME	BRAND NAME	AVAILABILITY	INITIAL DOSE (PO)	MAXIMUM DAILY DOSE (MG)
Benztropine mesylate	Cogentin,	Tablets: 0.5, 1, 2, mg Inj: 1 mg/ml in 2 ml amps	0.5-1 mg at bedtime	6
Biperiden hydrochloride	Akineton	Tablets: 2 mg	2 mg 1-3 times daily	10
Diphenhydramine hydrochloride	Benadryl, ✤ Insominal	Tablets: 50 mg Capsules: 25, 50 mg Elixir: 12.5 mg/5ml Syrup: 12.5 mg/5 ml		
Ethopropazine hydrochloride	Parsidol, ✤ Parsifan	Tablets: 10, 50 mg	50 mg 1-2 times daily	600
Orphenadrine hydrochloride	Orflagen, Norflex	Tablets: 100 mg Sustained release tablets: 100 mg Inj: 30 mg/ml in 2, 10 ml vials	50 mg 3 times daily	150-250
Procyclidine hydrochloride	Kemadrin, ✤ Procyclid	Tablets: 5 mg	2 mg 3 times daily	15-20
Trihexyphenidyl hydrochloride	Artane, Tremin, ✤ Aparkane	Tablets: 2, 5 mg Sustained release capsules: 5 mg Elixir: 2 mg/5 ml	1 mg daily	12-15

✤ Available in Canada only.

PALPITATIONS, ARRHYTHMIAS. Report for further evaluation.

Implementation

GLAUCOMA. All patients should be screened for the presence of angle-closure glaucoma *prior* to the initiation of therapy.

Patients with open-angle glaucoma can safely use anticholinergic agents. Monitoring of intraocular pressure should be performed on a regular basis.

PO. Administer medication with food or milk to reduce gastric irritation.

Drug interactions

AMANTADINE, TRICYCLIC ANTIDEPRESSANTS, PHENOTHIAZINES. These agents may enhance the anticholinergic side effects. Developing confusion and hallucinations are characteristic of excessive anticholinergic activity. Dosage reduction may be required.

LEVODOPA. Large doses of anticholinergic agents may slow gastric emptying and inhibit absorption of levodopa. An increase in the dosage of levodopa may be required.

PSYCHOTROPIC DISORDERS
OBJECTIVES

1. Define terminology associated with psychotropic agents and the illnesses treated.
2. Describe the essential components of a baseline assessment of a patient's mental status.
3. Cite the side effects of hydroxyzine therapy and identify those effects requiring close monitoring when used preoperatively.
4. Develop a teaching plan for patient education of persons taking minor tranquilizers (anxiolytics), major

tranquilizers (neuroleptics), antidepressant agents, antimanic agents, and monoamine oxidase inhibitors.
5. Cite monitoring parameters used for persons taking lithium carbonate, phenothiazines, haloperidol, or thioxanthenes.
6. Discuss psychological and physiological drug dependence.

KEY WORDS

psychotropic agents	apathy
coherency	euphoria
relevancy	phobias
delusions	anxiety
anxiolytics	tranquilizers
tardive dyskinesias	antidepressants
dystonias	akathisias
photosensitivity	antipsychotic agents
neuroleptic malignant syndrome (NMS)	

General Nursing Considerations for Patients Receiving Psychotropic Agents

Perform a baseline assessment of the individual's mental status. On succeeding occasions, repeat the evaluation and compare the findings to the original data.

Patients experiencing altered thinking, behavior, or feelings need careful evaluation of both verbal and nonverbal actions. Many times, the thoughts, feelings, and behaviors displayed are inconsistent with the so-called normal responses of individuals in similar circumstances.

A complete history of the patient's previous responses to crises can serve as a basis for anticipating response to current events. Evaluate the degree of reaction of the patient to the perceived threat and decide on the appropriateness of the reaction to the situation.

Try to identify the defense mechanisms currently being employed by the patient to cope with the circumstances. Ask yourself whether the coping mechanism is effective.

During periods of severe anxiety, as well as during periods of depression, the nurse should deal calmly and quietly with the individual and provide for personal well-being and safety.

At a time appropriate to the patient's ability to focus on the problems, alternative methods of handling the anxiety or depression may be explored.

Observe the patient during initial treatment with medications for increased anxiety and changes in levels of depression, or for oversedation, which would require a dosage adjustment.

Patient Concerns: Nursing Intervention/Rationale

General appearance. Observe the patient on admission and succeeding occasions for the following:

Personal grooming and appropriateness of dress to the occasion.

Posture: stooped, erect, slumped?

Facial expression: tense, worried, sad, angry, expressionless?

General motor activity: check gestures, gait, presence or absence of tremors, ability to perform gross or fine motor movements.

Speech: tone, clarity, pace, appropriateness; does the conversation flow in a logical sequence?

Level of consciousness. Assess the individual's orientation to time, place, and person.

Evaluate the coherency, relevancy, and organization of thoughts.

Mood (affect). State whether the mood being displayed is consistent with the circumstances being described (for example, the person is speaking of death yet is smiling).

Terms usually used to describe affect are euphoric, depressed, aggressive, blunted (lack of normal range of emotions). Note any disturbances in thoughts, such as hallucinations, phobias, or delusions.

Memory. Ask questions to ascertain the individual's memory of recent and past events.

Judgment. Observe the patient during social interactions for the appropriateness of the mannerisms and responses displayed.

Sensory perception. Ask questions to uncover any impairment of the five senses.

Developmental pattern. Compare the individual's behavior and responses with the "normals" for the patient's age.

Psychological assets. Does the individual have the ability to form close relationships? Can the patient function independently? What financial resources are available? Who forms the individual's support group?

Degree of depression. Assess for signs of depression: loneliness, apathy, withdrawal, or isolation.

Be particularly alert for statements of failure, hopelessness, or self-hatred.

Observe for appetite, symptoms of headache, fatigue, and activity levels. Ask questions to identify any particular sleep pattern being experienced.

If the individual is suspected of being suicidal, ask the patient if he or she has ever thought about suicide. If the response is yes, get more details. Is a specific plan formulated? How often do these thoughts occur?

Take all thoughts of suicide seriously and provide for the patient's personal safety. Record and *report* all findings promptly to the physician.

Patient Education Associated with Therapy for Psychotropic Disorders

Communication and responsibility. Encourage open communication with the patient concerning frustrations and anger as attempts are made to adjust to the diagnosis and need for treatment. The patient must be guided to insight into the disorder if he or she is to assume responsibility for the continuation of the treatment. Keep emphasizing those things the patient can do to alter the progression of disease, including maintenance of general health, nutritional needs, adequate rest and appropriate exercise, and continuation of prescribed medication therapy.

Expectations of therapy. Discuss the expectations of therapy (such as level of interaction and socialization, degree of depression relief, frequency of use of therapy, sexual activity, maintenance of mobility, ability to maintain activities of daily living and/or work).

Changes in expectations. Assess changes in expectations as therapy progresses and the patient gains understanding and skill in the management of the diagnosis.

Identify underlying stressors and appropriate coping mechanisms to reduce the effects of stress.

Changes in therapy through cooperative goal setting. Work cooperatively with the patient and family to encourage adherence to the treatment as prescribed. The need for long-term treatment should be discussed if appropriate to the circumstances.

When the patient feels that a change should be made in a treatment plan, encourage discussion with the physician. Side effects with psychotropic agents are often a deterrent to medication compliance. Management of side effects of prescribed medications must be an integral part of patient and family education.

Written record. Enlist the patient's and family's aid in developing and maintaining a written record (Figure

Patient Education and Monitoring of Therapeutic Outcomes for Patients Receiving Antianxiety Medication or Antidepressants

Medications	Color	To be taken

Name _____

Physician _____

Physician's phone _____

Next appt.* _____

Parameters	Day of discharge							Comments
Weight								
Blood pressure	AM / PM	AM / PM	AM / PM	AM / PM	AM / PM	AM / PM	AM / PM	
Resting pulse rate								
I would like to be alone? All the time — Some of the time — Not really 10 5 1								
How I feel about my children? Too much work — Fun to be with 10 5 1								
How I feel today? Poor — Fair — Okay 10 5 1								
Appetite? Poor — Fair — Good 10 5 1 B / L / D / ☆								
Has family noted any problems: Judgment? Socialization?								
Does patient dress daily (Yes/No)?								
Does patient take pride in appearance (yes/No)?								
Use of alcohol (Yes/No)? Amount (e.g., one drink)?								

*Please bring this record with you to your next appointment.
Use the back of this sheet for additional information.

Figure 9-3 *Patient education and monitoring of therapeutic outcomes for patients receiving antianxiety medication or antidepressants.*

9-3) of monitoring parameters (such as blood pressure, pulse, degree of socialization and interaction, general mood, judgments, memory, and daily or weekly weights, if a problem exists) and response to prescribed therapies for discussion with the physician. Patients should be encouraged to bring this record with them on follow-up visits.

Fostering compliance. Throughout the hospitalization, discuss medication information and how it will benefit the course of treatment. Seek cooperation on and understanding of the following points so that medication compliance may be enhanced:

1. Name
2. Dosage
3. Route and administration times
4. Anticipated therapeutic response
5. Side effects to expect
6. Side effects to report
7. What to do if a dosage is missed
8. When, how, or if to refill the medication

Difficulty in comprehension. If it is evident that the patient or family does not understand all aspects of continuing therapy being prescribed (such as administration and monitoring of medications, sedative effect, hypotensive episodes, need to monitor depressed patient's response), consider use of social service or visiting nurse agencies.

Associated teaching. Always inform the physician or dentist of any prescription or over-the-counter medication being taken.

Over-the-counter medications should not be taken without discussion first with the physician or pharmacist.

Always report side effects of rash, itching, or hives immediately. Nausea, vomiting, or diarrhea should be reported for the physician's evaluation if it is a new symptom.

Take all of the medication as prescribed for the full course of treatment. Do not discontinue use when feeling improved; do not save for future use or give medicine to another individual. Sudden discontinuation of certain medications may produce harmful effects.

Keep all medications out of the reach of children.

If pregnancy is suspected, consult an obstetrician as soon as possible about continuation of medication therapy.

At discharge. Items to be sent home with the patient should include the following:

1. Written instructions for the item's use
2. Labels in a level of language and size of print appropriate for the patient
3. If needed, identification cards or bracelets
4. A list of additional supplies to be purchased after discharge
5. A schedule for follow-up appointments

Drug Therapy for Psychotropic Disorders

Antianxiety agents

Anxiety is a normal human emotion, similar to fear. When it recurs too frequently or becomes uncontrollable, it is considered to be pathological. Its clinical manifestations include apprehension, irritability, nervousness, feelings of inadequacy, indecision, worry, tremor, insomnia, restlessness, headache, constipation, diarrhea, nausea, muscle tensions, and palpitations.

Anxiety is a primary symptom of many psychiatric disorders and a component of many medical and surgical conditions. When it is decided to treat the anxiety in addition to the other medical or psychiatric diagnoses, *antianxiety* medications, also known as *anxiolytics* or *minor tranquilizers,* are prescribed. It must be kept in mind that these agents are not cures for anxiety and should be used only for a short time to prevent the development of tolerance and dependence.

A great many medications have been used over the decades to treat anxiety. They range from the purely sedative effects of ethanol, bromides, chloral hydrate, and barbiturates to drugs with more specific antianxiety and less sedative activity, such as meprobamate, hydroxyzine, and the benzodiazepines.

Benzodiazepines

Benzodiazepines are most commonly used because they are more consistently effective, less likely to interact with other drugs, less likely to cause overdose, and have less potential for abuse than barbiturates and antianxiety agents. They now account for perhaps 75% of the 100 million prescriptions written annually for anxiety.

More than 2000 benzodiazepine derivatives have been identified, and more than 100 have been tested for sedative-hypnotic or other activity. Seven benzodiazepine derivatives are used as antianxiety agents (see Table 9-5). Patients with anxiety reactions to recent events and patients with a treatable medical illness that induces anxiety respond most readily to benzodiazepine therapy. Since all the benzodiazepines have similar mechanisms of action, selection of the appropriate derivative is dependent on how the benzodiazepine is metabolized. In patients with reduced hepatic function or in the elderly, alprazolam, lorazepam, or oxazepam may be most appropriate, because they have a relatively short duration of action and have no active metabolites. Oxazepam has been the most thoroughly investigated. The other benzodiazepines all have active metabolites that significantly prolong the duration of action and may accumulate to the point of excessive side effects with chronic administration. The primary active ingredient of both prazepam and clorazepate is desmethyldiazepam; therefore similar activity and patient response should be expected. Halazepam and diazepam are therapeutically active, but their major metabolite is

Table 9-5 *Benzodiazepines Used to Treat Anxiety*

GENERIC NAME	BRAND NAME	AVAILABILITY	INITIAL DOSE (PO)	MAXIMUM DAILY DOSE (MG)
Alprazolam	Xanax	Tablets: 0.25, 0.5, 1, 2 mg	0.25-0.5 mg 3 times daily	4
Clorazepate	Tranxene	Tablets: 3.75, 7.5, 15 mg Capsules: 3.75, 7.5, 15 mg	10 mg 1-3 times daily	60
Chlordiazepoxide	Librium, Mitran	Tablets: 5, 10, 25 mg Capsules: 5, 10, 25 mg	5-10 mg 3-4 times daily	300
Diazepam	Valium	Tablets: 2, 5, 10 mg Liquid: 5 mg/ml Inj.: 5 mg/ml in 1, 2, 10 ml vials	2-10 mg 2-4 times daily	—
Halazepam	Paxipam	Tablets: 20, 40 mg	20 mg 1-2 times daily	160
Lorazepam	Ativan	Inj.: 2, 4 mg/ml in 1, 10 ml vials; 1 ml prefilled syringe Tablets: 0.5, 1, 2 mg	2-3 mg 2-3 times daily	10
Oxazepam	Serax	Tablets: 15 mg Capsules: 10, 15, 30 mg	10-15 mg 3-4 times daily	120
Prazepam	Centrax	Tablets: 20 mg Capsules: 5, 10, 20 mg	20 mg at bedtime	60

again desmethyldiazepam, so similar response should be expected with chronic administration. Oxazepam, lorazepam, chlordiazepoxide, diazepam, and clorazepate are all approved for use in treating the anxiety associated with alcohol withdrawal. Oxazepam is the drug of choice because it has no active metabolites. Its use is somewhat limited, however, in patients who cannot tolerate oral administration because of nausea and vomiting. Chlordiazepoxide, diazepam, or lorazepam may be administered intramuscularly for this indication.

Side effects. The more common side effects of benzodiazepines are extensions of their pharmacologic properties. Drowsiness, fatigue, lethargy, and "morning hangover" are relatively common, dose-related adverse effects.

Paradoxic reactions occasionally occur within the first few weeks of therapy. These reactions are manifested by increased anxiety, hyperexcitation, hallucinations, acute rage, and insomnia.

The habitual use of benzodiazepines may result in physical and psychological dependence. Rapid discontinuance of benzodiazepines after long-term use may result in symptoms similar to alcohol withdrawal. These may vary from weakness and anxiety to delirium and grand mal seizures. The symptoms may not appear for several days after discontinuation. Treatment consists of gradual withdrawal of benzodiazepines over a 2- to 4-week period.

Benzodiazepines should be administered with caution to patients with a history of blood dyscrasias or hepatic damage.

It is generally recommended that benzodiazepines not be administered during at least the first trimester of pregnancy. There may be an increased incidence of birth defects because these agents readily cross the placenta and enter fetal circulation.

Mothers who are breastfeeding should not receive benzodiazepines regularly. The benzodiazepines readily cross into breastmilk and exert a pharmacologic effect on the infant.

Availability. See Table 9-5.

Dosage and administration. See Table 9-5.

• Nursing Interventions: Monitoring benzodiazepine therapy

See also General Nursing Considerations for Patients Receiving Psychotropic Agents (p. 184).

Side effects to expect

"HANGOVER," SEDATION, LETHARGY. Patients may complain of "morning hangover," blurred vision, and transient hypotension on arising.

Explain to the patient the need for arising first to a sitting position, equilibrating, and then standing. Assistance with ambulation may be required.

If "hangover" becomes troublesome, there should be a reduction in the dosage or a change in the medication or both.

Persons who are working around machinery, driving a car, pouring and giving medicines, or performing other duties in which they must remain mentally alert should not take these medications while working.

Side effects to report

EXCESSIVE USE OR ABUSE. Assist the patient to recognize the abuse problem.

Identify underlying needs and plan for more appropriate management of those needs.

Discuss the case with the physician and make plans to cooperatively approach gradual withdrawal of the medications being abused.

Provide for emotional support of the individual; display an accepting attitude—be kind but firm.

PARADOXIC RESPONSE. Report for further evaluation. Alternative therapy may be necessary.

BLOOD DYSCRASIAS. Routine laboratory studies (RBC, WBC, and differential counts) should be scheduled. Stress the importance of patient's returning for this laboratory work.

Monitor for the development of a sore throat, fever, purpura, jaundice, or excessive and progressive weakness.

HEPATOXICITY. The symptoms of hepatotoxicity are anorexia, nausea, vomiting, jaundice, hepatomegaly, splenomegaly, and abnormal liver function tests (elevated bilirubin, AST, ALT, GGT, alkaline phosphatase, prothrombin time).

Drug interactions

DRUGS THAT INCREASE TOXIC EFFECTS. Antihistamines, alcohol, analgesics, anesthetics, tranquilizers, narcotics, cimetidine, and other sedative-hypnotics.

Monitor the patient for excessive sedation and reduce the dosage of the benzodiazepine if necessary.

SMOKING. Smoking enhances the metabolism of the benzodiazepines. Larger dosages may be necessary to maintain sedative effects in patients who smoke.

buspirone (boos-peer'ohn)

BuSpar (bue-sphar')

Buspirone is an antianxiety agent chemically unrelated to the barbiturates, benzodiazepines, or other anxiolytic agents. It is approved for use in the treatment of anxiety disorders and for the short-term relief of the symptoms of anxiety. Its mechanism of action is unknown. Its advantage over other antianxiety agents is that it has less sedative properties. It requires 7 to 10 days of treatment before initial signs of improvement are evident, and 3 to 4 weeks of therapy for optimal effects. Since buspirone has shown minimal potential for abuse, it is not a controlled substance. Buspirone has no antipsychotic activity and should not be used in place of appropriate psychiatric treatment.

Side effects. The most common adverse effects of buspirone therapy are CNS disturbances (3.4%), which include dizziness, insomnia, nervousness, drowsiness, and lightheadedness; GI disturbances (1.2%), primarily nausea; and miscellaneous complaints (1.1%), primarily headache and fatigue. Approximately 10% of patients discontinue therapy within 3 to 4 weeks due to side effects.

In general, sedation with buspirone is minor compared to other anxiolytic agents. Individual patients, however, may be quite susceptible to lethargy and sedation with initial therapy.

Availability

PO—5 and 10 mg tablets.

Administration and dosage

Adult

PO—Initially, 5 mg three times daily. Doses may be increased by 5 mg every 2 to 3 days. Maintenance therapy often requires 20 to 30 mg daily in divided dosages. Do not exceed 60 mg daily.

• Nursing Interventions: Monitoring buspirone therapy

See also General Nursing Considerations for Patients Receiving Psychotropic Agents (p. 184).

Side effects to expect

SEDATION, LETHARGY. Persons who are working around machinery or performing other duties in which they must remain mentally alert should not take this medication while working.

Side effects to report

SLURRED SPEECH, DIZZINESS. These are signs of excessive dosage. Report to the physician for further evaluation. Provide for patient safety during these episodes.

Drug interactions

ALCOHOL. Buspirone and alcohol generally do not have additive CNS depressant effects, but individual patients may be susceptible to impairment. Use with extreme caution.

meprobamate (mep-ro-bam'ate)

Equanil (ek'wa-nil), Miltown (mil'-towhn)

Meprobamate acts on multiple sites within the central nervous system to produce mild sedation, antianxiety, and muscle relaxation. Meprobamate is used as an antianxiety agent and mild skeletal muscle relaxant for the short-term relief (less than 4 months) of anxiety and tension. It is of little use in the treatment of psychoses.

Side effects. Psychologic and physiologic dependence may occur in patients taking doses of 3.3 to 6.4 g per day for 40 or more days. Symptoms of chronic use and abuse of high doses include ataxia, slurred speech, and dizziness. Withdrawal reactions such as vomiting, tremors, confusion, hallucinations, and grand mal seizures may develop within 12 to 48 hours after abrupt discontinuation. Symptoms usually decline within the next 12 to 48 hours. Withdrawal from high and prolonged dosages should be completed gradually over 1 to 2 weeks.

Meprobamate may cause seizures in patients with epilepsy.

Adverse effects to meprobamate are generally mild and dose-related. They include dizziness, slurred speech, headache, paradoxic excitement, and allergic reactions that usually occur between the first and fourth dose in patients having no previous exposure to the drug.

Availability

PO—200, 400, and 600 mg tablets and capsules.

Dosage and administration

Adult

PO—400 mg 3 to 4 times daily. Smaller doses may work well in elderly and debilitated patients. Maximum daily doses should not exceed 2400 mg.

• **Nursing Interventions: Monitoring meprobamate therapy**

See also General Nursing Considerations for Patients Receiving Psychotropic Agents (p. 184).

Side effects to expect

SEDATION. Persons who are working around machinery, driving a car, pouring and giving medicines, or performing other duties in which they must remain mentally alert should not take these medications while working.

Side effects to report

SLURRED SPEECH, DIZZINESS. These are signs of excessive dosage. Report to the physician for further evaluation.

Provide for patient safety during these episodes.

EXCESSIVE USE OR ABUSE. Assist the patient to recognize the abuse problem.

Identify underlying needs and plan for more appropriate management of those needs.

Discuss the case with the physician and make plans cooperatively to approach gradual withdrawal of the medications being abused.

Provide for emotional support of the individual; display an accepting attitude—be kind but firm.

ORTHOSTATIC HYPOTENSION (DIZZINESS, WEAKNESS, FAINTNESS). Although this effect is infrequent and generally mild, meprobamate may cause some degree of orthostatic hypotension manifested by dizziness and weakness, particularly when therapy is being initiated.

Monitor the blood pressure daily in both the supine and standing positions.

Anticipate the development of postural hypotension and take measures to prevent an occurrence. Teach the patient to rise slowly from a supine or sitting position; encourage the patient to sit or lie down if feeling "faint."

PARADOXIC EXCITEMENT, ARRHYTHMIAS. Withhold further doses, report for further evaluation.

HIVES, PRURITUS, RASH. Report symptoms for further evaluation by the physician.

Pruritus may be relieved by adding baking soda in the bath water.

Drug interactions

DRUGS THAT INCREASE TOXIC EFFECTS. Antihistamines, alcohol, analgesics, tranquilizers, narcotics, and other sedative-hypnotics.

Monitor the patient for excessive sedation and reduce the dosage of the meprobamate if necessary.

hydroxyzine (hi-drox'ee-zeen)

Vistaril (vis-tar'il), **Atarax** (ah-tar-axe')

Defined strictly by chemical structure, hydroxyzine is an antihistamine. It acts within the central nervous system, however, to produce sedation, antiemetic, anticholinergic, antihistaminic, antianxiety, and antispasmodic activity. This variety of actions makes it a somewhat multipurpose agent. It is used as a mild tranquilizer in psychiatric conditions characterized by anxiety, tension, and agitation. It is also routinely used as a preoperative or postoperative sedative to control vomiting, diminish anxiety, and reduce the amount of narcotics needed for analgesia. Hydroxyzine may also be used as an antipruritic agent to relieve the itching associated with allergic reactions.

Side effects. The most common side effects are those associated with anticholinergic activity. These include dry mucous membranes, drowsiness, constipation, blurred vision, and nasal stuffiness.

Availability

PO—10, 25, 50, and 100 mg tablets and capsules, 10 mg/5 ml syrup, 25 mg/5 ml suspension.

IM—25 and 50 mg/ml.

Dosage and administration

Adult

ANTIANXIETY

PO—25 to 100 mg 3 to 4 times daily.

IM—50 to 100 mg every 4 to 6 hours.

PRE- AND POSTOPERATIVE

IM—25 to 100 mg.

ANTIEMETIC

IM—25 to 100 mg.

• **Nursing Interventions: Monitoring hydroxyzine therapy**

See also General Nursing Considerations for Patients Receiving Psychotropic Agents (p. 184).

Side effects to expect

BLURRED VISION, CONSTIPATION, DRYNESS OF MUCOSA OF THE MOUTH, THROAT, AND NOSE. These symptoms are the anticholinergic effects produced by hydroxyzine. Patients taking these medications should be monitored for the development of these side effects.

Dryness of the mucosa may be relieved by sucking hard candy or ice chips, or by chewing gum.

The use of stool softeners such as docusate may be required for constipation.

Caution the patient that blurred vision may occur and make appropriate suggestions for personal safety.

SEDATION. Persons who are working around machinery, driving a car, pouring and giving medicines, or performing other duties in which they must remain mentally alert should not take these medications while working.

Side effects to report

SLURRED SPEECH, DIZZINESS. These are signs of excessive dosage. Report to the physician for further evaluation.

Provide for patient safety during these episodes.

Drug interactions

DRUGS THAT INCREASE TOXIC EFFECTS. Antihistamines, alcohol, analgesics, anesthetics, tranquilizers, barbiturates, narcotics, and other sedative-hypnotics.

Monitor the patient for excessive sedation and reduce the dosage of the hydroxyzine if necessary.

Antidepressants

Monoamine oxidase inhibitors

In the early 1950s, isoniazid and iproniazid were released for the treatment of tuberculosis. It was soon reported that iproniazid has mood-elevating properties in tuberculosis patients. Further investigation discovered that iproniazid, in addition to its antitubercular properties, inhibited monoamine oxidase (MAO), whereas isoniazid did not. Other monoamine oxidase inhibitors were synthesized and used extensively to treat mental depression until the 1960s, when the tricyclic antidepressants became available.

Monoamine oxidase inhibitors (MAOI) (Table 9-6) are used now when tricyclic antidepressant therapy is unsatisfactory and when electroconvulsive therapy (ECT) is inappropriate or refused. They are most useful in atypical depressions accompanied by anxiety neuroses, phobias, hysteria, hypochondria, and/or obsessive-compulsive behavior.

The monoamine oxidase inhibitors act by blocking the metabolic destruction of biogenic amines (neurotransmitters) by the enzyme monoamine oxidase in the presynaptic neurons of the brain. According to the biogenic amine hypothesis of depression, the MAO in-

hibitors are effective because they prevent the degradation of norepinephrine and serotonin so that the concentration of these central nervous system neurotransmitters is increased. Although MAO inhibition occurs within a few days of initiating therapy, the antidepressant effects may be delayed for 2 to 4 weeks. Phenelzine and tranylcypromine are the two most commonly used MAOIs. Although earlier studies suggested that tranylcypromine was safer and more effective, phenelzine is now the preferred agent, because it has been more thoroughly studied.

Side effects. A major disadvantage of the MAOI is that they inhibit MAO not only in the brain, but elsewhere as well. Sedation, anticholinergic effects (blurred vision, dry mouth, weakness, difficulty in urination), and orthostatic hypotension are common side effects associated with the MAO inhibitors. Some patients report adverse effects associated with excessive central stimulation, consisting of tremors, insomnia, and hyperhidrosis.

A major potential complication with MAOI therapy is that of hypertensive crisis, particularly with tranylcypromine. Since MAO inhibitors block amine metabolism in tissues outside the brain, patients who consume foods or medications (see Drug Interactions) con-

Table 9-6 *Antidepressants*

GENERIC NAME	BRAND NAME	AVAILABILITY	INITIAL DOSE (PO)	DAILY MAINTENANCE DOSE (MG)	MAXIMUM DAILY DOSE (MG)
Monoamine oxidase inhibitors					
Isocarboxazid	Marplan	Tablets: 10 mg	30 mg daily	10-20	—
Phenelzine	Nardil	Tablets: 15 mg	15 mg 3 times daily	15-60	90
Tranylcypromine	Parnate	Tablets: 10 mg	10 mg 2 times daily	10-20	30
Tricyclic antidepressants					
Amitriptyline	Elavil, Endep	Tablets: 10, 25, 50, 75, 100, 150 mg IM: 10 mg/ml in 10 ml vials	25 mg 3 times daily	150-250	300
Amoxapine	Asendin	Tablets: 25, 50, 100, 150 mg	50 mg 3 times daily	200-300	400 (outpatients) 600 (inpatients)
Clomipramine	Anafranil	Capsules: 25, 50, 75 mg	25 mg 3 times daily	100-150	250
Desipramine	Norpramin, Pertofrane	Tablets: 10, 25, 50, 75, 100, 150 mg Capsules: 25, 50 mg	25 mg 3 times daily	75-200	300
Doxepin	Adapin, Sinequan, ♣Triadapin	Capsules: 10, 25, 50, 75, 100, 150 mg Oral concentrate 10 mg/ml	25 mg 3 times daily	at least 150	300
Imipramine	Tofranil, Janimine, ♣Impril	Tablets: 10, 25, 50 mg IM: 25 mg/2 ml	30-75 mg daily	150-250	300
Nortriptyline	Aventyl, Pamelor	Capsules: 10, 25, 75 mg	25 mg 3-4 times daily	50-75	100
Protriptyline	Vivactil, ♣Triptil	Tablets: 5, 10 mg	5-10 mg 3-4 times daily	20-40	60
Trimipramine	Surmontil	Capsules: 25, 50, 100 mg	25 mg 3 times daily	50-150	200 (outpatients) 300 (inpatients)

♣ Available in Canada.

taining indirect sympathomimetic amines are at considerable risk for a hypertensive crisis. Foods containing significant quantities of tyramine are well-ripened cheeses (Camembert, Edam, Roquefort, Parmesan, Mozzarella, cheddar); yeast extract; red wines; overripe bananas, figs, or avocadoes; chicken livers; and beer. Foods containing other vasopressors include fava beans, chocolate, and coffee, tea, and colas. Common prodromal symptoms of hypertensive crisis include severe occipital headache, stiff neck, sweating, nausea and vomiting, and sharply elevated blood pressure. The alpha blocking agent, phentolamine (or chlorpromazine, which also has alpha blocking properties) may be used to gain control of the crisis.

Drug interactions. The following drugs will potentiate the toxicity of MAOI by raising amine levels: amphetamines, ephedrine, methyldopa, mazindol, diethylpropion, levodopa, epinephrine, and norepinephrine.

MAOI and tricyclic antidepressants (especially imipramine and desipramine) should not be administered concurrently. It is recommended that at least 10 days elapse between the discontinuation of MAOIs and the initiation of another antidepressant.

Monoamine oxidase inhibitors may potentiate the hypotensive effects of general anesthesia, diuretics, and antihypertensive agents.

Monoamine oxidase inhibitors have an additive hypoglycemic effect in combination with insulin and oral sulfonylureas. Monitor blood glucose; lower hypoglycemic doses if necessary.

When used concurrently, meperidine and MAOI may cause hyperpyrexia, restlessness, hyper- /hypotension, convulsions, and coma. The effects of this interaction may occur for several weeks after the discontinuation of MAOI. Use morphine instead of meperidine.

Tricyclic antidepressants

The tricyclic antidepressants have become the most widely used medications in the treatment of depression. They produce antidepressant and mild tranquilizing effects. After 2 to 3 weeks of therapy, the tricyclic antidepressants elevate the mood, improve the appetite, and increase alertness in about 80% of patients with endogenous depression. Combination therapy with phenothiazine derivatives may be beneficial in the treatment of the depression of schizophrenia or moderate to severe anxiety and depression observed with psychosis or psychoneurosis.

The tricyclic antidepressants are equally effective in treating depression, assuming that appropriate dosages are used for an adequate duration of time. Consequently the selection of an antidepressant is based primarily on the characteristics of each individual agent. Sedation is more notable with amitriptyline, doxepin, and trimipramine, while protriptyline has no sedative properties and may actually produce mild stimulation in

some patients. All tricyclic compounds display anticholinergic activity, with amitriptyline displaying the most and desipramine the least. This factor should be considered in patients with cardiac disease, prostatic hypertrophy, or glaucoma. Other factors to consider are that men tend to respond better to imipramine than women do, and the elderly tend to respond better to amitriptyline than do younger patients.

Side effects. The most common side effects are those associated with anticholinergic activity. These include dry mucous membranes, constipation, blurred vision, nausea, and urinary retention.

About 10% of patients develop a fine rapid tremor of the hands. Occasionally, patients have reported numbness and tingling of arms and legs. Rarely, extrapyramidal side effects resembling parkinsonism develop.

Cardiovascular side effects such as arrhythmias, congestive heart failure, and tachycardia are rare, but orthostatic hypotension is fairly common with therapeutic dosages.

High doses of tricyclic antidepressants lower the seizure threshold. Seizures may occur in those with and without a history of seizure activity.

Availability. See Table 9-6.

Dosage and administration

Adult

PO—see Table 9-6.

• Nursing Interventions: Monitoring antidepressant therapy

See also General Nursing Considerations for Patients Receiving Psychotropic Agents (p. 184).

Side effects to expect

BLURRED VISION, CONSTIPATION, URINARY RETENTION, DRYNESS OF MUCOSA OF THE MOUTH, THROAT, AND NOSE. These symptoms are the anticholinergic effects produced by these agents. Patients taking these medications should be monitored for the development of these side effects.

Dryness of the mucosa may be relieved by sucking hard candy or ice chips, or by chewing gum.

The use of stool softeners such as docusate or the occasional use of a potent laxative such as bisacodyl may be required for constipation.

Caution the patient that blurred vision may occur and make appropriate suggestions for personal safety of the individual.

ORTHOSTATIC HYPOTENSION. All tricyclic antidepressants may cause some degree of orthostatic hypotension manifested by dizziness and weakness, particularly when therapy is being initiated.

Monitor the blood pressure daily in both the supine and standing positions.

Anticipate the development of postural hypotension and take measures to prevent an occurrence. Teach the patient to rise slowly from a supine or sitting position; encourage the patient to sit or lie down if feeling "faint."

SEDATIVE EFFECTS. Tell the patient of sedative effects, especially during the onset of therapy. Single doses at bedtime may diminish or relieve the sedative effects.

Side effects to report

TREMOR. About 10% of patients develop this adverse effect. The tremor can be controlled with small doses of propranolol.

NUMBNESS, TINGLING. Report for further evaluation.

PARKINSONIAN SYMPTOMS. If these symptoms develop, the tricyclic antidepressant dosage must be reduced or discontinued.

Antiparkinsonian medications will not control symptoms induced by tricyclic antidepressants.

ARRHYTHMIAS, TACHYCARDIA, CONGESTIVE HEART FAILURE. Report for further evaluation.

SEIZURE ACTIVITY. High doses of antidepressants lower the seizure threshold. Adjustment of anticonvulsant therapy may be required, especially in seizure-prone patients.

SUICIDAL ACTIONS. Monitor the patient for changes in thoughts, feelings, and behaviors during the initial stages of therapy.

Implementation

PO. Dosage should be initiated at a low level and increased gradually, particularly in elderly or debilitated patients. Increases in dosage should be made in the evening because increased sedation is often present.

OBSERVATION. Symptoms of depression may improve within a few days (for example, improved appetite, sleep, and psychomotor activity). The depression still exists, however, and it usually takes several weeks of the therapeutic doses before improvement is noted. Suicide precautions should be maintained during this time.

Drug interactions

ENHANCED ANTICHOLINERGIC ACTIVITY. The following drugs enhance the anticholinergic activity associated with tricyclic antidepressant therapy: antihistamines, phenothiazines, trihexyphenidyl, benztropine, and meperidine.

The side effects are usually not severe enough to cause discontinuation of therapy, but stool softeners may be required.

ENHANCED SEDATIVE ACTIVITY. The following drugs enhance the sedative activity associated with tricyclic antidepressant therapy: ethanol, barbiturates, narcotics, tranquilizers, antihistamines, anesthetics, and sedative-hypnotics. Concurrent therapy is not recommended.

BARBITURATES. Barbiturates may stimulate the metabolism of tricyclic antidepressants. Dosage adjustments of the antidepressant may be necessary.

METHYLPHENIDATE, THYROID HORMONES. These agents may increase serum levels of the tricyclic antidepressants. This reaction has been advantageous in attempts to gain a faster onset of antidepressant activity, but an increased incidence of arrhythmias also has been reported.

GUANETHIDINE, CLONIDINE. Tricyclic antidepressants inhibit the antihypertensive effects of these agents. Concurrent therapy is not recommended.

MONOAMINE OXIDASE INHIBITORS. Severe reactions including convulsions, hyperpyrexia, and death have been reported with concurrent use.

It is recommended that 2 weeks lapse between discontinuance of an MAO inhibitor and starting tricyclic antidepressants.

PHENOTHIAZINES. Concurrent therapy may increase serum levels of both drugs, causing an increase in anticholinergic and sedative activity. Dosages of both agents may be reduced.

bupropion hydrochloride (beuh-prop′e-on)

Wellbutrin (wel-beu′trinh)

Bupropion is chemically unrelated to other antidepressants. It is approved for use in patients unresponsive to the tricyclic antidepressants and in patients who cannot tolerate the adverse effects of the tricyclic antidepressants. Its mechanism of action is unknown.

Side effects. Bupropion has a low incidence of anticholinergic, sedative effects, and orthostatic hypotension in comparison to tricyclic antidepressants. In contrast, bupropion causes a significant degree of restlessness, agitation, anxiety, and insomnia.

Bupropion is associated with seizures in less than 1% of patients. The risk of seizure is strongly associated with dose and the presence of risk factors (previous seizure activity, history of head trauma, other medications that may lower seizure threshold). The risk of seizure increases substantially with dosages above 450 mg daily.

About 20% to 25% of patients report gastrointestinal disturbances such as constipation, nausea and vomiting, and anorexia.

Availability

PO—75 and 100 mg tablets

Dosage and administration

Adult

PO—Initially, 100 mg twice daily. This may be increased to 100 mg 3 times daily (at least every 6 hours) after several days of therapy. No single dose of bupropion should exceed 150 mg; do not exceed 450 mg daily.

• Nursing Interventions: Monitoring bupropion therapy

See also General Nursing Considerations for Patients Receiving Psychotropic Agents (p. 184).

Side effects to expect

GASTROINTESTINAL EFFECTS. Most of these effects may be minimized by temporary reduction in dosage, administration with food, and use of stool softeners for constipation.

RESTLESSNESS, AGITATION, ANXIETY, INSOMNIA. This usually occurs early in therapy and may require short term treatment with sedative/hypnotic agents. Avoiding bedtime doses may also help decrease the incidence of insomnia.

Side effects to report

SEIZURES. See General Nursing Considerations for Patients with Seizure Disorders (p. 201).

SUICIDAL ACTIONS. Monitor the patient for changes in thoughts, feelings, and behaviors during the initial stages of therapy.

Implementation

PO—Initiate therapy at lower doses to minimize adverse effects. No single dose of bupropion should exceed 150 mg; do not exceed 450 mg daily. Space dosages at least 6 hours apart, but avoid a dosage shortly before bedtime.

OBSERVATION. Symptoms of depression may improve within a few days (for example, improved appetite, sleep, and psychomotor activity). The depression still exists, however, and it usually takes several weeks of the therapeutic doses before improvement is noted. Suicide precautions should be maintained during this time.

Drug interactions

CARBAMAZEPINE, CIMETIDINE, PHENOBARBITAL, PHENYTOIN. Bupropion may be an inducer of hepatic enzymes that may metabolize these agents more quickly. The dosage of these medications may need to be increased if taken concurrently with bupropion.

LEVODOPA. Bupropion has some mild dopaminergic activity and may cause an increase in adverse effects from levodopa. If bupropion is to be added to levodopa therapy, it should be initiated in small doses with small increases in the dosage of bupropion.

fluoxetine hydrochloride (flu-ox′et-een)

> **Prozac** (pro-zak′)

Fluoxetine is an antidepressant that acts by inhibiting serotonin in certain parts of the brain. Fluoxetine is chemically unrelated to any other class of agents that demonstrate antidepressant activity, but has been shown to be equally as effective as tricyclic antidepressants. A particular advantage of fluoxetine is that it does not have the anticholinergic or cardiovascular side effects that often limit the use of the tricyclic antidepressants. As with other antidepressants, it takes a full 1 to 3 weeks of therapy to see the full therapeutic benefit in treating depression. Fluoxetine is also being studied for the treatment of obesity, bulimia nervosa, and obsessive-compulsive disorders.

Side effects. Fluoxetine has a low incidence of anticholinergic effects (constipation, blurred vision, dry mouth, urinary retention), sedative effects, and orthostatic hypotension in comparison to the tricyclic antidepressants. The most commonly observed adverse effects associated with the central nervous system are nervousness, anxiety, and insomnia; drowsiness and fa-

tigue; and dizziness or lightheadedness. Anorexia, nausea, and diarrhea are the most common gastrointestinal side effects.

Availability

PO—20 mg capsules.

Dosage and administration

PO—Initially, 20 mg daily as a single morning dose. After several weeks of therapy, the dose may be increased in 20 mg increments, given twice daily at morning and noon. Do not exceed 80 mg daily.

• Nursing Interventions: Monitoring fluoxetine therapy

See also General Nursing Considerations for Patients Receiving Psychotropic Agents (p. 184).

Side effects to report

RESTLESSNESS, AGITATION, ANXIETY, INSOMNIA. This usually occurs early in therapy and may require short term treatment with sedative/hypnotic agents. Avoiding bedtime doses may also help decrease the incidence of insomnia.

SEDATIVE EFFECTS. Tell the patient of possible sedative effects. The patient should use caution while driving or performing other tasks that require alertness. Consult with the physician to consider moving the daily dosage to bedtime if sedation continues to be a problem.

GASTROINTESTINAL EFFECTS. Most of these effects may be minimized by temporary reduction in dosage and administration with food. Encourage the patient not to discontinue therapy without consulting the physician first.

SUICIDAL ACTIONS. Monitor the patient for changes in thoughts, feelings and behaviors during the initial stages of therapy.

Implementation

PO—Initiate therapy at lower doses to minimize adverse effects.

OBSERVATION. Symptoms of depression may improve within a few days (e.g., improved appetite, sleep, and psychomotor activity). The depression still exists, however, and it usually takes several weeks of the therapeutic doses before improvement is noted. Suicide precautions should be maintained during this time.

Drug interactions

LITHIUM. Fluoxetine may induce lithium toxicity. Monitor your patients for lithium toxicity manifested by nausea, anorexia, fine tremors, persistent vomiting, profuse diarrhea, hyperreflexia, lethargy, and weakness.

MONOAMINE OXIDASE INHIBITORS. Severe reactions including convulsions, hyperpyrexia, and death have been reported with concurrent use. It is recommended that at least 14 days lapse between discontinuance of an MAO inhibitor and starting fluoxetine therapy.

DIAZEPAM. Fluoxetine prolongs the activity of diazepam, resulting in excessive sedation and impaired motor skills.

WARFARIN. Fluoxetine may enhance the anticoagulant effects of warfarin. Observe for the development of petechiae, ecchymoses, nosebleeds, bleeding gums, dark tarry stools, and bright red or "coffee-ground" emesis. Monitor the prothrombin time and reduce the dosage of warfarin if necessary.

maprotiline hydrochloride (ma-pro′til-een)

Ludiomil (lew-deo′mil)

Maprotiline is the first of the tetracyclic antidepressants to be released for clinical use. The tetracyclic agents are similar to the tricyclic antidepressants, but the frequency and severity of anticholinergic effects, cardiac arrhythmias, and orthostatic hypotension are reported to be lower with maprotiline. There is a slightly higher incidence of seizure activity and delirium associated with maprotiline therapy.

Side effects. Maprotiline shares the same adverse effects as those of the tricyclic antidepressants. See Tricyclic Antidepressants.

Availability

PO—25, 50, and 75 mg tablets.

Dosage and administration

Adult

PO—Initially, 75 mg daily. Increase in increments of 25 to 50 mg daily as needed and tolerated. The usual maintenance dose is 150 mg daily. The maximum dose is 300 mg daily. Therapeutic blood levels are 50 to 200 ng/ml.

Increases in dosage should be made in the evening because increased sedation is often present.

NOTE: Symptoms of depression may improve (for example, improved appetite, sleep, and psychomotor activity) within a few days. The depression still exists, however, and it usually takes several weeks of therapeutic doses before improvement in the depression is noted. Suicide precautions should be maintained during this time.

• Nursing Interventions

See Tricyclic Antidepressants (p. 192).

trazodone hydrochloride (traz-oh-doan′)

Desyrel (dez-er′el)

Trazodone is the first of the triazolopyridine antidepressants to be released for clinical use. They are chemically unrelated to the tricyclic and tetracyclic antidepressants. Trazodone has been shown to be as effective in treating depression as amitriptyline and imipramine. Compared with other antidepressants, it has a low incidence of anticholinergic side effects, making trazodone particularly useful in patients whose antidepressant dosages are limited by anticholinergic side effects and in patients with severe angle-closure glaucoma, prostatic hypertrophy, organic mental disorders, and cardiac arrhythmias.

Side effects. Drowsiness and decreased energy are the most commonly reported adverse effects. Other CNS effects reported are fatigue, light-headedness, dizziness, ataxia, mild confusion, and inability to think clearly.

Cardiovascular side effects reported are orthostatic hypotension, tachycardia, and palpitations.

Availability

PO—50, 100, 150, and 300 mg tablets.

Dosage and administration

Adult

PO—Initially, 150 mg in 3 divided doses. Increase in increments of 50 mg daily every 3 to 4 days while monitoring clinical response. Do not exceed 400 mg daily in outpatients or 600 mg daily in hospitalized patients.

• Nursing Interventions: Monitoring trazodone therapy

See also General Nursing Considerations for Patients Receiving Psychotropic Agents (p. 184).

Side effects to expect and report

CONFUSION. Perform a baseline assessment of the patient's degree of alertness and orientation to name, place, and time *prior* to initiating therapy. Make regularly scheduled subsequent evaluations of mental status and compare findings. Report development of alterations.

DIZZINESS, LIGHT-HEADEDNESS. Provide for patient safety during episodes of dizziness; report for further evaluation.

DROWSINESS. Persons who are working around machinery, driving a car, pouring and giving medicines, or performing other duties in which they must remain mentally alert should not take these medications while working.

ORTHOSTATIC HYPOTENSION. Although episodes are infrequent and generally mild, trazodone may cause some degree of orthostatic hypotension manifested by dizziness and weakness, particularly when therapy is being initiated.

Monitor the blood pressure daily in both the supine and standing positions.

Anticipate the development of postural hypotension and take measures to prevent an occurrence. Teach the patient to rise slowly from a supine or sitting position; encourage the patient to sit or lie down if feeling "faint."

ARRHYTHMIAS, TACHYCARDIA. Report for further evaluation.

Implementation

PO. Dosage should be initiated at a low level and increased gradually, particularly in elderly or debilitated patients.

Increases in dosage should be made in the evening because increased sedation is often present.

Administer medication shortly after a meal or with a light snack to reduce adverse effects.

OBSERVATION. Symptoms of depression may improve (for example, improved appetite, sleep, and psychomotor activity) within a few days. The depression still exists, however, and it usually takes several weeks of therapeutic doses before improvement is noted. Suicide precautions should be maintained during this time.

Drug interactions

ENHANCED SEDATIVE ACTIVITY. The following drugs enhance the sedative effects associated with trazodone therapy: ethanol, barbiturates, narcotics, tranquilizers, antihistamines, anesthetics, and sedative-hypnotics. Concurrent therapy is not recommended.

GUANETHIDINE, CLONIDINE. Trazodone inhibits the antihypertensive effects of these agents. Concurrent therapy is not recommended.

Antipsychotic agents

Phenothiazines, thioxanthenes, haloperidol, molindone, loxapine, and clozapine. Antipsychotic agents, also known as neuroleptic agents and major tranquilizers, are used to treat severe mental illnesses such as schizophrenia, mania, psychotic depression, and psychotic organic brain syndrome. Medications used to treat these disorders are grouped into two broad categories: the phenothiazines and the nonphenothiazines (thioxanthenes, haloperidol, molindone, loxapine and clozapine). Although each agent is from a distinctly different chemical class, all antipsychotic agents are similar in that they act by blocking the action of dopamine in the brain. Since they work at different sites within the brain, the side effects are observed on different systems throughout the body.

Side effects. The extrapyramidal effects are the most troublesome side effects associated with antipsychotic therapy. They include the following:

1. Parkinsonian symptoms (4% to 40%) of tremor, muscular rigidity, masklike expression, shuffling gait, and loss or weakness of motor function. These symptoms are often controlled by anticholinergic antiparkinsonian agents. (Levodopa does not control these adverse effects.)
2. Dystonias and dyskinesias (2% to 10%) are spasmodic movements of the body and limbs (dystonias) and coordinated, involuntary rhythmic movements (dyskinesias). Acute dystonic reactions may be controlled by diphenhydramine or benztropine.
3. Akathisias (7% to 10%) consist of involuntary motor restlessness, constant pacing, and the inability to sit still; they are often accompanied by fidgeting, with lip and limb movements. Occasionally, sedatives may be required.
4. All antipsychotic agents have the potential to produce tardive dyskinesias. This drug-induced neurologic disorder is noted for such symptoms as facial grimaces; involuntary movement of the lips, tongue, and jaw, producing smacking noises; and frequent, recurrent protrusions of the tongue. This adverse effect is usually irreversible and appears after several years of antipsychotic therapy. The frequency (15% to 45%) appears to be higher in patients taking both antiparkinsonian anticholinergic agents and antipsychotic agents together. It is thought that a fine tremor of the tongue may be an early indication of the disease. If the dosage is gradually reduced, where possible, the tardive dyskinesia may not develop.
5. Neuroleptic malignant syndrome (NMS) occurs in 0.5 to 1% of patients receiving antipsychotic therapy. It has been most frequently reported with high-potency antipsychotic agents given intramuscularly. It typically occurs after 3 to 9 days of treatment with antipsychotic agents and is not related to dose or previous drug exposure. Once NMS begins, symptoms rapidly progress over 24 to 72 hours. Symptoms usually last 5 to 10 days after discontinuing oral medications and 13 to 30 days with depot antipsychotic medicine. Most cases have occurred in patients under 40 years of age, and is twice as common in males. NMS is characterized by fever, severe extrapyramidal symptoms such as lead-pipe rigidity, trismus, choreiform movements, and opisthotonus; autonomic instability such as tachycardia, labile hypertension, diaphoresis, and incontinence; and alterations in consciousness such as stupor, mutism, and coma. Mortality rates have been as high as 20% to 30%, but prompt recognition of the symptoms has reduced the mortality to 4% in recent years. Treatment includes bromocriptine as a dopamine agonist, and dantrolene as a muscle relaxant. Fever is treated by using cooling blankets, adequate hydration, and antipyretics. Once the patient's condition is stabilized, a thorough evaluation of the medications being prescribed is made. Resumption of the antipsychotic agent may result in a recurrence of NMS; therefore, the lowest dosage possible of the antipsychotic agent is prescribed and close observation of the patient's response is required.

Side effects frequently observed with antipsychotic therapy, especially when initiating therapy, are chronic drowsiness and fatigue, hypotension, blurred vision, nasal stuffiness, constipation, and dry mouth. Use antipsychotic therapy with caution in patients with glaucoma, prostatic hypertrophy, or urinary retention.

Antipsychotic agents may lower the seizure threshold in patients with seizure disorders.

Antipsychotic agents may produce myriad side effects other than those already listed. These include hepatotoxicity, blood dyscrasias, allergic reactions, endocrine disorders, skin pigmentation, and reversible effects in the eyes. Patients receiving clozapine are particularly susceptible to developing agranulocytosis. Weekly WBC counts are mandatory.

Availability. See Table 9-7.

Dosage and administration. See Table 9-7. Dosages must be individualized according to the degree of mental and emotional disturbance. It will often take several weeks for a patient to show optimal improvement and become stabilized on an adequate maintenance dosage. As a result of the cumulative effects of antipsychotic agents, patients must be reevaluated periodically to determine the lowest effective dosage necessary to control psychiatric symptoms. Sedative effects associated with antipsychotic therapy can be minimized by giving the dose of medication at bedtime.

• **Nursing Interventions: Monitoring antipsychotic therapy**

See also General Nursing Considerations for Patients Receiving Psychotropic Agents (p. 184).

Side effects to expect

CHRONIC FATIGUE, DROWSINESS. Persons who are working around machinery, driving a car, pouring and giving medicines, or performing other duties in which they must remain mentally alert should not take these medications while working.

ORTHOSTATIC HYPOTENSION. All antipsychotic agents may cause some degree of orthostatic hypotension manifested by dizziness and weakness, particularly when therapy is being initiated.

Monitor the blood pressure daily in both the supine and standing positions.

Anticipate the development of postural hypotension and take measures to prevent an occurrence. Teach the patient to rise slowly from a supine or sitting position; encourage the patient to sit or lie down if feeling "faint."

BLURRED VISION, CONSTIPATION, URINARY RETENTION, DRYNESS OF THE MUCOSA OF THE MOUTH, THROAT, AND NOSE. These symptoms are the anticholinergic effects produced by these agents. Patients taking these medications should be monitored for the development of these side effects.

Dryness of the mucosa may be relieved by sucking hard candy or ice chips, or by chewing gum.

The use of stool softeners such as docusate or the occasional use of a potent laxative such as bisacodyl may be required for constipation.

Caution the patient that blurred vision may occur and make appropriate suggestions for personal safety of the individual.

Side effects to report

SEIZURE ACTIVITY. Provide for patient safety during episodes of seizures; report for further evaluation. Adjustment of anticonvulsant therapy may be required, especially in seizure-prone patients.

PARKINSONIAN SYMPTOMS. Report the development of drooling, cogwheel rigidity, shuffling gait, masklike expression, or tremors. Anticholinergic agents may be used to control these symptoms.

TARDIVE DYSKINESIA. Report the development of fine tremors of the tongue, "fly catching" tongue movements, and lipsmacking. This is particularly important in patients who have been receiving antipsychotic agents and anticholinergic agents for several years.

HEPATOTOXICITY. The symptoms of hepatotoxicity are anorexia, nausea, vomiting, jaundice, hepatomegaly, splenomegaly, and abnormal liver function tests (elevated bilirubin, AST, ALT, GGT, alkaline phosphatase, prothrombin time).

BLOOD DYSCRASIAS. Routine laboratory studies (RBC, WBC, and differential counts) should be scheduled. This is particularly important for clozapine.

Monitor for the development of sore throat, fever, purpura, jaundice, or excessive and progressive weakness.

HIVES, PRURITUS, RASH. Report symptoms for further evaluation by the physician.

PHOTOSENSITIVITY. The patient should be cautioned to avoid exposure to sunlight and ultraviolet light. Suggest wearing long-sleeved clothing, a hat, and sunglasses when going to be exposed to sunlight. Advise against using artificial "tanning" lamps. Notify the physician for the advisability of discontinuing therapy.

Implementation

DOSAGE ADJUSTMENT. Dosages must be individualized according to the degree of mental and emotional disturbance. It will often take several weeks for a patient to show optimal improvement and become stabilized on an adequate maintenance dosage.

Periodic evaluations should be made to make sure the patient is taking the smallest effective dose.

Drug interactions

DRUGS THAT INCREASE TOXIC EFFECTS. Antihistamines, alcohol, analgesics, anesthetics, tranquilizers, barbiturates, narcotics, and other sedative-hypnotics.

Monitor the patient for excessive sedation and reduce the dosage of the above agents if necessary.

GUANETHIDINE. Antipsychotic agents may inhibit the antihypertensive effect of guanethidine. Concurrent therapy is not recommended.

BETA ADRENERGIC BLOCKERS. Beta adrenergic blocking agents (propanolol, timolol, nadolol, pindolol, and others) will significantly enhance the hypotensive effects of antipsychotic agents. Concurrent therapy is not recommended.

BARBITURATES. Barbiturates may stimulate the rate of metabolism of phenothiazines. Dosage adjustments of the antipsychotic agent may be necessary.

INSULIN, ORAL HYPOGLYCEMIC AGENTS. Diabetic or prediabetic patients need to be monitored for the development of hyperglycemia, particularly during the early weeks of therapy.

Assess regularly for glycosuria and report if it occurs with any frequency.

Patients receiving oral hypoglycemic agents or insulin may require an adjustment in dosage.

Table 9-7 *Antipsychotic Agents*

GENERIC NAME	BRAND NAME	AVAILABILITY	ADULT DOSAGE RANGE (MG)	MAJOR SIDE EFFECTS			
				SEDATION	EPS*	HYPOTENSION	ACE†
Phenothiazines							
Acetophenazine	Tindal	Tablets: 20 mg	60-120	++	+++	+	++
Chlorpromazine	Thorazine, ♣Largactil	Tablets: 10, 25, 50, 100, 200 mg Sustained release capsules: 30, 75, 150, 200, 300 mg Syrup: 10 mg/5 ml; 30, 100 mg/ml Injection: 25 mg/ml Suppository: 25, 100 mg	30-1000	+++	++	+++	++
Fluphenazine	Prolixin, Permitil	Tablets: 1, 2.5, 5, 10 mg Elixir: 2.5 mg/5 ml Injection: 2.5 mg/ml	0.5-20	+	+++	+	+
Mesoridazine	Serentil	Tablets: 10, 25, 50, 100 mg Concentrate: 25 mg/ml Injection: 25 mg/ml	30-400	+++	+	++	++
Perphenazine	Trilafon ♣Phenazine	Tablets: 2, 4, 8, 16 mg Concentrate: 16 mg/5 ml Injection: 5 mg/ml	12-64	+	+++	+	++
Prochlorperazine	Compazine ♣Stemetil	Tablets: 5, 10, 25 mg Sustained release capsules: 10, 15, 30 mg Syrup: 5 mg/5 ml Injection: 5 mg/ml Suppository: 2.5, 5, 25 mg	15-150	+	+++	+	+
Promazine	Sparine, ♣Promanyl	Tablets: 25, 50, 100 mg Injection: 25, 50 mg/ml	40-1000	++	++	++	+++
Thioridazine	Mellaril, ♣Novoridazine	Tablets: 10, 15, 25, 50, 100, 150, 200 mg Suspension: 25, 100 mg/5 ml Concentrate: 30, 100 mg/ml	150-800	+++	+	++	++
Trifluoperazine	Stelazine, ♣Terfluzine	Tablets: 1, 2, 5, 10 mg Concentrate: 10 mg/ml Injection: 2 mg/ml	2-40	+	+++	+	+
Triflupromazine	Vesprin	Injection: 10, 20 mg/ml	60-150	+++	++	+++	++
Thioxanthenes							
Chlorprothixene	Taractan, ♣Tarasan	Tablets: 10, 25, 50, 100 mg Concentrate: 100 mg/5 ml Injection: 12.5 mg/ml	75-600	+++	++	+++	++
Thiothixene	Navane	Capsules: 1, 2, 5, 10, 20 mg Concentrate: 5 mg/ml Injection: 5 mg/ml	6-60	+	+++	+	+
Other							
Clozapine	Clozaril	Tablets: 125, 100 mg	300-900	+++	+	++	++
Haloperidol	Haldol	Tablets: 0.5, 1, 2, 5, 10, 20 mg Concentrate: 2 mg/ml Injection: 5, 50, 100 mg/ml	1-15	+	+++	+	+
Loxapine	Loxitane, ♣Loxapac	Capsules: 5, 10, 25, 50 mg Concentrate: 25 mg/ml Injection: 50 mg/ml	20-250	++	+++	+	+
Molindone	Moban	Tablets: 5, 10, 25, 50, 100 mg Concentrate: 20 mg/ml	15-225	++	++	++	+

Key to symbols: (+) low; (++) moderate; (+++) high.
*Extrapyramidal symptoms.
†Anticholinergic effects.
♣Available in Canada.

Antimanic agent

Bipolar disorder (previously known as manic-depression) is one of several mood (affective) disorders. It is typically characterized by distinct episodes of mania (elation) and depression separated by intervals without mood disturbances. At any one time, a bipolar patient may be manic, depressed, exhibit symptoms of both mania and depression (mixed), or be between episodes. Bipolar disorder occurs equally between men and women, and has a prevalence rate of 0.4% to 1.2% of the adult population. The onset of bipolar disorder is usually in late adolescence or early twenties. It is rare in preadolescence and may occur as late as 50 years of age.

lithium carbonate (lith-e'um)

Eskalith (esk-ah'lith), **Lithane** (lith'ahn)

Lithium carbonate is used to prevent reoccurrences of mania. It has no sedative, depressant, or euphoric properties, thus separating it from all other psychiatric agents.

Side effects. Side effects frequently include nausea, vomiting, anorexia, and abdominal cramps. During the first week of therapy, excessive thirst and urination and fine hand tremors may occur. Other side effects rarely reported include nephrotoxicity, hyperglycemia, generalized pruritus with and without rash, edematous swelling of the ankles and wrists, and metallic taste.

Lithium may enhance sodium depletion, and sodium depletion enhances lithium toxicity. Early signs of toxicity include nausea, vomiting, abdominal pain, diarrhea, lethargy, speech difficulty, mild dizziness, and tremor.

Rarely, long-term lithium therapy (longer than 6 months) produces hypothyroidism. The hypothyroidism is treated by thyroid replacement.

Availability

PO—150, 300, 600 mg capsules and tablets, 300 and 450 mg slow-release tablets, and 300 mg/5 ml syrup.

Dosage and administration. NOTE: Before the initiation of lithium therapy, the following laboratory tests should be completed for baseline information: electrolytes, fasting blood glucose, BUN, serum creatinine, creatinine clearance, urinalysis, and thyroid function tests.

Serum lithium levels are monitored once or twice weekly during initiation of therapy and monthly while on a maintenance dose. Blood should be drawn approximately 12 hours after the last dose was administered. The normal serum level is 0.9 to 1.5 mEq/L. Report serum levels above these values to the physician promptly.

Adult

PO—300 to 600 mg 3 to 4 times daily. Administer with food or milk. Adequate diet is important to maintain normal serum sodium levels and prevent the development of toxicity.

• Nursing Interventions: Monitoring lithium therapy

See also General Nursing Considerations for Patients Receiving Psychotropic Agents (p. 184).

Side effects to expect

NAUSEA, VOMITING, ANOREXIA, ABDOMINAL CRAMPS. These side effects are usually mild and tend to resolve with continued therapy. Encourage the patient not to discontinue therapy without first consulting the physician.

If gastric irritation occurs, administer medication with food or milk. If symptoms persist or increase in severity, report for physician evaluation. These may also be early signs of toxicity.

EXCESSIVE THIRST AND URINATION, FINE HAND TREMOR. These side effects are usually mild and tend to resolve within a week with continued therapy. Encourage the patient not to discontinue therapy without first consulting the physician.

If these symptoms persist or become severe, the patient should consult the physician.

Side effects to report

PROGRESSIVE FATIGUE, WEIGHT GAIN. These may be early signs of hypothyroidism. Report for further evaluation.

PRURITUS, ANKLE EDEMA, METALLIC TASTE, HYPERGLYCEMIA. These are all rare side effects from lithium therapy Report for further evaluation.

NEPHROTOXICITY. Monitor urinalysis and kidney function tests for abnormal results. Report on increasing BUN and creatinine, increasing or decreasing urine output and/or decreasing specific gravity (despite amount of fluid intake), casts or protein in the urine.

Implementation

PO. Nausea, vomiting, anorexia, and abdominal cramps are frequently reduced by administering medication with meals.

GOOD NUTRITION. Lithium may enhance sodium depletion, and sodium depletion enhances lithium toxicity. It is very important that patients maintain a normal dietary intake of sodium with adequate maintenance fluids (10 to 12 8-ounce glasses of water daily), especially during the initiation of therapy, to prevent toxicity.

Drug interactions

REDUCED SERUM SODIUM LEVELS. Therapeutic activity and toxicity of lithium are highly dependent on sodium concentrations. Decreased sodium levels significantly enhance the toxicity of lithium.

Patients who are to initiate diuretic therapy, a low-sodium diet, or activities that will produce excessive and prolonged sweating should be observed particularly closely.

METHYLDOPA. Monitor patients on concurrent, long-term therapy for signs (nausea, vomiting, abdominal pain, diarrhea, lethargy, speech difficulty, mild dizziness, and tremor) of the development of lithium toxicity.

INDOMETHACIN. Indomethacin reduces the renal excretion of lithium, allowing it to accumulate, potentially to toxic levels.

SEIZURE DISORDERS
OBJECTIVES

1. Prepare a chart to be used as a study guide that includes the following information:
   Name of seizure type
   Description of seizure
   Medications used to treat each type of seizure
   Nursing interventions and monitoring parameters
2. Describe the effects of the hydantoins on patients with diabetes and on persons receiving oral contraceptives, theophylline, folic acid, or antacids.
3. Cite precautions needed when administering phenytoin intravenously.
4. Explain the rationale for proper dental care for persons receiving hydantoin therapy.
5. Develop a teaching plan for patient education for persons diagnosed with a seizure disorder.

KEY WORDS

anticonvulsant agents	seizure threshold
postictal state	tonic-clonic phase
status epilepticus	nystagmus
gingival hyperplasia	urticaria
alopecia	

Seizures are a symptom of an abnormality in the nerve centers of the brain. Seizures may result from a fever, a head injury, brain tumor, meningitis, hypoglycemia, a drug overdose or withdrawal, or poisoning. It is estimated that 8% to 10% of all people will have a seizure during their lifetime. If the seizures are chronic and recurrent, the patient is diagnosed as having *epilepsy*. Epilepsy is the most common of all neurologic disorders. It is actually not a single disease but several different diseases that have one common characteristic: a sudden discharge of excessive electrical energy from nerve cells in the brain. An estimated 2 million Americans suffer from this disorder; an estimated 100,000 new cases are diagnosed annually. The cause of epilepsy may be unknown (idiopathic epilepsy), or it may be the result of a head injury, a brain tumor, meningitis, or a stroke.

Epilepsy has been classified in several different ways. Traditionally, the most important subdivisions have been *grand mal, petit mal, psychomotor,* and *Jacksonian* types. An international commission has recently classified epilepsies into two broad categories based on their clinical and electroencephalographic (EEG) patterns. These broad categories are (1) generalized and (2) focal (localized). Generalized seizures are subdivided into convulsive and nonconvulsive types; focal seizures may be subdivided into simple and complex symptom types. See Figure 9-4 for a classification of epilepsies. Because the traditional terms are still frequently used, they have been included in the figure in parentheses. Epilepsy is treated almost exclusively with medications (anticonvulsants).

Descriptions of Seizures
Generalized convulsive seizures

The most common generalized convulsive seizures are the tonic-clonic, atonic, and myoclonic seizures.

Tonic-clonic (grand mal) seizures. These seizures are the most common type and are what many people think of as epilepsy. In the first (tonic) phase, patients suddenly develop intense muscular contractions that cause the patient to fall to the ground, lose consciousness, and lie rigid. There may be arching of the back, flexion of the arms, extension of the legs, and clenching of the teeth. Air is forced up the larynx, extruding saliva as foam and producing an audible cry-like sound. Respirations stop and the patient may become cyanotic. The tonic phase usually lasts 20 to 60 seconds before a diffuse trembling sets in. The clonic phase,

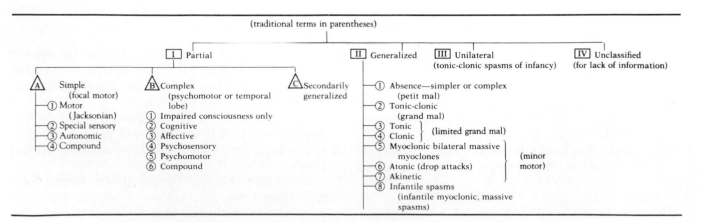

Figure 9-4 *International classification of common seizures. (From Hahn AG, Barkin RL, Oestreich SJ: Pharmacology in Nursing, ed 15, St Louis, 1982, Mosby–Year Book.)*

manifested by bilaterally symmetrical jerks alternating with relaxation of extremities, then begins. The clonic phase starts slightly first, then gradually becomes more violent and involves the whole body. Patients often bite their tongues and become incontinent of urine or feces. Usually within 60 seconds this phase proceeds to a resting, recovery phase of flaccid paralysis and sleep lasting 2 to 3 hours (post-ictal depression). The patient has no recollection of the attack upon awakening. The severity, frequency, and duration of attacks are highly variable. They may last from 1 to 30 minutes and occur as frequently as daily or every few years.

Atonic or akinetic seizures. A sudden loss of muscle tone is known as an atonic seizure or "drop attack." This may be described as a head drop, the dropping of a limb, or a slumping to the ground. There is a sudden loss of consciousness and muscle tone that results in a dramatic fall. Seated patients may slump forward violently. The attacks are short, but there is frequent injury from the uncontrolled falls. These patients often wear protective headware to minimize the trauma.

Myoclonic seizures. Myoclonic epilepsy involves lightning-like repetitive contractions of the voluntary muscles of the face, trunk, and extremities. The jerks may be isolated events or rapidly repetitive. It is not uncommon for patients to lose their balance and fall to the floor. These attacks occur most frequently at night as the patient enters sleep.

Generalized nonconvulsive seizures

By far the most common generalized nonconvulsive seizure disorder is *absence (petit mal) epilepsy*. These seizures occur primarily in children and usually disappear at puberty, although the patient may develop a second type of seizure. Attacks consist of paroxysmal episodes of altered consciousness lasting for 5 to 20 seconds. There are no prodromal or postictal phases. Patients appear to be staring into space and may exhibit a few rhythmic movements of the eyes or head, lip smacking, mumbling, chewing, or swallowing movements. Falling does not occur, patients do not convulse, and they will have no memory of events occurring during the seizures.

Focal (localized) seizures

The most common types of non-generalized seizures are unilateral seizures and partial seizures.

Unilateral seizures. These seizures involve seizure activity confined to one side of the brain. The seizures, which may last from several minutes to hours are manifested by one-sided clonus with or without loss of consciousness. Following an attack, the patient's affected side is usually left with a postictal paralysis that clears over time.

Partial seizures. Partial seizures are subdivided into partial simple motor seizures and partial complex seizures. *Partial simple motor (Jacksonian) seizures* involve localized convulsions of voluntary muscles. A single body part, such as a finger or an extremity, may start jerking. The muscle spasm may end spontaneously or spread over the whole body. The patient does not lose consciousness unless the seizure develops into a generalized convulsion. *Partial seizures with complex symptoms (psychomotor seizures)* are manifested by a vast array of possible symptoms. The patient's outward appearance may be normal or there may be aimless wandering, unusual and repeated chewing, lip smacking, or swallowing movements. The person is conscious, but may be in a confused, dream-like state. The attacks, which may occur several times daily and last several minutes, commonly end in sleep or with a clouded sensorium, with no recollection of the events of the attack.

General Nursing Considerations for Patients with Seizure Disorders

Nurses may play an important role in the correct diagnosis of seizure disorders. Accurate seizure diagnosis is crucial to selecting the most appropriate medications for each individual patient. Because physicians are not always able to observe patient seizures directly, nurses should learn to observe and record these events objectively. It is important that the patient's behavior prior to the onset of the seizure be recorded. For example, did the patient complain of feeling ill or describe an unusual sensation? The onset, duration, and characteristics of the seizure should also be described as completely as possible. For example, did the eyes deviate to one side, or was spastic muscle activity localized to one area of the body? Another important factor is the patient's behavior after the seizure. For example, did the patient continue as though nothing had happened, or was the patient groggy and confused (postictal state)? Close, accurate observation of these factors will be a tremendous aid in the proper diagnosis and selection of therapy.

> *Patient Concerns:*
> *Nursing Intervention/Rationale*

History of seizure activity. What activities was the individual engaging in immediately prior to the last seizure?

Has the individual noticed any particular activity that usually precedes attacks?

When was the last seizure before the current one?

Did the individual experience any changes in behavior prior to the onset (for example, increasing anxiety or depression)?

Is the individual aware of a pre-seizure "aura" (a particular feeling or odor that occurs prior to a seizure onset)?

Was there an "epileptic cry"?

Seizure description. Record the exact time of seizure onset and duration of each phase, a description of the specific body parts involved, and any progression of the affected parts. Did the individual lose consciousness? Was stiffening and jerking present? Describe the course of progression to various body parts.

Describe automatic responses usually seen during the clonic phase—alerted, jerky respirations or frothy salivation, dilated pupils and any eye movements, cyanosis, diaphoresis, incontinence.

Postictal behaviors. Record the level of consciousness—orientation to time, place, and person.

Assess the degree of alertness, fatigue, or headache present.

Evaluate the degree of weakness, alterations in speech, and memory loss.

Patients frequently experience muscle soreness and extreme need for sleep. Record the time spent sleeping.

Evaluate any bodily harm that occurred during the seizure—bruises, cuts, lacerations.

Management of seizure activity. Assist the patient during a seizure by doing the following:

1. Protect the patient from further injury. Place padding around or under the head; do not try to restrain; loosen tight clothing. If in a standing position initially, lower the patient to a flat position.
2. If possible, place a soft object such as a face cloth between the patient's teeth to prevent accidental biting of the tongue or breakage of the teeth.
3. Once the patient enters into the relaxation stage, turn slightly on the side to allow secretions to drain out of the mouth.
4. Remain calm and quiet and give reassurance to the patient when the seizure is over.
5. Provide for a place for the patient to rest immediately after a seizure. Summon appropriate assistance so that the individual can get home.
6. If the patient starts into another seizure, or if a seizure lasts longer than 4 minutes, immediately summon assistance; the patient may be going into status epilepticus.

Psychological implications

Lifestyle. Encourage maintenance of a normal lifestyle. Provide for appropriate limitations (such as on operating power equipment or a motor vehicle, on swimming) to ensure patient safety.

Expression of feelings. Allow for ventilation of feelings. Seizures may occur in public and may be accompanied by incontinence. Patients are usually very embarrassed about having a seizure in front of others.

Provide for ventilation of any discrimination the patient feels at the workplace.

School-age children. Acceptance by peers can present a problem to the patient. The school nurse can help teachers and other children to understand seizures.

Denial. Be alert for signs of denial of the disease. An indication of this is increased seizure activity in a previously well-controlled patient. Question compliance with the drug regimen.

Compliance. Determine the patient's current medication schedule: name of medication, dosage, when last dose was taken; have any doses been skipped, if so how many? If compliance appears to be a problem, try to find out the reasons for patient noncompliance so appropriate interventions can be implemented.

Complications

Status epilepticus. Status epilepticus is a rapidly recurring seizure that does not allow the individual to regain normal function between seizures.

Provide for patient protection and summon assistance for transportation of the patient to the emergency room.

Administer oxygen; have suction and resuscitation equipment available.

Establish an IV and have available drugs for treatment (such as phenytoin, phenobarbital, diazepam).

Monitor vital signs and neurologic status.

Insert a nasogastric tube if vomiting is present.

Patient Education Associated with Anticonvulsant Therapy

Communication and responsibility. Encourage open communication with the patient concerning frustrations and anger as attempts are made to adjust to the diagnosis and need for treatment. The patient must be guided to insight into the disorder if he or she is to assume responsibility for the continuation of the treatment. Keep emphasizing those things the patient can do to alter the progression of disease, including maintenance of general health, nutritional needs, adequate rest and appropriate exercise, and continuation of prescribed medication therapy.

Exercise and activity. Encourage maintenance of a regular lifestyle with moderate activity. Avoid excessive exercise and expenditures of energy that would lead to excessive fatigue.

Nutrition. Avoid excessive use of stimulants (e.g., caffeine-containing products). Seizures are also known to follow the significant intake of alcoholic beverages; therefore, ingestion should be avoided or limited.

Stress. Reduction of tension and stress within the individual's environment may reduce seizure activity in some patients.

Oral hygiene. Encourage maintenance of daily oral hygiene practices and scheduling of regular dental exams. Gingival hyperplasia, gum overgrowth associated with hydantoins (phenytoin, ethotoin, and mephenytoin) can be reduced by good oral hygiene, frequent gum massage, regular brushing, and proper dental care.

Expectations of therapy. Discuss the expectations of therapy (for example, level of seizure control, degree of lethargy, sedation, frequency of use of therapy, relief of symptoms, sexual activity, maintenance of mobility, ability to maintain activities of daily living and/or work, and limitations in operating power equipment or a motor vehicle).

Changes in expectations. Assess changes in expectations as therapy progresses and the patient gains understanding and skill in the management of the diagnosis.

Stress that once seizures are controlled, medication must be continued.

Changes in therapy through cooperative goal setting. Work cooperatively with the patient to encourage adherence to the treatment prescribed. When the patient feels that a change should be made in a treatment plan, encourage discussion with the physician.

Written record. Enlist the patient's aid in developing and maintaining a written record (Figure 9-5) of monitoring parameters (such as degree of lethargy; sedation; oral hygiene for gum disorders; degree of seizure relief; nausea, vomiting, or anorexia present) and response to prescribed therapies for discussion with the physician.

Have others record the date, time, duration, and frequency of any seizure episodes. Also record the behavior immediately prior to and following seizures.

Patients should be encouraged to bring this record with them on follow-up visits.

Fostering compliance. Throughout the hospitalization, discuss medication information and how it will benefit the course of treatment. Recognize that noncompliance may be a means of denial. Explore underlying problems in acceptance of disease and the need for strict compliance for maximum control. Seek cooperation and understanding of the following points so that medication compliance may be enhanced:

1. Name.
2. Dosage: Do not adjust the dosage without consulting the physician. Plasma drug levels will be performed periodically to determine therapeutic versus toxic drug level.
3. Route and administration times: If using the oral suspension, shake well and use an oral syringe for accurate measurement.
4. Anticipated therapeutic response: The eventual goal is to maintain the patient in a seizure-free state.
5. Side effects to expect: Drowsiness.
6. Side effects to report: Recurrence of seizures should always be reported. Other data to report are nausea and vomiting, sore throat, general malaise, mucosal ulcerations, gum swelling, lymph node swelling.
7. What to do if a dosage is missed; and when, how, or if to refill the medication: Always keep an adequate supply of medication on hand so that blood levels will be maintained by accurate, regular use.

Difficulty in comprehension. If it is evident that the patient or family does not understand all aspects of continuing therapy being prescribed (such as administration and monitoring of medications, management of seizure activity when present, diets, follow-up appointments, and the need for lifelong management), consider use of social service or visiting nurse agencies.

Associated teaching. Always inform the physician or dentist of any prescription or over-the-counter medication being taken.

Over-the-counter medications should not be taken without first discussing with the physician or pharmacist.

Always report side effects of rash, itching, or hives immediately. Nausea, vomiting, or diarrhea should be reported for the physician's evaluation if it is a new symptom.

Take all of the medication as prescribed for the full course of treatment. Do not discontinue use when feeling improved; do not save for future use or give medicine to another individual. Sudden discontinuation of certain medications may produce harmful effects.

Keep all medications out of the reach of children.

If pregnancy is suspected, consult an obstetrician as soon as possible about continuation of medication therapy.

The patient should carry an identification card or bracelet.

At discharge. Items to be sent home with the patient should include the following:

1. Written instructions for the item's use
2. Labels in a level of language and size of print appropriate for the patient
3. If needed, identification cards or bracelets
4. A list of additional supplies to be purchased after discharge (such as oral syringes)
5. Schedule for follow-up appointments
6. Stress the danger of suddenly discontinuing seizure medications. Always carry extra medications when traveling in the event the time away is extended.
7. The Epilepsy Foundation of America and State Vocational Rehabilitation Agencies can provide the patient with information about vocational rehabilitation and employment.

Drug Therapy for Seizure Disorders

Barbiturates

The long-acting barbiturates (phenobarbital, mephobarbital, methabarbital, amobarbital) are very effective anticonvulsants. They may be used to treat grand mal, petit mal, myoclonic, and mixed seizures, usually in combination with other anticonvulsants (see Table 9-8). Barbiturates are discussed in greater detail elsewhere in this chapter (p. 168).

Patient Education and Monitoring of Therapeutic Outcomes for Patients Receiving Anticonvulsants

Medications	Color	To be taken

Name _____

Physician _____

Physician's phone _____

Next appt.* _____

	Parameters	Day of discharge							Comments
Previous seizure activity	Number / day?								
	Lasted how long?								
	Type, describe								
Present seizure activity	Number / day?								
	Lasted how long?								
	Type, describe								
	Slept after?								
Compliance	I take my medication as ordered.								
	Sometimes I forget.								
	I don't like to take medication.								
Drowsiness: Feel like sleeping all day Feel like being active 10 5 1									
Disease acceptance: I don't want people to know I have epilepsy I have epilepsy and take medication 10 5 1									
Oral hygiene: brushing and flossing teeth	3 times a day								
	2 times a day								
	1 time per day								
	I forgot								
Condition of gums?	No bleeding								
	Some bleeding (#) times / day								
	Bleeding every time I brush								
Nausea and vomiting	All day								
	Sometimes (when?)								

*Please bring this record with you to your next appointment.
Use the back of this sheet for additional information.

Figure 9-5 *Patient education and monitoring of therapeutic outcomes for patients receiving anticonvulsants.*

Table 9-8 *Anticonvulsants*

GENERIC NAME	BRAND NAME	AVAILABILITY	ADULT DOSAGE RANGE	USE IN SEIZURES
Barbiturates				
Mephobarbital	Mebaral	Tablets: 32, 50, 100 mg	400-600 mg/day	Grand mal, petit mal
Metharbital	Gemonil	Tablets: 100 mg	Up to 600-800 mg/day	Grand mal, petit mal, myoclonic seizures, mixed seizures
Phenobarbital	Luminal, Solfoton, Barbita, ♣Gardenal	Tablets: 8, 16, 30, 65, 100 mg Capsules: 16 mg Elixir: 20 mg/5 ml	100-300 mg/day	All forms of epilepsy
Benzodiazepines				
Clonazepam	Klonopin, ♣Rivotril	Tablets: 0.5, 1, 2 mg	Up to 20 mg/day	Petit mal, myoclonic seizures
Clorazepate	Tranxene	Tablets: 3.75, 7.5, 11.25, 15, 22.5 mg Capsules: 3.75, 7.5, 15 mg	Up to 90 mg/day	Focal seizures
Diazepam	Valium, ♣Meval	Tablets: 2.5, 5, 10 mg IV: 5 mg/ml Liquid: 1, 5 mg/ml	Initially 5-10 mg, up to 30 mg	All forms of epilepsy; used in conjunction with other agents
Hydantoins				
Ethotoin	Peganone	Tablets: 250, 500 mg	2-3 g/day	Grand mal, psychomotor seizures
Mephenytoin	Mesantoin	Tablets: 100 mg	200-600 mg/day	Grand mal, psychomotor seizures, focal seizures, Jacksonian seizures
Phenytoin	Dilantin	Tablets: 50 mg Capsules: 30, 100 mg Suspension: 30, 125 mg/5 ml Inj: 50 mg/ml in 2 and 5 ml amps	300-600 mg/day	Grand mal, psychomotor seizures
Succinimides				
Ethosuximide	Zarontin	Capsules: 250 mg Syrup: 250 mg/5 ml	1000-1250 mg/day	Petit mal
Methsuximide	Celontin	Capsules: 150, 300 mg	900-1200 mg/day	Petit mal
Phensuximide	Milontin	Capsules: 500 mg	1-2 g/day	Petit mal

♣Available in Canada only.

Benzodiazepines

The three benzodiazepines approved for use as anticonvulsants are diazepam, clonazepam, and clorazepate. Clonazepam is useful in the oral treatment of absence seizures in children. Diazepam must be administered intravenously to control seizures but is the drug of choice for treatment of status epilepticus. Clorazepate is used with other antiepileptic agents to control partial seizures.

Side effects. The more common side effects of benzodiazepines are extensions of their pharmacologic properties. Drowsiness, fatigue, lethargy, and ataxia are relatively common, especially when other anticonvulsants with depressant effects are added to the therapy.

Behavioral disturbances such as aggressiveness and agitation have been reported, especially in patients who are mentally retarded or have psychiatric disturbances.

Rapid discontinuance of benzodiazepines after longterm use may result in symptoms similar to alcohol withdrawal. These may vary from weakness and anxiety to delirium and grand mal seizures. The symptoms may not appear for several days after discontinuation. Treatment consists of gradual withdrawal of benzodiazepines over a 2- to 4-week period.

Benzodiazepines should be administered with caution to patients with a history of blood dyscrasias or hepatic damage.

Availability. See Table 9-8.

Dosage and administration. See Table 9-8.

• **Nursing Interventions: Monitoring benzodiazepine therapy**

See also General Nursing Considerations for Patients with Seizure Disorders (p. 201).

Side effects to expect

SEDATION, DROWSINESS, DIZZINESS, BLURRED VISION, FATIGUE, LETHARGY. These symptoms tend to disappear with continued therapy and possible readjustment of the dosage. Encourage the patient not to discontinue therapy without first consulting the physician.

Persons who are working around machinery, driving a car, or performing other duties in which they must remain mentally alert should be particularly cautious. Provide for patient safety during episodes of dizziness and ataxia; report for further evaluation.

Caution the patient that blurred vision may occur and make appropriate suggestions for personal safety of the individual.

Side effects to report

BEHAVIORAL DISTURBANCES. Provide supportive physical care and safety during these responses.

Assess the level of excitement and deal calmly with the individual. During periods of excitement, protect persons from harm and provide for physical channeling of energy (for example, walk with them).

Seek change in the medication order.

BLOOD DYSCRASIAS. Routine laboratory studies (RBC, WBC, and differential counts) should be scheduled.

Monitor for the development of sore throat, fever, purpura, jaundice, or excessive and progressive weakness.

HEPATOTOXICITY. The symptoms of hepatotoxicity are anorexia, nausea, vomiting, jaundice, hepatomegaly, splenomegaly, and abnormal liver function tests (elevated bilirubin, AST, ALT, GGT, alkaline phosphatase, prothrombin time).

Implementation

IV. Do not mix parenteral diazepam in the same syringe with other medications; do not add to other IV solutions because of precipitate formation.

Administer slowly at a rate of at least 5 mg per minute. If at all possible, give under ECG monitoring and observe closely for bradycardia. Stop boluses until the heart rate returns to normal.

Drug interactions

DRUGS THAT INCREASE TOXIC EFFECTS. Antihistamines, alcohol, analgesics, anesthetics, tranquilizers, narcotics, cimetidine, sedative-hypnotics, and other anticonvulsants.

Monitor the patient for excessive sedation, and eliminate the nonanticonvulsants if possible.

SMOKING. Smoking enhances the metabolism of the benzodiazepines. Larger dosages may be necessary to maintain effects in patients who smoke.

Hydantoins

Hydantoins (phenytoin, ethotoin, and mephenytoin) are anticonvulsants used to control grand mal and psychomotor seizures. Mephenytoin may also be used to treat focal and Jacksonian seizures when less toxic anticonvulsants are unsuccessful. Phenytoin is by far the most commonly used anticonvulsant of the hydantoins.

Side effects. Common adverse effects include nausea and vomiting, nystagmus, slurred speech, dizziness, gingival hyperplasia, insomnia, mental confusion, and transient nervousness.

Rarely, hydantoins may cause rashes, blood dyscrasias, and hepatitis.

Hydantoins may elevate blood sugar levels, especially if higher doses are used; patients with diabetes mellitus are more susceptible to hyperglycemia.

Availability. See Table 9-8.

Dosage and administration. See Table 9-8.

• Nursing Interventions: Monitoring hydantoin therapy

See also General Nursing Considerations for Patients with Seizure Disorders (p. 201).

Side effects to expect

NAUSEA, VOMITING, INDIGESTION. These effects are common during initiation of therapy. Gradual increases in therapy and administration with food or milk will reduce gastric irritation.

SEDATION, DROWSINESS, DIZZINESS, BLURRED VISION, FATIGUE, LETHARGY. These symptoms tend to disappear with continued therapy and possible adjustment of dosage. Encourage the patient not to discontinue therapy without first consulting the physician.

Persons who are working around machinery, driving a car, or performing other duties in which they must remain mentally alert should be particularly cautious.

Provide for patient safety during episodes of dizziness; report for further evaluation.

Caution the patient that blurred vision may occur and make appropriate suggestions for personal safety of the individual.

CONFUSION. Perform a baseline assessment of the patient's degree of alertness and orientation to name, place, and time prior to initiating therapy. Make regularly scheduled subsequent evaluations of mental status and compare findings. Report development of alterations.

GINGIVAL HYPERPLASIA. The frequency of gum overgrowth may be reduced by good oral hygiene including gum massage, frequent brushing, and proper dental care.

Side effects to report

HYPERGLYCEMIA. Particularly during the early weeks of therapy, diabetic or prediabetic patients need to be monitored for the development of hyperglycemia.

Assess regularly for glycosuria and report if it occurs with any frequency.

Patients receiving oral hypoglycemic agents or insulin may require an adjustment in dosage.

BLOOD DYSCRASIAS. Routine laboratory studies (RBC, WBC, and differential counts) should be scheduled.

Monitor for the development of sore throat, fever, purpura, jaundice, or excessive and progressive weakness.

HEPATOTOXICITY. The symptoms of hepatotoxicity are anorexia, nausea, vomiting, jaundice, hepatomegaly, splenomegaly, and abnormal liver function tests (elevated bilirubin, AST, ALT, GGT, alkaline phosphatase, prothrombin time).

DERMATOLOGIC REACTIONS. Report a rash or pruritus immediately and withhold additional doses pending approval by the physician.

Implementation

PO. Administer medication with food or milk to reduce gastric irritation. If an oral suspension is used, shake well first. Encourage the use of an oral syringe for accurate measurement.

IM. If at all possible, avoid IM administration. Absorption is slow and painful.

IV. Do not mix parenteral phenytoin in the same syringe with other medications; because of precipitate formation, do not add to other IV solutions.

Administer slowly at a rate of 25 to 50 mg per minute. If at all possible, give under ECG monitoring and observe closely for bradycardia. Stop boluses until the heart rate returns to normal. Therapeutic blood levels are 10 to 20 mg/L.

Drug interactions

DRUGS THAT ENHANCE THERAPEUTIC AND TOXIC EFFECTS. Warfarin, carbamazepine, disulfiram, phenylbutazone, amiodarone, isoniazid, chloramphenicol, cimetidine, and sulfonamides.

Monitor patients with concurrent therapy for signs of phenytoin toxicity; nystagmus, sedation, lethargy. Serum levels may be ordered, and a reduced dosage of phenytoin may be required.

DRUGS THAT DECREASE THERAPEUTIC EFFECTS. Barbiturates, folic acid, and antacids.

Monitor patients with concurrent therapy for increased seizure activity. Monitoring changes in serum levels should help warn of possible increased seizure activity.

DISOPYRAMIDE, QUINIDINE, MEXILETINE. Phenytoin decreases serum levels of these agents. Monitor patients for redevelopment of arrhythmias.

PREDNISOLONE, DEXAMETHASONE. Phenytoin decreases serum levels of these agents. Monitor patients for reduced antiinflammatory activity.

ORAL CONTRACEPTIVES. Spotting or bleeding may be an indication of reduced contraceptive activity. Use of alternate forms of birth control is recommended.

THEOPHYLLINE. Phenytoin decreases serum levels of theophylline derivatives. Monitor patients for a greater frequency of respiratory difficulty. The theophylline dose may have to be increased 50% to 100% to maintain the same therapeutic response.

VALPROIC ACID. This agent may increase or decrease the activity of phenytoin.

Monitor for increased frequency of seizure activity. Monitoring changes in serum levels should help warn of possible increased seizure activity.

Monitor patients with concurrent therapy for signs of phenytoin toxicity: nystagmus, sedation, lethargy.

Serum levels may be ordered, and a reduced dosage of phenytoin may be required.

KETOCONAZOLE. Concurrent administration with ketoconazole may alter the metabolism of one or both drugs. Monitoring for both is recommended.

CYCLOSPORINE. Phenytoin enhances the metabolism of cyclosporine. Increased doses of cyclosporine may be necessary in patients receiving concomitant therapy.

Succinimides

Succinimides (ethosuximide, methsuximide, and phensuximide) are used for the control of absence (petit mal) seizures.

Side effects. Gastrointestinal symptoms of nausea, vomiting, indigestion, cramps, anorexia, diarrhea, and constipation occur frequently with this class of anticonvulsants.

As noted with other classes of anticonvulsants, drowsiness, ataxia, and dizziness are common side effects.

Availability. See Table 9-8.

Dosage and administration. See Table 9-8.

Drug interactions. The following drugs, when used concurrently with the succinimides, may enhance the toxic effects of the succinimides: antihistamines, alcohol, analgesics, anesthetics, tranquilizers, other anticonvulsants, and sedative-hypnotics.

Nursing interventions. See also General Nursing Considerations for Patients with Seizure Disorders (p. 201) and Hydantoins (p. 206).

Miscellaneous anticonvulsants

carbamazepine (kar-bah-maz'e-peen)

Tegretol (teg'reh-tol)

Carbamazepine is an anticonvulsant frequently used in combination with other anticonvulsants to control grand mal seizures. It is not effective in the control of absence seizures. Carbamazepine has also been used successfully to treat the pain associated with trigeminal neuralgia (tic douloureux). It may also be used to treat manic-depressive disorders when lithium therapy has not been optimal.

Side effects. Side effects frequently seen when therapy is started are drowsiness, nausea, vomiting, and dizziness.

As a result of serious adverse reactions, the manufacturer recommends that the following baseline studies be repeated at regular intervals: complete blood count, liver function tests, urinalysis, BUN and serum creatinine, and ophthalmologic examination.

Side effects based on organ systems are as follows:

Cardiovascular: hypotension, hypertension, congestive heart failure, edema, and aggravation of coronary artery disease.

Neurologic: incoordination, nystagmus, visual hallucinations, and speech disturbances.

Dermatologic: pruritus, rashes, skin pigmentation, urticaria, and alopecia (loss of hair).

Availability

PO—100 and 200 mg tablets; 100 mg/5 ml suspension.

Dosage and administration

Adult

PO—Initial dose is 200 mg 2 times daily in the first day. Increase gradually by 200 mg/day in divided doses at 6- to 8-hour intervals. Do not exceed 1200 mg daily. Therapeutic plasma levels are 4 to 10 mg/L.

• **Nursing Interventions: Monitoring carbamazepine therapy**

See also General Nursing Considerations for Patients with Seizure Disorders (p. 201).

Side effects to expect

NAUSEA, VOMITING, DROWSINESS, DIZZINESS. These effects can be reduced by slowly increasing the dose.

These effects are usually mild and tend to resolve with continued therapy. Encourage the patient not to discontinue therapy without first consulting the physician.

Provide for patient safety during episodes of dizziness.

Persons who are working around machinery, driving a car, or performing other duties in which they must remain mentally alert should not take these medications while working.

Side effects to report

ORTHOSTATIC HYPOTENSION, HYPERTENSION. Monitor the blood pressure daily in both the supine and standing positions.

Anticipate the development of postural hypotension and take measures to prevent an occurrence. Teach the patient to rise slowly from a supine or sitting position; encourage the patient to sit or lie down if feeling "faint."

DYSPNEA, EDEMA. If carbamazepine is used in patients with a history of congestive heart failure, monitor daily weights, lung sounds, and accumulation of edema.

NEUROLOGIC. Perform a baseline assessment of the patient's speech patterns and degree of alertness and orientation to name, place, and time *prior* to initiating therapy. Make regularly scheduled subsequent evaluations of mental status and compare findings. Report development of alterations.

NEPHROTOXICITY. Monitor urinalysis and kidney function tests for abnormal results. Report an increasing BUN and creatinine, decreasing urine output and/or decreasing specific gravity (despite amount of fluid intake), casts or protein in the urine, frank blood or smoky-colored urine, or RBCs in excess of 0 to 3 on the urinalysis report.

HEPATOTOXICITY. The symptoms of hepatotoxicity are anorexia, nausea, vomiting, jaundice, hepatomegaly, splenomegaly, and abnormal liver function tests (elevated bilirubin, AST, ALT, GGT, alkaline phosphatase, prothrombin time).

BLOOD DYSCRASIAS. Routine laboratory studies (RBC, WBC, and differential counts) should be scheduled.

Monitor for the development of sore throat, fever, purpura, jaundice, or excessive and progressive weakness.

DERMATOLOGIC REACTIONS. Report a rash or pruritus immediately and withhold additional doses pending approval by the physician.

Drug interactions

ISONIAZID. Isoniazid inhibits the metabolism of carbamazepine. Monitor for signs of toxicity: disorientation, ataxia, lethargy, headache, drowsiness, nausea, and vomiting.

PROPOXYPHENE, VERAPAMIL, DILTIAZEM. Propoxyphene, Verapamil, and Diltiazem increase serum levels of carbamazepine. Monitor for signs of toxicity: disorientation, ataxia, lethargy, headache, drowsiness, nausea, and vomiting. A 40% to 50% decrease in carbamazepine dosage may be necessary.

WARFARIN. Carbamazepine may diminish the anticoagulant effects of warfarin. Monitor the prothrombin time and increase the dosage of warfarin if necessary.

PHENOBARBITAL, PHENYTOIN, VALPROIC ACID, PRIMIDONE. Carbamazepine enhances the metabolism of these agents. Monitor for increased frequency of seizure activity. Monitoring changes in serum levels should help warn of possible increased seizure activity.

DOXYCYCLINE. Carbamazepine enhances the metabolism of this antibiotic. Monitor patients for signs of continued infection.

ORAL CONTRACEPTIVES. Carbamazepine enhances the metabolism of estrogens. Spotting or bleeding may be an indication of reduced contraceptive activity. Use of other forms of birth control is recommended.

primidone (prih′mih-doan)

Mysoline (my′so-leen)

Primidone is structurally related to the barbiturates. It is metabolized into phenobarbital and phenylethylmalonamide (PEMA), both of which are active anticonvulsants. Primidone is used in combination with other anticonvulsants to treat grand mal and psychomotor seizures.

Side effects. Common adverse effects include sedation, drowsiness, dizziness, blurred vision, and nystagmus.

Primidone may cause paradoxic excitability in children. Blood dyscrasias have rarely been reported with the use of primidone.

Availability

PO—50 and 250 mg tablets, and 250 mg/5 ml oral suspension.

Dosage and administration

Adult. PO—250 mg daily, with weekly increases of 250 mg until therapeutic response or intolerance develops. Usual dose is 750 to 1500 mg daily. Do not exceed 2000 mg daily.

• Nursing Interventions: Monitoring primidone therapy

See also General Nursing Considerations for Patients with Seizure Disorders (p. 201).

Side effects to expect

SEDATION, DROWSINESS, DIZZINESS, BLURRED VISION. These symptoms tend to disappear with continued therapy and possible adjustment of dosage. Encourage the patient not to discontinue therapy without first consulting the physician.

Persons who are working around machinery, driving a car, or performing other duties in which they must remain mentally alert should be particularly cautious while working.

Provide for patient safety during episodes of dizziness; report for further evaluation.

Caution the patient that blurred vision may occur and make appropriate suggestions for personal safety of the individual.

Side effects to report

BLOOD DYSCRASIAS. Routine laboratory studies (RBC, WBC, and differential counts) should be scheduled.

Monitor for the development of sore throat, fever, purpura, jaundice, or excessive and progressive weakness.

PARADOXICAL EXCITABILITY. During a period of excitement, protect persons from harm and provide for physical channeling of energy (for example, walk with them). Notify the physician for a possible change in medication.

Drug interactions

ORAL CONTRACEPTIVES. Spotting or bleeding may be an indication of reduced contraceptive activity. Use of alternate forms of birth control is recommended.

PHENYTOIN. Phenytoin may increase the phenobarbital serum levels when taken concurrently with primidone. Monitor patients for increased sedation.

valproic acid (val-pro'ik)

Depakene (dep'ah-keen)

Valproic acid is an anticonvulsant structurally unrelated to any other agent used to treat seizure disorders. It is most effective in treating petit mal seizure activity; it may be effective in treating other types of seizures when used in combination with other agents.

Side effects. Side effects include nausea, vomiting and indigestion, dizziness, blurred vision, nystagmus, and headache.

The manufacturer recommends that the following baseline studies be completed before therapy is initiated and at regular intervals thereafter: liver function tests, bleeding time determination, and platelet count.

One of the metabolites of valproic acid is a ketone. It is excreted in the urine and may produce a false-positive test (Ketostix, Acetest) for urine ketones.

Availability

PO—250 mg tablets; 125, 250, 500 mg enteric-coated tablets; 250 mg/5 ml syrup.

Dosage and administration

Adult. PO—5 mg/kg every 8 hours. Increase by 5 to 10 mg/kg/day at weekly intervals. The maximum daily dosage is 30 mg/kg/day. Therapeutic blood levels are 50 to 100 mg/L.

• Nursing Interventions: Monitoring valproic acid therapy

See also General Nursing Considerations for Patients with Seizure Disorders (p. 201).

Side effects to expect

NAUSEA, VOMITING, INDIGESTION. These effects are common during initiation of therapy. Gradual increases in therapy and administration with food or milk will reduce gastric irritation.

SEDATION, DROWSINESS, DIZZINESS, BLURRED VISION. These symptoms tend to disappear with continued therapy and possible adjustment of dosage. Encourage the patient not to discontinue therapy without first consulting the physician.

Persons who are working around machinery, driving a car, or performing other duties in which they must remain mentally alert should not take these medications while working.

Provide for patient safety during episodes of dizziness; report for further evaluation.

Caution the patient that blurred vision may occur and make appropriate suggestions for personal safety of the individual.

Side effects to report

BLOOD DYSCRASIAS. Routine laboratory studies (RBC, WBC, and differential counts) should be scheduled.

Monitor for the development of sore throat, fever, purpura, jaundice, or excessive and progressive weakness.

HEPATOTOXICITY. The symptoms of hepatotoxicity are anorexia, nausea, vomiting, jaundice, hepatomegaly, splenomegaly, and abnormal liver function tests (elevated bilirubin, AST, ALT, GGT, alkaline phosphatase, prothrombin time).

Implementation

PO. Administer medication with food or milk to reduce gastric irritation.

An enteric-coated tablet is available for those patients having persistent difficulty.

Drug interactions

ENHANCED SEDATION. CNS depressants, including sleeping aids, analgesics, tranquilizers, and alcohol, will enhance the sedative effects of valproic acid. Persons who are working around machinery, driving a car, or performing other duties in which they must remain mentally alert should not take these medications while working.

PHENOBARBITAL, PHENYTOIN, CARBAMAZEPINE. Monitor for increased frequency of seizure activity. Monitoring changes in serum levels should help warn of possible increased seizure activity.

MOTION SICKNESS
OBJECTIVES

1. Cite the side effects of antihistamines used to treat motion sickness.
2. Identify the most effective time to administer antihistamines to prevent motion sickness.

Drug Therapy for Motion Sickness

Anticholinergic agents

Nausea and vomiting associated with motion are thought to result from stimulation of the labyrinth system of the ear, with subsequent transmission of this stimulus to the vestibular network located near the vomiting center. When there is strong or frequent stimulation, such as from a rocking ship or airplane, the vestibular network is bombarded with an abnormally high number of impulses that radiate by cholinergic nerve impulses to the adjacent vomiting center. Thus drugs that inhibit the cholinergic nerve impulses from the vestibular network to the vomiting center should be effective in the treatment of motion sickness.

Most agents used to reduce nausea and vomiting from motion sickness are chemically related to antihistamines. The effectiveness of antihistamines in motion sickness probably results from their anticholinergic properties, not from their ability to block histamine. See Table 9-9. Drugs used for motion sickness should be initiated approximately 30 minutes in advance of embarking on a trip or undertaking activity that initiates motion sickness.

Side effects. The most common side effect of antihistamines used to control motion sickness is drowsiness. With prolonged therapy, most patients acquire a tolerance to this adverse effect. Reduction in dosage or a change to another antihistamine may occasionally be necessary.

The anticholinergic effects that are capitalized on for the treatment of motion sickness also cause dry mouth, stuffy nose, blurred vision, constipation, and urinary retention. Patients with asthma, prostatic enlargement, or glaucoma should take antihistamines only under a physician's supervision. The drying effects may also make respiratory mucus more viscous and tenacious.

Availability. See Table 9-9.

Dosage and administration. It is essential that the patient take the medication 30 to 60 minutes prior to the activity that is likely to produce motion sickness.

- **Nursing Interventions: Monitoring drug therapy for motion sickness**
  Side effects to expect

SEDATIVE EFFECTS. Tolerance may develop over a period of time, thus diminishing the effect.

The operation of power equipment or a motor vehicle may prove hazardous. Caution patients to provide for their personal safety in these situations.

FLUID INTAKE. Maintain fluid intake at 8 to 12 8-ounce glasses daily.

BLURRED VISION, CONSTIPATION, URINARY RETENTION, DRYNESS OF MUCOSA OF THE MOUTH, THROAT, AND NOSE. These symptoms are the anticholinergic effects produced by these agents. Patients taking these medications should be monitored for the development of these side effects.

Dryness of the mucosa may be relieved by sucking hard candy or ice chips, or by chewing gum.

The use of stool softeners such as docusate or the occasional use of a potent laxative such as bisacodyl may be required for constipation.

Caution the patient that blurred vision may occur and make appropriate suggestions for personal safety of the individual.

Patients who develop urinary hesitancy should discontinue the medication and contact their physician for further evaluation.

Implementation

PO. Administer 30 to 60 minutes prior to the activity that is likely to produce motion sickness.

Drug interactions

ENHANCED SEDATION. CNS depressants, including sleeping aids, analgesics, tranquilizers, and alcohol, will enhance the sedative effects of the antihistamines. Persons who are working around machinery, driving a car, or performing other duties in which they must remain mentally alert should not take these medications while working.

PAIN
OBJECTIVES

1. Differentiate among *opiate agonists, opiate partial agonists,* and *opiate antagonists.*
2. Describe monitoring parameters necessary for patients receiving opiate agonists.
3. Cite the side effects to expect when opiate agonists are administered.
4. Compare the analgesic effectiveness of opiate partial agonists when administered before or after opiate agonists.
5. Explain when naloxone can be used effectively to treat respiratory depression.

Table 9-9 *Anticholinergic Agents Used for Motion Sickness*

GENERIC NAME	BRAND NAME	AVAILABILITY	ADULT DOSAGE	PEDIATRIC DOSAGE
Buclizine	Bucladin-S Softabs	Tablets: 50 mg	PO: 50 mg, repeated in 4-6 hours; do not exceed 150 mg daily	Not approved for use by children
Cyclizine	Marezine, ♣Marzine	Tablets: 50 mg Inj: 50 mg/1 ml	PO: 50 mg, repeated in 4-6 hours; do not exceed 200 mg daily IM: 50 mg every 4-6 hours	PO: 6-12 years: 25 mg up to 3 times daily
Dimenhydrinate	Dramamine, ♣Travamine	Capsules: 50 mg Tablets: 50 mg Inj: 50 mg/ml Liquid: 12.5 mg/4 ml, 15.6 mg/5 ml	PO: 50-100 mg every 4-6 hours; do not exceed 400 mg in 24 hours IM: 50 mg, as needed	PO: 6-12 years: 25-50 mg every 6-8 hours; do not exceed 150 mg in 24 hours 2-6 years: up to 25 mg every 6-8 hours; do not exceed 75 mg in 24 hours
Diphenhydramine	Benadryl, Noradryl, ♣Insomnal	Tablets: 50 mg Capsules: 25, 50 mg Elixir: 12.5 mg/5 ml Syrup: 12.5, 13.3 mg/5 ml Inj: 10, 50 mg/ml	PO: 25-50 mg 3 or 4 times daily IM: 10-50 mg; do not exceed 400 mg/24 hours	PO: Over 20 lbs: 12.5-25 mg 3 or 4 times daily (5 mg/kg/24); do not exceed 300 mg/24 hours IM: 5 mg/kg/24 hours, in 4 divided doses; do not exceed 300 mg in 24 hours
Hydroxyzine	Atarax, Durrax, Vistaril, ♣Multi-pax	Tablets: 10, 25, 50, 100 mg Capsules: 25, 50, 100 mg Syrup: 10 mg/5 ml Oral Suspension: 25 mg/5 ml Inj: 25, 50 mg/ml	PO: 25-100 mg 3-4 times daily IM: As for PO	PO: Over 6 years: 10-25 mg every 4-6 hours; under 6 years: 10 mg every 4-6 hours IM: As for PO
Meclizine	Antivert, ♣Bonamine	Tablets: 12.5, 25, 50 mg Capsules: 25 mg	PO: 25-50 mg; may be repeated every 24 hours	PO: Not approved for use by children
Scopolamine, Transdermal	Transderm-Scōp	Transdermal patch: delivers 0.5 mg over three days	Patch: Apply to skin behind the ear at least 4 hours before antiemetic effect is required. Replace in 3 days if continued therapy is required.	Not approved for use by children

♣Available in Canada only.

6. State the three pharmacological effects of salicylates.
7. Prepare a list of side effects to expect, side effects to report, and drug interactions that are associated with salicylates.
8. Explain why synthetic nonopiate analgesics are not used for inflammatory disorders.
9. Prepare a patient education plan for a person being discharged with a continuing prescription for an analgesic.
10. Examine Table 9-10 and identify the active ingredients in commonly prescribed analgesic combination products. Identify products containing aspirin, and compare the analgesic properties of agents available in different strengths.

KEY WORDS

analgesics
opiate agonists
pain threshold
nonsteroidal antiinflammatory agents
pain perception
pain tolerance
salicylates
opiate partial agonists
opiate antagonists
addictive
projected pain
referred pain
local pain
radiating pain

Pain is an unpleasant sensation that is part of a larger experience called *pain experience*. The pain experience includes all the emotional sensations (attention, anxiety, fatigue, suggestion, prior conditioning) for a particular person under a certain set of circumstances. This accounts for the wide variation in individual responses to the sensation of pain.

Three terms used in relationship to the pain experience are: pain perception, pain threshold, and pain tolerance. *Pain perception* is the individual's awareness of the feeling or sensation of pain. *Pain threshold* is the point at which an individual first acknowledges or interprets a sensation as being painful. *Pain tolerance* is the individual's ability to endure the pain being experienced.

General Nursing Considerations for Patients with Pain

Nurses need to assist the patient in the management of pain. The first vital step in this process is to believe the patient's description of the pain being experienced. Pain brings with it a variety of feelings, such as anxiety, anger, loneliness, frustration, and depression. Part of the patient's response is tied to past experiences, sociocultural factors, current emotional state, and beliefs regarding pain.

Psychological, physical, and environmental factors all need consideration in the management of the pain. Never overlook the value of general comfort measures such as a back rub, repositioning, and the use of hot or cold applications. A variety of relaxation techniques, as well as diversional activities, may prove psychologically beneficial. Measures to decrease environmental stimuli and thereby provide for successful periods of rest are essential.

Patient Concerns: Nursing Intervention/Rationale

The patient's perception. In order to identify the cause(s) of an individual's pain a thorough assessment must be performed. The process can be initiated by having the patient describe his or her perception of the pain being experienced. Pain assessment tools such as The McGill-Melzack PAIN QUESTIONNAIRE may be used to assist the patient in describing subjective pain experience (Figure 9-6). This tool includes a number of descriptive words or phrases to identify the pain being experienced and is especially useful for individuals who have chronic pain. Whenever possible, chart the description in the patient's exact words. It may be necessary to seek additional data from significant others.

Listen to the patient and *believe the pain experience* being described regardless of whether the physical data substantiates the degree of discomfort described. DO NOT let your personal biases or values interfere with establishing interventions that provide for maximum pain relief for the individual.

Onset. When was the pain first noticed? When was the most recent attack? Is the onset slow or abrupt? Is there any particular activity that starts the pain?

Location. What is the exact location of the pain being experienced? Having the patient shade in a human figure with the areas where the pain is felt may be helpful, especially with pediatric patients who can be given different color crayons as a means of identifying different intensities in addition to the location. With acute pain the site of the pain can be more easily identified; however, with chronic pain this may be more difficult because the normal physiologic responses of the sympathetic nervous system are no longer present.

What is the depth of the pain? Does the pain radiate, having the sensation of spreading out or diffusing over an area, or is it confined or localized in a specific site?

It is important that the lack of physical symptoms comparable with the pain being described does not mean that the patient's complaints should be ignored.

Quality. What is the actual sensation felt when the pain is present—stabbing, dull, cramping, sore, burning, other? Is the pain always in the same place and of the same intensity?

Duration. Is the pain continuous or intermittent? How often does it occur, and once felt, how long does it last? Is there a cyclical pattern to the pain?

Severity. Scales (Figure 9-7) are frequently used to assess acute pain. The most common scale used has the patient rate the pain being experienced on a scale of 0 (no pain) to 10 (intense or excruciating). (The degree of relief for the pain after an analgesic is given is again rated using the same 0 to 10 scale.) When different potencies of analgesic agents are ordered for the same patient, the nurse can use this numerical rating data in combination with the other data gathered to determine whether a more or less potent analgesic agent should be administered.

Pain relief. Is there anything specific that relieves the pain? What has already been tried as pain relief measures and what, if anything, has been beneficial?

Nonverbal observations. Note the patient's general body position during an episode of pain. Be particularly observant about subtle clues such as facial grimaces, immobility of a particular part, holding or resisting movement of an extremity.

Physical data. Initially, the pain experienced activates the sympathetic nervous system resulting in an increase in the heart rate, pulse, respirations, and blood pressure. This also causes nausea, diaphoresis, dilated pupils, and an elevation in glucose. Over time and with the recurrence of pain, the parasympathetic nervous system reverses these findings and the pulse, respiration, and blood pressure decrease. In chronic, poorly controlled pain, these symptoms are generally absent and the predominate descriptors parallel those of depression.

In the presence of pain, always examine the affected

McGill-Melzack Pain Questionnaire

Patient's name _____ Age _____
File No. _____ Date _____
Clinical category (e.g., cardiac, neurologic)
Diagnosis: _____
_____

Analgesic (if already administered):
1. Type _____
2. Dosage _____
3. Time given in relation to this test _____
Patient's intelligence: circle number that represents best estimate.

1 (low) 2 3 4 5 (high)

This questionnaire had been designed to tell us more about your pain. Four major questions we ask are:

1. Where is your pain?
2. What does it feel like?
3. How does it change with time?
4. How strong is it?

It is important that you tell us how yur pain feels now. Please follow the instructions at the beginning of each part.

Part 1. Where Is Your Pain?
Please mark, on the drawing below, the areas where you feel pain. Put E if external, or I if internal, near the areas you mark. Put EI if both external and internal.

Part 2. What Does Your Pain Feel Like?
Some of the words below describe your present pain. Circle ONLY those words that best describe it. Leave out any category that is not suitable. Use only a single word in each appropriate category—the one that applies best.

1	6	11	16
Flickering	Tugging	Tiring	Annoying
Quivering	Pulling	Exhausting	Troublesome
Pulsing	Wrenching		Miserable
Throbbing		**12**	Intense
Beating	**7**	Sickening	Unbearable
Pounding	Hot	Suffocating	
	Burning		**117**
2	Scalding	**13**	Spreading
Jumping	Searing	Fearful	Radiating
Flashing		Frightful	Penetrating
Shooting	**8**	Terrifying	Piercing
	Tingling		
3	Itchy	**14**	**18**
Pricking	Smarting	Punishing	Tight
Boring	Stinging	Grueling	Numb
Drilling		Cruel	Drawing
Stabbing	**9**	Vicious	Squeezing
Lancinating	Dull	Killing	Tearing
	Sore		
4	Hurting	**15**	**19**
Sharp	Aching	Wretched	Cool
Cutting	Heavy	Blinding	Cold
Lacerating			Freezing
	10		
5	Tender		**20**
Pinching	Taut		Nagging
Pressing	Rasping		Nauseating
Gnawing	Splitting		Agonizing
Cramping			Dreadful
Crushing			Torturing

Part 3. How Does Your Pain Change with Time?
1. Which word or words would you use to describe the *pattern* of your pain?

1	2	3
Continuous	Rhythmic	Brief
Steady	Periodic	Momentary
Constant	Intermittent	Transient

2. What kind of things *relieve* your pain?

3. What kind of things *increase* your pain?

Part 4. How Strong Is Your Pain?
People agree that the following 5 words represent pain of increasing intensity. They are:

1	2	3	4	5
Mild	Discomforting	Distressing	Horrible	Excruciating

To answer each question below, write the number of the most appropriate word in the space beside the question.

1. Which word describes your pain right now? _____
2. Which word describes it at its worst? _____
3. Which word describes it when it is least? _____
4. Which word describes the worst toothache you ever had? _____
5. Which word describes the worst headache you ever had? _____
6. Which word describs the worst stomach ache you ever had? _____

Figure 9-6 *The McGill-Melzack Pain Questionnaire. (From Melzack R: The McGill Pain Questionnaire: major properties and scoring methods, Pain 1:277-299, 1975.*

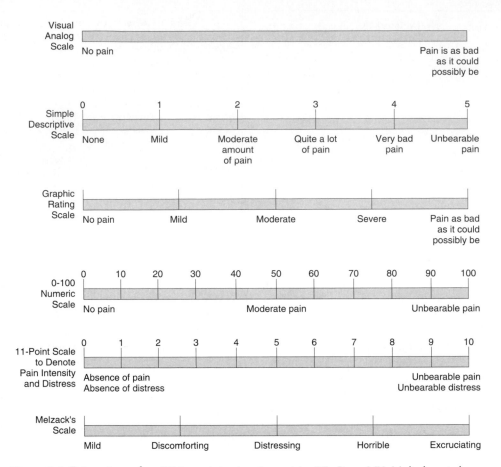

Figure 9-7 *Pain rating scales. (With permission from Ignatavicius DD, Bayne MV: Medical-surgical nursing: a nursing process approach, Philadelphia, 1991, WB Saunders, p. 123.)*

part for any alterations in appearance, change in sensation, or limitation in mobility or range of motion.

Behavioral response. Pain has both a physical and emotional component. Factors that decrease an individual's tolerance to pain include: prolonged pain that is insufficiently relieved, fatigue accompanied by the inability to sleep, an increase in anxiety or fear, unresolved anger, depression, and isolation. Patients with severe, intractable pain fear that the pain cannot be relieved and patients with cancer fear that new or increasing pain means the cancer is spreading to a new site or that a reoccurrence is present.

What are the patient's coping mechanisms used to handle the pain experience—crying, anger, withdrawal, depression, anxiety, fear, hopelessness? Does the individual continue to perform the activities of daily living despite the pain? Does the individual alter lifestyle patterns appropriately to enhance pain relief measures prescribed? Is the individual able to continue to work? Is the person seeing more than one physician in hope of obtaining an answer to the origin of the pain?

Comfort measures. Provide for the patient's basic hygiene and comfort. Utilize such techniques as back rubs, massage, hot and cold applications, or warm baths, as ordered.

Ask the patient what measures have been successful in the past in providing pain relief.

Relieve pain by doing any or all of the following, as appropriate:

- Support an affected part during movement.
- Provide appropriate assistance during movement or activities.
- Apply binders or splint an incisional area prior to initiating activities such as deep breathing and coughing.
- Give analgesics in advance of undertaking painful activities and plan for the activity to take place during the peak action of the medication given.

Environmental control. Provide for a quiet environment with as little distraction as possible during periods of rest. Modify hospital schedules such as routine vital signs and specimen collection so that the individual is not disturbed once asleep.

Provide for mental stimulation through the appropriate use of television, visitors, card games, and other patients to take the patient's mind off the pain.

Psychological interventions. Initiate relaxation techniques, use of distractions, hypnosis, biofeedback, or music therapy to assist the patient to relax and obtain pain relief. Try implementing these techniques at the same time the analgesic is administered to maximize the outcomes. Pain produces both a physical discomfort and an emotional component or "suffering"; therefore, instituting measures to diminish both factors simultaneously may be beneficial to the patient.

Involve the patient's support group in the plan for relief of chronic pain. Chronic pain can interfere with all facets of the individual's life. Financial losses can be significant due to the costs associated with repeated evaluations and treatment of the underlying causes of pain. The pain syndrome may progressively limit the individual's ability to continue employment or perform functions within the family unit. Family members or other persons within the patient's support group may have difficulty understanding why the individual is unable to function as in the past and, as a result of these interpersonal relationships, suffer major alterations. Therefore, it is important to include members of the patient's support group in the planning process for the effective management of the pain experience.

During the planning process it is important to stress to support persons that they can be involved in a positive way by expressing understanding, helping to provide diversional activities, and encouraging frequent rest periods especially after the administration of analgesics, antidepressants, and antianxiety medications.

Medication administration. The medication administration guide may list more than one analgesic order for the same patient. This requires the nurse to use judgement in choosing the correct medication for the patient based on pain assessment data collected.

Effective pain control must depend upon the degree of pain being experienced. The use of the previously described scale of 0 (no pain) to 10 (intense/unbearable pain) can prove useful. For a patient with mild to moderate acute pain, a non-narcotic agent may be successful in pain control. With severe, chronic pain, a potent analgesic such as morphine may be necessary. The route of administration chosen must be based on several factors. One major consideration is how soon the action of the drug is needed. The oral and rectal routes will have a longer onset of action than the parenteral route. It is sometimes erroneously felt that the oral route of administration is inadequate to treat pain. In truth, oral medications can provide very adequate pain relief if adequate dosages are provided. Generally, the oral route is used initially to treat pain if no nausea and vomiting is present. Patients may initially be treated effectively with administration via the oral route, however, the rectal, subcutaneous, intramuscular, intraspinal, epidural, and intravenous routes may be required depending upon the patient and the course of the underlying disease.

During the immediate postoperative period, assess all complaints thoroughly so that complications (e.g., wound dehiscence, heart attack) are not overlooked or masked. During the first 24 to 48 hours, the pain may be severe, and the patient will respond best to liberal medication so that rest, deep breathing and coughing, and ambulation can be accomplished effectively. (Plan these activities when the pain medication is at a peak.)

Some patients will not ask for pain medication; therefore, it is important to intervene for individuals who hold this belief. Whenever pain is being treated it is important not to make the patient wait unnecessarily for the pain medication.

The nurse must identify when the last dose of pain medication was administered by checking both the patient's chart/medication administration guide and the narcotic control record. It is common practice for analgesics to be ordered intermittently on a prn basis every 3 to 4 hours. However, in the case of chronic pain or intractable pain, it has been found that giving analgesics to persons on a scheduled basis every 3 to 4 hours will maintain a more constant plasma level of the drug, providing more effective analgesia. This approach can result in better control of the pain while using less of the analgesic ordered.

Patient-controlled analgesia (PCA) is gaining acceptance in both the inpatient and ambulatory setting. This method of administration allows the patient to control a small syringe pump containing an opiate agonist, usually morphine, which is connected to an intravenous indwelling catheter. When initiating the PCA pump, a loading dose is frequently given to gain rapid blood plasma levels necessary for analgesia. The patient then receives a slow, continuous infusion from the syringe pump. Depending upon the activity level and the level of analgesia needed, the patient may push a button, self-administering a small bolus of analgesic to meet the immediate need. A timing control on the device limits the amount and frequency of the dose that can be self-administered per hour. Additional adjustments in the dosing and frequency may be required as therapy continues. This approach allows the patient to have some control over the pain relief being provided and eliminates the need for the patient to wait for a nurse to answer the call light, check the last dosage of analgesics given, and the time required to prepare and administer the medication. After discharge from the hospital, this method of administration also allows significantly more freedom of movement for the patient and care giver.

Nurses need to evaluate and document in the patient's chart the effectiveness of the pain medications given. This requires careful assessments at intervals following the administration of the analgesics that will validate the duration and degree of pain relief attained from the analgesic. Recording the patient's rating of the degree of pain relief at one-, two-, and three-hour intervals after administration will provide useful information for evaluating future analgesic needs for the individual. Record and report all complaints of pain for analysis by the physician. The pattern of pain, particularly an increase in frequency or severity, may indicate new causes of pain. Major reasons for increased frequency and/or intensity of pain are: (1) pain from long-term immobility, (2) pain from the actual treatment modalities utilized—surgery, chemotherapy, and/or radiation therapy, (3) pain from direct extension of a tumor or metastases into bone, nerve, or viscera and, (4) pain unrelated to the original cause or the therapeutic modalities being utilized.

Patient Education Associated with Analgesic Therapy

Communication and responsibility. Encourage open communication with the patient concerning frustrations and anger as attempts are made to adjust to the diagnosis and need for prolonged treatment. The patient must be guided to insight into the disorder if he or she is to assume responsibility for the continuation of the treatment. Keep emphasizing those things the patient can do to alter progression of the disease, including maintenance of general health, nutritional needs, adequate rest and appropriate exercise, and continuation of prescribed medication therapy.

Nutritional aspects. The patient should eat a diet that is well balanced and high in B-complex vitamins; should limit or eliminate sugar, nicotine, caffeine, and alcoholic intake; and should drink 8 to 10 8-ounce glasses of water per day and maintain normal elimination patterns. To avoid or control the constipating effects of opiates, increase intake of fiber and fluids. If long-term use of opiates is planned, stool softeners may be necessary.

Exercise and activity. Unless contraindicated, moderate exercise should be encouraged.

Many times, pain causes the individual not to move the affected part or to position it in a manner that provides relief. Stress the need to prevent complications by utilizing a passive range of motion.

Relaxation. Teach the patient relaxation techniques and encourage use of the techniques simultaneously with the medication regimen.

Visualization techniques and biofeedback are also being utilized with some success.

Establish a schedule that provides for sufficient rest. Fatigue and anxiety may increase the perception of pain. Decrease noise; provide for a quiet environment.

Medication. Teach the patient to request pain medication before the pain escalates and becomes severe. Encourage open communications between the patient and health team regarding the effectiveness of the medications being utilized. Although the smallest dose possible to control the pain is the goal of therapy, it is also important that the dose be sufficient to provide adequate relief. Therefore, the patient must understand the importance of expressing the degree of relief being obtained so that appropriate adjustments in dosage and analgesics can be made.

Physical relief. Utilize hot or cold applications, massage, warm baths, pressure, and vibration as interventions for pain relief.

Cutaneous stimulation may be used alone or in conjunction with analgesic therapy for the relief of acute or chronic pain. Transcutaneous electrical nerve stimulation (TENS) units may be applied using electrodes at the pain site which are connected to a small battery box. The voltage delivered is adjusted by the patient to provide pain relief.

Expectations of therapy. Discuss the expectations of therapy (such as level of exercise attainable without severe pain, degree of pain relief, frequency of use of therapy, sexual activity, maintenance of mobility, ability to maintain activities of daily living and/or work).

Pain control without addiction is a goal for most patients, but for the terminally ill, comfort is the major priority. Concern for addiction is not a consideration.

Changes in expectations. Assess changes in expectations as therapy progresses and the patient gains understanding and skill in the management of the diagnosis.

In terminal illnesses, increasing pain needs careful management. The duration and intensity of the pain should be constantly reported to the physician for appropriate modifications of the medication regimen.

Assist the patient to learn to cope effectively with the pain. Include family members in discussion of pain management. Give praise when techniques are tried and success is achieved.

Changes in therapy through cooperative goal setting. Work mutually with the patient to encourage adherence to the treatment as prescribed. When the patient feels that a change should be made in a treatment plan, encourage discussion first with the physician.

Written record. Enlist the patient's aid in developing and maintaining a written record (Figure 9-8) of monitoring parameters (such as frequency of pain attacks, activity being performed when pain occurs, techniques being used to control pain, degree of pain relief, exercise tolerance) and response to prescribed therapies for discussion with the physician. Patients should be encouraged to bring this record with them on follow-up visits.

Fostering compliance. Throughout the hospitalization, discuss medication information and how it will benefit the course of treatment. Seek cooperation and understanding of the following points so that medication compliance may be enhanced:

1. Name
2. Dosage
3. Route and administration times
4. Anticipated therapeutic response
5. Side effects to expect
6. Side effects to report
7. What to do if a dosage is missed
8. When, how, or if to refill the medication

Patient Education and Monitoring of Therapeutic Outcomes for Patients Receiving Analgesics

Medications	Color	To be taken

Name _____

Physician _____

Physician's phone _____

Next appt.* _____

Parameters			Day of discharge														Comments
Pain: Onset:	*Example:*	8AM 3PM 9PM															
duration	Before taking medication																
relief	*Example:*	6hrs 3hrs															
Describe pain	Location																
	Check one: C = Constant I = Intermittent		C___ I___	C___ I___	C___ I___	C___ I___	C___ I___	C___ I___	C___ I___								
	Record: sharp, dull, throbbing																
Pain *before* medication Intense Moderate Low 10 5 1	Time: e.g. 8AM = 9																
Pain *after* medication Intense Moderate Low None 10 5 1 0	Time: e.g. 9AM = 5 9PM = 8 2AM = 1																
Sleep No Sleep Fair Sleep well 10 5 1																	
Appetite Poor Decreased Normal 10 5 1																	
I enjoy life? Yes Only when not in pain No 10 5 1																	
Activities of daily living: Check one: Perform without difficulty Perform with difficulty Unable to function adequately																	

*Please bring this record with you to your next appointment.
Use the back of this sheet for additional information.

Figure 9-8 *Patient education and monitoring of therapeutic outcomes for patients receiving analgesics.*

Difficulty in comprehension. If it is evident that the patient or family does not understand all aspects of continuing therapy being prescribed (such as administration and monitoring of medications, exercises, diets, follow-up appointments), consider use of social service or visiting nurse agencies.

Associated teaching. Always inform the physician or dentist of any prescription or over-the-counter medication being taken.

Over-the-counter medications should not be taken without prior discussion with a physician or pharmacist.

Always report side effects of rash, itching, or hives immediately. Nausea, vomiting, or diarrhea should be reported for the physician's evaluation if it is a new symptom.

Take all of the medication as prescribed for the full course of treatment. Do not discontinue use when feeling improved; do not save for future use or give medicine to another individual. Sudden discontinuation of certain medications may produce harmful effects.

Keep all medications out of the reach of children.

If pregnancy is suspected, consult an obstetrician as soon as possible about continuation of medication therapy.

At discharge. Items to be sent home with the patient should include the following:

1. Written instructions for the item's use
2. Labels in a level of language and size of print appropriate for the patient
3. If needed, identification cards or bracelets
4. A list of additional supplies to be purchased after discharge (such as syringes, dressings)
5. A schedule of follow-up appointments

Drug Therapy for Pain

Analgesics are drugs that relieve pain without producing loss of consciousness or reflex activity. The search for an ideal analgesic continues, but it is difficult to find one that does all that is desired of it. It should (1) be potent, so that it will afford maximum relief of pain; (2) not cause dependence; (3) exhibit a minimum of side effects such as constipation, hallucinations, respiratory depression, nausea, and vomiting; (4) not cause tolerance to develop; (5) act promptly and over a long period of time with a minimum amount of sedation so that the patient is able to remain conscious and responsive; and (6) be relatively inexpensive. Needless to say, no present-day analgesic has all these qualifications, so the search must continue.

There is, at present, no completely satisfactory classification of analgesics. Historically, we have categorized them based on potency (mild, moderate, and strong analgesics), by origin (opium, semisynthetic,

synthetic, coal-tar derivatives), or by addictive properties (narcotic and nonnarcotic agents).

Research into the control of pain over the past decade has given new insight into pathways of pain within the nervous system and a better understanding of precise mechanisms of action of analgesic agents. The new nomenclature for analgesics stems from these recent discoveries into mechanisms of actions. In this section the medications have been divided into (1) opiate agonists; (2) opiate partial agonists, opiate antagonists; (3) nonsteroidal antiinflammatory agents; and (4) miscellaneous analgesic agents.

Mild, acute pain is very effectively treated with analgesics such as aspirin or acetaminophen. Pain associated with inflammation (i.e., rheumatoid arthritis) responds well to the nonsteroidal antiinflammatory agents. Moderate pain is generally treated with a moderate potency opiate such as codeine or oxycodone. These two agents are often used in combination with acetaminophen or aspirin (e.g., Empirin with codeine #3, Tylenol #3, Percodan). Severe, acute pain is treated with the opiate partial agonists (e.g. buprenorphine, butorphanol) or the opiate agonists (e.g., morphine, meperidine, methadone). Morphine sulfate is usually the drug of choice for the treatment of severe, chronic pain. Other agents may be used as adjunctive therapy with analgesics such as chlorpromazine, antidepressants, and antianxiety agents. These agents are not analgesics, but may reduce the anxiety associated with chronic pain, thus allowing the analgesic to be more effective.

Opiate agonists

The term *opiate* was once used to refer to drugs derived from opium, such as heroin and morphine. It has been found that many other analgesics, not related to morphine, act at the same sites within the brain. It is now understood that when we refer to opiate agonists or opiate antagonists, we are referring to drugs that act at the same site as morphine either to stimulate analgesic effects (opiate agonists) or block the effects of opiate agonists (opiate antagonists).

Another outdated word is *narcotic*. Originally it referred to medications that induced a stupor or sleep. Over the past 80 years it has gradually come to refer to addictive, morphine-like analgesics. The Harrison Narcotic Act of 1914, which placed morphine-like products under governmental control, helped foster this association. With the development in recent years of analgesics that are as potent as morphine but that do not have the sedative or addictive properties of morphine, the word *narcotic* should be abandoned in exchange for *opiate agonists* and *opiate partial agonists*.

Opiate agonists are a group of naturally occurring, semisynthetic, and synthetic drugs that have the capa-

Table 9-10 *Opiate Agonists*

GENERIC NAME	BRAND NAME	AVAILABILITY	INITIAL ADULT DOSE	DURATION (HOURS)	DOSE EQUAL TO MORPHINE (10 MG)	
					IM (MG)	ORAL (MG)
Morphine-like derivatives						
Codeine	Codeine Sulfate Codeine Phosphate ♣Paveral	Tablets: 15, 30, 60 mg Inj: 30, 60 mg	PO, SC, IM, IV: Analgesic: 15-60 mg every 4-6 hours Antitussive: 10-20 mg every 4-6 hours	4-6	130	200
Hydromorphone	Dilaudid, Dilaudid-HP	Tablets: 1, 2, 3, 4 mg Suppositories: 3 mg Inj: 1, 2, 3, 4, 10 mg/ml	PO: 2 mg every 4-6 hours SC, IM: 2 mg every 4-6 hours Rectal: 3 mg every 6-8 hours	4-5	1.5	7.5
Levorphanol	Levo-Dromoran	Tablets: 2 mg Inj: 2 mg/ml	PO: 2 mg SC, IM, IV: 2 mg	4-8	2	4
Morphine	Roxanol, Morphine Sulfate, Duramorph, MS Contin	Tablets: 10, 15, 30 mg Sustained release tablets: 30, 60 mg Solution: 10, 20, 100 mg/5 ml; 20 mg/10 ml; 20 mg/ml Suppositories: 5, 10, 20, 30 mg Inj: 0.5, 1, 2, 3, 4, 5, 8, 10, 15 mg/ml	PO: 10-30 mg every 4 hours SC, IM: 10 mg/70 kg IV: 4-10 mg slowly Rectal: 10-20 mg every 4 hours	up to 7	10	60
Oxycodone	Roxicodone	Tablets: 5 mg Oral Solution: 5 mg/5ml	PO: 5 mg every 6 hours	4-5	15	30
Oxycodone	Percodan (with aspirin)	Tablets: 5 mg Solution: 5 mg/ml	PO: 5 mg every 6 hours	4-5	15	30
Oxymorphone	Numorphan	Inj: 1 mg/ml Suppositories: 5 mg	IV: 0.5 mg SC, IM: 1-1.5 mg every 4-6 hours Rectal: 5 mg every 4-6 hours	3-6	1	6
Meperidine-like derivatives						
Fentanyl	Sublimaze	Inj: 0.05 mg/ml	IM: 0.05-0.1 mg	1-2	0.1	—
Meperidine	Demerol	Tablets: 50, 100 mg Syrup: 50 mg/5 ml Inj: 10, 25, 50, 75, 100 mg/1 ml	PO, SC, IM: 50-150 mg every 3-4 hours IV: 25-100 mg very slowly	2-4	75	300
Methadone-like derivatives						
Methadone	Methadone, Dolophine	Tablets: 5, 10 mg Solution: 5, 10 mg/5 ml Inj: 10 mg/ml Oral Concentrate: 10 mg/ml	Analgesia: PO, SC, IM: 2.5-10 mg every 3-4 hours Maintenance: PO: 20-40 mg; up to 120 mg daily	4-6	10	20

♣ Available in Canada only.

bility to relieve severe pain without the loss of consciousness. These agents also have the ability to produce physical dependence and are thus considered controlled substances under the Federal Controlled Substances Act of 1970.

These agents can be subdivided into three groups: the morphine-like derivatives, the meperidine-like derivatives, and the methadone-like derivatives (see Table 9-10). Administration of these agents causes primary effects on the central nervous system; there are also significant effects on the respiratory, cardiovascular, gastrointestinal, and urinary tracts.

The opiate agonists are used to relieve acute or chronic moderate to severe pain such as that associated with acute injury, postoperative pain, renal or biliary colic, myocardial infarction, or terminal cancer. These agents may be used to provide preoperative sedation and supplement anesthesia. In patients with acute pulmonary edema, small doses of the opiate agonists are used to reduce anxiety and produce positive cardiovascular effects to control edema.

Side effects. The most frequently observed adverse reactions include light-headedness, dizziness, sedation, nausea, vomiting, and sweating. These effects generally occur more frequently in standing patients receiving parenteral administration and those not suffering severe pain.

The actions of the opiate agonists on the central nervous system are analgesia, suppression of the cough reflex, respiratory depression, drowsiness, sedation, mental clouding, euphoria, nausea, and vomiting.

The opiate agonists may produce orthostatic hypotension caused by peripheral vasodilation. This usually does not occur in patients who are supine, but it is commonly observed in ambulatory patients, particularly with the first dose.

Gastrointestinal effects include nausea and vomiting (usually limited to the first dose if it occurs) and constipation (with multiple doses). All opiate agonists may produce an increased pressure and spasm of the biliary tract, but the action depends somewhat on the agonist and the patient. Morphine appears to have the greatest effect, with meperidine and codeine having lesser effects. Nevertheless, the opiate agonists are frequently administered to patients with acute, painful, biliary colic because the spasm does not occur in all patients with therapeutic doses, and the sedation produced may contribute to the relief of pain.

Opiate agonists may produce spasms of the ureters and bladder, causing urinary retention. Patients may also have difficulty in starting the stream for urination.

With continued, prolonged use, opiate derivatives may produce tolerance or psychological and physical dependence (addiction). Tolerance is said to occur when a patient requires increases in dosages to receive the same analgesic relief. Development of tolerance seems to depend on the extent and duration of CNS depression. Patients who have prolonged depression by the continued use of opiate agonists have a higher incidence of developing tolerance. Patients who have developed tolerance to one opiate agonist usually require increased doses of all opiate agonists.

Physical and psychological dependence may develop with prolonged use and higher dosages of the opiate agonists. Patients who are physically dependent on opiate agonists remain asymptomatic as long as they are able to maintain their daily opiate agonist requirement. Addiction may develop after 3 to 6 weeks of continuous use of the opiate agonists. Early signs of withdrawal are restlessness, perspiration, gooseflesh, lacrimation, runny nose, and mydriasis. Over the next 24 hours, these symptoms intensify, and the patient develops muscular spasms; severe aches in the back, abdomen, and legs; abdominal and muscle cramps; hot and cold flashes; insomnia; nausea, vomiting, and diarrhea; severe sneezing; and increases in body temperature, blood pressure, respiratory rate, and heart rate. These symptoms reach a peak at 36 to 72 hours after discontinuation of the medication and disappear over the next 5 to 14 days.

Patients do not have to undergo the symptoms of withdrawal to be treated for addiction. Patients may be treated by gradual reduction of daily opiate agonist dosages. If withdrawal symptoms become severe, the patient may receive methadone. Temporary administration of tranquilizers and sedatives may aid in reducing patient anxiety and craving for the opiate agonist.

Availability. See Table 9-10.

Administration and dosage. See Table 9-10.

Antidote. Naloxone, Naltrexone.

• **Nursing Interventions: Monitoring opiate therapy**

See also General Nursing Consideration for Patients with Pain (p. 212).

Side effects to expect

LIGHT-HEADEDNESS, DIZZINESS, SEDATION, NAUSEA, VOMITING, SWEATING. These effects tend to occur most frequently with the initial dosage. Symptoms can be reduced by keeping the patient supine. Provide for patient safety, assurance, and comfort.

ORTHOSTATIC HYPOTENSION. Orthostatic hypotension, manifested by dizziness and weakness, occurs particularly when therapy is being initiated in a patient not in a supine position. Monitor blood pressure closely, especially if the patient complains of dizziness or faintness. Do not allow the patient to sit up.

CONSTIPATION. Continued use may cause constipation. Maintain the patient's state of hydration and obtain an order for stool softeners or bulk-forming laxatives if necessary. Encourage the inclusion of sufficient roughage, fresh fruits, vegetables, and whole-grain products in the diet.

CONFUSION, DISORIENTATION. Perform a baseline assessment of the patient's degree of alertness and orientation to name, place, and time *prior* to initiating therapy. Make regularly scheduled subsequent evaluations of mental status and compare findings. Report development of alterations. Provide for patient safety during these episodes.

Side effects to report

RESPIRATORY DEPRESSION. Opiate agonists make the respiratory centers less sensitive to carbon dioxide, causing respiratory depression. This may occur before either the reduction in respiratory rate or tidal volume is noticeable. Check the respiratory rate and depth frequently. Have equipment for respiratory assistance available.

URINARY RETENTION. If the patient develops urinary hesitancy, assess for distension of the bladder. Report to the physician for further evaluation. Try to stimulate urination by running water or placing hands in water; if permitted, have male patients stand to void; female patients should sit on a bedpan or toilet with receptacle.

EXCESSIVE USE OR ABUSE. Evaluate the *patient's* response to the analgesic and suggest a change to a milder analgesic when indicated.

Assist the patient to recognize the abuse problem.

Identify underlying needs and plan for more appropriate management of those needs.

Discuss the case with the physician and make plans to cooperatively approach gradual withdrawal of the medications being abused.

Provide for emotional support of the individual; display an accepting attitude—be kind but firm.

Drug interactions

CNS DEPRESSANTS. The following drugs may enhance the depressant effects of the opiate agonists: general anesthetics, phenothiazines, tranquilizers, sedative-hypnotics, tricyclic antidepressants, antihistamines, and alcohol.

Respiratory depression, hypotension, and profound sedation or coma may result from this interaction unless the dose of the opiate agonist has been reduced appropriately (usually by one third to one half the normal dose).

PHENOBARBITAL, PHENYTOIN, RIFAMPIN, CHLORPROMAZINE. These enzyme-inducing agents may enhance the metabolism of meperidine to normeperidine. Patients receiving long-term, large oral doses of meperidine, those with renal impairment, and those with a highly acidic urine are predisposed to accumulating normeperidine. Evidence of toxic levels of normeperidine are seizures, tremors, and excitation.

Opiate partial agonists

Opiate partial agonists (buprenorphine, butorphanol, nalbuphine, and pentazocine) are an interesting class of drugs in that their pharmacologic actions depend on whether an opiate agonist has been administered previously and the extent to which physical dependence has

developed to that opiate agonist. When used without prior administration of opiate agonists, the opiate partial agonists are quite effective analgesics. Their potency with the first few weeks of therapy is similar to that of morphine; however, after prolonged use, tolerance may develop. Increasing the dosage does not significantly increase the analgesia but definitely increases the incidence of side effects. This is called a "ceiling effect" in that, contrary to the action of the opiate agonists, a larger dose does not produce a significantly higher analgesic effect.

If an opiate partial agonist is administered to a patient addicted to an opiate agonist such as morphine or meperidine, the opiate partial agonist will induce withdrawal symptoms from the opiate agonist. If the patient is not addicted to the opiate agonist, there is no interaction and the patient will be relieved of pain.

Opiate partial agonists may be used for the short-term relief (up to 3 weeks) of moderate to severe pain associated with cancer, burns, renal colic, preoperative analgesia, and obstetric and surgical analgesia.

Side effects. The most commonly reported adverse effects to the opiate partial agonists are sedation, nausea, a clammy and sweaty sensation, dizziness, dry mouth, and headache.

The opiate partial agonists may cause respiratory depression. Dosage adjustments should be made in patients with bronchial asthma, obstructive respiratory conditions, cyanosis, or other respiratory depression from any other cause.

Butorphanol and pentazocine, and nalbuphine to a lesser degree, may produce hallucinations. Patients may complain of seeing multicolored flashing patterns or animals, with and without sound, or may have very vivid dreams. These adverse effects have been reported after only one or two doses of medication and may occur in as many as one-third of the patients taking butorphanol or pentazocine.

Repeated use may lead to tolerance, dependence, and addiction. Abrupt discontinuance following extended use may result in withdrawal symptoms. The withdrawal symptoms may be treated by restarting the partial agonist and then gradually reducing the dosage over the next several days to weeks to prevent recurrences and stop the addiction.

Opiate partial agonists have weak antagonist activity. When administered to patients who have been receiving opiate agonists such as morphine or meperidine on a regular basis, it may precipitate withdrawal symptoms.

Availability. See Table 9-11.
Dosage and administration. See Table 9-11.
Antidote. Naloxone, Naltrexone.

• Nursing Interventions: Monitoring opiate partial agonist therapy

See also General Nursing Considerations for Patients with Pain (p. 212).

Table 9-11 *Opiate Partial Agonists*

GENERIC NAME	BRAND NAME	AVAILABILITY	ADULT DOSAGE	DURATION (HOURS)	DOSE EQUAL TO MORPHINE 10 MG
Buprenorphine	Buprenex	Inj: 0.3 mg/ml in 1 ml ampules	0.3-0.6 mg repeated in 5-6 hours	6	0.3 mg
Butorphanol	Stadol	Inj: 1, 2 mg in 1, 2, 10 ml vials	IM: 2 mg, repeated in 3-4 hours; do not exceed single doses of 4 mg IV: 1 mg, repeated in 3-4 hours	(IM) 3-4	(IM) 2-3 mg
Dezocine	Dalgan	Inj: 5, 10, 15 mg/ml in 2 ml ampules	IM: 5-20 mg (usual, 10 mg) every 3-6 hours IV: 2.5-10 mg every 2-4 hours	3-4	20 mg
Nalbuphine	Nubain	Inj: 10, 20 mg/ml in 1, 2, 10 ml vials	SC, IM, IV: 10 mg/70 kg, repeat every 3-6 hours; do not exceed 160 mg daily	3-6	10 mg
Pentazocine	Talwin, Talwin Nx*	Inj: 30 mg/ml in 1, 2, 10 ml vials Tablets: 50 mg	PO: 50-100 mg every 3-4 hours; do not exceed 600 mg daily SC, IM, IV: 30 mg every 3-4 hours; do not exceed 360 mg daily	2-3	30-60 mg

*Tablets contain naloxone to prevent abuse.

Side effects to expect

CLAMMINESS, DIZZINESS, SEDATION, NAUSEA, VOMITING, DRY MOUTH, SWEATING. These effects tend to occur most frequently with the initial dosage. Symptoms can be reduced by keeping the patient supine. Provide for patient safety, assurance, and comfort.

CONSTIPATION. Continued use may cause constipation. Maintain the patient's state of hydration and obtain an order for stool softeners or bulk-forming laxatives if necessary. Encourage the inclusion of sufficient roughage, fresh fruits, vegetables, and whole-grain products in the diet.

Side effects to report

CONFUSION, DISORIENTATION, HALLUCINATIONS. Perform a baseline assessment of the patient's degree of alertness and orientation to name, place, and time *prior* to initiating therapy. Make regularly scheduled subsequent evaluations of mental status and compare findings. Report development of alterations. Provide for patient safety during these episodes. If recurring, seek a change in the medication order.

RESPIRATORY DEPRESSION. Opiate partial agonists make the respiratory centers less sensitive to carbon dioxide, causing respiratory depression. This may occur before either the reduction in respiratory rate or tidal volume is noticeable. Check the respiratory rate and depth frequently.

EXCESSIVE USE OR ABUSE. Evaluate the patient's response to the analgesic and suggest a change to a milder analgesic when indicated.

Assist the patient to recognize the abuse problem.

Identify underlying needs and plan for more appropriate management of those needs.

Discuss the case with the physician and make plans to cooperatively approach gradual withdrawal of the medications being abused.

Provide for emotional support of the individual; display an accepting attitude—be kind but firm.

Drug interactions

CNS DEPRESSANTS. The following drugs may enhance the depressant effects of the opiate partial agonists: general anesthetics, phenothiazines, tranquilizers, sedative-hypnotics, tricyclic antidepressants, antihistamines, and alcohol.

Respiratory depression, hypotension, and profound sedation or coma may result from this interaction unless the dose of the opiate partial agonist has been reduced appropriately (usually by one third to one half the normal dose).

Opiate antagonists

naloxone (nal-oks'own)

Narcan (nar'can)

Naloxone is a so-called pure opiate antagonist because it has no effect of its own other than its ability to reverse the CNS depressant effects of opiate agonists, opiate partial agonists, and propoxyphene. When administered to patients who have not recently received opiates, there is no respiratory depression, psychomimetic effect, circulatory changes, or other pharmacologic activity. If administered to a person addicted to the opiate agonists or the opiate partial agonists, withdrawal symptoms may be precipitated. Naloxone is not effective in CNS depression induced by tranquilizers or sedative-hypnotics. Naloxone is a drug of choice for treatment of respiratory depression when the causative agent is unknown.

Side effects. Naloxone rarely manifests any side effects. The following adverse effects have been reported very rarely when very high doses have been used: mental depression, apathy, inability to concentrate, sleepiness, irritability, anorexia, nausea, and vomiting. These adverse effects usually occurred in the first few days of treatment and dissipated rapidly with continued therapy.

Naloxone should be used with caution following the use of opiates during surgery because it may result in excitement, and increase in blood pressure, and clinically important reversal of analgesia. The early reversal of opiate effects may induce nausea, vomiting, sweating, and tachycardia.

Naloxone should be given with caution to patients known or suspected to be physically dependent on opiates (including neonates born to women who are opiate dependent) because the drug may precipitate severe withdrawal symptoms. The severity of the symptoms depends on the dose of the naloxone and the degree of dependence.

Availability. Injection—0.02 mg/ml (for neonatal use); 0.4 mg/ml and 1 mg/ml.

Dosage and administration

Adult

IV—Postoperative opiate depression: 0.1 to 0.2 mg every 2 to 3 minutes until the desired response is achieved.

Opiate overdose: 0.4 to 2 mg every 2 to 3 minutes. If no response is seen after 10 minutes, the depressive condition may be caused by a drug or disease process not responsive to naloxone.

Drug interactions. There are no drug interactions other than that of the antagonist activity toward opiate agonists, opiate partial agonists, and propoxyphene.

• **Nursing Interventions: Monitoring naloxone therapy**

See also General Nursing Considerations for Patients with Pain (p. 212).

---

naltrexone (nal-trex′own)

Trexan (trex′ahn)

Naltrexone is a pure opioid antagonist that is closely related to naloxone. It differs, however, in that it is active after oral administration and has a considerably longer duration of action. Naltrexone is used clinically to block the pharmacologic effects of exogenously administered opiates in patients who are enrolled in drug abuse treatment programs. The rationale for using naltrexone as an adjunct in treatment is that naltrexone may diminish or eliminate opiate-seeking behavior by blocking the euphoric reinforcement produced by self-administration of opiates and by preventing the conditioned abstinence syndrome (that is, opiate craving) that occurs following opiate withdrawal.

Side effects. Many adverse effects have been associated with naltrexone therapy, but it is difficult to know exactly which adverse effects are secondary to naltrexone alone because some patients may have been experiencing mild opiate withdrawal symptoms as well. The adverse effects of drug and alcohol abuse and poor nutritional states may also contribute to the patient's discomfort.

The most common complaints are gastrointestinal in nature, manifested by diarrhea, abdominal pain and cramps, nausea, vomiting, constipation, and anorexia. The second most frequent group of adverse effects include headache, lassitude, insomnia, anxiety, and nervousness.

A major adverse effect is hepatotoxicity, manifested by increases in serum hepatic enzyme concentrations. Following doses of 300 mg daily for 3 to 8 weeks, serum ALT concentrations increased up to 3 to 19 times the baseline values in about 20% of patients. The manufacturer recommends that baseline determinations of liver function should be performed in all patients prior in initiation of therapy and repeated monthly for the next 6 months.

Availability

PO—50 mg tablets.

Administration and dosage

PO—Induction regimen—25 mg. Observe for 1 hr for development of withdrawal symptoms. If none occur, administer another 25 mg.

Maintenance regimen—50 mg daily. Alternative regimens of 100 mg every other day or 150 mg every third day have been used to improve compliance during a behavior modification program.

• **Nursing Interventions: Monitoring naltrexone therapy**

See also General Nursing Considerations for Patients with Pain (p. 212).

Side effects to expect

NAUSEA, VOMITING, ANOREXIA, ABDOMINAL CRAMPS. These side effects are usually mild and tend to resolve with continued therapy. Encourage the patient not to discontinue therapy without first consulting the physician and treatment program.

Side effects to report

HEPATOTOXICITY. The symptoms of hepatotoxicity are: jaundice, nausea, vomiting, anorexia, hepatomegaly, splenomegaly, and abnormal liver functions tests (elevated bilirubin, AST, ALT, alkaline phosphatase, prothrombin time). Since many of these patients do not develop clinical symptoms, but do develop abnormal liver function tests, strongly encourage patients to report for blood tests as scheduled. Report abnormal values to the appropriate physician.

Implementation

WITHDRAWAL SYMPTOMS. Naltrexone may precipitate acute and severe withdrawal symptoms in patients who are physically dependent on opioids. Addicts must be completely detoxified and opioid-free before taking naltrexone. The manufacturer recommends a minimum of 7 to 10 days abstinence from all opiates, a urinalysis to confirm the absence of opiates, and the use of a naloxone challenge test to assure that the patient will not develop withdrawal symptoms.

BEHAVIOR MODIFICATION. Naltrexone therapy in combination with behavioral therapy has been shown to be more effective than naltrexone or behavioral therapy alone in prolonging opiate cessation in patients formerly physically dependent on opiates.

Patients undergoing naltrexone therapy must be carefully instructed about the expectations of behavioral modification associated with therapy. They should also be advised that self-administration of small doses of opiates (such as heroin) during naltrexone therapy will not result in any pharmacologic effect and that large doses may result in serious pharmacologic effects, including coma and death. They should also be given identification to notify medical personnel that they are taking a long-acting opiate antagonist.

Drug interactions

OPIATE-CONTAINING PRODUCTS. Patients taking naltrexone will probably not benefit from opioid-containing medicines such as analgesics, cough and cold preparations, and antidiarrheal preparations. Use of these products should be avoided during naltrexone therapy when nonopiate therapy is available.

CLONIDINE. Clonidine may be administered in patients to reduce the severity of withdrawal symptoms precipitated or exacerbated by naltrexone.

Antiinflammatory agents

Salicylates. The salicylates are the most common analgesics used for the relief of slight to moderate pain. The salicylates were introduced into medicine in the late nineteenth century because of their three primary pharmacologic effects as analgesic, antipyretic, and antiinflammatory agents.

Although the mechanisms of action are not fully known, it appears that most of the activity of the salicylates comes from inhibition of prostaglandin synthesis. Salicylates inhibit the formation of prostaglandins that sensitize pain receptors to stimulation (causing pain); they inhibit the prostaglandins that produce the signs and symptoms of inflammation (redness, swelling, warmth); and they inhibit the synthesis and release of prostaglandins in the brain that cause the elevation of body temperature. A major benefit of the salicylates is

that they do not dull the conscious level and do not cause mental sluggishness, memory disturbances, hallucinations, euphoria, or sedation.

The combination of pharmacologic effects makes the salicylates the drugs of choice for symptomatic relief of discomfort and pain associated with bacterial and viral infections, headache, muscle aches, and rheumatoid arthritis. Salicylates can be taken to relieve pain on a chronic basis without including drug dependence. Many patients have difficulty accepting aspirin as an acceptable approach to a serious disorder such as rheumatoid arthritis. Recurrent teaching may be necessary to foster compliance.

Side effects. As beneficial as the salicylates are, they are not without adverse effects. In normal therapeutic doses, salicylates may produce gastrointestinal irritation, occasional nausea, and gastric hemorrhage. Extreme caution should be used with administration to those patients with a history of peptic ulcer, liver disease, or coagulation disorders.

Patients receiving higher dosages on a continuing basis are susceptible to developing salicylate intoxication (salicylism). Symptoms include tinnitus (ringing in the ears), impaired hearing, dimness of vision, sweating, fever, lethargy, dizziness, mental confusion, nausea, and vomiting. This condition is reversible on reduction of the dosage. Massive overdoses may lead to respiratory depression and coma. There is no antidote; primary treatment is discontinuation of the drug, gastric lavage, forced IV fluids, and alkalinization of the urine with IV sodium bicarbonate.

Ingestion of 8 to 18 of the 325 mg tablets of aspirin daily may result in false-positive Clinitest and false-negative Tes-Tape urine glucose determinations.

Availability. See Tables 9-12 and 9-13.

Dosage and administration. See Tables 9-12 and 9-13.

• Nursing Interventions: Monitoring salicylate therapy

See also General Nursing Considerations for Patients with Pain (p. 212).

Side effects to expect

GASTRIC IRRITATION. If gastric irritation occurs, administer medication with food, milk, antacids (1 hour later), or large amounts of water. If symptoms persist or increase in severity, report for physician evaluation. Aspirin is available in enteric-coated form to reduce gastric irritation.

Side effects to report

GASTROINTESTINAL BLEEDING. Observe for the development of dark tarry stools and bright red or "coffee-ground" emesis.

Test any suspicious stools or emesis for presence of occult blood.

SALICYLISM. Patients who develop signs of salicylate toxicity should be reevaluated for other underlying dis-

Table 9-12 *Nonsteroidal Antiinflammatory Agents*

GENERIC NAME	BRAND NAME	AVAILABILITY	USES AND DOSAGES	MAXIMUM DAILY DOSE (MG)
Salicylates				
Aspirin	Easprin, Zorprin, A.S.A., Bayer, Empirin	Tablets: 65, 81, 325, 487.5, 650 mg Capsules: 325, 500 mg Suppositories: 60, 130, 195, 300, 325, 600, 625, 1200 mg	Minor aches and pains: 325-600 mg every 4 hours Arthritis: 2.6-5.2 g/day in divided doses Acute rheumatic fever: 7.8 g/day	—
Choline salicylate	Arthropan	Liquid: 870 mg/5 ml	Mild pain: 870 mg every 3-4 hours (fewer GI side effects)	7000
Diflunisal	Dolobid	Tablets: 250, 500 mg	Mild to moderate pain: Initially, 1000 mg, then 500 mg every 8 hours Osteoarthritis: 250-500 mg 2 times daily	1500
Magnesium salicylate	Magan, Mobidin	Tablets: 325, 500, 545, 600 mg	Mild aches and pains: 500-650 mg 3 or 4 times daily	9600
Salicylamide	Uromide, Salicylamide	Tablets: 325, 667 mg	Minor aches and pains: 325-667 mg 3 or 4 times daily (less effective than equal doses of aspirin)	4000
Salsalate	Disalcid Artha-G	Tablets: 500, 750 mg Capsules: 500 mg	Mild pain: 500-750 mg 4-6 times daily	3000
Sodium salicylate	Uracel 5, Sodium Salicylate ♣S-60	Tablets: 325, 650 mg Enteric-coated tablets: 325, 650 mg	Mild analgesia: 325-650 mg every 4-8 hours (less effective than equal doses of aspirin)	3900
Sodium thiosalicylate	Asproject, Tusal	Inj: 50 mg/ml in 2 and 30 ml vials	Acute gout: IM: 100 mg every 3-4 hours for 2 days, then 100 mg/day Rheumatic fever: IM: 100-150 mg every 4-6 hours for 3 days, then 100 mg twice daily	—
Nonsteroidal antiinflammatory agents				
Diclofenac	Voltaren	Tablets: 25, 50, 75 mg	Rheumatoid and osteoarthritis, ankylosing spondylitis: 25-75 mg 2-3 times daily	200
Etodolac	Lodine	Capsules: 200, 300 mg	Osteoarthritis, pain: 300-400 mg 3-4 times daily	1200
Fenoprofen	Nalfon	Capsules: 200, 300, 600 mg Tablets: 600 mg	Rheumatoid and osteoarthritis: 300-600 mg 3 or 4 times daily Mild to moderate pain: 200 mg every 4-6 hours	3200
Flurbiprofen	Ansaid	Tablets: 50, 100 mg	Rheumatoid and osteoarthritis: 50-100 mg 2-3 times daily	300
Ibuprofen	Motrin, Rufen, ♣Novoprofen	Tablets: 200, 300, 400, 600, 800 mg	Rheumatoid and osteoarthritis: 300-600 mg 3-4 times daily Mild to moderate pain: 400 mg every 4-6 hours Primary dysmenorrhea: 400 mg every 4 hours	2400
Indomethacin	Indocin, ♣Indocid	Capsules: 10, 25, 50, 75 mg Sustained release capsules: 75 mg Oral suspension: 25 mg/5 ml Inj: 1 mg in 1 ml vial Suppository: 50 mg	Rheumatoid and osteoarthritis, ankylosing spondylitis: 25-50 mg 3-4 times daily Acute painful shoulder: 25-50 mg 2-3 times daily Acute gouty arthritis: 50 mg 3 times daily Closure of patent ductus arteriosus: IV — 1-3 IV doses given at 12-24 hour intervals	200

♣Available in Canada only.

Continued.

Table 9-12 *Nonsteroidal Antiinflammatory Agents—cont'd*

GENERIC NAME	BRAND NAME	AVAILABILITY	USES AND DOSAGES	MAXIMUM DAILY DOSE (MG)
Nonsteroidal antiinflammatory agents—cont'd				
Ketoprofen	Orudis	Capsules: 25, 50, 75 mg	Rheumatoid and osteoarthritis: Initially, 75 mg 3 times daily or 50 mg 4 times daily; reduce initial dose by ½ to ⅓ in elderly patients or those with impaired renal function	300
Ketorolac	Toradol	Injection: 15, 30 mg/ml in 1, 2 ml prefilled syringes	Injectable analgesic, antiinflammatory, antipyretic used for acute, short-term pain management: 30-60 mg IM initially, 15-30 mg every 6 hours prn pain	120-150
Meclofenamate	Meclomen	Capsules: 50, 100 mg	Rheumatoid and osteoarthritis: 200-400 mg daily in 3-4 equal doses. Mild to moderate pain: 50-100 mg 3-4 times daily; primary dysmenorrhea: 100 mg 3 times daily	400
Mefenamic acid	Ponstel, ♣Ponstan	Capsules: 250 mg	Moderate pain or primary dysmenorrhea: Initially 500 mg, then 250 mg every 6 hours	1000
Naproxen	Naprosyn	Tablets: 250, 375, 500 mg Oral suspension: 125 mg/ml	Rheumatoid and osteoarthritis, ankylosing spondylitis: 250-375 mg 2 times daily	1000
Naproxen sodium	Anaprox, Anaprox DS	Tablets: 275 mg Tablets: 550 mg	Acute gout: 750-825 mg initially, followed by 250-275 mg every 8 hours. Moderate pain, primary dysmenorrhea, acute tendonitis, bursitis: 500-550 mg followed by 250-275 mg	1100
Phenylbutazone	Butazolidin, Azolid	Tablets: 100 mg Capsules: 100 mg	Rheumatoid and osteoarthritis, ankylosing spondylitis: 100 mg 4 times daily	600
Piroxicam	Feldene	Capsules: 10, 20 mg	Rheumatoid and osteoarthritis: 20 mg 1 time daily	20
Sulindac	Clinoril	Tablets: 150, 200 mg	Rheumatoid and osteoarthritis, ankylosing spondylitis: 150 mg 2 times daily. Acute painful shoulder: 200 mg 2 times daily	400
Tolmetin	Tolectin	Tablets: 200, 600 mg Capsules: 400 mg	Rheumatoid and osteoarthritis: 400-600 mg 3 times daily	2000

♣Available in Canada only.

ease and the possibility that other medication would be more effective.

Drug interactions

SULFINPYRAZONE, PROBENECID. Salicylates inhibit the excretion of uric acid by these agents. Although an occasional aspirin will not be sufficient to interfere with the effectiveness of these agents, regular use of salicylates or products containing salicylate should be discouraged. If analgesia is required, suggest acetaminophen.

WARFARIN. The salicylates may enhance the anticoagulant effects of warfarin. Observe for the development of petechiae, ecchymoses, nosebleeds, bleeding gums, dark tarry stools, and bright red or "coffeeground" emesis. Monitor the prothrombin time and reduce the dosage of warfarin if necessary.

PHENYTOIN. Monitor patients with concurrent therapy for signs of phenytoin toxicity: nystagmus, sedation, lethargy. Serum levels may be ordered, and a reduced dosage of phenytoin may be required.

ORAL HYPOGLYCEMIC AGENTS. The salicylates may enhance the hypoglycemic effects of these agents. Monitor for hypoglycemia: headache, weakness, decreased coordination, general apprehension, diaphoresis, hunger, blurred or double vision.

The dosage of the hypoglycemic agent may need to

Table 9-13 *Ingredients of Selected Analgesic Combination Products*

PRODUCT	NONCONTROLLED SUBSTANCE			CONTROLLED SUBSTANCE	
	ASPIRIN (MG)	ACETAMINOPHEN (MG)	OTHER (MG)	CODEINE (MG)	OTHER (MG)
Anacin Tablets	400		Caffeine 32		
Anacin Maximum Strength	500		Caffeine 32		
Buffets II	226.8	162	Caffeine 32.4 Aluminum Hydroxide 50		
BC Powder	650		Caffeine 32 Salacylamide 195		
Darvocet N 50		325			Propoxyphene Napsylate 50
Darvocet N 100		325			Propoxyphene Napsylate 50
Darvon					Propoxyphene HCl 65
Darvon-N					Propoxyphene Napsylate 100*
Darvon Compound 65	389		Caffeine 32		Propoxyphene HCl 65
Empirin					
Codeine #2	325			15	
Codeine #3	325			30	
Codeine #4	325			60	
Excedrin	250	250	Caffeine 65		
Fioricet		325	Caffeine 40		Butalbital 50
Fiorinal	325		Caffeine 40		Butalbital 50
Fiorinal w/Codeine #3	325		Caffeine 40	30	Butalbital 50
Percocet		325			Oxycodone 5
Percodan	325				Oxycodone 5
Percogesic		325	Phenyltoloxamine 30		
Tylenol		325			
Tylenol					
w/Codeine #1		300		7.5	
Codeine #2		300		15	
Codeine #3		300		30	
Codeine #4		300		60	

*Propoxyphene napsylate 100 mg is equipotent to propoxyphene HCl 65 mg.

be reduced. Notify the physician if any of the above symptoms appear.

METHOTREXATE. Monitor for methotrexate toxicity: bone marrow suppression, decreased WBCs, RBCs, sore throat, fever, lethargy.

CORTICOSTEROIDS. Although frequently used together, salicylates and corticosteroids may produce gastrointestinal ulceration. Monitor for signs of gastrointestinal bleeding: observe for the development of dark tarry stools and bright red or "coffee-ground" emesis.

ETHANOL. Patients should avoid aspirin within 8 to 10 hours of heavy alcohol use. Small amounts of gastrointestinal bleeding often occur. If aspirin therapy is absolutely necessary, an enteric-coated product should be used.

CLINITEST. This drug may produce false-positive Clinitest results. Blood glucose measurements may be required for an accurate reading.

Nonsteroidal antiinflammatory agents. The nonsteroidal antiinflammatory drugs (NSAIDs) are also known as "aspirin-like" drugs. They are chemically unrelated to the salicylates but are prostaglandin inhibitors and share many of the same therapeutic actions and side effects. They all have, to varying degrees, analgesic, antipyretic, and antiinflammatory activity. The antipyretic activity is low enough that they are not used clinically for the control of fever. In clinical studies, all these agents (see Table 9-12) are superior to placebos and approach aspirin in effectiveness, but none is superior to aspirin. Depending on the agent used, the dosage, and the patient, the side effects of therapy tend to be somewhat less than those associated with salicylate therapy. The cost of therapy with NSAIDs is considerably higher than with aspirin treatment. Thus these agents are most effectively used as alternates for patients who do not tolerate aspirin. These agents are used to relieve the pain and inflammation of rheumatoid arthritis, osteoarthritis, ankylosing spondylitis, and gout. Certain agents are also approved for use to control the discomfort of primary dysmenorrhea. See Table 9-12.

Side effects. The most frequent adverse effects associated with NSAID therapy are gastrointestinal complaints. Symptoms include nausea, abdominal pain, diarrhea, indigestion, constipation, and flatulence. The development of ulcers and gastrointestinal bleeding has been reported with all these agents.

Dizziness, lethargy, and headache may occur in up to 10% of patients taking these agents.

Other adverse effects that have been attributed to these agents include tinnitus, drowsiness, mental confusion, vision disturbances, and various rashes.

Many other side effects may be caused rarely by these agents. They include blood dyscrasias, such as anemia, thrombocytopenia, and agranulocytosis; various dermatoses, such as urticaria, purpura, pruritus, and rashes; and hepatotoxicity and renal toxicity. Therapy should be discontinued if these complications develop.

Availability. See Table 9-12.

Dosage and administration. NOTE: Do not administer to patients who are allergic to aspirin. See Table 9-12.

• Nursing Interventions: Monitoring nonsteroidal antiinflammatory agent therapy

See also General Nursing Considerations for Patients with Pain (p. 212).

Side effects to expect

GASTRIC IRRITATION. If gastric irritation occurs, administer medication with food, milk, antacids, or large amounts of water. If symptoms persist or increase in severity, report for physician evaluation.

CONSTIPATION. The use of stool softeners or bulk-forming laxatives may be necessary. Maintain the patient's state of hydration. Encourage the inclusion of sufficient roughage, fresh fruits, vegetables, and whole-grain products in the diet.

DIZZINESS. Provide for patient safety during episodes of dizziness.

DROWSINESS. Persons who are working around machinery, driving a car, or performing other duties in which they must remain mentally alert should not take these medications while working.

Side effects to report

GASTROINTESTINAL BLEEDING. Observe for the development of dark tarry stools and bright red or "coffee-ground" emesis.

CONFUSION. Perform a baseline assessment of the patient's degree of alertness and orientation to name, place, and time *prior* to initiating therapy. Make regularly scheduled subsequent evaluations of mental status and compare findings. Report development of alterations.

HIVES, PRURITUS, RASH. Report symptoms for further evaluation by the physician.

NEPHROTOXICITY. Monitor urinalysis and kidney function tests for abnormal results. Report an increasing BUN and creatinine, decreasing urine output and/or decreasing specific gravity (despite amount of fluid intake), casts or protein in the urine, frank blood or smoky-colored urine, or RBCs in excess of 0 to 3 on the urinalysis report.

HEPATOTOXICITY. The symptoms of hepatotoxicity are anorexia, nausea, vomiting, jaundice, hepatomegaly, splenomegaly, and abnormal liver function tests (elevated bilirubin, AST, ALT, alkaline phosphatase, prothrombin time).

BLOOD DYSCRASIAS. Routine laboratory studies (RBC, WBC, and differential counts) should be scheduled.

Monitor for the development of sore throat, fever, purpura, jaundice, or excessive and progressive weakness.

Drug interactions

WARFARIN. The NSAIDs may enhance the anticoagulant effects of warfarin. Observe for the development of petechiae, ecchymoses, nosebleeds, bleeding gums, dark tarry stools and bright red or "coffee-ground" emesis. Monitor the prothrombin time and reduce the dosage of warfarin if necessary.

PHENYTOIN. Monitor patients with concurrent therapy for signs of phenytoin toxicity: nystagmus, sedation, lethargy. Serum levels may be ordered, and a reduced dosage of phenytoin may be required.

ORAL HYPOGLYCEMIC AGENTS. Monitor for hypoglycemia: headache, weakness, decreased coordination, general apprehension, diaphoresis, hunger, blurred or double vision.

The dosage of the hypoglycemic agent may need to be reduced. Notify the physician if any of the above symptoms appear.

FUROSEMIDE, THIAZIDE DIURETICS. Indomethacin inhibits the diuretic activity of this agent. The dose of the diuretic agents may need to be increased or indomethacin discontinued. Maintain accurate I/O and blood pressure records and monitor for a decrease in diuretic and antihypertensive activity.

PROBENECID. Probenecid inhibits the excretion of indomethacin. Monitor patients for signs of indomethacin toxicity: headache, drowsiness, mental confusion.

LITHIUM. Indomethacin may induce lithium toxicity. Monitor patients for lithium toxicity manifested by nausea, anorexia, fine tremors, persistent vomiting, profuse diarrhea, hyperreflexia, lethargy, and weakness.

Miscellaneous analgesics

acetaminophen (a-seet-a-min′o-fen)

Tylenol (ty′le-nol), **Datril** (day′tril), **Tempra** (tem′prah)

Acetaminophen is a synthetic nonopiate analgesic used in the treatment of mild to moderate pain. Its antipyretic effectiveness and analgesic potency are similar to that of aspirin in equal doses. This drug has no antiinflammatory activity and is therefore ineffective (other than as an analgesic) in the relief of symptoms of rheumatoid arthritis or other inflammation.

It is an effective analgesic-antipyretic for fever and discomfort associated with bacterial and viral infections, headache, and conditions involving musculoskeletal pain. It is a good substitute for patients who cannot take products containing aspirin because of allergic reactions, hypersensitivities, anticoagulant therapy, or possible bleeding problems from gastric or duodenal ulcers, gastritis, and hiatus hernia.

Side effects. When used as directed, acetaminophen is essentially free of side effects.

During the past decade, acetaminophen has often been recommended as the drug of choice for the relief of mild pain and fever. Its acquisition does not require a prescription, and its use has climbed steadily. Unfortunately, overdosage due to acute and chronic ingestion has risen dramatically in the last few years. Severe, life-threatening hepatotoxicity has been reported in patients who either ingest 5 to 8 g daily for several weeks or attempt suicide by consuming large quantities at one time.

Early indications of toxicity include anorexia, nausea, and vomiting—symptoms often attributed to other causes. A few days later, the patient develops jaundice, and the AST and ALT levels and prothrombin time rise dramatically. If acetaminophen toxicity is suspected, consult the manufacturer, a university drug information center, or a poison-control center for the most current recommendations for therapy.

Blood dyscrasias are rare side effects that may occur from prolonged administration of large doses.

Availability

PO—80, 160, 325, 500, and 650 mg tablets; 500 mg capsules; 120 mg/5 ml, 160 mg/5 ml, 325 mg/5 ml elixir; 100 mg/ml, 120 mg/2.5 ml solution; 165 mg/5 ml liquid.

Rectal—120, 125, 300, 325, 650 mg suppositories.

Dosage and administration

Adult

PO—300 to 650 mg every 4 hours. Doses up to 100 mg may be given 4 times daily for short-term therapy. Do not exceed 2.6 g daily.

Pediatric

PO—Doses may be repeated 4 or 5 times daily, not to exceed 5 doses in 24 hours.

  0-3 months: 40 mg
  4-11 months: 80 mg
  12-24 months: 120 mg
  2-3 years: 160 mg
  4-5 years: 240 mg
  6-8 years: 320 mg
  9-10 years: 400 mg
  11-12 years: 480 mg

Rectal—as for oral doses

Antidote. Acetylcysteine.

• **Nursing Interventions: Monitoring acetaminophen therapy**

See also General Nursing Considerations for Patients with Pain (p. 212).

propoxyphene (pro-poxs′ee-feen)

  Darvon (dar′von)

Propoxyphene is an effective, well-tolerated, synthetic nonopiate analgesic similar to aspirin in potency and duration of analgesic effect. It is used for the relief of mild to moderate pain associated with muscular spasms, premenstrual cramps, bursitis, minor surgery and trauma, headache, and labor and delivery. Greater pain relief may be attained when used in combination with aspirin or acetaminophen.

Side effects. Side effects of propoxyphene include gastrointestinal disturbance, headache, dizziness, somnolence, and skin rashes. Tolerance and addiction have been reported.

Symptoms of acute overdose are coma, respiratory depression, pulmonary edema, and seizures. Symptoms of propoxyphene overdose may be complicated by salicylism, which may also develop as a result of an overdose of combination products containing both propoxyphene and aspirin.

Availability

PO—65 mg capsules, 50 and 100 mg tablets, and 10 mg/ml suspension. (The 65 mg capsules and the 100 mg tablets are equal in analgesic potency.) Propoxyphene is also available in combination: Darvocet (propoxyphene, acetaminophen), Darvon Compound (propoxyphene, aspirin, caffeine).

Dosage and administration

Adult

PO—65 mg (capsules) or 100 mg (tablets) every 4 hours as needed. Do not exceed 390 mg (capsules) or 600 mg (tablets) daily.

Antidote. Naloxone, Naltrexone.

• **Nursing Interventions: Monitoring propoxyphene therapy**

See also General Nursing Considerations for Patients with Pain (p. 212).

Side effects to expect

GASTRIC IRRITATION. If gastric irritation occurs, administer medication with food or milk. If symptoms persist or increase in severity, report for physician evaluation.

SEDATION. This side effect is usually mild and tends to resolve with continued therapy.

DIZZINESS. Provide for patient safety during episodes of dizziness.

Side effects to report

EXCESSIVE USE OR ABUSE. Assist the patient to recognize the abuse problem.

Identify underlying needs and plan for more appropriate management of those needs.

Discuss the case with the physician and make plans to approach cooperatively gradual withdrawal of the medications being abused.

Provide for emotional support of the individual; display an accepting attitude—be kind but firm.

SKIN RASHES. Report for further evaluation.

Implementation

PO. If gastric irritation occurs, administer medication with food or milk.

Drug interactions

ORPHENADRINE. Combined use with propoxyphene is not recommended. Cases of mental confusion, anxiety, and tremors have been reported.

CARBAMAZEPINE. Propoxyphene inhibits the metabolism of carbamazepine. Monitor patients for signs of carbamazepine toxicity: dizziness, nausea, drowsiness, headache. Carbamazepine dosages usually need to be reduced.

CEREBROSPINAL STIMULANT
OBJECTIVES

1. Describe the symptoms of caffeine overdose.
2. Identify commonly available drinks that are sources of caffeine.

caffeine (ka-feen′)

NoDoz, Vivarin

Caffeine may be one of the most frequently used drugs in the world because it is a natural ingredient in coffee, tea, cocoa, and cola beverages. The average cup of coffee contains 100 to 150 mg per cup, depending on the strength of the brew. Caffeine has several pharmacologic actions. It stimulates the central nervous system, the respiratory center (causing more rapid, deeper respirations), the heart (bringing about an increase in both cardiac rate and cardiac output), and the secretion of hydrochloric acid in the stomach; and it has weak diuretic activity. With chronic ingestion, tolerance to the cardiovascular, CNS, and diuretic effects develop. Caffeine is sold as an aid in staying awake and for restoring mental alertness.

Side effects. The adverse effects of caffeine are extensions of the pharmacologic effects of the drug. Overdose can cause nervousness, tremulousness (caffeine jitters), insomnia, heart palpitations, headache, nausea, stomach pains, and minor dehydration due to the diuretic effects.

Caffeine has minor "addictive" properties. Persons who regularly consume over 500 to 600 mg daily may develop headache, anxiety, and muscle tension about 18 hours after the last ingestion if consumption is suddenly stopped. A conscientious effort to reduce gradually the daily intake of caffeine will reduce these symptoms.

Availability

PO—65, 100, 150, and 200 mg tablets.

Dosage and administration

Adult

PO—100 to 200 mg every 4 hours, as needed.

• Nursing Interventions: Monitoring caffeine therapy
Side effects to expect

NERVOUSNESS, JITTERINESS, UPSET STOMACH, HEADACHE. These are the pharmacological effects of caffeine. The best way to minimize these symptoms is to reduce intake. Switch to decaffeinated coffee, tea, or beverages.

Drug interactions

CIMETIDINE, ORAL CONTRACEPTIVES. These agents inhibit the metabolism of caffeine, enhancing pharmacological activity. If excessive CNS stimulation occurs, reduce the amount of caffeine consumed.

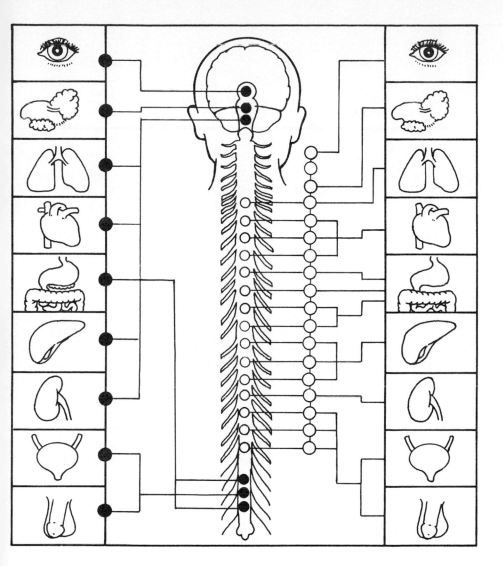

chapter 10

Drugs Affecting the Autonomic Nervous System

CHAPTER GOALS

After completing this chapter, the student should be able to do the following:

1. Explain the functions of the sympathetic and the parasympathetic nervous systems.
2. Identify the main actions (effects) of the adrenergic, cholinergic, and anticholinergic agents and the adrenergic blocking agents.
3. Describe patient data collection as it relates to each group of agents studied.
4. Identify essential components involved in planning patient education that will enhance compliance with the treatment regimen.

NURSING CONSIDERATIONS
AND DRUG THERAPY FOR:

Adrenergic agents
    (p. 232)

Adrenergic blocking agents   (p. 236)
Alpha-adrenergic blocking agents
Beta-adrenergic blocking agents

Cholinergic agents   (p. 238)
Anticholinergic agents   (p. 239)

THE AUTONOMIC NERVOUS SYSTEM

OBJECTIVES

1. Identify the two major neurotransmitters.
2. Cite the names of nerve endings liberating acetylcholine and those liberating norepinephrine.
3. Explain the action of drugs that inhibit the actions of the cholinergic and adrenergic fibers.

KEY WORDS

peripheral nervous
   system
autonomic nervous
   system
involuntary nervous
   system
cholinergic fibers

anticholinergic agents
motor nervous system
central nervous system
neurotransmitters
adrenergic fibers
adrenergic blocking
   agents

The brain and the spinal cord make up the *central nervous system*. Nerves that leave the central nervous system to conduct signals to other parts of the body (*efferent nerves*) and nerves that transmit signals from other parts of the body to the brain and spinal cord (*afferent nerves*) make up the *peripheral nervous system*. The peripheral nervous system further subdivides into the *motor nervous system* and the *autonomic nervous system*. The autonomic nervous system is an efferent motor system, which means that it relays information from the central nervous system to the rest of the body.

The autonomic nervous system controls the function of all tissues with the exception of striated muscle. This nervous system helps control blood pressure, gastrointestinal motility and secretion, urinary bladder function, sweating, and body temperature; in general it maintains a constant, internal environment (homeostasis) and responds to emergency situations. The word *autonomic* means "self-governing" or "automatic"; thus the autonomic nervous system has also been called the *involuntary* nervous system because we have little or no control over it. The *motor* nervous system controls skeletal muscle, and we can exercise control over much of it.

Studies have shown that the transmission of nerve impulses occurs because of the activity of chemical substances called *neurotransmitters* ("transmitters of nerve impulses"). A neurotransmitter is liberated at the end of one neuron, activating the next neuron in the chain, or at the end of the nerve chain, stimulating the "end organ" (the heart, smooth muscle, or gland). The

two major neurotransmitters are *norepinephrine* and *acetylcholine*. The nerve endings that liberate acetylcholine are called *cholinergic* fibers; the ones that secrete norepinephrine are called *adrenergic* fibers. Most organs are innervated by both adrenergic and cholinergic fibers, but they produce opposite responses. Examples of these opposing actions are in the heart, where adrenergic agents increase the heart rate and cholinergic agents slow the heart rate, and in the eyes, where adrenergic agents cause pupillary dilation and cholinergic agents cause pupillary constriction (see Table 10-1).

Drugs that cause effects in the body similar to those produced by acetylcholine are called *cholinergic* drugs because they mimic the action produced by stimulation of the parasympathetic division of the autonomic nervous system. Drugs that cause effects similar to those produced by the adrenergic neurotransmitter are called *adrenergic*, or sympathomimetic, drugs. Agents that block or inhibit cholinergic activity are called *anticholinergic agents*, and agents that inhibit the adrenergic system are referred to as *adrenergic blocking agents*. See Figure 10-1 for a diagram of the autonomic system and representative stimulants and inhibitors.

Adrenergic Agents

OBJECTIVES

1. Identify two broad classes of drugs used to stimulate the adrenergic nervous system.
2. Study the actions of the parasympathetic nervous system and correlate these with the actions of the cholinergic and anticholinergic agents.
3. Name the neurotransmitters called catecholamines.
4. List, analyze, and memorize the actions that result from stimulation of alpha, beta-1, beta-2, and dopaminergic receptors.
5. Review the actions of adrenergic agents to identify conditions that would be affected favorably and unfavorably by these medications.

KEY WORDS

catecholamines
beta receptors
dopaminergic receptors
sympathomimetic

alpha receptors
dopaminergic receptors
adrenergic activity

The adrenergic nervous system may be stimulated by two broad classes of drugs: catecholamines and noncat-

Table 10-1 *Actions of Autonomic Nerve Impulses on Specific Tissues*

TISSUE	RECEPTOR TYPE*	ADRENERGIC RECEPTORS (SYMPATHETIC)	CHOLINERGIC RECEPTORS (PARASYMPATHETIC)
Blood vessels			
Arterioles			
Coronary	$\alpha;\beta_2$	Constriction; dilation	Dilation
Skin	α	Constriction	Dilation
Renal	$\alpha_1;\beta_1$ & β_2	Constriction; dilation	—
Skeletal muscle	$\alpha;\beta_2$	Constriction; dilation	Dilation
Veins (systemic)	$\alpha_1;\beta_2$	Constriction; dilation	—
Eye			
Radial muscle, iris	α_1	Contraction (mydriasis)	—
Sphincter muscle, iris	—	—	Contraction (miosis)
Ciliary muscle	β	Relaxation for far vision	Contraction for near vision
Gastrointestinal tract			
Smooth muscle	$\alpha;\beta_1$ & β_2	Relaxation	Contraction
Sphincters	α	Contraction	Relaxation
Heart	β_1	Increased heartrate, force of contraction	Decreased heartrate
Kidney	Dopamine	Dilates renal vasculature, increasing renal perfusion	—
Lung			
Bronchial muscle	β_2	Smooth muscle relaxation (opens airways)	Smooth muscle contraction (closes airways)
Bronchial glands	$\alpha_1;\beta_2$	Decreased secretions; increased secretions	Stimulation
Metabolism	β_2	Glycogenolysis (increases blood glucose)	—
Urinary bladder			
Fundus (detrusor)	β	Relaxation	Contraction
Trigone and sphincter	α	Contraction	Relaxation
Uterus	$\alpha;\beta_2$	Pregnant: contraction (α); relaxation (β_2)	Variable

*α, Alpha receptors; β_1, Beta 1 receptors; β_2, Beta 2 receptors.

echolamines. The naturally occurring catecholamines that are neurotransmitters in the human body are norepinephrine, epinephrine, and dopamine. Norepinephrine is secreted primarily from nerve terminals, epinephrine primarily from the adrenal medulla, and dopamine at selected sites within the brain, kidneys, and gastrointestinal tract. All three agents are also synthetically manufactured and may be administered to produce the same effects as naturally secreted neurotransmitters. The noncatecholamines (see Table 10-2) have somewhat similar actions to those of the catecholamines but are more selective for certain types of receptors, are not quite as fast acting, and have a longer duration of action.

As illustrated in Figure 10-1, the autonomic nervous system can be subdivided into the alpha, beta, and dopaminergic receptors. These are specific types of receptors that, when stimulated by chemicals of certain shapes, produce a very specific action on that tissue. In general, stimulation of the alpha-1 receptors causes va-

soconstriction of blood vessels. The alpha-2 receptors appear to serve as mediators of negative feedback preventing further release of norepinephrine. Stimulation of beta-1 receptors causes an increase in the heartrate, while stimulation of beta-2 receptors causes relaxation of smooth muscle in the bronchi (bronchodilation), uterus (relaxation), and peripheral blood vessels (vasodilation). Stimulation of the dopaminergic receptors improves the symptoms associated with Parkinson's disease and increases urine output due to stimulation of specific receptors in the kidneys that result in better renal perfusion.

As noted in Table 10-2, many drugs act on more than one type of adrenergic receptor. Fortunately each agent acts to varying degrees, allowing a certain agent to be used for a specific purpose without many adverse effects. If recommended dosages are exceeded, however, certain receptors may be stimulated excessively, causing serious adverse effects. An example of this is terbutaline, which is primarily a beta stimulant. With

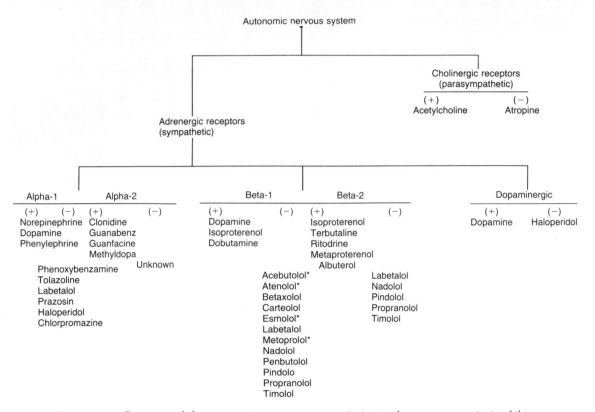

Figure 10-1 *Receptors of the autonomic nervous system. (+) stimulates receptors; (−) inhibits receptors; asterisks indicate representative examples only of selective beta-1 antagonists.*

normal doses, terbutaline is an effective bronchodilator. In addition to bronchodilation, terbutaline in higher doses causes central nervous system stimulation, resulting in insomnia and wakefulness. See Table 10-2 for clinical uses of the adrenergic agents.

Side effects. Side effects associated with the use of adrenergic agents are usually dosage-related and resolve when the dosage is reduced or discontinued. Palpitations, tachycardia, tremors, dizziness, and flushing of the skin are relatively common side effects when adrenergic agents are administered systemically. More serious adverse effects include arrhythmias, hypotension, severe hypertension, anginal pain, nausea, vomiting, and weakness. Reduce or discontinue therapy if these symptoms develop.

Patients who are potentially more sensitive to adrenergic agents are those with impaired hepatic function, thyroid disease, hypertension, and heart disease. Patients with diabetes mellitus may also have increased frequency of episodes of hyperglycemia.

Availability. See Table 10-2.

• Nursing Interventions: Monitoring adrenergic agent therapy

See also General Nursing Considerations for Patients with Respiratory Tract Disease; Nursing Interventions for Bronchodilators; Nursing Interventions for Decongestants.

Side effects to expect

PALPITATIONS, TACHYCARDIA, SKIN FLUSHING, TREMORS. These side effects are usually mild and tend to resolve with continued therapy. Encourage the patient not to discontinue therapy without first consulting the physician.

ORTHOSTATIC HYPOTENSION. Although infrequent and generally mild, adrenergic agents may cause some degree of orthostatic hypotension manifested by dizziness and weakness, particularly when therapy is being initiated.

Monitor the blood pressure daily in both the supine and standing positions.

Anticipate the development of postural hypotension and take measures to prevent an occurrence. Teach the patient to rise slowly from a supine or sitting position; encourage the patient to sit or lie down if feeling "faint."

Side effects to report

ARRHYTHMIAS, CHEST PAIN, SEVERE HYPOTENSION, HYPERTENSION, NAUSEA, AND VOMITING. Discontinue therapy immediately and notify the physician.

Implementation. See manufacturer's literature for each agent.

Drug interactions

AGENTS THAT MAY INCREASE THERAPEUTIC AND TOXIC EFFECTS. Monoamine oxidase inhibitors (isocarboxazid, pargyline, tranylcypromine); tricyclic antidepressants

Table 10-2 *Adrenergic Agents*

GENERIC NAME	BRAND NAME	AVAILABILITY	ADRENERGIC RECEPTOR	ACTION	CLINICAL USE
Albuterol*	Proventil, Ventolin	Aerosol: 90 mcg per puff Tablets: 2, 4 mg Syrup: 2 mg/5ml	$Beta_2$	Bronchodilator	Asthma, emphysema
Dopamine	Intropin, ♣Revimune	IV: 40, 80, 160 mg/ml in 5 ml ampules	Alpha, $beta_1$, dopaminergic	Vasopressor	Shock, hypotension, inotropic agent
Dobutamine	Dobutrex	IV: 250 mg/20 ml vials	$Beta_1$	Cardiac stimulant	Inotropic agent
Ephedrine*	Ephedrine	SC, IM, IV: 25, 50 mg/ml in 1 ml ampules	Alpha, beta	Bronchodilator, vasoconstrictor	Nasal decongestant, hypotension
Epinephrine*	Adrenalin	IV: 1:1000 in 1 and 2 ml ampules: 1:10,000 in 10 ml vials	Alpha, beta	Allergic reactions, vasoconstrictor, bronchodilator, cardiac stimulant	Anaphylaxis, cardiac arrest, topical vasoconstrictor
Isoetharine*	Bronkosol	Nebulization: 0.062, 0.08, 0.1, 0.125, 0.2, 0.25, 0.5, 1% solution	$Beta_2$	Bronchodilator	Inhalation therapy in bronchospasm, asthma
Isoproterenol	Isuprel	SC, IM, IV: 1:5000 solution, 1, 5, 10 ml vials Nebulization: 0.031, 0.065, 0.25, 0.5, 1% solution Aerosol: 0.2, 0.25% solution Sublingual tablets: 10, 15 mg	Beta	Bronchodilator, cardiac stimulant	Shock, digitalis toxicity, bronchospasm
Metaraminol	Aramine	SC, IM, IV: 10 mg/ml in 10 ml vials	$Alpha_1$	Vasoconstrictor	Shock, hypotension
Metaproterenol	Alupent, Metaprel	Aerosol: 15 ml vial Nebulization: 0.6, 5% solution Tablets: 10, 20 mg Syrup: 2 mg/ml	$Beta_2$	Bronchodilator	Bronchospasm
Norepinephrine (levarterenol)	Levophed	IV: 1 mg/ml in 4 ml ampules	$Alpha_1$	Vasoconstrictor	Shock, hypotension
Phenylephrine†	NeoSynephrine	SC, IM, IV: 1% in 1 ml ampules Ophthalmic drops: 0.12, 2.5, 10%	$Alpha_1$	Vasoconstrictor	Shock, hypotension, nasal decongestant, ophthalmic vasoconstrictor, mydriatic
Phenylpropanolamine†		Tablets: 25, 50 mg Capsules: 37.5 mg Timed release capsules and tablets: 75 mg	$Alpha_1$	Vasoconstrictor	Nasal decongestant, anorectic
Ritodrine	Yutopar	Tablets: 10 mg IV: 10, 15 mg/ml in 5 and 10 ml vials	$Beta_2$	Uterine relaxant	Premature labor
Terbutaline*	Brethine, Bricanyl, Brethaire	Tablets: 2.5, 5 mg SC: 1 mg/ml in 1 ml ampules Aerosol: 0.2 mg/puff	$Beta_2$	Bronchodilator, uterine relaxant	Emphysema, asthma, premature labor

♣Available in Canada only.
*See also Bronchodilators
†See also Decongestants

(amitriptyline, imipramine, others); guanethidine, atropine, and cyclopropane or halothane anesthesia.

Monitor patients for tachycardia, serious arrhythmias, hypotension, hypertension, chest pain.

AGENTS THAT INHIBIT THERAPEUTIC ACTIVITY. Beta adrenergic blocking agents (propranolol, nadolol, timolol, pindolol, atenolol, metoprolol); alpha adrenergic blocking agents (phenoxybenzamine, phentolamine, tolazoline); guanethidine, reserpine, bretylium tosylate.

Concurrent use of these agents with adrenergic agents is not recommended.

Adrenergic Blocking Agents

OBJECTIVES

1. Explain the rationale for use of adrenergic blocking agents for conditions that have vasoconstriction as part of the disease pathophysiology.
2. Describe the benefits of using beta adrenergic blocking agents for hypertension, angina pectoris, cardiac arrhythmias, and hyperthyroidism.
3. Identify disease conditions that would preclude the use of beta adrenergic blocking agents.
4. Describe the effects of the beta adrenergic blocking agents on respiratory conditions and diabetes mellitus.

KEY WORD

adrenergic blocking activity

Alpha adrenergic blocking agents

The alpha adrenergic blocking agents act by plugging the alpha receptors, which prevents other agents, usually the naturally occurring catecholamines, from stimulating the alpha receptors. Since a primary action of the alpha receptor stimulants is vasoconstriction, we would expect that alpha blocking agents would be indicated in patients with diseases associated with vasoconstriction. Indeed, phenoxybenzamine and tolazoline are used as vasodilators in peripheral vascular diseases such as Raynaud's phenomena and Buerger's disease. (See Chapter 11—"Cardiovascular Agents," for the clinical use of these agents.) Phentolamine is used in the diagnosis and treatment of pheochromocytoma, a tumor that secretes epinephrine.

Beta adrenergic blocking agents

The beta adrenergic blocking agents (beta blockers) are used extensively in the treatment of hypertension, angina pectoris, cardiac arrhythmias, symptoms of hyperthyroidism, and "stage fright." Beta blockers act by plugging beta adrenergic receptors so that beta receptor stimulants, usually the naturally occurring norepinephrine and epinephrine, cannot make contact with the receptor, thus preventing beta stimulation.

The beta blockers can be subdivided into nonselective and selective beta antagonists. The *nonselective blocking agents* have an equal affinity for and inhibit both beta-1 and beta-2 receptors. These agents are propranolol, nadolol, pindolol, and timolol. The *selective beta-1 blocking agents* exhibit action against the beta-1 receptors of the heart (cardioselective) and do not readily affect the beta-2 receptors of the bronchi. Selective beta-1 antagonists available are esmolol, metoprolol, acebutolol, and atenolol. This selective action is beneficial in patients, such as those with asthma, where nonselective beta blockers may induce bronchospasm. It is important to note, however, that the selectivity of these agents is only relative. In larger doses, these agents will also inhibit the beta-2 receptors. There are no selective beta-2 blockers available. Labetalol exhibits both selective alpha-1 and nonselective beta-adrenergic blocking activity.

Side effects. Most of the adverse effects associated with beta adrenergic blocking agents are dosage related. Potential side effects categorized by organ system are as follows:

- *Cardiovascular*—bradycardia, peripheral vascular insufficiency (Raynaud's phenomena).
- *Gastrointestinal*—diarrhea, nausea, vomiting, constipation, abdominal discomfort, anorexia, and flatulence.
- *Central nervous system*—dizziness, insomnia, and fatigue. Sedation, hallucinations, changes in behavior, and mental depression have been rarely reported.
- *Hematologic*—agranulocytosis and thrombocytopenic purpura have been reported very rarely.
- *Allergic*—rash, fever combined with aching and sore throat, laryngospasm, and respiratory distress.
- *Other adverse effects*—headache, dry mouth, eyes or skin; impotence or decreased libido, nasal stuffiness, sweating, tinnitus, and blurred vision.

Beta blockers must be used with extreme caution in patients with respiratory conditions such as bronchitis, emphysema, asthma, or allergic rhinitis. Beta blockage will produce severe bronchoconstriction and may aggravate wheezing, especially during the pollen season.

Use beta blockers with caution in diabetic patients and patients susceptible to hypoglycemia. The beta blockers will induce further hypoglycemic effects of insulin and will reduce the release of insulin in response to hyperglycemia. All beta blockers will mask most of the signs and symptoms of acute hypoglycemia.

Beta adrenergic blocking agents should be used in patients with controlled congestive heart failure. Further hypotension, bradycardia, and/or congestive heart failure may develop.

Availability. See Table 10-3.

Dosage and administration. See Table 10-3.

There is great interpatient variation in response to given dosages of the beta blockers. Dosages must be in-

Table 10-3 *Beta Adrenergic Blocking Agents*

GENERIC NAME	BRAND NAME	AVAILABILITY	CLINICAL USES	DOSAGE RANGE
Acebutolol	Sectral	Capsules: 200, 400 mg	Hypertension, ventricular arrhythmias	PO: Initial—400 mg daily Maintenance—1200-1600 mg daily
Atenolol	Tenormin	Tablets: 50, 100 mg Inj: 2 mg/ml in 10 ml amps	Hypertension, angina pectoris	PO: Initial—50 mg daily Maintenance—Up to 100 mg daily
Betaxolol	Kerlone	Tablets: 10, 20 mg	Hypertension	PO: Initial—10 mg daily Maintenance—20 mg daily
Carteolol	Cartrol	Tablets: 2.5, 5 mg	Hypertension	PO: Initial—2.5 mg daily Maintenance—2.5-5 mg daily
Esmolol	Brevibloc	Inj: 10, 250 mg/ml in 10 ml amps	Supraventricular tachycardia	IV: Initial—500 mcg/kg/min for 1 min, followed by 50 mcg/kg/min for 4 min; then adjust to patient's needs
Labetalol	Normodyne, Trandate	Tablets: 100, 200, 300 mg Inj: 5 mg/ml in 20, 40, 60 ml vials	Hypertension	PO: Initial—100 mg two times daily Maintenance—up to 2400 mg daily
Metoprolol	Lopressor, ✤Betaloc	Tablets: 50, 100 mg Inj: 1 mg/ml in 5 ml amps	Hypertension, myocardial infarction angina pectoris	PO: Initial—100 mg daily Maintenance—100-450 mg daily
Nadolol	Corgard	Tablets: 20, 40, 80, 120, 160 mg	Angina pectoris, hypertension	PO: Initial—40 mg once daily Maintenance—80-320 mg daily Maximum—640 mg/day
Penbutolol	Levatol	Tablets: 20 mg	Hypertension	PO: Initial—20 mg daily Maintenance—20 mg daily
Pindolol	Visken	Tablets: 5, 10 mg	Hypertension	PO: Initial—10 mg twice daily Maximum—60 mg/day
Propranolol	Inderal Inderal LA	Tablets: 10, 20, 40, 60, 80, 90 mg Solution 4, 8, 80 mg/ml Sustained Release Capsules: 60, 80, 120, 160 mg IV: 1 mg/ml in 1 ml ampules	Arrhythmias, hypertension, angina pectoris, myocardial infarction, migraine	PO: Initial—40 mg 2 times daily Maintenance—120-640 mg daily IV: 1-3 mg under very close ECG monitoring
Timolol	Blocadren	Tablets: 5, 10, 20 mg	Hypertension, myocardial infarction	PO: Initial—5 mg twice daily Maintenance—Up to 30 mg twice daily

✤Available in Canada only.

dividualized according to the pathologic condition being treated and the response of the patient.

It is extremely important that beta blocker therapy not be discontinued abruptly, especially in patients who are being treated for angina pectoris. Sudden discontinuation may result in an increased frequency of angina and possibly a myocardial infarction.

• **Nursing Interventions: Monitoring beta adrenergic blocking agent therapy**

See also General Nursing Considerations for Patients with Antiarrhythmic Therapy (p. 251) and for Patients with Hypertension (p. 280).

Side effects to expect or report. See introductory text above for adverse effects associated with specific organ systems.

Response by individual patients is highly variable. Many of these side effects may occur but may be transient. Strongly encourage patients to see their physician before discontinuing therapy. Minor dosage adjustment may be all that is required for most side effects.

BRONCHOSPASM, WHEEZING. Withhold additional doses until the patient has been evaluated by a physician.

DIABETIC PATIENTS. Monitor for hypoglycemia: headache, weakness, decreased coordination, general apprehension, diaphoresis, hunger, or blurred or double vision. Many of these symptoms may be masked by the beta adrenergic blocking agents. Notify the physician if you suspect that any of the above symptoms are appearing intermittently.

CONGESTIVE HEART FAILURE. Monitor patients for an increase in edema, dyspnea, rales, bradycardia, and orthopnea. Notify the physician if these symptoms are developing.

Implementation

INDIVIDUALIZATION OF DOSAGE. Although the onset of activity is fairly rapid, it may often take several days to weeks for a patient to show optimal improvement and become stabilized on an adequate maintenance dosage. Patients must be periodically reevaluated to determine the lowest effective dosage necessary to control the disorder being treated.

SUDDEN DISCONTINUATION. Sudden discontinuation of therapy has resulted in an exacerbation of anginal symptoms followed in some cases by myocardial infarction. When discontinuing chronically administered beta blockers, the dosage should be gradually reduced over a period of 1 to 2 weeks with careful monitoring of the patient. If anginal symptoms develop or become more frequent, beta blocker therapy should at least temporarily be restarted.

COMPLIANCE. Patients must be counseled against poor compliance or sudden discontinuation of therapy without a physician's advice.

Drug interactions

ANTIHYPERTENSIVE AGENTS. All the beta blocking agents have hypotensive properties that are additive with antihypertensive agents (guanethidine, methyldopa, hydralazine, clonidine, prazosin, minoxidil, captopril, saralasin, and reserpine).

If it is decided to discontinue therapy in patients receiving beta blockers and clonidine concurrently, the beta blocker should be withdrawn gradually and discontinued several days before the gradual withdrawal of the clonidine.

BETA ADRENERGIC AGENTS. Depending on the dosages used, the beta stimulants (isoproterenol, metaproterenol, terbutaline, albuterol, and ritodrine) may inhibit the action of the beta blocking agents, and vice versa.

LIDOCAINE, PROCAINAMIDE, PHENYTOIN, DISOPYRAMIDE, DIGITALIS GLYCOSIDES. Although these drugs are occasionally used concurrently, monitor patients very carefully for additional arrhythmias, bradycardia, and signs of congestive heart failure.

ENZYME-INDUCING AGENTS. Enzyme-inducing agents such as cimetidine, phenobarbital, Nembutal, and phenytoin enhance the metabolism of propranolol, metoprolol, pindolol, and timolol. This reaction probably does not occur with nadolol or atenolol since they are not metabolized, but excreted unchanged. The dosage of the beta blocker may have to be increased to provide therapeutic activity. If the enzyme-inducing agent is discontinued, the dosage of the beta blocking agent will also require reduction.

INDOMETHACIN AND SALICYLATES. Indomethacin and possibly other prostaglandin inhibitors inhibit the antihypertensive activity of propranolol and pindolol, resulting in loss of hypertensive control.

The dosage of the beta blocker may need to be increased to compensate for the antihypertensive inhibitory effect of indomethacin and perhaps other prostaglandin inhibitors.

Cholinergic Agents

OBJECTIVES

1. List the neurotransmitters responsible for cholinergic activity.
2. Identify the mechanisms of action of cholinergic agents.
3. List the predictable side effects of cholinergic agents.

KEY WORD

parasympathomimetic agents

Cholinergic agents, also known as parasympathomimetics, produce effects that are similar to those of acetylcholine. Some cholinergic agents act by directly stimulating the parasympathetic nervous system, whereas other agents act by inhibiting *acetylcholinesterase*, the enzyme that metabolizes acetylcholine once it is released by the nerve ending. These latter agents are known as *indirect-acting cholinergic agents*. Some of the cholinergic actions observed are the following: slowing of the heart, increased gastrointestinal motility and secretions, increased contractions of the urinary bladder with relaxation of muscle sphincter, increased secretions and contractility of bronchial smooth muscle, sweating, miosis of the eye reducing intraocular pressure, increased force of contraction of skeletal muscle, and sometimes a decrease in blood pressure. See Table 10-4.

Side effects. Because cholinergic fibers innervate the entire body, we can expect to see effects in most systems of the body. Fortunately, all receptors do not respond to the same dosage, so all adverse effects are not seen at all times. The higher the dosages used, however, the greater the likelihood for more adverse effects. Cholinergic side effects that may be observed are nausea, vomiting, diarrhea, abdominal cramping, increased bronchial secretions, bradycardia, sweating, and possible hypotension.

Availability. See Table 10-4.

• Nursing Interventions: Monitoring cholinergic agent therapy

See also General Nursing Considerations for Patients with Disorders of the Eyes, for Patients with Glaucoma, Patients with Urinary System Disease, and for Patients with Respiratory Tract Disease.

Table 10-4 *Cholinergic Agents*

GENERIC NAME	BRAND NAME	AVAILABILITY	CLINICAL USE
Ambenonium	Mytelase	Tablets: 10 mg	Treatment of myasthenia gravis
Bethanechol	Urecholine		See Chapter 15, "Drugs Affecting the Urinary System"
Edrophonium	Tensilon, Enlon	Inj: 10 mg/ml in 1, 10, 15 ml vials	Diagnosis of myasthenia gravis
			Reverse nondepolarizing muscle relaxants such as tubocurarine
Guanidine	Guanidine	Tablets: 125 mg	Treatment of myasthenia gravis
Neostigmine	Prostigmin	Tablets: 15 mg	Treatment of myasthenia gravis
		Inj: 1:1000, 1:2000, 1:4000	Reverse nondepolarizing muscle relaxants such as tubocurarine
Physostigmine	Antilirium	Inj: 1 mg/ml in 2 ml amp	Reverse toxicity of overdoses of anticholinergic agents (such as pesticides, insecticides)
Pilocarpine	Isopto-Carpine, Pilocar, Absorbocarpine		See Chapter 18, "Drugs Affecting the Eye"
Pyridostigmine	Mestinon, Regonol	Tablets: 60 mg	Treatment of myasthenia gravis
		Syrup: 60 mg/5 ml	Reverse nondepolarizing muscle relaxants such as tubocurarine
		Sustained Release tablets: 180 mg	
		Inj: 5 mg/ml in 2, 5 ml ampules	Reverse toxicity of overdoses of anticholinergic agents (such as pesticides, insecticides)

BRONCHOSPASM, WHEEZING, BRADYCARDIA. Withhold the next dose until the patient is evaluated by a physician.

Drug interactions

ATROPINE, ANTIHISTAMINES. Atropine, other anticholinergic agents, and most antihistamines antagonize the effects of the cholinergic agents.

Anticholinergic Agents

OBJECTIVES

1. List the effects of anticholinergic agents on parasympathetic activity.
2. Describe the clinical uses of anticholinergic agents.
3. List, analyze, and memorize the side effects observed with the use of anticholinergic agents.

KEY WORD

parasympatholytic agents

Anticholinergic agents, also known as cholinergic blocking agents or parasympatholytic agents, block the action of acetylcholine in the parasympathetic nervous system. These drugs act by occupying receptor sites at parasympathetic nerve endings, preventing the action of acetylcholine. The parasympathetic response is reduced depending on the amount of anticholinergic drug blocking the receptors. Inhibition of cholinergic activity (anticholinergic effects) includes mydriasis of the pupil with increased intraocular pressure in patients with glaucoma; dry, tenacious secretions of the mouth, nose, throat, and bronchi; decreased secretions and motility of the gastrointestinal tract; increased heartrate; decreased sweating. The anticholinergic agents are used clinically in treatment of gastrointesti-

nal and ophthalmic disorders, bradycardia, Parkinson's disease, and genitourinary disorders; as a preoperative drying agent; and to prevent vagal stimulation from skeletal muscle relaxants or placement of an endotracheal tube. See Table 10-5.

Side effects. Since cholinergic fibers innervate the entire body, we can expect to see effects from blocking this system throughout most systems in the body. Fortunately, all receptors do not respond to the same dosage, so all adverse effects are not seen to the same degree with all cholinergic blocking agents. The higher the dosages, however, the greater the likelihood for more adverse effects. Anticholinergic side effects that may be observed are: dryness and soreness of the mouth and tongue, blurring of vision, mild nausea, and nervousness. Other side effects include constipation, urinary hesitancy or retention, tachycardia, palpitation, mydriasis, muscle cramping, mental dullness, loss of memory, and mild and transient postural hypotension. Psychiatric disturbances such as mental confusion, delusions, nightmares, euphoria, paranoia, and hallucinations may be indications of overdosage.

All patients should be screened for the presence of closed-angle glaucoma. Anticholinergic agents may precipitate an acute attack of angle-closure glaucoma. Patients with open-angle glaucoma can safely use anticholinergic agents in conjunction with miotic therapy.

Availability. See Table 10-5.

• Nursing Interventions: Monitoring anticholinergic agent therapy

See also the General Nursing Considerations for Patients with Parkinson's Disease and for Patients with Disorders of the Eyes and the Nursing Interventions for Antihistamines.

Table 10-5 *Anticholinergic Agents*

GENERIC NAME	BRAND NAME	AVAILABILITY	CLINICAL USES
Anisotropine	Valpin	Tablets: 50 mg	See Chapter 14, "Drugs Affecting the Digestive System"
Atropine	Atropine Sulfate	Inj: 0.05, 0.1, 0.3, 0.4, 0.5, 0.8, 1.0 mg/ml	Presurgery—reduce salivation and bronchial secretions; minimizes bradycardia during intubation
		Tablets: 0.4, 0.6 mg	Treatment of pylorospasm and spastic conditions of the GI tract Treatment of urethral and biliary colic
Belladonna	Belladonna Tincture	Tincture: 30 mg/100 ml	Indigestion, peptic ulcer Nocturnal enuresis Parkinsonism
Clidinium bromide	Quarzan	Capsules: 2.5, 5 mg	Peptic ulcer diseases
Dicyclomine	Bentyl, Antispas, Dibent, ♣Bentylol	Tablets: 20 mg Capsules: 10, 20 mg Syrup: 10 mg/5 ml Inj: 10 mg/ml	Irritable bowel syndrome Infant colic
Glycopyrrolate	Robinul	Tablets: 1, 2 mg Inj: 0.2 mg/ml	Peptic ulcer disease Presurgery—reduce salivation and bronchial secretions; minimizes bradycardia during intubation
Isopropamide	Darbid	Tablets: 5 mg	Peptic ulcer disease
Mepenzolate	Cantil	Tablets: 25 mg	Peptic ulcer disease
Methantheline	Banthine	Tablets: 50 mg	Peptic ulcer disease
Oxyphencyclimine	Daricon	Tablets: 10 mg	Peptic ulcer disease
Propantheline	Probanthine, Norpanth	Tablets: 7.5, 15 mg	Peptic ulcer disease
Tridihexethyl Chloride	Pathilon	Tablets: 25 mg	Peptic ulcer disease

♣Available in Canada only.

Side effects to expect

BLURRED VISION, CONSTIPATION, URINARY RETENTION, DRYNESS OF THE MUCOSA OF THE MOUTH, NOSE, AND THROAT. These symptoms are the anticholinergic effects produced by these agents. Patients taking these medications should be monitored for the development of these side effects.

Dryness of the mucosa may be alleviated by sucking hard candy or ice chips, or by chewing gum.

If patients develop urinary hesitancy, assess for distension of the bladder. Report to the physician for further evaluation.

Give stool softeners as prescribed. Encourage adequate fluid intake and foods to provide sufficient bulk.

Caution the patient that blurred vision may occur and make appropriate suggestions for personal safety of the individual.

Side effects to report

CONFUSION, DEPRESSION, NIGHTMARES, HALLUCINATIONS. Perform a baseline assessment of the patient's degree of alertness and orientation to name, place, and time *prior* to initiating therapy. Make regularly scheduled subsequent evaluations of mental status and compare findings. Report development of alterations.

Provide for patient safety during these episodes.

Reduction in the daily dosage may control these adverse effects.

ORTHOSTATIC HYPOTENSION. Although the instance is infrequent and generally mild, all anticholinergic agents may cause some degree of orthostatic hypotension manifested by dizziness and weakness, particularly when therapy is being initiated.

Monitor the blood pressure daily in both the supine and standing positions.

Anticipate the development of postural hypotension and take measures to prevent an occurrence. Teach the patient to rise slowly from a supine or sitting position, and encourage the patient to sit or lie down if feeling "faint."

PALPITATIONS, ARRHYTHMIAS. Report for further evaluation.

Implementation

GLAUCOMA. All patients should be screened for the presence of angle-closure glaucoma *prior* to the initiation of therapy.

Patients with open-angle glaucoma can safely use anticholinergic agents. Monitoring of intraocular pressures should be performed on a regular basis.

PO. Administer medications with food or milk to minimize gastric irritation.

Drug interactions

AMANTADINE, TRICYCLIC ANTIDEPRESSANTS, PHENOTHIAZINES. These agents may potentiate the anticholinergic side effects. Developing confusion and hallucinations are characteristic of excessive anticholinergic activity.

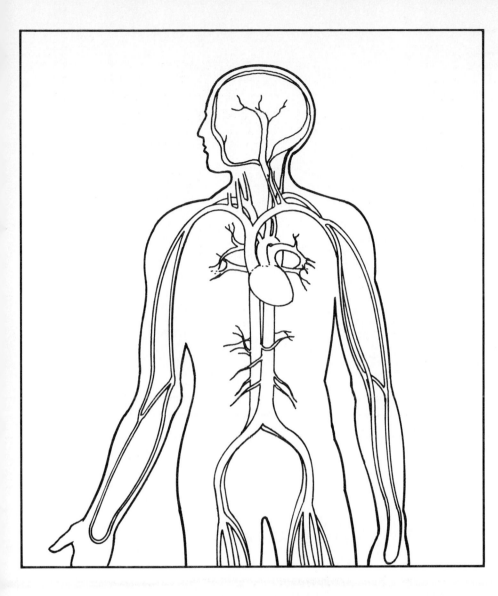

Drugs Affecting the Cardiovascular System

CHAPTER GOALS

After completing this chapter, the student should be able to do the following:

1. Explain the major actions and effects of drugs used to treat cardiovascular disorders.
2. Identify baseline data the nurse should collect on a continuous basis for comparison and evaluation of drug therapy.
3. Identify important nursing assessments and interventions associated with drug therapy and treatment of cardiovascular disorders.
4. Identify essential components involved in planning patient education that will enhance compliance with the treatment regimen.

CARDIOVASCULAR DISEASE

OBJECTIVES

1. Review the anatomical structures and conduction systems of the heart.
2. Cite nursing assessments used to evaluate the cardiovascular status of a patient.
3. Identify measures that can be suggested to the patient to alter, alleviate, or prevent the progression of the cardiovascular disorder being treated.
4. Develop measurable short- and long-term objectives for patient education for patients with cardiovascular disease.

KEY WORDS

syncopy	palpitations
clubbing	auscultation
percussion	pulse pressure
tachycardia	bradycardia

General Nursing Considerations for Patients with Cardiovascular Disease

The information the nurse assesses relative to the cardinal signs of cardiovascular disease can provide a basis for subsequent evaluation of the patient's response to the therapeutic modalities prescribed. Not all cardiovascular disorders exhibit every symptom.

Patient Concerns:
Nursing Intervention/Rationale

Cardinal signs of cardiovascular disease

Dyspnea (difficulty in breathing). If you are unfamiliar with the patient, first determine whether he or she has inhaled a foreign object.

Record if dyspnea is occurring upon exertion or while resting. Gather data relative to how the patient has been coping with any orthopneic problems.

Chest pain. Record data relative to the time of onset, frequency, duration, and quality of the chest pain.

Specifically note any conditions the patient has found that either aggravate or relieve the chest pain.

Fatigue. Determine whether fatigue occurs only at specific times of the day, such as toward evening.

Ask the patient if fatigue decreases in relation to a decrease in activity level.

Edema. Chart the time of day that the edema is present, such as when arising in the morning, and the specific parts on the body where present.

Always perform daily weights:

1. Using the same scale
2. In approximately the same weight of clothing
3. At the same time of day

Syncopy. Elicit from the patient conditions surrounding any episodes of syncopy. Record the degree of pre-

242

senting symptoms such as general muscle weakness, inability to stand upright, a feeling of "faintness," or loss of consciousness. Record what activities, if any, bring on these syncopal episodes.

Palpitations. Record the patient's description of palpitations, such as "my heart skips some beats" or "it began to feel like it was racing." Ask if these conditions are preceded by strenuous or mild exercise, and how long the palpitations last.

Indications of alterations in cardiovascular function

General mental status. Identify the individual's level of consciousness and clarity of thought. Both of these factors are indicators of adequate or inadequate cerebral perfusion.

Skin color. Note the color of the skin, mucous membranes, tongue, earlobes, and nailbeds. Chart the exact location of any cyanosis present.

Clubbing. Inspect the fingernails for clubbing and perform the blanching test on both the fingernails and toenails.

Neck vein distension. Record any neck vein distension present.

Respirations. Observe and chart the rate and depth of respirations.

Edema. Record the presence or absence of edema. If present, record location of edema, assessment data (e.g., degree of pitting present; ankle, mid-calf, or thigh circumference) and any measures the patient has employed in an attempt to bring relief. Weigh patient.

Pulse. Assess bilaterally the rhythm, quality, equality, and strength of the pulses (carotid, brachial, radial, femoral, popliteal, posterior tibial, and dorsalis pedis). If any pulse is diminished or absent, record the level where initial changes are noted. The usual words to describe the pulse are *absent, diminished,* or *average, full and brisk,* or *full bounding, frequently visible.*

Auscultation and percussion. Nurses with advanced skills can perform auscultation and percussion to note changes in heart size and heart and lung sounds. (See a medical-surgical nursing text for details of performing these advanced skills.)

Blood pressure. Blood pressure readings should be performed at least two times daily in stable cardiac patients and more frequently if indicated by the patient's symptoms or the physician's orders. Be sure to use the proper sized blood pressure cuff and have the patient's arm at heart level.

Initially record the blood pressure in both arms. A systolic pressure variance of 5-10 mm Hg is normal; readings reflecting a variance of more than 10 mm Hg should be reported for further evaluation. ALWAYS REPORT A NARROWING PULSE PRESSURE (difference between systolic and diastolic readings).

Laboratory tests. Review laboratory tests and report abnormal results to the physician promptly. Such tests may include (1) serum electrolytes, especially potassium, calcium, magnesium, and sodium, (2) arterial blood gases such as pH, pO_2, pCO_2, HCO_3^-, (3) coagulation studies to evaluate the bloods clotting, (4) serum enzymes (AST, CPK, LDH), (5) serum lipids (i.e. cholesterol, triglycerides), (6) electrocardiogram, (7) radiographic examinations, (8) nuclear cardiography, and (9) cardiac catheterization.

Examine urinalysis reports and perform hourly monitoring of intake and output (I&O). Report output that is less than intake or is below 30 to 50 ml per hour. Monitor other kidney function tests such as the blood urea nitrogen (BUN) and creatinine clearance. Abnormalities of these tests and/or insufficient hourly output may indicate inadequate renal perfusion.

Anxiety level. Patients experiencing cardiac disorders usually exhibit varying degrees of anxiety. Act in a calm manner when dealing with the person experiencing anxiety. Remember that hostility and anger are frequently employed as a means of dealing with loss of personal control of one's life.

It is essential that the nurse establish a trusting relationship with the patient and that he or she listen to the patient's concerns.

Work cooperatively with the patient to establish mutual goals that can effectively deal with expressed problems or needs. Be readily available to the patient and encourage discussion of personal *feelings.*

Administer appropriate medications and treatments that can best alleviate the patient's presenting symptoms and provide the maximum level of comfort.

Supportive health care measures

Prevention of skin breakdown. Many cardiovascular disorders require bedrest. Therefore, develop and follow a regular turning schedule that changes the patient's position every 2 hours around the clock.

Inspect pressure areas on the body for signs of skin breakdown each time you position the patient. Remember, when skin redness is seen and it does not subside rapidly, tissue damage is already extending into deeper tissue. In addition to assessing edema in the legs, feet, and abdomen, always check the sacral area of a patient on bedrest for the degree of edema present.

Facilitation of breathing. If the patient is experiencing dyspnea, position the patient in a semi-Fowler's to full Fowler's position to improve lung expansion. Always maintain good body alignment.

Oxygen may be administered by various methods (cannula, tent, mask) as ordered by the physician. Specific oxygen levels are monitored by measuring arterial blood gases (ABGs).

Elimination needs. Tell the patient to let the nurse know if he or she is experiencing constipation. It is extremely important that patients with cardiovascular disease not strain at stool. The physician usually orders a bulk laxative or stool softener to be taken on a scheduled basis.

Patient Education Associated with Cardiovascular Therapy

Communication and responsibility. Encourage open communication with the patient concerning frustrations and anger as the patient attempts to adjust to the diagnosis and need for prolonged treatment. The patient must be guided to gain insight into the condition in order to assume the responsibility for the continuation of treatment. Keep reemphasizing those factors the patient can control to alter the disease process.

Smoking. Smoking causes vasoconstriction of the vessels; therefore, drastic reduction and preferably total abstinence from smoking should be encouraged.

Hypertension. If the disease process is accompanied by hypertension, stress the importance of following prescribed emotional, dietary, and medicinal regimens to control the disease.

Nutrition. The physician usually prescribes dietary modifications aimed at decreasing the cholesterol level and a reducing program designed to maintain an ideal weight range.

Caffeine consumption should be drastically reduced or discontinued. Introduce the patient to decaffeinated products that can be substituted for previously used caffeine-containing foods.

Heavy alcohol consumption may contribute to hypertension.

Expectations of therapy. Discuss expectations of therapy with the patient.

Activities and exercise. Activities of daily living need to be resumed within the boundaries set by the physician. (Such activities as regular, moderate exercise, meal preparation, resumption of usual sexual activities, and social interaction all need to be fostered.) Generally patients can anticipate a decrease in anginal pain, decrease or absence of palpitations or dysrrhythmias, improvement in ability to breathe with activity or exercise, and improvement in edema.

Environment. Tell the patient the importance of dressing warmly, avoiding cold winds, and using a face mask in these conditions to prewarm inhaled air.

Pain relief. The degree of anginal pain relief with and without activity must be discussed.

Edema. Stress need to report weight gains of 2 or more pounds in a week, a return of symptoms of difficulty breathing or cough the patient may simply attribute to a "cold," and recurrence or increase in edema beyond limits described or present when discharged by the physician.

Stress management. Some stressors may be within the work environment; therefore, involvement of the industrial nurse, along with a thorough exploration of work factors that precipitate anginal attacks, may be appropriate.

Teach the patient relaxation techniques and personal comfort measures such as a warm bath to alleviate stress.

Referral for mastery of biofeedback or other techniques may be necessary to alter stress levels substantially.

Stress produced within the dynamics of the family may require professional counseling.

Encourage the patient to openly express *feelings* about this chronic illness. The adjustment to this situation involves working through great personal fears, frustrations, hostilities, and resentments associated with the loss of personal control within one's life.

Sexual activity. Encourage the patient to resume sexual activity. Discuss the use of medication or other adjustments for anginal pain before this activity.

Changes in expectations. Assess changes in expectations as therapy progresses and the patient gains understanding and skill in management of the diagnosis.

Changes in therapy through cooperative goal setting. Work with the patient to encourage adherence to the prescribed treatment. When the patient feels that a change should be made in a treatment plan, encourage a discussion first with the physician.

Written record. Enlist the patient's aid in developing and maintaining a written record of the monitoring parameters (that is blood pressure, pulse, daily weights, degree of pain relief, exercise tolerance) and response to prescribed therapies for discussion with the physician. Patients should be encouraged to take this record to follow-up visits.

Fostering compliance. Throughout the hospitalization, discuss medication information and how it will benefit the patient's course of treatment. Seek cooperation and understanding of the following points, so that medication compliance may be enhanced:

1. Name
2. Dosage
3. Route and administration times
4. Anticipated therapeutic response
5. Side effects to expect
6. Side effects to report
7. What to do if a dosage is missed
8. When, how, or if to refill the medication prescription

If it is evident that the patient and/or family does not understand all aspects of continuing therapy being prescribed (such as administration and monitoring of medications, exercises, diets, follow-up appointments), consider the use of social service or visiting nurse agencies.

Associated teaching. Give patients the following instructions:

Always inform the physician or dentist of any prescription or over-the-counter medication being taken. Over-the-counter medications should not be taken without first consulting the physician or pharmacist.

Always report side effects of rash, itching, or hives immediately. Nausea, vomiting, or diarrhea should also be reported for the physician's evaluation if it is a new symptom.

Take all of the medication as prescribed for the full course of treatment. Do not discontinue use when feeling improved; do not save for future use; do not give your medicine to another individual. Sudden discontinuation of certain medicines may produce harmful effects.

Keep all medications out of the reach of children.

If pregnancy is suspected, consult an obstetrician as soon as possible about continuation of medication therapy.

At discharge. Items to be sent home with the patient should:

1. Have written instructions for use
2. Be labeled in a level of language and size of print appropriate for the patient
3. If needed, include identification cards or bracelets
4. Include a list of additional supplies to be purchased after discharge (such as syringes, dressings)
5. Include a schedule for follow-up appointments

Drug Therapy for Cardiovascular Disease

Digitalis glycosides

OBJECTIVES

1. Identify the similarity in spelling of the generic names of the major cardiac glycosides.
2. List and memorize the brand name and generic name of each digitalis glycoside in this text.
3. State the two primary actions of digitalis glycosides.
4. Describe the effect of digitalis glycosides on cardiac output and renal function.
5. Compare the onset, peak, and duration of action and the methods of excretion of digoxin and digitoxin.
6. Explain the process of digitalizing a patient, including the initial dose, preparation and administration of the medication, and nursing assessments needed to monitor therapeutic response and digitalis toxicity.
7. Describe safety precautions associated with the preparation and administration of digitalis glycosides.
8. Describe the nurse's responsibilities associated with the timing of blood samples to determine digitalis glycoside serum levels.
9. Develop measurable short- and long-term objectives for patient education for patients receiving digitalis glycosides.

KEY WORDS

inotropy	chronotropy
digitalization	digitalis toxicity

The digitalis drugs are among the oldest and most effective therapeutic agents for the treatment of congestive heart failure. They are also used in the treatment of atrial fibrillation, atrial flutter, and paroxysmal tachycardia. Their use in medicine dates to the Eighteenth century. In 1785 William Withering, an English physician and botanist, published excellent observations on the treatment of various ailments with digitalis. Once derived naturally from the dried leaves of *Digitalis purpurea,* or purple foxglove, the drug is now synthetically prepared.

Digitalis glycosides have two primary actions on the heart: (1) digitalis increases the force of contraction (positive inotropy), and (2) slows the heart rate (negative chronotropy). The exact mechanisms of these actions are unknown, but the net result is that the heart is able to fill and empty more completely, thus improving circulation. With improved circulation, there is a reduction in systemic and pulmonary congestion, a reduction in heart size toward normal, and a reduction in peripheral edema due to better perfusion of blood through the kidneys.

The goal of treatment for heart failure is to give adequate doses of digitalis so that the best cardiac effects are achieved and cardiac output is increased, pulse rate is slowed, and vasoconstriction decreases resulting in the disappearance of many of the signs and symptoms of heart failure (i.e. dyspnea, orthopnea, and edema). The patient is often given a loading dose of the drug over a period of hours or days necessary to produce the desired cardiac effect. This is known as *digitalizing* the patient. A maintenance dose is then given, usually once daily. Many patients must continue to take digitalis preparations for the remainder of their lives.

Side effects. Common side effects of digitalis include weakness, fatigue, vomiting, diarrhea, arrhythmias, and pulse rate below 60 beats a minute (bradycardia). Headache, visual disturbances, and restlessness may also occur.

Adverse effects of digitalis may also be induced by electrolyte imbalance, resulting in hypokalemia, hypomagnesemia, and hypocalcemia. (See Drug Interactions for agents that may induce electrolyte imbalance.)

The patient's other clinical conditions may also induce digitalis intoxication. Patients who suffer from hypothyroidism, acute myocardial infarction, renal disease, severe respiratory disease, or far advanced heart failure may require lower than normal doses of the digitalis glycosides. It is important to remember that it is essential to treat the patient and the clinical symptomatology and that individual variation is frequently observed with the digitalis glycosides. Basic treatment of digitalis-induced arrhythmias consists of stopping the digitalis and any potassium-depleting diuretics, checking the potassium level (administering potassium as indicated), and administering antiarrhythmics (e.g., phenytoin and lidocaine). In some instances, atropine may be prescribed for sinus bradycardia. A pacemaker may be necessary for continuing bradycardia.

Antidote for severe digitalis intoxication. In cases of severe digitalis intoxication—as indicated by life-threatening arrhythmias such as ventricular tachycardia, fibrillation or severe sinus bradycardia, steady-state digoxin serum concentrations greater than 10 ng/ml, or a serum potassium concentration greater than 5 mEq/L in a known case of digitalis ingestion—treatment with an antidote, Digoxin Immune FAB (ovine) (DIGIBIND), is usually indicated. This product contains antigen binding fragments from sheep that have been injected with a digoxin-human albumin complex, against which the sheep makes antibodies. The antibodies are harvested and purified into the antigen binding fragments that have strong binding affinity for digoxin. When injected into humans who have received digoxin (or digitoxin), the fragments bind to molecules of digoxin, making them unavailable for binding at their site of action. The fragment-digoxin complex accumulates in the blood and is excreted by the kidneys. Improvement in signs and symptoms of digitalis intoxication begins in less than 30 minutes after injection of the antigen binding fragments.

• **Nursing Interventions: Monitoring digitalis glycoside therapy**

See General Nursing Considerations for Patients with Cardiovascular Disease (p. 242).

See also Nursing Interventions for digoxin and digitoxin (pp. 247, 248).

Side effects to report
DIGITALIS TOXICITY

Cardiac effects. Always observe your patient for the development of a pulse deficit, bradycardia, tachycardia, or bigeminy. These may be signs of developing heart block. Whenever the individual is attached to a monitor, the pattern should be closely watched for any type of abnormal cardiac arrhythmia.

In children, digitalis toxicity is usually detected by the development of atrial arrhythmias.

Noncardiac effects. Noncardiac symptoms of digitalis toxicity are often quite vague and are difficult to separate from symptoms of the heart disease. Any patient who is taking digitalis products who develop loss of appetite, nausea, extreme fatigue, weakness of the arms and legs, psychiatric disturbances (nightmares, agitation, listlessness, or hallucinations), or visual disturbances (hazy or blurred vision, difficulty in reading, and difficulty in red-green color perception) should be evaluated for digitalis toxicity.

Other diseases. Other diseases such as hypothyroidism, myocardial infarction, renal disease, or pulmonary disease may increase the potential for digitalis toxicity. Monitor closely.

ELECTROLYTE BALANCE. Monitor lab reports and notify the physician of deviations from the normal range of 4 to 5.4 mEq/liter of potassium. Always monitor the pulse carefully if potassium level is abnormal. Hypokalemia is especially likely to occur when the patient exhibits nausea, vomiting, diarrhea, or heavy diuresis.

Implementation
DIGITALIZATION. Digitalization is the administration of a larger dose of a digitalis preparation for an initial period of 24 to 48 hours. Following this initial "loading" period, the patient is switched to a daily maintenance dose. Be sure to monitor the patient carefully for signs of digitalis toxicity.

PULSE VARIATIONS. Always take the apical pulse 1 *full* minute *before* administering any digitalis preparation. Do not administer the drug when the pulse rate in an adult is below 60 beats per minute until the physician is consulted. In a child report findings below 90 beats per minute. The physician may decide to withhold the medication.

ACCURATE IDENTIFICATION. Digitalis glycosides are frequently given in minute amounts. *Always* have mathematical computations checked by another professional nurse.

Use the correct type of syringe to facilitate accuracy in dosage measurement.

Always question any order that is unusual *before* administration. Read the medication label carefully; *digoxin* and *digitoxin* are *not* the same.

SERUM LEVELS. Serum levels of digitalis are performed to measure the amount of digitalis in the bloodstream. Blood should be drawn prior to the daily dose of medication, or at least 6 hours after administration. It is important to be consistent in the time of drawing the blood and administering the dose if more than one serum level is to be drawn in the same patient.

ORAL ADMINISTRATION. Give digitalis glycosides after meals to minimize gastric irritation.

Drug interactions
DRUGS THAT ENHANCE THERAPEUTIC AND TOXIC EFFECTS. Verapamil, propafenone, beta adrenergic blocking agents (such as atenolol, esmolol, timolol, nadolol, propranolol, others), succinylcholine, calcium gluconate, and calcium chloride. Monitor for signs and symptoms of digitalis toxicity.

DRUGS THAT REDUCE THERAPEUTIC EFFECTS. *Cholestyramine:* Watch for an increase in the patient's disease symptomatology.

DRUGS THAT MAY ALTER ELECTROLYTE BALANCE, ALTERING DIGITALIS RESPONSE. Drugs that may alter digitalis response and the incidence of any of the side effects by alteration of electrolyte balance include the following:

Hypokalemia
  Amphotericin B (Fungizone)
  Bumetanide (Bumex)
  Chlorthalidone (Hygroton)
  Corticosteroids
  Ethacrynic acid (Edecrin)
  Furosemide (Lasix)
  Metolazone (Zaroxolyn)
  Thiazide diuretics
Hyperkalemia
  Amiloride (Midamor)
  Beta adrenergic blockers
  Heparin
  Mannitol infusions
  Potassium chloride

Potassium gluconate
Potassium penicillin G
Potassium supplements (K-Lyte, Kaon, K-Lore, others)
Salt substitutes
Succinylcholine
Hypomagnesemia
Chlorthalidone (Hygroton)
Ethacrynic acid (Edecrin)
Ethanol
Furosemide (Lasix)
Metolazone (Zaroxolyn)
Neomycin (Mycifradin)
Thiazide diuretics

See the individual agents for drug interactions specific to digoxin and digitoxin.

Digitalis preparations

digitoxin (dij-i-tok′-sin)

Crystodigin (kris-to-dij′in), **Purodigin** (pu-ro-dij′in)

Availability

PO—0.05, 0.1, 0.15, and 0.2 mg tablets.

Dosage and administration. NOTE: A baseline ECG is recommended before initiation of therapy. Assuming the patient has not ingested a digitalis preparation in the preceding 3 weeks, the following dosages apply:

Adult

PO—1. Digitalizing: 0.6 mg initially followed by 0.2 mg at intervals of 4 to 6 hours.
2. Maintenance: 0.05 to 0.3 mg once daily. The average dose is 0.1 to 0.15 mg daily.

IV—1. Digitalizing: 0.6 mg initially followed by 0.4 mg 4 to 6 hours later, then followed by 0.2 mg every 4 to 6 hours thereafter until therapeutic effects are apparent. These effects are usually observed within 8 to 12 hours.
2. Maintenance: Same as for PO maintenance therapy.

Pediatric

PO—1. Digitalizing
    a. Premature, full-term, and infants with impaired renal function: 0.022 mg/kg.
    b. Ages 2 weeks to 1 year: 0.045 mg/kg.
    c. Over 2 years of age: 0.03 mg/kg.

NOTE: Divide total digitalizing dose into 3 or more doses, administered at least 6 hours apart.
2. Maintenance: Give one-tenth the total digitalizing dose daily.

IV—As for PO therapy.

• Nursing Interventions: Monitoring digitoxin therapy

See General Nursing Considerations for Patients with Cardiovascular Disease (p. 242).

See also Nursing Interventions for digitalis glycosides (p. 246).

Drug interactions

DRUGS THAT REDUCE THERAPEUTIC EFFECTS. See also Digitalis Glycosides.

Phenobarbital, phenylbutazone, phenytoin, and cholestyramine.

Monitor patient symptoms for response to therapy; recurrence or intensification of patient's disease should be reported to the physician.

digoxin (di-joks′in)

Lanoxin (lah-noks′in)

Digoxin is the most commonly used member of the digitalis glycoside family. It digitalizes more rapidly than digitoxin. Oral administrations may digitalize within a few hours and IV injections within a few minutes.

Availability

PO—0.125, 0.25, and 0.5 mg tablets; 0.05, 0.1 and 0.2 mg Gelcaps; pediatric elixir, 0.05 mg/ml.

IV—0.25 mg/ml in 1 and 2 ml vials and ampules, and 0.1 mg/ml in 1 ml ampules.

Dosage and administration. NOTE: A baseline ECG is recommended before initiation of therapy. Assuming the patient has not ingested a digitalis preparation in the preceding 2 weeks, the following dosages apply:

Adult

PO—1. Digitalizing: 0.25 to 0.50 mg initially followed by 0.125 mg every 6 hours until adequate digitalization is achieved.
2. Maintenance: 0.125 to 0.25 mg daily. Some patients may require 0.375 to 0.5 mg daily.

IV—1. Digitalizing: 0.25 to 0.5 mg initially followed by 0.125 mg every 6 hours until adequate digitalization is achieved. Administer at a rate of 0.5 to 1 ml/minute.
2. Maintenance: Same as for PO administration. Adult therapeutic blood levels are 0.5 to 1.8 ng/ml.

Pediatric

PREMATURE

IM or IV—1. Digitalizing: 0.015 to 0.02 mg/kg initially followed by 0.01 mg every 6 to 8 hours for 2 doses (total digitalizing dose: 0.03 to 0.05 mg/kg).
2. Maintenance: 0.003 to 0.006 mg/kg every 12 hours.

AGES 2 WEEKS TO 2 YEARS

PO—1. Digitalizing: 0.03 to 0.04 mg/kg initially followed by 0.02 mg/kg every 6 to 8 hours for 2 doses (total digitalizing dose: 0.06 to 0.08 mg/kg).
2. Maintenance: 0.006 to 0.01 mg/kg every 12 hours.

IM or IV—1. Digitalizing: 0.02 to 0.03 mg/kg initially, followed by 0.01 to 0.015 mg/kg every 6 to 8 hours for 2 doses (total digitalizing dose: 0.04 to 0.06 mg/kg).
2. Maintenance: 0.003 to 0.006 mg/kg every 12 hours.

OVER 2 YEARS OF AGE

PO—1. Digitalizing: 0.02 to 0.03 mg/kg initially, followed by 0.01 to 0.015 mg every 6 to 8 hours for 2 doses (total digitalizing dose: 0.04 to 0.06 mg/kg).

2. Maintenance: 0.004 to 0.009 mg/kg every 12 hours.

IM or IV—1. Digitalizing: 0.01 to 0.02 mg/kg initially, followed by 0.005 to 0.01 mg/kg every 6 to 8 hours for 2 doses (total digitalizing dose: 0.02 to 0.04 mg/kg).

2. Maintenance: 0.002 to 0.004 mg/kg every 12 hours.

• Nursing Interventions: Monitoring digoxin therapy

See General Nursing Considerations for Patients with Cardiovascular Disease (p. 242).

See also Nursing Interventions for digitalis glycosides (p. 246).

Drug interactions. See also Digitalis Glycosides

DRUGS THAT INCREASE THERAPEUTIC AND TOXIC EFFECTS. Quinidine, nifedipine, verapamil, and antibiotics. Monitor for signs and symptoms of digitalis toxicity.

DRUGS THAT REDUCE THERAPEUTIC EFFECTS. Neomycin and antacids.

Monitor patient symptoms for response to therapy; recurrence or intensification of the patient's disease should be reported to the physician.

Inotropic agent

amrinone (am′rhin-own)

Inocor (aye′no-core)

Amrinone is an inotropic agent that increases the force and velocity of myocardial contractions. It also is a vascular smooth muscle relaxant that causes vasodilation, reducing preload and afterload. It is used for the short-term management of congestive heart failure in patients who have not responded adequately to digitalis, diuretics, and/or vasodilator therapy. The inotropic effects of amrinone are additive to those of digitalis, and can be used in fully digitalized patients.

Side effects. As would be expected, the cardiovascular side effects of arrhythmias (3%) and hypotension (1.3%) are the most commonly reported adverse effects.

Thrombocytopenia with platelet counts of less than 100,000/mm³ has been reported in 2.4% of patients. It appears to be dose-dependent, occurring within 48 to 72 hours after initiation of therapy. It is more frequent with higher-than-recommended dosages.

Nausea (1.7%), vomiting (0.9%), and abdominal pain (0.4%) have been experienced by some patients.

Hepatotoxicity has been reported in about 0.2% of patients following IV therapy.

Availability

IV—5 mg/ml in 20-ml ampules.

Dosage and administration

Adult

IV—Initiate therapy with a bolus of 0.75 mg/kg given slowly over 2 to 3 minutes.

Continue therapy with a maintenance infusion between 5 and 10 mcg/kg/min. This should place the amrinone serum level around the 3 mcg/ml level.

Based upon clinical response, an additional bolus injection of 0.75 mg/kg may be given 30 minutes after the initial bolus.

In general, the total daily dose should not exceed 10 mg/kg/24 hr.

• Nursing Interventions: Monitoring amrinone therapy

See also General Nursing Considerations for Patients with Cardiovascular Disease (p. 242).

Side effects to expect

NAUSEA, VOMITING, ABDOMINAL DISCOMFORT. These side effects are generally transient and subside with continued therapy. If discomfort becomes severe, reduce the dosage rate and call a physician immediately.

Side effects to report

ARRHYTHMIAS, HYPOTENSION. Monitor blood pressure, heart rate and rhythm closely during therapy. These adverse effects are often dose-related and will respond to a reduction in infusion rate. Contact a physician immediately if arrhythmias or significant hypotension develop.

THROMBOCYTOPENIA. Platelet counts should be performed prior to and periodically during therapy. If thrombocytopenia does occur, discontinuation of therapy should be considered, especially when platelet counts decrease to fewer than 50,000/mm³. The nadir in platelet count appears to be variable but occurs within 1 to 4 weeks.

HEPATOTOXICITY. The symptoms of hepatotoxicity are: anorexia, nausea, vomiting, jaundice, hepatomegaly, splenomegaly, and abnormal liver function tests (elevated bilirubin, AST, ALT, alkaline phosphatase, prothrombin time). If these symptoms appear, it is recommended that amrinone therapy be discontinued.

Implementation

INCOMPATIBILITY WITH DEXTROSE SOLUTIONS. Do not dilute amrinone with dextrose solutions. With time, the amrinone loses potency. Amrinone may be injected into running dextrose infusions through a Y-connector or directly into the tubing.

MONITORING PARAMETERS. Patient improvement should be observed by increases in cardiac output, reduction in pulmonary capillary wedge pressure, and reduced dyspnea, orthopnea and fatigue.

Drug interactions

DIGITALIS GLYCOSIDES. Concurrent administration of amrinone and digitalis glycosides produces additive inotropic effects.

FUROSEMIDE. Amrinone and furosemide are chemically incompatible. When furosemide is mixed with amrinone, a precipitate forms immediately. Do not infuse into the same intravenous line.

Antilipemic agents
OBJECTIVES

1. Identify the four major types of lipoproteins.
2. Describe the primary treatment modalities for lipid disorders.
3. State specific oral administration instructions needed with antilipemic agents.
4. Analyze Table 11-2 to identify the specific agents used to treat Type II and Type IV forms of hyperlipidemia.

KEY WORDS

atherosclerosis   lipoprotein
chylomicrons   triglycerides

A major cause of cardiovascular disease is *atherosclerosis*, a disease characterized by the accumulation of fatty deposits on the inner walls of arteries and arterioles throughout the body. These fatty substances eventually produce degenerative changes and obstruct blood flow to vital organs resulting in hypertension, strokes, myocardial infarctions, and peripheral vascular disease. Although other risk factors are involved, high levels of lipids (fatty substances) in the blood are major contributors to the development of atherosclerosis. The primary source of lipids is the fat content of our diet. Once absorbed from the gastrointestinal tract, the fats (lipids) are bound to circulating proteins and called lipoproteins. There are four major types of lipoproteins: chylomicrons, very low density lipoproteins (VLDL), low density lipoproteins (LDL), and high density lipoproteins (HDL). The four types differ in concentration of triglycerides, cholesterol, and proteins. Chylomicrons consist of about 90% triglycerides and 5% cholesterol, while the high density lipoproteins contain about 20% cholesterol and 1% to 7% triglycerides.

The lipid disorders are classified into six types (Table 11-1). The most common hyperlipidemias are Type II and IV. The primary treatment for hyperlipidemias is weight reduction, exercise, and a diet low in cholesterol and saturated fat and high in unsaturated fat. Studies now indicate that with reduction in elevated cholesterol and/or triglycerides, the frequency of heart attacks and strokes is substantially reduced. If a change in diet does not produce an acceptable decrease in blood lipid levels, an antilipemic agent (Table 11-2) may be added to the patient's regimen.

Table 11-1 *Classification of Hyperlipidemias*

TYPE	GENERIC NAME	ELEVATED LIPOPROTEINS PATTERNS	ELEVATED CHOLESTEROL	ELEVATED TRIGLYCERIDES	INCIDENCE	TREATMENT DIET	TREATMENT DRUGS
I	Exogenous hyperlipemia	Chylomicrons		↑	Rare	Very low fat: 25 to 35 g a day; high carbohydrate	None
IIa	Familial hypercholesterolemia	LDL (beta lipoproteins)	↑		Common	Low cholesterol (300 mg a day); low saturated fat; high unsaturated fat	Cholestyramine, colestipol, nicotinic acid, probucol, lovastatin
IIb	Combined hyperlipoproteinemia	LDL + VLDL	↑	↑	Common	Low cholesterol; high unsaturated fat. Reduce obesity	Nicotinic acid, probucol, lovastatin
III	Broad-beta hyperlipidemia (familial dysbetalipoproteinemia)	IDL (broad-beta lipoproteins)	↑	↑	Rare	See II-b	Clofibrate, nicotinic acid
IV	Endogenous hyperlipemia	VLDL (prebeta lipoproteins)		↑	Common	Low carbohydrate; high unsaturated fat; low cholesterol and alcohol. Reduce obesity	Clofibrate, gemfibrozil, nicotinic acid
V	Mixed hyperlipemia	VLDL + Chylomicrons		↑	Rare	Low fat and carbohydrate; high protein. Low alcohol	Clofibrate, nicotinic acid

Modified from Hahn, AB et al: *Mosby's Pharmacology in Nursing*, ed 16, St Louis, Mosby–Year Book, p. 471.

Table 11-2 *Antilipemic Agents*

GENERIC NAME	BRAND NAME	DOSAGE AND ADMINISTRATION	COMMENTS
Cholestyramine resin	Questran	ORAL: 1 tsp (about 4 gm of resin) 3-4 times daily with meals. The resin must be mixed with 2-6 oz water, fruit juices, soups, or applesauce and should be allowed to stand for a few minutes to allow absorption and dispersion. Do not attempt to swallow the dry powder. Follow administration with another glass of water.	Type II hyperlipidemia. This resin stays in the intestine, binding bile acids to be excreted. The liver enhances cholesterol degradation to make more bile acids. Administer at least 1-2 hours after medications to prevent binding of medications. May cause constipation; add roughage to the diet. Increase fluid intake, add stool softener. Potentiates warfarin anticoagulation.
Clofibrate	Atromid-S	ORAL: 2 gm daily divided into 2-4 doses. Administer with meals to reduce stomach upset.	Types III, IV, and V hyperlipidemia; Type II if VLDL elevated. Several mechanisms of action. May cause GI upset. Drug interactions with probenecid, warfarin, sulfonylureas.
Colestipol hydrochloride	Colestid	ORAL: 15-30 g daily in 2-4 divided doses. Mix as cited for cholestyramine.	As for cholestyramine.
Gemfibrozil	Lopid	ORAL: 600 mg 30 minutes before morning and evening meals. Dosage range is 900-1500 mg daily.	Type IV hyperlipidemia; lowers triglycerides in VLDL; may also lower cholesterol in LDL; increases HDL. Related to clofibrate. Potentiates warfarin anticoagulation.
Lovastatin	Mevacor	ORAL: Initially, 20 mg daily at evening meal. Adjust dose every 4 weeks. Dosage range: 20-80 mg daily.	Type II hyperlipidemia. Lowers triglyceride levels and VLDL and LDL cholesterol, while increasing HDL cholesterol. Test liver function every 4-6 weeks. Do not use in pregnant and nursing women.
Nicotinic acid (Niacin)	Nicobid	ORAL: 1 to 2 gm, 3 times daily, with or following meals.	Type II, III, IV, V hyperlipidemia, often used in conjunction with other antilipemic agents. May cause flushing and a sense of warmth to the face and upper body. If dizziness occurs, avoid sudden changes in posture.
Pravastatin	Pravachol	ORAL: 10 to 40 mg once daily at bedtime.	As for Lovastatin.
Probucol	Lorelco	ORAL: 500 mg twice daily with breakfast and dinner.	Type II hyperlipidemia. Lowers cholesterol probably by inhibiting biosynthesis in the liver. Transient diarrhea reported. Excessive and foul-smelling perspiration has also been reported.

ARRHYTHMIAS

OBJECTIVES

1. Describe the therapeutic response that should be observable when an antiarrhythmic agent is administered.
2. Identify baseline nursing assessments that should be implemented during the treatment of arrhythmias.
3. State signs and symptoms associated with myocardial toxicity.
4. List the dosage forms and precautions needed in the preparation of IV lidocaine for the treatment of arrhythmias.

5. Name the site of IM administration of lidocaine.
6. Cite the common side effects that may be observed with the administration of amiodarone, bretylium tosylate, disopyramide, lidocaine, flecainide, mexiletine, phenytoin, procainamide, quinidine, and tocainide.
7. Identify the potential effects of muscle relaxants used during surgical intervention when combined with antiarrhythmic therapy.
8. Develop measurable short- and long-term objectives for patient education for patients with antiarrhythmic therapy.

KEY WORDS

arrhythmias	atrial flutter
atrial fibrillation	paroxysmal tachycardia
tinnitus	cinchonism

Any patient with heart disease or a disease that affects cardiovascular function may experience arrhythmias. *Arrhythmias* are any heart rate and rhythm other than normal sinus rhythm. The more common causes of arrhythmias include electrolyte and acid-base imbalance, emotional stress, hypoxia, and congestive heart failure.

Patients may "sense" that they are having arrhythmias because they can feel the heart "flip-flop" or "race." Nurses may also suspect that a patient is having arrhythmias because of an irregular pulse. Arrhythmias, however, must be identified with the aid of an electrocardiogram (ECG), which provides a tracing of the electrical activity of the heart. When an arrhythmia is suspected, a patient is frequently admitted to a coronary care unit where wire leads are placed in appropriate locations to provide continuous ECG monitoring. A combination of the physical examination, patient history, and ECG pattern is used to diagnose the underlying cause of the arrhythmia. The goal of treatment is to restore normal sinus rhythm and normal cardiac function and to prevent recurrence of life-threatening arrhythmias.

Advanced coronary care classes are required for nurses in a coronary care unit because advanced training in the interpretation of data from ECG monitors and in drug therapy used in the management of life-threatening arrhythmias is required. However, the information nurses assess relative to the cardinal signs of cardiovascular disease can provide a basis for subsequent evaluation of the patient's response to the therapeutic modalities prescribed.

General Nursing Considerations for Patients with Arrhythmias

Patient Concerns: Nursing Intervention/Rationale

Baseline assessment

Vital signs. Vital signs should be taken as often as necessary to monitor the patient's status.

Chest pain. Not all patients with arrhythmias will have chest pain, but for those who do, record the time of onset, frequency, duration, and quality of the chest pain.

Specifically note any conditions the patient has found that either aggravate or relieve chest pain.

Mental status and anxiety level. Perform a baseline assessment of the patient's degree of anxiety, alertness, and agitation. Subsequent regular observations of this data should be made so that apparent improvement or deterioration can be assessed.

Patients experiencing cardiovascular disorders frequently exhibit varying degrees of anxiety. Act in a calm manner when dealing with the patient experiencing anxiety. Remember that hostility and anger are frequently employed as a means of dealing with loss of personal control of one's life.

It is essential that the nurse establish a trusting relationship with the patient and that he or she listen to the patient's concerns.

Arrhythmias. Arrhythmias are initially assessed by electrocardiographic monitoring. A 24 hour ambulatory electrocardiogram (Holter Monitor), electrophysiologic studies (EPS), exercise electrocardiography and laboratory values are used to analyze and diagnose the patient's myocardial status.

Patients are usually admitted to the coronary care unit where specialized monitoring equipment is available for continual surveillance of the patient. The nurses have advanced education in cardiac physiology and the nursing care needs of these individuals. (See a general medical-surgical nursing text for an in-depth explanation of care of the patient with arrhythmias.)

Cardinal signs of cardiovascular disease. See above, General Nursing Considerations for Patients with Cardiovascular Disease (p. 242).

Patient Education Associated with Antiarrhythmic Therapy

Communication and responsibility. Encourage open communication concerning frustrations and anger as the patient attempts to adjust to the diagnosis and need for prolonged treatment. The patient must be guided to gain insight into the condition in order to assume responsibility for the continuation of treatment. Keep emphasizing those factors the patient can control to alter the disease process, including maintenance of general health, elimination of smoking, meeting nutritional needs, adequate rest, and appropriate exercise, and continuation of prescribed medication therapy.

Expectations of therapy. Discuss expectations of therapy with the patient (such as level of exercise, degree of pain relief, frequency of use of therapy, sexual activity, maintenance of mobility, ability to maintain activities of daily living and/or work).

Changes in expectations. Assess changes in expectations as therapy progresses and the patient gains understanding and skill in management of the diagnosis.

Changes in therapy through cooperative goal-setting. Work with the patient to encourage adherence to the prescribed treatment. When the patient feels that a change should be made in a treatment plan, encourage discussion first with the physician.

Written record. Enlist the patient's aid in developing and maintaining a written record of monitoring parameters (such as blood pressure, pulse, daily weights, degree of pain relief, exercise tolerance) and response to prescribed therapies for discussion with the physician. Patients should be encouraged to take this record on follow-up visits.

Fostering compliance. Throughout the hospitalization, discuss medication information and how it will benefit the course of treatment. Seek cooperation and understanding of the following points so that medication compliance may be enhanced:

1. Name
2. Dosage
3. Route and administration times
4. Anticipated therapeutic response
5. Side effects to expect
6. Side effects to report
7. What to do if a dosage is missed
8. When, how, or if to refill the medication prescription

Difficulty in comprehension. If it is evident that the patient and/or family does not understand all aspects of continuing therapy being prescribed (such as administration and monitoring of medications, exercises, diets, follow-up appointments), consider the use of social service or visiting nurse agencies.

Associated teaching. Give the patient the following instructions:

Always inform the physician or dentist of any prescription or over-the-counter medication being taken. Over-the-counter medications should not be taken without first consulting the physician or pharmacist.

Always report side effects of rash, itching, or hives immediately. Nausea, vomiting, or diarrhea should also be reported for the physician's evaluation if it is a new symptom.

Take all of the medication as prescribed for the full course of treatment. Do not discontinue use when feeling improved; do not save for future use; do not give your medicine to another individual. Sudden discontinuation of certain medications may produce harmful effects.

Keep all medications out of reach of children.

If pregnancy is suspected, consult an obstetrician as soon as possible about continuation of medication therapy.

At discharge. Items to be sent home with the patient should:

1. Have written instructions for use
2. Be labeled in a level of language and size of print appropriate for the patient
3. If needed, include identification cards or bracelets
4. Include a list of additional supplies to be purchased after discharge
5. Include a schedule for follow-up appointments

Classification of Antiarrhythmic Agents

In the normal heart, a contraction of the heart muscle begins in the sino-atrial (SA) node. The electrical

Table 11-3 *Classification of Antiarrhythmic Agents*

CLASS	GENERIC NAME	BRAND NAME
I	Moricizine*	Ethmozine
Ia	Disopyramide	Norpace
	Procainamide	Pronestyl, Procan-SR
	Quinidine	Quinidex, Quinaglute
Ib	Lidocaine	Xylocaine
	Mexiletine	Mexitil
	Phenytoin	Dilantin
	Tocainide	Tonocard
Ic	Flecainide	Tambocor
	Propafenone	Rythmol
II	Beta Adrenergic Blocking Agents (see p. 255)	
III	Amiodarone	Cordarone
	Bretylium	Bretylol
IV	Verapamil	Calan, Isoptin
—	Adenosine	Adenocard

*Does not belong to the subclasses (A,B,C), but has properties of all three subclasses.

wave passes through the electrical system in the atrial muscle causing it to contract, forcing blood in the atrial chambers into the ventricles below. The electrical current then triggers the atrio-ventricular (AV) node, which sends an electrical current through the Bundle of His and the Purkinje fibers to the ventricular muscle tissue. The muscle contracts from the apex upward, causing blood to be pumped from the ventricles into the pulmonary artery and the aorta. The tissues of the electrical system can be classified into two types: The SA and AV nodes are dependent upon calcium for electrical conduction, and the atria, His-Purkinje system and the ventricular muscle are dependent upon sodium for contraction.

Antiarrhythmic agents are complex agents with multiple mechanisms of action. They are classified according to their effects on the electrical conduction system of the heart. Class I agents are sodium channel blockers. Class II agents are beta adrenergic blocking agents (many arrhythmias are caused by stimulation of the beta cells of the sympathetic nervous system of the heart). Class III agents slow the rate of electrical conduction, and Class IV agents block calcium channels, slowing AV conduction. See Table 11-3, Classification of Antiarrhythmic Agents.

Drug Therapy for Arrhythmias

adenosine (aden'oh-seen)

Adenocard (aden'oh-card)

Adenosine is a naturally-occurring chemical found in every cell within the body. It has a variety of physiological roles including energy transfer, promotion of prostaglandin release, inhibition of platelet aggregation, antiadrenergic effects, coronary vasodilation, and suppression of heart rate. Because of its strong depressant effects on the SA and AV nodes, adenosine is recommended for the treatment of paroxysmal supraventricular tachycardia that involves conduction in the SA node, atrium, or AV node.

Side effects. The most commonly reported adverse reactions with adenosine include flushing of the face (18%), shortness of breath (12%), chest pressure (7%), nausea (3%), headache and lightheadedness (2%). Due to the short duration of action of the medicine, most adverse effects last for less than 1 minute.

Availability

IV—3 mg in 2 ml vials

Dosage and administration

IV—6 mg administered by rapid IV bolus injection (over 1 to 2 seconds) followed by a saline flush. A follow-up dose of 12 mg rapid IV bolus is recommended if the initial dose is unsuccessful in restoring a normal heart rate. The 12 mg dose may be repeated once if required.

• Nursing Interventions: Monitoring adenosine therapy

See also General Nursing Considerations for Patients with Cardiovascular Disease (p. 242) and Arrhythmias (p. 251).

Side effects to expect. Since the half-life of adenosine is less than 10 seconds, adverse effects are very short-lived. Treatment of any prolonged adverse effect would include oxygen and, possibly, other antiarrhythmic agents.

Drug interactions

DRUGS THAT ENHANCE THERAPEUTIC AND TOXIC EFFECTS. Dipyridamole and carbamazepine potentiate the effects of adenosine. Smaller doses of adenosine should be used if therapy is required.

DRUGS THAT REDUCE THERAPEUTIC EFFECTS. Theophylline, aminophylline, and caffeine competitively antagonize adenosine, thus larger doses of adenosine are required with concurrent use.

amiodarone hydrochloride (am e-o'dahr-own)

Cordarone (cor-dahr'own)

Amiodarone is a member of a new chemical class of antiarrhythmic agents and is not related to any other available antiarrhythmic product. Although its mechanism of action is unknown, it is a class III agent that acts by prolonging the action potential of atrial and ventricular tissue and by increasing the refractory period without altering the resting membrane potential, thus delaying repolarization. In addition, amiodarone has been shown to antagonize noncompetitively both alpha and beta adrenergic receptors causing systemic and coronary vasodilatation. Amiodarone is being used in the management of life-threatening supraventricular tachyarrhythmias, atrial fibrillation and flutter, bradycardia-tachycardia syndromes, ventricular tachycardia and fibrillation, and hypertrophic cardiomyopathy resistant to currently available therapy.

Side effects. Adverse reactions are very common with the use of amiodarone, particularly in patients receiving greater than 400 mg/day. Fifteen to twenty percent of patients discontinue therapy due to adverse effects.

Availability

PO—200 mg tablets.

Dosage and administration. NOTE: Amiodarone is contraindicated in patients with severe sinus-node dysfunction causing sinus bradycardia; with second-degree and third-degree AV block; and when episodes of bradycardia have caused syncope (except in the presence of a pacemaker).

The difficulty of using amiodarone effectively and safely itself poses a significant risk to patients. Patients must be hospitalized while the loading dose is given, and the response often takes 2 weeks or more. Because absorption and elimination are variable, maintenance-dose selection is difficult, and it is not unusual to require a reduction in dosage or a discontinuation of treatment. The time at which a previously controlled life-threatening arrhythmia will recur after discontinuation or dosage adjustment is unpredictable, ranging from weeks to months. Attempts to substitute other antiarrhythmic agents when amiodarone is discontinued are made difficult by the gradually, but unpredictably, changing amiodarone body store. A similar problem exists when amiodarone is not effective; it still poses the risk of a drug interaction with whatever subsequent treatment is tried.

PO: Loading dose—800 to 1600 mg daily in divided doses for 1 to 3 weeks until an initial therapeutic response occurs. Following the loading dose, a dosage of 600 to 800 mg daily is given for about one month.

Maintenance—The lowest effective dose should be used, usually 400 mg daily.

• Nursing Interventions: Monitoring amiodarone therapy

See also General Nursing Considerations for Patients with Cardiovascular Disease (p. 242) and with Arrhythmias (p. 251).

Side effects to report

FATIGUE, TREMORS, INVOLUNTARY MOVEMENTS, SLEEP DISTURBANCES, NUMBNESS AND TINGLING, DIZZINESS, ATAXIA, CONFUSION. Many of these symptoms are dose-related and resolve with reduction of dosage or discontinuation of therapy. Peripheral neuropathy may be associated with long-term therapy, although the onset and presentation of symptoms is variable. Symptoms usually resolve 1 to 4 months after the discontinuation of therapy.

Teach the patient to rise slowly from a supine or sitting position, and encourage the patient to sit or lie down if feeling faint.

Perform a baseline assessment of the patient's degree of alertness and orientation to name, place, and time *prior* to initiating therapy. Make regularly scheduled subsequent mental status evaluations and compare findings. Report development of alterations.

Provide for patient safety during episodes of dizziness.

EXERTIONAL DYSPNEA, NONPRODUCTIVE COUGH, PLEURITIC CHEST PAIN. Pulmonary interstitial pneumonitis/alveolitis has been reported in 10% to 15% of patients. Particular care should be taken not to assume that such symptoms are related to cardiac failure. Tests for diffusion capacity are most likely to show abnormality. Symptoms gradually resolve upon discontinuation of therapy. Periodic chest X-rays and clinical evaluation are recommended every 3 to 6 months.

THYROID DISORDERS. Administration of amiodarone has been associated with the development of hypothyroidism (2% to 10%) and hyperthyroidism (1% to 3%). Patients with a history of thyroid disorders appear to be more susceptible to this complication. Baseline and periodic thyroid function tests should be completed in all patients.

YELLOW-BROWN PIGMENTATIONS IN THE CORNEA, BLURRED VISION, HALOS. Corneal microdeposits have been observed by slit lamp examination as early as 2 weeks after the initiation of therapy. Symptoms of blurred vision or visual halos develop in about 10% of patients. This complication is reversible upon drug withdrawal. Use of methylcellulose ophthalmic solution and a minimization of the maintenance doses may limit this complication. Provide for patient safety during temporary visual impairment. Instruct the patient not to rub the eyes with force when tearing.

NAUSEA, VOMITING, CONSTIPATION, ABDOMINAL PAIN, ANOREXIA. Gastrointestinal complaints occur in about 25% of patients but rarely require discontinuation of therapy. These adverse effects commonly occur during high dosage administration and usually respond to dosage reduction or divided dosages.

ARRHYTHMIAS. Amiodarone can cause an exacerbation of the preexisting arrhythmias and, in 2% to 4% of patients, induce others as well.

PHOTOSENSITIVITY. Amiodarone has produced photosensitivity in about 10% of patients. The severity of the rash may be dependent on the degree of sun exposure. Symptoms such as burning, tingling, erythema, and blistering may occur as early as 2 hours after exposure to the sun. The use of sunscreens may minimize this adverse effect. Patients should be encouraged to wear long-sleeved shirts and to avoid wearing shorts outdoors. Photosensitivity may persist for up to 4 months after discontinuation of therapy. With long-term treatment, a blue-gray discoloration of the exposed skin may occur. The risk is increased in patients of fair complexion or those with excessive sun exposure, and may be related to cumulative dose and duration of therapy. This effect gradually subsides after discontinuation of therapy. The patient should also be instructed not to use artificial tanning lamps.

HEPATOTOXICITY. Abnormal liver function tests AST and ALT occur in 4% to 9% of patients. Liver enzymes in patients on relatively high maintenance doses should be monitored on a regular basis. Persistent significant elevations in the liver enzymes or hepatomegaly are indications for considering a reduction in dosage or discontinuation of therapy. Hepatitis and other liver abnormalities may develop in 1% to 3% of patients. The symptoms of hepatotoxicity are: anorexia, nausea, vomiting, jaundice, hepatomegaly, splenomegaly, and abnormal liver function tests.

Implementation

BASELINE TESTS. Before initiation of therapy, baseline pulmonary, thyroid, and liver function tests should be completed.

GASTRIC IRRITATION. If gastric irritation occurs, administer with food or milk. If symptoms persist or increase in severity, report for physician evaluation.

Drug interactions

DIGOXIN, DIGITOXIN. Administration of amiodarone to patients receiving digoxin or digitoxin therapy regularly results in an increase in the serum digitalis concentration. The dose of digitalis should be reduced by 50% or discontinued. Digitalis serum levels should be closely monitored and patients observed for clinical evidence of toxicity (anorexia, nausea, fatigue, blurred or colored vision, bradycardia, arrhythmias).

WARFARIN. Potentiation of warfarin is almost always seen within 3 to 4 days in patients receiving concomitant therapy. The dose of the anticoagulant should be reduced by one-third to one-half and prothrombin times should be monitored closely. Observe for the development of petechiae, ecchymoses, nosebleeds, bleeding gums, dark tarry stools, and bright red or "coffee-ground" emesis.

QUINIDINE. Elevation of quinidine serum levels (32% to 50%) is often observed within 2 to 3 days. The dose of quinidine should be reduced by one-third to one-half or discontinued.

PROCAINAMIDE. Elevation of procainamide serum levels (50%) is often observed in less than 7 days. The dose of procainamide should be reduced by one-third or discontinued.

PHENYTOIN. Elevation of phenytoin levels (200% to 300%) is observed over several weeks. The dose of phenytoin must be gradually reduced based upon patient response. Monitor patients with concurrent therapy for signs of phenytoin toxicity: nystagmus, sedation, and lethargy. Serum levels should be monitored periodically.

BETA BLOCKING AGENTS (PROPRANOLOL, TIMOLOL, NADOLOL, PINDOLOL, OTHERS); CALCIUM ANTAGONISTS (DILTIAZEM, VERAPAMIL, NIFEDIPINE). Amiodarone should be used with caution in patients receiving beta adrenergic blocking agents or calcium antagonists because of the possible potentiation of bradycardia, sinus arrest, and AV block. If necessary, amiodarone can be used after insertion of a pacemaker in patients with severe bradycardia or sinus arrest.

beta adrenergic blocking agents

The beta adrenergic blocking agents (acebutolol, atenolol, betaxolol, carteolol, esmolol, labetolol, metoprolol, nadolol, penbutolol, pindolol, propranolol, and timolol), are widely used as antiarrhythmic agents. These agents inhibit cardiac response to sympathetic nerve stimulation by blocking the beta receptors. As a result, the heart rate, systolic blood pressure, and cardiac output are reduced. These agents are effective in the treatment of various ventricular arrhythmias, sinus tachycardia, paroxysmal atrial tachycardia, premature ventricular contractions, and tachycardia associated with atrial flutter or fibrillation because atrioventricular conduction is diminished. See Chapter 10, "The Autonomic Nervous System," for further discussion of patient education and nursing interventions associated with beta adrenergic inhibition.

bretylium tosylate (bre-til'ee-um tahs'e-layt)

Bretylol (bre'ti-lol) ✦Bretylate (bre'til-ate)

Bretylium, an adrenergic blocking agent, inhibits the release of norepinephrine. It is a class III antiarrhythmic agent used for short-term suppression of life-threatening ventricular arrhythmias, primarily tachycardia and fibrillation, that have not responded to other widely used antiarrhythmic drugs. Bretylium is not a cardiac depressant, so it is particularly useful in patients with poor myocardial contractility and low cardiac output.

Side effects. Side effects include postural hypotension in most patients and often nausea and vomiting after rapid IV infusion. Other symptoms that may occur include vertigo, light-headedness, slow heart rate, syncope, increased premature ventricular contractions, increased arrhythmias, transient hypertension, substernal discomfort, and anginal attacks.

Availability
IV—50 mg/ml in 10 ml ampules.

Dosage and administration. For ventricular fibrillation: After failure of electrical cardioversion, 5 mg/kg IV undiluted. Repeat cardioversion. If fibrillation persists, the dosage may be increased to 10 mg/kg and repeated every 15 to 30 minutes. Dosages up to 40 mg/kg/day have been reported.

For other ventricular arrhythmias: Administer 5 to 10 mg/kg IV over 8 to 10 minutes. The dose may be repeated in 1 to 2 hours if the arrhythmia persists.

IV—Continuous infusion: Recommended dosage is 1 to 2 mg/minute.

IM—5 to 10 mg/kg. Dosage may be repeated in 1 to 2 hours if the arrhythmia still persists. Thereafter repeat every 6 to 8 hours.

• Nursing Interventions: Monitoring bretylium therapy

See also General Nursing Considerations for Patients with Cardiovascular Disease (p. 242) and Arrhythmias (p. 251).

Side effects to expect

DIZZINESS, LIGHTHEADEDNESS. These symptoms are transient and may be reduced by keeping the patient in a supine position. When changing positions, encourage the patient to move slowly and to lie down if feeling faint.

HYPERTENSION, HYPOTENSION. Transient hypertension followed by hypotension is frequently observed when therapy is initiated. Avoid the use of subtherapeutic doses (less than 5 mg/kg), as hypotension frequently occurs. Systolic blood pressures below 75 mm Hg may be treated with infusions of dopamine. Initiate dopamine at low doses and titrate as needed based on frequent blood pressure readings.

Drug interactions

DIGITALIS GLYCOSIDES. Bretylium is not recommended in the treatment of arrhythmias associated with digitalis toxicity. The sudden release of norepinephrine caused by the initiation of bretylium therapy may seriously aggravate the digitalis toxicity.

disopyramide (die-so-peer'ah-myd)

Norpace (nor'pace)

Disopyramide is a class Ia antiarrhythmic agent effective in the treatment of primary cardiac arrhythmias and those that occur in association with organic heart disease, including coronary artery disease. It may be used in both digitalized and non-digitalized patients. It is usually a useful drug as an alternative to quinidine or procainamide when patients develop an intolerance to or serious side effects from these agents.

Side effects. The more common adverse effects of therapy include dry mouth, nose, and throat; urinary hesitancy and retention; constipation with bloating and gas; and occasional diarrhea.

The myocardial toxicities of disopyramide may be manifested by premature ventricular contractions, bradycardia, atrioventricular block, ventricular tachycardia, ventricular fibrillation, or an increase in congestive heart failure.

Disopyramide generally has fewer side effects than quinidine and is comparable to quinidine in treatment of atrial and ventricular arrhythmias.

Availability
PO—100 and 150 mg capsules; 100 and 150 mg controlled release capsules

Dosage and administration
PO—Dosage is individualized. Recommended adult dosage schedule is 150 mg every 6 hours. If body weight is less than 110 pounds (50 kg), the recommended dose is 100 mg every 6 hours. Therapeutic blood levels are 2 to 6 mg/L.

• Nursing Interventions: Monitoring disopyramide therapy

See also General Nursing Considerations for Patients with Cardiovascular Disease (p. 242) and Arrhythmias (p. 251).

Side effects to expect

DRY MOUTH, NOSE, THROAT. Suggest frequent mouth rinses or sucking on ice chips or hard candy to relieve symptoms.

Side effects to report

MYOCARDIAL TOXICITY. Report bradycardia or increasing signs of congestive heart disease.

Monitoring of the ECG for various types of arrhythmias may be indicated as ordered by the physician.

URINARY HESITANCY. Tell the patient that hesitancy in starting to urinate may occur. Suggest running tap water or immersing hands in water as means to stimulate urination. Report decreased urinary output and bladder distention.

In the hospitalized patient, record I/O. Palpate the area of the symphysis pubis to assess for actual distention.

CONSTIPATION WITH DISTENSION AND FLATUS. Report difficulties in defecation to the physician. Assess distension by measuring abdominal girth, as appropriate. Assess ability to expel flatus.

Drug interactions

DRUGS THAT ENHANCE THERAPEUTIC AND TOXIC EFFECTS. Procainamide, quinidine, digitalis, and beta adrenergic blocking agents (propranolol, atenolol, timolol, others): Monitor for increases in severity of drug effects such as bradycardia and hypotension.

DRUGS THAT REDUCE THERAPEUTIC EFFECTS. Phenytoin, barbiturates, glutethimide, primidone, and rifampin.

Monitor for an increase in frequency of the patient's arrhythmias.

DRUGS THAT INCREASE HYPOTENSIVE EFFECTS. Diuretics and antihypertensive agents.

Instruct patients to rise slowly from a supine position. If symptoms become more severe, report to the physician.

flecainide acetate (fleh-kayn′ayd)

Tambocor (tam-boh′kor)

Flecainide acetate is a class Ic antiarrhythmic agent that may be taken orally. It may be used in the treatment of sustained ventricular tachycardia, and nonsustained ventricular tachycardia, and frequent premature ventricular contractions. Flecainide is generally used for more serious ventricular arrhythmias that have not responded to more traditional therapy. In addition to its therapeutic activity, a particular advantage is its dosing schedule of twice daily.

Side effects. The more frequent adverse effects that occur with flecainide therapy are dizziness, lightheadedness, faintness, and unsteadiness (19%); visual disturbances such as blurred vision, difficulty in focusing, and spots before the eyes (16%); dyspnea (1%); headache (10%); nausea (9%); fatigue (8%); constipation (5%); edema (3%); and abdominal pain.

Flecainide has a negative inotropic effect and may cause or worsen congestive heart failure, particularly in patients with preexisting severe heart failure. This adverse effect may take hours to months to develop. New or worsened congestive heart failure occurs in approximately 5% of patients.

Flecainide may aggravate existing arrhythmias and precipitate new ones, especially in patients with underlying heart disease.

Availability

PO—100 mg tablets.

Dosage and administration. NOTE: Flecainide should not be used in patients with second or third degree atrioventricular block in the absence of an artificial ventricular pacemaker and must be used with caution in patients with known heart failure. Monitor the electrocardiogram before and during initiation of therapy.

Adult. Sustained ventricular tachycardia:

PO—Initially, 100 mg every 12 hours. Increase in 50 mg increments twice daily every 4 days. Most patients respond at 150 mg twice daily. Maximum daily dose is 400 mg daily.

Nonsustained ventricular tachycardia or premature ventricular contractions:

PO—Initially, 100 mg every 12 hours. Increase in 50 mg increments twice daily every 4 days. Most patients are treated at less than 200 mg every 12 hours. If a patient is still symptomatic at 400 mg/day with plasma levels less than 0.6 mg/ml, cautiously increase to a maximum of 600 mg daily.

• Nursing Interventions: Monitoring flecainide therapy

See also General Nursing Considerations for Patients with Cardiovascular Disease (p. 242) and Arrhythmias (p. 251).

Side effects to expect

DIZZINESS, HEADACHE, CONSTIPATION, NAUSEA. These side effects are usually mild and tend to resolve with continued therapy. Encourage the patient not to discontinue therapy without first consulting a physician.

Side effects to report

VISUAL DISTURBANCES. Provide for patient safety during temporary visual impairment. Caution the patient to avoid temporarily tasks that require visual acuity, such as driving or operating power machinery. Instruct the patient not to rub the eyes with force when tearing. These side effects are usually mild and tend to resolve with continued therapy. Encourage the patient not to discontinue therapy without consulting the physician first.

INCREASING DYSPNEA, EXERCISE INTOLERANCE, EDEMA. Flecainide may induce or aggravate preexisting congestive heart failure. If these symptoms become more pronounced, the patient should be instructed to contact the physician for further evaluation.

ARRHYTHMIAS. Flecainide may induce or aggravate preexisting arrhythmias. The patient should be instructed to contact the physician for further evaluation if sensations of a "jumping" or "racing" heart develop.

Drug interactions

DIGOXIN. When multiple doses of flecainide are administered to patients stabilized on a dose of digoxin, there is a 10% to 20% increase in serum digoxin concentrations. This increase may result in signs of digitalis toxicity, such as anorexia, nausea, fatigue, blurred or colored vision, bradycardia, and arrhythmias. Monitor serum digoxin levels, ECG readings, and the clinical course of the patient closely.

PROPRANOLOL. When flecainide and propranolol are administered concurrently, there is a 20% increase in serum flecainide levels and a 30% increase in propranolol levels, with additive pharmacological effects. Monitor serum levels, ECG readings, and the clinical course of the patient closely. Dosage reductions of either one or both agents may be required.

lidocaine (li'do-kayn)

Xylocaine (zi'lo-kayn)

Lidocaine has become one of the most frequently used drugs in the treatment of ventricular arrhythmias. It is a class Ib agent and the drug of choice for the treatment of ventricular arrhythmias associated with acute myocardial infarction and ventricular tachycardia.

Side effects. Side effects tend to be dose-related and are usually fairly minor. Adverse effects include light-headedness, tinnitus, muscle twitches, and blurred or double vision. When higher doses are used, patients may develop CNS stimulation, hypotension, restlessness, euphoria, and, rarely, convulsions. These side effects may be controlled by reducing the dosage.

Availability

IM—300 mg/3 ml; 10% (100 mg/ml) in 5 ml ampules.

Direct IV—1% (10 mg/ml) in 5 and 10 ml disposable syringes; 2% (20 mg/ml) in 5 ml disposable syringes and ampules.

IV Admixtures—4% (40 mg/ml) in 25 and 50 ml vials and additive syringes; 20% (200 mg/ml) in 5 ml and 10 ml additive syringes.

IV Infusion—0.2% (2 mg/ml) in 500 ml of 5% dextrose; 0.4% (4 mg/ml) in 500 ml of 5% dextrose; 0.8% (8 mg/ml) in 250 and 500 ml of 5% dextrose.

Dosage and administration. NOTE: Lidocaine should not be used in patients with complete heart block.

Adult

IM—200 to 300 mg in the deltoid muscle.

IV—The initial dose (bolus) is 50 to 100 mg (1 mg/kg) at a rate of 25 to 50 mg/minute. Boluses of 50 to 100 mg may be given every 3 to 5 minutes until the desired effect is achieved or side effects appear. Do not exceed 300 mg by intermittent bolus. To maintain the antiarrhythmic effect, an IV infusion must be initiated. The usual rate of administration is 1 to 4 mg/minute. For routine lidocaine administration for

cardiac arrhythmias, add 50 ml of 40 mg/ml (2 g) of lidocaine to dextrose 5%. Therapeutic blood levels are 1 to 5 mg/L.

Pediatric

IV—Initial bolus: 1 mg/kg up to 15 mg if under 25 kg (55 pounds); up to 25 mg if over 25 kg (55 pounds). Continous infusion: 20 to 40 μg/kg/minute (maximum total dose 5 mg/kg).

• Nursing Interventions: Monitoring lidocaine therapy

See also General Nursing Considerations for Patients with Cardiovascular Disease (p. 242) and Arrhythmias (p. 251).

Side effects to report

LIGHT-HEADEDNESS, MUSCLE TWITCHING, HALLUCINATIONS, AGITATION, EUPHORIA. Monitor patients carefully for progressive symptoms of restlessness, agitation, anxiety, hallucinations, and euphoria.

Act calmly with the excited, anxious, or euphoric patient. Provide for safety and fulfillment of patient's needs. Report patient's alteration in response to the physician as soon as possible.

RESPIRATORY DEPRESSION. Observe the rate and depth of respiratory effort. Monitor for cyanosis and increasing frequency of arrhythmias.

Implementation

IV. Lidocaine for IV use for arrhythmias is *different* from lidocaine used as a local anesthetic. For use with arrhythmias, check the label carefully to be certain it says: "Xylocaine for Arrhythmias" or "Lidocaine without Preservatives." Severe arrhythmias could result if "Lidocaine with Preservatives" or "Lidocaine with Epinephrine" were accidentally administered to these patients.

IM. Intramuscular injections of lidocaine should be given in the deltoid. The IM route should be used only in emergency situations until an IV can be established.

Drug interactions

DRUGS THAT ENHANCE THERAPEUTIC AND TOXIC EFFECTS. Phenytoin and beta adrenergic blocking agents (nadolol, atenolol, timolol, propranolol, others).

Monitor for an increase in severity of side effects such as bradycardia and hypotension.

NEUROMUSCULAR BLOCKING ACTION. When lidocaine is administered in conjunction with succinylcholine, observe for respiratory depression. Patients who are on respirators may require additional time to be weaned off ventilatory assistance.

mexiletine (mehx-ihl'et-een)

Mexitil (mehx-it'ihl)

Mexiletine is a class Ib antiarrhythmic agent similar in many respects to lidocaine. It has the advantage of good oral absorption with minimal initial hepatic metabolism, thus allowing it to be administered orally.

Mexiletine can be effective therapy in the treatment of unifocal and multifocal premature ventricular contractions, couplets, and ventricular tachycardia, but is usually ineffective in the therapy of drug-resistant ventricular tachycardia. It is generally more effective against drug-resistant ventricular tachycardia when used in combination with other antiarrhythmic agents.

Side effects. Adverse effects have required the discontinuation of mexiletine in 5% to 30% of patients.

Mexiletine has dose-related effects on the central nervous system. At higher serum levels (greater than 2.0 mcg/ml) mexiletine may precipitate neurologic toxicity and, occasionally, paradoxical seizure activity.

Mexiletine may cause gastrointestinal adverse effects such as nausea, vomiting, dyspepsia, or anorexia in approximately 40% of patients. These adverse effects are usually not serious and do not correlate well with high serum levels, but are more prevalent with large orally administered doses.

Availability

PO—150, 200, 250 mg capsules.

Dosage and administration. NOTE: Mexiletine should not be used in patients with second or third degree heart block if a pacemaker is not present. NOTE: Dosage adjustment is necessary in patients with severe renal dysfunction (creatinine clearance less than 10 ml/min) and in patients with severe congestive heart failure or acute myocardial infarction.

PO—200 to 400 mg every 8 hours, or 10-14 mg/kg/ day.

• **Nursing Interventions: Monitoring mexiletine therapy**

See also General Nursing Considerations for Patients with Cardiovascular Disease (p. 242) and Arrhythmias (p. 251).

Side effects to report

ARRHYTHMIAS. Mexiletine may induce or aggravate arrhythmias. This is uncommon in patients with less serious arrhythmias, such as frequent premature beats or nonsustained ventricular tachycardia. Patients with more serious arrhythmias, such as sustained ventricular tachycardia, are more susceptible to myocardial toxicity.

NEUROTOXICITY, SEIZURES. The initial manifestation of mexiletine neurotoxicity is usually a fine hand tremor, but ataxia, dizziness, lightheadedness, nystagmus, paresthesia, blurred vision, diplopia, dysarthria, confusion, and drowsiness are other signs of impending toxicity. Provide for patient safety during these episodes.

CONFUSION. Some patients have been reported to experience serious side effects such as seizures, severe ataxia, or mental confusion without manifestation of early warning signs. Perform a baseline assessment of the patient's degree of alertness and orientation to name, place, and time *prior* to initiating therapy. Make regularly scheduled subsequent mental status evaluations and compare findings. Report development of alterations.

Implementation

GASTRIC IRRITATION. Administration with food or antacids may minimize gastric irritation without significantly inhibiting absorption. If symptoms persist or increase in severity, report for physician evaluation.

Drug interactions

DRUGS THAT REDUCE THERAPEUTIC EFFECTS (PHENYTOIN, RIFAMPIN). The hepatic metabolism of mexiletine is enhanced by rifampin and phenytoin. Patients should be observed for redevelopment of arrhythmias, which may require an increase in dosage of mexiletine.

URINARY ACIDIFIERS. These agents may lower the urine pH, causing an increase in the urinary excretion of mexiletine. Patients should be observed for redevelopment of arrhythmias, which may require an increase in dosage of mexiletine.

moricizine (mor-is'ih-zeen)

Ethmozine (eth-moh'zeen)

Moricizine is an antiarrhythmic agent chemically unrelated to other medicines used to treat arrhythmias. It acts by inhibition of influx of sodium ions into myocardial cells, making it a class I agent. It cannot be subclassified into the A, B, or C groups because it contains properties of each of the subcategories. It is used for the treatment of life-threatening ventricular arrhythmias. Because of its ability to cause additional arrhythmias, its use is reserved for those patients in whom the benefits outweigh the potential risks.

Side effects. The most frequently cited adverse reactions associated with moricizine therapy involve the CNS and include dizziness (10% to 40%), perioral numbness (18%), euphoria (15%), headache (8%), and fatigue (6%). Many of these effects occur only early in therapy. The need to discontinue therapy for causes other than arrhythmias is quite rare.

About 3% of patients receiving moricizine will experience an increase in serious arrhythmias. Other significant cardiovascular adverse effects include palpitations and hypotension.

Availability

PO—200, 250, and 300 mg tablets.

Dosage and administration

PO—Initially, 200 mg every 8 hours. Dosages may be adjusted every three days in increments of 150 mg/ day. The usual adult dosage is between 600 and 900 mg daily.

• **Nursing Interventions: Monitoring moricizine therapy**

See also General Nursing Considerations for Patients with Cardiovascular Disease (p. 242) and Arrhythmias (p. 251).

Side effects to expect

HYPOTENSION, DIZZINESS. This may occur, particularly during initiation of therapy. It usually subsides within a few days. Instruct the patient to rise slowly from a supine position. Monitor the patient's blood pressure.

NAUSEA. Gastrointestinal complaints occur in about 10% of patients but rarely require discontinuation of therapy. Administer with food or milk to alleviate nausea. Encourage the patient not to discontinue therapy without first consulting a physician.

Side effects to report

ARRHYTHMIAS. Moricizine may induce or aggravate arrhythmias. Patients with more serious arrhythmias, such as sustained ventricular tachycardia, are more susceptible to myocardial toxicity. The patient should be instructed to contact the physician for further evaluation if sensations of a "jumping" or "racing" heart develop.

EUPHORIA, CONFUSION. Perform a baseline assessment of the patient's degree of alertness and orientation to name, place, and time prior to initiating therapy. Make regularly scheduled subsequent mental status evaluations and compare findings. Report development of alterations. Provide for patient safety during episodes of dizziness. After discharge, caution the patient about operating machinery or driving if this is a recurrent problem.

Implementation

ORAL. Administer in divided dosages around the clock. If gastric irritation is a problem, administer with food or milk.

Drug interactions

DRUGS THAT ENHANCE THERAPEUTIC AND TOXIC EFFECTS. Digoxin, cimetidine. Monitor for an increase in severity of side effects such as emesis, lethargy, hypotension, arrhythmias, and bradycardia.

THEOPHYLLINE. Moricizine, when given with theophylline, may result in theophylline toxicity. Observe for vomiting, dizziness, restlessness, and cardiac arrhythmias. Monitor theophylline serum levels. The dosage of theophylline may have to be reduced.

phenytoin (fen'e-toe-in)

DPH, Dilantin (di-lan'tin)

Phenytoin was introduced about 50 years ago for the treatment of epilepsy, but it is also effective in controlling paroxysmal atrial tachycardia and ventricular arrhythmias, particularly those induced by digitalis toxicity. It is classified as a class Ib antiarrhythmic agent. (For seizure disorders, see p. 200.)

Side effects. Phenytoin has a wide variety of side effects associated with therapy, but most occur following long-term use. Sedation, lethargy, dizziness, blurred vision, hypotension, and bradycardia are the most common adverse effects observed when phenytoin is used as a short-term antiarrhythmic agent. Occasionally, anti-

arrhythmic therapy may be continued on a chronic basis. See below for adverse effects and nursing interventions associated with long-term treatment with phenytoin.

Availability

PO—30, 100 mg capsules, 50 mg chewable tablets.
Oral suspension—30, 125 mg/5ml.
IV—50 mg/ml in 2 and 5 ml ampules, 2 ml syringes.

Dosage and administration

Adults

PO—250 mg 4 times during the first day, 500 mg daily on days 2 and 3, and 300 to 400 mg on subsequent days.

IM—Not recommended because of erratic absorption and pain on injection.

IV—250 mg initially, at a rate no faster than 50 mg/min until the arrhythmia is abolished, a total of 1000 mg has been given, or side effects appear.

• Nursing Interventions: Monitoring phenytoin therapy

See also General Nursing Considerations for Patients with Cardiovascular Disease (p. 242) and Arrhythmias (p. 251).

Side effects to expect

NAUSEA, VOMITING, INDIGESTION. These effects are common during initiation of therapy. Gradual increases in therapy and administration with food or milk will minimize gastric irritation.

SEDATION, DROWSINESS, DIZZINESS, BLURRED VISION. These symptoms tend to disappear with continued therapy and possible readjustment of dosage. Encourage the patient not to discontinue therapy without first consulting the physician.

Provide for patient safety during episodes of dizziness; report for further evaluation.

Caution the patient that blurred vision may occur and make appropriate suggestions for personal safety.

CONFUSION. Perform a baseline assessment of the patient's degree of alertness and orientation to name, place, and time *prior* to initiating therapy. Make regularly scheduled subsequent mental status evaluations and compare findings. Report development of alterations.

Side effects to report

DERMATOLOGIC REACTIONS. Report a rash or pruritis immediately and withhold additional doses pending approval by the physician.

Implementation

PO. Administer with food or milk to minimize gastric irritation. If an oral suspension is used, shake well first. Encourage the use of an oral syringe for accurate measurement.

IM. If at all possible, avoid IM administration. Absorption is slow and painful.

IV RATE OF INFUSION. Administer no faster than 50 mg/minute. If given too rapidly, bradycardia and severe hypotension may result. The diluent, propylene glycol, will also potentiate the hypotensive effect of phenytoin and cause ECG changes. Cardiac and respiratory arrest may occur with excessive dosage and speed of administration. Blood pressure and the ECG should be monitored carefully, especially during administration.

MIXTURE WITH IV SOLUTIONS. Phenytoin should not be mixed with any drugs or added to any IV infusion solutions. The solubility is very pH dependent, and use with other medications or solutions will result in a white precipitate. Each IV injection should be followed by an injection of sterile saline through the same needle or IV catheter to avoid local venous irritation.

Drug interactions

DRUGS THAT ENHANCE THERAPEUTIC AND TOXIC EFFECTS. Warfarin, disulfiram, phenylbutazone, isoniazid, carbamazepine, amiodarone, chloramphenicol, cimetidine, and the sulfonamide antimicrobial agents.

Monitor patients with concurrent therapy for signs of phenytoin toxicity: nystagmus, sedation, lethargy. Serum levels may be ordered, and a reduced dosage of phenytoin may be required.

DRUGS THAT DECREASE THERAPEUTIC EFFECTS. Barbiturates, folic acid, antacids.

Monitor patients with concurrent therapy for increased seizure activity. Monitoring changes in serum levels should help warn of possible increased seizure activity.

DISOPYRAMIDE, QUINIDINE, MEXILETINE. Phenytoin decreases serum levels of these agents. Monitor patients for redevelopment of arrhythmias.

PREDNISOLONE, DEXAMETHASONE. Phenytoin decreases serum levels of these agents. Monitor patients for reduced antiinflammatory activity.

ORAL CONTRACEPTIVES. Spotting or bleeding may be an indication of reduced contraceptive activity. Use of alternative forms of birth control is recommended.

THEOPHYLLINE. Phenytoin decreases serum levels of theophylline derivatives. Monitor patients for a greater frequency of respiratory difficulty. The theophylline dose may have to be increased 50% to 100% to maintain the same therapeutic response.

VALPROIC ACID. This agent may increase or decrease the activity of phenytoin. Monitor for increased frequency of seizure activity. Monitoring changes in serum levels should help warn of possible increased seizure activity. Monitor patients with concurrent therapy for signs of phenytoin toxicity: nystagmus, sedation, lethargy. Serum levels may be ordered, and a reduced dosage of phenytoin may be required.

KETOCONAZOLE. Concurrent administration with ketoconazole may alter the metabolism of one or both drugs. Monitoring for both is recommended.

CYCLOSPORINE. Phenytoin enhances the metabolism of cyclosporine. Increased doses of cyclosporine may be necessary in patients receiving concomitant therapy.

procainamide hydrochloride (pro'kane'ah-myd)
Pronestyl (pro-nes'til)

Procainamide is an effective synthetic class Ia antiarrhythmic agent that has many cardiac effects similar to those of quinidine, but generally with fewer side effects. It is used to treat a wide variety of ventricular and supraventricular arrhythmias, atrial fibrillation, and flutter. It is usually not as effective in the last two disorders as quinidine.

Side effects. When taken orally, the most common side effects include anorexia, nausea, vomiting, bitter taste, flushing, and diarrhea.

Hypotension may be observed while therapy is being initiated, particularly by the intravenous route.

Hypersensitivity reactions including chills, fever, joint and muscle pain, pruritus, urticarial or maculopapular skin rashes, photosensitivity, and anaphylaxis have been reported.

Availability

PO—250, 375, 500 mg tablets and capsules; 250, 500, 750, 1000 mg sustained release tablets.

IV—100 mg/ml in 10 ml ampules, 500 mg/ml in 2 ml ampules.

Dosage and administration. NOTE: Do not use in complete atrioventricular block, and use with extreme caution in partial atrioventricular block.

Adult

PO—Loading dose: 1 to 1.25 g. Follow with 750 mg 1 hour later if the arrhythmia is still present. Maintain the dosage at 0.5 to 1 g every 4 to 6 hours. Some patients may require maintenance doses every 3 to 4 hours to maintain adequate control of arrhythmias.

IM—0.5 to 1 g every 6 hours until PO therapy is possible.

IV—100 mg every 5 minutes at 25 to 50 mg/minute until arrhythmias are suppressed, a maximum of 1 g has been administered, or side effects develop. Once arrhythmias are suppressed, a continuous infusion may be started at 25 to 30 µg/kg/minute. If arrhythmias recur, suppress the arrhythmias with bolus therapy as above and increase the rate of infusion.

Therapeutic blood levels are 4 to 8 mg/L.

• Nursing Interventions: Monitoring procainamide therapy

See also General Nursing Considerations for Patients with Cardiovascular Disease (p. 242) and Arrhythmias (p. 251).

Side effects to expect

DROWSINESS, SEDATION, DIZZINESS. Tell patients they may experience these symptoms early in therapy, as the dosage is being adjusted. Use caution in operating power equipment or driving.

HYPOTENSION. Hypotension is usually transient. Patients can avoid this complication by rising slowly from supine and sitting positions.

Side effects to report

FEVER, CHILLS, JOINT AND MUSCLE PAIN, SKIN ERUPTIONS. Tell patients to report the development of these symptoms.

Monitor laboratory reports for leukocyte counts and the antinuclear antibody (ANA) titer.

Implementation

ORAL. Administer in divided doses around the clock. If gastric irritation is a problem administer with food or milk.

IV. Patients should have ECG and blood pressure monitoring when receiving intravenous doses of procainamide.

SERUM LEVELS. Serum levels of procainamide are performed to measure the amount of digitalis in the bloodstream. Blood should be drawn prior to the daily dose of medication, or at least 6 hours after administration. It is important to be consistent in the time of drawing the blood and administering the dose if more than one serum level is to be drawn in the same patient.

Drug interactions

DRUGS THAT ENHANCE THERAPEUTIC AND TOXIC EFFECTS. Digitalis, quinidine, and beta adrenergic blocking agents (timolol, nadolol, propranolol, and others). Monitor for an increase in severity of side effects such as bradycardia and hypotension.

NEUROMUSCULAR BLOCKAGE, RESPIRATORY DEPRESSION. Surgical muscle relaxants (tubocurarine, succinylcholine, gallamine triethiodide) and aminoglycoside antibiotics (gentamicin, streptomycin, amikacin, kanamycin, netilmycin, others). Monitor the patient's respiratory rate and depth. Observe for signs of cyanosis and additional arrhythmias.

Patients who are on respirators may require additional time to be weaned off ventilatory assistance.

HYPOTENSION. Diuretics and antihypertensive agents: Instruct patients to rise slowly from a supine position. If symptoms are becoming more recurrent, report to the physician.

propafenone (pro-pah'fen-own)

Rythmol (rith'mohl)

Propafenone is classified as a class 1c antiarrhythmic agent based upon its electrophysiologic effects, acting primarily by inhibition of sodium ion influx into the myocardial cells. It also has weak beta-blocking and calcium channel-blocking effects. It is used for the treatment of life-threatening ventricular arrhythmias such as ventricular tachycardia. Because of its ability to cause additional arrhythmias, its use is reserved for those patients in whom the benefits outweigh the potential risks.

Side effects. The most common adverse reactions associated with propafenone therapy involve the cardiovascular, gastrointestinal, and central nervous systems. Propafenone may worsen arrhythmias or cause new ones (proarrhythmic effect) in about 5% of patients. Gastrointestinal effects include nausea and vomiting (11%), metallic taste (9%), and constipation. The central nervous system reactions include dizziness (13%) and fatigue (6%). Approximately 20% of patients receiving propafenone discontinue therapy because of adverse effects.

Since propafenone has mild beta-adrenergic blocking properties, it should not be used in patients with bronchospastic diseases (e.g., asthma).

Availability

PO—150 and 300 mg tablets

Dosage and administration

PO—Initially, 150 mg every 8 hours. At 3- to 4-day intervals, the dosage may be increased to 225 mg every 8 hours, then 300 mg every 8 hours (900 mg/day).

• **Nursing Interventions: Monitoring propafenone therapy**

See also General Nursing Considerations for Patients with Cardiovascular Disease (p. 242) and Arrhythmias (p. 251).

Side effects to expect

DIZZINESS. This may occur, particularly during initiation of therapy. It usually subsides within a few days.

Instruct the patient to rise slowly from a supine position.

Monitor the patient's blood pressure.

NAUSEA, VOMITING, CONSTIPATION. Gastrointestinal complaints occur in about 11% of patients but rarely require discontinuation of therapy. Administer with food or milk to alleviate nausea. Encourage the patient not to discontinue therapy without first consulting a physician.

Side effects to report

ARRHYTHMIAS. Propafenone may induce or aggravate arrhythmias. Patients with more serious arrhythmias, such as sustained ventricular tachycardia, are more susceptible to myocardial toxicity. The patient should be instructed to contact the physician for further evaluation if sensations of a "jumping" or "racing" heart develop.

Implementation

ORAL. Administer in divided dosages around the clock. If a patient misses a dose of propafenone, the next dose should not be doubled because of an increased risk of adverse reactions.

Drug interactions

DRUGS THAT ENHANCE THERAPEUTIC AND TOXIC EFFECTS. Quinidine, cimetidine. Monitor for an increase in severity of side effects from propafenone such as hypotension, somnolence, bradycardia, and arrhythmias.

DIGOXIN. Propafenone produces dose-related increases in serum digoxin levels. Measure plasma digoxin levels and reduce digoxin dosage when propafenone is started.

PROPRANOLOL, METOPROLOL. Propafenone appears to inhibit the metabolism of these beta blocking agents. A reduction in beta-blocker dosage may be necessary during concurrent therapy with propafenone.

WARFARIN. Propafenone increases plasma warfarin concentrations by inhibiting warfarin metabolism, thus prolonging prothrombin time. Observe for the development of petechiae, ecchymoses, nosebleeds, bleeding gums, dark tarry stools, and bright red or "coffee-ground" emesis. Monitor the prothrombin time and reduce the dosage of warfarin if necessary.

quinidine (kwin'i-din)

Quinidine, originally obtained from cinchona bark, has been used as an antiarrhythmic agent for several decades. It is classified as a class 1a antiarrhythmic agent, working on the muscle of the heart, stabilizing the rate of conduction of impulses. It slows the heart and changes a rapid, irregular pulse to a slow, regular pulse. Quinidine is used most frequently to suppress atrial fibrillation, atrial flutter, paroxysmal supraventricular and ventricular tachycardia, and premature ventricular contractions. Use with extreme caution in patients with digitalis intoxication or heart block.

Side effects. The most common side effects are diarrhea, nausea, and vomiting. Other side effects include hypotension, headache, facial flushing, hypersensitivity manifested by rash and fever, and arrhythmias.

Cinchonism (quinidine toxicity) is dose-related and will subside with reduction in dosage. It is manifested by salivation, tinnitus, vertigo, headache, visual disturbances, and confusion.

Availability
Quinidine sulfate
PO—100, 200, 300 mg tablets; 200, 300 mg capsules; 300 mg sustained release tablets.
IM, IV—200 mg/ml in 1 ml ampules.
Quinidine gluconate
PO—324 mg, 330 mg sustained release tablets.
IM, IV—80 mg/ml in 10 ml vials.
Dosage and administration
Adult
PO—Quinidine sulfate: 200 to 400 mg 3 to 5 times daily. Higher doses may be used, but the maximum single dose should not exceed 600 to 800 mg.
IM—Quinidine gluconate: 600 mg initially, then 400 mg every 2 hours as needed.
IV—Quinidine gluconate: 800 mg diluted to 40 ml with dextrose 5% and infused at a rate of 1 ml/minute.
NOTE: IV administration is extremely hazardous. Blood pressure and ECG readings should be monitored continuously as hypotension and arrhythmias may occur. Therapeutic blood levels are 1.5 to 3 mg/L.

Pediatric
PO—Quinidine sulfate: 30 mg/kg/24 hours divided into 4 to 6 doses.
IM—Quinidine gluconate: As for PO administration.

• Nursing Interventions: Monitoring quinidine therapy

See also General Nursing Considerations for Patients with Cardiovascular Disease (p. 242) and Arrhythmias (p. 251).

Side effects to expect
DIARRHEA. Diarrhea is fairly common during initiation of therapy. It usually subsides, but occasionally a patient will have to change to another medication due to this adverse effect.

Chart the frequency and consistency of the diarrhea, and monitor the patient for dehydration and electrolyte imbalance.

DIZZINESS, FAINTNESS. This may occur, particularly during initiation of therapy. It usually subsides within a few days.

Instruct the patient to rise slowly from a supine position.

Monitor the patient's blood pressure.
Side effects to report
CINCHONISM. Monitor patients for signs of cinchonism and report the development of rash, chills, fever, ringing in the ears, and increasing mental confusion.
Implementation
IDENTIFICATION AND ACCURACY. Read labels carefully. Quinidine and quinine are *not* the same.

GASTRIC IRRITATION. Administer with food or milk if gastric irritation develops.

SERUM LEVELS. Serum levels of quinidine are performed to measure the amount of guinidine in the bloodstream. Blood should be drawn prior to the daily dose of medication, or at least 6 hours after administration. It is important to be consistent in the time of drawing the blood and administering the dose if more than one serum level is to be drawn in the same patient.
Drug interactions
DRUGS THAT ENHANCE THERAPEUTIC AND TOXIC EFFECTS. Cimetidine, phenothiazines, procainamide, digitalis, and beta adrenergic blocking agents (propranolol, atenolol, timolol, others). Monitor for increases in severity of drug effects such as bradycardia, tachycardia, and hypotension.

DRUGS THAT REDUCE THERAPEUTIC EFFECTS. Rifampin. Monitor for an increase in the patient's arrhythmias.
Other interactions
NEUROMUSCULAR BLOCKADE, RESPIRATORY DEPRESSION. Surgical muscle relaxants (tubocurarine, succinylcholine, gallamine triethiodide) and aminoglycoside antibiotics (gentamicin, streptomycin, kanamycin, netilmycin, others). Monitor the patient's respiratory rate and depth. Observe for signs of cyanosis and additional arrhythmias.

Patients who are on respirators may require additional time to be weaned off ventilatory assistance.

DIGITALIS. Quinidine may increase the effects of digitalis.

Monitor the patient for symptoms of anorexia, nausea, vomiting, headaches, blurred or colored vision, and bradycardia. A digitalis serum level and quinidine serum level may be ordered by the physician.

BLEEDING. Quinidine may increase the anticoagulant effects of warfarin.

Monitor for signs of increased bleeding: bleeding gums, increased menstrual flow, petechiae, bruises.

Monitor the laboratory report and notify the physician immediately if the prothrombin time is abnormally high.

HYPOTENSION. Diuretics and antihypertensive agents: Instruct the patient to rise slowly from a supine position. If symptoms become excessive, report to the physician.

tocainide (toe-kayn′ayd)

Tonocard (toe-no′kard)

Tocainide hydrochloride is the first available derivative of lidocaine with antiarrhythmic activity when taken orally. Like lidocaine, it is a class Ib antiarrhythmic agent. It is indicated for the suppression of ventricular arrhythmias, including frequent premature ventricular contractions, unifocal or multifocal couplets, and ventricular tachycardia. Most patients who respond to lidocaine will also respond to tocainide. It is useful in patients whose arrhythmias have been initially controlled with intravenously administered lidocaine.

Side effects. Adverse effects occur quite frequently in patients receiving tocainide, and may force 16% to 20% of patients to discontinue therapy. Gastrointestinal (nausea, vomiting, anorexia) and neurologic (lightheadedness, restlessness, dizziness, paresthesia, tremor, confusion) reactions predominate and are the primary reasons for discontinuation in 80% of cases.

Although very rare, pulmonary fibrosis has been reported.

Adverse cardiovascular effects include aggravation of ventricular arrhythmias in up to 16% of patients, worsening of heart failure in less than 5%, and exacerbation of preexisting cardiac conduction disturbances in less than 2%.

Hematologic effects such as anemia, leukopenia, agranulocytosis, and thrombocytopenia have occurred in less than 1% of patients.

Availability

PO—400 and 600 mg tablets.

Dosage and administration. NOTE: Tocainide should not be used in patients with second or third degree atrioventricular block in the absence of an artificial ventricular pacemaker and must be used with caution in patients with known heart failure. Monitor the ECG readings before and during therapy.

PO—Initially, 400 mg every 8 hours. The usual maintenance dose is 1200 to 1800 mg daily given in equally divided doses every 8 hours. Maximum daily doses are usually less than 2400 mg.

Conversion from lidocaine—A 600 mg oral dose of tocainide is given 6 hours before cessation of lidocaine therapy and repeated 6 hours later, at the time of lidocaine discontinuation. Maintenance doses may be started 6 to 8 hours later. Patients should be monitored closely during this transition.

• Nursing Interventions: Monitoring tocainide therapy

See also General Nursing Considerations for Patients with Cardiovascular Disease (p. 242) and Arrhythmias (p. 251).

Side effects to expect

NAUSEA, VOMITING, ANOREXIA, ABDOMINAL PAIN. These side effects are usually mild and tend to resolve with continued therapy. Encourage the patient not to discontinue therapy without first consulting a physician.

Side effects to report

DIZZINESS, CONFUSION, NUMBNESS, AND TINGLING. Perform a baseline assessment of the patient's degree of alertness and orientation to name, place, and time *prior* to initiating therapy. Make regularly scheduled subsequent mental status evaluations and compare findings. Report development of alterations. Provide for patient safety during episodes of dizziness.

DYSPNEA, WHEEZING, COUGH. Adverse pulmonary effects associated with tocainide therapy are usually characterized by pulmonary radiographic changes, including bilateral infiltrates, and are clinically manifested by dyspnea, wheezing, and cough. Symptoms usually occur within 3 to 18 weeks of initiating therapy. If these adverse effects develop, tocainide therapy should be discontinued.

THROMBOCYTOPENIA, LEUKOPENIA, ANEMIA. These effects usually occur 2 to 12 weeks after initiation of therapy. Blood cell counts usually return to normal within 1 month following discontinuation of therapy.

Routine laboratory studies (RBC, platelets, WBC, and differential counts) should be scheduled. Stress the importance of returning for this laboratory work.

Monitor patients for the development of a sore throat, fever, purpura, jaundice, or excessive, progressive weakness.

Drug interactions

DRUGS THAT ENHANCE THERAPEUTIC AND TOXIC EFFECTS. Procainamide, disopyramide, quinidine, phenytoin, and beta adrenergic blocking agents. Monitor for an increase in severity of side effects such as bradycardia and hypotension.

CALCIUM ION ANTAGONISTS
OBJECTIVES

1. Cite the primary action of the calcium ion antagonists.
2. Cite the common side effects that may be observed with the administration of calcium ion antagonists.
3. Discuss the essential patient education needed regarding the management of anginal attacks during the initiation of nifedipine.
4. Develop measurable short- and long-term objectives for patient education for patients receiving calcium ion antagonists.

KEY WORDS

hypotension
peripheral vascular resistance
syncopy

This class of chemicals represents a new approach to controlling heart disease. These agents are known variously as *calcium antagonists, slow channel blockers,* and *calcium ion influx inhibitors.* Regardless of their names, they all share the ability to inhibit the movement of calcium ions across a cell membrane. This results in fewer arrhythmias, a slower rate of contraction of the heart, and relaxation of smooth muscle of blood vessels, resulting in vasodilation. Although each of these agents act by calcium ion inhibition, there are significant differences in their clinical use. This is because they act somewhat differently on coronary blood vessels, systemic blood vessels, the pacemaker cells of the heart and the conducting tissue of the heart. Their clinical effects are also dependent upon the type and severity of the patient's disease. The calcium ion antagonists are classified by structure: benzthiazepines—diltiazem; diaminopropanol ether—bepridil; diphenylalkylamines—Verapamil; and dihydropyridines—felodipine, isradipine, nicardipine, nifedipine, and nimodipine.

bepridil (bhep-rid'il)

Vascor (vas-cohr')

Bepredil is the first of a new chemical class of calcium ion antagonists, the diaminopropanol ether group. It is unique among calcium ion antagonists in that it also slows sodium ion influx into the cells. Bepridil produces significant coronary artery vasodilation and modest peripheral vasodilation, while slowing heart rate and force of contraction. Since it improves coronary blood flow, decreases heart rate, and has no effect on cardiac output, blood pressure, or systemic peripheral resistance, it is used as an antianginal agent. Because it may induce serious ventricular arrhythmias, and because cases of agranulocytosis have been reported, the use of bepridil is reserved for patients who have failed to respond effectively to the nitrates and beta blocker therapy for angina pectoris.

Side effects. The most frequently reported adverse reactions associated with bepridil therapy include nausea, dyspepsia, diarrhea, dizziness, headache, tremor, and nervousness.

Potentially life-threatening arrhythmias have developed in patients receiving bepridil. Hypokalemia was also often present. It is recommended that if diuretic therapy is required, low doses be used, the use of a potassium-sparing diuretic be considered, and the serum potassium be monitored closely.

Although the frequency of agranulocytosis is quite low, the potential for life-threatening infections is quite significant. Routine laboratory studies (WBC with differential) must be regularly scheduled and monitored.

Availability

PO—200, 300, and 400 mg tablets.

Dosage and administration

Adult

PO—Initially, 200 mg daily with a meal or at bedtime. After 10 days, adjust upward to a maximum of 400 mg daily. Most patients require 300 mg daily.

- **Nursing Interventions: Monitoring bepridil therapy**

See also General Nursing Considerations for Patients with Cardiovascular Disease (p. 242) and Monitoring Patients Receiving Calcium Ion Antagonists (p. 267).

diltiazem (dil'ty'az-em)

Cardizem (kar'dih-zem)

Diltiazem is a calcium antagonist chemically unrelated to other members of this class of therapeutic agents. Its mechanisms of action are unknown, but it slows the heart rate and causes vasodilation of coronary and peripheral blood vessels, improving oxygenation to these tissues. Diltiazem is currently being used to treat angina pectoris in patients who do not receive therapeutic relief from nitrates or beta adrenergic blocker therapy. The sustained release capsule is also approved for treatment of essential hypertension.

Side effects. The following side effects, although relatively infrequent (less than 3%), have been reported: nausea, swelling and edema, arrhythmias, headache, rash, and fatigue. Bradycardia, hypotension, congestive heart failure, mental depression, confusion, hallucinations, pruritus, petechiae, urticaria, photosensitivity, and paresthesias have all been reported but with an incidence of less than 1%.

Availability

PO—30, 60, 90, and 120 mg tablets; 60, 90, and 120 mg sustained-release capsules.

Dosage and administration

Adult

ANGINA PECTORIS

PO—Initially 30 mg 4 times daily before meals and at bedtime. The dosage is gradually increased to 60 mg 4 times daily at 1 to 2 day intervals.

NOTE: Patients may continue nitroglycerin therapy for acute anginal attacks while being stabilized on diltiazem therapy.

HYPERTENSION

PO—Initially, 60 to 120 mg sustained release capsule twice daily. Adjust as needed after 14 days. Optimum dosage range is 240 to 360 mg daily.

• **Nursing Interventions: Monitoring diltiazem therapy**

See also General Nursing Considerations for Patients with Cardiovascular Disease (p. 242) and Monitoring Patients Receiving Calcium Ion Antagonists (p. 267).

felodipine (fehl-od'ih-peen)

Plendil (plen-dil')

Felodipine is a member of the dihydropyridine class of calcium ion antagonists. It is approved for use in the treatment of essential hypertension, either alone or in combination with other antihypertensive agents.

Side effects. The most frequently reported adverse reactions associated with felodipine therapy include pheripheral edema and headache.

Availability

PO—5 and 10 mg tablets.

Dosage and administration

Adult

PO—Initially, 5 mg daily. After 14 days, adjust upward to a maximum of 20 mg one time daily. Most patients require 5 to 10 mg daily. Swallow the tablet whole, do not crush. Mild gingival hyperplasia has been reported; good oral hygiene will minimize incidence and severity.

• **Nursing Interventions: Monitoring felodipine therapy**

See also General Nursing Considerations for Patients with Cardiovascular Disease (p. 242) and Monitoring Patients Receiving Calcium Ion Antagonists (p. 267).

isradipine (iz-rad'ih-peen)

DynaCirc (dyn-ah-serk')

Isradipine is a member of the dihydropyridine class of calcium ion antagonists. It has a particular affinity for the calcium channels of the peripheral vascular smooth muscle causing vasodilation. Since it has a minimal effect on cardiac conduction and contractility, it does not produce myocardial depression to the extent that other calcium ion antagonists such as verapamil do. It is approved for use in the treatment of essential hypertension, either alone or in combination with thiazide diuretics.

Side effects. The most frequently reported adverse reactions associated with isradipine therapy include flushing, headache, tachycardia, dizziness, and ankle edema.

Availability

PO—2.5 and 5 mg tablets.

Dosage and administration

Adult

PO—Initially, 2.5 mg two times daily. Maximal response may require 2 to 4 weeks of therapy. If the desired response is not achieved in this time period, the dose may be adjusted in increments of 5 mg per day at 2- to 4-week intervals. Maximum daily dose is 20 mg, but most patients respond well to 10 mg daily.

• **Nursing Interventions: Monitoring isradipine therapy**

See also General Nursing Considerations for Patients with Cardiovascular Disease (p. 242) and Monitoring Patients Receiving Calcium Ion Antagonists (p. 267).

nicardipine (neye-card'ih-peen)

Cardene (car-deen')

Nicardipine is a member of the dihydropyridine class of calcium ion antagonists. It reduces coronary artery vascular resistance and peripheral vascular resistance, making it effective for the treatment of both angina pectoris and hypertension.

Side effects. Most of the adverse effects of nicardipine therapy are related to its potent peripheral vasodilator properties and include flushing, headache, tachycardia, dizziness, diaphoresis, and ankle edema. These adverse effects are more common within the first few weeks of therapy and diminish with continued therapy.

Due to peripheral vasodilation, nicardipine produces a reflex increase in heart rate. This tachycardia may actually induce more angina pectoris. Dosage reduction or a change to other therapy may be required.

Availability

PO—20 and 30 mg capsules

Dosage and administration

Adult

ANGINA PECTORIS AND ESSENTIAL HYPERTENSION

PO—Initially, 20 mg three times daily. Maximal response may require 2 weeks of therapy. If the desired response is not achieved in this time period, an increase to 30 or 40 mg three times daily may be instituted. The dose of nicardipine should be determined by measuring the patient's blood pressure at trough (about 8 hours after the last dose). Peak effect is determined by measuring blood pressure 1 to 2 hours after dosage administration.

• **Nursing Interventions: Monitoring nicardipine therapy**

See also General Nursing Considerations for Patients with Cardiovascular Disease (p. 242) and Monitoring Patients Receiving Calcium Ion Antagonists (p. 267).

nifedipine (ny-fed'i-peen)

Procardia (pro-kar'dee-ah)

Nifedipine is a calcium ion antagonist structurally related to the dihydropyridines. Its mechanisms of action are unknown, but it is a potent vasodilator of coronary and peripheral arteries. It reduces peripheral vascular resistance, thus reducing systolic and diastolic blood pressure, and improves blood flow and oxygenation to the coronary tissues. Nifedipine is currently being used to treat patients with angina pectoris who do not respond adequately to nitrates or beta adrenergic agents. Nifedipine has the advantage of not slowing the heart rate and thus can be used more effectively in patients with a reduced heart rate and in combination with digitalis and beta adrenergic blocking agents. It is also being tested investigationally as treatment for migraine headaches, Raynaud's syndrome and congestive heart failure.

Side effects. When starting therapy or increasing doses, patients report an increased frequency of angina pectoris. The cause of this is unknown. Sublingual nitroglycerin therapy should be continued until the dosage is stabilized.

The following are the most common side effects and occur in about 10% of patients: dizziness, light-headedness, peripheral edema, nausea, weakness, headache, and flushing. Transient hypotension develops in about 5%, palpitations in 2%, and syncope in 0.5% of patients. Hypotension and peripheral edema occur more frequently in patients receiving higher dosages of nifedipine.

Other adverse effects that develop in less than 2% of patients include nasal and chest congestion, constipation, cramps, fever and chills, sweating, urticaria, pruritus, nervousness, and sleep disturbances.

Availability

PO—10 and 20 mg capsules; 30, 60, and 90 mg sustained-release tablets.

Dosage and administration

Adult

PO—Initially 10 mg 3 times daily. Adjust the dosage upward over the next 7 to 14 days to balance between antianginal and hypotensive activity. The usual effective dose is 10 to 20 mg 3 times daily. Dosages above 180 mg are not recommended. Sustained release tablets may be administered once daily. Do not exceed 120 mg daily. Sublingual nitroglycerin therapy may be continued for acute anginal attacks, especially during adjustment of dosages.

• Nursing Interventions: Monitoring nifedipine therapy

See also General Nursing Considerations for Patients with Cardiovascular Disease (p. 242) and Monitoring Patients Receiving Calcium Ion Antagonists (p. 267).

nimodipine (nim-od'ih-peen)

Nimotop (nim-oh'top)

Nimodipine is a member of the dihydropyridine class of calcium ion antagonists. Due to high lipid solubility, it readily crosses the blood-brain barrier where it has a high affinity for cerebral blood vessels. It has been found to be effective in reducing the complications associated with subarachnoid hemorrhage secondary to a ruptured intracranial aneurysm. The exact mechanism is not known, but it is hypothesized that dilation of small cerebral resistance vessels, with a resultant increase in collateral circulation, and/or a direct effect involving prevention of calcium overload in neurons causes the beneficial effects.

Side effects. Adverse effects of nimodipine therapy occur in about 11% of patients receiving oral therapy. The most common adverse effects of nimodipine is decreased blood pressure, headache, and peripheral edema.

Availability

PO—30 mg liquid capsules.

Dosage and administration

PO—Begin therapy within 96 hours of subarachnoid hemorrhage; administer 60 mg every 4 hours for 21 consecutive days. If the patient cannot swallow the capsule, the contents of the liquid capsule may be extracted using an 18 gauge needle on a syringe. The contents can then be injected into a nasogastric tube and rinsed in with 30 ml of normal saline solution.

• Nursing Interventions: Monitoring nimodipine therapy

See also General Nursing Considerations for Patients with Cardiovascular Disease (p. 242) and Monitoring Patients Receiving Calcium Ion Antagonists (p. 267).

verapamil hydrochloride (ver-ap'a-mil)

Calan, Isoptin (ka'lan, ice-op'tin)

Verapamil is a calcium ion antagonist structurally unrelated to other available calcium antagonists. Its mechanisms of action are unknown, but it slows electrical conduction across the atrioventricular node, reducing rapid ventricular rate caused by atrial flutter or atrial fibrillation. It also produces coronary and peripheral arterial vasodilation, resulting in improved myocardial oxygenation. Verapamil is currently being used to treat angina pectoris and arrhythmias that are initiated within atrial tissue. It is a class IV antiarrhythmic agent. It is also approved for use in treating essential hypertension and is also being studied for treatment of migraine headaches.

Side effects. The following side effects have been reported with oral verapamil therapy: constipation (6.3%), dizziness (3.6%), hypotension (2.9%), headache (1.8%), peripheral edema (1.7%), nausea (1.6%), fatigue (1.1%), bradycardia (1.1%), and complete atrioventricular heart block (0.8%).

The following side effects have been reported with IV verapamil therapy: hypotension (1.5%), bradycardia (1.2%), dizziness and headache (1.2%), severe tachycardia (1.0%), nausea (0.9%), and abdominal discomfort (0.6%).

Availability

PO—40, 80, and 120 mg tablets; 180, 240 mg sustained-release tablets.

IV—2.5 mg/ml in 2 and 4 ml ampules and prefilled syringes.

Dosage and administration

Adult

PO—Initially 80 mg 3 to 4 times daily. Increase weekly until an optimal clinical response is achieved. The total daily dose ranges from 240 to 480 mg. Most patients will require 320 to 480 mg daily. Sustained-release tablets are initiated at 120 to 240 mg once daily in the morning. As dosages are adjusted, an additional 120 to 240 mg may be required in the evening. Give dosages with food.

IV—Initially 5 to 10 mg administered over 2 to 3 minutes with continuous ECG monitoring. Additional doses of 10 mg every 30 minutes may be administered if therapeutic activity has not been achieved. Administer each dose over 3 minutes.

NOTE: Sublingual nitroglycerin therapy may be continued for acute anginal attacks.

Pediatric

IV—Newborn to 1 year of age: 0.1 to 0.2 mg/kg over 2 minutes with continuous ECG monitoring. 1 to 15 years of age: 0.1 to 0.3 mg/kg over 2 minutes with continuous ECG monitoring. Do not exceed 5 mg. Repeat above doses 30 minutes after the first dose if the initial response is not adequate.

• Nursing Interventions: Monitoring verapamil therapy

See also General Nursing Considerations for Patients with Cardiovascular Disease (p. 242) and Monitoring Patients Receiving Calcium Ion Antagonists (below).

Monitoring patients receiving calcium ion antagonists

Side effects to report

ANGINAL ATTACKS. Monitor patients taking calcium ion antagonists for an increase in anginal attacks during initiation of the medication or during dosage adjustments. Reduce patients' fears by assuring them that once the dosage is stabilized, the frequency of these attacks will subside.

Assess for frequency, location, duration, and intensity of anginal pain and have the patient *continue* to take the nitroglycerin sublingually when attacks occur.

HYPOTENSION AND SYNCOPY. Caution the patient that for the first week or so he may experience hypotension and syncopy. These side effects decline once the dosage is stabilized.

Take blood pressure readings every shift in the hospitalized patient and stress the need for the patient to monitor it after discharge.

Prevent hypotensive episodes by having the patient rise slowly from a supine or sitting position and perform exercises to prevent blood pooling when standing or sitting in one position for prolonged periods. If the patient feels "faint," have him or her sit or lie down.

EDEMA. Assess the patient for development of edema. Perform daily weights:

1. At the same time
2. In similar clothing
3. On the same scale

Report increases in weight to the physician for further evaluation.

AGRANULOCYTOSIS. (Bepridil) Routine laboratory studies (WBC with differential counts) should be scheduled. Stress that the patient return for this laboratory work.

Monitor for the development of a sore throat, fever, purpura, jaundice, or excessive, progressive weakness.

Implementation

DOSAGE ADJUSTMENTS. See individual drugs for dosage parameters. Adjustments are made based upon the individual patient's response to therapy.

Remember that anginal attacks may increase during dosage adjustments; sublingual nitroglycerin should be continued for these episodes.

Drug interactions

DRUGS THAT ENHANCE THERAPEUTIC AND TOXIC EFFECTS. Beta adrenergic blocking agents (propranolol, atenolol, nadolol, pindolol, others). Histamine H_2 antagonists (cimetidine, ranitidine). Assess the patient for hypotension, light-headedness, dizziness, and bradycardia.

Provide for patient safety; prevent falls.

OTHER INTERACTIONS. Digitalis glycosides. Calcium ion antagonists may increase serum levels of digitalis glycosides.

Monitor the patient for symptoms of anorexia, nausea, vomiting, headaches, blurred or colored vision, and bradycardia. The physician may order a digitalis serum level.

Antihypertensive agents. The vasodilating action of the calcium ion antagonists and antihypertensive agents may result in excessive hypotensive effects. Assess blood pressure at regular intervals to monitor the combined effects.

Glucose metabolism. The dosage of oral hypoglycemic agents may require adjustment in non-insulin-dependent diabetes mellitus (NIDDM) patients.

Assess for signs of hyperglycemia.

Perform urine testing for glucose 4 times per day; report results 1% or above.

Verapamil and disopyramide. DO NOT administer disopyramide 48 hours before or 24 hours after the administration of verapamil.

ANGINA PECTORIS
OBJECTIVES

1. State the major goal of antianginal therapy.
2. Identify the systemic effects to expect when vasodilation of blood vessels occurs.
3. Cite the nursing assessments and interventions needed in caring for patients with angina pectoris.
4. Explain how to evaluate the therapeutic effectiveness of anginal medication and the actions that are needed when an insufficient response occurs.
5. Describe the effect of smoking, hypertension, and obesity on the cardiovascular system.
6. Identify the dosage forms available for administration of vasodilators.
7. Describe the nursing assessments and anticipated side effects that occur with the administration of vasodilator products.
8. Describe procedures for administration of the various forms of nitroglycerin therapy: ointment, topical disk, sublingual tablets, translingual spray, and buccal tablets.
9. Explain the correct storage and handling of nitroglycerin tablets to minimize deterioration.
10. Develop measurable short- and long-term objectives for patient education for patients with angina pectoris.

General Nursing Considerations for Patients with Angina Pectoris

The patient experiencing anginal episodes is apprehensive and frequently becomes discouraged if unable to tolerate exercise or participate in activities of daily living at a pre-illness level. Appropriate use of medications can help these patients approach this goal.

The nurse must carefully perform a baseline assessment of the individual's pattern of anginal pain and the responses exhibited to medical management. Fostering compliance with the patient's total treatment plan is essential to his or her attainment of optimal response. See General Nursing Considerations for Patients with Cardiovascular Disease (p. 242) for further details of assessment.

Patient Concerns: Nursing Intervention/Rationale

Degree of anginal pain relief. Monitor and record the following data relative to the pain relief achieved from the medication:

1. Number of pain attacks per day (per shift while hospitalized)
2. Length of time between taking the medication and relief of anginal symptoms
3. Degree of pain relief achieved (partial or complete)
4. Number of times sublingual doses were repeated before relief was achieved
5. Any particular activities that usually precipitate the anginal pain; suggest taking sublingual nitroglycerin, if ordered, prior to undertaking the activity

Patient Education Associated with Therapy for Angina Pectoris

Communication and responsibility. Encourage open communication concerning frustrations and anger as the patient attempts to adjust to the diagnosis and need for prolonged treatment. The patient must be guided to gain insight into the condition in order to assume responsibility for the continuation of treatment. Keep emphasizing those factors the patient can control to alter progression of the disease.

Smoking. Smoking causes vasoconstriction; therefore, encourage drastic reduction and preferably total abstinence from smoking.

Hypertension. If the disease process is accompanied by hypertension, stress the importance of following prescribed emotional, dietary, and medicinal regimens to control the disease.

Nutrition. The physician usually prescribes dietary modifications aimed at decreasing the cholesterol level and a reducing program to maintain an ideal weight.

Caffeine consumption should be drastically reduced or discontinued. Introduce the patient to decaffeinated products that can substitute for foods containing caffeine.

Expectations of therapy. Discuss the following expectations of therapy with the patient:

Activities and exercise. The patient must resume activities of daily living *within the boundaries* set by the physician. (Such activities as regular, moderate exercise, meal preparation, resumption of usual sexual activities, and social interaction all need to be fostered.)

Individuals who are unable to attain the degree of activity they hoped the drug would allow them to achieve may become frustrated.

Caution the patient *not* to attempt more exercise than recommended once pain relief is attained.

Environment. Tell the patient the importance of dressing warmly, avoiding cold winds, and using a face mask in these conditions to prewarm inhaled air.

Pain relief. The degree of anginal pain relief with and without activity needs to be discussed.

Sexual activity. Encourage the patient to resume sexual activity. Discuss the use of medication or other adjustments for anginal pain before this activity.

Changes in expectations. Assess changes in expectations as therapy progresses and the patient gains understanding and skill in the management of the diagnosis.

Changes in therapy through cooperative goal setting. Work with the patient to encourage adherence to the prescribed treatment. When the patient feels that a change should be made in a treatment plan, encourage discussion first with the physician.

Written record. Enlist the patient's aid in developing and maintaining a written record (Figure 11-1) of monitoring parameters (such as blood pressure, pulse, degree of pain relief, exercise tolerance, and side effects experienced) and response to prescribed therapies for discussion with the physician. Patients should be encouraged to take this record on follow-up visits.

Fostering compliance. Throughout the hospitalization, discuss medication information and how it will benefit the course of treatment. Seek cooperation and understanding of the following points so that medication compliance may be enhanced:

1. Name
2. Dosage
3. Route and administration times
4. Anticipated therapeutic response: Relief of anginal pain
5. Side effects to expect: Flushing of the face and neck, transient throbbing headache. Hypotension: Have the patient rise slowly from a sitting and/or lying position. Weakness, dizziness, or "faintness" can usually be relieved by increasing muscular activity or by sitting or lying down. Resting for 10 to 15 minutes after taking medication may also assist in management of the hypotension.
6. Side effects to report: Always report poor response to medication. The patient may exhibit tolerance to the medication or may need further evaluation of the progression of the disease or re-education on the proper use of the medication (such as proper application of ointment, use of sublingual nitroglycerin prior to undertaking an activity known to precipitate an anginal attack).

   Report episodes of severe hypotension, prolonged headache, and blurred vision.
7. What to do if a dosage is missed
8. When, how, or if to refill the medication prescription

If it is evident that the patient and/or family does not understand all aspects of continuing therapy being prescribed (such as administration and monitoring of medications, exercises, diets, follow-up appointments), consider the use of social service or visiting nurse agencies.

Associated teaching. Give patients the following instructions:

Always inform the physician or dentist of any prescription or over-the-counter medication being taken.

Over-the-counter medications should not be taken without first discussing them with the physician or pharmacist.

Always report side effects of rash, itching, or hives immediately. Nausea, vomiting, or diarrhea should also be reported for the physician's evaluation if it is a new symptom.

Take all of the medication as prescribed for the full course of treatment. Do not discontinue use when feeling improved; do not save for future use; do not give your medicine to another individual. Sudden discontinuation of certain medications may produce harmful effects.

Keep all medications out of the reach of children.

If pregnancy is suspected, consult an obstetrician as soon as possible about continuation of medication therapy.

At discharge. Items to be sent home with the patient should:

1. Have written instructions for use
2. Be labeled in a level of language and size of print appropriate for the patient
3. If needed, include identification cards or bracelets
4. Include a list of additional supplies to be purchased after discharge (such as protective covering, clear plastic, tape)
5. Include a schedule for follow-up appointments

Drug Therapy for Angina Pectoris

The goals in treatment of angina pectoris are: to relieve symptoms; to improve the quality of life; to prevent complications such as sudden death, myocardial infarction, and arrhythmias; and to prolong life expectancy. At the present time, three classes of drugs are used to treat angina: (1) nitrates, (2) beta adrenergic blocking agents (p. 255), and (3) calcium ion antagonists (p. 264). Combination therapy is beneficial in many patients.

The nitrates

The nitrates are the oldest effective therapy for angina pectoris. Although they have been known as *coronary vasodilators*, these agents do not increase total coronary blood flow. First, nitrates relieve angina pectoris by inducing relaxation of peripheral vascular smooth muscles, resulting in dilation of arteries and veins. This results in a diminished venous blood return, which in turn leads to decreased oxygen demands on the heart. Second, nitrates increase myocardial oxygen supply by dilating large coronary arteries and by redistributing blood flow, enhancing oxygen supply to ischemic areas.

Sublingual nitroglycerin is the treatment of choice for an acute anginal episode, but other dosage forms of

Patient Education and Monitoring of Therapeutic Outcomes for Patients Receiving Cardiovascular Agents

Medications	Color	To be taken

Name _____

Physician _____

Physician's phone _____

Next appt.* _____

Parameters		Day of discharge								Comments
Weight	AM / PM									
Blood pressure	AM / PM									
Pulse	AM / PM									
Chest pain	Activity Lasting how long? How many nitroglycerin taken?									
Bowel movements	Normal (times) Diarrhea (times) Constipation									
Fatigue All day ⊢10 ⊢5 After exercise ⊣1 Normal										
Edema	Morning									
	Evening									
	Other									
	Can wear shoes, slippers?									
Visual changes	Clear, hazy, blurred, colored haloes?									
Fainting and dizziness	Standing, sitting, or lying									
Heart beat ("Skips a beat," "racing" feeling or irregular)	Times per day At rest Activity Asleep									
Difficulty breathing	Times per day At rest Activity Asleep (_#_) of pillows?									
Exercise: Degree of tiredness:	Walk across room Walk (_#_) stairs Walk (_#_) blocks									
Extremely ⊢10 ⊢5 Very ⊣1 Normal										
Sexual activity (Note pain experienced in comments at right side.)										
Very tired ⊢10 ⊢5 Tired ⊣1 Normal										

*Please bring this record with you to your next appointment.
Use the back of this sheet for additional information.

Figure 11-1 *Patient education and monitoring of therapeutic outcomes for patients receiving cardio-vascular agents.*

nitrates are available to provide a long duration of action in prophylaxis against anginal attacks.

Side effects. The side effects of the nitrates are an extension of its pharmacologic activity. The most common side effect of the nitrate therapy is headache. This can range from a very mild sensation of fullness in the head to an intense and severe generalized headache. Other possible side effects include dizziness, nausea, flushing, and rarely, syncope or hypotension. Tolerance to the nitrate dosages can develop rapidly, particularly if large doses are administered frequently. Tolerance can appear within a few days and may be well established within a few weeks. The smallest dose to give satisfactory results should be used to minimize the development of tolerance. Tolerance is broken by withdrawing the drug for a short period.

Nitrate preparations

amyl nitrite (am'il ny'tryt)

Amyl nitrite is a volatile liquid, available in small glass ampules. The ampules are encased in a loosely woven material so that the ampule can be easily crushed under the patient's nostrils for inhalation. The onset of action is less than 1 minute, but the duration is only about 10 minutes.

Availability
Inhalation—0.18 ml and 0.3 ml ampules in a woven sack for crushing.

• Nursing Interventions: Monitoring amyl nitrite therapy

See also General Nursing Considerations for Patients with Cardiovascular Disease (p. 242) and see also General Nursing Considerations for Patients with Angina Pectoris (p. 268).

erythrityl tetranitrate (e-rith'ri-til tet-rah-ny'trayt)

Cardilate (kar'di-layt)

Availability
PO—5, 10 mg oral/sublingual tablets

Dosage and administration
Adult
PO—Sublingual: 5 to 10 mg tablet placed under the tongue before anticipated physical or emotional stress.

Oral: If the patient is able to swallow the tablet, therapy should be initiated with 10 mg before each meal, as well as midmorning and midafternoon if needed, and at bedtime for patients subject to nocturnal attacks. The dose may be increased or decreased as needed.

Dosage may be increased up to 100 mg daily, but temporary headache is more apt to occur with increasing doses. If headache occurs, the dose should be reduced for a few days.

• Nursing Interventions: Monitoring eythrityl tetranitrate therapy

See also General Nursing Considerations for Patients with Cardiovascular Disease (p. 242) and Angina Pectoris (p. 268).

isosorbide dinitrate (i-so-sor'byd)

Isordil (i'sor-dil)

Availability
PO—2.5, 5, 10 mg sublingual tablets; 5, 10, 20, 30, 40 mg oral tablets; 5, 10 mg chewable tablets; and 40 mg long-acting oral tablets and capsules.

Dosage and administration
Adult
PO—Sublingual: 5 to 10 mg every 3 hours.
Chewable: Initially 5 mg every 2 to 3 hours.
Oral: Initially 10 mg 4 times daily. Dosage may range up to 30 mg 4 times daily.
Long-acting: Initially 40 mg every 6 hours.

• Nursing Interventions: Monitoring isosorbide therapy

See also General Nursing Considerations for Patients with Cardiovascular Disease (p. 242) and Angina Pectoris (p. 268).

nitroglycerin (ny-tro-glis'er-in)

Glyceryl trinitrate (glis'er-il try-ny'trayt)

Nitroglycerin is currently the drug of choice for treating angina pectoris. It is available in different dosages for adjustment to the patient's needs. Sublingual tablets dissolve quite rapidly and are used primarily for acute attacks of angina. The sustained release tablets and capsules, ointment, transmucosal tablets, and transdermal patches are used prophylactically to prevent anginal attacks. The translingual spray may be used for both acute treatment and prophylaxis of anginal attacks.

Availability
Sublingual—0.15, 0.3, 0.4, and 0.6 mg tablets.
PO—2.5, 6.5, and 9 mg sustained-release tablets and capsules.
Ointment—2%.
Transmucosal—1, 2, and 3 mg tablets.
Transdermal—2.5, 5, 7.5, 10, and 15 mg/24 hr patches.
Translingual—0.4 mg metered spray.
Intravenous—0.5, 0.8, 5, and 10 ml/ml in 5, 10, and 20 ml vials and ampules.

Dosage and administration
Sublingual. 0.15, 0.3, 0.4, or 0.6 mg for prophylactic use before the initiation of activity that may induce angina pectoris, or at the time of an acute anginal attack.

PO. Sustained release tablets or capsules: 1.3, 2.5, or 6.5 mg 2 to 3 times daily at 8 and 12 hour intervals.

Transmucosal tablets. 1 to 2 mg 3 to 6 times daily.

Translingual spray. At the onset of an attack, one or two metered doses are sprayed onto the oral mucosa. The spray may be used to prevent anginal attack by spraying one to two doses onto the oral mucosa 5 to 10 minutes prior to engaging in activities that might precipitate an attack.

Topical ointment. This dosage form is more suitable for patients who suffer from the fear of nocturnal attacks of angina pectoris. If the dosage is adjusted properly, the ointment may be used every 3 to 4 hours and at bedtime.

Transdermal disks. This dosage form provides a controlled release of nitroglycerin through a semipermeable membrane for 24 hours when applied to intact skin. The dosage released is dependent upon the surface area of the disk. Therapeutic effect can be observed about 30 minutes after attachment, and is maintained for about 30 minutes after removal.

Intravenous. This dosage form is diluted and then administered by continuous infusion to treat high blood pressure during surgery, congestive heart failure associated with acute myocardial infarction, angina pectoris in patients who have not responded to other dosage forms of nitroglycerin, and to produce controlled hypotension during certain surgical procedures.

• **Nursing Interventions: Monitoring nitroglycerin therapy**

See also General Nursing Considerations for Patients with Cardiovascular Disease (p. 242) and Angina Pectoris (p. 268).

Side effects to report

PROLONGED HEADACHE, EXCESSIVE HYPOTENSION, TOLERANCE (INCREASING DOSES TO ATTAIN RELIEF). Report these adverse effects so that more appropriate dosage adjustment may be made.

Implementation

SUBLINGUAL

1. Have the patient sit or lie down at the first sign of an oncoming anginal attack.
2. Place a tablet under the tongue and allow it to dissolve; encourage the patient not to swallow the saliva immediately.
3. If more than 3 tablets within 15 minutes are required to control pain, the patient should seek medical attention.
4. One or two tablets may be taken prophylactically a few minutes before engaging in activities that may trigger an anginal attack.
5. Chart the patient's ability to place the sublingual medication under the tongue correctly.

Medication deterioration. Every 3 months, the nitroglycerin prescription should be refilled and the old tablets safely discarded. (Be sure the patient knows how to refill the prescription.)

Medication storage. Store nitroglycerin in the original, dark-colored glass container with a tight lid.

Medication accessibility. Nonhospitalized patients should carry nitroglycerin with them at all times, but not in a pocket directly next to the body, because heat hastens the deterioration of the medication. When taken, the drug should produce a slight "stinging" or "burning" sensation, which usually indicates the drug is still potent.

Allow the hospitalized patient to keep the nitroglycerin at bedside, or on his or her person, if ambulatory. Check hospital policy to see if a fresh supply of medicine should be issued, rather than using the agents brought from home. (Remember, the nurse is still responsible for gathering and charting relevant data regarding all medication taken by the patient when the medication is left at bedside.)

SUSTAINED RELEASE TABLETS. This type of nitroglycerin is best taken on an empty stomach every 8 to 12 hours, as prescribed.

If gastritis develops, it may be necessary to take the sustained release tablet with food.

TRANSMUCOSAL TABLETS. When placed under the upper lip or buccal pouch, it releases nitroglycerin for absorption by the oral mucosa over the next 3 to 5 hours.

Patients may eat, drink, and talk while the tablet is in place.

The usual initial dose is one tablet 3 times daily upon arising, after lunch, and after the evening meal.

Do not administer more than one tablet every 2 hours.

Development of headache, dizziness, and hypotension are indications of overdose.

TRANSLINGUAL SPRAY. Patients should be instructed to familiarize themselves with the position of the spray orifice, which can be identified by the finger rest on top of the valve. This can be particularly helpful for administration at night.

The spray is highly flammable. Do not use it where it might be ignited.

1. At the time of administration, the patient should preferably be in a sitting position.
2. The canister should be held vertically with the valve head uppermost and the spray orifice as close to the mouth as possible.
3. The dose should be sprayed onto the tongue by pressing the button firmly.
4. The mouth should be closed immediately after each dose. THE SPRAY SHOULD NOT BE INHALED.

If more than three doses are required within 15 minutes, medical attention should be sought.

TOPICAL OINTMENT

1. Lay the dose-measuring applicator paper with the printed side down.
2. Squeeze the proper amount of ointment onto the applicator paper.
3. Place the measuring applicator on the skin, ointment down, spreading in a thin, uniform layer. Do

not massage or rub in. Any area without hair may be used; however, many people prefer the chest, flank, or upper arm. (Because of the potential for skin irritation, do not shave an area to apply the medication.)

4. Help the patient develop a site rotation schedule to prevent skin irritation. Stress not applying the ointment to an area that still shows signs of irritation. Use of the applicator allows measuring of the proper dose and also prevents absorption through the fingertips.
5. Cover the area where the patch is placed with a clear plastic wrap and tape in place. (Caution the patient that the medication may discolor clothing.)
6. Close the tube tightly and store in a cool place.
7. When terminating the use of the topical ointment, gradually reduce the dose and frequency of application over 4 to 6 weeks.

TRANSDERMAL DISKS. This dosage form provides a controlled release of nitroglycerin through a semipermeable membrane for 24 hours when applied to intact skin. The dosage released is dependent upon the surface area of the disk. Therapeutic effect can be observed in about 30 minutes after attachment and continues for about 30 minutes after removal.

1. The disk should be applied to a hairless and clean-shaven area of skin on the upper chest or side, pelvis, or inner, upper arm. Avoid scars, skin folds, or wounds. Rotate skin sites daily. (Help the patient develop a rotation chart.)
2. Wash hands before applying and after removing the product.
3. Transderm-Nitro and Nitro-Dur may be worn while showering; Nitrodisc should be replaced after bathing.
4. If a disk becomes partially dislodged, discard it and replace with a new disk.
5. Sublingual nitroglycerin may be necessary for anginal attacks, especially while the dosage is being adjusted.

INTRAVENOUS NITROGLYCERIN. This drug is used in an intensive care setting and requires continuous monitoring of vital signs: blood pressure, pulse, respirations, and central venous pressure.

Use an infusion pump to monitor the precise delivery of the infusion. Dose is titrated to achieve the desired clinical response. Gradual weaning is needed under controlled conditions to prevent a rebound action.

This medication is never mixed with other medications and is administered only with administration sets made specially for nitroglycerin, since most plastic administration sets absorb the drug. See the manufacturer's literature for exact directions recommended for preparation and administration.

Drug interactions
ALCOHOL. Alcohol accentuates the vasodilation and postural hypotension of the nitrates and nitrites. Patients should be warned that drinking alcohol while on therapy may cause hypotension.

pentaerythritol tetranitrate
(pen-tah-e-rith'ri-tol tet-rah-ny'trayt)

❧ **Peritrate** (per'i-trayt) **Pentritol** (pen'tri-tol)

Pentaerythritol tetranitrate is a nitrate derivative that is used for the relief of angina pectoris. It does not relieve the acute anginal episode, but it is widely regarded as useful in the prophylactic treatment of angina pectoris.

Availability
PO—10, 20, 40, and 80 mg tablets; 30, 45, and 80 mg sustained release tablets and capsules.

Dosage and administration
Adult
PO—Initially 10 to 20 mg 4 times daily. Dosage may be adjusted up to 40 mg 4 times daily. Take one-half hour before meals. Tablets may be chewed or swallowed whole.

Alternatively, Peritrate SA (sustained action) can be administered every 12 hours. It should be taken on an empty stomach and *not* chewed.

• **Nursing Interventions: Monitoring pentaerythritol tetranitrate therapy**

See also General Nursing Considerations for Patients with Cardiovascular Disease (p. 242) and Angina Pectoris (p. 268).

PERIPHERAL VASCULAR DISEASE
OBJECTIVES

1. List the baseline assessments needed to evaluate a patient with peripheral vascular disease.
2. Identify specific measures the patient can use to improve peripheral circulation and prevent complications from peripheral vascular disease.
3. Identify the systemic effects to expect when peripheral vasodilating agents are administered.
4. Explain why hypotension and tachycardia occur frequently with the use of peripheral vasodilators.
5. Develop measurable short- and long-term objectives for patient education for patients with peripheral vascular disease.

KEY WORDS

intermittent claudication
vasospasm
Raynaud's disease
arteriosclerosis
thrombophlebitis

The use of vasodilating agents for chronic occlusive arterial disease or peripheral vascular disease has not been encouraging to date. However, several drugs have been used with some success in the treatment of these diseases.

General Nursing Considerations for Patients with Peripheral Vascular Disease

A baseline assessment of the individual patient should be completed. It should include the following data to evaluate the degree of oxygenation that exists in the extremities. Subsequent *regular* assessments should be performed for comparison and analysis of therapeutic effectiveness or lack of response to *all* treatment modalities instituted.

Patient Concerns: Nursing Intervention/Rationale

Assessment of tissue

Oxygenation. Observe the color of each hand, finger, leg, and foot; report cyanosis or reddish-blue locations.

Examine the skin of the extremities for any signs of ulceration.

Temperature. Feel the temperature in each hand, finger, leg, and foot. Report paleness and coldness. (Note that these symptoms will be increased if the limb is elevated above the level of the heart.)

Edema. Report edema and its extent, and whether relieved or unchanged when the limb is in a dependent position.

Peripheral pulses. Record the pedal and radial pulses at least every 4 hours if circulatory impairment is found in that limb. Compare findings between each of the extremities; report diminished or absent pulses immediately. When pulses are difficult to palpate or are absent, use of a Doppler ultrasound device may aid in determining peripheral blood flow.

Limb pain. Monitor pain in the patient carefully. Pain upon exercise that is relieved by rest may be from claudication. Conversely, pain when the patient is at rest may be from sudden obstruction by a thrombus or embolus. Check the apprehension level of the patient, pedal and radial pulses, details of onset and location of pain, vital signs, and whether pain is increased by dorsiflexion of the foot. Until status of patient's limb pain is established, have the patient remain on bedrest, administer analgesic if ordered. Notify physician of findings.

Patient Education for Patients with Peripheral Vascular Therapy

Communication and responsibility. Encourage open communication concerning frustrations and anger as the patient attempts to adjust to the diagnosis and need for prolonged treatment. The patient must be guided to gain insight into the condition in order to assume responsibility for the continuation of treatment. Keep emphasizing those factors that the patient can control to alter the progression of the disease.

Smoking. Smoking causes vasoconstriction of the blood vessels. Therefore, encourage drastic reduction and preferably total abstinence from smoking.

Promoting peripheral circulation. Patients should be taught to maintain posture that will maximize peripheral circulation.

Encourage patients not to wear anything that constricts peripheral blood flow, such as tight-fitting anklets, socks, or garters. Always check with the physician before initiating elevation of the extremities. It is *contraindicated* in patients with *arterial* insufficiency. Tell the patient *not* to elevate the extremities above the level of the heart without specific orders to do so from the physician.

Sitting or standing. Standing or sitting for prolonged periods should be avoided.

Persons who must sit for extended periods of time must have a properly fitting chair. The seat must be of the correct depth so that no pressure is exerted on the popliteal space.

Encourage individuals not to sit with knees or ankles crossed and to take frequent short breaks for walks.

Persons who must stand for long periods of time should seek aspects of the job that can be performed sitting down in a properly fitting chair or other alternatives.

For the hospitalized patient, do not place pillows in the popliteal space or flex the knee-rest on the bed.

Limb pain. Meticulous foot and hand care are essential. The need to inspect the extremities for possible skin breakdown or signs of infection must be stressed. Notify the physician immediately of sudden changes in color, such as mottling or a more purplish color. Cold temperatures will increase pain or decrease sensations in the extremities.

Areas of discoloration in nails, cracking of skin, callouses, or blisters on the extremities need complete follow-up. Listen to the patient's description of changes he or she has noted. Tell the patient that going barefoot can be dangerous because of potential injuries to the feet.

Because of the possible decrease in sensation in the extremities, encourage the patient to test the water temperature prior to immersing the hands or feet. Following bathing, gently pat, do not vigorously rub, the feet and hands to dry them.

Patients should alternate pairs of shoes to allow for thorough drying between wearings, change socks or hose daily, and avoid rubber-soled shoes.

If the patient is hospitalized, use a cradle or footboard to prevent bedsheets from constricting the circulation. Show the patient or family how to improvise a footboard at home.

The physician may order the foot of the patient's bed elevated at night. Encourage the patient to maintain good posture and to sleep on a firm mattress.

UNABOOT or TED stockings may also be employed to promote circulation.

Activity and exercise. Maximum mobility should be maintained. Devise a daily activity plan that includes walks and usual activities of daily living, such as shopping and housework.

Environment. During periods of exposure to cold temperature, the patient should wear several layers of lightweight clothing. Caution needs to be exercised during exposure to the cold to avoid frostbite. Because of decreased sensations in the extremities, frostbite can occur without the patient's awareness.

Pain relief. Pain management and the psychological aspects of dealing with a prolonged illness with persistent symptoms are a major challenge to the patient and the nurse. (See Chapter 9 for pain management information.)

Nutritional status. Dietary education is indicated in the treatment of peripheral vascular disease. It is particularly important to control obesity and cholesterol and triglyceride levels.

When ulcerations are present, encourage a high protein diet with adequate intake of vitamins to promote the healing process.

Unless other medical conditions contraindicate, have the patient drink eight 8-ounce glasses of water daily to promote adequate hydration of body tissues. This will help reduce peripheral vasoconstriction.

Caffeine does not necessarily have to be limited unless other coexisting conditions warrant it.

Expectations of therapy. Discuss expectations of therapy with the patient: degree of pain relief, ability to work, maintenance of mobility, and exercise tolerance that the drug regimen and preventive measures will permit.

Encourage the patient to express *feelings* with regard to this chronic illness. The adjustment to this situation involves working through great personal fears, frustrations, hostilities, and resentments associated with the loss of control within one's life.

Changes in expectations. Assess changes in expectations as therapy progresses and the patient gains understanding and skill in the management of the diagnosis.

Changes in therapy through cooperative goal setting. Work with the patient to encourage adherence to the prescribed treatment. When the patient feels that a change should be made in a treatment plan, encourage discussion first with the physician.

Written record. Enlist the patient's aid in developing and maintaining a written record of monitoring parameters (Figure 11-2) (such as degree of numbness, color, and temperature of extremities, degree of pain relief, exercise tolerance), and response to prescribed therapies for discussion with the physician. Encourage patients to take this record on follow-up visits.

Fostering compliance. Throughout the hospitaliza-

tion, discuss medication information and how it will benefit the course of treatment.

Stress the importance of all measures taught (stopping smoking, promotion of peripheral circulation, activity and exercise, and nutritional actions) to promote maximum peripheral vascular circulation and prevention of further tissue damage.

Seek cooperation and understanding of the following points so that medication compliance may be enhanced:

1. Name
2. Dosage
3. Route and administration times
4. Anticipated therapeutic response
5. Side effects to expect
6. Side effects to report
7. What to do if a dosage is missed
8. When, how, or if to refill the prescription

Difficulty in comprehension. If it is evident that the patient and/or family does not understand all aspects of continuing therapy being prescribed (such as administration and monitoring of medications, exercises, diets, follow-up appointments), consider the use of social service or visiting nurse agencies.

Associated teaching. Give patients the following instructions:

Always inform the physician or dentist of any prescription or over-the-counter medication being taken. Over-the-counter medications should not be taken without first discussing them with the physician or pharmacist.

Always report side effects of rash, itching, or hives immediately. Nausea, vomiting, or diarrhea should also be reported for the physician's evaluation if it is a new symptom.

Take all of the medication as prescribed for the full course of treatment. Do not discontinue use when feeling improved; do not save for future use; do not give your medicine to another individual. Sudden discontinuation of certain medications may produce harmful effects.

Keep all medications out of the reach of children.

If pregnancy is suspected, consult an obstetrician as soon as possible about continuation of medication therapy.

At discharge. Items to be sent home with the patient should:

1. Have written instructions for use
2. Be labeled in a level of language and size of print appropriate for the patient
3. If needed, include identification cards or bracelets
4. Include a list of additional supplies to be purchased after discharge

Patient Education and Monitoring of Therapeutic Outcomes for Patients Receiving Vasodilators

Medications	Color	To be taken

Name _____

Physician _____

Physician's phone _____

Next appt.* _____

Parameters			Day of discharge								Comments
Weight											
Blood pressure											
Pulse (take for 1 full minute)											
Color of limbs	N = Normal P = Pale M = Mottled B = Blue	Left hand / Right hand Left foot / Right foot									
Pain in limb	Stress										
	Exercise										
	Resting										
	When cold										
	Dull ache										
	Sharp pain										
Intense 10	Moderate 5	Slight 1									
Limb pulse	Feel every beat; can count										
	Feel beats; cannot count										
	No pulse felt										
Temperature in normal position											
Cold, pale 10	Cooler than rest of limb 5	Warm 1									
Edema	More if hanging down										
	Present all the time										
Exercise	Normal Walk (_#_) stairs Walk (_#_) blocks										

*Please bring this record with you to your next appointment.
Use the back of this sheet for additional information.

Figure 11-2 *Patient education and monitoring of therapeutic outcomes for patients receiving vasodilators.*

5. Include a schedule of appointments for follow-up visits

Drug Therapy for Peripheral Vascular Disease

cyclandelate (si-klan′de-layt)

Cyclospasmol (si-klo-spaz′mol)

Cyclandelate has a direct relaxation effect on the smooth muscles of peripheral arterial blood vessels, increasing circulation to the extremities. It is considered "possibly" effective in treating patients with intermittent claudication, arteriosclerosis obliterans, vasospasm associated with thrombophlebitis, nocturnal leg cramps, and Raynaud's disease.

Side effects. Side effects include flushing, tingling, sweating, dizziness, headache, feeling of weakness, and tachycardia. These side effects tend to be more common during the first weeks of therapy and to resolve with continued therapy.

Since cyclandelate is a vasodilator, it should be used with caution in patients with glaucoma.

Availability

PO—200 and 400 mg capsules.

Dosage and administration

PO—It is often advantageous to initiate therapy at higher dosages: 1200 to 1600 mg daily in divided doses before meals and at bedtime. When a clinical response is noted, the dosage can be decreased in 200 mg increments until the maintenance dosage is reached. The usual maintenance dose is between 400 and 800 mg per day in 2 to 4 divided doses.

• Nursing Interventions: Monitoring cyclandelate therapy

See also General Nursing Considerations for Patients with Peripheral Vascular Disease (p. 274).

Side effects to expect

FLUSHING, TINGLING, SWEATING. Explain to the patient that these side effects may occur during the initial phase of therapy; however, these symptoms resolve with continued therapy.

Implementation

PO. Administer at meals or with milk to decrease gastric irritation.

Drug interactions. None specifically associated with cyclandelate have been reported.

isoxsuprine hydrochloride (i-sok′su-preen)

Vasodilan (vas-o-dy′lan)

Isoxsuprine hydrochloride is a sympathomimetic agent that causes relaxation of the smooth muscles of the blood vessels. It is used to treat the symptoms of peripheral vascular spasm, cerebral vascular insufficiency, Raynaud's and Buerger's diseases, and arteriosclerosis obliterans.

Side effects. Adverse effects are quite infrequent, but occasionally a patient may complain of flushing, hypotension, tachycardia, nausea, vomiting, dizziness, abdominal distress, or a severe rash. If a rash does appear, discontinue the medication. As the dosage is increased, more patients tend to complain of nervousness and weakness.

Dosage and administration

Adult

PO—10 to 20 mg 3 or 4 times daily.

IM—5 to 10 mg 2 or 3 times daily. Intramuscular administration may be used initially in acute conditions.

• Nursing Interventions: Monitoring isoxsuprine therapy

See also General Nursing Considerations for Patients with Peripheral Vascular Disease (p. 274).

Side effects to expect

FLUSHING, TINGLING, SWEATING, NAUSEA, VOMITING. Explain to the patient that these side effects may occur during the initial phase of therapy; however, these symptoms resolve with continued therapy.

Side effects to report

HYPOTENSION, TACHYCARDIA. Monitor blood pressure and pulse throughout the course of therapy.

Prevent hypotensive episodes by having the patient rise slowly from a supine or sitting position, and perform exercises to prevent blood pooling when standing or sitting in one position for prolonged periods. Have the patient sit or lie down if feeling "faint."

SEVERE RASH. Discontinue medication if a severe rash develops. Notify the physician so that appropriate alternate agents may be prescribed.

NERVOUSNESS AND WEAKNESS. As therapy progresses, these symptoms may develop. Tell the patient to discuss them with the physician if they become a problem.

Drug interactions

DRUGS THAT ENHANCE THERAPEUTIC AND TOXIC EFFECTS. Antihypertensive agents:

The vasodilating action of isoxsuprine and antihypertensive agents may result in excessive hypotensive effects.

Assess the blood pressure at regular intervals to monitor the combined effects.

Monitor the patient for hypotension, light-headedness, dizziness, and tachycardia.

Provide for patient safety; prevent falls.

DRUGS THAT REDUCE THERAPEUTIC EFFECTS. Warn the patient against taking over-the-counter cough and cold preparations without first consulting the physician or pharmacist. Many of these products will counteract the effects of isoxsuprine.

papaverine hydrochloride (pah-pav′er-in)

Pavabid (pah-vah′bid)

Papaverine is a drug that has been tried for many illnesses for many years. Even so, there is very little objective evidence to indicate that it has any therapeutic value. Pharmacologically, it relaxes smooth muscle, vasodilates cerebral and coronary blood vessels, and inhibits atrial and ventricular premature contractions, and ventricular arrhythmias.

Papaverine is used orally as a smooth muscle relaxant to treat cerebral and peripheral ischemia associated with arterial spasm, and myocardial ischemia complicated by arrhythmias.

Side effects. Side effects are usually quite mild and are dose-related. Most common are facial flushing, sweating, nausea, abdominal distress, tachycardia, vertigo, drowsiness, headache, and sedation.

Availability

PO—30, 60, 100, 150, 200, and 300 mg tablets 150 mg timed release capsules; 200 mg timed release tablets.

IV—30 mg/ml in 2 ml ampules and 10 ml vials.

Dosage and administration

Adult

PO—60 to 300 mg 1 to 5 times daily. Timed release products: 150 mg every 12 hours. In difficult cases, increase to 150 mg every 8 hours, or 300 mg every 12 hours.

- **Nursing Interventions: Monitoring papaverine therapy**

See also General Nursing Considerations for Patients with Peripheral Vascular Disease (p. 274).

Side effects to expect and report

FLUSHING, SWEATING, NAUSEA, ABDOMINAL DISTRESS, TACHYCARDIA, VERTIGO, DROWSINESS, HEADACHE. These side effects are usually quite mild and are dose related.

Monitor vital signs (blood pressure, pulse, and respirations) and report deviations from baseline data for the physician's evaluation.

Drug interactions

DRUGS THAT ENHANCE THERAPEUTIC AND TOXIC EFFECTS. Antihypertensive agents:

The vasodilating action of papaverine and antihypertensive agents may result in excessive hypotensive effects.

Assess the blood pressure at regular intervals to monitor the combined effects.

Monitor the patient for hypotension, light-headedness, dizziness, and tachycardia.

Provide for patient safety; prevent falls.

DRUGS THAT REDUCE THERAPEUTIC EFFECTS. Warn the patient against taking over-the-counter cough and cold preparations without first consulting the physician or pharmacist. Many of these products will counteract the effects of papaverine.

phenoxybenzamine hydrochloride
(fe-nok-se-ben′zah-meen)

Dibenzyline (di-ben′zi-leen)

Phenoxybenzamine is an alpha adrenergic blocking agent that relaxes the smooth muscle of blood vessels,

resulting in vasodilation and improved blood flow to peripheral tissues. It is used in blood vessel disorders, such as Raynaud's disease, leg ulceration, and the complications of frostbite.

Side effects. Severity of side effects is usually dependent upon the dosage administered. Common side effects include nasal stuffiness, miosis, hypotension, and tachycardia. Nausea and vomiting occasionally occur.

Availability

PO—10 mg capsules.

Dosage and administration

Adult

PO—Initially 10 mg per day. After determining response for 4 or more days, increase the dose by 10 mg increments every few days to a maximum of 60 mg per day. Several weeks of therapy are usually needed to observe full therapeutic benefits.

- **Nursing Interventions: Monitoring phenoxybenzamine therapy**

See also General Nursing Considerations for Patients with Peripheral Vascular Disease (p. 274).

Side effects to expect and report

NASAL STUFFINESS, MIOSIS, HYPOTENSION, AND TACHYCARDIA. Monitor blood pressure and pulse.

Prevent hypotensive episodes by having the patient rise slowly from a supine or sitting position, and perform exercises to prevent blood pooling when standing or sitting in one position for prolonged periods. Have the patient sit or lie down if feeling "faint."

Report increasing episodes so that dosage is adjusted accordingly.

Drug interactions

DRUGS THAT ENHANCE THERAPEUTIC AND TOXIC EFFECTS. Antihypertensive agents and alcohol:

The vasodilating action of phenoxybenzamine and antihypertensive agents may result in excessive hypotensive effects.

Assess the blood pressure at regular intervals to monitor the combined effects.

Monitor the patient for hypotension, light-headedness, dizziness, and tachycardia.

Provide for patient safety; prevent falls.

DRUGS THAT REDUCE THERAPEUTIC EFFECTS. Warn the patient against taking over-the-counter cough and cold preparations without first consulting the physician or pharmacist. Many of these products will counteract the effects of phenoxybenzamine.

tolazoline (tol-az′o-leen)

Priscoline (pris′ko-leen)

Tolazoline acts directly on the smooth muscle of the blood vessels to produce vasodilation and increased blood flow. It is used to improve the circulation of patients with diabetes, Raynaud's disease, chronic ulcers, gangrene, frostbite, and other spastic peripheral vascular diseases. It should be used cautiously in patients with ulcers, because it also causes stimulation of gastric secretions that might aggravate the ulcers.

Side effects. Side effects are generally mild and usually decrease progressively during continued therapy. The most common response is flushing of the face, neck, chest, and back as a result of dilation of blood vessels. Other infrequent reactions include arrhythmias, tachycardia, anginal pain, nausea, vomiting, diarrhea, and, rarely, psychiatric reactions characterized by confusion or hallucinations.

Availability

Parenteral—25 mg/ml in 4 ml ampules.

Dosage and administration

Adult

IV, SC, IM—Dosage must be individualized. General dosage requirements are 10 to 50 mg 4 times daily. Start with lower dosages, increasing gradually until therapeutic response (localized flushing) is observed. Keeping the patient warm will often increase effectiveness of the medication.

• **Nursing Interventions: Monitoring tolazoline therapy**

See also General Nursing Considerations for Patients with Peripheral Vascular Disease (p. 274).

Side effects to expect

FLUSHING OF THE FACE, NECK, CHEST, AND BACK. Tell the patient to expect that these areas will become increasingly red; this is a desirable effect.

Keeping the patient warm enhances the effectiveness of the drug.

TINGLING, SWEATING, NAUSEA, VOMITING. Explain to the patient that these side effects may occur during the initial phase of therapy; however, these symptoms are self-limiting.

Side effects to report

ARRHYTHMIAS, TACHYCARDIA, ANGINAL PAIN. Monitor the pulse rate and report changes in rhythm.

Anginal pain should be reported and the time of onset, frequency, duration, and intensity documented in the nurse's notes for hospitalized patients.

CONFUSION, HALLUCINATIONS. These adverse effects are quite rare, but monitor patients carefully for progressive symptoms of restlessness, agitation, anxiety, hallucinations, and euphoria.

Act calmly with the excited, anxious, or euphoric patient. Provide safety and fulfillment of his or her needs.

Report this alteration in the patient's response to the physician as soon as possible.

Drug interactions

DRUGS THAT ENHANCE THERAPEUTIC AND TOXIC EFFECTS. Antihypertensive agents and alcohol:

The vasodilating action of tolazoline and antihypertensive agents may result in excessive hypotensive effects.

Assess the blood pressure at regular intervals to monitor the combined effects.

Monitor the patient for hypotension, light-headedness, dizziness, and tachycardia.

Provide for patient safety; prevent falls.

DRUGS THAT REDUCE THERAPEUTIC EFFECTS. Warn the patient against taking over-the-counter cough and cold preparations without first consulting the physician or pharmacist. Many of these products will counteract the effects of tolazoline.

HYPERTENSION
OBJECTIVES

1. Differentiate among mild, moderate, and severe hypertension.
2. Identify four types of drugs used to treat hypertension.
3. Define the *stepped-care* approach used for treatment of hypertension.
4. Identify specific factors the hypertensive patient can use to assist in the management of the disease.
5. Develop measurable short- and long-term objectives for patient education for patients with hypertension.

KEY WORDS

primary hypertension
stepped-care therapy

Hypertension is a disease characterized by an elevation of the blood pressure above values considered normal for patients of similar racial backgrounds, age, and environment. Statistics in North America show that blood pressures above 140/90 to 150/90 mm Hg are associated with premature death, which results from accelerated vascular disease of the brain, heart, and kidneys.

Primary, or *essential*, hypertension accounts for 80% to 90% of all clinical cases of high blood pressure. The following stratification of hypertension by diastolic blood pressure has become standard:

• Mild—90 to 104 mm Hg
• Moderate—105 to 114 mm Hg
• Severe—115 mm Hg or greater

The etiology of hypertension is unknown. It is uncurable at present, but it is certainly controllable. It is estimated that as many as 58 million people in the United States have hypertension. The prevalence increases steadily with advancing age. In every age group, the incidence of hypertension is higher for black persons than for white persons of both sexes. Other factors associated with high blood pressure are a family history of hypertension, obesity, spikes of high blood pressure in young adult years, cigarette smoking, hyperglycemia, hypercholesterolemia, preexisting cardiovascular disease (angina, congestive heart failure), abnormal renal function, retinopathies, and a history of a previous stroke.

The goal of antihypertensive therapy is to prolong a useful life by preventing cardiovascular complications.

To accomplish this goal, the blood pressure must be reduced and maintained below 140/90 mm Hg, if possible. Treatment schedules should interfere as little as possible with the patient's lifestyle. Nonpharmacologic therapy must include elimination of smoking, weight control, routine activity, restriction of alcohol intake, stress reduction, and sodium control. If this therapy is successful in controlling high blood pressure, drug therapy is often not necessary.

Many drugs are used in the treatment of hypertension, but, in general, only four classes of drugs are used: (1) direct vasodilators, such as hydralazine, minoxidil, and diazoxide; (2) diuretics, such as the thiazides, bumetanide, furosemide, and ethacrynic acid; (3) sympathetic nervous system stimulants and inhibitors, such as guanethidine, reserpine, methyldopa, prazosin, the beta blocking agents, guanabenz, guanfacine, and clonidine; and (4) inhibitors of the renin-angiotensin system, such as captopril and enalapril.

All of these agents act either directly or indirectly to reduce the peripheral vascular resistance, therefore lowering blood pressure. It is routine practice to use two or more antihypertensive medications at a time; using drugs that act by different mechanisms to reduce peripheral vascular resistance provides the benefit of using lower doses of each drug, so that the patient suffers fewer side effects. This is known as the *stepped-care approach*, as recommended by the Joint National Committee on Detection, Evaluation, and Treatment of High Blood Pressure. The first step of treatment after nonpharmacologic measures is the initiation of small doses of a diuretic, a beta blocker, a calcium channel blocker, or an ACE inhibitor together with dietary and exercise instructions. The dose is gradually increased, and then other drugs are sequentially added until the hypertension is controlled (see Figure 11-3).

Addition of subsequent agents is often not necessary because 70% of the adult hypertensive population will respond to diuretics alone. See Table 11-4 for a list of the ingredients of the common antihypertensive combination products.

Patient education is vitally important in treating hypertension. This education should be emphasized and reiterated frequently by the physician, pharmacist, and nurse.

General Nursing Considerations for Patients with Hypertension

Patient Education Associated with Antihypertensive Therapy

Communication and responsibility. Encourage open communication concerning frustrations and anger as the patient attempts to adjust to the diagnosis and need for prolonged treatment. Since the disease process is frequently asymptomatic, the patient usually has difficulty accepting the diagnosis. The patient must be guided to insight into the condition in order to assume responsibility for the continuation of treatment. Keep emphasizing those factors the patient can control to alter the progression of the disease.

Smoking. Suggest that the patient stop smoking entirely. Explain the increased risk of coronary artery disease if the habit is continued. It may be necessary to settle for a drastic decrease in smoking in some persons, although total abstinence should be the goal.

Nutritional status. Dietary counseling is essential in the treatment of hypertension. Control of obesity alone may be sufficient to alter the hypertensive condition. Most patients are placed on a reduced sodium, low fat, and low calorie diet. The goal of dietary therapy is a reduction of cholesterol, lipids, saturated fats, caffeine, and alcohol consumpton. Foods high in potassium and calcium are encouraged to decrease blood pressure. (Refer to Appendix J for foods high in potassium and/or low in sodium.)

Dietary planning should always involve the patient in menu planning so that personal preferences, availability of food products, and cost are discussed. Also include the person who actually purchases as well as prepares the meals in the dietary counseling.

Show the patient various food labels and explain which words to watch for that would indicate a high sodium content (such as salt, sodium, sodium chloride, sodium bicarbonate, sodium aluminum sulfate). Suggest the use of a variety of spices as substitutes for sodium when cooking. Explain foods that should be avoided in large quantities (such as bacon, smoked meats, crabmeat, tuna, crackers, processed cheeses, ham).

Stress management. Identify stress-producing situations in the patient's life and seek means to reduce these factors significantly. In some cases, referral for training in stress management, relaxation techniques, meditation, or biofeedback may be necessary. If stress is produced in the work setting, it may be appropriate to involve the industrial nurse.

Stress within the family is often significant and may require professional counseling for the family and patient.

Exercise and activity. Develop a plan for moderate exercise to improve the patient's general condition. Consult the physician for any individual modifications deemed appropriate. Suggest including activities that the patient finds help reduce stress.

Blood pressure monitoring. Demonstrate the correct procedure for taking blood pressure. Validate the patient's and family's understanding by having them perform this task on several occasions under supervision.

Expectations of therapy. Discuss expectations of therapy with the patient. Because the disease process is frequently asymptomatic, the patient usually has difficulty accepting the diagnosis.

Always suggest a hopeful course of treatment. Although there is no known cure at this point, there are

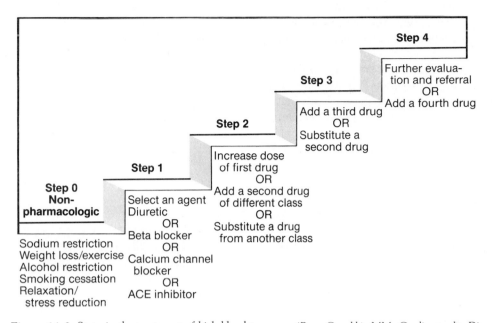

Figure 11-3 *Steps in the treatment of high blood pressure. (From Canobbia MM: Cardiovascular Disorders: Mosby's clinical nursing series, St Louis, 1990, Mosby–Year Book; based on the 1988 Report of Joint National Committee on Detection, Evaluation, and Treatment of High Blood Pressure. Arch Intern Med 1988;148).*

Table 11-4 *Ingredients of Common Antihypertensive Combination Products**

PRODUCT	DIURETIC (MG)	ANTIHYPERTENSIVE (MG)	OTHER (MG)
Aldoclor-150	Chlorothiazide (150)	Methyldopa (250)	
Aldoril-15	Hydrochlorothiazide (15)	Methyldopa (250)	
Apresazide 100/50	Hydrochlorothiazide (50)	Hydralazine (100)	
Apresoline-Esidrix	Hydrochlorothiazide (15)	Hydralazine (25)	
Capozide 25/25	Hydrochlorothiazide (25)	Captopril (25)	
Combipres 0.1	Chlorthalidone (15)	Clonidine (0.1)	
Combipres 0.2	Chlorthalidone (15)	Clonidine (0.2)	
Corzide 40/5	Bendroflumethiazide (5)	Nadolol (40)	
Diupres-250	Chlorothiazide (250)	Reserpine (0.125)	
Diutensen-R	Methyclothiazide (2.5)	Reserpine (0.1)	
Enduronyl	Methyclothiazide (5)	Deserpidine (0.25)	
Hydropres-25	Hydrochlorothiazide (25)	Reserpine (0.125)	
Inderide LA 120/50	Hydrochlorothiazide (50)	Propranolol (120)	
Lopressor HCT 100/50	Hydrochlorothiazide (50)	Metoprolol (100)	
Minizide 1	Polythiazide (0.5)	Prazosin (1)	
Normozide	Hydrochlorothiazide (25)	Labetalol (300)	
Oreticyl-25	Hydrochlorothiazide (25)	Deserpidine (0.125)	
Regroton	Chlorthalidone (50)	Reserpine (0.25)	
Renese-R	Polythiazide (2)	Reserpine (0.25)	
Salutensin	Hydroflumethiazide (50)	Reserpine (0.125)	
Ser-Ap-Es	Hydrochlorothiazide (15)	Reserpine (0.1)	Hydralazine (25)
Serpasil-Apresoline		Reserpine (0.1)	Hydralazine (25)
Tenoretic 50	Chlorthalidone (25)	Atenolol (50)	
Timolide 10-25	Hydrochlorothiazide (25)		Timolol (10)
Unipres	Hydrochlorothiazide (15)	Reserpine (0.1)	Hydralazine (25)
Vaseretic 10-25	Hydrochlorothiazide (25)	Enalapril (10)	

*This is a representative listing. Other strengths of these products, as well as products not listed, are available.

several important treatments that are successful in the control of hypertension.

Changes in expectations. Assess changes in expectations as therapy progresses and the patient gains understanding and skill in the management of hypertension.

Changes in therapy through cooperative goal setting. Work with the patient to encourage adherence to the prescribed treatment. When the patient feels that a change should be made in a treatment plan, encourage discussion first with the physician.

Written record. Enlist the patient's aid in developing and maintaining a written record of monitoring parameters (blood pressure, pulse, daily weights, exercise tolerance) and response to prescribed therapies for discussion with the physician. Patients should be encouraged to take this record on follow-up visits.

Fostering compliance. Throughout the hospitalization, discuss medication information and how it will benefit the patient's course of treatment. Seek cooperation and understanding of the following points, so that medication compliance may be enhanced:

1. Name
2. Dosage
3. Route and administration times
4. Anticipated therapeutic response: Gradual reduction and maintenance of blood pressure at an optimal level for the individual
5. Side effects to expect:
   - When initiating antihypertensive therapy in the hospitalized patients, protect from possible falls by assisting during ambulation and by carefully assessing for faintness. Take blood pressure in lying and standing positions to identify hypotensive responses.
   - Caution the patient that for the first 2 weeks of antihypertensive therapy, he or she may often experience drowsiness. Patients should be told that this side effect is self-limiting. They should be cautious in operating power equipment and driving as long as this symptom exists.
   - A common side effect of antihypertensive medications is hypotension. Have the patient rise slowly from a sitting or lying position. Tell him or her to avoid standing for long periods, especially within 2 hours of taking antihypertensive medication. Weakness, dizziness, or faintness can usually be relieved by increasing muscular activity or by sitting or lying down.
   - Have the person perform exercises that prevent blood pooling in the extremities when sitting or standing for long periods of time. These exercises include flexing the calf muscles, wiggling the toes, rising on the toes and then returning to the feet in a flat position.
6. Side effects to report:
   - See specific agents for further details.
   - The patient should always report a lack of response to the medication prescribed and/or a blood pressure that continues to rise after medications have been taken.
7. What to do if a dosage is missed:
   - Generally, the patient should not take an extra dose of medication if there is a question of a missed dose, but should resume a normal schedule.
   - If forgotten doses become a common occurrence, additional teaching aids should be provided to the patient.
   - Individual agents may require specific instructions.
8. When, how, or if to refill the medication prescription:
   - Stress that sudden discontinuation of medications can be dangerous. Have the patient explain to you how to refill the prescriptions.
   - You may want to determine if paying for medications is a problem; approach the issue with sensitivity. Also, try to find out if the person has insurance that may cover some of the medication costs. The patient may need assistance in filling out the insurance forms. Involve a social worker in this process if necessary.

Difficulty in comprehension. If it is evident that the patient and/or family does not understand all aspects of continuing therapy being prescribed (such as administration and monitoring of medications, exercises, diets, follow-up appointments), consider the use of social service or visiting nurse agencies.

Associated teaching. Give patients the following instructions:

Always inform the physician or dentist of any prescription or over-the-counter medication being taken. Over-the-counter medications should not be taken without first discussing them with the physician or pharmacist.

Always report side effects of rash, itching, or hives immediately. Nausea, vomiting, or diarrhea should also be reported for the physician's evaluation if it is a new symptom.

Take all of the medication as prescribed for the full course of treatment. Do not discontinue use when feeling improved; do not save for future use; do not give your medicine to another individual. Sudden discontinuation of certain medications may produce harmful effects.

Keep all medications out of reach of children.

If pregnancy is suspected, consult an obstetrician as soon as possible about continuation of medication therapy.

At discharge. Items to be sent home with the patient should:

1. Have written instructions for use
2. Be labeled in a level of language and size of print appropriate for the patient

3. If needed, include identification cards or bracelets
4. Include a list of additional supplies to be purchased after discharge
5. Include a schedule of follow-up visits

Drug Therapy for Hypertension

Sympathetic nervous system stimulants and inhibitors
OBJECTIVES

1. Review Figure 10-1 (p. 234) to identify the actions of the sympathetic nervous system. Analyze to determine the effects of stimulation or blockade in body functions and compare these findings with the actions of each drug studied in this category.
2. Discuss the essential patient education needed regarding the initiation of therapy with prazosin.
3. State the nursing assessments needed to monitor therapeutic response and/or the development of side effects to expect or report from sympathetic nervous system stimulants and inhibitors.

beta adrenergic blocking agents

The beta adrenergic blocking agents (acebutolol, atenolol, esmolol, labetolol, metoprolol, nadolol, pindolol, propranolol, and timolol) are widely used as antihypertensive agents. These agents inhibit cardiac response to sympathetic nerve stimulation by blocking the beta receptors. As a result, the heart rate, cardiac output, and renin released from the kidneys—and thus the blood pressure—are reduced. The clinical advantages of the beta adrenergic blocking agents in treating hypertension include minimal postural or exercise hypotension, no effect on sexual function, blood pressure reduction in the supine position, and little or no slowing of the central nervous system. See Chapter 10, "The Autonomic Nervous System," for further discussion of patient education and nursing interventions associated with beta adrenergic inhibition.

clonidine hydrochloride (Klo′ni-deen)

Catapres (Cat′ah-pres)

Clonidine is a potent antihypertensive agent that acts within the central nervous system to reduce both cardiac output and peripheral vascular resistance, thus reducing both systolic and diastolic blood pressure. After prolonged therapy, the lowered blood pressure is a result mainly of reduced peripheral vascular resistance. Clonidine is now used in the treatment of mild to moderate hypertension. Its effectiveness is generally improved when used in combination with diuretics and other antihypertensive agents.

Side effects. Patients must be warned of the need to continue this medication therapy. Abrupt discontinuation of clonidine may cause a rapid increase in diastolic and systolic blood pressure, nervousness, agitation, restlessness, tremor, headache, nausea, and increased salivation.

The most frequent adverse effects are dry mouth, drowsiness and sedation, constipation, headache, and dizziness.

Patients on long-term clonidine therapy should have periodic eye examinations. Laboratory animals have developed degenerative retinal changes, although none have been reported in humans.

Those patients having a diagnosis of mental depression may be more susceptible to further depressive activity.

Availability
PO—0.1, 0.2, and 0.3 mg tablets.
Transdermal—2.5, 5, and 7.5 mg patches.

Dosage and administration
Adult
PO—Initially 0.1 mg twice daily. Maintenance dose: add 0.1 to 0.2 mg daily until desired effect is achieved. Average daily doses range from 0.2 to 0.8 mg in divided doses daily. Maximum recommended daily dose is 2.4 mg.

Transdermal—Apply patch to a hairless area of intact skin on the upper arm or torso once every 7 days. Each new application should be on a different skin site from the previous location. Initially, apply 0.1 mg patch weekly. If after 1 to 2 weeks the desired reduction is not achieved, increase the dosage by adding an additional 0.1 mg patch or switching to a 0.2 or 0.3 mg patch. Maximum dosage is two 0.3 mg patches weekly.

Clonidine may be administered together with other antihypertensive agents without interactions, but the antihypertensive effects of these agents will be enhanced, requiring careful adjustment of dosage.

• Nursing Intervention: Monitoring clonidine therapy

See also General Nursing Considerations for Patients with Hypertension (p. 280).

Side effects to expect
DROWSINESS, DRY MOUTH, DIZZINESS. Tell the patient these symptoms may occur but that they tend to be self-limiting. Tell him or her not to stop taking the medication, and to consult the physician if the side effects become an unacceptable problem.

Side effects to report
DEPRESSION. Assess the patient's affective (loneliness, sadness, anxiety, anger), cognitive (confusion, ambivalence, loss of interest), and other behavioral responses (agitation, irritability, altered activity level, withdrawal) before initiating therapy. After initiating therapy with clonidine, carefully monitor the patient for changes in usual response patterns. Assess otherwise normal emotions for an increase in duration or intensity.

Note the patient's degree of socialization, response to stimulation, and changes in interactions with others. All individuals taking this drug should be monitored for development of depression, especially those with a history of depression.

RASH. Patients who develop moderate or severe erythema and/or vesicle formation at the site of application should consult their physician about the possible need to remove the patch and alternative therapy.

Implementation. Never suddenly discontinue the medication, as it may cause a rebound effect and a rapid increase in blood pressure, manifested by nervousness, agitation, restlessness, tremors, headache, nausea, and increased salivation.

Rebound symptoms are most pronounced after 1 to 2 months of therapy, and may begin to appear within a few hours of a missed dose. Within 8 to 24 hours, severe symptoms may develop.

When therapy is to be discontinued, a gradual reduction in dosage is necessary over 2 to 4 days, during which blood pressure must be carefully monitored.

If the transdermal patch becomes loose during the 7 day wearing, the adhesive overlay should be applied directly over the patch to ensure good adhesion.

Drug interactions

DRUGS THAT ENHANCE THERAPEUTIC AND TOXIC EFFECTS. Guanethidine, digitalis glycosides, barbiturates, tranquilizers, antihistamines, alcohol, and beta adrenergic blocking agents (such as propranolol, atenolol, pindolol, others) and other antihypertensive agents: Monitor the blood pressure response to the cumulative effects of antihypertensive agents. Take the blood pressures in supine and erect positions.

Monitor for an increase in severity of side effects such as sedation, hypotension, and bradycardia or tachycardia.

DRUGS THAT REDUCE THERAPEUTIC EFFECTS. Tricyclic antidepressants (amitriptyline, imipramine, desipramine) and trazodone. Monitor carefully for poor blood pressure control or a gradually increasing blood pressure.

guanabenz (gwan'ah-benz)

Wytensin (y-ten'sin)

Guanabenz is an alpha-2 adrenergic receptor stimulant that acts as an antihypertensive agent by reducing the outflow of sympathetic nervous system impulses to the peripheral blood vessels. This causes a drop in peripheral vascular resistance. It may be used alone or in combination with a diuretic.

Side effects. The most common side effects are drowsiness and sedation. Other relatively common adverse effects reported include dry mouth, dizziness, weakness, and headache.

Patients must be warned to continue therapy. Abrupt discontinuance may result in a rapid increase in systolic and diastolic pressure. If therapy is to be discontinued, the patient's dose should be tapered down over 1 to 2 weeks, if possible.

Availability

PO—4 and 8 mg tablets.

Dosage and administration

Adult

PO—Initially 4 mg twice daily. Doses may be increased every 1 to 2 weeks in increments of 4 to 8 mg daily. Maximum dose is 64 mg per day.

• **Nursing Interventions: Monitoring guanabenz therapy**

See also General Nursing Considerations for Patients with Hypertension (p. 280).

Side effects to expect

DROWSINESS, DRY MOUTH, DIZZINESS. Tell the patient these side effects may occur, but that they tend to be self-limiting. Tell the patient not to stop taking the medication and to consult the physician if side effects become an unacceptable problem.

Caution the patient against driving or performing hazardous tasks until adjusted to the sedative effects of the medication.

Implementation. Never suddenly discontinue the medication, as it may cause a rebound effect and a rapid increase in blood pressure, manifested by nervousness, agitation, restlessness, tremors, headache, nausea, and increased salivation.

When therapy is to be discontinued, a gradual reduction in dosage is necessary over 2 to 4 days, during which blood pressure must be carefully monitored.

Drug interactions

SEDATIVE EFFECTS. Alcohol, barbiturates, phenothiazines, benzodiazepines, and antihistamines all potentiate the sedative effects of guanabenz. Patients should be warned that their tolerance to alcohol and other depressants may be diminished.

guanadrel (gwan'a-drel)

Hylorel (hi-lor'el)

Guanadrel is quite similar to guanethidine as an antihypertensive agent in that it causes a release and subsequent depletion of norepinephrine from adrenergic nerve endings. It is recommended for use in moderate to severe hypertension, usually in combination with a thiazide diuretic.

Side effects. Orthostatic hypotension occurs frequently, especially with sudden changes in posture.

Some patients will develop significant salt and water retention, causing edema and congestive heart failure.

Sedation and lethargy commonly occur when guanadrel therapy is initiated or during adjustment to higher doses. These effects are most notable during the first few days and tend to dissipate with time.

Availability

PO—10 and 25 mg tablets.

Dosage and administration

Adult

PO—Initially 10 mg daily in two divided doses. Adjust the dosages weekly to monthly until the therapeutic goal has been attained. The usual dosage range is 20 to 75 mg divided into 2 to 3 daily doses.

- **Nursing Interventions: Monitoring guanadrel therapy**

See also General Nursing Considerations for Patients with Hypertension (p. 280).

Side effects to expect

ORTHOSTATIC HYPOTENSION. This may occur, particularly during initiation of therapy. Patients can generally avoid this complication by rising slowly from supine and sitting positions.

Side effects to report

EDEMA. Salt and water retention may cause edema.

Weigh patients daily, using the same scale, at the same time of day, in similar clothing. Report increases of 2 pounds or more per week.

Report edema of the extremities, and increase in dyspnea, pallor, tachycardia, wheezing, and frothy or blood-tinged sputum.

Drug interactions

DRUGS THAT ENHANCE THERAPEUTIC AND TOXIC EFFECTS. Guanethidine, barbiturates, disopyramide, quinidine, diuretics, tranquilizers, antihistamines, alcohol, and beta adrenergic blocking agents (such as propanolol, atenolol, pindolol, others), diuretics, and other antihypertensive agents. Monitor the blood pressure response to the cumulative effects of antihypertensive agents. Take the blood pressures in supine and erect positions.

Monitor for an increase in severity of side effects such as sedation, hypotension, and bradycardia or tachycardia.

DRUGS THAT REDUCE THERAPEUTIC EFFECTS. Tricyclic antidepressants (amitriptyline, imipramine, others), amphetamines, ephedrine, phenothiazines, monoamine oxidase inhibitors, haloperidol. Monitor carefully for poor blood pressure control or a gradually increasing blood pressure.

guanethidine sulfate (gwan-eth'i-deen)

Ismelin (is'meh-lin)

Guanethidine is an antihypertensive agent that causes a release and subsequent depletion to norepinephrine from postganglionic or adrenergic nerve endings. It is recommended for treatment of moderate to severe hypertension.

Side effects. Side effects include fatigue, nausea, nasal stuffiness, abdominal distress, weight gain, bradycardia, diarrhea, and light-headedness and weakness, especially when first getting out of bed.

Availability

PO—10 and 25 mg tablets.

Dosage and administration

Adult

PO—Initially 10 mg daily. Increase the dose 10 mg every 5 to 7 days, if the blood pressure measurements so

indicate and side effects are tolerable. Maintenance doses range between 25 and 50 mg daily; however, much higher doses are occasionally required.

- **Nursing Interventions: Monitoring guanethidine therapy**

See also General Nursing Considerations for Patients with Hypertension (p. 280).

Side effects to expect

LIGHT-HEADEDNESS, WEAKNESS. Guanethidine causes arteriolar and venous dilation that permits pools of blood to collect in the lower extremities, causing a reduction in cerebral blood flow. These symptoms often disappear during the day and can be lessened by rising slowly, sitting on the edge of the bed for a few minutes, and performing leg, foot, and toe exercises before standing.

These orthostatic effects are increased with alcohol consumption or prolonged standing with little movement.

Drug interactions

DRUGS THAT ENHANCE THERAPEUTIC AND TOXIC EFFECTS. Barbiturates, disopyramide, quinidine, diuretics, tranquilizers, antihistamines, alcohol, and beta adrenergic blocking agents (propranolol, atenolol, pindolol, others), and other antihypertensive agents: Monitor the blood pressure response to the cumulative effects of antihypertensive agents. Take the blood pressure in supine and erect positions.

Monitor for an increase in severity of side effects, such as sedation, hypotension, and bradycardia or tachycardia.

DRUGS THAT REDUCE THERAPEUTIC EFFECTS. Tricyclic antidepressants (amitriptyline, imipramine, others), amphetamines, ephedrine, phenothiazines, and haloperidol. Monitor carefully for poor blood pressure control or a gradually increasing blood pressure.

OTHER INTERACTIONS. Insulin and oral hypoglycemic agents. Guanethidine may increase the hypoglycemic effects of insulin and oral hypoglycemic agents.

Monitor these patients for headache, weakness, decreasing muscle coordination, diaphoresis. (Onset of hypoglycemic symptoms may be quite rapid.)

Give orange juice with two teaspoonfuls of sugar if the patient is still alert and responsive.

guanfacine (gwan'fah-seen)

Tenex (ten-ex')

Guanfacine is an alpha-2 adrenergic receptor stimulant similar to clonidine, guanabenz, and methyldopa. The onset of antihypertensive activity of guanfacine is slower but of longer duration than that of clonidine, thus allowing dosage administration once daily. Guanfacine is used for the management of mild to moderate hypertension, usually with a thiazide diuretic. Clinical studies have shown it to be equally effective as methyldopa and clonidine in controlling hypertension.

Side effects. The most common side effects are drowsiness, sedation, fatigue, and constipation. Orthostatic hypotension has been reported infrequently.

Availability

PO—1 mg tablets.

Dosage and administration

Adult

PO—Initially, 0.5 to 1 mg daily, usually at bedtime. Maintenance therapy is 1 to 3 mg daily. Much higher doses may be used, but the frequency of side effects usually becomes unacceptable.

• Nursing Interventions: Monitoring guanfacine therapy

See also General Nursing Considerations for Patients with Hypertension (p. 280). See Clonidine and Guanabenz.

methyldopa (meth'il-do'pah)

Aldomet (al'do-met)

Methyldopa is an antihypertensive agent whose mechanism of action has never been fully determined. It is recommended for mild to moderate hypertension.

Side effects. The most common side effects that occur with methyldopa are sedation, lethargy, and dizziness.

Methyldopa or its metabolites may discolor the urine, causing it to darken on exposure to air.

Methyldopa may cause a false-positive Clinitest reaction for urine glucose. It does not affect Tes-tape or Diastix, however.

Availability

PO—125, 250, and 500 mg tablets; 250 mg/5 ml suspension.

IV—250 mg/5 ml in 5 ml vials.

Dosage and administration

Adult

PO—250 to 500 mg 3 times a day. Maximum recommended dose is 3 g daily.

IV—250 to 500 mg every 6 hours as needed. Add the desired dose of methyldopa to 100 ml of dextrose 5% and infuse IV over 30 to 60 minutes.

• Nursing Interventions: Monitoring methyldopa therapy

See also General Nursing Considerations for Patients with Hypertension (p. 280).

Side effects to expect

DROWSINESS, DRY MOUTH, DIZZINESS. Tell the patient these side effects may occur, but that they tend to be self-limiting. Tell the patient not to stop taking the medication and to consult the physician if side effects become an unacceptable problem.

ALTERED URINE COLOR. Discoloration of the urine is to be expected and is not harmful. The darkened color usually occurs with prolonged exposure to air.

ALTERED TEST REACTIONS. A false-positive urine glucose test may occur when using Clinitest; Diastix and Tes-tape are not affected by methyldopa.

Methyldopa may cause up to 20% of patients to develop a positive reaction to the direct Coombs' test. Less than 0.2% of these patients will develop hemolytic anemia, however. Blood counts should be determined annually during therapy to detect hemolytic anemia.

Side effects to report

DEPRESSION. Assess the patient's affective (loneliness, sadness, anxiety, anger), cognitive (confusion, ambivalence, loss of interest), and other behavioral responses (agitation, irritability, altered activity level, withdrawal) before initiating therapy. After initiating therapy with methyldopa, carefully monitor the patient for changes in usual response patterns. Assess otherwise normal emotions for an increase in duration or intensity.

Note the patient's degree of socialization, responses to stimulation, and changes in interactions with others. All individuals taking this drug should be monitored for development of depression, especially those with a history of depression.

Drug interactions

DRUGS THAT ENHANCE THERAPEUTIC AND TOXIC EFFECTS. Disopyramide, quinidine, procainamide, diuretics, levodopa, tranquilizers, phenothiazines, alcohol, and beta adrenergic blocking agents (propranolol, atenolol, pindolol, others), and other antihypertensive agents. Monitor the blood pressure response to the cumulative effects of antihypertensive agents. Take the blood pressures in supine and erect positions.

Monitor for an increase in severity of side effects such as sedation, lethargy, hypotension, and bradycardia or tachycardia.

DRUGS THAT REDUCE THERAPEUTIC EFFECTS. Tricyclic antidepressants (amitriptyline, imipramine, desipramine, doxepine, others). Monitor carefully for poor blood pressure control or a gradually increasing blood pressure.

OTHER INTERACTIONS. Tolbutamide. Methyldopa may increase the hypoglycemic effects of tolbutamide.

Monitor these patients for headache, weakness, decreasing muscle coordination, diaphoresis. (Onset of hypoglycemic symptoms may be quite rapid.)

Give orange juice with two teaspoonfuls of sugar if the patient is still alert and responsive.

HALOPERIDOL. Methyldopa used concurrently with haloperidol may produce irritability, aggressiveness, assaultiveness, and dementia. Concurrent use is generally not recommended.

prazosin hydrochloride (pray'zo-sin)

Minipress (min'ee-pres)

Prazosin acts directly on the smooth muscle of arterioles to produce peripheral vasodilation and a reduction in diastolic blood pressure. Prazosin is used in combination with other antihypertensive agents in the treatment of mild to moderate hypertension.

Side effects. The most common adverse effects reported with prazosin include dizziness, headache, drowsiness, nausea, weakness, and lethargy. All are transient and disappear with continued therapy.

Availability

PO—1, 2, and 5 mg capsules.

Dosage and administration

Adult

PO—Initially, 1 mg 3 times daily. Gradually increase until desired therapeutic response is achieved. The usual maintenance dose is 10 mg twice daily. Do not exceed 40 mg daily.

NOTE: The initial doses of prazosin may cause dizziness, tachycardia, and fainting, but these adverse effects occur in less than 1% of patients starting therapy. Symptoms occur 15 to 90 minutes after initial dosages and occur most frequently in patients who are already receiving propranolol (and presumably other beta adrenergic blocking agents). This effect may be minimized by giving the first doses with food and limiting the initial dose to 1 mg. Patients should be warned that this side effect may occur, that it is transient, and that they should lie down immediately if symptoms develop.

• Nursing Interventions: Monitoring prazosin therapy

See also General Nursing Considerations for Patients with Hypertension (p. 280).

Side effects to expect

DROWSINESS, HEADACHE, DIZZINESS, WEAKNESS, LETHARGY. Tell the patient that these side effects may occur, but that they tend to be self-limiting. Tell the patient not to stop taking the medication and to consult the physician if they become an unacceptable problem.

Implementation

DIZZINESS, TACHYCARDIA, AND FAINTING. These side effects occur in about 1% of patients when therapy is initiated. They develop 15 to 90 minutes after the first dosage is taken. To decrease their incidence, administer the first dose with food and limit the initial dose to 1 mg.

Tell the patient to lie down immediately if these symptoms occur.

Provide for the patient's safety.

Drug interactions

DRUGS THAT ENHANCE THERAPEUTIC AND TOXIC EFFECTS. Diuretics, tranquilizers, alcohol, barbiturates, antihistamines, beta adrenergic blocking agents (propranolol, atenolol, pindolol, others), and other antihypertensive agents. Monitor the blood pressure response to the cumulative effects of antihypertensive agents. Take the blood pressures in supine and erect positions.

Monitor for an increase in severity of side effects such as sedation, hypotension, and bradycardia or tachycardia.

reserpine (res′er-peen)

 Serpasil (ser′pah-sil)

Reserpine is an alkaloid obtained from the root of a certain species of *Rauwolfia*. It is one of the oldest antihypertensive agents available. Reserpine acts as an antihypertensive agent by reducing norepinephrine levels in peripheral nerve endings, thus reducing peripheral vascular resistance. Reserpine also depletes norepinephrine from various other organs, including the brain. Brain depletion of norepinephrine may be the cause of the sedative and depressive actions of reserpine. Reserpine is used to treat mild hypertension.

Side effects. Side effects include nasal stuffiness, weight gain, diarrhea, dryness of the mouth, nosebleeds, itching, skin eruptions, insomnia, mental depression, and, occasionally, gastric irritation, and reactivation of old ulcers or formation of new ones.

Availability

PO—0.1, 0.25, and 1 mg tablets;

Dosage and administration

Adult

PO—Initially 0.5 mg daily for 1 to 2 weeks. Maintenance: 0.1 to 0.25 mg daily.

IM—Hypertensive crisis: Initially 0.5 to 1 mg, followed by 2 to 4 mg every 3 hours as needed.

• Nursing Interventions: Monitoring reserpine therapy

See also General Nursing Considerations for Patients with Hypertension (p. 280).

Side effects to expect

NASAL STUFFINESS. Encourage the patient not to treat this symptom with over-the-counter nasal decongestants. (They aggravate the hypertension.) Fortunately, this side effect tends to be self-limiting, but have the patient consult the physician if it becomes a serious problem.

DIARRHEA. Diarrhea and stomach cramps may be associated with depressed sympathetic activity. These side effects tend to be self-limiting, but if they persist, or if there is an increase in abdominal pain, the physician should be notified.

Side effects to report

DEPRESSION. Depression caused by this medication may progress to the point of the individual's becoming suicidal.

Assess the patient's affective (loneliness, sadness, anxiety, anger), cognitive (confusion, ambivalence, loss of interest), and other behavioral responses (agitation, irritability, altered activity level, withdrawal) before initiating therapy. After initiating medication therapy with reserpine, carefully monitor the patient for changes in usual response patterns. Assess otherwise normal emotions for an increase in duration or intensity.

Note the patient's degree of socialization, responses to stimulation, and changes in interactions with others.

All individuals taking this drug should be monitored for development of depression, especially those with a history of depression.

NIGHTMARES AND INSOMNIA. If these symptoms occur, report them to the physician for evaluation. Drug therapy may need to be changed.

GASTRIC SYMPTOMS. Patients experiencing gastric symptoms such as burning, pain, nausea, or vomiting should report them immediately as this medication can cause formation of new or exacerbation of old ulcers.

Drug interactions

DRUGS THAT ENHANCE THERAPEUTIC AND TOXIC EFFECTS. Phenothiazines, procainamide, disopyramide, thiothixene, quinidine, diuretics, tranquilizers, antihistamines, alcohol, and beta adrenergic blocking agents (propranolol, atenolol, pindolol, others), and other antihypertensive agents. Monitor the blood pressure response to cumulative effects of antihypertensive agents. Take the blood pressures in supine and erect positions.

Monitor for an increase in severity of side effects, such as sedation, hypotension, and bradycardia or tachycardia.

DRUGS THAT REDUCE THERAPEUTIC EFFECTS. Tricyclic antidepressants (amitriptyline, imipramine, doxepin, others). Monitor carefully for poor blood pressure control or a gradually increasing blood pressure.

Direct vasodilators
OBJECTIVES

1. Cite the effects of vasodilation on blood pressure, smooth muscle structures, and peripheral resistance.
2. State the compensatory mechanism that occurs with a drop in the peripheral vascular resistance.
3. Explain why a potent diuretic may be required in conjunction with minoxidil therapy.
4. State the nursing assessments needed to monitor therapeutic response and/or the development of side effects to expect or report from direct vasodilator therapy.

diazoxide (dy-az-ok′syd)

Hyperstat IV Injection

Diazoxide is used for emergency reduction of blood pressure in hospitalized patients with severe hypertension. It is administered undiluted in a peripheral vein in a dosage of 300 mg in 30 seconds or less. The blood pressure must be continuously monitored.

Availability

IV—300 mg/20 ml ampule.

hydralazine (hy-dral′ah-zeen)

Apresoline (ah-pres′o-leen)

This antihypertensive agent is used to treat moderate to severe essential hypertension and hypertension associated with renal disease and toxemia of pregnancy. It acts directly on the smooth muscle of arteries and veins to cause vasodilation.

Side effects. Early side effects that are sometimes observed and that usually disappear as the drug is continued include nausea, vomiting, dizziness, palpitations, tachycardia, numbness and tingling of legs and feet, nasal congestion, and postural hypotension. The nasal congestion can be treated with an antihistamine, such as pyribenzamine or diphenhydramine. If arthritic symptoms occur, the drug should be discontinued.

Availability

PO—10, 25, 50, and 100 mg tablets.
IV—20 mg/ml in 1 ml ampules.

Dosage and administration
Adult

PO—Initially, 10 mg 4 times daily for the first 2 to 4 days, then 25 mg 4 times daily. The second week, increase the dosage to 50 mg 4 times daily as the patient tolerates the dosage and the blood pressure is brought under control.

IM, IV—20 to 40 mg repeated as necessary. Monitor blood pressure frequently. Results usually become evident within 10 to 20 minutes.

• Nursing Interventions: Monitoring hydralazine therapy

See also General Nursing Considerations for Patients with Hypertension (p. 280).

Side effects to expect

NAUSEA, DIZZINESS, PALPITATIONS, TACHYCARDIA, NUMBNESS AND TINGLING IN THE LEGS, NASAL CONGESTION. Although these symptoms may be anticipated, they do require monitoring. If severe, they should be reported so that the dosage can be adjusted appropriately.

ORTHOSTATIC HYPOTENSION. This may occur particularly during initiation of therapy. Patients can generally avoid this complication by rising slowly from supine and sitting positions.

Side effects to report

FEVER, CHILLS, JOINT AND MUSCLE PAIN, SKIN ERUPTIONS. Tell patients to report the development of these symptoms.

Monitor laboratory reports for leukocyte counts and the antinuclear antibody (ANA) titer.

Drug interactions

DRUGS THAT ENHANCE THERAPEUTIC AND TOXIC EFFECTS. Diuretics, alcohol, beta adrenergic blocking agents (propranolol, atenolol, pindolol, others), and other antihypertensive agents. Monitor the blood pressure response to the cumulative effects of antihypertensive agents. Take the blood pressures in supine and erect positions.

Monitor for an increase in severity of side effects, such as sedation, hypotension, and bradycardia or tachycardia.

minoxidil (min-ox'i-dil)

Loniten (lon'-i-ten) Minodyl (min-oh'dil)

Minoxidil acts by direct relaxation of the smooth muscle of arterioles, reducing peripheral vascular resistance. Due to the drop in peripheral vascular resistance, there is a compensatory increase in heart rate and sodium and water retention. For this reason, minoxidil is usually administered in conjunction with a beta adrenergic blocking agent and a potent diuretic such as furosemide or bumetanide. Minoxidil is used only for severely hypertensive patients who do not respond adequately to maximum therapeutic doses of a diuretic and two other antihypertensive agents.

Side effects. Due to salt and water retention, about 10% of patients develop edema, tachycardia, and possible congestive heart failure.

Within 3 to 6 weeks after initiating therapy, about 80% of patients will start developing *hypertrichosis*—an elongation, thickening, and increased pigmentation of fine body hair. It is usually noticed first on the face and later extends to the back, arms, legs, and scalp.

Other adverse effects that have been reported include breast tenderness and gynecomastia, changes in skin pigmentation, polymenorrhea, thrombocytopenia, leukopenia, bullous lesions on the legs, and hypersensitivity rash.

Availability

PO—2.5 and 10 mg tablets.

Dosage and administration

Adult

PO—Initially 5 mg daily. Dosage may be gradually increased after at least 3-day intervals to 10 mg, 20 mg, and then 40 mg daily in 1 to 2 doses. Maintenance dosage: 10 to 40 mg daily. Maximum dosage is 100 mg daily.

• Nursing Interventions: Monitoring minoxidil therapy

See also General Nursing Considerations for Patients with Hypertension (p. 280).

Side effects to expect

HAIR GROWTH. A gradual increase and thickening of body hair can be anticipated approximately 3 to 6 weeks after initiating therapy.

Growth may be controlled by shaving or by hair-removing creams. Upon discontinuation, new hair growth stops, but it may take up to 6 months for complete return to pretreatment appearance.

Side effects to report

GYNECOMASTIA. Swelling or tenderness of the breasts may develop in men.

SALT AND WATER RETENTION. This drug is usually administered with a diuretic and a beta adrenergic blocking agent to reduce the incidence of fluid retention, and for additive antihypertensive effects.

Perform daily weights using the same scale, in similar clothing, and at approximately the same time of day. Report gains of more than 2 pounds per week and swelling or puffiness of the face, ankles, or hands to the physician.

INCREASED RESTING PULSE. Instruct and validate the patient's ability to take own pulse.

A resting pulse that increases 20 or more beats per minute above normal should be reported.

LIGHT-HEADEDNESS, FAINTING, DIZZINESS. These symptoms require reporting to the physician. If possible, the individual's blood pressure during these episodes should be taken and reported.

ORTHOSTATIC HYPOTENSION. This may occur, particularly during initiation of therapy. Patients can generally avoid this complication by rising slowly from supine and sitting positions.

CONGESTIVE HEART FAILURE. Assess for development of: dyspnea, orthopnea, edema, weight gain.

Drug interactions

DRUGS THAT ENHANCE THERAPEUTIC AND TOXIC EFFECTS. Diuretics, alcohol, beta adrenergic blocking agents (propanolol, atenolol, pindolol, others), guanethidine, guanadrel, and other antihypertensive agents. Monitor the blood pressure response due to the cumulative effects of antihypertensive agents. Take the blood pressures in supine and erect positions.

Monitor for increase in severity of side effects, such as sedation, hypotension, and bradycardia or tachycardia.

nitroprusside sodium (ny-tro-prus'yd)

Nipride (ny'pryd)

Nitroprusside is a potent vasodilator that acts directly on the smooth muscle of blood vessels to produce vasodilation. It is used in patients with sudden severe hypertensive crisis, and in those with refractory congestive heart failure.

Side effects. Adverse effects are usually dose-related and dissipate rapidly with dosage reduction. Side effects reported include nausea, retching, abdominal pain, diaphoresis, restlessness, apprehension, headache, muscle twitching, palpitations, and retrosternal discomfort. Keeping the patient in a supine position will also reduce the incidence of adverse effects.

Availability

IV—10 mg/ml in 5 ml vials.

Renin-angiotensin inhibitors

OBJECTIVES

1. State the action of renin-angiotensin II on blood vessels.
2. Explain how to monitor for proteinuria.
3. Name the laboratory studies that should be completed before renin-angiotensin inhibitor therapy is initiated.

4. State the nursing assessments needed to monitor therapeutic response and/or the development of side effects to expect or report from renin-angiotensin inhibitor therapy.

Angiotensin-converting enzyme (ACE) inhibitors represent a major breakthrough in the treatment of hypertension. These agents inhibit angiotensin I-converting enzyme, the enzyme responsible for the conversion of angiotensin I to angiotensin II in the renin-angiotensin-aldosterone system. It is thought that blood pressure is reduced by inhibiting the formation of angiotensin II, a potent vasoconstrictor of peripheral blood vessels.

ACE inhibitors reduce blood pressure, preserve cardiac output, and increase renal blood flow. They are effective as single therapy for mild-to-moderate hypertension as well as effective in severe accelerated hypertension and renal hypertension. Although they may be used alone, they tend to be more effective when combined with diuretic therapy. Advantages of ACE inhibitors are the infrequency of orthostatic hypotension, lack of CNS depression and sexual dysfunction side effects; the lack of aggravation of asthma, obstructive pulmonary disease, or diabetes; and an additive effect with diuretics. The ACE inhibitors are also effective in the treatment of congestive heart failure and may also be used to slow the progression of diabetic nephropathy.

Side effects. The most frequent clinical adverse effects are headache, dizziness, and fatigue. Other adverse effects include diarrhea, rash, hypotension, cough, nausea, and orthostatic hypotension.

Angioedema has been reported to occur in a few patients, especially after the first dose of therapy. Patients should be cautioned to discontinue further therapy and seek medical attention immediately.

Neutropenia (300 neutrophils/mm^3) and agranulocytosis (drug-induced bone marrow suppression) have been observed in patients receiving ACE inhibitors. The neutropenia appears within the first 3 to 12 weeks of therapy and develops slowly; the white count falls to its nadir in 10 to 30 days. The white count returns to normal in about 2 weeks after discontinuation of enalapril therapy.

A few hypertensive patients who are receiving ACE inhibitors, particularly those with preexisting renal impairment, have developed increases in blood urea and serum creatinine. These elevations have usually been minor and transient, especially when the ACE inhibitor was administered concomitantly with a diuretic.

Because ACE inhibitors inhibit aldosterone, patients may develop slight increases in serum potassium. Approximately 1% of patients may develop hyperkalemia (greater than 5.7 mEq/L). Most cases resolve without discontinuing therapy. Risk factors for development of hyperkalemia include diabetes mellitus, renal insufficiency, and the use of potassium supplements or potassium-sparing diuretics.

There is concern about the potential for birth defects in neonates whose mothers received ACE inhibitors during pregnancy. Women who wish to become pregnant or become pregnant while receiving ACE inhibitors should discuss alternative therapies to the ACE inhibitors with their physician.

Availability. See Table 11-5.

• **Nursing Interventions: Monitoring ACE inhibitor therapy**

See also General Nursing Considerations for Patients with Hypertension (p. 280).

Side effects to expect

NAUSEA, FATIGUE, HEADACHE, DIARRHEA. These side effects are usually mild and tend to resolve with continued therapy. Encourage the patient not to discontinue therapy without first consulting a physician.

ORTHOSTATIC HYPOTENSION (DIZZINESS, WEAKNESS, FAINTNESS). Although these side effects are infrequent and generally mild, certain patients, particularly those also receiving diuretics, may suffer some degree of orthostatic hypotension, particularly when therapy is initiated. Observe the patient closely for at least 2 hours after the initial dose and until blood pressure has stabilized for at least an additional hour.

Monitor the blood pressure in both the supine and standing positions.

Anticipate the development of postural hypotension and take measures to prevent an occurrence. Teach the patient to rise slowly from a supine or sitting position, and to sit or lie down if feeling faint.

Side effects to report

SWELLING OF THE FACE, EYES, LIPS, TONGUE; DIFFICULTY IN BREATHING. Angioedema has been reported to occur in a small number of patients, especially after the first dose. Patients should be cautioned to discontinue further therapy and seek medical attention immediately.

NEUTROPENIA. Neutropenia appears within the first 3 to 12 weeks and develops slowly over the next 10 to 30 days. The white count returns to normal in about 2 weeks after discontinuing the ACE inhibitor.

The patients most susceptible are those receiving captopril who also have impaired renal function, serious autoimmune diseases (such as lupus erythematosus), or who are exposed to drugs known to affect the white cells or immune response (such as corticosteroids).

Patients at risk should have differential and total white cell counts before initiation of therapy and then every 2 weeks thereafter for the first 3 months of therapy. Stress the importance of returning for this laboratory work. Patients should be told to notify their physician promptly if any evidence of infection such as sore throat or fever (which may be an indicator of neutropenia) should develop.

NEPHROTOXICITY. Renal function should be monitored during the first few weeks of therapy. Report an increasing BUN and creatinine level. Dosage reduction of the

Table 11-5 *Angiotensin Converting Enzyme (ACE) Inhibitors*

GENERIC NAME	BRAND NAME	AVAILABILITY	APPROVED USES	DOSAGE RANGE
Benazepril	Lotensin	Tablets: 5, 10, 20, 40 mg	Hypertension	PO: Initial—2.5-5 mg once daily Maintenance: 20-40 mg daily
Captopril	Capoten	Tablets: 12.5, 25, 50, 100 mg	Hypertension; heart failure	PO: Initial—25 mg 2 to 3× daily Maintenance: 75-450 mg daily
Enalapril	Vasotec	Tablets: 2.5, 5, 10, 20 mg	Hypertension; heart failure	PO: Initial—2.5-5 mg once daily Maintenance: 10-40 mg daily
Enalaprilat	Vasotec I.V.	Inj.: 1.25 mg/ml	Hypertension	IV: 1.25 mg every 6 hr over 5 min.
Fosinopril	Monopril	Tablets: 10, 20 mg	Hypertension	PO: Initial—10 mg once daily Maintenance: 20-80 mg daily
Lisinopril	Prinivil, Zestril	Tablets: 5, 10, 20, 40 mg	Hypertension	PO: Initial—5-10 mg once daily Maintenance: 20-80 mg daily
Ramipril	Altace	Capsules: 1.25, 2.5, 5, 10 mg	Hypertension	PO: Initial—1.25-2.5 mg daily Maintenance: 2.5-20 mg daily

ACE inhibitor or possible discontinuation of the diuretic may be required.

HYPERKALEMIA. Many symptoms associated with altered fluid and electrolyte balance are subtle and interspersed with general symptoms of drug toxicity or the disease process itself. Patients most susceptible to the development of hyperkalemia are those with renal impairment, diabetes mellitus, and those patients already receiving a potassium supplement.

Gather data relative to *changes* in the patient's mental status (such as alertness, orientation, confusion), muscle strength, muscle cramps, tremors, nausea, and general appearance (drowsy, anxious, lethargic).

Always check the electrolyte reports for early indications of electrolyte imbalance.

Keep accurate records of intake and output, daily weights and vital signs.

CHRONIC COUGH. As many as one-third of patients receiving ACE inhibitors may develop a chronic, dry, nonproductive, persistent cough. Women appear to be more susceptible than men. Patients should be told to contact their physician if the cough becomes troublesome. The cough resolves after discontinuation of therapy.

Drug interactions

DRUGS THAT ENHANCE THERAPEUTIC AND TOXIC EFFECTS. Diuretics, phenothiazines, alcohol, beta adrenergic blocking agents (propranolol, atenolol, pindolol, others), and other antihypertensive agents. Probenecid blocks the excretion of captopril, causing an increased antihypertensive effect. Monitor the blood pressure response to the cumulative effects of antihypertensive agents. Take the blood pressures in supine and erect positions.

DRUGS THAT REDUCE THERAPEUTIC EFFECTS. Antacids may diminish absorption of ACE inhibitors. Separate the administration times by 1 to 2 hours. Indomethacin may reduce the antihypertensive effects of the ACE inhibitors. Rifampin may decrease the antihypertensive effects of enalapril. Monitor carefully for poor blood pressure control or a gradually increasing blood pressure.

Other drug interactions

DIGOXIN. ACE inhibitors may increase the serum levels of digoxin. Monitor the patient for symptoms of anorexia, nausea, vomiting, headaches, blurred or colored vision, and bradycardia. A digoxin serum level may be ordered by the physician.

LITHIUM. ACE inhibitors may induce lithium toxicity. Monitor for lithium toxicity manifested by nausea, anorexia, fine tremors, persistent vomiting, profuse diarrhea, hyperreflexia, lethargy, and weakness.

HYPERKALEMIA. ACE inhibitors may cause small increases in potassium levels by inhibiting aldosterone secretion. Patients should not take dietary supplements of potassium or potassium-sparing diuretics (triamterene, spironolactone, amiloride) without specific approval from the physician. If a patient has received spironolactone up to several months before ACE inhibitor therapy, the serum potassium level should be monitored closely, because the potassium-sparing effect of spironolactone persists.

Diuretics

OBJECTIVES

1. Identify the action of diuretics that results in a reduction of blood pressure.
2. State the nursing assessments needed to monitor therapeutic response and/or the development of side effects to expect or report from diuretic therapy.

The diuretics, including the thiazides, chlorthalidone, bumetanide, metolazone, furosemide, and ethacrynic acid, are mainstays in antihypertensive therapy. They have a low incidence of adverse effects, they potentiate the hypotensive activity of the nondiuretic antihypertensive agents, and they are often the least expensive of the antihypertensive agents.

The diuretics act as antihypertensive agents by causing volume depletion, sodium excretion, and direct vasodilation of peripheral arterioles. Diuretics are used to treat mild, moderate, and severe hypertension and are most effective when used in combination with other antihypertensive agents (see Table 11-4, page 281). The agents are discussed under the urinary system drugs (see Chapter 15).

ANTICOAGULATION

OBJECTIVES

1. State the primary purposes of anticoagulant therapy.
2. Identify the effects of anticoagulant therapy on existing blood clots.
3. Describe conditions that place an individual at risk for developing blood clots.
4. Identify specific nursing interventions that can prevent clot formation.
5. Explain laboratory data used to establish dosing of anticoagulant medications.
6. Describe specific monitoring procedures to detect hemorrhage in the anticoagulated patient.
7. Describe procedures used to insure that the correct dose of an anticoagulant is prepared and administered.
8. Explain the specific procedures and techniques used to administer heparin subcutaneously, via intermittent administration through a heparin lock, and via intravenous infusion.
9. Identify the purpose, dosing determination, and scheduling factors associated with the use of protamine sulfate.
10. State the nursing assessments needed to monitor therapeutic response and/or the development of side effects to expect or report from anticoagulant therapy.
11. Develop measurable short- and long-term objectives for patient education for patients receiving anticoagulant therapy.

KEY WORDS

thrombophlebitis	hemodialysis
prophylactic	petechiae
anticoagulation	pulmonary embolism
venous thrombosis	ecchymoses
coronary occlusion	

Diseases associated with abnormal clotting within blood vessels are a frequent cause of death. Diseases caused by intravascular clotting are major causes of death from cardiovascular sources, such as coronary occlusion and thromboembolisms secondary to thrombophlebitis. Drugs that inhibit clotting are, therefore, most important.

Anticoagulant therapy is used during and after certain types of surgery, in the treatment of thrombophlebitis, in conjunction with hemodialysis, and in the management of certain heart valve disorders. Anticoagulants are used prophylactically; they cannot dissolve an existing clot. The primary purpose of anticoagulants is to prevent new clot formation or the extension of existing clots.

General Nursing Considerations for Patients Receiving Anticoagulant Therapy

Patient Concerns:
Nursing Intervention/Rationale

Patients at risk. Patients at greater risk for clot formation are those with a history of clot formation, those with recent abdominal, thoracic, or orthopedic surgery, and those at prolonged bedrest.

Techniques for preventing clot formation. Provide early, regular ambulation after surgery. Use active or passive leg exercises for patients at bedrest or restricted activity.

Develop and follow a specific turning schedule for persons at complete bedrest to prevent tissue breakdown and blood stasis. Implement good back care, deep breathing, and coughing exercises as part of general nursing care.

Do not flex the knees or place pressure against the popliteal space with pillows.

Do not allow the patient to stand or sit motionless for prolonged periods of time.

Use elastic hose, such as TED stockings. Remove stockings and inspect the skin on every shift. Make sure they are being worn properly and not becoming bunched around the knees or ankles.

Nutritional status. The dietary regimen will depend on the individual's diagnosis and current clinical status.

Adequate hydration to promote fluidity of the blood is important. Unless coexisting diagnoses prohibit, give at least six to eight 8-ounce glasses of fluid daily.

Laboratory data. Monitoring and reporting to the physician laboratory results is essential during anticoagulant therapy. Coagulation tests that might be ordered include the following: whole blood clotting time (WBCT); prothrombin time (PT); partial thromboplastin time (PTT); activated partial thromboplastin time (APTT); activated coagulation time (ACT). The prothrombin time (PT) is routinely used to monitor warfarin therapy, and the activated partial thromboplastin time (APTT) is most commonly used to monitor heparin therapy.

Never administer an anticoagulant without first checking the chart for the most recent laboratory results. Be certain that the anticoagulant to be administered has been ordered *since* the most recent results have been reported to the physician. Follow policy statements regarding checking of anticoagulant doses with other qualified professionals.

Patient Education Associated with Anticoagulant Therapy

Communication and responsibility. Encourage open communication concerning frustrations and anger as the patient attempts to adjust to the diagnosis and need for treatment. The patient must be guided to gain insight into the condition in order to assume responsibility for the continuation of treatment. Keep emphasizing those factors the patient can control to alter the progress of the disease, including maintenance of general health, nutritional needs, adequate rest and appropriate exercise, and continuation of prescribed medication therapy.

Stress the need to prevent bodily injury: avoid use of power equipment; use care in stepping up or down from curbs; do not participate in contact sports; use only an electric razor; and brush teeth gently with a soft-bristled toothbrush.

Expectations of therapy. Discuss expectations of therapy with the patient:

• Level of exercise specified by the physician.
• Ability to maintain activities of daily living and work.
• Pain relief, if appropriate to the etiology of clot formation.

Changes in expectations. Assess changes in expectations as therapy progresses and the patient gains understanding and skill in the management of the diagnosis.

Changes in therapy through cooperative goal setting. Work with the patient to encourage adherence to the prescribed treatment. When the patient feels that a change should be made in a treatment plan, encourage him or her to discuss it first with the physician.

Written record. Enlist the patient's aid in developing and maintaining a written record of monitoring parameters (Figure 11-4) (such as blood pressure, pulse, daily weights, degree of pain relief, exercise tolerance) and response to prescribed therapies for discussion with the physician. Patients should be encouraged to take this record on follow-up visits.

Fostering compliance. Throughout the hospitalization, discuss medication information and how it will benefit the patient's course of treatment. Seek cooperation and understanding of the following points, so that medication compliance may be enhanced:

1. Name
2. Dosage
3. Route and administration times

• Take medications at the same time each day or alternate days as prescribed. Have the patient record times on a calendar when taken to prevent inadvertently repeating a dose.

4. Anticipated therapeutic response
5. Side effects to expect
6. Side effects to report

• Nosebleeds, tarry stools, "coffee-ground" or blood-tinged vomitus; petechiae (tiny purple or red spots occurring in various sites on the skin); ecchymoses (bruises); hematuria (blood in the urine); or bleeding from the gums or any other body opening; cuts or injuries from which the bleeding is difficult to control. If a dressing is on, check periodically for bleeding.
• Tell the patient that not all bleeding is clearly visible; therefore, report immediately a rapid, weak pulse; deep, rapid respirations; moist, clammy skin; and a general feeling of weakness or faintness.
• In some cases the physician may want the patient to perform guaiac testing to detect blood in the stool. If ordered, specific patient education should be done to teach the patient or support person how to perform the test.

7. What to do if a dosage is missed: If a dose is missed, take it as soon as possible. If it is almost time for the next dose, do not take the missed dose. Instead, continue with the regular dosing schedule. Ask the patient to record the date of the missed dose and inform the doctor at the next scheduled blood test. If more than one dose is missed, the patient should contact the doctor.
8. When, how, or if to refill the medication prescription. Follow-up visits to the physician and laboratory are essential during anticoagulant therapy. Failure to keep these appointments may lead to serious complications.

Difficulty in comprehension. If it is evident that the patient and/or family does not understand all aspects of continuing therapy being prescribed (such as administration and monitoring of medications, exercises, diets,

Patient Education and Monitoring of Therapeutic Outcomes for Patients Receiving Anticoagulants

Medications	Color	To be taken

Name _____

Physician _____

Physician's phone _____

Next appt.* _____

Parameters		Day of discharge							Comments
Weight									
Blood pressure									
Pulse									
Color of urine	Normal								
	Red								
	Orange								
Mouth	Gums bleed with brushing								
Shaving	Bleeding — difficulty stopping blood								
Bruising	Nosebleeds — (#) of times?								
	Bruising to light touch								
Pain relief	Name limb (e.g., left leg, right leg)								
	Color of limb								
	Temperature								
Activities of daily living	Able to do								
	Done with difficulty								
	Too difficult to do								
Bowel movements	Normal								
	Diarrhea								
	Color — normal or black, tarry								
	Smell — normal or foul								
Report immediately									
	Chest pain								
	Faintness								
	Dizziness								
	Red vomitus								
	Black stools								

*Please bring this record with you to your next appointment.
Use the back of this sheet for additional information.

Figure 11-4 *Patient education and monitoring of therapeutic outcomes for patients receiving anti-coagulants.*

follow-up appointments), consider the use of social service or visiting nurse agencies.

Associated teaching. Give patients the following instructions:

Always inform the physician or dentist of any prescription or over-the-counter medication being taken. While receiving anticoagulant therapy, no prescription or over-the-counter medications should be taken without first discussing them with the physician or pharmacist.

Always report side effects of rash, itching or hives immediately. Nausea, vomiting, or diarrhea should also be reported for the physician's evaluation, if it is a new symptom.

Take all of the medication as prescribed for the full course of treatment. Do not discontinue use when feeling improved; do not save for future use; do not give your medicine to another individual. Sudden discontinuation of certain medications may produce harmful effects.

Keep all medications out of the reach of children.

If pregnancy is suspected, consult an obstetrician as soon as possible about continuation of medication therapy.

At discharge. Items to be sent home with the patient should:

1. Have written instructions for use
2. Be labeled in a level of language and size of print appropriate for the patient
3. If needed, include identification cards or bracelets
4. Include a list of additional supplies to be purchased after discharge
5. Include a schedule for follow-up appointments

Drug Therapy for Anticoagulation

heparin (hep'ah-rin)

Heparin is a natural substance that is commercially extracted from gut and lung tissue of pigs and cattle. It acts directly on several plasma protein molecules within the blood to prevent coagulation. It is used to treat deep venous thrombosis, pulmonary embolism, cerebral embolism, and acute peripheral arterial embolism; it is also used in the treatment of patients with heart valve prostheses. It is also used prophylactically before and during cardiovascular surgery and hemodialysis.

Side effects. Adverse effects of heparin therapy are most commonly due to inappropriate administration technique or overdosage. Factors that can influence the incidence of complications include age, weight, sex, and recent trauma. The most common signs of overdosage are petechiae, hematomas, hematuria, bleeding gums, and melena.

Availability

SC, IV—1000, 5000, 10,000, 20,000, and 40,000 units/ml in various sizes of ampules and vials.

Dosage and administration

Adult

SC—Prophylactic: 5000 units every 8 to 12 hours. Therapeutic: Initially 10,000 to 15,000 units. Maintenance: 5000 to 10,000 units every 8 to 12 hours (see Figure 11-4).

IM—Not recommended because of the development of hematomas.

IV—Intermittent: Initially 10,000 unit bolus; maintenance: 5000 to 10,000 units every 4 to 6 hours.

IV—Continuous infusion: Initially 5000 unit bolus; Maintenance, 700 to 1200 units/hour. (Patient variation may require as little as 200 units/hour or as much as 2000 or more units/hour.)

Antidote. One mg of protamine sulfate will neutralize approximately 120 units of heparin. If protamine sulfate is given more than one-half hour after the heparin was administered, then give only one-half the dose of protamine sulfate. Excessive doses of protamine may also cause excessive anticoagulation, so it must be used judiciously.

• Nursing Interventions: Monitoring heparin therapy

See also General Nursing Considerations for Patients Receiving Anticoagulant Therapy (p. 292).

Side effects to expect

HEMATOMA FORMATION, BLEEDING AT INJECTION SITE. Inappropriate administration techniques lead to hematoma formation at the site of injection. USE PROPER TECHNIQUE!

Side effects to report

BLEEDING. Inspect the skin and mucous membranes for petechiae, ecchymoses, or hematomas. Also monitor for hematuria, bleeding gums, and melena.

Always monitor menstrual flow to be certain that it is not excessive or prolonged.

Assess and record vital signs at regular intervals. Report signs and symptoms of internal bleeding (decreasing blood pressure; increasing pulse, cold, clammy skin, feelings of faintness; or disoriented sensorium).

Check urine and stools for blood. Urine may appear red, smoke-colored, or brownish. Stools may appear to be dark and tarry. Perform a Hemocult test on the stool, if necessary.

Vomitus may contain bright red blood or may be coffee-ground in appearance.

Postoperative patients need assessment or dressings or drainage tubes for any signs of bleeding.

Implementation

INTRAMUSCULAR INJECTIONS. DO NOT INJECT INTRAMUSCULARLY!

DOSAGE ADJUSTMENT. Blood samples for laboratory studies are usually drawn 4 to 6 hours after each subcutaneous dose, or just before each intravenous dose. It may be drawn every 6 to 8 hours during a continuous intravenous infusion.

ACCURACY OF DOSE. Always confirm the dosage calcu-

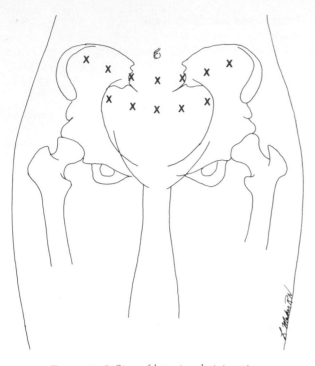

Figure 11-5 *Sites of heparin administration.*

lations with two nurses before subcutaneous or intravenous administration.

Be certain the strength is correct. There is a *drastic difference* in clinical response from 1 ml of 1:1,000 units and 1 ml of 1:10,000 units of heparin.

SUBCUTANEOUS ADMINISTRATION. Subcutaneous injection is usually made into the tissue over the abdomen, the upper arm, or lateral thigh (see Figure 11-5).

Needle length and angle need to be adapted to the patient's size so that the drug will be deposited into the subcutaneous tissue. (Usually a 26 or 27 gauge, ½-inch needle is used.) The injection is usually made at a 90° angle to the skin.

Always use a tuberculin syringe so that the dosage can be accurately measured.

DO NOT aspirate, because this will increase local tissue damage and the possibility of hematoma formation.

DO NOT inject into a hematoma or an area with any infection present.

Follow a planned site rotation schedule.

After injection, apply gentle pressure for 1 to 2 minutes to control local bleeding.

Ice packs on the site following injection may be used; check your hospital policy. At this time, there is little documented evidence that ice packs prevent hematoma formation or affect drug absorption.

INTERMITTENT INTRAVENOUS ADMINISTRATION. A heparin lock, consisting of a 22-25 gauge scalp vein needle attached to a 3½-inch tubing ending in a resealing rubber diaphragm, may be used to administer intermittent IV doses of heparin. (See Figure 6-10.)

Advantages of a heparin lock are the mobility that it provides the patient and the fewer venipunctures.

After injecting a bolus of heparin through the rubber diaphragm, flush the line with 1 ml of a solution containing 10 units of heparin/ml of saline solution. The heparin flush solution ensures that the patient will receive the entire heparin bolus and it prevents the formation of a clot in the scalp vein needle.

INTRAVENOUS INFUSION. Continuous infusions of heparin provide the advantage of steady heparin levels in the blood, but do require periodic dosage adjustment based upon the response of the patient.

When making a solution for infusion, always have two nurses confirm your calculations and the strength of the heparin to be used. As a safety measure, never make infusions to run more than 6 to 8 hours. This protects patients from receiving massive doses of heparin should the infusion "run away."

Always use an electronic control device for infusion, but the nurse should monitor the infusion at least every 30 to 60 minutes.

Drug interactions

INCREASED THERAPEUTIC AND TOXIC EFFECTS. Concurrent use of aspirin, dipyridamole, and glyceryl gualacolate may predispose the patient to hemorrhage.

---

warfarin (war'fah-rin)

Coumadin (koo'mah-din), **Panwarfin** (pan-war'fin)

Warfarin is a very potent anticoagulant that acts by inhibiting the activity of vitamin K, which is required to produce certain blood coagulation factors in the blood. Warfarin is used to treat or prophylactically prevent venous thrombosis, atrial fibrillation with embolism, pulmonary embolism, and coronary occlusion.

Side effects. Adverse reactions to warfarin, other than the possibility of hemorrhage due to overdosage, are quite rare. Evidence of hemorrhage is usually seen as petechiae, hematuria, bleeding gums, melena, or the development of hematomas after minor trauma.

Availability

PO—2, 2.5, 5, 7.5, and 10 mg tablets.

IV—50 mg vial with a 2 ml ampule of diluent.

Dosage and administration

Adult

PO—10 to 15 mg daily for 3 days; maintenance: 2 to 15 mg daily as determined by the prothrombin time.

IV—As for PO administration; onset of action is similar to that of PO administration because of dependence on individual coagulation factor synthesis.

• **Antidote.** Vitamin K is a specific antidote for warfarin-induced hemorrhage, but is rarely needed. Most cases of bleeding induced by warfarin overdose can be controlled by discontinuing warfarin therapy. An alternative in severe hemorrhage is a transfusion with plasma or whole blood.

• Nursing Interventions: Monitoring warfarin therapy

See also General Nursing Considerations for Patients Receiving Anticoagulant Therapy (p. 292).

Side effects to report

BLEEDING. Inspect the skin and mucous membranes for petechiae, ecchymoses, or hematomas. Also monitor for hematuria, bleeding gums, and melena.

Always monitor menstrual flow to be certain that it is not excessive or prolonged.

Assess and record vital signs at regular intervals. Report signs and symptoms of internal bleeding (decreasing blood pressure; increasing pulse; cold, clammy skin; feelings of faintness; or disoriented sensorium).

Check urine and stools for blood. Urine may appear red, smoke-colored, or brownish. Stools may appear to be dark and tarry. Perform a Hemocult test on the stool, if necessary.

Vomitus may contain bright red blood or may be coffee-ground in appearance.

Postoperative patients need assessment of dressings or drainage tubes for any signs of bleeding.

Implementation

DOSAGE ADJUSTMENT. Dosage during initial therapy is based on prothrombin times. The optimal dosage is that which maintains PT at 1.3 to 1.6 times the control value.

When warfarin therapy is initiated, the patient should be monitored closely for evidence of hemorrhage, because of the drug's accumulative effects.

Stress the need to comply with the prescribed regimen and the need for laboratory data to determine the correct maintenance dose.

Tell the patient to resume a regular schedule if one dose is missed. If more than two doses are missed, he or she should consult the physician.

Drug interactions. The following drugs, when used concurrently with warfarin, may enhance the therapeutic and toxic effects of warfarin:

allopurinol	aminoglycoside antibiotics	amiodarone
anabolic steroids	cephalosporins	chloral hydrate
chloramphenicol	cimetidine	clofibrate
co-trimoxazole	danazol	dextrothyroxine
diazoxide	diflunisal	disulfiram
erythromycin	ethacrynic acid	ethanol
fluoxetine	glucagon	indomethacin
isoniazid	meclofenamate	mefenamic acid
metronidazole	miconazole	nalidixic acid
phenylbutazone	phenytoin	propafenone
propoxyphene	quinidine	salicylates
sulfinpyrazone	sulindac	sulfonamides
tetracyclines	thyroid hormones	vitamin E

The following drugs, when used concurrently with warfarin, may decrease the therapeutic activity of warfarin:

barbiturates	disopyramide	mercaptopurine
carbamazepine	ethchlorvynol	rifampin
cholestyramine	gluthethimide	spironolactone
cyclophosphamide	griseofulvin	vitamin K

ALL PRESCRIPTION AND NONPRESCRIPTION MEDICATIONS. Caution the patient *not* to take *any* over-the-counter or prescription medication without first discussing them with the physician or pharmacist.

HEMORRHEOLOGIC AGENT

pentoxifylline (pen-tox-e'fi-leen)

Trental (tren-tahl)

Pentoxifylline is the first available agent that is specifically indicated for the treatment of intermittent claudication caused by chronic occlusive arterial disease of the limbs. It is not an anticoagulant but is thought to increase erythrocyte flexibility, decrease the concentration of fibrinogen in blood, and prevent aggregation of red blood cells and platelets. These actions decrease the viscosity of blood and improve its flow properties, resulting in increased blood flow to the affected microcirculation and enhanced tissue oxygenation. Pentoxifylline therapy should be considered an adjunct to, and not a replacement for, smoking cessation, weight loss, exercise therapy, or surgical bypass or removal of arterial obstructions.

Side effects. The most frequent adverse effects of therapy involve the GI tract. Dyspepsia, nausea, and vomiting occur in about 1% to 3% of patients, while belching and/or flatus occur in less than 1% of patients. Adverse effects from all categories required discontinuation of therapy in less than 5% of patients.

Central nervous system disturbances characterized by dizziness occurred in about 2% of patients, while headache and tremor occurred less frequently.

Adverse cardiovascular effects such as angina, chest pain, arrhythmia, tachycardia, flushing, and dyspnea have been reported in less than 1% of patients.

Pentoxifylline is a xanthine derivative. It is contraindicated in patients who have a history of intolerance to other xanthine derivatives such as caffeine, theophylline, or theobromine.

Availability
PO—400 mg tablets.

Dosage and administration
PO—400 mg three times daily. If adverse GI and/or CNS effects develop, dosage should be reduced to 400 mg twice daily. If adverse effects persist, therapy should be discontinued. Symptomatic relief may start within 2 to 4 weeks, but treatment should be continued for at least 8 weeks to determine maximal efficacy.

• **Nursing Interventions: Monitoring pentoxifylline therapy**

Side effects to expect

NAUSEA, VOMITING, DYSPEPSIA. These side effects are usually mild and tend to resolve with continued therapy. Administration with food or milk may help minimize discomfort. Encourage the patient not to discontinue therapy without first consulting a physician.

DIZZINESS, HEADACHE. These side effects are usually mild and tend to resolve with continued therapy. Provide for patient safety during episodes of dizziness. Encourage the patient to sit down if feelings of faintness develop. Encourage the patient not to discontinue therapy without first consulting a physician.

Side effects to report

CHEST PAIN, ARRHYTHMIAS, SHORTNESS OF BREATH. Without causing undue alarm, strongly encourage the patient to seek a physician's attention for further evaluation.

INTOLERANCE TO CAFFEINE, THEOPHYLLINE, THEOBROMINE. Pentoxifylline is a xanthine derivative. Patients should be asked specifically about intolerance to xanthine derivatives prior to initiating therapy.

Drug interactions

ANTIHYPERTENSIVE AGENTS. Although pentoxifylline is not an antihypertensive agent, patients receiving pentoxifylline therapy frequently display a small reduction in systemic blood pressure. Blood pressure should be monitored to observe for hypotension. The dosage of antihypertensive therapy may have to be reduced to minimize adverse effects.

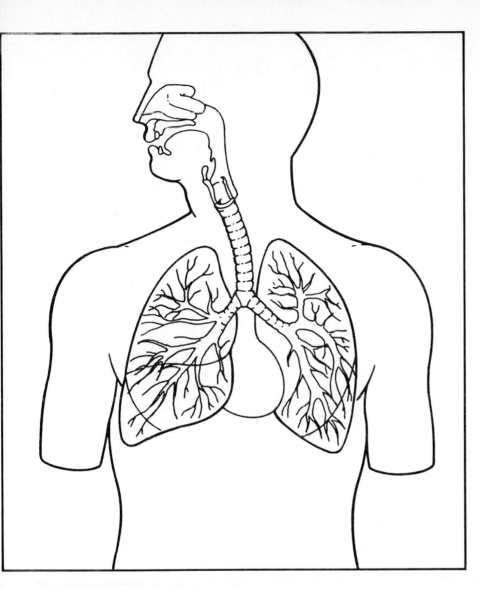

CHAPTER GOALS

After completing this chapter, the student should be able to do the following:

1. Explain the major actions (effects) of drugs used to treat disorders of the respiratory tract.
2. Identify baseline data the nurse should collect on a continuous basis for comparison and evaluation of drug effectiveness.
3. Identify important nursing assessments and interventions associated with the drug therapy and treatment of diseases of the respiratory tract.
4. Identify essential components involved in planning patient education that will enhance compliance with the treatment regimen.

RESPIRATORY TRACT DISEASE
OBJECTIVES

1. Identify components of blood gases.
2. Cite nursing assessments used to evaluate the respiratory status of a patient.
3. Develop measurable short- and long-term objectives for patient education for patients with respiratory disease.

KEY WORDS

perfusion   diffusion
blood gases   cyanosis
clubbing   auscultation
percussion   asthma
bronchitis   emphysema
COPD   pneumonia
bronchospasm

General Nursing Considerations for Patients with Respiratory Tract Disease

Nursing assessment of the signs of respiratory dysfunction can provide a baseline for subsequent evaluation of the patient's response to therapy. Assessment may range from the "common cold," of limited severity and duration, to chronic and progressively more debilitating disorders, such as emphysema.

Throughout the course of managing the respiratory disorder, adequate oxygenation of the individual body cells is essential to maintain the body functions. *Ventilation,* the movement of the air in and out of the lungs, is affected by a number of complex mechanisms. To be effective, air must reach the alveoli. This allows atmospheric air, with a fresh supply of oxygen, to be exchanged with carbon dioxide and "stale" air from the lungs by inspiration and expiration. Any blockage in the respiratory pathway prevents this process from occurring. Diseases that affect the tracheobronchial tree or the ability of the lungs to expand can affect the ventilation process.

Blood flow through the pulmonary vessels, where gas exchange between the alveoli and pulmonary vessels occurs, is called *perfusion. Diffusion* is the point at which oxygen (O_2) enters and carbon dioxide (CO_2) leaves the cells. Blood circulation provides *distribution* of oxygen to the body's cells for the sustenance of life. Ventilation and perfusion must be equal to maintain homeostasis. Dysfunction of one or more of the processes that interfere with the gaseous exchange results in difficult breathing.

Oxygen is transported to the individual tissue cells either by combining with the hemoglobin or by dissolving in the blood plasma. Arterial blood gas (ABG) determinations indicate the effectiveness of pulmonary function. ABGs are a measurement for assessing ventilation and external respiratory effectiveness. They measure the amount of oxygen dissolved in blood plasma. ABGs are done to assist in the management of patients with acute and chronic pulmonary disorders.

Five main diagnostic tests are used to evaluate the patient's status. Beginning nurses need to know the normal range of the laboratory studies (see Table 12-1). Deviations from normal need to be reported to facilitate effective management of the patient with a respiratory disorder.

Patient Concerns:
Nursing Intervention/Rationale

Normal respiratory activity
Respirations

RATE. Throughout the course of therapy, monitor the respiratory pattern at regularly scheduled intervals. Normal values are as follows:

- Infants—26-34/minute
- Adult—14-25/minute

Report increasing or decreasing respiratory rate.

DEPTH. Shallow breathing may lead to hypercapnea, hypoxemia, hypoxia, and acidosis. Rapid, deep breathing (Kussmaul breathing) is one sign of metabolic acidosis. Report *changes* in the patient's depth of respirations.

Table 12-1 *Laboratory Tests Used to Assess Respiratory Function*

TEST	NORMAL VALUE	RESULTS
pH	7.35-7.45 (arterial)	>7.45 = alkalosis <7.35 = acidosis
pCO$_2$	35-45 mm Hg	Abnormalities indicate respiratory acid-base imbalance. > = hypercapnea = respiratory acidosis < = hypocapnea = respiratory alkalosis
HCO$_3$	21-28 mEq/L	Abnormalities indicate metabolic acid-base imbalance. > = metabolic alkalosis < = metabolic acidosis
pO$_2$	80-100 mm Hg	Measures the amount of oxygen moving through pulmonary alveoli into blood for transport to other tissues. It is dependent upon the amount of inspired oxygen. < = hypoxemia, hypoventilation > = hyperventilation
SaO$_2$	95%	Measures the ratio of actual oxygen content of hemoglobin compared to the hemoglobin's carrying capacity. When decreased, either there is an impairment of oxygen binding to hemoglobin (e.g., metabolic acidosis) or inadequate amounts of oxygen are being inspired.

Indications of respiratory impairment

Dyspnea (difficult or labored respirations). Complete respiratory obstruction is evidenced by such signs as the inability to cough or speak, the lack of chest movement, or cyanosis; the patient may be clutching the throat in a state of panic.

Incomplete or partial respiratory obstruction is evidenced by weak cough, cyanosis, shortness of breath, frequent respirations, and use of accessory muscles.

Always check the patient for possible inhalation of a foreign object if you are unfamiliar with the individual's diagnosis or the conditions surrounding the onset of respiratory difficulty.

Respiratory distress. Assess the patient for the following:

Early signs and symptoms of respiratory distress, including: increased blood pressure, pulse, and respiratory rate; anxiety; restlessness; headache; slight confusion or impaired judgment; possible sweating.

Late signs and symptoms, including: flaring nostrils; cyanosis; dyspnea; use of accessory chest, abdominal and neck muscles; confusion progressing to coma; gradual reduction in pulse and blood pressure.

Cyanosis. Peripheral cyanosis is defined as a bluish coloring of an isolated area of the body (such as the earlobes, toes, feet, or fingers).

Central cyanosis indicates a general lack of oxygenated hemoglobin. The entire body has a slight bluish-white tinge. It is most readily observed on the lips and mucous membranes of the mouth.

Muscle involvement. Elevations of the shoulders, retraction of the neck and intercostal muscles, and use of the abdominal muscles is associated with advanced respiratory disease; report new observations immediately.

Changes in mental status. As the oxygen level in the body diminishes, the mental status will deteriorate from alertness to progressively lower levels of function (alert →anxious →restless →drowsy →unconscious →dead).

Breath sounds. Auscultation for rales, rhonchi, and lung clarity should be performed at appropriate intervals based on the patient's diagnosis and current status.

Posture. Dyspneic patients usually sit upright or lean forward from the waist, resting the elbows on the knees. Position patients experiencing dyspnea in the high Fowler's position, or place a pillow on table over the bed and allow them to rest with their head forward on the pillow.

Pain. Chest discomfort may result from lying on the affected side too long.

Chest contour. Note changes in contour of the chest, such as "barrel chest," kyphosis, or scoliosis.

Clubbing of fingernails and toenails. Assess for a decrease in the angle between the nailbeds and the fingers or toes.

Fatigue. Check for the degree of fatigue the patient is experiencing. Ask specific questions regarding the correlation of the activity level with the onset and degree of fatigue.

Cough. Note whether a cough is productive or nonproductive. Record sputum color, consistency, amount, and any appearance of frothiness or blood (hemoptysis).

Patient Education Associated with Respiratory Therapy

Communication and responsibility. Encourage open communication concerning frustrations and anger as the patient attempts to adjust to diagnosis and the need for prolonged treatment. The patient must be guided to insight into the condition in order to assume responsibility for the continuation of treatment. Keep emphasizing those factors the patient can control to alter the progression of the disease, including the following:

Avoiding irritants. Smoking, pollen, and environmental pollutants frequently aggravate respiratory disorders.

Activity and exercise. Fatigue and resulting dyspnea

may require alterations in physical activity and employment. Support the patient's concerns. Plan for rest periods to alternate with activity.

Nutritional status. A well-balanced diet that avoids weight loss or excessive gains is important. Encourage patients with dyspnea to eat small bites, with several small servings throughout the day.

Preventing infections. Encourage patients to avoid exposure to persons with infection; to practice good hygiene, such as handwashing; to get adequate rest; and to dispose of secretions properly. Patients should seek medical attention at the earliest sign of suspected infection.

Increased fluid intake. Unless contraindicated, encourage patients to increase fluid intake. This will aid in decreasing the viscosity of secretions.

Environmental elements. People experiencing difficulty in breathing can benefit from proper temperature, humidification of the air, or ventilation of their immediate surroundings. Moist air from a humidifier or vaporizer can readily relieve dryness of the nose or throat.

Breathing techniques. If ordered by the physician, teach postural drainage and pursed-lip breathing or abdominal breathing and coughing. Encourage the use of blow-bottles.

See a general medical-surgical nursing text for details of these treatment modalities.

Expectations of therapy. Discuss expectations of therapy with the patient (such as level of exercise; degree of pain relief, if present; tolerance; frequency of use of therapy; relief of dyspnea; ability to maintain activities of daily living and work; and others as indicated by the underlying pathology).

Changes in expectations. Assess changes in expectations as therapy progresses and the patient gains understanding and skill in the management of the diagnosis.

Changes in therapy through cooperative goal setting. Work with the patient to encourage adherence to the prescribed treatment. When the patient feels that a change should be made in a treatment plan, encourage discussion first with the physician.

Written record. Enlist the patient's aid in developing and maintaining a written record (see Figure 12-1) of monitoring parameters (such as respirations, pulse, daily weights, degree of dyspnea relief, exercise tolerance, secretions being expectorated) and response to prescribed therapies for discussion with the physician. Patients should be encouraged to take this record with them on follow-up visits.

Fostering compliance. Throughout the hospitalization, discuss medication information and how it will benefit the course of treatment. Seek cooperation and understanding of the following points so that medication compliance may be enhanced:

1. Name
2. Dosage
3. Route and administration times
4. Anticipated therapeutic response
5. Side effects to expect
6. Side effects to report
7. What to do if a dose is missed
8. When, how, or if to refill the medication prescription

Difficulty in comprehension. If it is evident that the patient and/or family does not understand all aspects of the continuing therapy being prescribed (such as administration and monitoring of medications, exercise, diet, or follow-up appointments) consider the use of social service or visiting nurse agencies.

Associated teaching. Give patients the following instructions: Always inform the physician or dentist of any prescription or over-the-counter medication being taken. Over-the-counter medications should not be taken without first discussing them with a physician or pharmacist.

Always report side effects of rash, itching, or hives immediately. Nausea, vomiting, and diarrhea should also be reported for the physician's evaluation if it is a new symptom.

Take all of the medication as prescribed for the full course of treatment. Do not discontinue use when feeling improved; do not save for future use; do not give your medicine to another individual. Sudden discontinuation of certain medications may produce harmful effects.

Keep all medications out of reach of children.

If pregnancy is suspected, consult an obstetrician as soon as possible about continuation of medication therapy.

If medications are ordered for inhalation, be certain the individual understands the proper method of administration and operation of the nebulizer he or she will be using at home.

At discharge. Items to be sent home with the patient should include the following:

1. Written instructions for use
2. Labels in language and size of print appropriate for the patient
3. If needed, identification cards or bracelets
4. A list of additional supplies to be purchased after discharge (such as nebulizers or vaporizers)
5. A schedule for follow-up appointments

Expectorant, Antitussive, and Mucolytic Therapy

Secretions of the respiratory tract
OBJECTIVES

1. Explain the effects of exposure to irritants on respiratory tract function.
2. Differentiate between a *productive* and a *nonproductive* cough.

Patient Education and Monitoring of Patients Receiving Respiratory Agents

Medications	Color	To be taken

Name _____

Physician _____

Physician's phone _____

Next appt.* _____

Parameters		Day of discharge									Comments
Blow bottles	AM # Liters										
	Noon										
	PM										
Postural drainage	Times of day performed (e.g., 8AM, 2PM)										
	Response: productive cough, non-productive										
Describe cough	Frequent, intermittent										
	Secretions: Color:										
	Thickness of secretions: thick, thin										
How do you feel today? (Record 2 times per day.) Awful — Improving — Good 10 — 5 — 1		AM / PM	AM / PM	AM / PM	AM / PM	AM / PM	AM / PM	AM / PM			
Exercise level: degree of tiredness with exercise. Extremely — Moderate — Normal 10 — 5 — 1											
Activities of daily living	Walk (#) of stairs										
	Walk (#) of blocks										
	Can or cannot perform daily activities Yes/No										
Pain pattern	Pain is on L (left) or R (right) side										
	Pain on inspiration=I Pain on expiration=E										
Difficulty breathing	Sleep with (#) pillows										
	Difficulty on exertion										
	Difficulty during stress										
	Difficulty when resting										
Appetite Poor — Decreased — Normal 10 — 5 — 1											

*Please bring this record with you to your next appointment.
Use the back of this sheet for additional information.

Figure 12-1 *Patient education and monitoring of therapeutic outcomes for patients receiving respiratory agents.*

3. Distinguish the mechanisms of action of expectorants, antitussives, and mucolytic agents.
4. Name three drugs used as expectorants.
5. Describe the procedure for administering iodine products to prevent staining of the teeth.
6. Cite potential complications of the long-term use of iodine products.
7. Compare the effects of hypotonic, hypertonic, and isotonic saline solutions administered by nebulizers.
8. Review the procedures for administration of medication by inhalation.
9. State the nursing assessments needed to monitor therapeutic response and/or the development of side effects to expect or report from expectorant, antitussive, and mucolytic therapy.

KEY WORDS

tracheostomy	goblet cells
viscous	phlegm
expectorants	antitussive
mucolytic	

The fluids of the respiratory tract originate from specialized cells called *goblet cells* that line the respiratory tract and form the bronchial glands. The goblet cells produce a gelatinous mucus that forms a thin layer over the interior surfaces of the trachea, bronchi, and bronchioles. Factors that control the secretion of mucus from the goblet cells are not known, but exposure to irritants such as smoke, airborne particulate matter, and bacteria increases the mucus output of the cells. The bronchial glands are controlled by the cholinergic nervous system. When stimulated, the bronchial glands secrete a watery fluid to the interior surface of the bronchial tract. There, the mucus secretions of the goblet cells and the watery secretions of the bronchial glands combine to form respiratory tract fluid.

Normally, respiratory tract fluid forms a protective layer over the trachea, bronchi, and bronchioles. Foreign bodies such as smoke particles and bacteria are caught in the respiratory tract fluid and are pushed upward by ciliary hairs that line the passages to the throat, where it is swallowed. This ciliary action cleanses the pulmonary system of foreign matter. The mucus becomes viscous, forming thick plugs in the bronchiolar airways, if too much mucus is secreted, the cilia are destroyed by chronic ingestion of smoke and alcohol, dehydration dries the mucus, or if anticholinergic agents inhibit watery secretions from the bronchial glands (Figure 12-2). These thick plugs are quite difficult to eliminate. They allow the colonization of pathogenic microorganisms in the lower respiratory tract, which causes additional mucus secretions and the possible development of pneumonia from trapped bacteria.

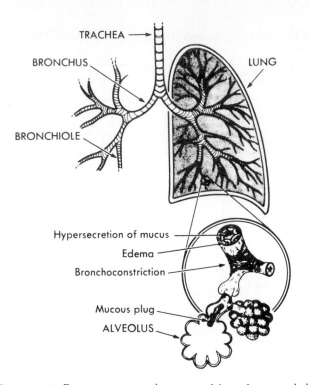

Figure 12-2 *Factors restricting the airway. Major factors include hypersecretion of mucus, mucosal edema, and bronchoconstriction. Mucous plugs may form in the alveoli.* (*From Clark JB, Queener SF, Karb VB: Pharmacological Basis of Nursing Practice, ed 3, St Louis, 1982, Mosby–Year Book.*)

Cough

A cough is a reflex initiated by irritation of the airway. It is a protective, beneficial mechanism for clearing excess secretions from the tracheobronchial tree. The same irritants responsible for asthma or allergy may stimulate the cough receptors, or congestion of the nasal mucosa from a cold may cause a postnasal drip into the back of the throat, stimulating the cough.

A cough is *productive* if it helps remove accumulated secretions and phlegm from the tracheobronchial tree. A *nonproductive* cough results when irritants repeatedly stimulate the cough receptors, but are not removed by the coughing reflex. Excessive coughing, particularly if it is dry and nonproductive, is not only discomforting, but also tends to be self-perpetuating because the rapid air expulsion further irritates the tracheobronchial mucosa.

Treatment of the cough is of secondary importance; primary treatment is aimed at the underlying disorder. If the air is dry, a vaporizer may be used to liquefy the secretions so that they do not become irritating. A dehydrated state thickens respiratory secretions, so drinking plenty of fluids will help reduce the viscosity (thickness) of the secretions. Patients can also suck on hard candies to increase the flow of saliva to coat the throat, thus reducing irritation. If these simple measures do not

Table 12-2 *Antitussive Agents*

GENERIC NAME	BRAND NAMES	AVAILABILITY	ADULT ORAL DOSAGE RANGE
Benzonatate	Tessalon Perles	Capsules: 100 mg	100 mg 3 times daily
Codeine*		Tablets: 15, 30, 60 mg	10-20 mg every 4-6 hours
Dextromethorphan	Sucrets, Delsym, Benylin DM	Lozenges: 5, 15 mg Syrup: 5, 7.5, 10, 15 mg/5 ml Liquid: 30 mg/5 ml	10-30 mg every 4-8 hours. Do not exceed 60-120 mg/24 hours
Diphenhydramine	Benylin, Diphen, Tusstat, Valdrene	Syrup: 12.5, 13.3 mg/5 ml	25 mg every 4 hours. Do not exceed 150 mg/24 hours
Hydrocodone*			5 mg every 4-6 hours

*Often an ingredient in combination antitussive products.

reduce the frequency of the cough, expectorants or cough suppressants (antitussives) may be used. The therapeutic objective is to decrease the intensity and frequency of the cough yet permit adequate elimination of tracheobronchial secretions. In severe cases of pulmonary congestion, a mucolytic agent may be required.

Expectorants are agents that liquefy mucus by stimulating the secretion of natural lubricant fluids from the bronchial glands. This flow of natural secretions helps to liquefy thick mucous masses that may plug the narrow bronchioles. A combination of ciliary action and coughing will then expel the debris from the pulmonary system. Expectorants are used to treat nonproductive coughs, bronchitis, and pneumonia where mucus plugs inhibit the expulsion of irritants and bacteria causing the bronchitis or pneumonia.

Cough suppressants (antitussives) act by suppressing the cough center in the brain. They are used when the patient has a bothersome dry, hacking, nonproductive cough. These agents will not stop the cough completely, but should decrease the frequency of the cough and suppress the severe spasms which prevent adequate rest at night. Under normal circumstances, it is not appropriate to suppress a productive cough. See Table 12-2 for available antitussive agents.

Mucolytic agents reduce the thickness and stickiness of pulmonary secretions by acting directly on the mucous plugs to dissolve them. This eases the removal of the secretions by suction, postural drainage, or coughing. Mucolytic agents are most effective in removing mucous plugs obstructing the tracheobronchial airway. They are used in the treatment of patients with acute and chronic pulmonary disorders, as well as before and after bronchoscopy, following chest surgery, and as a part of the treatment of tracheostomy care.

Expectorants

guaifenesin (gwi-feh-neh′sin)

   Robitussin (row-bih-tus′sin)

Guaifenesin, formerly known as glyceryl guaiacolate, is an expectorant that acts by enhancing the output of respiratory tract fluid. The increased flow of secretions promotes ciliary action and facilitates the removal of mucus. It is used for the symptomatic relief of conditions characterized by a dry, nonproductive cough, as well as to remove mucus plugs from the respiratory tract.

Guaifenesin should not be used with a dry, persistent cough that lasts more than 1 week. The patient should seek medical attention if the cough does not subside.

Guaifenesin should be used with caution in patients with cardiovascular disorders, diabetes mellitus, hyperthyroidism, and people sensitive to sympathomimetic amines.

Side effects. Side effects are infrequent, but gastrointestinal upsets, nausea, and vomiting have been reported.

Availability

PO—100, 200, 600 mg tablets, 200, 300 mg capsules, 100, 200 mg/5 ml liquid. It is also available in individual products in combination with pseudoephedrine, dextromethorphan, codeine phosphate, and phenylpropanolamine.

Dosage and administration

Adult

PO—100 to 400 mg every 4 to 6 hours. Do not exceed 2400 mg/day.

Pediatric

PO—Ages 6 to 12: 100 to 200 mg every 4 hours. Do not exceed 1200 mg/day. Ages 2 to 6: 50 to 100 mg every 4 hours. Do not exceed 600 mg/day.

• **Nursing Interventions: Monitoring guaifenesin therapy**

See also General Nursing Considerations for Patients with Respiratory Tract Disease (p. 300).

Side effects to expect

GASTROINTESTINAL UPSET, NAUSEA, VOMITING. Development of these side effects is rare.

Implementation

FLUID INTAKE. Maintain fluid intake at 8 to 12 8-ounce glasses daily.

HUMIDIFICATION. Suggest the concurrent use of a humidifier.

Drug interactions. No significant drug interactions have been reported.

iodine products (SSKI, potassium iodide, others)

The iodides are the most commonly used expectorants. They act by stimulating increased secretions from the bronchial glands to decrease the viscosity of mucous plugs, making it easier for patients to cough up the dry, hardened plugs blocking the bronchial tubes. Iodides are used as expectorants in the symptomatic treatment of chronic pulmonary diseases where tenacious mucus is present.

Side effects. Side effects are quite mild and infrequent. Oral and gastric irritation, with nausea, have been reported.

Patients with a hypersensitivity to iodides, hyperthyroidism, hyperkalemia, and acute bronchitis should not use iodide products. An early indication of hypersensitivity is development of a rash.

Long-term, chronic use may induce goiter, particularly in children with cystic fibrosis.

Availability

PO—liquids, tablets, syrups, and elixirs of varying strengths.

Dosage and administration

Adult

PO—See individual products.

• Nursing Interventions: Monitoring iodine therapy

See also General Nursing Considerations for Patients with Respiratory Tract Disease (p. 300).

Side effects to expect

NAUSEA. Symptoms are usually mild; if they become bothersome, report to a physician.

Implementation

PREGNANCY. Ask if the patient is pregnant prior to administration. Excessive use of iodine-containing products may result in goiter in the newborn.

THYROID FUNCTION TESTS. Always inform the physician of the use of this product if thyroid function tests are to be scheduled.

Drug interactions

POTASSIUM SUPPLEMENTS, SALT SUBSTITUTES, POTASSIUM-SPARING DIURETICS. DO NOT administer with potassium-sparing diuretics (amiloride, triamterene, spironolactone). Do not use potassium supplements or salt substitutes high in potassium because of potentially dangerous effects from hyperkalemia.

LITHIUM, ANTITHYROID AGENTS. Concurrent use with lithium and antithyroid medications (methimazole, propylthiouracil) may result in hypothyroidism.

saline solutions

Saline solutions of varying concentrations can be very effective expectorants when administered by nebuliza-

tion. They act by hydrating mucus, reducing its viscosity. When administered by inhalation, hypotonic solutions (0.45% sodium chloride) are thought to provide deeper penetration into the more distant airways, while a hypertonic solution (1.8% sodium chloride) hydrates as well as stimulates a productive cough by irritating the respiratory passages. Isotonic saline solutions (0.9% sodium chloride), administered by nebulization, are used to hydrate respiratory secretions.

Saline nose drops are sometimes ordered for infants experiencing nasal congestion to clear the nasal passage and aid in breathing. Administration is usually immediately before giving them a bottle or breast feeding, since infants are nasal breathers.

Mucolytic agents

acetylcysteine (a-see'-til-cist-een)

Mucomyst (mu'-co-mist)

Acetylcysteine is currently the only mucolytic agent available that acts by dissolving chemical bonds within the mucus itself, thus causing it to separate and liquefy. It is used to dissolve abnormally viscous mucus secretions that may occur in chronic emphysema, emphysema with bronchitis, asthmatic bronchitis, and pneumonia.

Side effects. The most common adverse effects of acetylcysteine are mouth and throat irritation, nausea, vomiting, chest tightness, bronchoconstriction and runny nose (rhinorrhea).

Availability

Inhalation—10% and 20% solutions in 4, 10, and 30 ml vials.

Dosage and administration

Adult

Inhalation—The recommended dosage for most patients is 3 to 5 ml of the 20% solution 3 to 4 times daily. It may be administered by nebulization, direct application, or intratracheal instillation.

NOTE: After administration, the volume of bronchial secretions may increase. Some patients with inadequate cough reflex may require mechanical suctioning to maintain an open airway.

• Nursing Interventions: Monitoring acetylcysteine therapy

See also General Nursing Considerations for Patients with Respiratory Tract Disease (p. 300).

Side effects to expect

NAUSEA, VOMITING. This drug has a pungent odor (similar to rotten eggs) which may cause nausea and vomiting. Have an emesis basin available in case vomiting should occur. (Do not, however, suggest it by having it in clear view.)

Side effects to report

BRONCHOSPASM. This agent may occasionally cause

bronchoconstriction and bronchospasm. Concurrent use of a bronchodilator may be necessary.

Implementation

NEBULIZER. This solution tends to concentrate as the solution is used. When three-fourths of the original amount in the nebulizer is used, dilute the remaining solution with sterile water.

After therapy, wash the patient's face and hands because the drug is sticky and irritating. Thoroughly cleanse equipment used.

STORAGE. Store the opened solution of the drug in a refrigerator for up to 48 hours. Discard the unused portion after that time.

DISCOLORATION. Use this medication only in plastic or glass containers. Contact with metals other than stainless steel can cause discoloration of the solution.

Drug interactions

ANTIBIOTICS. Acetylcysteine inactivates most antibiotics. Do not mix together for aerosol administration. Schedule administration of inhalation antibiotics 1 hour after administration of acetylcysteine.

Side effects to report

TACHYCARDIA, PALPITATIONS. Since most symptoms are dose-related, alterations should be reported to the physician. Monitor the patient's heart rate and rhythm at regular intervals throughout therapy with bronchodilators.

Report heart rates significantly higher than baseline values.

Always report palpitations and suspected arrhythmias.

TREMORS. Tell the patient to notify the physician if tremors develop after starting any of these medications. A dosage adjustment may be necessary.

NERVOUSNESS, ANXIETY, RESTLESSNESS, HEADACHE. Perform a baseline assessment of the patient's mental status—degree of anxiety, nervousness, alertness; compare subsequent, regular assessments to the findings obtained. Report escalation of tension.

NAUSEA, VOMITING. Monitor all aspects of the development of these symptoms. Question the patient concerning other medications being taken and any other symptoms that have also developed.

Administer the medication with food and a full glass of water or milk. Report if the symptoms are not relieved.

DIZZINESS. Provide for patient safety during episodes of dizziness; report for further evaluation.

OBSTRUCTIVE AIRWAY DISEASE

Asthma and bronchitis are diseases that cause a reversible obstruction of the airways, while the airway constriction associated with emphysema is reversible in varying degrees depending on the severity and duration of the disease. Bronchodilators are agents that relax the smooth muscle of the tracheobronchial tree. This allows an increase in the opening of the bronchioles and alveolar ducts and a decrease in resistance to airflow into the alveolar sacs. The primary agents used in the treatment of airway-obstructive diseases include sympathomimetic agents, a new anticholinergic aerosol, xanthine derivatives, and corticosteroid inhalants.

Drug Therapy for Obstructive Airway Disease

Sympathomimetic bronchodilating agents

OBJECTIVES

1. Review the actions of the sympathetic nervous system in Table 9-1.
2. Compare the common side effects of sympathomimetic agents with the actions of the sympathetic nervous system.
3. Identify disease processes that increase a patient's sensitivity to sympathomimetic bronchodilating agents.
4. State the nursing assessments needed to monitor therapeutic response and/or the development of side effects to expect or report from sympathomimetic bronchodilator therapy.

Sympathomimetic agents are used as bronchodilators because they stimulate receptors within the smooth muscle of the tracheobronchial tree to relax, thus opening the airway passages to greater volumes of air. The primary sympathomimetic agents used as bronchodilators are listed in Table 12-3. They are used to reverse airway constriction caused by acute and chronic bronchial asthma, bronchitis, and emphysema. Those agents with more selective beta-2 receptor activity (such as albuterol and terbutaline) have more direct bronchodilating activity with fewer other systemic side effects. See also Chapter 10, "Drugs Affecting the Autonomic System," on selective beta-receptor activity.

Side effects. Unfortunately, the receptors stimulated by sympathomimetic agents, causing relaxation of the smooth muscle in the tracheobronchial tree, are found in other tissues as well as the pulmonary system. The receptors are also found in the muscles of the heart, blood vessels, uterus, gastrointestinal, urinary, and central nervous systems. They also help regulate fat and carbohydrate metabolism. For this reason, there are many side effects from these agents, particularly if used too frequently or in higher doses than recommended.

The most common side effects are dose-related. These include tachycardia, tremor, nervousness, heart palpitations, and dizziness. Other, less frequent, side effects may include nausea, vomiting, headache, restlessness, drowsiness, sweating, and tinnitus.

Patients who receive these medications by inhalation therapy may experience an unusual taste, heartburn, and dry throat leading to throat irritation.

Table 12-3 *Bronchodilators*

GENERIC NAME	BRAND NAMES	AVAILABILITY	ADULT DOSAGE RANGE
Sympathomimetics			
Albuterol	Proventil, Ventolin	Tablets: 2, 4 mg Aerosol: 90 mcg Syrup: 2 mg/5 ml	PO: 2-4 mg 3-4 times daily Inhale: 2 inhalations every 4-6 hours
Bitolterol	Tornalate	Aerosol: 0.37 mg/puff	Inhale: 2-3 inhalations every 8 hours Wait 2-3 minutes between each inhalation
Ephedrine	Ephedrine	Tablets: 25 mg Capsules: 25, 50 mg Syrup: 11, 20 mg/5 ml Injection: 25, 50 mg/ml	PO: 25-50 mg every 3-4 hours SC, IM, IV: 25-50 mg
Epinephrine	Primatene, Vaponefrin, Bronkaid Mist	Nebulization: 1:100 Aerosol: 0.2, 0.25, 0.3 mg Injection: 1:200, 1:100	See Manufacturer's Recommendations
Ethylnorepinephrine	Bronkephrine	Injection: 2 mg/ml in 1 ml amps	SC or IM: 0.5-1 ml
Isoetharine	Bronkosol, Beta-2, Bronkometer	Nebulization: 0.125, 0.2, 0.5, 1% Aerosol: 0.61%	See Manufacturer's Recommendations
Isoproterenol	Isuprel, Aerolone	Nebulization: 0.25, 0.5, 1% Aerosol: 0.2, 0.25% Injection: 0.02, 0.2 mg/ml SL: 10, 15 mg tabs	See Manufacturer's Recommendations
Metaproterenol	Alupent, Metaprel	Tablets: 10, 20 mg Syrup: 10 mg/5 ml Aerosol: 225 mg Nebulization: 0.6, 5%	See Manufacturer's Recommendations
Pirbuterol	Maxair	Aerosol: 0.2 mg/puff	Inhale: 1-2 inhalations every 4-6 hours
Terbutaline	Brethine, Bricanyl, Brethaire	Tablets: 2.5, 5 mg Injection: 1 mg/ml Aerosol: 0.2 mg/puff	PO: 5 mg every 6 hours SC: 0.25 mg; repeat, if needed, in 30 minutes Aerosol: 2 inhalations every 4-6 hours
Xanthine derivatives			
Aminophylline		Tablets: 100, 200 mg Elixir: 250 mg/15 ml Liquid: 105 mg/5 ml Suppositories: 250, 500 mg Injection: 250, 500 ml Others	See Manufacturer's Recommendations
Dyphylline	Dilor, Dyflex, Lufyllin, ♣ Protophylline	Tablets: 200, 400 mg Liquid: 100 mg/5 ml Elixir: 100, 160 mg/15 ml Injection: 250 mg/ml	PO: 15 mg/kg, 5 times daily IM: 250-500 mg slowly
Oxtriphylline	Choledyl	Tablets: 100, 200 mg Elixir: 100 mg/5 ml Syrup: 50 mg/5 ml	200 mg 4 times daily
Theophylline	Bronkodyl, Elixophyllin, Theolair, others	Tablets: 125, 200, 225, 300 mg Capsules: 100, 200, 250 mg Elixir: 26.7, 50 mg/5 ml Liquid: 26.7, 50 mg/5 ml Syrup: 26.7, 50 mg/5 ml Others	9-20 mg/kg/24 hours in 4 divided doses

♣ Available in Canada only.

Patients known to have hypertension, hyperthyroidism, diabetes mellitus, or cardiac disease with arrhythmias may be particularly sensitive to adverse reactions and must be observed closely.

Availability. See Table 12-3 for available sympathomimetic bronchodilator products and recommended dosage ranges.

• Nursing Interventions: Monitoring bronchodilator therapy

See also General Nursing Considerations for Patients with Respiratory Tract Disease (p. 300).

Side effects to report

TACHYCARDIA, PALPITATIONS. Since most symptoms are dose-related, alterations should be reported to the physician. Monitor the patient's heart rate and rhythm at regular intervals throughout therapy with bronchodilators. An increase of 20 beats or more per minute after treatment should be reported to the physician.

Always report palpitations and suspected arrhythmias.

TREMORS. Tell the patient to notify the physician if tremors develop after starting any of these medications. A dosage adjustment may be necessary.

NERVOUSNESS, ANXIETY, RESTLESSNESS, HEADACHE. Perform a baseline assessment of the patient's mental status—degree of anxiety, nervousness, alertness; compare subsequent, regular assessments to the findings obtained. Report escalation of tension.

NAUSEA, VOMITING. Monitor all aspects of the development of these symptoms. Question the patient concerning other medications being taken and any other symptoms that have also developed.

Administer the medication with food and a full glass of water or milk. Report if the symptoms are not relieved.

DIZZINESS. Provide for patient safety during episodes of dizziness; report for further evaluation.

Drug interactions

DRUGS THAT ENHANCE TOXIC EFFECTS. Tricyclic antidepressants (imipramine, amitriptyline, nortriptyline, doxepin, others), monoamine oxidase inhibitors (tranylcypromine, isocarboxazid, pargyline) and other sympathomimetic agents (metaproterenol, isoproterenol, others). Monitor for increases in severity of drug effects such as nervousness, tachycardia, tremors, and arrhythmias.

DRUGS THAT REDUCE THERAPEUTIC EFFECTS. Beta adrenergic blocking agents (propanolol, timolol, nadolol, pindolol, others). Higher doses, or use of another class of bronchodilator, may be required.

ANTIHYPERTENSIVE AGENTS. Sympathomimetic agents may reduce the therapeutic effects of antihypertensive agents. Monitor blood pressure for an indication of loss of antihypertensive control.

Anticholinergic bronchodilating agents

OBJECTIVES

1. Review the actions of the anticholinergic agents on the cholinergic nervous system.
2. Review the procedures for administration of medication by inhalation.
3. State the nursing assessments needed to monitor therapeutic response and/or the development of side effects to expect or report from anticholinergic bronchodilator therapy.

ipratropium bromide (ihp-rah'trop-eum)

Atrovent (at'roh-vent)

Anticholinergic agents have been used as bronchodilators in the treatment of chronic obstructive pulmonary disease for more than 200 years, but the potent anticholinergic adverse effects of throat irritation, dry mouth, reduced mucous secretions, increased viscosity of secretions, mydriasis, cycloplegia, urinary retention, and tachycardia and the availability of selective sympathomimetic agents have limited their use in pulmonary disorders. In 1987, a new anticholinergic agent with significantly fewer side effects became available. Ipra-tropium bromide is administered by aerosol inhalation and produces bronchodilation by competitive inhibition of cholinergic receptors on bronchial smooth muscle. It has minimal effect on ciliary activity, mucous secretion, sputum volume or viscosity. Initial bronchodilation is evident within the first few minutes following inhalation, but maximal effects are seen in 1 to 2 hours. The duration of significant bronchodilation is 4 to 6 hours with usual doses. Since its maximal effects are not felt immediately, the drug is more appropriately used for prophylaxis and maintenance treatment of bronchospasm associated with chronic obstructive lung disease than for acute episodes of bronchospasm associated with asthma.

Side effects. The adverse effects of ipratropium therapy are quite mild because there is minimal systemic absorption of the active ingredient. Transient dryness of the mouth and scratching of the throat are reported in up to 15% of patients, while a bitter taste was noted in 20% to 30% of patients.

Rare systemic effects such as visual disturbances, tachycardia, blurred vision, drowsiness and dizziness have been reported.

Availability. Inhalation—Aerosol canister containing approximately 200 inhalations (18 mcg/metered dose) with metered dose inhaler mouthpiece.

Dosage and administration. NOTE: Ipratropium bromide should not be used in the initial treatment of acute episodes of bronchospasm where rapid response is required. Use with caution in patients with the potential for narrow angle glaucoma.

Inhalation—The usual dose is two inhalations (36 mcg) four times a day. Patients may take additional inhalations as required, but should not exceed 12 inhalations in 24 hours.

Drug interactions. No significant interactions have been reported.

• **Nursing Interventions: Monitoring ipratropium therapy**

See also General Nursing Considerations for Patients with Respiratory Diseases (p. 300).

Side effects to expect

DRYNESS OF MOUTH AND THROAT, IRRITATION. These side effects are usually mild and tend to resolve with continued therapy. Encourage the patient not to discontinue therapy without first consulting the physician.

Ensure that regular oral hygiene measures are continued. Suggest the use of 1 teaspoon of hydrogen peroxide in 6 to 8 ounces of water as a mouthwash. Commercial mouthwashes contain alcohol, which may cause further drying and oral irritation.

Other measures to alleviate dryness include sucking on ice chips or hard candy.

Side effects to report

TACHYCARDIA, URINARY RETENTION, EXACERBATION OF PULMONARY SYMPTOMS. Request that the patient consult a physician before continuing with further therapy.

Implementation

ENSURE THAT PATIENT UNDERSTANDS HOW TO INHALE MEDICATION

1. Clear throat and mouth of sputum.
2. Insert the metal canister into the clear end of the mouthpiece.
3. Remove the protective cap, invert the canister, and shake thoroughly.
4. Enclose the mouthpiece with the lips. The base of the canister should be held vertically. (Keep the eyes closed because temporary blurring of vision may result if the aerosol is sprayed into the eyes.)
5. Exhale deeply, then inhale slowly through the mouthpiece and at the same time firmly press once on the upended canister base; continue to inhale deeply.
6. Hold breath for a few seconds, then remove the mouthpiece from the mouth and exhale slowly. Wait approximately 15 seconds and repeat the second inhalation as outlined above.
7. Replace the protective cap after use.
8. Keep the mouthpiece clean. Wash with hot water. If soap is used, rinse thoroughly with plain water.

Xanthine derivative bronchodilating agents
OBJECTIVES

1. Cite the action of xanthine derivatives on the smooth muscle of the tracheobronchial tree.
2. State the desired action of xanthine derivatives when used in combination with sympathomimetic bronchodilators.

3. Recall the signs and symptoms of central nervous system stimulation.
4. List side effects known to occur with the use of xanthine derivatives and correlate these with the needed nursing assessments and interventions.
5. State the type of schedule that should be maintained for administration of these agents to maintain a therapeutic blood plasma level and to prevent gastric irritation.

Methylxanthines, more commonly known as the xanthine derivatives, act directly on the smooth muscle of the tracheobronchial tree to dilate the bronchi, thus increasing airflow in and out of the alveolar sacs. The primary xanthine derivatives used as bronchodilators are listed in Table 12-3. They are frequently used in combination with sympathomimetic bronchodilators to reverse airway constriction caused by acute and chronic bronchial asthma, bronchitis, and emphysema.

Side effects. In addition to relaxing pulmonary smooth muscle, the xanthine derivatives stimulate the central nervous system, induce diuresis, increase gastric acid secretions, and stimulate the heart to beat more rapidly. Consequently, side effects associated with bronchodilator therapy, particularly in higher doses, include nervousness, agitation, insomnia, nausea, vomiting, abdominal cramps, epigastric pain, and tachycardia, possibly with arrhythmias. All of these side effects are dose-dependent and may diminish with a reduction in dosage.

Xanthine derivatives should be administered cautiously to patients with congestive heart failure, chronic obstructive pulmonary disease, or renal or hepatic disease. These patients metabolize xanthine derivatives much more slowly and may develop toxicities more easily.

Xanthine derivatives should also be used with caution in patients with angina pectoris, peptic ulcer disease, hyperthyroidism, glaucoma, and diabetes mellitus.

Availability. See Table 12-3 for available xanthine derivative bronchodilator products and recommended dosage ranges.

• **Nursing Interventions: Monitoring xanthine therapy**

See also General Nursing Considerations for Patients with Respiratory Tract Disease (p. 300).

Side effects to report

TACHYCARDIA, PALPITATIONS. Since most symptoms are dose-related, alterations should be reported to the physician. Monitor the patient's heart rate and rhythm at regular intervals throughout therapy with bronchodilators.

Report heart rates significantly higher than baseline values.

Always report palpitations and suspected arrhythmias.

TREMORS. Tell the patient to notify the physician if

tremors develop after starting any of these medications. A dosage adjustment may be necessary.

NERVOUSNESS, ANXIETY, RESTLESSNESS, HEADACHE. Perform a baseline assessment of the patient's mental status—degree of anxiety, nervousness, alertness; compare subsequent, regular assessments to the findings obtained. Report escalation of tension.

Implementation

NAUSEA, VOMITING, EPIGASTRIC PAIN, AND ABDOMINAL CRAMPS. These symptoms may occur from gastric irritation caused by increased gastric acid secretions stimulated by these agents.

If gastric irritation occurs, administer with food or milk. If symptoms persist or increase in severity, report for physician evaluation.

PLASMA LEVELS. To maintain consistent plasma levels, administer the medication around the clock.

Drug interactions

DRUGS THAT ENHANCE TOXIC EFFECTS. Cimetidine, erythromycin, troleandomycin, diltiazem, nifedipine, verapamil, moricizine, thiabendazole, influenza vaccine, propranolol, and allopurinol. Monitor for increases in severity of drug effects such as nervousness, agitation, nausea, tachycardia, and arrhythmias.

DRUGS THAT REDUCE THERAPEUTIC EFFECTS. Tobacco or marijuana smoking. Higher doses of the bronchodilator may be required.

LITHIUM. Xanthine derivatives may increase the renal excretion of lithium carbonate. Higher doses of lithium are required to maintain therapeutic effects. Monitor for the return of manic or depressive activity. Enlist the aid of family and friends to help identify early symptoms.

BETA ADRENERGIC BLOCKING AGENTS. Xanthine derivatives and beta adrenergic blocking agents (propranolol, timolol, nadolol, atenolol, others) may be mutually antagonistic in their actions. Patients must be observed for inhibition of either drug.

Corticosteroids used for obstructive airway disease
OBJECTIVES

1. Review the procedures for administration of medication by inhalation.
2. State the nursing assessments needed to monitor therapeutic response and/or the development of side effects to expect or report from corticosteroid inhalant therapy.

Patients with severe asthma or chronic obstructive lung disease who are losing response to sympathomimetic agents or xanthine derivatives may have corticosteroids added to their medication regimen to provide enhanced bronchodilation. Corticosteroids (see Chapter 17, "Drugs Affecting the Immune System") whether applied by aerosol or administered systemically, have been shown to be highly effective for the treatment of obstructive lung disease. The mechanisms of action are not completely known, but corticosteroids have a direct effect on smooth muscle relaxation; they enhance the effect of beta-adrenergic bronchodilators and inhibit inflammatory responses that may result in bronchoconstriction.

Side effects vary with the duration and timing of the administration as well as with the type of steroid preparation used. The first therapy is often a short course (5 to 7 days) of systemic corticosteroids (such as prednisone), with intervals of several weeks or months without steroid treatment. Alternate-day therapy (that is, a single morning dose every other day) is the next preferable program. Aerosolized corticosteroids may be used daily in certain patients in place of alternate-day therapy. If the patient has not previously been receiving corticosteroid therapy, several weeks may pass before the full benefits from the aerosolized medication are achieved, but a single aerosol "burst" does produce noticeable benefits in reduced bronchoconstriction. It is important to remember that the corticosteroid aerosols should not be regarded as true bronchodilators and should not be used for rapid relief of bronchospasm.

Side effects. On initiation of aerosol therapy, some patients will complain of mild, transient hoarseness or dry mouth.

Oral, laryngeal, and pharyngeal fungal infections (thrush) have been reported with varying degrees of frequency.

Availability. See Table 12-4 for available inhalant corticosteroid products and recommended dosage ranges.

Dosage and administration. The adverse effects of corticosteroids can be significant. Therefore, all efforts must be made to minimize these adverse effects. After symptoms are controlled, the initial corticosteroid doses should always be reduced to the lowest possible dose that is still compatible with continued control.

• Nursing Interventions: Monitoring corticosteroid therapy

See also General Nursing Considerations for Patients with Respiratory Tract Disease (p. 300).

Side effects to expect

HOARSENESS, DRY MOUTH. These side effects are usually mild and tend to resolve with continued therapy. Encourage the patient not to discontinue therapy without consulting the physician first.

Side effects to report

FUNGAL INFECTIONS (THRUSH). Increased risk factors for the development of oral thrush include concomitant antibiotic use, diabetes, improper aerosol administration, large oral doses of corticosteroids, and poor dental hygiene.

Patients should be instructed on good oral hygiene technique and should be instructed to gargle and rinse their mouths after each aerosol treatment with a mouthwash such as 1 teaspoon of hydrogen peroxide in 6 to 8 ounces of water. Commercial mouthwashes con-

Table 12-4 *Inhalant Corticosteroids*

GENERIC NAME	BRAND NAME	AVAILABILITY	ADULT DOSAGE RANGE
Beclomethasone dipropionate	Beclovent, Vanceril	Aerosol: 200 doses/inhaler	2 inhalations (84 mcg) 3-4 times daily; maximum of 840 mcg (20 inhalations) daily
Dexamethasone sodium phosphate	Decadron Respihaler	Aerosol: 170 doses/container	3 inhalations (150 mcg) 3-4 times daily; maximum of 12 inhalations daily
Flunisolide	AeroBid, ♣Bronalide	Aerosol: 50 doses/inhaler	2 inhalations (500 mcg) twice daily; do not exceed 2 mg (8 inhalations) daily
Triamcinolone acetonide	Azmacort	Aerosol: 50 doses/inhaler	2 inhalations (200 mcg) 3-4 times daily; do not exceed 1600 mcg (16 inhalations) daily

♣Available in Canada only.

tain alcohol, which may cause further drying and oral irritation.

If thrush should develop, it is usually not sufficiently troublesome to require discontinuation of the steroid aerosol therapy. An antifungal mouthwash such as nystatin (Mycostatin, Nilstat) will usually eradicate the oral candidiasis.

Implementation

COUNSELING, COMPLIANCE. The therapeutic effects, unlike those of sympathomimetic bronchodilators, are not immediate. This should be explained to the patient in advance to ensure cooperation and continuation of treatment with the prescribed dosage regimen, even when asymptomatic. Full therapeutic benefit requires regular use, and may require up to 4 weeks of therapy for maximum benefit.

PREPARATION BEFORE ADMINISTRATION. Patients receiving bronchodilators by inhalation should be advised to use the bronchodilator before the corticosteroid inhalant in order to enhance penetration of the corticosteroid into the bronchial tree. Wait several minutes to allow the time for the bronchodilator to relax the smooth muscle.

MAINTENANCE THERAPY. After the desired clinical effect is obtained, the maintenance dose should be reduced to the smallest amount necessary to control the symptoms.

SEVERE STRESS OR ASTHMA ATTACK. During periods of stress or a severe asthma attack, patients may require treatment with systemic steroids. Exacerbation of asthma that occurs during the course of corticosteroid inhalant therapy should be treated with a short course of systemic steroid. Do not attempt to use the inhaler, because the aerosol not only may cause irritation and exacerbate symptoms, but may not penetrate deeply into the bronchial tree for maximal effect.

NASAL CONGESTION
OBJECTIVES

1. State the two major causes of allergic rhinitis.
2. Identify the three classes of nasal decongestants.

KEY WORDS

allergic rhinitis   rebound effect
rhinorrhea

Nasal stuffiness and congestion are caused by swelling of the nasal mucous membranes. Two major causes of a stuffy nose are allergic rhinitis (in which the nasal passages swell because of an allergic reaction, most commonly due to dust or pollen) and symptoms of the common cold. Symptomatic relief of nasal congestion is a result of reduced swelling of the nasal passages. The three classes of nasal decongestants are the sympathomimetics, antihistamines, and corticosteroids.

Drug Therapy for Nasal Congestion

Sympathomimetic decongestants
OBJECTIVES

1. Review the actions of adrenergic agents on body systems (see Table 9-1).
2. Define *rebound effect* and describe the patient education needed to prevent it.
3. Review procedures for administration of medications by nose drops and sprays.
4. Explain why all decongestant products should be used cautiously in persons with hypertension, hyperthyroidism, diabetes mellitus, cardiac disease, increased intraocular pressure, or prostatic disease.
5. State the nursing assessments needed to monitor therapeutic response and/or the development of side effects to expect or report from sympathomimetic decongestants.

Sympathomimetic nasal decongestants (Table 12-5) stimulate the alpha adrenergic receptors of the vascular smooth muscle of the nasal passages, causing constriction of the blood vessels within the nasal passages. This constriction reduces blood flow in the engorged nasal area, resulting in shrinkage of the engorged membranes, thus promoting drainage, improving nasal air passage, and relieving the feeling of stuffiness.

The use of nasal decongestants provides temporary

Table 12-5 *Nasal Decongestants*

GENERIC NAME	BRAND NAMES	AVAILABILITY	ADULT DOSAGE RANGE
Ephedrine	Efedron, Vatronol	Solution: 0.5% Jelly: 0.6%	Nasal: 2-3 drops 2-3 times daily
Epinephrine	Adrenalin	Solution: 0.1%	Nasal: 1-2 drops in each nostril every 4-6 hours
Naphazoline	Privine	Solution: 0.05%	Nasal: 2-3 drops or sprays no more than every 3 hours (drops) or 4-6 hours (spray).
Phenylephrine	Neo-Synephrine, Sinex	Solution: 0.125, 0.16, 0.2, 0.25, 0.5, 1% Jelly: 0.5%	Nasal: 0.25% every 3-4 hours
Phenylpropanolamine	Rhindecon, Propagest	Tablets: 25, 50 mg Capsules: 75 mg	PO: 25 mg every 3-4 hours or 50 mg every 6-8 hours. Do not exceed 150 mg daily
Pseudoephedrine	Sudafed, Neofed, Novafed	Tablets: 30, 60, 120 mg Liquid: 15, 30 mg/5 ml Drops: 7.5 mg/0.8 ml	PO: 60 mg every 6 hours. Do not exceed 240 mg/24 hours
Oxymetazoline	Afrin, Duration	Solution: 0.025-0.05%	Nasal: 2-3 drops or sprays of 0.05% solution twice daily
Tetrahydrozoline	Tyzine	Solution: 0.05-0.1%	Nasal: 2-4 drops of 0.1% solution every 4-6 hours
Xylometazoline	Otrivin	Solution: 0.05, 0.1%	Nasal: 2-3 sprays every 8-10 hours

relief of the symptoms. Initially, the "stuffiness" or "blocked" sensation exhibits relief. However, as the constricting action diminishes, the symptoms return. Prolonged use can cause irritation of the narcs; excessive use may result in a *rebound effect* caused by swelling of the nasal passages. Instill drops or sprays appropriately. (See "Administration by Inhalation" in Chapter 7.)

Side effects. Products used as nasal decongestants have the ability to stimulate alpha receptors at other sites in the body as well. Therefore, they should be used with caution in patients with hypertension, hyperthyroidism, diabetes mellitus, cardiac disease, increased intraocular pressure, or prostatic hypertrophy.

It is important for the patient to follow directions on the label carefully. Misuse by patients, including excessive use or frequency of administration, may cause a rebound swelling of the nasal passages. This secondary congestion is thought to be caused by excessive vasoconstriction of the blood vessels and by direct irritation of the nasal membranes by the solution. When the vasoconstrictor effects wear off, the irritation causes excessive blood flow to the passages, causing them to swell and become engorged again; the nose feels more stuffy and congested than before treatment. Rebound effects are minimal if decongestants are used for only 3 to 5 days.

Availability. See Table 12-5 for available decongestant products.

- **Nursing Interventions: Monitoring nasal decongestant therapy**

See also General Nursing Considerations for Patients with Respiratory Tract Disease (p. 300).

Side effects to expect

MILD NASAL IRRITATION. A burning or stinging sensation may be experienced. This may be alleviated by using a weaker strength of solution.

Drug interactions

DRUGS THAT ENHANCE TOXIC EFFECTS. Beta adrenergic blocking agents (such as propanolol, timolol, atenolol, nadolol, others) and monoamine oxidase inhibitors (tranylcypromine, isocarboxazid, pargyline).

Excessive use may result in significant hypertension.

Patients already receiving antihypertensive therapy should avoid the use of decongestants.

METHYLDOPA, RESERPINE. Frequent use of decongestants inhibits the antihypertensive activity of these agents. Concurrent therapy is not recommended.

Antihistaminic decongestants
OBJECTIVES

1. Define an antigen-antibody response.
2. Cite specific signs and symptoms seen when histamine is released.
3. State two types of drugs used to antagonize histamine responses.
4. Explain the action of antihistamines.

5. List the anticholinergic side effects displayed with antihistamine therapy.
6. State the nursing assessments needed to monitor therapeutic response and/or the development of side effects to expect or report with antihistamine therapy.
7. Identify the anticholinergic side effects displayed with antihistamine therapy.

KEY WORDS

histamine   allergen
antigen   antibody

Histamine is a compound derived from an amino acid called *histidine*. It is stored in small granules in most body tissues. Its physiologic functions are not completely known, but it is released in response to allergic reactions and tissue damage from trauma or infection. When histamine is released in the area of tissue damage or at the site of an *antigen-antibody reaction* (such as a pollen being inhaled into the nose of a patient allergic to that specific pollen) the following reactions take place: (1) arterioles and capillaries in the region dilate, allowing an increased blood flow to the area, resulting in redness; (2) capillaries become more permeable, resulting in the outward passage of fluid into the extracellular spaces and, thus, edema; this edema is manifested by congestion in the mucous membranes of the patient's nose and lungs; (3) nasal, lacrimal, and bronchial secretions are released, resulting in the running nose and eyes noted in patients with allergies.

When large amounts of histamine are released, such as in a severe allergic reaction, there is extensive arteriolar dilatation. The blood pressure drops (hypotension), and the skin becomes flushed and edematous with severe itching (urticaria). Constriction and spasm of the bronchial tubes makes respiratory effort more difficult (dyspnea), and copious amounts of pulmonary and gastric secretions are released.

Histamine response can be antagonized by two types of drugs, rapidly acting epinephrine and the more slowly acting group of antihistamines. Epinephrine is used only in severe, acute allergic reactions.

Antihistamines can reduce the severity of the symptoms observed in the allergic patient. *Antihistamines* are chemical agents that act by competing with the allergy-liberated histamine for receptor sites in the patient's arterioles, capillaries, and glands. Antihistamines do not prevent histamine release, but will reduce the symptoms of an allergic reaction if the concentration of the antihistamine exceeds the concentration of histamine at the receptor site. Antihistamines are, therefore, more effective if taken when the symptoms are first appearing.

Antihistamines treat only the symptoms of allergy and do not immunize the patient against allergic reactions. Relief of various allergic symptoms is obtained only while the drug is being taken. There is no cumulative action, so these drugs can be taken for prolonged periods of time. Some patients, requiring frequent antihistamine use, find that they do not obtain the same degree of relief after several weeks or months of therapy. If tolerance does develop, patients may easily switch to another antihistamine that does provide relief.

Side effects. The most common side effect of many of the antihistaminic drugs is drowsiness. Most patients acquire a tolerance to this adverse effect with continued therapy. Reduction in dosage or a change to another antihistamine may occasionally be necessary, however.

All antihistamines display anticholinergic side effects, particularly when higher dosages are used. Symptoms include dry mouth, stuffy nose, blurred vision, constipation, and urinary retention. Patients with asthma, prostatic enlargement, or glaucoma should take antihistamines only under a physician's supervision. The drying effects may also make respiratory mucus more viscous and tenacious. Use antihistamines with caution in patients who have a productive cough. If the cough continues but becomes nonproductive, consider additional hydration of the patient and discontinuation of the antihistamine.

Availability. See Table 12-6 for available antihistamine products and recommended dosage ranges.

• **Nursing Interventions: Monitoring antihistamine therapy**

See also General Nursing Considerations for Patients with Respiratory Tract Disease (p. 300).

Because antihistamines are prescribed for a variety of symptoms, such as hay fever, dermatological reactions, drug hypersensitivity, rhinitis, and transfusion reactions, it is necessary for the nurse to individualize the patient assessments with the underlying pathology. Identification of the trigger mechanism, or allergens, that initiate an allergic response is imperative to treatment. Repeated exposure to the conditions that precipitate an attack will again initiate an allergic response.

Side effects to expect

SEDATIVE EFFECTS. The types of antihistamines ordered can produce varying degrees of sedation. Tolerance may be produced over a period of time, thus diminishing the effect.

Operating power equipment or driving may be hazardous. Caution patients to provide for their personal safety in these situations.

DRYING EFFECTS. Monitor the patient's cough and degree of sputum production when antihistamines are administered. Because of their drying effects, antihistamines may impair expectoration.

FLUID INTAKE. Give adequate fluids concurrently with the use of antihistamines. Maintain fluid intake at 8 to 12 8-ounce glasses daily.

Table 12-6 *Antihistamines**

GENERIC NAME	BRAND NAMES	AVAILABILITY	ADULT DOSAGE RANGE	MAXIMUM DAILY DOSE (MG)
Astemizole	Hismanal	Tablets	10 mg daily	10
Azatadine maleate	Optimine	Tablets	1-2 mg twice daily	4
Brompheniramine maleate	Veltane, Dimetane, Bromphen	Injection, tablets, elixir	4 mg four to six times daily	24
Carbinoxamine maleate	Clistin	Tablets	4-8 mg three to four times daily	24
Clemastine fumarate	Tavist	Tablets, syrup	1.34-2.68 mg three times daily	8
Chlorpheniramine maleate	Chlor-tab-4, Chlor-Trimeton, Trymegen	Tablets, capsules, syrup	4 mg three to six times daily	24
Cyproheptadine hydrochloride	Periactin	Tablets, syrup	4 mg three times daily	32
Diphenhydramine hydrochloride	Benadryl, Allermax, Nordryl	Injection, capsules, tablets, syrup, elixir	25-50 mg three or four times daily	300
Doxylamine succinate	Decapryn	Tablets, syrup	12.5-25 mg every 4-6 hours	150
Promethazine hydrochloride†	Phenergan, Prorex	Injection, tablets, syrup, suppository	12.5-25 mg three or four times daily	100
Pyrilamine maleate	Nisaval	Tablets	25-50 mg four times daily	200
Terfenadine	Seldane	Tablets	60 mg twice daily	120
Tripelennamine	PBZ, Pelamine	Tablets, elixir	25-50 mg every 4-6 hours	300
Triprolidine	Actidil	Tablets, syrup	2.5 mg every 4-6 hours	15

*Many of these antihistamines are also available in combination with decongestants and analgesics for relief of cold and flu symptoms.
†Promethazine is a phenothiazine with antihistaminic properties.

BLURRED VISION, CONSTIPATION, URINARY RETENTION, DRYNESS OF MUCOSA OF THE MOUTH, THROAT, AND NOSE. These symptoms are the anticholinergic effects produced by antihistamines. Patients taking these medications should be monitored for the development of these side effects.

Dryness of the mucosa may be alleviated by sucking hard candy or ice chips, or chewing gum.

Caution the patient that blurred vision may occur and make appropriate suggestions for personal safety of the individual.

Drug interactions

CNS DEPRESSANTS. CNS depressants, including sleep aids, analgesics, tranquilizers, and alcohol will potentiate the sedative effects of antihistamines. People who work around machinery, drive a car, pour and give medicines, or perform other duties in which they must remain mentally alert should not take these medications while working.

Corticosteroid decongestants
OBJECTIVE

1. State the nursing assessments needed to monitor therapeutic response and/or the development of side effects to expect or report from corticosteroid inhalant therapy.

Patients with severe allergic seasonal rhinitis who do not respond to sympathomimetic agents or antihistamines may be placed on corticosteroids to provide relief of symptoms of the allergy. Corticosteroids (see also Chapter 17, "Drugs Affecting the Immune System"), whether applied topically or administered systemically, have been shown to be highly effective for the treatment of allergic rhinitis. Intranasal hydrocortisone, prednisolone, and dexamethasone have been reported to be successful in controlling nasal symptoms, but they also produce systemic side effects, including significant adrenal suppression. The newer topically active aerosol steroids, such as beclomethasone dipropionate and flunisolide, have been shown to be highly effective with minimal incidence of side effects. The therapeutic effect (reduction of sneezing, nasal itching, stuffiness, and rhinorrhea) is usually observed by the third day, although the maximal effects may not be evident for 2 weeks. To minimize the development of adrenal suppression, these corticosteroids should be used only for short courses of therapy for acute seasonal allergies.

Side effects. Approximately half of patients who receive intranasal steroid therapy complain of a mild, transient nasal burning and stinging. This adverse effect diminishes with continued therapy, and only about 3% of patients discontinue therapy due to adverse effects.

Availability. See Table 12-7 for available intranasal corticosteroid products and recommended dosage ranges.

Table 12-7 *Intranasal Corticosteroids*

GENERIC NAME	BRAND NAME	AVAILABILITY	ADULT DOSAGE RANGE
Beclomethasone dipropionate	Beconase, Vancerase	Nasal aerosol: 200 doses/canister	1 inhalation (42 mcg) in each nostril 2 to 4 times daily
Beclomethasone dipropionate, monohydrate	Beconase AQ	Nasal spray	1-2 sprays (42-84 mcg) in each nostril 2 times daily
Dexamethasone sodium phosphate	Decadron, Tubinaire	Nasal aerosol: 170 doses/cartridge	2 sprays (168 mcg) in each nostril 2 to 3 times daily; maximum daily dose is 12 sprays (1008 mcg) in 24 hours
Flunisolide	Nasalide, ✦Rhinalar	Nasal spray: 200 doses/bottle	2 sprays (50 mcg) in each nostril 2 times daily; maximum daily dose is 8 sprays (400 mcg) in 24 hours
Triamcinolone	Nasacort	Nasal spray: 100 doses/bottle	2 sprays in each nostril once daily. Maximum daily dose is 4 sprays in 24 hours

✦Available in Canada only.

• **Nursing Interventions: Monitoring nasal corticosteroid therapy**

See also General Nursing Considerations for Patients with Respiratory Tract Disease (p. 300).

Side effects to expect

NASAL BURNING. This side effect is usually mild and tends to resolve with continued therapy. Encourage the patient not to discontinue therapy without first consulting the physician.

Implementation

COUNSELING. The therapeutic effects, unlike those of sympathomimetic decongestants, are not immediate. This should be explained to the patient in advance to ensure cooperation and continuation of treatment with the prescribed dosage regimen. Full therapeutic benefit requires regular use and is usually evident within a few days, although a few patients may require up to 3 weeks of therapy for maximum benefit.

PREPARATION BEFORE ADMINISTRATION. Patients with blocked nasal passages should be encouraged to use a decongestant just before intranasal corticosteroid administration to ensure adequate penetration. Patients should also be advised to clear their nasal passages of secretions prior to use.

MAINTENANCE THERAPY. After desired clinical effect is obtained, the maintenance dose should be reduced to the smallest amount necessary to control the symptoms.

Other agents

OBJECTIVES

1. State the action of cromolyn sodium on histamine.
2. Compare the action of antihistamine preparations and cromolyn sodium on histamine.
3. Review the procedure of intranasal and inhalation administration of cromolyn.

4. State the nursing assessments needed to monitor therapeutic response and/or the development of side effects to expect or report from cromolyn therapy.

cromolyn sodium (kro'mo-lin)

Intal (in-tahl') **(Nasalcrom)**

Cromolyn sodium is a unique medication that is administered to prevent the release of histamine from its storage sites, the mast cells. It must be administered before the body receives a stimulus to release histamine, such as an antigen that initiates an antigen-antibody allergic reaction. Cromolyn is recommended for use in conjunction with other medications in the treatment of patients with severe bronchial asthma or allergic rhinitis to prevent the release of histamine that results in asthmatic attacks or symptoms of allergic rhinitis.

Cromolyn has no direct bronchodilatory, antihistaminic, anticholinergic, or antiinflammatory activity. The concomitant use of antihistamines or nasal decongestants may be necessary during initial treatment with cromolyn. A 2- to 4-week course of therapy is usually required to determine clinical response. Therapy should be continued only if there is a decrease in the severity of asthmatic symptoms during treatment.

Side effects. The most common side effect is irritation of the throat and trachea caused by inhalation of the dry powder. This irritation may be manifested by nasal itching and burning, nasal stuffiness, sneezing, coughing, and bronchospasm. Other side effects that infrequently arise are nausea, drowsiness, dizziness, and headache.

Availability

Inhalation—20 mg capsules, 20 mg/2ml solution for nebulizer, and 112 and 200 metered spray aerosols.

Nasal solution—40 mg/ml in 13 ml metered spray device.

Dosage and administration

Adult

PO—Patients must be advised that the capsules are not absorbed when swallowed and that the drug is inactive when administered by this route.

Inhalation—40 mg (2 capsule), via inhaler, 4 times daily.

Nasal spray—1 spray in each nostril 3 to 4 times daily at regular intervals. Maximum is 6 sprays in each nostril daily.

Aerosol—2 metered sprays inhaled 4 times daily at regular intervals.

Drug interactions. No significant drug interactions have been reported.

• Nursing Interventions: Monitoring cromolyn therapy

See also General Nursing Considerations for Patients with Respiratory Tract Disease (p. 300).

Side effects to expect

ORAL IRRITATION, DRY MOUTH. Start regular oral hygiene measures when the therapy is initiated. Suggest the use of 1 teaspoon of hydrogen peroxide in 6 to 8 ounces of water as a mouthwash. Commercial mouthwashes contain alcohol, which may cause further drying and oral irritation.

Other measures to alleviate dryness include sucking on ice chips or hard candy.

Side effects to report

BRONCHOSPASM, COUGHING. Notify the physician if inhalation causes these symptoms.

Implementation

COUNSELING. The therapeutic effects, unlike those of sympathomimetic decongestants, are not immediate. This should be explained to the patient in advance to ensure cooperation and continuation of treatment with the prescribed dosage regimen. Full therapeutic benefit requires regular use and is usually evident within 2 to 4 weeks.

INHALATION. Inhalation during an acute asthma attack may aggravate symptoms since the powder form of the drug can increase the irritation in the respiratory passage causing more bronchospasm.

Proper technique is quite important to the success of therapy. Document and verify that the patient can do the following:

1. Load the inhaler with a capsule and pierce (only once) the capsule immediately before use.
2. Hold the inhaler away from the mouth and exhale, emptying as much air from the lungs as possible.
3. With the head tilted back and teeth apart, close lips around the mouthpiece.
4. Inhale deeply and rapidly through the inhaler with a steady, even breath.
5. Remove the inhaler and hold the breath for a few seconds, then exhale. (Do not exhale through the inhaler, because moisture from the breath will interfere with proper function of the inhaler.)
6. Repeat several times until the powder is inhaled. (A light dusting of powder remaining in the capsule is normal.)

NASAL SOLUTION. Patients with blocked nasal passages should be encouraged to use a decongestant just before intranasal cromolyn administration to ensure adequate penetration. Patients should also be advised to clear their nasal passages of secretions and then inhale through the nose during administration.

Drug interactions. No significant drug interactions have been reported.

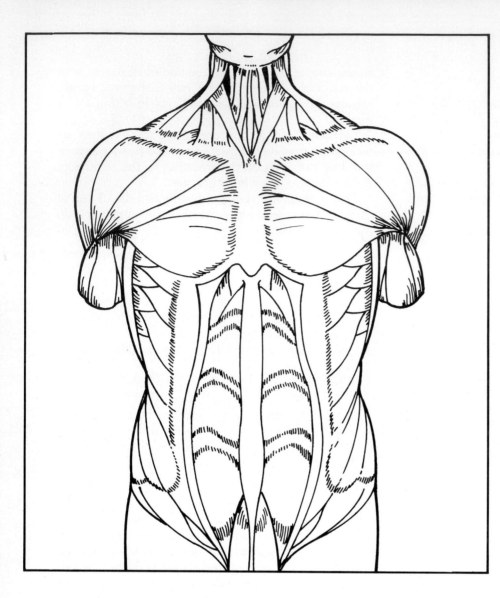

CHAPTER GOALS

After completing this chapter, the student should be able to do the following:

1. Explain the major actions and effects of drugs used to treat disorders of the muscular system.

2. Identify baseline data the nurse should collect on a continuous basis for comparison and evaluation of drug effectiveness.

3. Identify important nursing assessments and interventions associated with drug therapy and treatment of diseases associated with the muscular system.

4. Identify essential components involved in planning patient education that will enhance compliance with the treatment regimen.

SKELETAL MUSCLE DISORDERS
OBJECTIVES

1. Prepare a list of assessment data needed to evaluate a patient with a skeletal muscle disorder.
2. State the nursing assessments needed to monitor therapeutic response and/or the development of side effects to expect or report from skeletal muscle relaxant therapy.
3. Develop measurable short- and long-term objectives for patient education for patients with skeletal muscle relaxant therapy.

KEY WORD

muscle spasticity

General Nursing Considerations for Patients Receiving Muscle Relaxants

Musculoskeletal disorders may produce varying degrees of pain, immobility, and effect on the individual's daily activities of living. The nursing assessments performed are individualized to the muscles affected and the disease processes involved.

Patient Concerns:
Nursing Intervention/Rationale

Assessment of skeletal muscle disorders

Muscle spasticity. Assess the extent of the spasticity and the muscle groups affected.

History. Obtain a brief history of injury and details of the areas involved.

Degree of impairment. Seek information relative to the degree of impairment being experienced (strength, gait, conservation effect, compensatory action).

Activities of daily living. Determine which activities of daily living the individual can perform independently and those which require assistance.

Pain level. Determine the pain level and extent, frequency of analgesic use, precipitating factors, and any measures the patient has identified that alleviate it.

Examination. Inspect the affected part for swelling, edema, bruises, redness, localized tenderness, deformities, or malalignments. (Be gentle during the inspection.)

Patient Education Associated with Muscle Relaxants

Communication and responsibility. Encourage open communication concerning frustrations and anger as the patient attempts to adjust to the diagnosis and need for prolonged treatment. The patient must be guided to insight into the condition in order to assume responsibility for continuation of treatment. Keep emphasizing those factors the patient can control to alter the progression of the disease, including the following:

Hot or cold applications. Provide specific instructions regarding the application of heat or cold. Generally, ice packs alleviate swelling immediately after muscle injury. Later in the course of treatment, application of heat provides comfort.

Elevation. Elevating the extremity immediately following injury decreases swelling and, to some degree, alleviates pain.

Activity and exercise. During the initial phase of treatment, immobilizing the affected part will decrease muscle spasms and thereby decrease pain. Various approaches may be used for immobilization, including Ace bandages, splinting, casts, bedrest, or modified activity levels.

Range of motion exercises may be prescribed to maintain joint function and to prevent muscle atrophy and contractures. The activity plan prescribed will be individualized to the diagnosis and should be carefully followed for maximum effectiveness.

Pain management. Analgesic and antiinflammatory agents may be given, if appropriate to the underlying pathology, to relieve pain and reduce inflammation.

Positioning. Maintenance of proper alignment and immobility of the affected part will also relieve pain and swelling.

The following measures are appropriate for persons with lower back pain: (1) Bedrest with the head of the bed elevated 15 to 20° and the knees slightly flexed will provide relief to muscles of the lower back area. (2) Proper body alignment during sleep is important. (3) Maintenance of optimal body weight will prevent undue stress on lower back musculature. (4) Proper techniques of lifting to avoid future injury must be taught.

Anxiety. Increased anxiety produces stress on the body's muscles. Implement measures to produce relaxation and provide for the psychological needs of the individual.

Expectations of therapy. Discuss expectations of therapy with the patient.

Activities and exercises. The patient must resume activities of daily living within the boundaries set by the physician. (Such activities as regular moderate exercise, meal preparation, resumption of usual sexual activities, and social interaction all need to be fostered once specific orders are obtained.)

Pain relief. The degree of musculoskeletal pain relief with and without activity needs to be discussed. Make modifications appropriate to the diagnosis and degree of impairment (see Drug Therapy for Pain, p. 218).

Emotional support. For disorders of a chronic nature, encourage the patient to express openly feelings regarding chronic illness. The adjustment to this situation involves working through great personal fears, frustrations, hostilities, and resentments associated with the loss of personal control within one's life.

Changes in expectations. Assess changes in expectations as therapy progresses and the patient gains understanding of the diagnosis. Areas to assess include pain relief, resumption of daily activities, and increasing mobility.

Changes in therapy through cooperative goal setting. Work with the patient to encourage adherence to the prescribed treatment. When the patient feels that a change should be made in a treatment plan, encourage discussion first with the physician.

Written record. Enlist the patient's aid in developing and maintaining a written record of monitoring parameters (Figure 13-1) (such as level, location, and duration of pain; areas or muscles affected; degree of impairment with improvement in mobility; exercise tolerance) and response to prescribed therapies for discussion with the physician. Patients should be encouraged to take this record on follow-up visits.

Fostering compliance. Throughout hospitalization, discuss medication information and how it will benefit the course of treatment. Seek cooperation and understanding of the following points so that medication compliance may be enhanced:

1. Name
2. Dosage
3. Route and administration times
4. Anticipated therapeutic response; increased ability to participate in activities of daily living as a result of pain relief and increased degree of mobility; increased tolerance of exercise
5. Side effects to expect: sedation, weakness, lethargy, dizziness, light-headedness
6. Side effects to report
7. What to do if a dosage is missed
8. When, how, or if to refill medication prescription

Difficulty in comprehension. If it is evident that the patient and/or family does not comprehend all aspects of the prescribed continuing therapy (such as administration and monitoring of medications, exercises, diets, follow-up appointments), consider use of social service or visiting nurse agencies.

Associated teaching. Give patients the following instructions:

Always inform the physician or dentist of any prescription or over-the-counter medication being taken.

Over-the-counter medications should not be taken without first discussing them with a physician or pharmacist.

Always report side effects of rash, itching, or hives immediately. Nausea, vomiting, or diarrhea should also be reported for the physician's evaluation if it is a new symptom.

Take all of the medication as prescribed for the full course of treatment. Do not discontinue use when feeling improved; do not save for future use; do not give your medicine to another individual. Sudden discontinuation of certain medications may produce harmful effects.

Keep all medications out of reach of children.

If pregnancy is suspected, consult an obstetrician as soon as possible about continuation of medication therapy.

At discharge. Items to be sent home with the patient should include the following:

1. Written instructions for use
2. Labels in language and size of print appropriate for the patient
3. If needed, identification cards or bracelets
4. A list of additional supplies to be purchased after discharge (such as elastic bandages or dressings)
5. A schedule of follow-up appointments

Drug Therapy

Centrally acting skeletal muscle relaxants
OBJECTIVES

1. Describe the effect of centrally acting skeletal muscle relaxants on the central nervous system.
2. List the side effects to expect from use of these agents and the safety precautions required during use.
3. Identify laboratory data and patient assessments needed to monitor for possible development of hepatotoxicity or blood dyscrasias.
4. State the rationale for cautioning patients not to combine use of these agents with other central nervous system depressants.

KEY WORDS

hyperflexia	clonus
cerebral palsy	multiple sclerosis
stroke syndrome	

Patient Education and Monitoring of Therapeutic Outcomes for Patients Receiving Muscle Relaxants

Medications	Color	To be taken

Name _____

Physician _____

Physician's phone _____

Next appt.* _____

Parameters			Day of discharge								Comments
Muscle areas affected	List areas:		AM	AM	AM	AM	AM	AM	AM		
	1.										
	2.										
	3.										
	4.										
Chart areas affected 2 times per day	Example: 1. Arm, lower 2. Lower back 3. 4.	AM 1,2 / PM 1,2	PM	PM	PM	PM	PM	PM	PM		
Exercise and range of motion pain	No improvement — Moderate improvement — Much improvement / 10 — 5 — 1										
Pattern of pain	Location										
	Time of day pain occurs										
	Relieved by										
	Made worse by										
Impairment(s) and improvement	Example: Could not comb hair — can now. Could not turn head without pain — can now.										
Physical therapy prescribed	Example: Application of cold packs at 8AM – 4PM and bedtime	Therapy									
		Time of day									
		Feeling, response									

*Please bring this record with you to your next appointment.
Use the back of this sheet for additional information.

Figure 13-1 *Patient education and monitoring of therapeutic outcomes for patients receiving muscle relaxants.*

The centrally acting skeletal muscle relaxants are a class of compounds used to relieve acute muscle spasm. The exact mechanism of action of the centrally acting skeletal muscle relaxants is not known, except that they act by CNS depression. They do not have any direct effect on muscles, nerve conduction, or myoneural junctions. All of these muscle relaxants produce some degree of sedation, and most physicians think that the benefits of these agents come from their sedative effects rather than from actual muscle relaxation. These agents are used in combination with physical therapy, rest, and analgesics to relieve muscle spasm associated with acute, painful musculoskeletal conditions. They should not be used in muscle spasticity associated with cerebral or spinal cord disease, as they may reduce the strength of remaining active muscle fibers and produce further impairment and debilitation. The centrally acting skeletal muscle relaxants are listed in Table 13-1.

Side effects. These relaxants have many side effects. Mild symptoms include drowsiness, blurred vision, headache, dizziness, light-headedness, and feelings of weakness, lethargy, and lassitude. Abdominal distress, heartburn, diarrhea, and constipation are common.

Rarely, these centrally acting relaxants may produce hepatotoxicity or blood dyscrasias. Periodic laboratory tests, including blood counts and liver function tests, are recommended to avoid complications.

Availability. See Table 13-1 for available products and recommended dosage ranges.

• **Nursing Interventions: Monitoring centrally acting skeletal muscle relaxants**

See also General Nursing Considerations for Patients Receiving Muscle Relaxants.

Side effects to expect

SEDATION, WEAKNESS, LETHARGY, GASTROINTESTINAL COMPLAINTS. These side effects are usually mild and tend to resolve with continued therapy. Encourage the patient not to discontinue therapy without first consulting the physician.

Provide for patient safety for the duration of these symptoms. Patients must avoid operating power equipment or driving.

DIZZINESS. Provide for patient safety during episodes of dizziness; report for further evaluation.

Side effects to report

HEPATOTOXICITY. The symptoms of hepatotoxicity are anorexia, nausea, vomiting, jaundice, hepatomegaly, splenomegaly, and abnormal liver function tests (elevated bilirubin, AST, ALT, GGT, alkaline phosphatase, prothrombin time).

BLOOD DYSCRASIAS. Routine laboratory studies (RBC, WBC, and differential counts) are scheduled for patients taking these agents for 30 days or longer. Stress returning for this laboratory work.

Monitor for the development of sore throat, fever, purpura, jaundice, or excessive progressive weakness.

Drug interactions

CNS DEPRESSANTS. Alcohol, narcotics, barbiturates, anticonvulsants, sedative-hypnotics, tranquilizers, phenothiazines, antidepressants. Persons who are working around machinery, driving a car, pouring and giving medicines, or performing other duties in which they must remain mentally alert should not take these medications while working.

baclofen (bak'lo-fen)

Lioresal (ly-or'e-sahl)

Baclofen is a skeletal muscle relaxant that apparently acts somewhat differently from the centrally acting musculoskeletal agents. Its complete mechanism of action is unknown, although reflex activity at the spinal cord is partially inhibited. Baclofen is used in the management of spasticity resulting from multiple sclerosis,

Table 13-1 *Centrally Acting Muscle Relaxants*

GENERIC NAME	BRAND NAME	ADULT DOSAGE (PO)	COMMENTS
Carisoprodol	Rela, Soma	350 mg 4 times daily	Onset of action—30 minutes; duration—4 to 6 hours
Chlorphenesin carbamate	Maolate	400-800 mg 3 to 4 times daily	Recommended only for short-term treatment (8 weeks) of muscle spasm induced by trauma or inflammation; may cause blood dyscrasias
Chlorzoxazone	Paraflex	250-750 mg 3 to 4 times daily	Commonly causes gastrointestinal discomfort; may be hepatotoxic
Cyclobenzaprine	Flexeril	10 mg 3 times daily; do not exceed 60 mg daily	Recommended only for short-term treatment (2-3 weeks) of painful musculoskeletal conditions
Metaxalone	Skelaxin	800 mg 3 to 4 times daily	Use with caution in patients with liver disease; causes false-positive Clinitest reaction
Methocarbamol	Robaxin, Delaxin	1-1.5 g 4 times daily	Parenteral forms also available
Orphenadrine citrate	Norflex, Flexon, Myolin	100 mg 2 times daily	Also has analgesic properties; do not use in patients with glaucoma or prostatic hypertrophy

spinal cord injuries, and other spinal cord diseases. It is not recommended for use in spasticity associated with Parkinson's disease, cerebral palsy, stroke, or rheumatic disorders. Use with caution in patients who must use spasticity to maintain an upright posture and balance in moving.

Side effects. The most common side effects associated with baclofen therapy are drowsiness, fatigue, nausea, mental depression, headache, and muscle weakness. These side effects are usually transient and may be minimized by starting therapy with low dosages. Increases in dosage should be made as tolerated.

Availability

PO—10 and 20 mg tablets

Dosage and administration

Adult

NOTE: Do not abruptly discontinue therapy. Severe exacerbation of spasticity and hallucinations may result.

PO—Initially 5 mg 3 times daily. Increase the dosage by 5 mg every 3 to 7 days based on response. Optimum effects are usually noted at dosages of 40 to 80 mg daily but may take several weeks to achieve.

- **Nursing Interventions: Monitoring baclofen therapy**

See also General Nursing Considerations for Patients Receiving Muscle Relaxants.

Side effects to expect

NAUSEA, FATIGUE, HEADACHE, DROWSINESS. These side effects are usually mild and tend to resolve with continued therapy. Encourage the patient not to discontinue therapy without first consulting the physician.

DIZZINESS. Provide for patient safety during episodes of dizziness; report for further evaluation.

Drug interactions

CNS DEPRESSANTS. CNS depressants, including sleeping aids, analgesics, tranquilizers, and alcohol, will potentiate the sedative effects of baclofen. Persons who are working around machinery, driving a car, pouring and giving medicines, or performing other duties in which they must remain mentally alert should not take these medications while working.

Direct-acting skeletal muscle relaxant

OBJECTIVE

1. Identify the site of action and generalized response of the direct-acting skeletal muscle relaxant.

dantrolene (dan'tro-leen)

Dantrium (dan'tree-um)

Dantrolene is a muscle relaxant that acts directly on skeletal muscle. It produces generalized mild weakness of skeletal muscles and decreases the force of reflex muscle contractions, hyperflexia, clonus, muscle stiffness, involuntary muscle movements, and spasticity. Dantrolene is used to control the spasticity of chronic disorders such as cerebral palsy, multiple sclerosis, spinal cord injury, and stroke syndrome. It is also used to treat neuroleptic malignant syndrome associated with the use of antipsychotic agents (see p. 196).

Side effects. Common side effects include muscle weakness, drowsiness, dizziness, light-headedness, and diarrhea. These effects occur early in treatment and may be prevented by initiating treatment with low doses. If symptoms persist or recur after temporary discontinuation of the drug, dantrolene may have to be permanently discontinued.

Dantrolene must not be used in patients whose spasticity is needed to obtain or maintain an upright posture and balance or body function.

Drug-induced photosensitivity may occur, so patients should refrain from excessive or unnecessary exposure to sunlight.

Dantrolene must be used with caution in patients with chronic lung disease, liver disease, or impaired myocardial function. Dantrolene has been implicated as a causative factor in reported cases of hepatitis.

Availability

PO—25, 50, and 100 mg capsules.

IV—0.32 mg/ml in 70 ml vials.

Dosage and administration

Adult

PO—Initially 25 mg daily. Increase to 25 mg two, three, or four times daily at 4 to 7 day intervals, then gradually increase the dosage up to 100 mg two, three, or four times daily. A few patients may require 200 mg four times daily.

- **Nursing Interventions: Monitoring dantrolene therapy**

See also General Nursing Considerations for Patients Receiving Muscle Relaxants.

Side effects to expect

WEAKNESS, DIARRHEA, DROWSINESS. These side effects are usually mild and tend to resolve with continued therapy. Encourage the patient not to discontinue therapy without first consulting the physician.

DIZZINESS, LIGHT-HEADEDNESS. Provide for patient safety during episodes of dizziness; report for further evaluation.

RESPONSE TO THERAPY. Tell the patient that effectiveness of the drug may not be apparent for 1 week or longer. Encourage the patient not to discontinue therapy without first consulting the physician.

Side effects to report

PHOTOSENSITIVITY. The patient should be cautioned to avoid exposure to sunlight and ultraviolet light. Suggest wearing long-sleeved clothing, hat, and sunglasses while exposed to sunlight. The patient must not use artificial "tanning" lamps. The patient should not discontinue therapy without advising the physician.

HEPATOTOXICITY. The symptoms of hepatotoxicity are anorexia, nausea, vomiting, jaundice, hepatomegaly, splenomegaly, and abnormal liver function tests (elevated bilirubin, AST, ALT, GGT, alkaline phosphatase, prothrombin time).

Drug interactions

CNS DEPRESSANTS. CNS depressants, including sleeping aids, analgesics, tranquilizers, and alcohol, will potentiate the sedative effects of dantrolene. Persons who are working around machinery, driving a car, pouring and giving medicines, or performing other duties in which they must remain mentally alert should not take these medications while working.

Skeletal Muscle Relaxants Used during Surgery

OBJECTIVES

1. Describe essential components of patient assessment used for patients receiving neuromuscular blocking agents.
2. Identify where information on the use of these agents is found in the patient's chart.
3. Name the equipment that should be available in the immediate patient care area when neuromuscular blocking agents have been administered.
4. Describe the physiological effects of neuromuscular blocking agents.

KEY WORDS

neuromuscular blockade
hypercapnia

General Nursing Considerations for Patients Receiving Neuromuscular Blocking Agents

See also General Nursing Considerations for Patients with Respiratory Tract Disease.

Patient Concerns: Nursing Intervention/Rationale

Assessment. Assessment of the patient's vital signs, mental status, and in particular, respiratory function, is mandatory for persons having received neuromuscular blocking agents. The side effects associated with these drugs may occur 48 hours or more after their administration; therefore, close observation of respiratory function, ability to swallow (handle secretions), and cough reflex is necessary. Suction, oxygen, mechanical ventilators, and resuscitation equipment should be available in the immediate area.

Detection of respiratory depression

RESTLESSNESS, LETHARGY, DECREASED MENTAL ALERTNESS. Early signs of diminished ventilation are difficult to detect, particularly in the immediate postoperative period. Often the signs of restlessness, anxiety, decreased mental alertness, and headache are early, subtle clues to distress.

BLOOD PRESSURE, PULSE, AND RESPIRATIONS. Know the baseline readings of your patient's vital signs before administration of anesthetic and neuromuscular blocking agents.

Generally, *changes* from the baseline should be reported.

Monitor your patient closely for clinical signs (tachycardia, hypotension, cyanosis) of hypoxia and hypercapnia. Arterial blood gases (ABGs) may be drawn to accurately confirm your clinical observations.

USE OF ACCESSORY MUSCLES. Use of the abdominal, intercostal, or neck muscles is an indication of respiratory distress. Flaring of the nostrils may be present in severe cases.

RESPIRATORY RATE, DEPTH. As respiratory distress progresses, respirations become shallow and rapid; assess for asymmetrical chest movements as well.

CYANOSIS. The development of cyanosis is a late sign of respiratory complications. Respiratory distress should be detected early through close observation before cyanosis develops.

VENTILATED RESPIRATIONS. The use of various mechanical ventilators may be employed to improve alveolar ventilation and oxygenation of the patient. See a general medical-surgical nursing text for a detailed discussion of nursing care while the patient is on mechanical ventilation.

Nursing measures associated with neuromuscular blockade therapy

RESPIRATORY SECRETIONS. The histamine release caused by these drugs may produce increased salivation. In patients who are paralyzed or who have incomplete return of control over swallowing, coughing, and deep breathing, these secretions may obstruct the airway.

Assess for dyspnea and loud or gurgling sounds with respirations. Suction secretions according to hospital policies and procedures. If qualified, palpate for coarse chest wall vibrations and listen for rales or rhonchi.

COUGH REFLEX. In order to cough effectively, the patient must be able to breathe deeply, contract the abdominal and diaphragmatic muscles, and control the closing and opening of the epiglottis so that air can be trapped in the lung and then forcefully expelled.

DEEP BREATHING. Deep-breathing exercises can allow the opportunity to assess the patient's cough reflex. Assist the patient by splinting any abdominal or thoracic incisions. Have the patient take 3 or 4 deep breaths, then cough. During this process, assess the ability to breathe deeply. Cupping your hand and holding it a few inches from the mouth while the patient breathes allows you to feel the air being exhaled.

POSITIONING. Patients can usually cough better in a semi-Fowler's or high Fowler's position; therefore, depending on the situation and stability of the patient's vital signs, elevating the head of the bed may assist coughing and breathing. For unconscious or semiconscious individuals, position them, using good body alignment, on the side. Keep the siderails up.

PAIN MANAGEMENT. Persons still paralyzed by the effects of these agents may experience pain and be unable to speak to request medication. Make sure analgesics are scheduled on a regular basis and administered on time.

ANXIETY. Deal calmly with the patient experiencing respiratory dysfunction. The inability to breathe may cause the patient to panic. Give reassurance while initiating measures to assist the patient.

Drug Therapy

Neuromuscular blocking agents
OBJECTIVES

1. Name the neuromuscular blocking agents and identify the agents routinely used in your practice setting.
2. Cite four uses of neuromuscular blocking agents.
3. Identify the effect of neuromuscular blocking agents on consciousness, memory, and the pain threshold.
4. Describe disease conditions that may affect the patient's ability to tolerate the use of neuromuscular blocking agents.
5. Review the drugs listed as enhancing the therapeutic and toxic effects of these agents; identify appropriate nursing actions to prevent concurrent administration of these agents.
6. Identify steps required to treat respiratory depression.

Neuromuscular blocking agents are important skeletal muscle relaxants. These agents are used to (1) produce adequate muscle relaxation during anesthesia to reduce the use (and side effects) of general anesthetics, (2) ease endotracheal intubation and prevent laryngospasm, (3) decrease muscular activity in electroshock therapy, and (4) aid in the muscle spasms associated with tetanus. The neuromuscular blocking agents are listed in Table 13-2.

Neuromuscular blocking agents act by interrupting transmission of impulses from motor nerves to muscles at the skeletal neuromuscular junction. Neuromuscular blocking agents have no effect on consciousness, memory, or the pain threshold. Reassurance by nursing personnel is essential to paralyzed patients (such as those on respirators), and analgesics must be administered on schedule. These patients may suffer extreme pain without being able to ask for analgesics.

Side effects. Side effects shared by all neuromuscular blocking agents are residual muscle weakness, hypersensitivity reactions, and interference with respiratory function. They also cause histamine release, which may cause bronchospasm, bronchial and salivary secretions, flushing, edema, and urticaria.

Patients with hepatic, pulmonary, or renal disease, or neurologic disorders such as myasthenia gravis, spinal cord injury, or multiple sclerosis must be fully evaluated to assess their ability to tolerate neuromuscular blocking agents. Much smaller doses are often necessary when these diseases are present. Neonates and elderly patients also require adjustments in dosage because of the insensitivity of their neuromuscular junction.

Availability. See Table 13-2.

Administration. These agents are usually given intravenously but may also be given intramuscularly. They are potent drugs, so they should be used only by persons thoroughly familiar with their effects, such as an anesthetist or anesthesiologist, and under conditions where the patient can receive constant, close attention for signs of respiratory failure. Adequate equipment for artificial respiration, antidotes, and other measures for prompt treatment of toxicity must be readily available.

Treatment of overdose. Treatment of overdose includes artificial respiration with oxygen and antidotes such as neostigmine methylsulfate (Prostigmin), pyridostigmine bromide (Mestinon, Regonal), and edrophonium chloride (Tensilon). Atropine sulfate is usually administered with neostigmine or pyridostigmine to block bradycardia, hypotension, and salivation induced by these agents. There is no antidote for the early blockade induced by succinylcholine. Fortunately, it is of short duration and does not require reversal.

Table 13-2 *Neuromuscular Blocking Agents*

GENERIC NAME	BRAND NAME	AVAILABILITY
Atacurium besylate	Tracrium	10 mg/ml in 5 ml ampules
Doxacurium chloride	Nuromax	1 mg/ml in 5 ml vials
Gallamine triethiodide	Flaxedil	20 mg/ml in 10 ml vials
Metocurine iodide	Metubine Iodide	2 mg/ml in 20 vials
Pancuronium bromide	Pavulon	1 mg/ml in 10 ml vials; 2 mg/ml in 2 and 5 ml ampules
Pipecuronium bromide	Arduan	1 mg/ml in 10 ml vials
Succinylcholine	Anectine, Quelicin, Sux-Cert	20 mg/ml in 5 and 10 ml vials, 50 mg/ml in 10 ml ampules, 100 mg/ml in 10 ml vials and ampules
Tubocurarine chloride	Tubocurarine Chloride	3 mg/ml in 10 and 20 mg vials
Vecuronium bromide	Norcuron	10 mg/5 ml vial

• **Nursing Interventions: Monitoring neuromuscular blocking agent therapy**

See also General Nursing Considerations for Patients Receiving Neuromuscular Blocking Agents.

Side effects to expect

MILD DISCOMFORT. Mild to moderate discomfort, particularly in the neck, upper back, lower intercostal, and abdominal muscles, will be noted when first ambulating following use.

Side effects to report

SIGNS OF RESPIRATORY DISTRESS. Monitor vital signs for a prolonged period following administration of neuromuscular blocking agents.

DIMINISHED COUGH REFLEX, INABILITY TO SWALLOW. Assess deep breathing and coughing at regular intervals. Have suction and oxygen equipment available and be familiar with emergency code practices at your hospital.

Drug interactions

DRUGS THAT ENHANCE THERAPEUTIC AND TOXIC EFFECTS. General anesthetics (ether, fluroxene, methoxyflurane, enflurane, halothane, cyclopropane), aminoglycoside antibiotics (kanamycin, gentamicin, neomycin, streptomycin, netilmycin, tobramycin, amikacin), quinidine, quinine, beta adrenergic blocking agents (propranolol, timolol, pindolol, nadolol, others), and agents that deplete potassium (thiazide diuretics, furosemide, bumetanide, ethacrynic acid, chlorthalidone, amphotericin B, corticosteroids), thus prolonging neuromuscular blockage.

Label charts of patients scheduled for surgery who are taking any of these agents. These combinations may potentiate respiratory depression. Check the anesthetist's records of surgical patients; monitor post-operative patients for a prolonged period for respiratory depression. This may occur 48 hours or more after drug administration.

DRUGS THAT REDUCE THERAPEUTIC EFFECTS. Neostigmine methylsulfate, pyridostigmine bromide, and edrophonium chloride.

These agents are used as antidotes in case of overdosage of the neuromuscular blocking agents.

RESPIRATORY DEPRESSANTS. Analgesics, sedatives, tranquilizers.

These agents, in combination with muscle relaxants, may potentiate respiratory depression. Check the anesthetist's records of surgical patients. Monitor postoperative patients for a prolonged period for respiratory depression. This may occur 48 hours or more after drug administration.

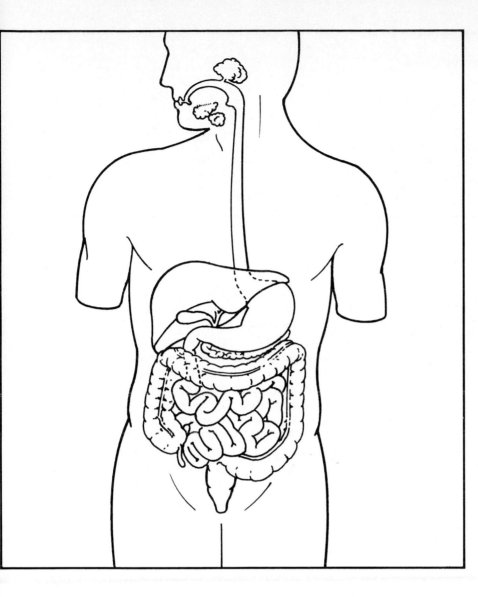

14

Drugs Affecting the Digestive System

CHAPTER GOALS

After completing this chapter, the student should be able to do the following:

1. Explain the major action and effects of drugs used to treat disorders of the digestive tract.

2. Identify baseline data the nurse should collect on a continuous basis for comparison and evaluation of drug effectiveness.

3. Identify important nursing assessments and interventions associated with the drug therapy and treatment of diseases of the digestive system.

4. Identify essential components involved in planning patient education that will enhance compliance with the treatment regimen.

GASTROINTESTINAL DISORDERS

OBJECTIVES

1. Cite nursing assessments needed to evaluate a patient's gastrointestinal status.
2. Identify measures that can be suggested to alleviate or prevent gastrointestinal symptoms (such as constipation, diarrhea, or "gas").
3. Develop measurable short- and long-term objectives for patient education for patients with a gastrointestinal disorder.

KEY WORDS

coffee ground emesis	hyperresonance
bruit	ascites
paralytic ileus	hiatal hernia
regurgitation	reflux esophagitis

General Nursing Considerations for Patients with Gastrointestinal Disorders

The nurse should assess the following areas to form a baseline for comparison with subsequent observations.

> ### Patient Concerns:
> ### Nursing Intervention/Rationale

Assessment of patients with gastrointestinal disorders

Nutritional assessment. Obtain the patient's data relating to current height, weight, and any recent weight gains or losses. Identify normal pattern of eating. Utilize the four food groups as a guide while asking specific questions to distinguish the usual foods eaten by the individual.

Oral cavity. Assessment of the mouth indicates the patient's ability to salivate, chew, and swallow, and provides signs of disease that can interfere with nutrition. Examine the tongue, lips, and mucous membranes for color, cyanosis, sores (describe location, size, and characteristics), moisture (dryness may indicate dehydration), swelling, or inflammation.

Assess for the presence of teeth, dental caries, plaque, inflamed or receding gums, and sores from poorly fitting dentures.

Foul-smelling breath may indicate poor dental hygiene or oral infection. Odors may occur after certain foods, such as garlic or alcohol, are consumed, or with some systemic diseases (acetone for diabetes, ammonia for liver disease).

Esophagus, stomach. Ask patients to describe any symptoms in their own words. Question in detail what is meant by their use of the terms *indigestion, heartburn, upset stomach, nausea,* or *pain.*

Pain, discomfort. Have the patient give specific details of the onset, duration, location, and characteristics of pain or discomfort. Determine whether there is a relationship between ingestion of certain types of food or drinks and the onset of pain. Find out what the patient has done in the past to relieve the pain or discomfort.

Emesis. Has the patient vomited? What is the frequency, color, consistency, and duration of current symptoms? Has there been any bright red or "coffee-ground" colored emesis? What initiates the vomiting episodes, and what causes them to stop? How many episodes of vomiting has the patient experienced over what time span?

In the postoperative patient always check the following: patency of the nasogastric tube; that the abdomen is splinted when vomiting; that dressings and wound sites are checked frequently for possible increases in drainage or wound dehiscence.

Prevent possible aspiration while a patient is vomiting by placing the person in a high Fowler's position and/or on the side, if not fully alert.

Always give regular oral hygiene to patients experiencing nausea and vomiting.

Skin alterations. Ask about any changes in skin coloration (for example, jaundice, rashes, bruising) and if any rashes or itching of the skin has occurred.

Bowels. Ask patients to describe any changes they have noted in their abdomen (such as distension, "swelling or bloating," loud gurgling sounds, or the presence of any lumps).

Using a stethoscope, listen for hyperresonance (loud tingling and rushing), absence of bowel sounds, or the presence of a bruit (similar to a systolic murmur).

Measure and record the abdominal girth. Continue

measurements in the same location daily, especially if ascites or paralytic ileus are suspected.

Record any changes in abdominal contour (such as hernia, enlarged spleen or liver).

Record any sharp pain felt when fingers are withdrawn suddenly after palpation of the abdomen.

Constipation. *Constipation* is the formation of dry, hard stools that are difficult and sometimes painful to pass.

The underlying cause of constipation must be determined.

ELIMINATION PATTERN. Determine whether the onset of constipation is recent and can be associated with a change in diet or new environment (from travel or undue stress). Ask patients to describe their "normal" elimination pattern—number of stools per day, color, and consistency. Has there been any change in the "normal" pattern of bowel movements? It is important for patients to understand that not all people defecate daily; every 2 to 3 days is normal for some people.

FLUID INTAKE. Ask patients to describe fluid intake: how much water, coffee (caffeinated, decaffeinated), tea, soft drinks, fruit juice, and alcoholic beverages are consumed daily?

EATING PATTERN. Ask patients for a description of their diet over the past 24 hours. Evaluate the data for types of foods from each of the four food groups eaten, the quantity eaten, and the amount of time spent in eating. Ask if the eating pattern has changed over recent months and to what the patients attribute any identified changes.

Ask whether certain foods cause bloating, indigestion, or constipation; ask how much seasoning and spices are put on foods.

EXERCISE. Ask the patient about exercise levels and activity. Does the patient play vigorous sports, take walks, jog, or have a sedentary job and hobby?

NURSING MEASURES. Explain the benefits of trying dietary and exercise modification to treat constipation, prior to initiating the use of laxatives.

Nurses may facilitate defecation in hospitalized patients by encouraging ambulation (if possible), providing privacy, and having the individual sit in an upright position. If possible, sitting on the actual toilet or bedside commode is best.

Encourage the patient to attempt to defecate as soon as the urge arises and not to suppress this urge until a later time. The urge to defecate occurs most frequently following meals, particularly breakfast.

If an enema or laxative is ordered, explain the purpose to the patient and how long it will take before action is expected.

Diarrhea. *Diarrhea* is an increased frequency and/or fluid content of bowel movements. Diarrhea may result from disturbances in either the small or large intestine caused by a change in the fecal contents or a decrease in intestinal transit time, so that less fluid is reab-sorbed. The result is passage of feces that are high in water content.

Since diarrhea is usually caused by a pathologic condition or is a side effect of medications, medical treatment usually consists of correcting the underlying cause.

HISTORY. Ask the patient experiencing diarrhea if there has been a recent change in eating habits or a change in water source, if there has been additional stress, or if medications (especially laxatives or antibiotics) are being taken.

Obtain a detailed history of the illness, including the onset and duration of the diarrhea, characteristics of the stool, and associated symptoms.

DEHYDRATION AND ELECTROLYTE IMBALANCE. Monitor patients with prolonged or severe diarrhea for dehydration and electrolyte imbalance. (See Chapter 15, "Drugs Affecting the Urinary System.")

SKIN BREAKDOWN. Provide for protection of the tissue surrounding the anal area when the symptoms of diarrhea start, *prior to skin breakdown.* Cleanse the anal area thoroughly, dry gently, and apply protective products such as Desitin or A & D Ointment. Repeat this process after *every* defecation.

Patient Education Associated with Gastrointestinal Drug Therapy

Communication and responsibility. Encourage open communication concerning frustrations and anger as the patient attempts to adjust to the diagnosis and need for prolonged treatment. The patient must be guided to gain insight into the disorder in order to assume responsibility for the continuation of the treatment. Keep emphasizing those factors the patient can control to alter the progress of the disease, including maintenance of general health, nutritional needs, adequate rest, appropriate exercise, and continuation of the prescribed medication therapy.

Self-treatment. Millions of patients treat their own gastrointestinal symptoms with over-the-counter products each year. Patients must understand that symptoms that are not relieved by self-treatment, usually within 1 to 2 weeks, require a physician's evaluation. Many people consider gastrointestinal symptoms to be minor and do not realize that chronic symptoms may be an indication of a serious underlying disease.

Alternative therapies

FOR GASTROINTESTINAL DISTRESS. Avoid foods known to cause gas such as cabbage, cauliflower, Brussels sprouts, and bran products.

Avoid irritating foods and beverages such as spices, alcohol, coffee, chocolate, citrus fruits, fried foods, and gravies. Occasionally, foods high in roughage (such as lettuce, celery, raw fruits, and vegetables) can aggravate an inflamed mucosa.

Elevation of the head of the bed at night may help

patients who have developed a hiatus hernia, night regurgitation, or reflux esophagitis.

Antacids may be used to neutralize stomach acid, thus reducing gastric irritation, but continued use may mask a more serious underlying disorder.

Contrary to popular opinion, large glasses of milk or baking soda used as an antacid will actually stimulate more acid production, causing further gastric irritation. Occasional use of an antacid is more appropriate.

Other measures to reduce gastrointestinal distress include the ingestion of frequent, small feedings, taking a walk after meals, and remaining upright after meals rather than sitting or lying down.

FOR NAUSEA, VOMITING. Before using antiemetics, try more simple measures such as a cup of warm tea or carbonated beverages served at room temperature.

FOR CONSTIPATION. Before making any suggestions, the underlying cause of the constipation must be established. Determine whether the onset of constipation is recent and if it can be associated with a change in diet, a new environment from travel, or undue stress. Constipation from these causes is usually self-limiting and resolves with the one-time use of a mild laxative.

People with chronic constipation frequently drink an inadequate amount of water daily. Initially, encourage patients to drink 6 to 8 8-ounce glasses of water daily, gradually increasing to 8 to 12 glasses daily.

A regular diet containing sufficient roughage, in the form of fresh fruits and vegetables and whole grain breads and cereals, should be encouraged unless coexisting medical problems prohibit these foods.

A plan of regular exercise can be helpful, particularly if the person leads a sedentary life. Exercise promotes bowel activity and improves the abdominal muscle tone necessary for defecation. Straight-leg raises also promote increased abdominal muscle strength.

If the above measures fail, or if the patient has a medical indication to prevent straining at the stool, medications such as stool softeners or bulk-forming laxatives may be suggested. It is *essential* that *adequate water* be taken with these products.

Also stress personal hygiene by having patients wash their hands after each defecation and urination. For females, teach the importance of wiping from front to back (urethra to rectum) to prevent development of urinary tract infections.

FOR DIARRHEA. Ask patients experiencing diarrhea if they have an idea of what is causing the diarrhea (such as a change in food or water sources, travel, recent undue stress, or the initiation of a new medication).

Explain what medications have been ordered, how often they are repeated, and when to discontinue therapy, in order to prevent constipation.

Initiate protection of the tissue surrounding the anal area when diarrhea symptoms start, *prior to skin breakdown.* Cleanse the anal area thoroughly, dry gently, and apply protective skin products such as Desitin or A & D Ointment. Repeat this procedure after *every* defecation.

Expectations of therapy. Discuss the expectations of therapy: relief of heartburn, indigestion, nausea and vomiting, or diarrhea.

(Occasionally a patient may have the unrealistic expectation that a medication will change a lifelong pattern of defecation from once every 3 or 4 days to daily, even though there was no change in dietary and fluid intake or activity.)

Changes in expectations. Assess changes in expectations as therapy progresses and the patient gains understanding and skill in the management of the diagnosis.

Symptoms of recurrent gastrointestinal discomfort need thorough diagnosis to identify any underlying pathology.

Changes in therapy through cooperative goal setting. Work with the patient to encourage adherence to the prescribed treatment. When the patient feels that a change should be made in a treatment plan, encourage discussion with the physician.

A definite plan to alleviate the gastrointestinal symptoms should be developed and the patient's response carefully evaluated.

Cooperatively explore any conditions the patient feels may be precipitating these episodes. Set goals together to eliminate underlying stressors. Simpler approaches such as dietary modification should be used *before* the initiation of medications.

Written record. Enlist the patient's aid in developing and maintaining a written record of monitoring parameters (Figure 14-1) (such as diet diary, onset of pain, nausea or vomiting in relation to mealtime or type of foods eaten, frequency and characteristics of stools during diarrhea) and response to prescribed therapies for discussion with the physician. Patients should be encouraged to take this record on follow-up visits.

Fostering compliance. Throughout the hospitalization, discuss medication information and how it will benefit the course of treatment. Seek cooperation and understanding of the following points so that medication compliance may be enhanced:

1. Name
2. Dosage (be certain specific instructions are given for each medication)
3. Route and administration times; if the patient is taking more than one medication, be sure that the patient knows when to take each one (for example, with meals, 1 hour before or 2 hours after antacids)
   - For antidiarrheal medication, be sure that the patient understands how much and how often the prescription is to be taken, and when to discontinue the medication
   - For constipation, stress the use of diet, exercise, and adequate fluid intake prior to the initiation of

Patient Education and Monitoring of Therapeutic Outcomes for Patients Receiving Agents Affecting the Digestive System

Medications	Color	To be taken

Name _____

Physician _____

Physician's phone _____

Next appt.* _____

Parameters		Day of discharge							Comments
Bloating	Time it occurs — night, after eating, midday								
	Causes, eg., food eaten								
Pain: Severity of pain severe ——— Moderate ——— Dull 10 ——— 5 ——— 0	Time — before/after meals								
	Location								
Nausea	Vomiting — describe amount, color, time of day								
	Nausea — no vomiting								
Bowels	Color?								
	No. of stools per day?								
	Soft, watery, or hard?								
Diet: List foods that cause problems									
Degree of relief from medications? Great ——— Good ——— Poor 10 ——— .5 ——— 1									
Appetite? Excellent ——— Good ——— Poor 10 ——— 5 ——— 1									

*Please bring this record with you to your next appointment.
Use the back of this sheet for additional information.

Figure 14-1 *Patient education and monitoring of therapeutic outcomes for patients receiving agents affecting the digestive system.*

a laxative; ensure that the individual understands that bulk-forming laxatives and stool softeners must be taken with a full glass of water to be safe and effective

4. Anticipated therapeutic responses include the following:
   - Antidiarrheal products—Relief of diarrhea
   - Antacids—Relief of heartburn or pain
   - Laxatives—Relief of constipation
   - Stool softeners—Smooth, consistent bowel movement with no straining or gripping

5. Side effects to expect: see individual product information

6. Side effects to report: lack of improvement in the symptoms for which the medication was prescribed, or excessive adverse effects; patients should be told to report immediately any vomitus that looks like "coffee grounds" or contains bright red blood, any bloody or tarry-colored stools, or any recurrent abdominal pains; patients must not attempt to treat these symptoms by themselves

7. When, how, or if to refill the medication

Difficulty in comprehension. If it is evident that the patient and/or family does not understand all aspects of continuing therapy being prescribed (such as administration and monitoring of medications, exercises, diets, follow-up appointments) consider the use of social service or visiting nurse agencies.

Associated teaching. Give patients the following instructions: Always inform the physician or dentist of any prescription or over-the-counter medication being taken. Over-the-counter medications should not be taken without first discussing them with the physician or pharmacist.

Always report side effects of rash, itching, or hives immediately. Nausea, vomiting, or diarrhea should also be reported for the physician's evaluation if it is a new symptom.

Take all of the medication, as prescribed, for the full course of treatment. Do not discontinue use when feeling improved; do not save for future use; do not give your medicine to another individual. Sudden discontinuation of certain medications may produce harmful effects.

Keep all medications out of reach of children.

If pregnancy is suspected, consult an obstetrician as soon as possible about continuation of medication therapy.

At discharge. Items to be sent home with the patient should include the following:

1. Written instructions for use
2. Label in language and size of print appropriate for the patient
3. If needed, identification cards or bracelets
4. A list of additional supplies to be purchased after discharge (such as syringes or dressings)
5. A schedule for follow-up appointments

Drug Therapy for Gastrointestinal Disorders

OBJECTIVES

1. Identify mouthwashes that can be used full strength and those that require dilution (see also oral stomatitis.
2. Describe the precautions that should be taken when lidocaine mouthwash is prescribed.
3. List dentifrices containing fluoride.
4. Identify dentifrices that will help control gum disease.
5. Compare the actions of antacids on the secretion and buffering of hydrochloric acid.
6. Describe precautions that must be emphasized to lay persons regarding the excessive or prolonged use of antacids.
7. Define the meaning of *combined products* when used in relation to antacid therapy.
8. Identify the actions of the following ingredients of combination product antacids: simethicone, alginic acid, and bismuth.
9. Compare the side effects from prolonged use of products containing aluminum hydroxide and calcium carbonate.
10. Identify antacid products that are low in sodium content.
11. Identify antacid products that persons with renal failure should avoid.
12. Prepare a chart of medications that interact with antacids.
13. Explain the scheduling adjustments that may be needed to avoid interactions of antacids and other drugs.
14. Identify the drug interaction between antacids and levodopa; include monitoring parameters that should be implemented to observe for and avoid this interaction.
15. Identify the effect of an increased urinary pH on quinidine and amphetamines.

KEY WORDS

peptic ulcer disease   gastritis
rebound hyperacidity   hyperchlorhydria

Mouthwashes and gargles

A common personal need in the hospitalized patient is oral hygiene. The most effective treatment of oral discomfort is mechanical cleansing of the teeth with a toothbrush and dentifrice followed by flossing and rinsing. However, this may not be possible for the patient who has undergone oral surgery or who has suffered facial trauma. Although mouthwashes and gargles cannot be used in strong enough concentrations to ensure germicidal effects, they may be temporarily effective in removing disagreeable tastes and reducing halitosis.

Cepacol mouthwash is used in many hospitals and is available commercially in liquid and lozenge form. It is used full strength. Chloraseptic mouthwash maintains oral hygiene and also provides surface anesthesia when needed to alleviate pharyngeal discomfort. It is diluted with equal parts of water or sprayed full strength.

Occasionally, certain mouthwashes are recommended for specific purposes. Products containing zinc chloride are used as astringents for temporary decrease of bleeding or irritation. A 0.9% solution of sodium chloride (normal saline) is an effective gargle. It can be used to provide temporary, soothing relief of pharyngeal irritation from nasogastric tubes, endotracheal tubes, sore throat, or oral surgery. Solutions containing hydrogen peroxide may be used to cleanse and debride minor lesions. However, their use should be limited to 7 to 10 days in order to prevent further tissue irritation. Mouthwashes containing 0.05% fluoride have been shown significantly to reduce tooth decay. Lidocaine, a local anesthetic, is available in both an oral spray solution (Xylocaine 10% oral spray) and an oral viscous solution (Xylocaine 2% viscous solution). The spray solution is used as a short-term, topical anesthetic for the mucous membranes in the mouth. The viscous solution has a much longer-lasting local anesthesia and can be used as a gargle for patients with sore throats. This product is frequently used in immunosuppressed patients with painful candidal infections of the mouth and throat. It is extremely important that the recommended dosages of both products not be exceeded, as lidocaine is readily absorbed into the body. (See adverse effects associated with lidocaine therapy.)

Dentifrices

The primary purpose for brushing teeth is to promote dental health. Dentifrices contain one or more mild abrasives, a foaming agent, and flavoring materials. They are available in powder or paste form and are used as an aid in the mechanical cleansing provided by a soft nylon toothbrush. The essential requirement of toothpaste or toothpowder is that it must not injure the teeth or surrounding tissues. For children and teenagers, who are most susceptible to tooth decay, the best dentifrices are those that contain fluoride. The American Dental Association recognizes Crest, Colgate with MFP, Macleans Fluoride, Regular Strength Aim, Aqua-Fresh Fluoride, and Gleem as toothpastes having proven caries-inhibiting properties.

Adults should use toothpastes that are the least abrasive to the teeth while controlling gum disease as well as decay. This is especially important to patients with receding gums. Colgate Regular and Peak toothpastes are the least abrasive, while smokers' products such as Pearl Drops and Zact are the most abrasive. Baking soda is a very mild abrasive agent and can be very effective and inexpensive as a dentifrice. The only disadvantages to baking soda are its slightly bitter taste and lack of fluoride. Denquel is a mildly abrasive toothpaste that also contains a desensitizing agent. The American Dental Association states that it is a toothpaste that "has been shown to be an effective desensitizing dentifrice that with regular brushing can be of significant value in relieving sensitivity to hot and cold in otherwise normal teeth."

Antacids

Antacids are chemical substances used in the treatment of hyperchlorhydria and peptic ulcer disease. Peptic ulcer disease is thought to be the result of several pathogenic processes. The control of hyperacidity is one of the therapeutic measures used in its treatment.

The main digestive substances secreted by the stomach are *hydrochloric acid* and *pepsin*. Hydrochloric acid activates the secretion of pepsin, and pepsin then begins protein digestion. Excess secretion of hydrochloric acid may result in erosion, ulceration, and possible perforation of the gastric walls. Antacids lower the acidity of gastric secretions by buffering the hydrochloric acid (normally pH 1 or 2) to a lower hydrogen ion concentration. Buffering hydrochloric acid to a pH of 3 or 4 is highly desired, as then the proteolytic action of pepsin is reduced and the gastric juice loses its corrosive effect.

Antacid products account for one of the largest sales volumes of medication that may be purchased without prescription. Antacids are commonly used for treatment of heartburn, excessive eating and drinking, and peptic ulcer disease. However, nurses and patients must be aware that not all antacids are alike. They should be used judiciously, particularly by certain types of patients. Long-term self-medication with antacids may also mask symptoms of serious underlying diseases, such as a bleeding ulcer.

The most effective antacids available are combinations of aluminum hydroxide, magnesium oxide or hydroxide, magnesium trisilicate, and calcium carbonate (Table 14-1). All act by neutralizing gastric acid. Combinations of these compounds must be used because any compound used alone in therapeutic quantities may also produce severe systemic side effects. Other ingredients found in antacid combination products include simethicone, oxethazaine, alginic acid, and bismuth. *Simethicone* is a defoaming agent that breaks up gas bubbles in the stomach, reducing stomach distension and heartburn. It is effective for use in patients who have overeaten or who suffer from heartburn, but it is not effective in the treatment of ulcer disease. *Alginic acid* produces a highly viscous solution of sodium alginate that floats on top of the gastric contents. It may be effective only in the patient who suffers from esophageal reflux or hiatal hernia and should not be used in the patient with acute gastritis or ulcer disease. *Bismuth* compounds have little acid-neutralizing capacity and are therefore poor antacids.

Side effects. A common complaint of patients consuming large quantities of calcium carbonate or alumi-

Table 14-1 *Ingredients of Commonly Used Antacids*

PRODUCT	FORM	CALCIUM CARBONATE	ALUMINUM HYDROXIDE	ALUMINUM CARBONATE	MAGNESIUM OXIDE OR HYDROXIDE	MAGNESIUM TRISILICATE	MAGNESIUM CARBONATE	SODIUM BICARBONATE	SIMETHICONE	OTHER INGREDIENTS
Aludrox	Tablet, suspension		X		X				X	
Amphojel	Tablet, suspension		X							
Basaljel	Tablet, capsule, suspension			X						
BiSoDol	Tablet, powder					X	X			
Di-Gel	Tablet, liquid		X		X				X	
Gelusil II	Tablet, suspension		X		X				X	
Maalox	Tablet, suspension		X		X					
Maalox Plus	Tablet, suspension		X		X				X	
Mylanta	Tablet, suspension		X		X				X	
Mylanta II	Tablet, suspension		X		X				X	
Phillips' Milk of Magnesia	Tablet, suspension				X					
Phosphaljel*	Suspension									Aluminum phosphate
Riopan	Tablet, suspension									Magaldrate
Riopan Plus	Tablet, suspension								X	Magaldrate
Rolaids	Tablet									Dihydroxyaluminum sodium carbonate
Titralac	Tablet, suspension	X								Glycine
Tums	Tablet	X								
WinGel	Tablet, suspension		X		X					

*No longer classified as an antacid. Used to reduce fecal excretion of phosphates.

num hydroxide is constipation, while excess magnesium results in diarrhea.

Calcium carbonate and sodium bicarbonate may cause rebound hyperacidity.

Patients with renal failure should not use large quantities of antacids containing magnesium. The magnesium ions cannot be excreted and may produce hypermagnesemia and toxicity.

Availability. See Table 14-1.

Dosage and administration. Follow directions on the product container.

Drug interactions. The absorption of tetracycline antibiotics, digoxin, digitoxin, and iron compounds is inhibited by antacids. These medications should be administered 1 hour before or 2 hours after the administration of antacids.

Levodopa absorption is increased by antacids. When antacid therapy is added, toxicity may result in the parkinsonian patient who is well controlled taking a certain dosage of levodopa. If the patient's parkinsonism is well controlled on levodopa *and* antacid therapy, withdrawal of antacids may result in a recurrence of parkinsonian symptomatology.

Frequent use of antacid therapy may result in increased urinary pH. Renal excretion of quinidine and amphetamines may be inhibited, and toxicity may occur.

• **Nursing Interventions: Monitoring antacid therapy**

See General Nursing Considerations for Patients with Gastrointestinal Disorders.

Nurses are frequently asked by patients and friends to recommend antacid products. Before recommending antacid therapy, several questions should be asked to help ascertain whether there is a serious underlying medical condition:

1. How long has the pain been present?
2. When and where does the pain occur? Immediately after meals, or several hours after meals?
3. Have you vomited blood or black "coffee grounds" material?
4. Have you noticed blood in the stool or have the stools been black?
5. Are you on any dietary restrictions, such as a low-salt diet?
6. Are you under a physician's care?

If the answers to these questions suggest an underlying disease, patients should be referred immediately to a physician.

The following principles should be considered when antacid therapy is being planned:

1. For indigestion, antacids should not be administered for more than 2 weeks. If, after this time, the pa-

tient is still experiencing discomfort, a physician should be contacted.

2. Patients with edema, congestive heart failure, hypertension, renal failure, pregnancy, or salt-restricted diets should use low-sodium antacids. These products include Riopan, Maalox, and Mylanta II. Therapy should continue only on the recommendation of a physician.

3. Antacid tablets should be used only for the patient with an occasional case of indigestion or heartburn. Tablets *do not* contain enough antacid to be effective in treating peptic ulcer disease.

4. Excessive use of antacids frequently results in either constipation or diarrhea. If a patient experiences these symptoms and is still suffering from stomach discomfort, a physician should be consulted.

5. Effective management of *acute* ulcer disease requires large volumes of antacids. The selection of an antacid, and the quantity to be taken, depend on the neutralizing capacity of the antacid. Any patient with "coffee grounds" hematemesis, bloody stools, or recurrent abdominal pain should seek medical attention immediately and must not attempt to self-treat the disorder.

6. Most antacids have similar ingredients (see Table 14-1). Selection of an antacid for occasional use should be determined by quantity of each ingredient, cost, taste, and frequency of side effects. Patients may need to try more than one product and to weigh the advantages and disadvantages of each.

Histamine H₂ antagonists

OBJECTIVES

1. Identify diseases treated with histamine antagonists.
2. Describe drug scheduling used when antacids and histamine antagonists are prescribed concurrently.
3. Review the list of drug classes affected by the concurrent use of cimetidine, and identify monitoring parameters needed to detect adverse effects.

KEY WORDS

Zollinger-Ellison syndrome   gynecomastia

Stimulation of H_2 receptors on the parietal cells of the stomach by food, caffeine, histamine, and insulin causes gastric acid secretion. The H_2 antagonists—cimetidine, ranitidine, nizatidine, and famotidine—act by blocking H_2 receptors on parietal cells, thus decreasing the volume and increasing the pH of gastric acid secreted during both the day and the night.

The H_2 antagonists are now being used to treat duodenal ulcers and pathologic hypersecretory conditions, such as Zollinger-Ellison syndrome, and for the prevention and treatment of stress ulcers. Other unapproved uses include prevention of aspiration pneumonitis, gastroesophageal reflux, acute upper-GI bleeding, and hyperparathyroidism. Due to the diversity of adverse effects, dosage schedules, and drug interactions among the H_2 antagonists, they are discussed separately below.

cimetidine (si-me′ti-deen)

Tagamet (tag′ah-met)

Side effects. Most side effects are quite mild and transient. About 1% of patients develop diarrhea, dizziness, headaches, or somnolence.

If high dosages are used in patients with liver or renal disease or in patients over 50 years of age, mental confusion, slurred speech, disorientation, and hallucinations may occur. This adverse effect dissipates over 3 to 4 days after therapy has been discontinued.

Mild bilateral gynecomastia and breast soreness may occur with long-term use (greater than 1 month) but resolves after discontinuation of therapy.

Other rare adverse effects include transient hyperthermia, maculopapular rashes, urticaria, muscular pain, transient neutropenia, hypotension, and bradycardia.

Availability

PO—200, 300, 400, and 800 mg tablets, 300 mg per 5 ml liquid.

Injection—300 mg per 2 ml in 2 and 8 ml vials and 50 ml piggybacks.

Dosage and administration

Adult

PO—300 mg 4 times daily with meals and at bedtime. Do not exceed 2400 mg daily. Antacid therapy may be continued for relief of pain but should be administered 1 to 2 hours before or after the cimetidine dosage.

IV—300 mg every 6 hours.

• Nursing Interventions: Monitoring cimetidine therapy

See also General Nursing Considerations for Patients with Gastrointestinal Disorders.

Side effects to expect

DIZZINESS, HEADACHES, DIARRHEA, SOMNOLENCE. These side effects are usually mild and resolve with continued therapy. Encourage the patient not to discontinue therapy without first consulting the physician.

Provide for patient safety during episodes of dizziness.

If patients develop somnolence and lethargy, encourage them to use caution when working around machinery or driving a car.

Side effects to report

CONFUSION, DISORIENTATION, HALLUCINATIONS. Perform a baseline assessment of the patient's degree of alertness and orientation to name, place and time *prior* to initiating therapy. Make regularly scheduled subsequent mental status evaluations and compare findings. Report development of alterations.

GYNECOMASTIA, RASHES, NEUTROPENIA, HYPOTENSION, BRADYCARDIA. Report for further observation and possible laboratory tests.

Implementation
PO. Administer with food.

ANTACIDS. Because antacid therapy is often continued during early therapy of ulcer disease, administer 1 hour before or 2 hours after the cimetidine dose.

IV. Dilute in 20 ml of saline solution or D5W and administer over 1 to 2 minutes *or* dilute in 100 ml of IV fluid and infuse over 15 to 20 minutes.

Drug interactions
BENZODIAZEPINES. Cimetidine inhibits the metabolism and/or excretion of the following benzodiazepines: alprazolam, chlordiazepoxide, diazepam, clorazepate, flurazepam, halazepam, prazepam, and triazolam.

Patients taking cimetidine and a benzodiazepine concurrently should be observed for increased sedation and may require a reduction in dosage of the benzodiazepine. The metabolism of temazepam, and lorazepam does not appear to be affected.

THEOPHYLLINE DERIVATIVES. Cimetidine inhibits the metabolism and/or excretion of the following xanthine derivatives: aminophylline, oxtriphylline, dyphylline, and theophylline.

Patients at greater risk include those receiving larger doses of theophylline and those with liver disease. Observe for restlessness, vomiting, dizziness, and cardiac arrhythmias. The dosage of theophylline may need to be reduced.

BETA ADRENERGIC BLOCKING AGENTS. Beta adrenergic blocking agents (propranolol, labetalol, metoprolol) may accumulate due to inhibited metabolism. Monitor for signs of toxicity, such as hypotension and bradycardia.

PHENYTOIN. Cimetidine inhibits the metabolism of phenytoin. Monitor patients with concurrent therapy for signs of phenytoin toxicity: nystagmus, sedation, lethargy. Serum levels may be ordered, and a reduced dosage of phenytoin may be required.

LIDOCAINE, QUINIDINE, PROCAINAMIDE. Cimetidine may inhibit the metabolism of these agents. Monitor patients for signs of toxicity (bradycardia, additional arrhythmias, hyperactivity, sedation) and reduce the dose if necessary.

ANTACIDS. Administer 1 hour before or 2 hours after administration of cimetidine.

WARFARIN. This medication may enhance the anticoagulant effects of warfarin. Observe for the development of petechiae, ecchymoses, nosebleeds, bleeding gums, dark tarry stools and bright red or "coffee ground" emesis. Monitor the prothrombin time and reduce the dosage of warfarin if necessary.

CALCIUM ANTAGONISTS. Cimetidine may inhibit the metabolism of diltiazem, nifedipine, and verapamil. Patients should be monitored for increased effects from the calcium antagonists (bradycardia, hypotension, arrhythmias, fatigue).

TRICYCLIC ANTIDEPRESSANTS. Cimetidine may inhibit the excretion of imipramine, desipramine, and nortriptyline, usually within 3 to 5 days of starting cimetidine. If anticholinergic effects or toxicity of these agents become apparent, a decreased dose of the antidepressant may be necessary. If cimetidine is discontinued, the patient should be monitored for a decreased response to the antidepressant.

famotidine (fam-ot'ih-deen)

Pepcid (pehp'sid)

Famotidine is another histamine H_2 antagonist. It is similar in action and use to cimetidine, but has the apparent advantages of one dose daily, fewer drug interactions, and no antiandrogenic effect (which causes gynecomastia).

Side effects. Side effects reported with famotidine include headache (4.7%), diarrhea (1.7%), dizziness (1.3%), and constipation (1.2%).

Availability
PO—20, 40 mg tablets; 40 mg/5 ml oral suspension.
INJ—10 mg/ml in 2 and 4 ml vials.

Dosage and administration
Adult
PO—Initially, 40 mg once daily at bedtime for 6 to 8 weeks. Maintenance therapy is 20 mg daily at bedtime. Patients with severe Zollinger-Ellison syndrome may require up to 160 mg every 6 hours.
IV—20 mg every 12 hours.

• Nursing Interventions: Monitoring famotidine therapy

See General Nursing Considerations for Patients with Gastrointestinal Disorders.

Side effects to expect
DIZZINESS, HEADACHES, CONSTIPATION, DIARRHEA. These side effects are usually mild and resolve with continued therapy. Encourage the patient not to discontinue therapy without first consulting the physician.

Provide for patient safety during episodes of dizziness.

Maintain the patient's state of hydration, and obtain an order for stool softeners or bulk-forming laxatives, if necessary. Encourage the inclusion of sufficient roughage, fresh fruits, vegetables, and whole-grain products in the diet.

Implementation
PO. Administer with food.

ANTACIDS. Because antacid therapy is often continued during early therapy of ulcer disease, administer 1 hour before or 2 hours after the famotidine dose.

IV. Dilute in 5 to 10 ml of saline solution or D5W and administer over at least 2 minutes *or* dilute in 100 ml of IV fluid and infuse over 15 to 30 minutes.

Drug interactions. No significant drug interactions have been reported.

nizatidine (nye-zaht'ih-deen)

Axid (axe-id')

Nizatidine is another histamine H_2 antagonist. It is similar in action and use to cimetidine, famotidine, and ranitidine, but has the apparent advantages of one- to two-times daily administration, no antiandrogenic effects, and fewer drug interactions. In contrast to the other agents, it is not available in a parenteral dosage form.

Side effects. The most commonly reported adverse effects of nizatidine include headache, abdominal pain, diarrhea, and rhinitis.

Availability

PO—150 and 300 mg capsules.

Dosage and administration

Adult

PO—300 mg once daily at bedtime or 150 mg 2 times daily.

• Nursing Interventions: Monitoring nizatidine therapy

Side effects to expect

HEADACHES, ABDOMINAL PAIN, DIARRHEA, RHINITIS. These side effects are usually mild and resolve with continued therapy. Encourage the patient not to discontinue therapy without first consulting the physician.

Maintain the patient's state of hydration. Encourage the inclusion of sufficient roughage, fresh fruits, vegetables, and whole-grain products in the diet.

Implementation

PO. Nizatidine may be administered with or without food.

Drug interactions. No significant drug interactions have been reported.

ranitidine (ran-it'ih-deen)

Zantac (zahn'tack)

Ranitidine is another histamine H_2 antagonist. It is similar in action and use to cimetidine, but has the apparent advantages of fewer drug interactions and no antiandrogenic effect (which causes gynecomastia).

Side effects. Up to 1% of patients may develop mild and transient lethargy, dizziness, constipation, nausea, abdominal pain, and rash. About 3% of patients develop headaches with ranitidine therapy.

Cases of hepatitis have been associated with ranitidine.

Availability

PO—150 and 300 mg tablets; 15 mg/ml syrup

INJ—0.5 mg/ml in 100 ml containers; 25 mg/ml in 2, 10, and 40 ml vials.

Dosage and administration

Adult

PO—150 mg 2 times daily. Absorption is not affected by food; thus, medication may be taken without regard to meals. However, do not administer within 1 hour of taking an antacid.

IM, IV—50 mg every 6 to 8 hours.

• Nursing Interventions: Monitoring ranitidine therapy

See General Nursing Considerations for Patients with Gastrointestinal Disorders.

Side effects to expect

DIZZINESS, HEADACHES, CONSTIPATION, LETHARGY. These side effects are usually mild and resolve with continued therapy. Encourage the patient not to discontinue therapy without first consulting the physician.

Provide for patient safety during episodes of dizziness.

If patients develop somnolence and lethargy, encourage them to use caution when working around machinery or driving a car.

Maintain the patient's state of hydration, and obtain an order for stool softeners or bulk-forming laxatives, if necessary. Encourage the inclusion of sufficient roughage, fresh fruits, vegetables, and whole-grain products in the diet.

Side effects to report

HEPATOTOXICITY. The symptoms of hepatotoxicity are anorexia, nausea, vomiting, jaundice, hepatomegaly, splenomegaly, and abnormal liver function tests (elevated bilirubin, AST, ALT, GGT, alkaline phosphatase, prothrombin time).

Implementation

PO. Administer with food.

ANTACIDS. Because antacid therapy is often continued during early therapy of ulcer disease, administer 1 hour before or 2 hours after the ranitidine dose.

IV. Dilute in 20 ml of saline solution or D5W and administer over at least 5 minutes *or* dilute in 100 ml of IV fluid and infuse over 15 to 20 minutes. Do not exceed 400 mg/day.

Drug interactions. In general, there appear to be no interactions with ranitidine. There are conflicting data, however. Studies indicate that patients receiving higher doses of ranitidine may be more susceptible to drug interactions with ranitidine. When used concurrently, monitor for toxic effects of warfarin, theophylline, procainamide, and glipizide.

Gastrointestinal prostaglandin

OBJECTIVES

1. Identify the class of medicines that induce gastric ulcerations that may be treated by gastrointestinal prostaglandins.
2. List the contraindication to misoprostol use.

misoprostol (mis-oh'pros-tohl)

Cytotec (site-oh'tech)

Misoprostol is the first of a new synthetic prostaglandin E series to be used to treat gastrointestinal disorders. Prostaglandins are normally present in the gastrointestinal tract and act to stimulate motility, gastric acid, and pepsin secretion and to protect the stomach and duodenal lining against ulceration. The prostaglandin E analogues may also induce uterine contractions.

Misoprostol is used to prevent and treat gastric ulcers caused by nonsteroidal antiinflammatory agents (NSAIDs), including aspirin. The NSAIDs are prostaglandin inhibitors used to treat pain and inflammation. Whereas prostaglandin inhibition is effective in reducing pain and inflammation, especially in arthritis, the prostaglandin inhibition in the stomach makes the patient more predisposed to gastric ulcers.

Side effects. As a gastrointestinal stimulant, it is not surprising that the most common side effect of misoprostol therapy is diarrhea. Other gastrointestinal effects include loose stools, vomiting, flatulence, and anorexia.

Misoprostol is contraindicated during pregnancy and in women at risk of becoming pregnant. As a uterine stimulant, it may induce miscarriage.

Availability

PO—100 and 200 mcg tablets.

Dosage and administration

Adult

PO—100 to 200 mcg tablets 4 times daily with food during NSAID therapy.

- **Nursing Interventions: Monitoring misoprostol therapy**

Side effects to expect

DIARRHEA. Diarrhea associated with misoprostol therapy is dose-related and usually develops after about 2 weeks of therapy. It often resolves after about 8 days, but a few patients will require discontinuation of misoprostol therapy. Diarrhea can be minimized by taking misoprostol with meals and at bedtime, and by avoiding magnesium-containing antacids (Maalox, Mylanta).

Encourage the patient not to discontinue therapy without first consulting the physician.

Encourage the inclusion of sufficient roughage, fresh fruits, vegetables, and whole-grain products in the diet.

Side effects to report

PREGNANCY. While pregnancy is not a side effect of misoprostol therapy, it is crucial that misoprostol therapy be discontinued. The patient must receive care from the physician who prescribed the misoprostol and an obstetrician. The question of alternative therapies to NSAIDs must also be considered.

Implementation

PO. Administer with meals and at bedtime.

Do not administer misoprostol if the patient is pregnant or may become pregnant while taking this medication.

Drug interactions. No significant drug interactions have been reported.

Gastric acid pump inhibitor
OBJECTIVES

1. Identify the name of the cells that secrete acid in the stomach.

2. List the types of diseases for which omeprazole may be used.
3. List the drug interactions associated with omeprazole therapy and the monitoring required to prevent serious complications.

omeprazole (oh-mep′rah-zol)

Prilosec (pril-oh′sec)

Omeprazole is the first of a new class of drugs that inhibit gastric secretion by inhibiting the gastric acid pump of the parietal cells of the stomach. Omeprazole is used to treat severe esophagitis, gastroesophageal reflux disease (GERD), gastric and duodenal ulcers, and hypersecretory disorders such as Zollinger-Ellison (ZE) syndrome.

Side effects. The most commonly reported adverse effects during clinical trials were diarrhea, headache, itching, rash, muscle pain, and fatigue.

Availability

PO—20 mg sustained release capsules.

Dosage and administration

PO—Initially, 20 mg once daily. Dosages up to 120 mg daily in divided doses may be required for certain hypersecretory conditions.

- **Nursing Interventions: Monitoring omeprazole therapy**

Side effects to expect

DIARRHEA, HEADACHE, MUSCLE PAIN, FATIGUE. These symptoms are relatively mild and rarely cause the discontinuation of therapy. Encourage the patient not to discontinue therapy without first consulting the physician.

Maintain the patient's state of hydration. Encourage the inclusion of sufficient roughage, fresh fruits, vegetables, and whole-grain products in the diet.

Side effects to report

RASH. Persistent vesicular rash may be cause for discontinuation of therapy. Report for further observation and possible laboratory tests.

Implementation

PO. Administer before a meal. Swallow the capsule whole; do not open, chew, or crush.

Drug interactions

DIAZEPAM. Omeprazole significantly increases the half-life of diazepam by inhibiting its metabolism. Observe patients for increased sedative effect of diazepam. Caution against hazardous tasks such as driving and operating machinery. The dosage of diazepam may have to be reduced.

PHENYTOIN. Omeprazole slows the metabolism of phenytoin. Observe for nystagmus, sedation, lethargy. The dosage of phenytoin may have to be reduced.

WARFARIN. Omeprazole may reduce the rate of metabolism of warfarin. Monitor the patient closely for signs of bleeding tendencies and monitor the prothrombin time closely. The dosage of warfarin may have to be reduced.

Coating agent
OBJECTIVE

1. Compare the actions of sucralfate, histamine antagonists, misoprostol, omeprazole, and antacids.

sucralfate (sook-rahl'fate)
Carafate (kair-ah'fate)

Sucralfate is an agent that, when swallowed, forms a complex that adheres to the crater of an ulcer, protecting it from aggravators such as acid, pepsin, and bile salts. Sucralfate does not inhibit gastric secretions (like the H_2 antagonists), or alter gastric pH (like antacids). It is used to treat duodenal ulcers, particularly in those patients who do not tolerate other forms of therapy.

Side effects. Since there is very little absorption of sucralfate, there are very few side effects associated with its use. The most common complaints are constipation (2.2%) and dry mouth. Other very infrequently reported side effects are nausea, stomach discomfort, and dizziness.

Availability

PO—1 g tablets.

Dosage and administration

Adult

PO—1 tablet 1 hour before each meal and at bedtime, all on an empty stomach. Antacids may be used, but should not be administered within half an hour before, or after, sucralfate.

• Nursing Interventions: Monitoring sucralfate therapy

See also General Nursing Considerations for Patients with Gastrointestinal Disorders.

Side effects to expect

CONSTIPATION, DRY MOUTH, DIZZINESS. These side effects are usually mild and tend to resolve with continued therapy. Encourage the patient not to discontinue therapy without first consulting the physician.

Measures to alleviate dry mouth include sucking on ice chips or hard candy. Avoid mouthwashes that contain alcohol, as it causes further drying and irritation.

Maintain the patient's state of hydration, and obtain an order for stool softeners or bulk-forming laxatives, if necessary. Encourage the inclusion of sufficient roughage, fresh fruits, vegetables, and whole-grain products in the diet.

Provide for patient safety during episodes of dizziness.

Implementation

PO. Administer on an empty stomach.

ANTACIDS. Administer antacids at least one half hour before or after sucralfate.

Drug interactions

TETRACYCLINES. Sucralfate may interfere with the absorption of tetracycline.

Administer tetracyclines 1 hour before or 2 hours after sucralfate.

Gastric stimulant
OBJECTIVES

1. Describe the actions of metoclopramide.
2. Explain precautions in using metoclopramide for persons with epilepsy or for those receiving antipsychotic agents.

KEY WORDS

gastroparesis	extrapyramidal symptoms
oculogyric crisis	torticollis

metoclopramide (met-oh-klo'prah-myd)
Reglan (reg'lan)

Metoclopramide is a gastric stimulant that has an unknown mechanism of action. It increases stomach contractions, relaxes the pyloric valve, and increases peristalsis in the gastrointestinal tract, resulting in an increased rate of gastric emptying and intestinal transit. Metoclopramide is used to relieve the symptoms of diabetic gastroparesis, as an antiemetic for vomiting associated with cancer chemotherapy, as an aid in small bowel intubation, and to stimulate gastric emptying and intestinal transit of barium after radiologic examination of the upper GI tract.

Side effects. Common side effects are drowsiness, fatigue, and lethargy. Other less frequent adverse effects include insomnia, headache, dizziness, nausea, and bowel disturbances.

About 1 in 500 patients may develop extrapyramidal symptoms manifested by restlessness, involuntary movements, facial grimacing, and possibly oculogyric crisis, torticollis, or rhythmic protrusion of the tongue. Children and young adults are most susceptible, as are those receiving higher doses of metoclopramide as an antiemetic. Metoclopramide should not be used in patients with epilepsy or in patients receiving drugs that are likely to cause extrapyramidal reactions (such as phenothiazines), as the frequency and severity of seizures or extrapyramidal reactions may be increased.

Metoclopramide must not be used in patients when increased gastric motility may be dangerous, such as in cases of gastrointestinal perforation, mechanical obstruction, or hemorrhage.

Availability

PO—5 and 10 mg tablets and 5 mg/5 ml syrup.

Injection—5 mg/ml in 2 and 10 ml ampules.

Dosage and administration

Adult

PO—Diabetic gastroparesis: 10 mg 30 minutes before each meal and at bedtime. Duration of therapy is dependent on response and continued well-being after discontinuation of therapy.

IV—Antiemesis: Initial 2 doses: 2 mg/kg. If vomiting is suppressed, follow with 1 mg/kg.

NOTE: Rapid IV infusion may cause sudden, intense anxiety and restlessness, followed by drowsiness.

NOTE: If extrapyramidal symptoms should develop, treat with diphenhydramine.

• Nursing Interventions: Monitoring metoclopramide therapy

See also General Nursing Considerations for Patients with Gastrointestinal Disorders.

Side effects to expect

DROWSINESS, FATIGUE, LETHARGY, DIZZINESS, NAUSEA. These side effects are usually mild and tend to resolve with continued therapy. Encourage the patient not to discontinue therapy without first consulting the physician.

People who are working around machinery, driving a car, or performing other duties that require mental alertness should be particularly cautious.

Provide for patient safety during episodes of dizziness.

Side effects to report

EXTRAPYRAMIDAL SYMPTOMS. Provide for patient safety, then report immediately.

Implementation

IV. Dilute the dose in 50 ml of parenteral solution (D_5W, N.S. 0.9%, D_5/.45 N.S., Ringer's solution, or lactated Ringer's solution).

Infuse over at least 15 minutes, 30 minutes before beginning chemotherapy. Repeat every 2 hours for 2 doses, followed by 1 dose every 3 hours for 3 doses.

Drug interactions

DRUGS THAT INCREASE SEDATIVE EFFECTS. Antihistamine, alcohol, analgesics, tranquilizers, sedative-hypnotics.

Monitor the patient for excessive sedation, and reduce the dosage of the above agents, if necessary.

DRUGS THAT DECREASE THERAPEUTIC EFFECTS. Anticholinergic agents (atropine, benztropine, antihistamines, dicyclomine) and narcotic analgesics (meperidine, morphine, oxycodone, others). Try to avoid the use of these agents while using metoclopramide.

ALTERED ABSORPTION. The gastrointestinal stimulatory effects of metoclopramide may alter absorption of food and drugs as follows:

DIGOXIN. Monitor for signs of decreased activity (for example, return of edema, weight gain, congestive heart failure).

LEVODOPA. Monitor for signs of increased activity (for example, restlessness, nightmares, hallucinations, additional involuntary movements such as bobbing of head and neck, facial grimacing, and active tongue movements).

ALCOHOL. Monitor for signs of sedation, drunkenness with smaller amounts of alcohol.

INSULIN. The absorption of food may be altered, requiring an adjustment in timing or dosage of insulin in patients with diabetes mellitus.

Antispasmodic agents

OBJECTIVES

1. State the action of stimulation of cholinergic fibers on the gastrointestinal tract.
2. Explain the rationale for anticholinergic agents also being referred to as *antispasmodic agents*.
3. Describe diseases that may respond favorably to antispasmodic agent therapy.
4. Identify principles underlying the safe use of anticholinergic agents in patients with open-angle glaucoma.
5. List the side effects to expect and report for anticholinergic agents.
6. Explain why stool softeners are frequently prescribed in conjunction with anticholinergic agent therapy.

KEY WORDS

mydriasis	peristalsis
open-angle glaucoma	closed-angle glaucoma

Drugs used as antispasmodic agents are actually anticholinergic agents. The GI tract is heavily innervated by the cholinergic branch of the autonomic nervous system. Cholinergic fibers stimulate the GI tract causing (1) secretion of saliva, hydrochloric acid, pepsin, bile, and other enzymatic fluids necessary for digestion; (2) relaxation of sphincter muscles; and (3) peristalsis to move the contents of the stomach and bowel through the GI tract. The antispasmodic agents act by preventing acetylcholine from attaching to the cholinergic receptors in the GI tract. The extent of reduction of cholinergic activity depends upon the amount of anticholinergic drug blocking the receptors. Inhibition of cholinergic nerve conduction results in decreased GI motility and reduced secretions.

Antispasmodic agents are used to treat irritable bowel syndrome, biliary spasm, mild ulcerative colitis, diverticulitis, pancreatitis, infant colic, and, in conjunction with diet and antacids, peptic ulcer disease. Since the advent of the histamine H_2 antagonists, antispasmodic agents are used much less frequently in the treatment of ulcers.

Side effects. Because cholinergic fibers innervate the entire body, and because these agents are not selective in their actions to the GI tract, we can expect to see the effects of blocking this system throughout the body. In order to provide adequate doses to inhibit gastrointestinal motility and secretions, we should also expect a reduction in perspiration and in oral and bronchial secretions; *mydriasis* (dilation of the pupils) with blurring of vision; constipation; urinary hesitancy or retention; tachycardia, possibly with palpitations; and mild, transient postural hypotension. Psychiatric disturbances such as mental confusion, delusions, nightmares, euphoria, paranoia, and hallucinations may be indications of overdosage.

Table 14-2 *Antispasmodic Agents*

GENERIC NAME	BRAND NAME	AVAILABILITY	CLINICAL USES	INITIAL DOSAGE
Anisotropine	Valpin 50	Tablets: 50 mg	Peptic ulcer disease	PO: 50 mg 3 times daily
Atropine	Atropine Sulfate	Inj: 0.05, 0.1, 0.3, 0.4, 0.5, 0.8, 1 mg/ml Tablets: 0.4 mg	Treatment of pylorospasm and spastic conditions of the GI tract	PO: 0.4-0.6 mg
Belladonna	Belladonna Tincture	Tincture: 30 mg/100 ml	Indigestion, peptic ulcer Nocturnal enuresis Parkinsonism	Tincture—PO: 0.6-1 mg 3-4 times daily
Clidinium bromide	Quarzan	Capsules: 2.5, 5 mg	Peptic ulcer disease	PO: 2.5-5 mg 3-4 times daily
Dicyclomine	Bentyl, Antispas, Dibent, ✦Bentylol	Tablets: 20 mg Capsules: 10, 20 mg Syrup: 10 mg/5 ml Inj: 10 mg/ml	Irritable bowel syndrome Infant colic	Adults—PO: 20-40 mg 3-4 times daily Infants—PO: 5 mg 3-4 times daily
Glycopyrrolate	Robinul	Tablets: 1, 2 mg Inj: 0.2 mg/ml	Peptic ulcer disease	PO: 1 mg 2-3 times daily
Hexocyclium	Tral	Tablets: 25 mg	Peptic ulcer disease	PO: 25 mg 4 times daily
Isopropamide	Darbid	Tablets: 5 mg	Peptic ulcer disease	PO: 5 mg every 12 hours
Mepenzolate	Cantil	Tablets: 25 mg	Peptic ulcer disease	PO: 25-50 mg 4 times daily
Methantheline	Banthine	Tablets: 50 mg	Peptic ulcer disease	PO: 50-100 mg every 6 hours
Methscopolamine	Pamine	Tablets: 2.5 mg	Peptic ulcer disease	PO: 2.5 mg 30 min before meals and 2.5-5 mg at bedtime
Oxyphencyclimine	Daricon	Tablets: 10 mg	Peptic ulcer disease	PO: 10 mg 2 or 3 times daily, morning and bedtime
Propantheline	ProBanthine	Tablets: 7.5, 15 mg	Peptic ulcer disease	PO: 15 mg before meals and 30 mg at bedtime
Scopolamine	Scopolamine, ✦Buscopan	Inj: 0.3, 0.4, 0.86, 1 mg/ml	GI hypermotility, pylorospasm, irritable colon syndrome	SC or IM: 0.32-0.65 mg
Tridihexethyl chloride	Pathilon	Tablets: 25 mg	Peptic ulcer disease	PO: 25-50 mg 3-4 times daily before meals and at bedtime

✦Available in Canada only.

All patients should be screened for the presence of closed-angle glaucoma. Anticholinergic agents may precipitate an acute attack of closed-angle glaucoma. Patients with open-angle glaucoma can safely use anticholinergic agents in conjunction with miotic therapy.

Availability. See Table 14-2.

Dosage and administration. See Table 14-2.

• **Nursing Interventions: Monitoring antispasmodic agent therapy**

See also General Nursing Considerations for Patients with Gastrointestinal Disorders.

Side effects to expect

BLURRED VISION, CONSTIPATION, URINARY RETENTION, DRYNESS OF THE MOUTH, NOSE, AND THROAT. These symptoms are the anticholinergic effects produced by these agents. Patients taking these medications should be monitored for the development of these side effects.

Dryness of the mucosa may be alleviated by sucking hard candy or ice chips or by chewing gum.

If patients develop urinary hesitancy, assess for distension of the bladder. Report to the physician for further evaluation.

Give stool softeners as prescribed. Encourage adequate fluid intake and foods to provide sufficient bulk.

Caution the patient that blurred vision may occur and make appropriate suggestions for personal safety of the individual.

Side effects to report

CONFUSION, DEPRESSION, NIGHTMARES, HALLUCINATIONS. Perform a baseline assessment of the patient's degree of alertness and orientation to name, place, and time *before* initiating therapy. Make regularly scheduled subsequent mental status evaluations and compare findings. Report development of alterations.

Provide for patient safety during these episodes.

Reduction in the daily dosage may control these adverse effects.

ORTHOSTATIC HYPOTENSION. All antispasmodic agents may cause some degree of orthostatic hypotension, although it is infrequent and generally mild. It is manifested by dizziness and weakness, particularly when therapy is being initiated.

Monitor the blood pressure daily in both the supine and standing positions.

Anticipate the development of postural hypotension and take measures to prevent an occurrence. Teach the patient to rise slowly from a supine or sitting position. Encourage the patient to sit or lie down if feeling faint.

PALPITATIONS, ARRHYTHMIAS. Report for further evaluation.

Implementation

GLAUCOMA. All patients should be screened for the presence of closed-angle glaucoma before the initiation of therapy.

Patients with open-angle glaucoma can safely use anticholinergic agents. Intraocular pressure should be monitored on a regular basis.

PO. Administer with food or milk to minimize gastric irritation.

Drug interactions

AMANTADINE, TRICYCLIC ANTIDEPRESSANTS, PHENOTHIAZINES. These agents may potentiate the anticholinergic side effects. Developing confusion and hallucinations are characteristic of excessive anticholinergic activity.

Digestants
OBJECTIVE

1. State the purpose for prescribing digestants.

Digestants are combination products used to treat various digestive disorders and supplement deficiencies of natural digestive enzymes. They are taken orally to aid digestion and absorption of dietary carbohydrates, proteins, and fats.

These products usually contain a wide variety of ingredients, each supposedly serving a purpose. See Table 14-3 for a list of components and their intended purposes.

Table 14-3 *Digestants*

INGREDIENT	PURPOSE
Bile extracts	Activation of lipase, emulsification of fats, absorption of food
Glutamic acid and betaine	Acidifiers
Simethicone and ginger	Antiflatulents
Activated charcoal	Adsorbant
Calcium carbonate or sodium bicarbonate	Antacids
Dehydrocholic acid and desoxycholic acid	Increase secretion of bile and aid in digestion of fats
Digestive enzymes:	
Pepsin, papain, protease	Digest protein
Lipase, amylase	Digest starch, fat, protein
Diastase	Digest starch
Cellulase	Digest cellulose
Anticholinergic agents	Relieve spasm and reduce hypermotility
Barbiturates, antihistamines	Sedatives
Berberis and hydrastis	Astringents used in inflammation of the mucosa

Dosage and administration
Adult

PO—Take one or two tablets or capsules with or after meals.

Drug interactions. Concurrent administration of antacids containing calcium carbonate or magnesium hydroxide interferes with the action of the digestive enzymes.

Emetics
OBJECTIVES

1. Compare the purposes of using emetic and antiemetic products.
2. Identify the location of the nearest poison control center.
3. State conditions under which the use of ipecac syrup is contraindicated.
4. Describe the monitoring required following the administration of ipecac syrup.
5. State the therapeutic classes of antiemetics.
6. Discuss scheduling of antiemetics for maximum benefit.

KEY WORD

emesis

ipecac syrup (ip'e-kak)

Syrup of ipecac is used to induce vomiting in cases of ingested noncorrosive poisons. It probably acts by irritating the gastric mucosa and by stimulating the vomiting center in the brain. Vomiting usually occurs within 20 to 30 minutes.

Availability

PO—15 and 30 ml syrup.

Dosage and administration. NOTE: Before giving a dose of ipecac to induce vomiting, *call a physician, poison control center, or hospital emergency room for advice!*

Do not use ipecac if any of the following have been ingested: corrosives, such as alkalies (lye) and strong acids; strychnine; petroleum distillates, such as gasoline, coal oil, fuel oil, kerosene, cleaning fluid, or paint thinner.

Adult

PO—15 to 30 ml, followed by 200 to 300 ml of water or fruit juice. Do not administer with milk or carbonated beverages.

Pediatric

PO—Over 1 year of age: 10 to 15 ml followed by 200 ml of liquid. Under 1 year of age: 5 to 10 ml followed by as much liquid as the patient will take.

The dosages may be repeated once after 20 minutes if the first dose is not effective. If vomiting does not occur within 30 minutes, gastric lavage should be performed.

• Nursing Interventions: Monitoring ipecac therapy

Side effects to expect

VOMITING. Vomiting should appear within 20 minutes. Report failure to vomit after 20 additional minutes following a second dose.

Side effects to report

CARDIOTOXIC EFFECTS, SHOCK, ARRHYTHMIAS. Monitor pulse, respirations, and blood pressure. Report alterations in vital signs or developing symptoms of shock or cardiac arrhythmias.

Implementation

PO. See above.

Read the label carefully. Syrup of ipecac is not the same as fluid extract of ipecac.

Antiemetics

Nausea is the sensation of abdominal discomfort that is intermittently accompanied by a desire to vomit. *Vomiting* is the forceful expulsion of gastric contents up the esophagus and out the mouth. Nausea may occur without vomiting, and sudden vomiting may occur without prior nausea, but the two symptoms often occur together.

Nausea and vomiting are common symptoms experienced by virtually everyone at one time or another. They are symptoms that accompany almost any illness. Nausea and vomiting may be due to a wide variety of causes, including the following:

• Infection
• Gastrointestinal disorders such as gastritis, liver, gallbladder, or pancreatic disease
• Overeating or irritation of the stomach by certain foods or liquids

• Motion sickness (see Chapter 9)
• Drug therapy (nausea and vomiting are the most common side effects of drug therapy)
• Emotional disturbances and mental stress
• Pregnancy
• Pain and unpleasant sights and odors
• Radiation therapy

There are several physiologic mechanisms of nausea and vomiting and none are well understood. It is known that the vomiting center in the brain transmits impulses after receiving certain stimuli such as those listed, and that the stomach and duodenum respond to these impulses in the form of nausea and vomiting.

Control of vomiting is important, not only to relieve the obvious distress associated with vomiting, but also to prevent aspiration of gastric contents into the lungs, dehydration, and electrolyte imbalance. Primary treatment of nausea and vomiting should be directed at the underlying cause. Since this is not always possible, treatment with both nondrug and drug measures is appropriate. Most drugs (antiemetics) used to treat nausea and vomiting act either by suppressing the action of the vomiting center or by inhibiting the impulses going to or coming from the center. These agents are generally more effective if administered before the onset of nausea, rather than after the vomiting has already started.

Since there are several nerve pathways associated with nausea and vomiting, it stands to reason that more than one class of medicinal agents will prevent nausea and vomiting. The six classes of agents used as antiemetics (Table 14-4) are: dopamine antagonists, serotonin antagonists, anticholinergic agents, corticosteroids, benzodiazepines, and cannabinoids.

Dopamine antagonists. The dopamine antagonists include the phenothiazines, the butyrophenones, benzquinamide, and metoclopramide. These drugs inhibit dopamine receptors that are part of the pathway to the vomiting center. Unfortunately, dopamine receptors in other parts of the brain are also blocked, producing extrapyramidal symptoms of dystonia, parkinsonism, and tardive dyskinesia in some patients, especially when higher doses are required.

The phenothiazines are primarily used as antiemetics for the treatment of mild-to-moderate nausea and vomiting associated with anesthesia and surgery, radiation therapy, and cancer chemotherapy. Prochlorperazine is the phenothiazine most widely used as an antiemetic.

The butyrophenones are also used as antiemetics in surgery and cancer chemotherapy. These agents tend to cause less hypotension than the phenothiazines, but do produce more sedation. The most widely used butyrophenone is haloperidol. Droperidol must be administered parenterally.

Metoclopramide is an antagonist of both dopamine and serotonin receptors. In addition to acting on receptors in the brain, it also acts on similar receptors in the

Table 14-4 *Antiemetic Agents*

GENERIC NAME	BRAND NAME	AVAILABILITY	ANTIEMETIC DOSAGE		COMMENTS
			ADULTS	CHILDREN	
Dopamine antagonists					*Comments for all phenothiazines*
Phenothiazines					
Chlorpromazine	Thorazine, ✦Largactil	Tablets: 10, 25, 50, 100, 200 mg Capsules: 30, 75, 150, 200, 300 mg Syrup: 10 mg/5 ml Concentrate: 30, 100 mg/ml Suppositories: 25, 100 mg Injection: 25 mg/ml	PO: 10-25 mg every 4-6 hr Rectal: 50-100 mg every 6-8 hr IM: 25 mg	PO: 0.25 mg/lb every 4-6 hr Rectal: 0.5 mg/lb every 6-8 hr IM: 0.25 mg/lb every 6-8 hr (Maximum IM dose: up to age 5: 40 mg/day; ages 5-12: 75 mg/day)	Phenothiazines may suppress the cough reflex. Ensure that the patient does not aspirate vomitus. Use with caution in patients, especially children, with undiagnosed vomiting. The phenothiazines can mask signs of toxicity of other drugs, or mask symptoms of other diseases such as brain tumor, Reye Syndrome, or intestinal obstruction. Use with extreme caution in patients with seizure disorders. Discontinue if rashes develop. May cause orthostatic hypotension. See Chapter 9, "Drugs Affecting the Central Nervous System," for a complete list of adverse effects, drug interactions, and nursing interventions.
Perphenazine	Trilafon, ✦Phenazine	Tablets: 2, 4, 8, 16 mg Concentrate: 16 mg/5 ml Injection: 5 mg/ml	PO: 4 mg every 4-6 hr IM: 5 mg	Not recommended	
Prochlorperazine	Compazine, ✦Stemetil	Tablets: 5, 10, 25 mg Capsules: 10, 15, 30 mg Syrup: 5 mg/5 ml Suppositories: 2.5, 5, 25 mg	PO: 5-10 mg every 6-8 hr Rectal: 25 mg 2 times daily IM: 5-10 mg	PO or Rectal: 20-29 lb—2.5 mg 1-2 times daily 30-39 lb—2.5 mg 2-3 times daily 40-85 lb—2.5 mg 3 times daily IM: 0.06 mg/lb	
Thiethylperazine	Torecan	Tablets: 10 mg Suppositories: 10 mg Injection: 5 mg/ml	PO, Rectal, IM: 10-30 mg daily in divided doses	Not recommended	
Triflupromazine	Vesprin	Injection: 10-20 mg/ml	IM: 5-15 mg every 4 hr	IM: 0.2-0.25 mg/kg up to 10 mg/day	

Table 14-4 *Antiemetic Agents—cont'd*

| GENERIC NAME | BRAND NAME | AVAILABILITY | ANTIEMETIC DOSAGE | | COMMENTS |
			ADULTS	CHILDREN	
Dopamine antagonists—cont'd					
Butyrophenones					
Haloperidol (see index)					
Metoclopramide (see index)					
Benzquinamide	Emete-Con	Injection: 50 mg/ vial	IM: 0.5-1 mg/kg; repeat in 1 hr, then every 3-4 hr IV: 25 mg at a rate of 1 ml/min	Not recommended	Recommended for nausea and vomiting associated with anesthesia and surgery. Reconstitute with sterile water. IM route preferred.
Trimethobenza- mide	Tigan	Capsules: 100, 250 mg Suppositories: 100, 200 mg Injection: 100 mg/ml	PO: 250 mg 3-4 times daily Rectal: 200 mg 3-4 times daily IM: 200 mg 3-4 times daily	PO: 30-90 lb; 100-200 mg 3-4 times daily Rectal: <30 lb: 100 mg 3-4 times daily 30-90 lb: 100-200 mg 3-4 times daily	Injectible form contains benzocaine. Do not use in patients allergic to benzocaine or local anesthetics. Inject in upper, outer quadrant of gluteal region. Avoid escape of solution along the route. May cause burning, stinging, pain, on injection.
Serotonin antagonist					
Ondansetron	Zofran	Injection: 2 mg/ml	IV: 3-0.15 mg/kg doses; (1) 30 min before chemotherapy, (2) 4 hours later, (3) 4 more hours later	As for adults	Recommended for prevention of nausea and vomiting associated with cancer chemotherapy.
Anticholinergic agents					
(See Motion Sickness in Index)					
Corticosteroids					
Dexamethasone	Decadron	Tablets: 0.25, 0.5, 0.75, 1, 1.5, 2, 4, 6 mg Elixir: 0.5 mg/5 ml Injection: 4, 10, 20, 24 mg/ml	PO: 4-25 mg every 4-6 hr for 1-2 days IV: as for PO	As for adults	Recommended for prevention of nausea and vomiting associated with chemotherapy.

Continued.

Table 14-4 *Antiemetic Agents—cont'd*

| GENERIC NAME | BRAND NAME | AVAILABILITY | ANTIEMETIC DOSAGE | | COMMENTS |
			ADULTS	CHILDREN	
Benzodiazepines					
Lorazepam	Ativan	Tablets: 0.5, 1, 2 mg Injection: 2, 4 mg/ml	PO: 1-4 mg q 4-6 hr IV: As for PO	Not recommended	Recommended for prevention of nausea and vomiting associated with chemotherapy.
Cannabinoids					
Dronabinol (THC)	Marinol	Capsules: 2.5, 5, 10 mg	PO: Initial 5-10 mg/m^2 1-3 hrs before chemotherapy, then every 2-4 hr for a total of 4-6 doses/day Maximum—15 mg/m^2/dose	Not recommended	Used for patients who have not responded to other antiemetics. Schedule II controlled substance. Common adverse effects include drowsiness, dizziness, muddled thinking, and possible impairment of coordination, sensory, and perceptual functions. Use with caution in hypertension or heart disease.

GI tract, thus making it particularly useful in treating nausea and vomiting associated with GI cancers, gastritis, peptic ulcer, radiation sickness, and migraine. High-dose metoclopramide is now routinely used to treat nausea and vomiting associated with certain cancer chemotherapies. In these higher doses, extrapyramidal symptoms are more common, so many cancer chemotherapy protocols now include both high-dose metoclopramide and routine doses of diphenhydramine when highly emetogenic anticancer agents are used. Metoclopramide appears to be of little value in treating motion sickness.

Serotonin antagonists. The serotonin antagonist, ondansetron, has been shown to actively control nausea and vomiting associated with several emetogenic chemotherapeutic agents. Side effects include mild-to-moderate diarrhea, headache and sedation, and dry mouth. A particular advantage to this agent is that there is no dopaminergic blockade and thus no extrapyramidal adverse effects.

Anticholinergic agents. Anticholinergic agents such as scopolamine and the antihistamines (diphenhydramine, cyclizine, meclizine, and promethazine) are used in the treatment of motion sickness and, in the case of the antihistamines, nausea and vomiting associated with pregnancy. The choice of drug depends on the period for which antinausea protection is required and the side effects. Scopolamine is the drug of choice for short periods of motion, and an antihistamine for longer periods. Of the antihistamines, promethazine is the drug of choice. Higher doses act longer, but usually sedation is a problem. Cyclizine and meclizine have fewer side effects than promethazine but have a shorter duration of action and are less effective for severe conditions. Diphenhydramine has a long duration, but excessive sedation is usually a problem. For very severe conditions, sympathomimetic drugs such as ephedrine are used in combination with scopolamine or antihistamines. Anticholinergic agents are usually not effective in chemotherapy-induced nausea and vomiting.

Corticosteroids. Several studies have shown that dexamethasone and methylprednisolone can be effective antiemetics either as single agents or in combination with other antiemetics. The mechanism of action is unknown. Other actions of the corticosteroids such as mood elevation, increased appetite, and a sense of well-being may also help in patient acceptance and control of emesis. A particular advantage of the steroids, apart from their efficacy, is their relative lack of side effects. Since only a few doses are administered, the usual complications associated with long-term therapy do not arise.

Benzodiazepines. The benzodiazepines (diazepam, lorazepam, and midazolam) are quite effective in reducing not only the frequency of nausea and vomiting but the anxiety often associated with chemotherapy. The benzodiazepines act through a combination of effects, including sedation, reduction in anxiety, possible depression of the vomiting center and an amnesic effect. Of these actions, the amnesic effect appears to be most important as far as treating cancer patients is concerned, and in this respect, lorazepam and midazolam are superior to diazepam. Clinically, the benzodiazepines are most useful in combination with other antiemetics such as metoclopramide, dexamethasone, and ondansetron.

Cannabinoids. Following numerous reports that smoking marijuana reduced nausea, the antiemetic properties of the active ingredients, tetrahydrocannabinol (THC), and synthetic analogs such as nabilone and levonantradol have been studied. The cannabinoids act through several mechanisms to inhibit pathways to the vomiting center. There is no dopaminergic activity. The cannabinoids have been shown to be more effective than placebo and equally as effective as prochlorperazine in patients receiving moderately emetogenic chemotherapy. They are less effective than metoclopramide. Most common adverse effects include dry mouth, sedation, orthostatic hypotension, dizziness, and confusion. Dysphoric effects such as depressed mood, dreaming or fantasizing, distortion of perception, and elated mood are more frequent with moderate to high doses. Younger patients appear to tolerate these side effects better than older patients or patients who have not used marijuana. Because of the mind-altering effects and the potential for abuse, the cannabinoids serve as antiemetics only in patients receiving chemotherapy. The cannabinoids are of more use in those younger patients who are refractory to other antiemetic regiments and in whom combination therapy may be more effective.

Treatment of Selected Causes of Nausea and Vomiting

Nausea and vomiting in pregnancy

The frequency of women reporting vomiting after the first 16 weeks of gestation is relatively constant at about 40%, decreasing to 20% during the 17- to 20-week interval, with only 9% of women complaining of vomiting after 20 weeks of pregnancy. Vomiting is significantly more common among primigravidas, younger women, women with less education, nonsmokers, blacks, and obese women. Contrary to commonly held beliefs, vomiting is not more common among women experiencing prior fetal losses, or among women with hypertension, proteinuria, diabetes, or those who used diethylstilbestrol. There is also no association with vomiting and cohabitation, unplanned pregnancy, or gallbladder, liver, or thyroid disease.

Although traditionally described as "morning sickness," the majority of women report that symptoms of nausea and vomiting tend to persist to varying degrees throughout the day. The cause of morning sickness is unknown, but its occurrence and severity appear to be related to the levels of free and bound estradiol and sex hormone-binding globulin binding capacity.

A woman with severe persistent vomiting that interferes with nutrition, fluid, and electrolyte balance may be suffering from *hyperemesis gravidarum*, a condition in which starvation, dehydration, and acidosis are superimposed on the vomiting syndrome. Hospitalization for fluid, electrolyte, and nutritional therapy may be required.

In most cases, morning sickness can be controlled by dietary measures alone. The woman should be advised to eat small, frequent, dry meals and to avoid fatty foods and other foods found to cause problems. Sometimes it may be very difficult or impossible to work in the kitchen, and assistance in this area may be required.

In about 15% of cases, dietary measures alone will be insufficient and drug therapy should be considered. Drugs that have been extensively used for the treatment of morning sickness are the phenothiazines, such as promethazine and prochlorperazine, and the antihistamines, such as diphenhydramine, dimenhydrinate, meclizine, and cyclizine. From a safety standpoint, meclizine, cyclizine, or dimenhydrinate is generally recommended first. If persistent vomiting threatens maternal nutrition, promethazine may be considered. If antidopaminergic antiemetic therapy is required, prochlorperazine is the most time-tested from a safety standpoint. Metoclopramide has been shown to be an effective antiemetic in treating *hyperemesis gravidarum*, and no teratogenic effects have been reported to date.

Psychogenic vomiting

Psychogenic vomiting can be self-induced or it can occur involuntarily in response to situations that the person considers threatening or distasteful (for example, eating food whose origin is considered repulsive).

When a person presents with chronic or recurrent vomiting, a diagnosis of psychogenic vomiting is made after elimination of all other possible causes. The person with psychogenic vomiting usually does not lose weight and is able to control vomiting in certain situations (for example, in public). The identification of the causes of psychogenic vomiting and the successful resolution of the problem may not be possible. After an extensive workup eliminates other potential causes, a short course of an antiemetic drug such as metoclopramide or antianxiety drugs may be prescribed, along with counseling.

Motion sickness (see index)

Chemotherapy-induced emesis

Chemotherapy-induced emesis (CIE) is the most unpleasant adverse effect associated with the use of cancer chemotherapy. Many patients regard it as the most stressful aspect of their disease, more so even than the prospect of dying. Since the object of therapy is to prolong life for a relatively short period, the effect of CIE on the quality of life must be considered.

Three types of emesis have been identified in patients receiving antineoplastic therapy: (1) anticipatory nausea and vomiting; (2) acute chemotherapy-induced emesis; and (3) delayed emesis.

Anticipatory nausea and vomiting is a conditioned response triggered by the sight or smell of the clinic or hospital or by the knowledge that treatment is imminent. The onset of anticipatory nausea and vomiting is usually 2 to 4 hours before treatment and is most severe at the time of chemotherapy administration. Patients who experience anticipatory nausea and vomiting are more likely to be younger and to have received about twice as many courses of chemotherapy with more drugs for about three times as long as patients who do not experience the complication. Persons with a negative attitude towards therapy, such as the belief that it will be of no benefit, are more likely to develop anticipatory nausea and vomiting. It tends to become more severe as treatments progress unless behavior therapy modifies the conditioned response. Such treatments include progressive muscle relaxation, mind diversion, hypnosis, self-hypnosis, and systematic desensitization. Nurses can play a significant role by maintaining a positive, supportive attitude with the patient and making sure the patient receives antiemetic therapy prior to each course of chemotherapy.

Antiemetic therapy to minimize acute chemotherapy-induced emesis is based upon the emetogenic potential of the antineoplastic agents being used. Combinations of antiemetics are often used, based on the assumption that antineoplastic agents produce emesis by more than one mechanism. In general, all patients being treated with chemotherapeutic agents of moderate to very high emetogenic potential should receive prophylactic antiemetic therapy before chemotherapy is started. Combinations of ondansetron, high-dose metoclopramide, dexamethasone, lorazepam, and/or diphenhydramine are often used. Haloperidol may be substituted for metoclopramide if the latter is not tolerated by the patient. Antiemetic therapy should be continued for 4 to 7 days to prevent delayed vomiting. Emesis induced by moderately emetogenic agents may be treated prophylactically with metoclopramide and dexamethasone, and therapy should be continued for 24 hours. A phenothiazine (prochlorperazine) or dexa-

methasone alone is recommended if the chemotherapy is of low emetic potential. All antiemetics should be administered an adequate time before chemotherapy is initiated and should be continued an appropriate time after the antineoplastic agent has been discontinued.

Delayed emesis occurs 24 to 120 hours after the administration of chemotherapy. The mechanism is not known, but it may be induced by metabolic by-products of the chemotherapeutic agent or by destruction of malignant cells. The emesis experienced is usually less severe than that which occurs acutely, but it can still be of significance in reducing activity, nutrition, and hydration. Events that often trigger delayed nausea and vomiting are brushing teeth, using mouthwash, manipulation of dentures, seeing food, and, in the morning, quickly standing up after getting out of bed. A combination of prochlorperazine, lorazepam, and diphenhydramine given orally 1 hour before meals has been successful in controlling delayed emesis.

• Nursing Interventions: Monitoring antiemetic therapy

See also General Nursing Considerations For Patients With Gastrointestinal Disorders. See also General Nursing Considerations for Patients With Cancer.

The nurse needs to analyze data collected on a continuum and adjust interventions to meet the individual patient's needs.

Administer antiemetic therapy at scheduled times when the agent(s) are prescribed on a specific schedule or at a specified time in relation to the administration of chemotherapy or radiation therapy.

Postoperative nausea and vomiting is usually handled with a p.r.n. order. The first step in treating the nausea and vomiting is to identify the cause. If a nasogastric tube is in place, check its patency and placement. Do not move a nasogastric tube that was inserted during surgery (for example, gastric resection); in such cases there is a danger of penetrating the suture line. Irrigations of a blocked nasogastric tube may alleviate the nausea and vomiting. (A physician's order to irrigate the nasogastric tube is required.) Administration of p.r.n. antiemetics when the patient first complains of nausea will often prevent actual vomiting.

Regardless of the underlying cause, all patients experiencing nausea and vomiting require close monitoring of weight, fluid intake and output, state of hydration, electrolyte status, bowel sounds, and pattern of eating —include foods being eaten and retained, foods that appear to precipitate an attack of nausea and vomiting, or other triggers for the vomiting experience.

After giving the prescribed medication the degree of response and overall effectiveness of the antiemetic therapy should be assessed, recorded, and reported to the members of the health team.

Laxatives

1. State the underlying causes of constipation.
2. Explain the meaning of normal bowel habits.
3. Identify the indications for use, method of action, and onset of action for contact or stimulant laxatives, saline laxatives, lubricant or emollient laxatives, bulk-forming laxatives, and fecal softeners.
4. State the principle involved in giving adequate fluids when bulk-forming laxatives are administered.
5. Describe medical conditions in which laxatives should *not* be used.

Constipation. Constipation is the infrequent, incomplete, or painful elimination of feces. It may result from decreased motility of the colon or from retention of feces in the lower colon or rectum. In either case, the longer the feces remain in the colon, the greater the reabsorption of water and the drier the stool becomes. The stool is then more difficult to expel from the anus. Causes of constipation are (1) improper diet— too little residue, too little fluid, or not enough vitamins; (2) muscular weakness of the colon; (3) sedentary habits; (4) failure to respond to the normal defecation impulses; (5) diseases such as anemia and hypothyroidism; (6) addiction to heroin, morphine, or codeine; (7) tumors of the bowel or pressure on the bowel from tumors; (8) diseases of the rectum.

Occasional constipation is not detrimental to a person's health, although it can cause a feeling of general discomfort or abdominal fullness, anorexia, and anxiety in some persons. Habitual constipation leads to decreased intestinal muscle tone, increased straining at stool as the person bears down in the attempt to pass the hardened stool, and an increased incidence of hemorrhoids. The daily use of laxatives or enemas should be avoided, as these decrease the muscular tone and mucus production of the rectum and may result in water and electrolyte imbalance. They also become habit-forming: the weakened muscle tone adds to the inability to expel the fecal contents, which leads to the continued use of enemas or laxatives.

Drugs have been used for centuries to overcome constipation. Today, many people believe that even occasional failure of the bowel to move daily should be treated with a laxative. Daily bowel movements are frequently not necessary. Many people have "normal" bowel habits even though they have one or two bowel movements per week. As long as the patient's health is good, and the stool is not hardened or impacted, this schedule is acceptable.

Types of laxatives. *Laxatives* are chemicals that act to promote the evacuation of the bowel. They are usually subclassified, based upon the mechanism of action, as follows:

Contact or stimulant laxatives. These agents act directly on the intestine, causing an irritation that promotes peristalsis and evacuation. If given orally, these agents act within 6 to 10 hours. If administered rectally, they act within 60 to 90 minutes. These products should be used only intermittently, because chronic use may cause loss of normal bowel function and dependency on the agent for bowel evacuation.

Saline laxatives. These are hypertonic compounds that attract water into the intestine from surrounding tissues. The accumulated water affects stool consistency and distends the bowel, causing peristalsis. These agents usually act within 1 to 3 hours. Continued use of these products significantly alters electrolyte balance and may cause dehydration.

Polyethylene glycol-electrolyte solution is a relatively new approach to saline laxative therapy. It is a mixture of a nonabsorbable ion-exchange solution and electrolytes that acts as an osmotic agent. When taken orally, it pulls electrolytes and water into the solution in lumen of the bowel and exchanges sodium ions to replace those removed from the body. The net result is a diarrhea that cleanses the bowel for colonoscopy and barium enema x-ray examination with no significant dehydration or loss of electrolytes.

Lubricant or emollient laxatives. These lubricate the intestinal wall and soften the stool, allowing a smooth passage of fecal contents. Onset of action is 6 to 8 hours, but is highly dependent upon the individual patient's normal gastrointestinal transit time. Peristaltic activity does not appear to be increased. If used frequently, these oils may inhibit the absorption of fat-soluble vitamins.

Bulk-producing laxatives. These must be administered with a full glass of water. The laxative causes water to be retained within the stool, increasing bulk that stimulates peristalsis. Onset of action is usually 12 to 24 hours, but may be as long as 72 hours, depending upon the patient's gastrointestinal transit time. Bulk-forming agents are usually considered to be the safest laxative, even when taken routinely. Fresh fruits, vegetables, and cereals such as bran are natural bulk-forming products.

Fecal softeners. These "wetting agents" draw water into the stool, causing it to soften. They do not stimulate peristalsis and may require up to 72 hours to aid in a soft bowel movement. Action from these agents depends upon the patient's state of hydration and the gastrointestinal transit time.

Indications. Laxatives may be indicated as follows: (1) contact or saline laxatives may be used to relieve acute constipation; (2) contact or saline laxatives are used to remove gas and feces before radiologic examination of the kidneys, colon, intestine, or gall bladder; (3) stool softeners are routinely used for prophylactic purposes to prevent constipation or straining at stool (for example, in patients recovering from myocardial infarction or abdominal surgery); (4) bulk-forming laxatives may be used in patients with irritable bowel syndrome to provide a softer consistency to the stools if a high-fiber diet is not adequate; and (5) bulk-forming laxatives are used to control certain types of diarrhea by absorbance of the irritating substance, thus allowing its removal from the bowel during defecation.

Side effects. The most common adverse effects are excessive bowel stimulation resulting in gripping, diarrhea, nausea, vomiting, and rectal irritation. Patients who are severely constipated may develop abdominal cramps.

Obstruction within the gastrointestinal tract may result from a bulk laxative that forms a sticky mass. This is usually due to inadequate mixing with water before ingestion.

Mineral oil may cause lipid pneumonia if inhaled into the lungs. Do not administer to debilitated patients who are constantly in a recumbent position.

Do not administer laxatives to patients with undiagnosed abdominal pain, or patients with inflammation of the gastrointestinal tract such as gastritis, appendicitis, or colitis.

Do not administer when fecal impaction exists or when there is intestinal obstruction, hemorrhage, severe spasm, diarrhea, or intestinal perforation.

Availability. See Table 14-5.
Dosage and administration. See product label.

• Nursing Interventions: Monitoring laxative therapy

See also General Nursing Considerations for Patients with Gastrointestinal Disorders.

Side effects to expect
GRIPPING, MINOR ABDOMINAL DISCOMFORT. The patient should first experience the urge to defecate, then defecate and feel a sense of relief.

Side effects to report
ABDOMINAL TENDERNESS, PAIN, BLEEDING, VOMITING, DIARRHEA, INCREASING ABDOMINAL GIRTH. Failure to defecate or defecation of only a small amount may be an indication of an impaction. These symptoms may indicate an "acute abdomen."

Dosage and administration
PO. Follow directions on the container. Be sure to give adequate water with bulk-forming agents to prevent esophageal, gastric, intestinal, or rectal obstruction.

Drug interactions
DULCOLAX. Do not administer with milk, antacids, cimetidine, famotidine, or ranitidine. These products may allow the enteric coating to dissolve prematurely causing nausea, vomiting, and cramping.

Table 14-5 *Laxatives*

PRODUCT	CONTACT	SALINE	BULK-FORMING	LUBRICANT	FECAL SOFTENER	OTHER
Agoral	Phenolphthalein		Agar, Tragacanth, Acacia, Egg albumin	Mineral oil		
Citrate of Magnesia		Magnesium citrate				
Colace					Docusate sodium	
Colyte						Polyethylene glycol, electrolyte solution
Dialose					Docusate potassium	
Dialose Plus	Casanthranol				Docusate potassium	
Doxidan	Phenolphthalein				Docusate calcium	
Dulcolax	Bisacodyl					
Ex-lax	Phenolphthalein					
GOLYTELY						Polyethylene glycol, electrolyte solution
Haley's MO		Magnesium hydroxide		Mineral oil		
Metamucil			Psyllium hydrophlic mucilloid			
Modane	Phenolphthalein					
Peri-Colace	Casanthranol				Docusate sodium	
Phillips' Milk of Magnesia		Magnesium hydroxide				
Phospho-Soda		Sodium phosphates				
Surfak					Docusate calcium	
X-Prep	Senna concentrate					

PSYLLIUM. Do not administer products containing psyllium (Metamucil, Siblin, others) at the same time as salicylates, nitrofurantoin, or digitalis glycosides. The psyllium may inhibit absorption. Administer these tablets at least 1 hour before or 2 hours after the psyllium.

MINERAL OIL. Daily administration of mineral oil for more than 1 to 2 weeks may cause a deficiency of the fat-soluble vitamins.

DOCUSATE. Docusate enhances the absorption of mineral oil. Concurrent use is not recommended in order to prevent granuloma formation in the liver, lymph nodes, and intestinal lining.

Antidiarrheal agents
OBJECTIVES

1. Cite nine causes of diarrhea.
2. State the differences between locally acting and systemically acting antidiarrheal agents.
3. Identify electrolytes that should be monitored whenever prolonged or severe diarrhea is present.
4. Describe nursing assessments needed to evaluate the patient's state of hydration.
5. Cite conditions that generally will respond favorably to antidiarrheal agents.
6. Review medications studied to date and prepare a list of those that may cause diarrhea.

Diarrhea. *Diarrhea* is an increase in the frequency and/or fluid content of bowel movements. Because normal patterns of defecation and the patient's perception of bowel function vary, a careful history must be obtained to determine the change in a particular patient's bowel elimination pattern. An important fact to remember about diarrhea is that diarrhea is a symptom, rather than a disease. It may be caused by any of the following:

- Intestinal infections. These are most frequently associated with ingestion of food contaminated with bacteria or protozoa (food poisoning), or eating or drinking water that contains bacteria that is foreign to the patient's gastrointestinal tract. People traveling, often to other countries, develop what is known as *traveler's diarrhea* due to ingestion of microorganisms that are pathogenic to their gastrointestinal tracts, but not to those of the local residents.
- Spicy foods may produce diarrhea by irritating the lining of the gastrointestinal tract. Diarrhea occurs particularly when the patient does not routinely eat spicy foods.
- Patients with deficiencies of digestive enzymes such as lactase or amylase have difficulty digesting foods. Diarrhea usually develops due to irritation from undigested food.
- Excessive use of laxatives.
- Drug therapy. Diarrhea is a common side effect caused by the irritation of the gastrointestinal lining by ingested medication. Diarrhea may also result from the use of antibiotics that may kill certain normal bacteria living in the gastrointestinal tract that help digest food.
- Emotional stress. Diarrhea is a common symptom of stress and anxiety.
- Hyperthyroidism induces increased gastrointestinal motility, resulting in diarrhea.
- Inflammatory bowel diseases such as diverticulitis, ulcerative colitis, gastroenteritis, and Crohn's disease cause inflammation of the gastrointestinal lining, resulting in diarrhea.
- Surgical-bypass procedures of the intestine often result in chronic diarrhea because of the decreased absorptive area remaining after surgery. Incompletely digested food and water rapidly pass through the gastrointestinal tract.

Types of antidiarrheal agents. Antidiarrheal agents include a wide variety of drugs, but they can be divided into two broad categories: (1) locally acting agents and (2) systemic agents. Locally acting agents such as activated charcoal, kaolin, pectin, psyllium, and activated attapulgite adsorb excess water to cause a formed stool and to adsorb irritants or bacteria that are causing the diarrhea. The systemic agents act through the autonomic nervous system to reduce peristalsis and motility of the gastrointestinal tract, allowing the mucosal lining to absorb nutrients, water, and electrolytes, leaving a formed stool from the residue remaining in the colon. Representatives of the systemically acting agents are paregoric, diphenoxylate, loperamide, and certain anticholinergic agents (Table 14-6).

Diarrhea may be acute or chronic, mild or severe. Since diarrhea may be a defense mechanism to rid the body of infecting organisms or irritants, it is usually self-limiting. If severe or prolonged, diarrhea may cause dehydration, electrolyte depletion, and exhaustion. Specific antidiarrheal therapy depends on the cause of the diarrhea. Antidiarrheal products are usually indicated when the following conditions prevail:

- The diarrhea is of sudden onset, has lasted more than 2 or 3 days, and is causing significant fluid and water loss. Young children and elderly patients are more susceptible to rapid dehydration and electrolyte imbalance and therefore should start antidiarrheal therapy earlier.
- Patients with inflammatory bowel disease develop diarrhea. Rapid treatment allows the patient to live a more normal lifestyle. Other agents such as adrenocortical steroids or sulfonamides may also be used to control the underlying bowel disease.
- Postgastrointestinal surgery patients develop diarrhea. These patients may require chronic antidiarrheal therapy to allow adequate absorption of fluids and electrolytes.

Table 14-6 *Antidiarrheal Agents*

GENERIC NAME	BRAND NAME	AVAILABILITY	ADULT DOSAGE	COMMENTS
Systemic action				
Diphenoxylate with atropine	Lomotil, Diphenatol, Lofene	Tablets: 2.5 mg diphenoxylate with 0.025 mg atropine Liquid: 2.5 mg diphenoxylate, with 0.025 mg atropine per 5 ml	PO: 5 mg 4 times daily	Inhibits peristalsis Atropine added to minimize potential overdose or abuse May cause drowsiness or dizziness; use caution in performing tasks requiring alertness Do not use in children less than 2 years of age
Loperamide	Imodium	Capsules: 2 mg Liquid: 1 mg/5 ml	PO: 4 mg initially, followed by 2 mg after each unformed movement. Do not exceed 16 mg/day	Inhibits peristalsis Used in acute nonspecific diarrhea and to reduce the volume of discharge from ileostomy
Camphorated tincture of opium	Paregoric	Liquid	PO: 5-10 ml 4 times daily	Inhibits peristalsis and pain of diarrhea 5 ml of liquid = 2 mg morphine
Local action				
Kaolin/pectin	Kapectolin, K-P	Suspension	PO: 60-120 mg after each loose bowel movement	Used as adsorbent
Attapulgite, pectin	Diar-Aid, Kaopectate tablets	Tablets	PO: 2 tablets after each loose bowel movement	Used as adsorbent
Lactobacillus acidophilus	Lactinex, Bacid	Capsules, granules, tablets	PO: 2-4 tablets or capsules, 2-4 times daily, with milk. Granules: 1 packet added to cereal, fruit juice, milk 3-4 times daily	Bacteria used to recolonize the gastrointestinal tract in an attempt to treat chronic diarrhea Do not use in acute diarrhea
Bismuth subsalicylate	Pepto-Bismol	Tablets, suspension	PO: 30 ml or 2 tablets chewed every 30-60 minutes up to 8 doses	Used as adsorbent
Combination action				
Opium, kaolin, pectin	Parepectolin	Suspension	PO: 15-30 ml after each loose bowel movement	Opium inhibits peristalsis and pain of diarrhea; Kaolin and pectin act as adsorbents
Kaolin, pectin, hyoscyamine, atropine, scopolamine	Donnagel, Quiagel	Suspension	PO: Initially, 30 ml, followed by 15 ml every 3 hr	Hyoscyamine, atropine and scopolamine are used to inhibit peristalsis and reduce gastrointestinal secretions Kaolin and pectin act as adsorbents
Kaolin, pectin, codeine, bismuth subsalicylate, carboxymethylcellulose	Kaodene with Codeine	Suspension	PO: Initially, 15 ml, followed by 10 ml every 30 min as needed	Codeine inhibits peristalsis and pain of diarrhea Other ingredients act as adsorbents

• The cause of the diarrhea has been diagnosed and the physician determines that an antidiarrheal product is appropriate for therapy. Since many cases of diarrhea are self-limiting, therapy may not be necessary.

Side effects. The locally acting agents have essentially no adverse effects, but if used excessively, they may cause abdominal distension, nausea, and constipation.

The systemically acting agents are associated with more adverse effects (see Table 14-6). These agents should not be used to treat diarrhea caused by substances toxic to the gastrointestinal tract, such as bacterial contaminants or other irritants. Because these agents act by reducing GI motility, they tend to allow the toxin to remain in the GI tract longer, causing further irritation.

Availability. See Table 14-6.

Dosage and administration. See Table 14-6.

• **Nursing Interventions: Monitoring antidiarrheal therapy**

See General Nursing Considerations for Patients with Gastrointestinal Disorders.

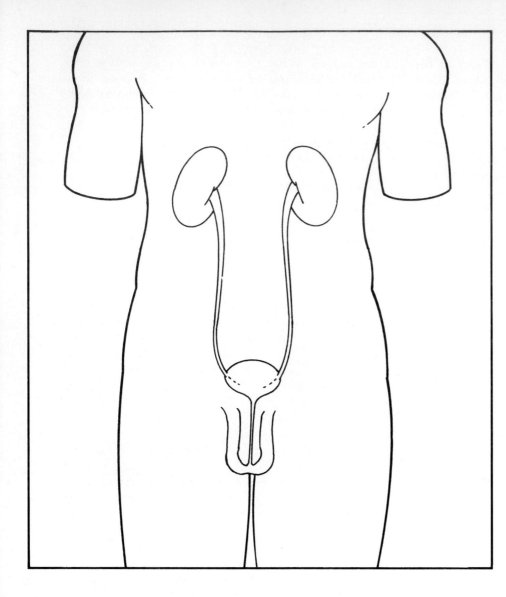

CHAPTER 15

Drugs Affecting the Urinary System

Chapter Goals

After completing this chapter, the student should be able to do the following:

1. Explain the major action and effects of drugs used to treat disorders of the urinary tract.

2. Identify baseline data the nurse should collect on a continuous basis for comparison and evaluation of drug effectiveness.

3. Identify important nursing assessments and interventions associated with the drug therapy and treatment of diseases of the urinary system.

4. Identify essential components involved in planning patient education that will enhance compliance with the treatment regimen.

URINARY SYSTEM DISEASE
OBJECTIVES

1. Cite nursing assessments used to evaluate renal function.
2. Identify specific factors the nurse can assess to evaluate a patient's hydration status.
3. Analyze Table 15-1 and identify specific portions of a urinalysis report that would indicate (1) proteinuria, (2) dehydration, (3) infection, and (4) renal disease.
4. State which electrolytes may be altered by diuretic therapy.
5. Identify the effects of diuretics on blood pressure, on electrolytes, and on diabetic or prediabetic patients.
6. Review the signs and symptoms of electrolyte imbalance and normal laboratory values of potassium, sodium, and chloride.
7. Develop measurable short- and long-term objectives for patient education for patients using loop, thiazide, and potassium-sparing diuretics.

General Nursing Considerations for Patients with Urinary System Disease

The information the nurse assesses relative to the patient's general clinical symptoms is important to the physician when analyzing data for diagnosis. In addition to assessing overall clinical symptoms, the nurse should include the following data for subsequent evaluation of the patient's response to prescribed therapeutic modalities that act upon the urinary system.

Patient Concerns:
Nursing Intervention/Rationale

Alterations in renal function

Pattern of pain. Record the details of any pain the patient describes: frequency, intensity, duration, and location. Pain associated with renal pathology usually occurs at the groin, flank, and suprapubic area and on urination (dysuria).

Pattern of urination. Ask the patient to describe his or her current urination pattern and to cite changes. Such details as frequency, dysuria, incontinence, changes in the stream, hesitancy in starting to void, hematuria, nocturia, and urgency are all of significance.

Intake and output. Intake and output should be recorded accurately every shift and totaled every 24 hours for all patients having renal evaluations or receiving diuretics.

Intake. Measure and record *accurately* all fluids taken (oral, parenteral, rectal, and via tubes). Ice chips and foods such as Jell-O that turn to a liquid state must be included. Irrigation solutions should be carefully measured so that the difference between that instilled and that returned can be recorded as intake.

Remember to enlist the patient, family, and other visitors' help in this process. Ask them to keep a record of how many water glasses, juice glasses, or coffee cups were consumed. You then convert the household measurements to milliliters.

Output. Record all output from the mouth, urethra, rectum, wounds, and tubes (surgical drains, nasogastric tubes, indwelling catheters).

Liquid stools should be recorded according to consistency, color, and quantity.

Urine output should include information on quantity, color, pH, odor, and specific gravity.

All other secretions should be characterized by color, consistency, volume, and changes from previous collections, if possible.

Daily output is usually 1200 to 1500 cc, or 30 to 50 cc per hour. Always report urine output below this hourly rate. Low hourly output may indicate dehydration, renal failure, or cardiac disease.

Keep the urinal or bedpan readily available.

Tell patients and their visitors the importance of not "helping" by dumping the bedpan or urinal, but rather to use the call light and allow the hospital personnel to empty and record all output.

States of hydration

Dehydration. Assess, report, and record significant signs of dehydration in the patient. Observe for poor

Table 15-1 *Urinalysis*

	NORMAL DATA	ABNORMAL DATA
Color	Straw, clear yellow, or amber	Dark smoky color, reddish, or brown may indicate blood. White or cloudy may indicate urinary tract infection or chyluria. Dark yellow to amber may indicate dehydration. Green, deep yellow, or brown may indicate liver or biliary disease. Some drugs may also alter urine color: Pyridium—orange; methylene blue—blue.
Odor	Ammonialike on standing	Foul smell may indicate an infection. The dehydrated patient's urine is concentrated and the ammonia smell is apparent.
Protein	0	Foamy or frothy-appearing urine may indicate protein. Proteinuria is associated with kidney disease and toxemia of pregnancy; it may be present following vigorous exercise.
Glucose	0-trace	Presence is usually associated with diabetes mellitus or low renal threshold with glucose "spillage." Also seen at times of stress, such as major infection, or following a high-carbohydrate meal.
pH	4.6-8.0	Medications can be prescribed to produce an alkaline or acid urine. pH of urine increases if urine is tested after standing four hours or more.
RBC	0-3	Indicative of bleeding at some location in the urinary tract: infection, obstruction, calculi, renal failure, or tumors. (Be sure urine is not contaminated by menses.)
Casts	Rare	May indicate dehydration, possible infection within renal tubules, or other types of renal disease.
WBC	0-4	An increase indicates infection somewhere in the urinary tract.
Specific gravity	1.003-1.030	Used as an indicator of the state of hydration (in absence of renal pathology). Above 1.018 is early sign of dehydration; below 1.010 is "dilute urine" and may indicate fluid accumulation. A fixed specific gravity at around 1.010 may indicate renal disease.
Bacteria	0	May indicate urinary tract infection.

skin turgor, sticky oral mucous membranes, a shrunken or deeply-furrowed tongue, crusted lips, weight loss, deteriorating vital signs, soft or sunken eyeballs, weak pedal pulses, delayed capillary filling, excessive thirst, high urine specific gravity (or no urine output), and possible mental confusion.

SKIN TURGOR. Check skin turgor by *gently* pinching the skin together over the sternum, on the forehead, or on the forearm.

Elasticity is present and the skin rapidly returns to a flat position in the well-hydrated patient. With dehydration, the skin will remain in a "peaked" or "pinched" position and returns very slowly to the flat, normal position.

ORAL MUCOUS MEMBRANES. With adequate hydration, the membranes of the mouth feel smooth and glisten. With dehydration, they appear dull and are sticky.

LABORATORY CHANGES. The values of the hematocrit, hemoglobin, blood urea nitrogen (BUN), and electrolytes will appear to fluctuate, based on the state of hydration. When a patient is overhydrated, the values appear to drop due to "hemodilution." A dehydrated patient will show higher values due to "hemoconcentration."

Overhydration. Increases in abdominal girth, weight gain, neck vein engorgement, and circumference of the medial malleolus are indications of overhydration.

Measure the abdominal girth daily at the umbilical level.

Measure the extremities bilaterally daily at a level approximately 5 cc above the medial malleolus.

Weigh the patient daily using the same scale, at the same time, in similar clothing.

Edema. Edema is a term used to describe excess fluid accumulation in the extracellular spaces. Edema is considered "pitting" when an indentation remains in the tissue after pressure is exerted against a bony part such as the shin, ankle, or sacrum. The degree is usually recorded as 1+ (slight) to 4+ (deep).

Pale, cool, tight, shiny skin is another sign of edema. Also listen to lung sounds to detect the presence of excess fluid.

Electrolyte imbalance. Because the symptoms of most electrolyte imbalances are similar, the nurse should gather data relative to changes in the patient's mental status (alertness, orientation, confusion), muscle strength, muscle cramps, tremors, nausea, and general appearance.

Susceptible persons. Those who are particularly susceptible to the development of electrolyte disturbances frequently have a history of renal or cardiac disease, hormonal disorders, massive trauma or burns, or are on diuretic or steroid therapy.

Serum electrolytes. Monitor serum electrolyte reports; notify physicians of deviations from normal values.

Hypokalemia. Serum potassium (K^+) levels below 3.5 mEq/L.

Hypokalemia is especially likely to occur when a patient exhibits vomiting, diarrhea, or heavy diuresis. All diuretics, except the potassium-sparing type, are likely to cause hypokalemia.

Hyperkalemia. Serum potassium (K^+) levels above 5.5 mEq/L.

Hyperkalemia occurs most commonly when a patient is given excessive amounts of potassium supplementation, either intravenously or orally. It may also occur as an adverse effect of potassium-sparing diuretics.

Hyponatremia. Serum sodium (Na^+) below 135 mEq/L.

Remember the phrase, "Where sodium goes, water goes." Since diuretics act by excreting sodium, monitor your patient for hyponatremia during and after diuresis.

Hypernatremia. Serum sodium (Na^+) above 145 mEq/liter.

Hypernatremia occurs most frequently when a patient is given intravenous fluids in excess of fluid excreted.

Nutrition

Edema. Patients are routinely placed on a restricted sodium diet to help control edema associated with congestive heart failure.

Renal disease. Diet therapy for renal disease is directed at keeping a normal equilibrium of the body while decreasing the excretory load on the kidneys. See a nutrition text for modifications specific to acute and chronic renal failure.

Renal diagnostics. Many laboratory tests are ordered throughout the treatment of renal dysfunction (BUN, serum creatinine, creatinine clearance, urine culture, serum osmolalities, and renal concentration tests).

Urinalysis. The urinalysis is the most basic test the nurse encounters, and an understanding of the significant data this routine test can reveal is imperative to monitoring the patient. Refer to Table 15-1 for a description of the data. See a general medical-surgical text for details of collecting urine samples correctly.

Patient Education Associated with Diuretic Therapy

Communication and responsibility. Encourage open communication concerning frustrations and anger as the patient attempts to adjust to the diagnosis and need for treatment. The patient must be guided to insight into the condition in order to assume responsibility for the continuation of treatment. Keep emphasizing those factors the patient can control to alter the progression of the disease, including maintenance of general health, nutritional needs, adequate rest and appropriate exercise, and continuation of prescribed medication therapy.

Hypertension. If the disease process is hypertension, stress the importance of following prescribed ways to deal with emotions and the dietary and medicinal regimens that can control the disease. (See General Nurs-

ing Considerations for Patients with Hypertension in Chapter 11.)

Nutrition. The physician usually prescribes dietary modifications aimed at weight reduction, if necessary, and sodium restrictions.

Do not suggest salt substitutes without physician approval. See Appendix J for sodium and potassium contents of common salt substitutes.

Patients receiving potassium-sparing diuretics should be taught which foods are high in potassium content. These foods should be moderately restricted but not withheld from the diet.

Expectations of therapy. Discuss expectations of therapy with the patient. This discussion should be individualized to the patient and to the underlying diagnosis for which diuretic therapy is prescribed (such as hypertension or congestive heart failure).

Changes in expectations. Assess changes in expectations as therapy progresses and the patient gains understanding and skill in the management of the diagnosis.

Changes in therapy through cooperative goal setting. Work with the patient to encourage adherence to the prescribed treatment. When the patient feels that a change should be made in a treatment plan, encourage discussion first with the physician.

Written record. Enlist the patient's aid in developing and maintaining a written record of monitoring parameters (Figure 15-1) (such as blood pressure, pulse, daily weights, exercise tolerance, and urine glucose, if appropriate) and response to prescribed therapies for discussion with the physician. Patients should be encouraged to take this record on follow-up visits.

Fostering compliance. Throughout the hospitalization, discuss medication information and how it will benefit the course of treatment. Seek cooperation and understanding of the following points so that medication compliance may be enhanced:

1. Name.
2. Dosage.
3. Route and administration times. Tell patients to take their diuretic in the morning so that the diuresis will not keep them up at night. They can reduce gastric irritation by taking it with food or milk.
4. Anticipated therapeutic response: When administered for edema: diuresis. During initial therapy, the individual can anticipate a 1- to 2-pound daily weight loss. Tell the patient who will be discharged with diuretics to weigh and keep a record of his or her weight at home and to report weight gains or losses of more than 2 pounds per week. When administered for hypertension: a gradual reduction in blood pressure toward mutually set goals.
5. Side effects to expect: Increased frequency and amount of urination; possible orthostatic hypotension, which can be avoided by rising slowly from supine and sitting positions.

Patient Education and Monitoring of Therapeutic Outcomes for Patients Receiving Diuretics or Urinary Antibiotics

Medications	Color	To be taken

Name _____

Physician _____

Physician's phone _____

Next appt.* _____

Parameters		Day of discharge								Comments
Weight										
Blood pressure										
Pulse										
Faintness, dizziness	At rest									
	On exertion									
	No. of occurrences									
Muscle weakness	With exertion									
	When at rest									
Pain pattern and severity Severe Moderate Low 10 5 1										
Description: On urination Without urination Flank area Suprapubic area										
Voiding and frequency	# times voiding per day									
	# times voiding per hour									
Fluid intake	# glasses per day									
	# cups per day									
Urine	Color (check one)	Straw								
		Dark								
		Red								
	Odor: usual or unusual									

*Please bring this record with you to your next appointment.
Use the back of this sheet for additional information.

Figure 15-1 *Patient education and monitoring of therapeutic outcomes for patients receiving diuretics or urinary antibiotics.*

6. Side effects to report: Tell the patient to notify the physician if experiencing changes in muscle strength, tremors, visible edema, nausea, vomiting, diarrhea, excessive thirst, or changes in normal behavior (progressively feeling more exhausted, becoming confused). Since so many electrolyte changes can be involved in diuretic therapy, it is best to use general terms when teaching the lay person.
7. What to do if a dose is missed.
8. When, how, or if to refill the medication.

Difficulty in comprehension. If it is evident that the patient and/or family does not understand all aspects of continuing therapy being prescribed (such as administration and monitoring of medications, exercises, diets, follow-up appointments), consider the use of social service or visiting nurse agencies.

Associated teaching. Give the following instructions:

Always inform the physician or dentist of any prescription or over-the-counter medication being taken. Over-the-counter medications should not be taken without first discussing them with your physician or pharmacist.

Always report side effects of rash, itching, or hives immediately. Nausea, vomiting, or diarrhea should also be reported for the physician's evaluation if it is a new symptom.

Take all of the medication as prescribed for the full course of treatment. Do not discontinue use when feeling improved; do not save for future use; do not give your medicine to another individual. Sudden discontinuation of certain medications may produce harmful effects.

Keep all medications out of the reach of children.

If pregnancy is suspected, consult your obstetrician as soon as possible about continuation of medication therapy.

At discharge. Items to be sent home with the patient should include the following:

1. Written instructions for use
2. Labels in a level of language and size of print appropriate for the patient
3. If needed, identification cards or bracelets
4. A list of additional supplies to be purchased after discharge

Drug Therapy for Urinary System Disorders

Diuretic agents

OBJECTIVES

1. Identify the action of diuretics.
2. Explain the rationale for administering diuretics cautiously to elderly patients, persons with impaired renal function, cirrhosis of the liver, or diabetes mellitus.
3. Describe the goal of administering diuretics to treat hypertension, congestive heart failure, or increased intraocular pressure, or prior to vascular surgery in the brain.
4. List side effects that can be anticipated whenever a diuretic is administered.
5. Cite alterations in diet that may be prescribed concurrently with loop, thiazide, or potassium-sparing diuretic therapy.
6. State the nursing assessments needed to monitor therapeutic response and/or the development of side effects to expect or report from diuretic therapy.

KEY WORDS

tubule	nephron
Loop of Henle	aldosterone

Diuretics are drugs that act to increase the flow of urine. The purpose of diuretics is to increase the net loss of water. To achieve this, they act on the kidneys in different locations to enhance the excretion of sodium. The methylxanthines increase glomerular filtration; spironolactone inhibits tubular reabsorption of sodium by inhibiting aldosterone; and the thiazides, furosemide, bumetanide, and ethacrynic acid act directly on the kidney tubules to inhibit the reabsorption of sodium and chloride from the lumen of the tubule. Sodium and chloride that are not reabsorbed are excreted into the collecting ducts and then into the ureters to the bladder, taking with them large volumes of water to be excreted from the body through urination (Figure 15-2).

Side effects. All diuretics may cause electrolyte abnormalities, including hyponatremia, hypochloremia, hyperkalemia, and hypokalemia.

Diuretics should be administered with particular caution to the elderly and to any patients with impaired renal function, cirrhosis of the liver, or diabetes mellitus. These types of patients are at greater risk for developing hyperkalemia.

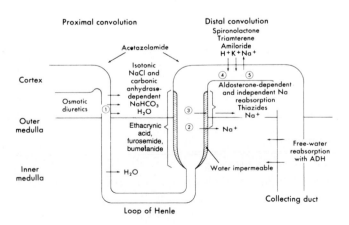

Figure 15-2 *Sites of actions of diuretics.*

Carbonic anhydrase inhibitor

acetazolamide (ah-see-tah-zol'a-myd)

Diamox (dy'ah-moks)

Acetazolamide is a rather weak diuretic that acts by inhibiting the enzyme carbonic anhydrase within the kidney, brain, and eye. As a diuretic, it promotes the excretion of sodium, potassium, water, and bicarbonate. This agent is now infrequently used as a diuretic due to the availability of more effective medications; however, it is used to reduce intraocular pressure in patients with glaucoma and to reduce seizure activity in patients with certain types of epilepsy (see Index).

Methylxanthine

aminophylline (ah-mi-noff'ih-lin)

Aminophylline is a methylxanthine derivative used for its diuretic effects in cardiorenal disease and as a bronchodilator in patients with pulmonary disease. The methylxanthine derivatives include theophylline, caffeine, and theobromine, all of which display weak diuretic properties. All act by improving blood flow to the kidneys.

Aminophylline is now rarely used as a diuretic because of the availability of more effective diuretic agents. However, a diuresis is occasionally noted when aminophylline is used in the treatment of asthma. For discussion of aminophylline as a bronchodilator, see Index.

Loop diuretics
OBJECTIVES

1. Compare the onset and duration of action of bumetanide, ethacrynic acid, and furosemide.
2. Explain scheduling of diuretic therapy.
3. State electrolytes altered by loop diuretic therapy.
4. Recall the signs and symptoms of digitalis toxicity. Discuss the possibility of this occurring when diuretic therapy is administered concurrently with a digitalis glycoside.
5. Identify potential complications of combining diuretics with aminoglycosides (gentamicin, amikacin, tobramycin, kanamycin, netilmicin).

KEY WORDS

asterixis   orthostatic hypotension
hyperuricemia   electrolyte imbalance

bumetanide (bu-met'an'-eyd)

Bumex (bu'mex)

Bumetanide is the newest of the potent diuretics. Its diuretic activity starts within 30 to 60 minutes after administration, and lasts for about 4 hours. It is used to treat edema due to congestive heart failure, cirrhosis of the liver, and renal disease, including nephrotic syndrome.

Side effects. If given in excessive dosages or to patients with massive fluid accumulation, treatment with bumetanide may lead to excessive diuresis and thus to water dehydration and electrolyte imbalance.

The most common side effects are oral and gastric irritation, abdominal pain, upset stomach, and dry mouth. Other generalized side effects include muscle weakness, fatigue, dizziness, dehydration, hives, pruritus, and asterixis.

Availability

PO—0.5, 1, and 2 mg tablets.
IV—0.25 mg/ml in 2 ml ampules.

Dosage and administration

Adult

PO—Initially 0.5 to 2 mg is administered as a single, daily dose. If additional diuresis is required, additional doses may be administered at 4 to 5 hour intervals. Do not exceed a maximum daily dose of 10 mg.
IM or IV—Initially, 0.5 to 1 ml administered over 1 to 2 minutes. Additional doses may be administered at 2 to 3 hour intervals, as necessary. Do not exceed 10 mg per 24 hours.

• Nursing Interventions: Monitoring bumetanide therapy

See also General Nursing Considerations for Patients with Urinary System Disease (p. 355).

Side effects to expect

ORAL IRRITATION, DRY MOUTH. Start regular oral hygiene measures when the therapy is initiated. Suggest the use of 1 teaspoon of hydrogen peroxide in 6 to 8 ounces of water as a mouthwash. Commercial mouthwashes contain alcohol which may cause further drying and oral irritation.

Other measures to alleviate dryness include sucking on ice chips or hard candy.

ORTHOSTATIC HYPOTENSION (DIZZINESS, WEAKNESS, FAINTNESS). Although this effect is infrequent and generally mild, all diuretics may cause some degree of orthostatic hypotension manifested by dizziness and weakness, particularly when therapy is being initiated.

Monitor the blood pressure daily in both the supine and erect positions.

Anticipate the development of postural hypotension and take measures to prevent an occurrence. Teach the patient to rise slowly from a supine or sitting position, and encourage the patient to sit or lie down if feeling faint.

Side effects to report

GASTRIC IRRITATION, ABDOMINAL PAIN. If gastric irritation occurs, administer with food or milk, if symptoms persist or increase in severity, report for physician evaluation.

ELECTROLYTE IMBALANCE, DEHYDRATION. The electrolytes most commonly altered are potassium (K^+), sodium (Na$^+$), and chloride (Cl$^-$). *Hypokalemia* is most likely to occur.

Many symptoms associated with altered fluid and electrolyte balance are subtle and interspersed with general symptoms of drug toxicity or the disease process itself.

Gather data relative to *changes* in the patient's mental status (that is, alertness, orientation, confusion), muscle strength, muscle cramps, tremors, nausea, and general appearance.

Always check the electrolyte reports for early indications of electrolyte imbalance.

Keep accurate records of intake and output, daily weights, and vital signs.

HIVES, PRURITUS, RASH. Report symptoms for further evaluation by the physician.

Pruritus may be relieved by adding baking soda in the bath water.

Implementation

PO. DO NOT administer after midafternoon so the diuresis will not keep the patient awake at night.

Administer with food or milk to reduce gastric irritation.

Drug interactions

ALCOHOL, BARBITURATES, NARCOTICS. Orthostatic hypotension associated with bumetanide therapy may be aggravated by these agents.

DIGITALIS GLYCOSIDES. This diuretic may excrete excess potassium, leading to hypokalemia. If your patient is also receiving a digitalis glycoside, monitor closely for digitalis toxicity (anorexia, nausea, fatigue, blurred or colored vision, bradycardia, arrhythmias).

AMINOGLYCOSIDES (GENTAMICIN, AMIKACIN, NETILMICIN, OTHERS). The potential for ototoxicity from the aminoglycosides is increased. Assess the patient for gradual, often subtle changes in hearing. Note if the patient seems to speak more loudly, asks for statements to be repeated, and turns the TV or radio progressively louder.

INDOMETHACIN. Indomethacin inhibits the diuretic activity of this agent. The dose of bumetanide may need to be increased, or indomethacin discontinued. Maintain accurate I/O records and monitor for a decrease in diuretic activity.

CORTICOSTEROIDS (PREDNISONE, OTHERS). Corticosteroids may enhance the loss of potassium. Check potassium levels and monitor more closely for hypokalemia when these two agents are used concurrently.

PROBENECID. Probenecid inhibits the diuretic activity of bumetanide. In general, do not use concurrently.

ethacrynic acid (eth-ah-krin'ik)

Edecrin (e'deh-krin)

Ethacrynic acid is another diuretic more potent than the thiazides. Its diuretic activity begins in about 30 minutes, and lasts 6 to 8 hours. Ethacrynic acid is used to treat edema due to congestive heart failure, cirrhosis of the liver, renal disease, and malignancy and for hospitalized pediatric patients with congenital heart disease.

Side effects. If given in excessive dosages or to patients with massive fluid accumulation, treatment with ethacrynic acid may lead to excessive diuresis and thus to water dehydration and electrolyte imbalance.

Dizziness, deafness, ringing, and a sense of fullness in the ears may occur in patients with severe impairment of renal function.

Gastrointestinal bleeding has been reported, particularly in patients receiving intravenous dose.

Sudden profuse watery diarrhea has been reported. Discontinue therapy if the diarrhea becomes severe and monitor the patient's electrolytes and state of hydration.

Ethacrynic acid may induce hyperglycemia and aggravate preexisting diabetes mellitus. Dosages of oral hypoglycemic agents and insulin may need adjustment in patients with diabetes mellitus who also require diuretic therapy.

Availability

PO—25 and 50 mg tablets.

IV—50 mg per vial.

Dosage and administration

Adult

PO—50 to 100 mg initially followed by 50 to 200 mg daily.

IV—50 mg or 0.5 to 1 mg/kg. Add 50 ml of dextrose 5% or saline solution to 50 mg of ethacrynic acid. This solution is stable for 24 hours.

• Administer over several minutes through the tubing of a running infusion or by direct IV.

• Occasionally the addition of a diluent may result in an opalescent solution. These solutions should not be used. Do not mix with blood derivatives.

Pediatric

PO—Initially 25 mg daily. Increase the dosage in increments of 25 mg to the desired effects.

IV—1 mg/kg. Dilute with dextrose 5% and administer over 5 minutes through a running infusion.

• **Nursing Interventions: Monitoring ethacrynic acid therapy**

See also General Nursing Considerations for Patients with Urinary System Disease (p. 355).

Side effects to expect

ORTHOSTATIC HYPOTENSION (DIZZINESS, WEAKNESS, FAINTNESS). Although this effect is infrequent and generally mild, all diuretics may cause some degree of orthostatic hypotension manifested by dizziness and weakness, particularly when therapy is being initiated.

Monitor the blood pressure daily in both the supine and erect positions.

Anticipate the development of postural hypotension

and take measures to prevent its occurrence. Teach the patient to rise slowly from a supine or sitting position, and encourage him or her to sit or lie down if feeling faint.

Side effects to report

ELECTROLYTE IMBALANCE, DEHYDRATION. The electrolytes most commonly altered are potassium (K^+), sodium (Na^+), and chloride (Cl^-). *Hypokalemia* is most likely to occur.

Many symptoms associated with electrolyte imbalance are subtle and interspersed with general symptoms of drug toxicity or the disease process itself.

Gather data relative to *changes* in the patient's mental status (that is, alertness, orientation, confusion), muscle strength, muscle cramps, tremors, nausea, and general appearance.

Always check the electrolyte reports for early indications of electrolyte imbalance.

Keep accurate records of intake and output, daily weights, and vital signs.

GASTROINTESTINAL BLEEDING. Observe for "coffee-ground" vomitus or dark tarry stools, particularly in patients receiving intravenous therapy.

DIZZINESS, DEAFNESS, TINNITUS. Persons with impaired renal function may experience these symptoms. Assess the patient for gradual, often subtle changes in balance and hearing. Note if the patient seems more unsteady when standing, speaks loudly, asks for statements to be repeated, and turns the TV or radio progressively louder.

DIARRHEA. Diarrhea may become severe; report to the physician and monitor the patient for dehydration and fluid and electrolyte imbalance.

HYPERGLYCEMIA. Diabetic or prediabetic patients need to be monitored for the development of hyperglycemia, particularly during the early weeks of therapy.

Assess regularly for glycosuria and report if it occurs with any frequency.

Patients receiving oral hypoglycemia agents or insulin may require an adjustment in dosage.

Implementation

PO. DO NOT administer after midafternoon so the diuresis will not keep the patient awake at night.

Administer with food or milk to reduce gastric irritation.

IV. Always monitor vital signs and I/O at regular intervals when administering this agent intravenously. Report blood pressure that decreases steadily or a narrowing pulse pressure, which may indicate hypovolemia.

DO NOT use IV solution if it turns opalescent when the diluent is added.

Follow the manufacturer's recommended procedure for mixing the solution. It is stable for 24 hours.

Drug interactions

AMINOGLYCOSIDES (GENTAMICIN, AMIKACIN, NETILMICIN, TOBRAMYCIN, OTHERS). The potential for ototoxicity

from the aminoglycosides is increased. Assess the patient for gradual, often subtle changes in hearing.

Note if the patient seems to speak loudly, asks for statements to be repeated, or turns the TV or radio progressively louder.

DIGITALIS GLYCOSIDES. This diuretic may cause excess potassium excretion, leading to hypokalemia. If your patient is also receiving a digitalis glycoside, monitor closely for digitalis toxicity (anorexia, nausea, fatigue, blurred or colored vision, bradycardia, arrhythmias).

WARFARIN. Ethacrynic acid may enhance the anticoagulant effects of warfarin. Monitor for the development of petechiae, ecchymosis, bleeding gums, nosebleeds, dark tarry stools.

CORTICOSTEROIDS (PREDNISONE, OTHERS). Corticosteroids may enhance the loss of potassium. Check potassium levels and monitor more closely for hypokalemia when these two agents are used concurrently.

furosemide (fu-ro'se-myd)

Lasix (lay'siks)

Furosemide is one of the most potent and effective diuretics currently available. Maximum effect occurs within 1 hour after oral administration and lasts up to 4 hours. In addition to treating edema caused by congestive heart failure, renal disease, and cirrhosis of the liver, it may also be used for the treatment of hypertension, alone or in combination with other antihypertensive therapy.

Side effects. The most common side effects are oral and gastric irritation, and constipation. Flushing, pruritus, postural hypotension, weakness, dizziness, blurred vision, and dermatitis may also occur.

If given in excessive dosages or to patients with massive fluid accumulation, treatment with furosemide may lead to excessive diuresis with water dehydration and electrolyte imbalance.

Patients who are allergic to sulfonamides may also be allergic to furosemide.

With long-term use, furosemide may inhibit the urinary secretion of uric acid, resulting in hyperuricemia. This may exacerbate an attack of gouty arthritis.

Furosemide may induce hyperglycemia and aggravate cases of preexisting diabetes mellitus. Dosages of oral hypoglycemia agents and insulin may need adjustment in patients with diabetes mellitus who also require diuretic therapy.

Availability
PO—20, 40, and 80 mg tablets; 10 mg/ml oral solution.
IV—10 mg/ml in 2, 4, and 10 ml ampules, vials, and prefilled syringes.

Dosage and administration
Adult
PO—20 to 80 mg as a single dose given preferably in the morning. If a second dose is necessary, administer 6 to 8 hours later.

IV—20 to 40 mg given over 1 to 2 minutes. Much larger doses are frequently administered IV. The rate of administration should not exceed 4 mg per minute.

Pediatric

PO—Initially 2 mg/kg. If the response is not satisfactory, increase by 1 to 2 mg/kg every 6 hours.

IV—Initially 1 mg/kg. If diuresis is not satisfactory, increase by 1 mg/kg every 2 hours to a maximum of 6 mg/kg.

• Nursing Interventions: Monitoring furosemide therapy

See also General Nursing Considerations for Patients with Urinary System Disease (p. 355).

Side effects to expect

ORAL IRRITATION, DRY MOUTH. Start regular oral hygiene measures when therapy is initiated. Suggest the use of 1 teaspoon of hydrogen peroxide in 6 to 8 ounces of water as a mouthwash. Commercial mouthwashes contain alcohol and may cause further drying and oral irritation.

Other measures to alleviate dryness include sucking on ice chips or hard candy.

ORTHOSTATIC HYPOTENSION (DIZZINESS, WEAKNESS, FAINTNESS). Although this effect is infrequent and generally mild, all diuretics may cause some degree of orthostatic hypotension manifested by dizziness and weakness, particularly when therapy is being initiated.

Monitor the blood pressure daily in both the supine and erect positions.

Anticipate the development of postural hypotension and take measures to prevent an occurrence. Teach the patient to rise slowly from a supine or sitting position, and encourage the patient to sit or lie down if feeling faint.

Side effects to report

ELECTROLYTE IMBALANCE, DEHYDRATION. The electrolytes most commonly altered are potassium (K^+), sodium (Na^+), and chloride (Cl^-). *Hypokalemia* is most likely to occur.

Many symptoms associated with altered fluid and electrolyte balance are subtle and interspersed with general symptoms of drug toxicity or the disease process itself.

Gather data relative to *changes* in the patient's mental status (that is, alertness, orientation, confusion), muscle strength, muscle cramps, tremors, nausea, and general appearance.

Always check the electrolyte reports for early indications of electrolyte imbalance.

Keep accurate records of I/O, daily weights, and vital signs.

HIVES, PRURITUS, RASH. Report symptoms for further evaluation by the physician.

Pruritus may be relieved by adding baking soda to the bath water.

HYPERURICEMIA. This diuretic may inhibit the excretion of uric acid, resulting in hyperuricemia. Patients who have had previous attacks of gouty arthritis are particularly susceptible to additional attacks due to hyperuricemia.

Monitor the laboratory reports for early indications of hyperuricemia. Report to the physician, who may then add a uricosuric agent or allopurinol to the patient's medication regimen.

HYPERGLYCEMIA. Diabetic or prediabetic patients need to be monitored for the development of hyperglycemia, particularly during the early weeks of therapy.

Assess regularly for glycosuria and report if it occurs with any frequency.

Patients receiving oral hypoglycemic agents or insulin may require an adjustment in dosage.

Implementation

PO. DO NOT administer after midafternoon so that diuresis will not keep the patient awake at night.

Administer with food or milk to reduce gastric irritation.

IV. Always monitor vital signs and I/O at regular intervals with the IV administration of this agent. Report blood pressure that decreases steadily or a narrowing pulse pressure, which may indicate hypovolemia.

Administer at a rate no greater than 4 mg per minute.

Drug interactions

DIGITALIS GLYCOSIDES. This diuretic may excrete excess potassium, leading to hypokalemia. If your patient is also receiving a digitalis glycoside, monitor closely for digitalis toxicity (anorexia, nausea, fatigue, blurred or colored vision, bradycardia, arrhythmias).

PROPRANOLOL. The action of propranolol may be increased. Monitor for hypotension and bradycardia. Dosage adjustment may be necessary.

THEOPHYLLINE DERIVATIVES. The action of theophylline derivatives may be increased. Assess patients for signs of theophylline toxicity (restlessness, irritability, insomnia, nausea, vomiting, tachycardia, arrhythmias). Serum levels of theophylline may be beneficial in dosage adjustment.

AMINOGLYCOSIDES (GENTAMICIN, AMIKACIN, NETILMICIN, TOBRAMYCIN, OTHERS). The potential for ototoxicity from the aminoglycosides is increased. Assess the patient for gradual, often subtle, changes in balance and hearing. Note if patient seems more unsteady when standing, or speaks loudly, asks for statements to be repeated, or turns the TV or radio progressively louder.

SALICYLATES. The potential for salicylate toxicity may be increased if taken concurrently for several days. Monitor patients for nausea, tinnitus, fever, sweating, dizziness, mental confusion, lethargy, and impaired hearing. Serum levels of salicylates may be beneficial in determining the amounts of salicylate dosage reduction.

INDOMETHACIN. Indomethacin inhibits the diuretic activity of this agent. The dose of furosemide may need to be increased, or indomethacin discontinued. Maintain accurate I/O records and monitor for a decrease in diuretic activity.

METOLAZONE. When used concurrently, there is a considerably greater diuresis than when either agent is used alone. Monitor closely for dehydration and electrolyte imbalance.

PHENYTOIN. Phenytoin may inhibit the absorption of orally administered furosemide. The dosage of furosemide may need to be increased based upon the clinical response of the patient to normal doses.

Thiazides

OBJECTIVES

1. Identify the primary site of action of thiazide diuretics.
2. Describe the effects of thiazides on the gastric mucosa.
3. Identify the effects of thiazide diuretics on the uric acid levels.

KEY WORDS

gouty arthritis	leukopenia
thrombocytopenia	agranulocytosis

The benzothiadiazides, better known as the thiazides, have been an important and useful class of diuretic and antihypertensive agents for the past two decades. As diuretics, thiazides act primarily on the distal tubules of the kidney to block the reabsorption of sodium and chloride ions from the tubule. The unreabsorbed sodium and chloride ions are passed into the collecting ducts, taking molecules of water with them, thus resulting in a diuresis. The thiazides are used as diuretics in the treatment of edema associated with congestive heart failure, renal disease, hepatic disease, pregnancy, obesity, premenstrual syndrome, and administration of adrenocortical steroids. The antihypertensive properties of the thiazides result from a direct vasodilatory action on the peripheral arterioles. (See Index for antihypertensive therapy.)

Side effects. Mild side effects, such as gastrointestinal disorders, dizziness, weakness, fatigue, and rash may occur.

Use of thiazides may cause or aggravate electrolyte imbalance, so patients should be observed regularly for signs such as dry mouth, drowsiness, confusion, muscular weakness, and nausea. Hypokalemia is the most likely of the electrolyte imbalances to occur, and supplementary potassium is often prescribed to prevent or treat hypokalemia.

The thiazides may induce hyperglycemia and aggravate cases of preexisting diabetes mellitus. Dosages of oral hypoglycemic agents and insulin may need adjustment in patients with diabetes mellitus who also require diuretic therapy.

The plasma uric acid is frequently elevated by the thiazides. Patients prone to hyperuricemia and acute attacks of gouty arthritis should also be placed on thiazide therapy with caution.

Patients should be observed for rare occurrences of leukopenia, thrombocytopenia, agranulocytosis, and aplastic anemia.

The thiazide diuretics should be used with caution in pregnant patients, because depression of bone marrow and thrombocytopenia are possible effects on the newborn.

Availability. Tables 15-2 and 15-3 provide a list of thiazide diuretics and those diuretics chemically related to the thiazides. Most of the diuretics listed are administered in divided daily doses for the treatment of hypertension. However, single daily dosages may be most effective for mobilization of edema fluid.

• Nursing Interventions: Monitoring thiazide therapy

See also General Nursing Considerations for Patients with Urinary System Disease (p. 355).

Side effects to expect

ORTHOSTATIC HYPOTENSION (DIZZINESS, WEAKNESS, FAINTNESS). Although this effect is infrequent and generally mild, all diuretics may cause some degree of orthostatic hypotension manifested by dizziness and weakness, particularly when therapy is being initiated.

Monitor the blood pressure daily in both the supine and erect positions.

Anticipate the development of postural hypotension and take measures to prevent an occurrence. Teach the patient to rise slowly from a supine or sitting position, and encourage him or her to sit or lie down if feeling "faint."

Side effects to report

GASTRIC IRRITATION, NAUSEA, VOMITING, CONSTIPATION. If gastric irritation occurs, administer with food or milk. If symptoms persist or increase in severity, report to the physician for evaluation.

ELECTROLYTE IMBALANCE, DEHYDRATION. The electrolytes most commonly altered are potassium (K^+), sodium (Na^+), and chloride (Cl^-). *Hypokalemia* is most likely to occur.

Many symptoms associated with altered fluid and electrolyte balance are subtle and interspersed with general symptoms of drug toxicity or the disease process itself.

Gather data relative to changes in the patient's mental status (that is, alertness, orientation, confusion), muscle strength, muscle cramps, tremors, nausea, and general appearance.

Always check the electrolyte reports for early indications of electrolyte imbalance.

Keep accurate records of I/O, daily weights, and vital signs.

HIVES, PRURITUS, RASH. Report symptoms for further evaluation by the physician.

Table 15-2 *Thiazide Diuretic Products*

THIAZIDE	BRAND NAME	DOSAGE RANGE (MG)	DOSAGE FORMS AVAILABLE
Bendroflumethiazide	Naturetin	2.5-15	Tablets: 5 and 10 mg
Benzthiazide	Exna, Hydrex, Proaqua	50-150	Tablets: 50 mg
Chlorothiazide	Diuril, Diachlor	1,000-2,000	Tablets: 250 and 500 mg Oral suspension: 250 mg/5 ml Injection: 500 mg/20 ml
Cyclothiazide	Anhydron	1-2	Tablets: 2 mg
Hydrochlorothiazide	Esidrix, HydroDiuril, Oretic, Hydromal	25-100	Tablets: 25, 50, and 100 mg
Hydroflumethiazide	Saluron, Diucardin	25-100	Tablets: 50 mg
Methyclothiazide	Enduron, Aquatensen	2.5-5	Tablets: 2.5 and 5 mg
Polythiazide	Renese	1-4	Tablets: 1, 2, and 4 mg
Trichlormethiazide	Naqua, Metahydrin, Aquazide, Diurese	1-4	Tablets: 2 and 4 mg

Table 15-3 *Thiazide-Related Products*

DIURETIC	BRAND NAME	DOSAGE RANGE (MG)	DOSAGE FORMS AVAILABLE
Chlorthalidone	Hygroton	50-200	Tablets: 25, 50, and 100 mg
Indapamide	Lozol	2.5-5	Tablets: 2.5 mg
Metolazone	Zaroxolyn, Diulo, Microx	2.5-10	Tablets: 2.5, 5, and 10 mg
Quinethazone	Hydromox	50-100	Tablets: 50 mg

Pruritus may be relieved by adding baking soda to the bath water.

HYPERURICEMIA. This diuretic may inhibit the excretion of uric acid, resulting in hyperuricemia. Patients who have had previous attacks of gouty arthritis are particularly susceptible to additional attacks due to hyperuricemia.

Monitor the laboratory reports for early indications of hyperuricemia. Report to the physician, who then may add a uricosuric agent or allopurinol to the patient's medication regimen.

HYPERGLYCEMIA. Diabetic or prediabetic patients need to be monitored for the development of hyperglycemia, particularly during the early weeks of therapy.

Assess regularly for glycosuria and report if it occurs with any frequency.

Patients receiving oral hypoglycemic agents or insulin may require an adjustment in dosage.

Implementation

PO. DO NOT administer after midafternoon so that diuresis will not keep the patient awake at night.

Administer with food or milk to reduce gastric irritation.

Drug interactions

DIGITALIS GLYCOSIDES. This diuretic may excrete excess potassium, leading to hypokalemia. If your patient is also receiving a digitalis glycoside, monitor closely for digitalis toxicity (anorexia, nausea, fatigue, blurred or colored vision, bradycardia, arrhythmias).

CORTICOSTEROIDS (PREDNISONE, OTHERS). Corticoster-

oids may enhance the loss of potassium. Check potassium levels and monitor more closely for hypokalemia when these two agents are used concurrently.

LITHIUM. Thiazide diuretics may induce lithium toxicity. Monitor your patients for lithium toxicity manifested by nausea, anorexia, fine tremors, persistent vomiting, profuse diarrhea, hyperreflexia, lethargy, and weakness.

INDOMETHACIN. Indomethacin inhibits the diuretic activity of this agent. The dose of thiazide may need to be increased, or indomethacin discontinued.

Maintain accurate I/O records and monitor for a decrease in diuretic activity.

ORAL HYPOGLYCEMIC AGENTS, INSULIN. Due to the hyperglycemic effects of the thiazide diuretics, dosages of insulin and oral hypoglycemic agents are frequently required.

WARFARIN. Thiazide diuretics may antagonize the anticoagulant activity of warfarin. Monitor the prothrombin activity at regular intervals.

Potassium-sparing diuretics
OBJECTIVES

1. Name three potassium-sparing diuretics.
2. Correlate the effects of potassium-sparing diuretics with the assessments needed to monitor for alteration in potassium levels.
3. Describe the effect of spironolactone and amiloride on sexual function.

KEY WORDS
gynecomastia   aldosterone

amiloride (am-il-or′eyd)

Midamor (my-da′mor)

Amiloride is a relatively new potassium-sparing diuretic that also has weak antihypertensive activity. Its mechanism of action is unknown, but it acts at the distal renal tubule to retain potassium and excrete sodium, resulting in a mild diuresis. Amiloride is usually used in combination with other diuretics in patients with hypertension or congestive heart failure to help prevent hypokalemia that may result from other diuretics.

Side effects. Side effects are usually quite mild and include anorexia, nausea, abdominal pain, flatulence, headache, and skin rash. Other side effects infrequently reported include muscle cramps, dizziness, constipation, fatigability, and impotence.

Availability
PO—5 mg.

Dosage and administration
Adult
PO—Initially 5 mg daily. Dosages may be increased in 5 mg increments up to 20 mg daily with close monitoring of electrolytes.

Administer with food.

• Nursing Interventions: Monitoring amiloride therapy

See also General Nursing Considerations for Patients with Urinary System Disease (p. 355).

Side effects to expect
ANOREXIA, NAUSEA, VOMITING, FLATULENCE. These side effects should be mild, particularly if the dose is administered with food. Persistent nausea and vomiting need to be evaluated for other causes, as well as for the development of electrolyte imbalance.

HEADACHE. Monitor the blood pressure at regularly scheduled intervals, since this agent is used for hypertension. Additional readings should be taken during headaches to determine if headaches are caused by the agents or by the hypertension.

Report persistence of headaches.

Side effects to report
ELECTROLYTE IMBALANCE, DEHYDRATION. The electrolytes most commonly altered are potassium (K^+), sodium (Na^+), and chloride (Cl^-). *Hyperkalemia* is most likely to occur. Report potassium levels above 5 mEq/liter.

Many symptoms associated with altered fluid and electrolyte balance are subtle and interspersed with general symptoms of drug toxicity or the disease process itself.

Gather data relative to *changes* in the patient's mental status (that is, alertness, orientation, confusion), muscle strength, muscle cramps, tremors, nausea, and general appearance.

Always check the electrolyte reports for early indications of electrolyte imbalance.

Keep accurate records of I/O, daily weights, and vital signs.

Implementation
PO. DO NOT administer after midafternoon so that diuresis will not keep the patient awake at night.

Administer with food or milk to reduce gastric irritation.

Drug interactions
LITHIUM. Amiloride may induce lithium toxicity. Monitor your patients for lithium toxicity manifested by nausea, anorexia, fine tremors, persistent vomiting, profuse diarrhea, hyperreflexia, lethargy, and weakness.

POTASSIUM SUPPLEMENTS, SALT SUBSTITUTES. Amiloride inhibits potassium excretion. DO NOT administer with potassium supplements or use salt substitutes high in potassium because of the potentially dangerous effects of hyperkalemia.

spironolactone (spy-ro-no-lak′tone)

Aldactone (al-dak′tone)

Spironolactone is a diuretic that is particularly useful in relieving edema and ascites that do not respond to the usual diuretics. It blocks the sodium-retaining and potassium-excreting properties of aldosterone, resulting in a loss of water with the increased sodium excretion. This drug may be given with thiazide diuretics to increase the effect of spironolactone and reduce the hypokalemia often induced by the thiazides.

Side effects. Side effects are usually quite mild with spironolactone therapy but include drowsiness, lethargy, headache, cramping and diarrhea, and mental confusion.

Since the chemical structure of spironolactone is similar to that of certain hormones, an occasional male patient will report gynecomastia, reduced libido, and diminished erection, and females may complain of breast soreness and menstrual irregularities. These effects are quite reversible upon discontinuation of therapy.

Availability
PO—25, 50, and 100 mg tablets.

Dosage and administration
Adult
PO—Initially 50 to 100 mg daily. Maintenance dosage is usually 100 to 200 mg daily, but doses up to 400 mg may be prescribed.

Pediatric
PO—3.3 mg/kg/day. Readjust the dosage every 3 to 5 days.

• Nursing Interventions: Monitoring spironolactone therapy

See also General Nursing Considerations for Patients with Urinary System Disease (p. 355).

Side effects to expect and report

MENTAL CONFUSION. Perform a baseline assessment of the patient's alertness, drowsiness, lethargy, and orientation to time, date, and place before initiating drug therapy. Compare subsequent mental status and analyze on a regular basis.

HEADACHE. Monitor the blood pressure at regularly scheduled intervals since this agent is used for hypertension. Additional readings should be taken during headaches to determine if headaches are caused by the agent or the hypertension. Report persistence of headaches.

DIARRHEA. The onset of new symptoms since initiation of the drug therapy requires evaluation if persistent.

ELECTROLYTE IMBALANCE, DEHYDRATION. The electrolytes most commonly altered are potassium (K^+), sodium (Na^+), and chloride (Cl^-). *Hyperkalemia* is most likely to occur. Report potassium levels above 5 mEq/liter.

Many symptoms associated with altered fluid and electrolyte balance are subtle and interspersed with general symptoms of drug toxicity or the disease process itself.

Gather data relative to *changes* in the patient's mental status (that is, alertness, orientation, confusion), muscle strength, muscle cramps, tremors, nausea, and general appearance.

Always check the electrolyte reports for early indications of electrolyte imbalance.

Keep accurate records of intake and output, daily weights and vital signs.

Dosage and administration

PO. DO NOT administer after midafternoon so that diuresis will not keep the patient awake at night.

Administer with food or milk to reduce gastric irritation.

Drug interactions

POTASSIUM SUPPLEMENTS, SALT SUBSTITUTES. Spironolactone inhibits potassium excretion. DO NOT administer with potassium supplements or use salt substitutes high in potassium because of potentially dangerous effects from hyperkalemia.

triamterene (try-am′ter-een)

Dyrenium (dy-reen′ee-um)

Triamterene is a very mild diuretic that acts by blocking the exchange of potassium for sodium in the distal tubule of the kidney. Potassium is retained, making it an effective agent to use in conjunction with the potassium-excreting diuretics such as the thiazides and furosemide.

Side effects. Side effects of triamterene are generally quite mild. Those reported include dry mouth, leg cramps, photosensitivity, rash, nausea, vomiting, diarrhea, and weakness.

Availability

PO—50 and 100 mg capsules.

Dosage and administration

Adult

PO—50 to 150 mg 2 times daily.

• Nursing Interventions: Monitoring triamterene therapy

See also General Nursing Considerations for Patients with Urinary System Disease (p. 355).

Side effects to expect and report

ELECTROLYTE IMBALANCE, DEHYDRATION, LEG CRAMPS, NAUSEA, VOMITING, WEAKNESS. The electrolytes most commonly altered are potassium (K^+), sodium (Na^+), and chloride (Cl^-). *Hyperkalemia* is most likely to occur. Report potassium levels above 5 mEq/liter.

Many symptoms associated with altered fluid and electrolyte balance are subtle and interspersed with general symptoms of drug toxicity or the disease process itself.

Gather data relative to *changes* in the patient's mental status (that is, alertness, orientation, confusion), muscle strength, muscle cramps, tremors, nausea, and general appearance (drowsy, anxious, lethargic).

Always check the electrolyte reports for early indications of electrolyte imbalance.

Keep accurate records of I/O, daily weights, and vital signs.

HIVES, PRURITUS, RASH. Report symptoms for further evaluation by the physician.

Pruritus may be relieved by adding baking soda to the bath water.

Drug interactions. Triamterene inhibits potassium excretion. DO NOT administer with potassium supplements or use salt substitutes high in potassium because of the potentially dangerous effects from hyperkalemia.

Combination diuretic products

A common problem associated with thiazide diuretic therapy is hypokalemia. In an attempt to minimize this adverse effect, several products have been manufactured that contain a potassium-sparing diuretic with a thiazide diuretic (see Table 15-4). The goal of the combination products is to promote diuresis and antihypertensive effect through different mechanisms of action while maintaining normal serum potassium levels. Patients receiving a combination product are at risk for side effects resulting from any of the component drugs. Many cases of *hyperkalemia* and hyponatremia have been reported following the use of the combination products.

Combination products should not be used as initial therapy for edema or hypertension. Therapy with individual products should be adjusted for each patient. If the fixed combination represents the appropriate dosage for each component, then the use of a combination product may be more convenient for patient compliance. Patients must be reevaluated periodically for ap-

Table 15-4 *Combination Diuretic Products*

DIURETICS	BRAND NAME	DOSAGE RANGE
Spironolactone 25 mg, Hydrochlorothiazide 25 mg	Aldactazide, Spirozide, Spironazide	1 to 8 tablets daily
Spironolactone 50 mg, Hydrochlorothiazide 50 mg	Aldactazide	1 to 4 tablets daily
Triamterene 50 mg, Hydrochlorothiazide 25 mg	Dyazide	1 to 2 capsules twice daily, after meals
Triamterene 75 mg, Hydrochlorothiazide 50 mg	Maxzide	1 tablet daily
Amiloride 5 mg, Hydrochlorothiazide 50 mg	Moduretic	1 to 2 tablets daily with meals

propriateness of therapy and to prevent electrolyte imbalance.

Drugs that act on the bladder

OBJECTIVE

1. State the effects of oxybutynin chloride and bethanechol chloride on the bladder and bladder function.

KEY WORDS

antispasmodic agent   neurogenic bladder

oxybutynin chloride (ok-se-bu′ti-nin)

Ditropan (di′trow-pan)

Oxybutynin chloride is an antispasmodic agent that acts directly on the smooth muscle of the bladder to reduce the frequency of bladder contractions and delay the initial desire to void in patients with neurogenic bladder.

Oxybutynin should not be used in patients with glaucoma, myasthenia gravis, bowel disease such as ulcerative colitis, or obstructive uropathy such as prostatitis.

Side effects. Side effects are usually dose-related and respond to a reduction in dosage. Routine side effects are dry mouth, decreased sweating, urinary hesitance and retention, blurred vision, tachycardia, palpitations, dilation of the pupil, cycloplegia, drowsiness, insomnia, nausea, vomiting, constipation, and a bloated feeling. Allergic reactions have also been reported.

Availability

PO—5 mg tablets; 5 mg/5 ml syrup.

Dosage and administration

Adult

PO—5 mg 2 or 3 times daily. Maximum dose is 20 mg daily.

Pediatric (over 5 years of age)

PO—5 mg twice daily. Maximum dose is 15 mg daily.

• **Nursing Interventions: Monitoring oxybutynin therapy**

See also General Nursing Considerations for Patients with Urinary System Disease (p. 355).

Side effects to expect

DRY MOUTH, URINARY HESITANCE, RETENTION. These side effects are usually dose-related and respond to a reduction in dose.

Relieve dry mouth by sucking on ice chips or hard candy or by chewing gum.

CONSTIPATION, BLOATING. Encourage balanced nutrition and inclusion of fresh fruits and vegetables, for roughage, and an adequate fluid intake to help alleviate this complication. If this approach is unsuccessful, suggest a stool softener or bulk-forming supplement. Avoid laxatives.

BLURRED VISION. Caution patients not to drive or operate power equipment until they have adjusted to this side effect.

Side effects to report

ABOVE SYMPTOMS. If any of the above symptoms intensifies, it should be reported to the physician for evaluation.

Drug interactions. No clinically significant interactions have been reported.

bethanechol chloride (be-tha′ne-kol)

Urecholine (u-re-ko′leen)

Bethanechol is a parasympathetic nerve stimulant that causes contraction of the detrusor urinae muscle in the bladder, usually resulting in urination. It also may stimulate gastric motility, increase gastric tone, and restore impaired rhythmic peristalsis. Bethanechol is used in nonobstructive urinary retention, particularly in postoperative and postpartum patients.

Side effects. Side effects are infrequent, but are usually extensions of the pharmacologic activity of parasympathetic stimulants. These include flushing of the skin, sweating, nausea, vomiting, headache, colicky pain, abdominal cramps, diarrhea, belching, and involuntary defecation.

Availability

PO—5, 10, 25, and 50 mg tablets.

SC—5 mg/ml in 1 ml vials.

Dosage and administration

Adult

PO—10 to 50 mg 2 to 4 times daily. The maximum daily dose is 120 mg.

SC—2.5 to 5 mg.

NOTE: If overdosage occurs, the pharmacologic actions of the drug can immediately be abolished by atropine.

• Nursing Interventions: Monitoring bethanechol therapy

See also General Nursing Considerations for Patients with Urinary System Disease (p. 355).

Side effects to expect

FLUSHING OF SKIN, HEADACHE. A pharmacologic property of the drug results in dilated blood vessels.

Side effects to report

NAUSEA, VOMITING, SWEATING, COLICKY PAIN, ABDOMINAL CRAMPS, DIARRHEA, BELCHING, INVOLUNTARY DEFECATION. These effects are caused by a pharmacologic property of the drug. Consult the physician; a dosage adjustment may control these adverse effects.

Support the patient with diarrhea or involuntary defecation.

Implementation

SC. Have atropine sulfate available to counteract serious adverse effects.

Drug interactions

QUINIDINE, PROCAINAMIDE. Do not use concurrently with bethanechol. The pharmacologic properties of these agents counteract those of bethanechol.

Urinary analgesic
OBJECTIVES

1. Identify the onset of action and purposes of administering a urinary analgesic.
2. State the effect of phenazopyridine on urine color.

phenazopyridine hydrochloride (fen-ay-zo-peer′i-deen)

Pyridium (py-rid′ee-um)

Phenazopyridine is an agent that, as it is excreted through the urinary tract, produces a local anesthetic effect on the mucosa of the ureters and bladder. It acts within about 30 minutes after oral administration and relieves burning, pain, urgency, and frequency associated with urinary tract infections. It also lessens bladder spasm, thus relieving the resulting urinary retention.

Phenazopyridine is also used for preoperative and postoperative surface analgesia in urologic surgical procedures and after diagnostic tests in which instrumentation was necessary. It is occasionally used to relieve the discomfort caused by the presence of an indwelling catheter.

Side effects. Phenazopyridine produces a reddish-orange discoloration of the urine.

A yellowish tinge to the sclera or the skin may indicate accumulation caused by reduced renal function. The drug should be discontinued if this manifestation results.

Phenazopyridine is frequently used in combination with sulfonamides (Azo-Gantanol and Azo-Gantrisin).

The same side effects apply, as well as those of the sulfonamides (see Index).

Availability

PO—100 and 200 mg tablets.

Dosage and administration

Adult

PO—200 mg 3 times daily.

Pediatric (6 to 12 years of age)

PO—100 mg 3 times daily.

• Nursing Interventions: Monitoring phenazopyridine therapy

See General Nursing Considerations for Patients with Urinary System Disease (p. 355).

Side effects to expect

REDDISH-ORANGE URINE DISCOLORATION. Be certain the patient understands that the color of the urine will become reddish-orange when this drug is used. There is no need for alarm.

Side effects to report

YELLOW SCLERA OR SKIN. The patient should report any yellowish tinge developing in the sclera (white portion) of the eye.

Drug interactions

URINE COLORIMETRIC PROCEDURES. This medication will interfere with colorimetric diagnostic tests performed on urine. Consult your hospital laboratory for alternative measures.

URINARY TRACT INFECTIONS
OBJECTIVES

1. Identify which tissues are infected in a pyelonephritis, cystitis, prostatitis, and urethritis.
2. Name the most common pathogens that cause urinary tract infections.
3. Describe factors to be considered in the selection of an antimicrobial agent to treat urinary tract infections.
4. State the rationale for maintaining an increased intake of fluid when a urinary tract infection is present.
5. Explain patient education necessary to prevent urinary tract infections.
6. Cite the signs and symptoms of a urinary tract infection.
7. Describe appropriate interventions for perineal irritation.
8. State methods used to maintain urine acidity.
9. Compare the effectiveness of methenamine mandelate in the treatment of initial as opposed to recurrent urinary tract infections.
10. Explain the action of methenamine mandelate and conditions necessary for maximum effectiveness.
11. Prepare a chart of antimicrobial agents used to treat urinary tract infections and give the drug names, the organisms treated, and special consider-

ations (such as the need for acidic urine, changes in urine color, effect on urine tests).

KEY WORDS

acidification   catheterization
prostatitis   urethritis
pyelonephritis   cystitis

Urinary tract infections are one of the most common infectious diseases in humans, second only to upper respiratory tract infection as a cause of morbidity from infection. Urinary tract infections actually encompass several different types of infection of local tissue: pyelonephritis (the kidney), cystitis (the bladder), prostatitis (the prostate gland), and urethritis (the urethra).

The incidence of urinary tract infections is about 10 times higher in women than men. The incidence increases in women with age, so that by 60 years of age, up to 20% of women will have suffered from at least one urinary tract infection in their lives.

Most urinary tract infections are caused by gram-negative aerobic bacilli from the gastrointestinal tract. *E. coli* accounts for about 80% of noninstitutionally-acquired uncomplicated urinary tract infections. Other common infecting organisms are *Klebsiella, Enterobacter, Proteus mirabilis* and *Pseudomonas aeruginosa.* Hospital-acquired urinary tract infections and those associated with urinary tract pathological abnormalities are considered to be complicated urinary tract infections. The pathogens tend to be the same types of bacteria, but they are frequently more resistant to the antibiotics commonly used. This requires the use of more potent antibiotics for longer courses of therapy, placing the patient at a greater risk for complications secondary to drug therapy.

The use of an indwelling urinary catheter should be avoided, if possible. When used, adherence to strict aseptic technique and attachment to a closed drainage system is necessary to reduce the rate of infection.

General Nursing Considerations for Patients with Urinary Tract Infections

See also General Nursing Considerations for Patients with Urinary System Disease (p. 355) and Patients with Infectious Disease (p. 457).

Patient Education Associated with Urinary Antimicrobial Therapy

Communication and responsibility. Encourage open communication concerning frustrations and anger as the patient attempts to adjust to the diagnosis and need for treatment.

The patient must be guided to insight into the condition in order to assume responsibility for the continu-

ation of treatment. Keep emphasizing those factors the patient can control to alter the progression of the disease, including maintenance of general health, nutritional needs, adequate rest and appropriate exercise, and continuation of prescribed medication therapy.

Prevention. Emphasize that permanent kidney damage and renal failure is a consequence of repeated urinary tract infections. *Prevention* is the key to avoiding this complication.

Adequate I/O, personal hygiene, completing all medications, and negative follow-up cultures are equally important.

Teach the female patient the following factors that may aid in preventing reinfection:

- Avoid nylon underwear (use cotton) and very tight, constricting clothing in the perineal area.
- Avoid frequent use of bubble bath.
- Avoid colored toilet paper, because the dye may cause irritations.
- Wash the perineal area immediately before and after sexual intercourse.
- Urinate immediately after intercourse.

Fluid intake. All patients with urinary tract infections or calculi, or those patients undergoing urologic procedures, need increased intake of fluids, especially water. Unless co-existing medical problems prohibit, have patients drink a minimum of eight 8-ounce glasses daily.

Perineal irritation. If the patient complains of irritation or itching of the perineal area, request an order for protective or anesthetic ointments. Also consider the possibility of a secondary yeast infection, especially if the patient is taking antibiotics.

Expectations of therapy. Discuss expectations of therapy with the patient:

Pain and discomfort are usually relieved within 30 minutes after the administration of a urinary analgesic.

The symptoms of burning, frequency, urgency, and even incontinence improve steadily after antimicrobial therapy is initiated. Stress previously cited hygiene measures to prevent recurrence.

Changes in expectations. Assess changes in expectations as therapy progresses and the patient gains understanding and skill in the management of the diagnosis. Recurrence of symptoms should be reported immediately.

Changes in therapy through cooperative goal setting. Work with the patient to encourage adherence to the prescribed treatment. When the patient feels that a change should be made in a treatment plan, encourage a discussion first with the physician.

Written record. Enlist the patient's aid in developing and maintaining a written record (Figure 15-1) of the monitoring parameters (such as burning, frequency or urgency of voiding, daily fluid intake, and temperature, if present) and response to prescribed therapies for discussion with the physician. Patients should be encouraged to take this record with them on follow-up visits.

Fostering compliance. Discuss medication information and how it will benefit the patient's course of treatment. Seek cooperation and understanding of the following points, so that medication compliance may be enhanced:

1. Name
2. Dosage
3. Route and administration times
4. Anticipated therapeutic response
5. Side effects to expect
6. Side effects to report
7. What to do if a dose is missed
8. When, how, or if to refill the medication prescription

Difficulty in comprehension. If it is evident that the patient and/or family does not understand all aspects of continuing therapy being prescribed (such as administration and monitoring of medications, need for increased fluid intake, follow-up appointments), consider the use of social service or visiting nurse agencies.

Associated teaching. Give patients the following instructions:

Always inform the physician or dentist of any prescription or over-the-counter medication being taken. Over-the-counter medications should not be taken without first discussing them with your physician or pharmacist.

Always report side effects of rash, itching, or hives immediately. Nausea, vomiting, or diarrhea should also be reported for the physician's evaluation if it is a new symptom.

Take all of the medication as prescribed for the full course of treatment. Do not discontinue use when feeling improved; do not save for future use; do not give your medicine to another individual. Sudden discontinuation of certain medications may produce harmful effects.

Emphasize the importance of antibiotic therapy being continued until urine samples at follow-up visits have been negative for organisms.

Keep all medications out of the reach of children.

If pregnancy is suspected, consult an obstetrician as soon as possible about continuation of medication therapy.

At discharge. Items to be sent home with the patient should include the following:

1. Written instructions for use
2. Labels in a level of language and size of print appropriate for the patient
3. If needed, identification cards or bracelets
4. List of additional supplies to be purchased after discharge
5. A schedule of follow-up appointments

Drug Therapy for Urinary Tract Infections

Urinary antimicrobial agents

Urinary antimicrobial agents are substances that are excreted and concentrated in the urine in sufficient amounts to have an antiseptic effect on the urine and the urinary tract. Selection of the product to be used is based upon identification of the pathogens by the Gram stain or by urine culture in severe, recurrent, or chronic infections. Fluid intake should be encouraged so that there will be at least 2000 ml of urinary output daily. Treatment should be continued for at least a week after symptoms have subsided or the results of cultures have been negative.

Cinoxacin, methenamine mandelate, nitrofurantoin, and nalidixic acid are used only for urinary tract infections. Other antibiotics that are also used to treat urinary infections are ampicillin, sulfisoxazole, co-trimoxazole, sulfamethazole, norfloxacin, gentamicin, and carbenicillin. These agents are effective in a variety of tissue infections against many different microorganisms. Because of their use in multiple organ systems, they are discussed in detail (with nursing interventions) in Chapter 19, "Antimicrobial Agents."

cinoxacin (sin-ox'ah-sin)

Cinobac (sin-oh'bak)

Cinoxacin is an organic acid that is chemically related to nalidixic acid. Cinoxacin is effective in treating initial and recurrent urinary tract infections caused by *E. coli, Proteus mirabilis,* and other gram-negative microorganisms. It is not effective against *Pseudomonas* species, common pathogens in chronic urinary tract infections. Clinical studies indicate that cinoxacin may have milder side effects than nalidixic acid.

Side effects. About 10% of patients will suffer reversible adverse effects from cinoxacin therapy. Most frequent are nausea (3%), vomiting, anorexia, diarrhea, and abdominal cramps (1%). Up to 3% of patients develop rash, perineal burning, urticaria, pruritus, or hives. Less than 2% of patients report headache and dizziness, and less than 1% report insomnia, photophobia, tingling sensations, and tinnitus.

Although it has not been reported, structural similarities with nalidixic acid indicate that hemolysis may occur in patients with glucose-6-phosphate dehydrogenase deficiency. Cinoxacin should be used with caution in these patients.

Although it has not been reported, structural similarities with nalidixic acid indicate that cinoxacin may produce false positive results with Clinitest. Clinistix or Tes-Tape may be used instead.

Availability

PO—250 and 500 mg capsules.

Dosage and administration

Adult

PO—1 g daily in 2 to 4 divided doses for 7 to 14 days.

Pediatric

Not recommended for children under 12 years of age.

• **Nursing Interventions: Monitoring cinoxacin therapy**

See also General Nursing Considerations for Patients with Urinary Tract Infections (p. 355) and Patients with Infectious Disease (p. 457).

Side effects to expect

NAUSEA, VOMITING, ANOREXIA, ABDOMINAL CRAMPS. These side effects are usually mild and tend to resolve with continued therapy. Encourage the patient not to discontinue therapy without first consulting his or her physician.

Side effects to report

PERINEAL BURNING, URTICARIA, PRURITUS, HIVES. Burning with urination may be produced by the infection itself.

Notify the physician if any of these symptoms develop. Symptomatic relief may be obtained by the use of cornstarch or bicarbonate of soda to the bath water. The use of antihistamines or topical steroids is rarely required.

HEADACHE, TINNITUS, DIZZINESS, TINGLING SENSATIONS, PHOTOPHOBIA. Report these symptoms for further evaluation.

Implementation

PO. Schedule medication administration to coincide with mealtime if gastrointestinal symptoms develop.

Drug interactions

PROBENECID. Probenecid may reduce urinary excretion of cinoxacin, thereby producing inadequate antimicrobial therapy and the possibility of developing resistant strains of microorganisms.

CLINITEST. This drug may produce false-positive Clinitest results. Use Clinistix or Tes-Tape to measure urine glucose.

methenamine mandelate (me-the′na-min man-del′ate)

Mandelamine (man-del′-ah-min)

Methenamine mandelate combines the action of methenamine and mandelic acid. Methenamine yields formaldehyde in the presence of an acidic urine. The formaldehyde released helps suppress the growth and multiplication of bacteria that may cause recurrent infection. Mandelic acid is present to help maintain the acidic urine. Ascorbic acid (vitamin C) is also frequently prescribed to help maintain the acidity of the urine.

Methenamine mandelate is used only in patients susceptible to chronic, recurrent urinary tract infections. It is not potent enough to be effective in patients suffering from a preexisting infection. The infection should be treated with antibiotics until the urine is sterile; then methenamine is started to help prevent recurrence of the infection.

Side effects. Side effects are rare, but when they do occur, the most common are nausea, vomiting, belching, skin rash, and pruritus.

Availability

PO—0.5 and 1 g enteric-coated tablets; 0.25 and 0.5 g/5 ml suspension; 1 g packets of granules.

Dosage and administration

Adult

PO—1 g 4 times daily after meals and at bedtime.

• **Nursing Interventions: Monitoring methenamine therapy**

See also General Nursing Considerations for Patients with Urinary Tract Infections (p. 355) and Patients with Infectious Disease (p. 457).

Side effects to expect

NAUSEA, VOMITING, BELCHING. These side effects are usually mild and tend to resolve with continued therapy. Encourage the patient not to discontinue therapy without first consulting his or her physician.

Side effects to report

HIVES, PRURITUS, RASH. Report symptoms for further evaluation by the physician.

Pruritus may be relieved by adding baking soda to the bath water.

BLADDER IRRITATION, DYSURIA, FREQUENCY. Notify the physician of these symptoms, as they may indicate the presence of another urinary tract infection.

Implementation

pH TESTING. Perform urine testing for pH at regular intervals. Report values above 5.5.

PO. Gastrointestinal symptoms may be minimized by administering with meals.

DO NOT crush the tablets! This will allow the formation of formaldehyde in the stomach, resulting in nausea and belching.

Drug interactions

ACETAZOLAMIDE, SODIUM BICARBONATE. Acetazolamide and sodium bicarbonate produce an alkaline urine, preventing the conversion of methenamine to formaldehyde, thus inactivating the medication.

SULFAMETHIZOLE. Sulfamethizole may form an insoluble precipitate in acidic urine. Therefore, concurrent treatment with sulfamethizole and methenamine should be avoided.

nalidixic acid (nal-ih-diks′ik)

NegGram (neg′gram)

Nalidixic acid is a urinary antiseptic chemically related to cinoxacin. As indicated by its brand name, Neg-Gram, it has antibacterial activity against gram-negative bacteria. It may be used to treat initial and recurrent urinary tract infections caused by *E. coli*, *Proteus mirabilis*, and other gram-negative microorganisms. It is not effective against *Pseudomonas* species, common pathogens in chronic urinary tract infections. Nalidixic acid may produce false-positive results with Clinitest. Clinistix or Tes-Tape may be used instead.

Side effects. The most common side effects of nalidixic acid include nausea and vomiting, drowsiness, headache, dizziness, and weakness.

Visual disturbances such as overbrightness of lights, changes in color perception, difficulty in focusing, and double vision may occur shortly after administration of each dose during the first few days of therapy.

Patients receiving nalidixic acid therapy should avoid undue exposure to sunlight, as photosensitivity may occur.

Nalidixic acid may induce hemolysis in patients with glucose-6-phosphate dehydrogenase deficiency. Nalidixic acid should not be used in these patients.

Nalidixic acid may produce false-positive results with Clinitest. Clinistix or Tes-Tape may be used instead.

Availability

PO—0.25, 0.5, and 1 g tablets; 250 mg/5 ml suspension.

Dosage and administration

Adult

PO—1 g 4 times daily for 1 to 2 weeks. If therapy is to be prolonged for prophylaxis, administer 500 mg 4 times daily.

Pediatric

PO—55 mg/kg/24 hours in 4 divided doses. If therapy is to be prolonged for prophylaxis, administer 33 mg/kg/24 hours in 4 divided doses.

• DO NOT administer to infants under 3 months of age.

• **Nursing Interventions: Monitoring nalidixic acid therapy**

See also General Nursing Considerations for Patients with Urinary Tract Infections (p. 355) and Patients with Infectious Disease (p. 457).

Side effects to report

NAUSEA, VOMITING. These side effects are usually mild and tend to resolve with continued therapy. Encourage the patient not to discontinue therapy without first consulting the physician.

VISUAL DISTURBANCES. During the first few days of therapy, difficulty focusing, double vision, and changes in brightness and colors may occur shortly after each dose is given. If these symptoms persist or occur later in therapy, notify the physician for further evaluation.

PHOTOSENSITIVITY. Patients should avoid exposure to direct sunlight and wear sunshades and long-sleeved garments outdoors while taking this medication. A severe burn requires medical attention.

DROWSINESS, HEADACHE, DIZZINESS, WEAKNESS. These side effects are usually mild and tend to resolve with continued therapy. Encourage the patient not to discontinue therapy without first consulting the physician.

Implementation

PO. Administer with food or milk if gastrointestinal symptoms are evident.

Drug interactions

WARFARIN. This medication may enhance the anticoagulant effects of warfarin. Observe for the development of petechiae, ecchymoses, nosebleeds, bleeding gums, dark tarry stools, and bright red or coffee ground emesis. Monitor the prothrombin time and reduce the dosage of warfarin if necessary.

CLINITEST. This drug may produce false-positive Clinitest results. Use Clinistix or Tes-Tape to measure urine glucose.

nitrofurantoin (ny-tro-fu-ran′to-in)

Furadantin (fur-ah-dan′tin), **Macrodantin** (mak-ro-dan′tin)

Nitrofurantoin is an antibiotic that acts by interfering with several bacterial enzyme systems. It is active against many gram-positive and gram-negative organisms, such as *Streptococcus faecalis*, *E. coli*, and *Proteus* species. Nitrofurantoin is not active against *Pseudomonas aeruginosa* or *Serratia* species. This antibiotic is not effective against microorganisms in the blood or in tissues outside the urinary tract.

Side effects. The most frequent side effects of nitrofurantoin are nausea, vomiting, and anorexia. This complication to therapy can be reduced by administration with food or milk.

Nitrofurantoin may tint the urine rust-brown to yellow.

Allergic reactions manifested by dyspnea, chills, fever, erythematous rash, and pruritus have been reported. Acute reactions usually develop within 8 hours in previously sensitized patients and within 7 to 10 days in patients who develop sensitivity during the course of therapy.

Nitrofurantoin may induce hemolysis in patients with glucose-6-phosphate dehydrogenase deficiency. Nitrofurantoin should not be used in these patients.

Nitrofurantoin may cause peripheral neuropathies, particularly in patients with renal impairment, anemia, diabetes, electrolyte imbalance, or vitamin B deficiency. Nitrofurantoin should be discontinued at the first sign of numbness or tingling in the extremities.

Availability

PO—50 and 100 mg tablets and capsules; 25 mg per 5 ml suspension.

Dosage and administration. NOTE: Nitrofurantoin must be in the bladder in sufficient concentrations to be therapeutically effective. Nitrofurantoin therapy is *not* recommended for use in patients with a creatinine clearance of less than 40 ml/min.

Adult

PO—50 to 100 mg 4 times daily for 10 to 14 days.

Pediatric

NOTE: Do not administer to infants under 1 month of age.

PO—5 to 7 mg/kg/24 hours in four divided doses.

• **Nursing Interventions: Monitoring nitrofurantoin therapy**

See also General Nursing Considerations for Patients with Urinary Tract Infections (p. 355) and Patients with Infectious Disease (p. 457).

Side effects to expect

NAUSEA, VOMITING, ANOREXIA. Administer with food or milk to reduce gastric irritation.

URINE DISCOLORATION. Tell the patient that urine may be tinted rust-brown to yellow. This should be no cause for alarm.

Side effects to report

DYSPNEA, CHILLS, FEVER, ERYTHEMATOUS RASH, PRURITUS. These symptoms are the early indications of an allergic reaction to nitrofurantoin.

Acute reactions usually occur within 8 hours in previously sensitized individuals, and within 7 to 10 days in patients who develop sensitivity during the course of therapy.

Discontinue the drug and notify the physician.

PERIPHERAL NEUROPATHIES. Discontinue the medication at the first sign of numbness or tingling in the extremities.

SECOND INFECTION. Report immediately the development of dysuria, pungent-smelling urine, or fever. These symptoms may be the early indication of a second infection due to an organism resistant to nitrofurantoin.

Implementation

PO. Administer with food or milk to reduce gastrointestinal side effects.

To maintain adequate urine concentrations, space the dosage at even intervals around the clock.

SUSPENSION. Store in a dark amber container away from bright light.

INTRAVENOUS. Always read and follow the manufacturer's recommendations:

Reconstitution: Just before use, add 20 ml of dextrose 5% or sterile water to the vial and shake well. Each milliliter of this initial solution should be further diluted with an additional 25 ml of fluid. Therefore, 180 mg in 20 ml must be diluted to at least 500 ml of parenteral fluid for infusion.

• DO NOT dilute with solutions containing methyl- or pro-pylparabens, phenol, or cresol as preservatives. These may cause nitrofurantoin to precipitate out of solution. Do not administer if a precipitate develops.

Drug interactions

CLINITEST. This drug may produce false-positive Clinitest results. Use Clinistix or Tes-Tape to measure urine glucose.

ANTACIDS. Encourage the patient *not* to take products containing magnesium trisilicate (Escot Capsules, Gaviscon, Gelusil) concurrently with nitrofurantoin because the antacid may inhibit absorption of the nitrofurantoin.

norfloxacin (nor-flocs'ah-sin)

Noroxin (nor-ox'in)

Norfloxacin is a broad spectrum antibiotic chemically related to cinoxacin and nalidixic acid. It has the ad-

vantage over these agents of having a much broader spectrum of activity against gram-positive and gram-negative microorganisms. Due to its expense, it should be reserved to treat resistant, recurrent urinary tract infections caused by *E. coli, Proteus mirabilis, Pseudomonas, Staphylococcus aureus, Staphylococcus epidermidis,* and other gram-positive and gram-negative microorganisms no longer sensitive to the penicillins, cephalosporins, or sulfonamides. Because this antibiotic is administered orally, it may also be useful in treating patients on an outpatient basis who would have required hospitalization for parenteral therapy.

Side effects. The most common side effects of norfloxacin include nausea (2.8%), headache (2.7%), and dizziness (1.8%). Other adverse effects reported (0.3% to 1%) include rash, abdominal pain, dyspepsia, constipation, flatulence, and heartburn.

Needle-shaped crystals have been found in the urine (crystalluria) of patients who were receiving higher than recommended dosages of norfloxacin or who were dehydrated.

Availability

PO—400 mg tablets.

Dosage and administration

Adult

PO—Uncomplicated urinary tract infections: 400 mg twice daily for 7 to 10 days. Take 1 hour before or 2 hours after meals with a large glass of fluid. Do not exceed 800 mg daily.

Complicated urinary tract infections: 400 mg twice daily for 10 to 21 days. Take 1 hour before or 2 hours after meals with a large glass of fluid. Do not exceed 800 mg daily.

• **Nursing Interventions: Monitoring norfloxacin therapy**

See also General Nursing Considerations for Patients with Urinary Tract Infections (p. 355) and Patients with Infectious Disease (p. 457).

Side effects to expect

NAUSEA, DYSPEPSIA, FLATULENCE. These side effects are usually mild and tend to resolve with continued therapy. Encourage the patient not to discontinue therapy without first consulting the physician.

DROWSINESS, HEADACHE, DIZZINESS. These side effects are usually mild and tend to resolve with continued therapy. Encourage the patient not to discontinue therapy without first consulting the physician.

Provide for patient safety during episodes of dizziness; report for further evaluation if recurrent.

Side effects to report

HEMATURIA. Although very rare, crystal formation has been reported when high doses have been used or when the patient is dehydrated. The crystals may cause hematuria. Report bloody urine to your physician immediately. Encourage the patient to drink 8 to 12 glasses of water daily.

Implementation

PO. Administer 1 hour before or 2 hours after meals. Food inhibits absorption of norfloxacin.

Drug interactions

PROBENECID. Probenecid may reduce urinary excretion of norfloxacin, thereby producing inadequate antimicrobial therapy and the possibility of resistant strains of microorganisms.

ANTACIDS. Antacids will decrease absorption of norfloxacin. Administer norfloxacin 1 hour before or 2 hours after antacid therapy.

NITROFURANTOIN. Nitrofurantoin may antagonize the antibacterial effects of norfloxacin. Do not use concurrently.

HYPERURICEMIA

OBJECTIVES

1. Describe two methods that are effective in the treatment of hyperuricemia.
2. Cite the nutritional aspects of treating gout.
3. Explain the rationale for maintaining an alkaline urine during the treatment of gout.
4. Explain probenecid dosages, requirements for fluid intake during administration, and effect on gouty arthritis.
5. State the nursing assessments needed to monitor therapeutic response and/or the development of side effects to expect or report from agents used to treat hyperuricemia.
6. Develop measurable short- and long-term objectives for patient education for patients with hyperuricemia.

Uric acid is a normal metabolite of cellular metabolism and is excreted by the kidneys under normal circumstances. For several reasons, however, uric acid can accumulate, resulting in acute attacks of gout, gouty arthritis, and deposits of urate tophi in joints. Hyperuricemia may be treated by inhibiting the production of uric acid with an agent known as allopurinol or by enhancing the excretion of uric acid by the kidneys. Two agents effective in enhancing the excretion of uric acid are probenecid and sulfinpyrazone.

General Nursing Considerations for Patients with Gout

Gout requires prolonged medical management to prevent the long-term progression of debilitating joint disease and renal dysfunction. The nurse must carefully assess the individual, initially for the presenting symptoms of the attack, and over a longer period for compliance with the therapeutic modalities prescribed. Baseline data need to be obtained so that symptoms, course of recovery, and degree of understanding and compliance with the management prescribed can be assessed in the future.

Assessment of current gout attack

Obtain data relative to the onset of this attack of gout.

Joint involvement. Describe the specific location of involvement.

Pain. State the degree, location, intensity, duration, and radiation of joint pain being experienced.

Warmth, color. Note the color and feel the warmth of affected areas.

Pain relief. Is the pain relieved by hot or cold compresses? Or have these proven intolerable?

Swelling. Inspect the affected areas for swelling.

Additional symptoms. Ask about additional symptoms such as general malaise, headache, fatigue, fever, or anorexia.

Nutritional compliance

In most cases, certain foods or alcoholic beverages may precipitate an attack. Ask for a food history, noting particularly whether the patient has eaten larger quantities of organ meats (liver, kidney), meat-based dishes (broth), seafood, or dried beans than usual.

Regimen compliance

If previously treated for gout, obtain details of the prescribed treatment to assess for compliance.

Medication. What medications are being taken?

Fluid intake. How much fluid is routinely ingested?

Diet. What type of diet had been prescribed? Ask the patient to describe his or her routine diet.

Patient Education Associated with Uricosuric Therapy

Communication and responsibility. Encourage open communication concerning frustrations and anger as the patient attempts to adjust to the diagnosis and need for prolonged treatment. The patient must be guided to insight into the condition in order to assume responsibility for the continuation of treatment. Keep emphasizing those factors the patient can control to alter the disease process, including maintenance of general health, nutritional needs, adequate rest and appropriate exercise, and continuation of prescribed medication therapy.

Nutrition. It is suggested, but not proven, that dietary alterations can relieve the symptoms of gout. Organ meats, meat-based dishes, seafood, and dried beans should be restricted from the diet until the desired uric acid level has been achieved.

Encourage the avoidance of specific foods or alcoholic beverages that may precipitate attacks.

Medication. If the patient is taking uricosuric agents, maintaining the urine alkalinity can enhance uric acid excretion. The doctor may prescribe agents to increase urine alkalinity.

Hydration. Drink 8 to 12 8-ounce glasses of fluid daily while receiving uricosuric agents.

Expectations of therapy. Discuss with the patient his or her expectations of therapy.

Activities and exercise. Activities of daily living should be resumed within the boundaries set by the patient and the physician.

During the acute attack, the patient may require bedrest.

Pain relief. Discuss the degree of joint pain relief with and without activity. Since effects on the joints are progressive, the degree of pain and associated activity will vary based on the individual's presenting symptoms and degree of joint involvement.

Stress management. Encourage the patient to openly express feelings with regard to this chronic illness. The adjustment to this situation involves working through great personal fears, frustrations, hostilities, and resentments associated with the loss of control in one's life.

Changes in expectations. Assess changes in expectations as therapy progresses and the patient gains understanding and skill in the management of the diagnosis.

Changes in therapy through cooperative goal setting. Work with the patient to encourage adherence to the prescribed treatment. When the patient feels that a change should be made in a treatment plan, encourage a discussion first with the physician.

Written record. Enlist the patient's aid in developing and maintaining a written record (Figure 15-3) of monitoring parameters (such as swelling, warmth, tenderness of particular joints, identification of foods that precipitate an attack, degree of pain relief, exercise tolerance) and response to prescribed therapies for discussion with the physician. Patients should be encouraged to take this record on follow-up visits.

Fostering compliance. Throughout the hospitalization, discuss medication information and how it will benefit the course of treatment. Seek cooperation and understanding of the following points, so that medication compliance may be enhanced:

1. Name
2. Dosage
3. Route and administration times
4. Anticipated therapeutic response
5. Side effects to expect
6. Side effects to report
7. What to do if a dosage is missed
8. When, how, or if to refill the medication prescription

Difficulty in comprehension. If it is evident that the patient and/or family does not understand all aspects of

continuing therapy being prescribed (such as administration and monitoring of medications, diets, follow-up appointments), consider the use of social service or visiting nurse agencies.

Associated teaching. Give the patients the following instructions:

Always inform the physician or dentist of any prescription or over-the-counter medication being taken. Over-the-counter medications should not be taken without first discussing them with a physician or pharmacist.

Always report side effects of rash, itching, or hives immediately. Nausea, vomiting, or diarrhea should also be reported for the physician's evaluation if it is a new symptom.

Take all of the medication as prescribed for the full course of treatment. Do not discontinue use when feeling improved; do not save for further use; do not give your medicine to another individual. Sudden discontinuation of certain medications may produce harmful effects.

Keep all medications out of the reach of children.

If pregnancy is suspected, consult an obstetrician as soon as possible about continuation of medication therapy.

At discharge. Items to be sent home with the patient should include the following:

1. Written instructions for use
2. Labels in a level of language and size of print appropriate for the patient
3. If needed, identification cards or bracelets
4. A list of additional supplies to be purchased after discharge
5. A schedule of follow-up appointments

Drug Therapy for Gout

Uricosuric agents

Uricosuric agents act on the tubules of the kidneys to enhance the excretion of uric acid.

probenecid (pro-ben′eh-sid)

Benemid (ben-′eh-mid)

Probenecid promotes renal excretion of a number of substances, including uric acid. It inhibits the reabsorption of urate in the kidney, which results in reduction of uric acid in the blood. Thus, probenecid is used to treat hyperuricemia and chronic gouty arthritis. It is not effective in acute attacks of gout and is not an analgesic.

Side effects. The number of gouty attacks may increase during the first 6 to 12 months of treatment. Continue probenecid therapy without changing doses during these attacks. Treat the acute attack with colchicine or antiinflammatory agents.

The most common adverse effects of probenecid

Patient Education and Monitoring of Therapeutic Outcomes for Patients Receiving Medication for Gout

Medications	Color	To be taken

Name _____

Physician _____

Physician's phone _____

Next appt.* _____

	Parameters	Day of discharge							Comments
Joint swelling	Location								
	Amount: Small, moderate, large								
Pain relief Poor Improved No pain 10 5 1									
Ability to perform exercise	No problem								
	Too painful								
	Produces discomfort								
Temperature of affected area	Red hot								
	Warm								
	Normal								
Color of joint	Red								
	White								
	Normal								
Sleep pattern	Cannot stand covers								
	Can sleep with covers								
Overall sleep evaluation: Poor Okay Good 10 5 1									
Fluid intake per day: Record # glasses per day									
List foods that generally cause an attack									

*Please bring this record with you to your next appointment.
Use the back of this sheet for additional information.

Figure 15-3 *Patient education and monitoring of therapeutic outcomes for patients receiving medication for gout.*

therapy are gastrointestinal in nature. About 8% of patients will complain of anorexia, nausea, and vomiting. Use with caution in patients with a history of peptic ulcer disease.

About 5% of patients develop a hypersensitivity to probenecid, manifested by fever, pruritus, and rashes. If these symptoms develop, discontinue therapy.

A false-positive reaction for glucose in the urine may occur with Clinitest tablets, but not with Clinistix or Tes-Tape.

Availability

PO—500 mg tablets.

Dosage and administration. NOTE: Do not start probenecid therapy during an acute attack of gout; wait 2 to 3 weeks.

Adult

PO—Initially 250 mg twice daily for 1 week, then 500 mg twice daily. The dosage may be increased by 500 mg every few weeks to a maximum of 2 to 3 g daily. Administer with food or milk to diminish gastric irritation.

- Maintain fluid intake at 2 to 3 liters daily.
- Do not administer to patients with a creatinine clearance of less than 40 ml/minute or a BUN greater than 40 mg/100 ml.
- Do not administer to patients with a history of blood dyscrasias or uric acid kidney stones.

- **Nursing Interventions: Monitoring probenecid therapy**

See also General Nursing Considerations for Patients with Gout (p. 375).

Side effects to expect

ACUTE GOUT ATTACKS. Patients should be told that the frequency of gout attacks may increase for the first few months of therapy. The patient should continue therapy without changing the doses during the attacks.

Side effects to report

NAUSEA, ANOREXIA, VOMITING. Use with caution in patients with a history of peptic ulcer disease. Individuals who experience symptoms of ulcers, and are yet undiagnosed, should be encouraged to report gastrointestinal symptoms if they increase in intensity or frequency. Always report bright bloody or coffee ground vomitus or dark, tarry stools.

HIVES, PRURITUS, RASH. Therapy may have to be discontinued.

Implementation

ACUTE ATTACKS. DO NOT start therapy during an acute attack of gout; wait 2 to 3 weeks.

GASTRIC IRRITATION. Give oral medication with food or milk to diminish gastric irritation.

FLUID INTAKE. Maintain fluid intake at 8 to 12 8-ounce glasses daily.

CONTRAINDICATION. DO NOT administer to patients with a history of blood dyscrasias or uric acid kidney stones.

Drug interactions

ORAL HYPOGLYCEMIC AGENTS. Monitor for hypoglycemia: headache, weakness, decreased coordination, general apprehension, diaphoresis, hunger, blurred or double vision.

The dosage of the hypoglycemic agent may need to be reduced. Notify the physician if any of the above symptoms appear.

DAPSONE, INDOMETHACIN, SULFINPYRAZONE, RIFAMPIN, SULFONAMIDES, NAPROXEN, PENICILLINS, CEPHALOSPORINS, METHOTREXATE, AND CLOFIBRATE. Probenecid blocks the renal excretion of these agents. See individual drugs listed for side effects to report that may indicate development of toxicity.

SALICYLATES. Although an occasional aspirin will not interfere with the effectiveness of probenecid, regular use of aspirin or aspirin-containing products should be discouraged. If analgesia is required, suggest acetaminophen.

ANTINEOPLASTIC AGENTS. Probenecid is not recommended for increased uric acid levels caused by antineoplastic therapy because of the potential development of renal uric acid stones.

CLINITEST. This drug may produce false-positive Clinitest results. Use Clinistix or Tes-Tape to measure urine glucose.

sulfinpyrazone (sul-fin-py'rah-zone)

Anturane (an'tu-rayn)

Sulfinpyrazone is a renal tubular blocking agent that inhibits the reabsorption of urate from the renal tubules, increasing the urinary excretion of uric acid and decreasing serum urate levels. It is used for long-term treatment of hyperuricemia associated with gout and gouty arthritis.

Side effects. The number of gouty attacks may increase during the first 6 to 12 months of treatment. Continue sulfinpyrazone therapy without changing doses during these attacks. Treat the acute attack with colchicine or antiinflammatory agents.

The most common adverse effects of sulfinpyrazone therapy are gastrointestinal in nature. Some patients will complain of anorexia, nausea, and vomiting. Use with caution in patients with a history of peptic ulcer disease.

About 3% of patients develop hypersensitivity to sulfinpyrazone, manifested by fever, pruritus, and rashes. If these symptoms develop, discontinue therapy. Patients who have developed hypersensitivities to oxyphenbutazone or phenylbutazone should not be placed on sulfinpyrazone therapy due to the possibility of cross-sensitivity.

Serious, potentially fatal blood dyscrasias including anemia, agranulocytosis, and thrombocytopenia have been associated with sulfinpyrazone therapy. Although the development of blood dyscrasias is quite rare, periodic differential blood counts are recommended.

Availability

PO—100 mg tablets, and 200 mg capsules.

Dosage and administration. NOTE: Do not start sulfinpyrazone therapy during an acute attack of gout; wait 2 to 3 weeks.

Adult

PO—Initially 100 to 200 mg twice daily during the first week of therapy. The maintenance dose is usually 200 to 400 mg twice daily. Administer with food or milk to diminish gastric irritation.

- Maintain fluid intake at 2 to 3 liters daily.
- DO NOT administer to patients with a creatinine clearance of less than 40 ml/minute or a BUN greater than 40 mg/100 ml.
- *Do not* administer to patients with a history of blood dyscrasias or uric acid kidney stones.

- **Nursing Interventions: Monitoring sulfinpyrazone therapy**

See also General Nursing Considerations for Patients with Gout (p. 375).

Side effects to expect

ACUTE GOUT ATTACKS. Patients should be told that the frequency of gout attacks may increase for the first few months of therapy. The patient should continue therapy without changing the doses during the attacks.

Side effects to report

NAUSEA, ANOREXIA, VOMITING. Use with caution in patients with a history of peptic ulcer disease. Individuals who experience symptoms of ulcers, and are yet undiagnosed, should be encouraged to report gastrointestinal symptoms if they increase in intensity or frequency. Always report bright bloody or coffee ground vomitus or dark, tarry stools.

HIVES, PRURITUS, RASH. Therapy may have to be discontinued.

Implementation

ACUTE ATTACKS. DO NOT start therapy during an acute attack of gout; wait 2 to 3 weeks.

GASTRIC IRRITATION. Give oral medication with food or milk to diminish gastric irritation.

FLUID INTAKE. Maintain fluid intake at 8 to 12 8-ounce glasses daily.

CONTRAINDICATIONS. DO NOT administer to patients with a creatinine clearance of less than 40 ml/minute or a BUN greater than 40 mg/100 ml.

DO NOT administer to patients with a history of blood dyscrasias or uric acid kidney stones.

Drug interactions

SALICYLATES. Although an occasional aspirin will not interfere with the effectiveness of sulfinpyrazone, discourage regular use of aspirin or aspirin-containing products. If analgesia is required, suggest acetaminophen.

ANTINEOPLASTIC AGENTS. Sulfinpyrazone is not recommended for increased uric acid levels caused by antineoplastic therapy because of the potential development of renal uric acid stones.

WARFARIN. This medication may enhance the anticoagulant effects of warfarin. Observe for the development of petechiae, ecchymoses, nosebleeds, bleeding gums, dark tarry stools, and bright red or coffee ground emesis.

Monitor the prothrombin time and reduce the dosage of warfarin if necessary.

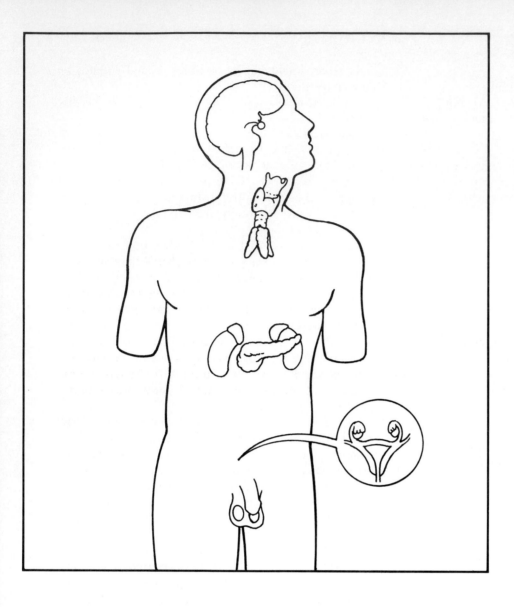

Drugs Affecting the Endocrine System

CHAPTER GOALS

After completing this chapter, the student should be able to do the following:

1. Explain the major action and effects of drugs used to treat disorders of the endocrine system.

2. Identify baseline data the nurse should collect on a continuous basis for comparison and evaluation of drug effectiveness.

3. Identify important nursing assessments and interventions associated with the drug therapy and treatment of diseases associated with the endocrine system.

4. Identify essential components involved in planning patient education that will enhance compliance with the treatment regimen.

DIABETES MELLITUS

OBJECTIVES

1. State the current definition of diabetes mellitus.
2. Identify the extent of the disease within the United States.
3. Describe the three clinical classes of diabetes mellitus.
4. Differentiate between the symptoms of Type I (IDDM) and Type II (NIDMM) diabetes mellitus.
5. Identify the objectives of dietary control of diabetes mellitus.
6. Discuss the use of insulin as opposed to oral hypoglycemic agents to control diabetes mellitus.
7. Identify the major nursing considerations associated with the management of the patient with diabetes (such as nutritional evaluation, dietary prescription, activity and exercise, psychological considerations).
8. Differentiate between the signs, symptoms, and management of hypoglycemia and hyperglycemia.
9. Discuss the contributing factors, nursing assessments, and nursing interventions needed for patients exhibiting complications associated with diabetes mellitus.
10. Develop measurable short- and long-term objectives for patient education for persons taking any type of insulin or oral hypoglycemic agent.

KEY WORDS

hypoglycemia	hyperglycemia
glucose tolerance	diabetic retinopathy
neuropathies	parasthesia
pheochromocytoma	neurogenic bladder
acromegaly	Cushing syndrome
gestational diabetes	

Diabetes mellitus has traditionally been defined as a chronic, progressive disease manifested by abnormalities in carbohydrate, protein, and fat metabolism resulting from a lack of insulin. It has now been redefined as a group of diseases that have glucose intolerance (hyperglycemia) in common. The causes of these diseases are still unknown, but it is now recognized that different pathologic mechanisms are involved for different diseases.

Diabetes mellitus is appearing with increasing frequency in the United States as the number of older people in the population increases. In the U.S., approximately 4.5 million people are being treated for diabetes. Another 2 million have undiagnosed diabetes, and 5 million more will develop diabetes during their lives. Undiagnosed diabetic adults, with few or no symptoms, present a major challenge to the health profession. Because early symptoms of diabetes are minimal, the patient does not seek medical advice. Indications of the disease are discovered only at the time of routine physical examination. Those with a predisposition to developing diabetes include (1) people who have relatives with diabetes (they have two and one half times greater incidence of developing the disease), (2) obese people (85% of all diabetic patients are overweight), and (3) older people (four out of five diabetics are over 45 years of age).

In 1979, the National Diabetes Data Group of the National Institutes of Health published a new classification system for diabetes that more accurately categorizes the various mechanisms associated with the diseases. The classification includes three clinical classes, characterized by either fasting hyperglycemia or abnormalities of glucose tolerance, and two statistical risk classes, with normal glucose tolerance, that are thought to be stages in the natural course of diabetes (see Table 16-1).

Type I, *insulin-dependent diabetes mellitus* (IDDM), is present in 5% to 10% of the diabetic population. It frequently occurs in juveniles, but it is now recognized that patients can become symptomatic for the first time at any age. The onset of this form of diabetes usually has a rapid progression of symptoms (a few days to a few weeks) characterized by polydipsia (increased thirst), polyphagia (increased appetite), polyuria (increased urination), increased frequency of infections, loss of weight and strength, irritability, and often ketoacidosis. There is no insulin secretion from the pancreas, and patients require administration of exogenous insulin. Insulin dosage adjustment is easily influenced by inconsistent patterns of physical activity and dietary irregularities.

Type II, *non–insulin-dependent diabetes mellitus* (NIDDM), represents about 90% of the diabetic popu-

Table 16-1 *National Diabetes Group Classification of Glucose Intolerance*

CLASS	FORMER TERMINOLOGY
Clinical classes	
Diabetes mellitus (DM)	
Type I: Insulin-dependent (IDDM)	Juvenile diabetes, juvenile-onset diabetes (JOD), ketosis prone diabetes, brittle diabetes
Type II: Non–insulin-dependent (NIDDM)	Adult-onset diabetes, maturity-onset diabetes (MOD), ketosis resistant diabetes, stable diabetes
Nonobese NIDDM	
Obese NIDDM	
Other types associated with certain conditions and syndromes:	Secondary diabetes
1. Pancreatic disease	
2. Hormonal	
3. Drug or chemical induced	
4. Insulin receptor abnormalities	
5. Certain genetic syndromes	
6. Other types	
Gestational diabetes (GDM)	Gestational diabetes
Impaired glucose tolerance (IGT)	Asymptomatic diabetes, chemical diabetes, borderline diabetes, latent diabetes
Nonobese IGT	
Obese IGT	
IGT associated with certain conditions and syndromes:	
1. Pancreatic disease	
2. Hormonal	
3. Drug or chemical induced	
4. Insulin receptor abnormalities	
5. Certain genetic syndromes	
Statistical risk classes	
Previous abnormality of glucose tolerance (PrevAGT)	Latent diabetes
Potential abnormality of glucose tolerance (PotAGT)	Prediabetes, potential diabetes

(Modified from National Diabetes Data Group, *Diabetes* 28:1039-1057, Dec. 1979.)

lation. It usually has a more insidious onset. The pancreas still maintains some capability to produce and secrete insulin. Consequently, symptoms are minimal or absent for a prolonged period of time. The patient may seek medical attention several years later only after symptoms of the disease are apparent. Patients may complain of weight gain or loss. Blurred vision may indicate diabetic retinopathy. Neuropathies may be first observed as numbness or tingling of the extremities (paresthesia), loss of sensation, orthostatic hypotention, impotence, and difficulty in controlling urination (neurogenic bladder). Nonhealing ulcers of the lower extremities may indicate chronic vascular disease. Fasting hyperglycemia can be controlled by diet in some patients, but other patients will require the use of supplemental insulin or oral hypoglycemic agents, such as tolbutamide or acetohexamide. Although the onset is usually after the fourth decade of life, NIDDM can occur in younger patients who do not require insulin for control.

The third subclass of diabetes mellitus includes additional types of diabetes that are a part of other diseases having features not generally associated with the diabetic state. Diseases that may have a diabetic component include pheochromocytoma, acromegaly, and Cushing syndrome. Other disorders included in this category are malnutrition, drugs and chemicals that induce hyperglycemia, defects in insulin receptors, and certain genetic syndromes.

The second clinical class, known as *gestational diabetes* (GDM), is reserved for women who show abnormal glucose tolerance during pregnancy. It does not include diabetic women who become pregnant. The majority of gestational diabetics will have a normal glucose tolerance postpartum. Gestational diabetics must be reclassified after delivery into the category of diabetes mellitus, impaired glucose tolerance, or previous abnormality of glucose tolerance. Gestational diabetics have been put into a separate category because of the special clinical features of diabetes that develop during pregnancy and the complications associated with fetal involvement. These women are also at a higher risk of developing diabetes 5 to 10 years after pregnancy.

The third and last clinical class is for those patients found to have an *impaired glucose tolerance* (IGT). It is now thought that patients with IGT are at a higher risk for developing NIDDM or IDDM in the future. In many of these patients, however, the glucose tolerance returns to normal or persists in the intermediate range for years. Studies indicate that these patients have an increased susceptibility to atherosclerotic disease.

There are two groups of patients at risk for diabetes or impaired glucose tolerance—those with a previous abnormality and those with a potential abnormality of glucose tolerance. Therefore, the National Diabetes Data Group included two statistical risk classes in the new classification. The first risk class is for patients with a *previous abnormality of glucose tolerance* (Prev-AGT). This class includes patients who now have normal glucose tolerance but who have a history of previous diabetes mellitus or impaired glucose tolerance. Representative of this class might be the gestational diabetic who has a normal glucose tolerance after delivery or an obese patient whose glucose tolerance has returned to normal because of diet control and weight loss. It is important to realize that PrevAGT patients are not diabetics and should not be labeled as such, but should be tested periodically for the development of diabetes.

The second statistical risk class is *potential abnormality of glucose tolerance* (PotAGT). This class is for patients who have never exhibited abnormal glucose tolerance but who are at an increased risk for developing abnormalities. Risk factors for the development of non-insulin-dependent diabetes include being the monozygotic twin of this type of diabetic, having a close relative (such as sibling, parent, or child) who is a non–insulin-dependent diabetic, and being obese. A person with islet cell antibodies, or who is a monozygotic twin of an insulin-dependent diabetic, or who is a sibling of an insulin-dependent diabetic has an increased probability of becoming an insulin-dependent diabetic.

Although the classification system of the National Diabetes Data Group was developed to facilitate clinical and epidemiologic investigation, the categorization of patients can also be helpful in determining general principles for therapy. As a cure for diabetes mellitus is unknown at present, the minimal purpose of treatment is to prevent ketoacidosis and symptoms resulting from hyperglycemia. The long-term objective of control of the disease must involve mechanisms to stop the progression of the complications of the disease. Major determinants involve a balanced diet, insulin or oral hypoglycemic therapy, routine exercise, and good hygiene. Patient education and reinforcement are extremely important to successful therapy. The intelligence and motivation of the diabetic patient, and his or her awareness of the potential complications, contribute significantly to the ultimate outcome of the disease and the quality of life the patient may lead.

Control of diabetes mellitus. Patients with diabetes can lead full and satisfying lives. However, unrestricted diets and activities are not possible. Dietary treatment of diabetes constitutes the basis for management of most patients, especially those with the Type II (NIDDM) form of the disease. With adequate weight reduction and dietary control, patients may not require the use of exogenous insulin or oral hypoglycemic drug therapy. Type I (IDDM) diabetics will always require exogenous insulin as well as dietary control because the pancreas has lost the capacity to produce and secrete

insulin. The aims of dietary control are (1) the prevention of excessive postprandial hyperglycemia, (2) the prevention of hypoglycemia in those patients being treated with hypoglycemic agents or insulin, (3) the achievement and maintenance of an ideal body weight, and (4) a reduction of lipids and cholesterol. A return to normal weight is often accompanied by a reduction in hyperglycemia. The diet should also be adjusted to reduce elevated cholesterol and triglyceride levels in an attempt to retard the progression of atherosclerosis.

To help maintain adherence to dietary restrictions, the diet should be planned in relation to the patient's food preferences, economic status, occupation, and physical activity. Emphasis should be placed on what food the patient may have and what exchanges are acceptable. Food should be measured for balanced portions, and the patient should be cautioned not to omit meals or between-meal and bedtime snacks.

All diabetic patients must receive adequate instruction on personal hygiene, especially regarding care of the feet, skin, and teeth. Infection is a common precipitating cause of ketosis and acidosis, and must be treated promptly.

Insulin is required to control Type I diabetes and for those patients whose diabetes cannot be controlled by diet, weight reduction, or oral hypoglycemic agents. Patients normally controlled with oral hypoglycemic agents will require insulin during situations of increased physiologic and psychologic stress, such as pregnancy, surgery, and infections. The dosage of insulin is usually adjusted according to the blood glucose levels and the degree of glucosuria. The patient should test blood or urine glucose before each meal and at bedtime while the insulin is being regulated.

Another adjunct in the therapy of Type II diabetes is the use of oral hypoglycemic agents. They are recommended only in those patients who cannot be controlled by diet alone and who are not prone to develop ketosis, acidosis, and/or infections. Patients most likely to benefit from treatment are those who have developed diabetes after 40 years of age and who require less than 40 units of insulin per day.

General Nursing Considerations for Patients with Diabetes Mellitus

A major challenge in nursing is to teach the newly diagnosed diabetic patient all the necessary information to manage self-care and the disease process and to prevent complications. The patient must be taught the entire therapeutic regimen—diet, activity level, urine or blood testing, the medication, self-injection techniques, prevention of complications, and the effective management of hypoglycemia or hyperglycemia. Many diabetics have difficulty understanding the critical balance among the dietary prescription, the prescribed medication, and the maintenance of general health.

All are important to the control and effective management of the disease process.

Patient Concerns: Nursing Intervention/Rationale

Management of patients with diabetes mellitus

Nutritional status. Diet is used alone or in combination with insulin or oral hypoglycemic agents to control diabetes mellitus. The diabetic patient, whether non–insulin-dependent or insulin-dependent, must follow a prescribed diet to achieve optimal control of the disease.

Nutritional evaluation. The newly diagnosed diabetic requires a thorough nutritional evaluation. Information collected by the nurse or dietitian should include identification of the patient's average daily diet, the ability and willingness to prepare foods, food budget, and level of daily exercise.

People who are readmitted for treatment should be reevaluated for both nutritional knowledge and compliance with the prescribed dietary plan.

Dietary prescription. The dietary prescription is based on providing the patient with the nutritional and energy requirements necessary to maintain an appropriate weight and lifestyle. Diabetics are encouraged to maintain a body weight slightly below an ideal weight based on height, gender, and frame size.

The diet for the obese diabetic, regardless of age, is calculated to achieve weight loss over the next several weeks to months. Even a small weight loss of 15, 20, or 25 pounds can improve the non–insulin-dependent diabetic's ability to control the blood glucose level. Weight loss and exercise can enhance the ability of the body to utilize insulin. Once the optimal weight is attained, these patients are placed on a maintenance diet. Small meals containing high-fiber foods can have the same effect in the nonobese Type II diabetic.

Meals for Type I diabetics are usually divided into three meals plus snacks. Decisions regarding the distribution of foods throughout the day are coordinated to provide sufficient foods when the existing exercise/activity or medication/insulin levels are high.

The American Diabetic Association (ADA) recommends that the diet be composed of 55% to 60% carbohydrates, 30% fats (primarily unsaturated; cholesterol intake of 300 mg/day or less), and 12% to 20% proteins (in adults 0.8 g/kg of body weight can be used to calculate the individual's protein needs). Including high-fiber foods (e.g., legumes, oats, and barley) has been found to assist in lowering both blood glucose levels and blood cholesterol. Low sodium, alcohol, and caffeine consumption is also advisable. (See a medical-surgical nursing text or a nutrition text for details on dietary calculations using the exchange list, point, constant carbohydrate, or total available glucose [TAG] systems.)

Activity and exercise. Maintenance of a normal life style is to be encouraged. This includes exercise and activities the individual enjoys. The normal daily energy level is used in determining the dietary and medication requirements for the patient.

Just as it is important for the patient to maintain a diet, it is equally important to maintain a certain activity level. Patients who suddenly increase or decrease activity levels are susceptible to developing episodes of hyperglycemia or hypoglycemia. Both dietary and medication prescriptions may require adjustment if the patient does not plan to resume the previous exercise level. The patient should consult with the physician prior to initiation of an exercise program. Additional self-monitoring of the blood glucose level may be advisable before, during, and approximately 30 minutes after exercise to provide the physician with data to analyze regarding the effects of exercise on the individual's blood glucose level.

Psychological considerations. When first diagnosed, the patient may experience varying degrees of grief, anger, denial, or acceptance. Let the patient express these concerns and address those items that are considered to be of greatest importance first.

Foster the idea that the patient can control most aspects of diabetes by careful management of diet, medications, and activities. Having a sense of control is important to all people. Stress that learning to manage the disease process is the best means of preventing complications.

Medication. As stated in the introduction, insulin or oral hypoglycemic agent therapy may be required to control diabetes mellitus. No changes in therapy should be made without medical supervision.

A variety of combinations of insulin or insulin and oral hypoglycemic agents may be used to provide control of the blood glucose level. The goal of therapy is to consistently maintain the blood glucose level within the normal range. A variety of administration schedules have evolved over the years to accomplish this goal. The schedules most commonly used are:

1. Divided doses of intermediate-acting insulin (two thirds in the morning, one third in the evening).
2. Combinations of short-acting and intermediate-acting insulin in the morning, followed by short-acting and long-acting insulin before dinner.
3. Long-acting insulin in the evening with small doses of short-acting regular insulin just before each meal.
4. Continuous infusion of regular insulin using a small, portable insulin infusion pump.

The regimen chosen depends upon each person's response to medications, schedule of daily activities, and compliance with blood glucose monitoring, insulin injections, and diet.

Hypoglycemia. Hypoglycemia, or low blood sugar, can occur from too much insulin, insufficient food intake to cover the insulin given, imbalances caused by vomiting and diarrhea, and excessive exercise without additional carbohydrate intake.

SYMPTOMS. Recognize and assess early symptoms of hypoglycemia: nervousness, tremors, headache, apprehension, sweating, cold, clammy skin, and hunger. If uncorrected, hypoglycemia progresses to blurring of vision, lack of coordination, incoherence, coma, and death.

TREATMENT. If the patient is conscious and *able to swallow*, give 2 to 4 ounces of fruit juice with two teaspoons of sugar or honey in it, or give a piece of candy such as Life-Savers or gum drops or carry a tube of cake frosting to squeeze in the mouth. (Chocolate contains fats that are utilized more slowly.) Repeat in 15 to 20 minutes if relief of symptoms is not evident.

If the patient is unconscious, having a seizure, or *unable to swallow*, administer 20 to 50 ml of glucose 50%, IV (only by a qualified individual).

With any hypoglycemic reaction, notify the team leader, primary nurse, or head nurse, who will then contact the physician. The underlying cause of the hypoglycemia must be identified to prevent further occurrences. If in doubt about whether the individual is hypoglycemic or hyperglycemic, the nurse should always proceed to treat the individual for hypoglycemia to prevent neurologic damage from prolonged reduction in glucose to the nerve cells (e.g., brain cells).

Hyperglycemia. *Hyperglycemia* (elevated blood sugar) occurs when the glucose available in the body cannot be transported into the cells for use, because of a lack of insulin necessary for the transport mechanism.

SYMPTOMS. Symptoms of hyperglycemia are headache, nausea and vomiting, abdominal pain, dizziness, rapid pulse, rapid shallow respirations, and a fruity odor to the breath from acetone. If untreated, hyperglycemia may also cause coma and death.

TREATMENT. Treatment of hyperglycemia requires hospitalization, insulin, and close monitoring of the blood and urine glucose and ketones. Since hyperglycemia usually occurs due to another cause, the problem, often an infection, must also be identified and treated to control the hyperglycemia.

PREVENTION. The risk of hyperglycemia can be minimized by taking the prescribed dose of insulin or oral hypoglycemic agent; by adhering to the prescribed diet and exercise; by reporting fevers, infection, or prolonged vomiting and/or diarrhea to the physician; and by maintaining an accurate written record for the physician to analyze to determine the individual patient's needs. Self-monitoring of blood glucose results (urine glucose is not a reliable means of assessing blood glucose) and evaluation of urine ketones can provide the physician with valuable data to effectively manage the treatment of the individual.

Complications associated with diabetes mellitus

Peripheral vascular disease. The person with diabetes mellitus is more likely to suffer from peripheral vascular disease than the general population. Reduced blood supply to the extremities may result in intermittent claudication, numbness and tingling, and a greater likelihood of foot infections, chronic skin ulcers, and gangrene.

Assessment of tissue oxygenation. Observe the color of each hand, finger, leg, and foot; report cyanosis or reddish-blue discolorations. Inspect the skin of the extremities for any signs of ulceration.

TEMPERATURE. Feel the temperature in each hand, finger, leg, and foot. Report paleness and coldness. Note that these symptoms will be increased if the limbs are elevated above the level of the heart.

EDEMA. Report edema, its extent, and whether relieved or unchanged when in a dependent position.

PERIPHERAL PULSES. Record the pedal and radial pulses at least every 4 hours if circulatory impairment is found in that limb. Compare findings between each of the extremities. Report diminished or absent pulses immediately.

LIMB PAIN. Monitor pain in the patient carefully. Pain with exercise that is relieved by rest may be from claudication.

CARE. Prevent ulcers, injury, and infection in the lower extremities with meticulous, regular care. See also General Nursing Consideration for Patients with Peripheral Vascular Disease in Chapter 11.

Visual alterations. Visual changes are common in the patient with diabetes mellitus. These individuals frequently suffer from blurred vision associated with an elevated blood sugar. People known to be diabetic who complain to the nurse of intermittently blurred vision should be referred to their physician for a check of the blood sugar level. Once the hyperglycemia is controlled, the blurred vision usually clears.

Ask specific questions to elicit information on any visual problems that the patient may be experiencing. If visual impairment is present, plan for an appropriate degree of intervention. Special equipment is available for the visually impaired diabetic patient.

BLINDNESS. In advanced stages of diabetes mellitus, the patient may suffer from changes (microangiopathies) in the small blood vessels of the eyes. Retinal hemorrhages, degeneration of retinal vascular tissue, cataracts, and eventual blindness may occur. The diabetic patient should have regular eye exams to allow early treatment of any apparent alterations.

Renal disease. Patients with diabetes may develop microangiopathies in the kidneys. Be alert for the development of proteinuria and elevations in serum creatinine and blood urea nitrogen levels. Report these to the physician. Persons with diabetes mellitus are also more susceptible to urinary tract infections; therefore, symptoms such as burning on urination should be evaluated promptly.

Infection. Any type of infection can cause a significant loss of control of diabetes mellitus. Observe carefully for any signs of redness, tenderness, swelling, or drainage which occurs when there is any break in the skin. Patients should be taught to report immediately early signs of infection, such as fever or sore throat.

During an infection, the dosage of insulin may require an adjustment to compensate for a change in metabolic rate, diet, and exercise.

Neuropathies. A complication of diabetes mellitus is degeneration of nerves, usually in the extremities. Ask the patient to describe any sensations, such as numbness or tingling, being experienced in the extremities. Inspect the feet for blisters, ingrown toenails, or sores. Occasionally the patient will not be aware of these lesions due to the degeneration of nerves in the area.

Always test the water temperature before immersing a limb of a diabetic patient. Due to impaired sensation, the patient may be easily burned and unaware of it until later.

Neuropathies can also affect the autonomic nervous system. Patients with diabetes mellitus should always be closely assessed if nausea, diarrhea, constipation, or visual disturbances develop.

Discharge planning

Before discharge, the patient must achieve a high degree of understanding of diabetes mellitus and its management. The patient and family members need to be included in the total educational program.

With the advent of shorter hospitalizations, it may be necessary to incorporate follow-up care by a visiting nurse association or a home health agency in the discharge planning.

The patient must understand the following:

- Recognition of the symptoms of hyperglycemia and hypoglycemia
- How to properly substitute foods to maintain a balance between nutritional requirements and insulin administration
- Self-monitoring of blood glucose and testing of urine for glucose and ketones; time, recording, and interpretation of the results
- Injection technique and care of the equipment
- Medication preparation, dosage, frequency, storage, and refilling
- Appropriate hygiene and care of minor wounds
- Importance of continual follow-up care to evaluate the degree of blood glucose control
- Management of insulin and/or oral hypoglycemic agent, food, and fluids during illness

Provide psychological support and guidance for the patient and family. Give them every opportunity to ask questions concerning the patient's care. Reassess and reinforce the analysis of symptoms they should watch for and appropriate actions to take for complications that may develop.

Support the family members as they learn to cope with the integration of the diabetic's needs into the family, the job setting, or school.

Patient Education Associated with the Control of Diabetes Mellitus

Communication and responsibility. Encourage open communication concerning frustrations and anger as the patient attempts to adjust to the diagnosis and the need for prolonged treatment. The patient must be guided to insight into the disorder in order to assume responsibility for the continuation of treatment. Keep emphasizing those factors the patient can control to alter progression of the disease, including maintenance of general health, nutritional needs, adequate rest and appropriate exercise, and continuation of the prescribed medication therapy.

Smoking. Smoking causes vasoconstriction of blood vessels, aggravating microangiopathies associated with diabetes mellitus. Patients who smoke should be encouraged to quit.

Nutritional needs. Explain the entire dietary prescription to the patient and family. Be certain to teach the dietary requirements of the patient to the person who will prepare the food.

Emphasize to the patient the importance of eating all of the prescribed foods at the proper times in order to cover the peak action of insulin or oral hypoglycemic therapy. Patients must understand how to properly substitute foods from the exchange lists to maintain a balance between nutritional requirements and insulin administration. Review with the patient the most common time when their particular drug regimen may cause hypoglycemia.

People who are readmitted for treatment should be reevaluated for both nutritional knowledge as well as for general understanding of all aspects of diabetic management. Never presume compliance or competence simply because the patient has long been diagnosed as a diabetic.

Activity and exercise. The prescribed diet and medication are carefully calculated to maintain the individual's lifestyle. Encourage the patient to report any major change in planned activity level so that appropriate adjustment can be made. Activities, such as changing from a sedentary job to one with physical labor, or starting to participate regularly in a strenuous sport, should be reported. The patient should also report discontinuation of a vigorous sport or a change to a more sedentary job.

Personal hygiene. Explain the importance of maintaining personal hygiene. Encourage the patient to cleanse even a slight injury with soap and water and apply a topical antibiotic to the area. Instruct the patient not to use antiseptics that could cause skin irritations.

Teach patients to inspect their feet for developing callouses, blisters, sores, and ingrown toenails. Emphasize the importance of good foot care and properly fitting shoes to minimize complications.

Encourage the patient not to self-treat corns, callouses, or ingrown toenails. Products used for these problems may cause further damage due to vasoconstriction and are specifically contraindicated in patients with diabetes mellitus. (See also General Nursing Considerations for Patients with Peripheral Vascular Disease in Chapter 11.)

Infections. Encourage the patient to report immediately any signs of redness, tenderness, swelling, or draining which might occur where any break in the skin is located. Also report wounds that are slow in healing.

Avoid exposure to people known to have infections.

Psychological considerations. Stress that learning to manage the entire disease process is the best means of preventing complications. Foster the idea that the individual can control many aspects of the disease by careful management of diet, medications, and activities.

Encourage individuals to return to as normal a lifestyle as possible. Help patients develop schedules that fit their pattern of life: are the patients late risers or early risers; do they work the midnight shift; do they play a vigorous sport three or four times a week?

Urine testing for ketones. Teach the patient to perform urine testing for ketones. The patient should test the urine for ketones at least four times daily during times of stress, infection, or when signs or symptoms of hyperglycemia are present or suspected. (Ketone testing should be done when the blood glucose level is 240 mg/dl or above.) The physician may suggest additional times when ketones should be monitored depending on the type of regimen prescribed for control of the blood glucose. An accurate written record of the results should be maintained. Guidelines for reporting abnormal results to the physician should be discussed at the time of discharge.

Self-monitoring of blood glucose. Home blood glucose monitoring (self-monitoring) is an accepted practice for the management of diabetes mellitus. It is used to evaluate the degree of control of the blood glucose being obtained. It can also be used to evaluate when additional insulin needs to be taken or to determine the effect of exercise on insulin needs.

A small sample of capillary blood is obtained, generally using an automatic finger-sticking lancet. The blood sample is applied to a reagent strip, which is then placed in an electronic device that "reads" the amount of color change and converts this into a numerical value representing the blood glucose level present. There also are meters and sensors (that do not use reagent strips) for delivering the glucose results. "Talking" glucometers are on the market for persons who are visually impaired. Written records of the blood glucose results should be maintained and taken to all follow-up visits with the physician for analysis.

Before leaving the hospital, the patient should be taught to perform the blood testing according to the directions accompanying the glucose monitor that will be used at home.

Additional testing for the degree of control of the blood glucose will be evaluated through periodic scheduling of the following tests:

1. Glycosylated hemoglobin (hemoglobin A_{1c}, or glycohemoglobin). This test measures the percent of hemoglobin that has been irreversibly glycosylated due to high blood sugar levels. This provides a reflection of the average blood sugar level attained over the past 8 to 10 weeks.
2. Fructosamine test that measures amount of glucose bonded to a protein, fructosamine. This reflects the average blood level attained over the past 1 to 3 weeks.

Expectations of therapy. Discuss the expectations of therapy (such as level of exercise, expectations for relief of symptoms, frequency of therapy use, degree of limitations, ability to maintain activities of daily living and/or work). If permanent visual impairment, atherosclerosis, or neuropathy are evident, discuss measures to control these factors.

Changes in expectations. Assess changes in expectations as therapy progresses and the patient gains understanding and skill in the management of the diagnosis.

Role-play aspects of the patient's care with the patient or family (such as insulin preparation, urine tests, self-injection, control of hypoglycemic or hyperglycemic reactions). Have the participants practice by repeating the appropriate intervention for the presenting problem.

Changes in therapy through cooperative goalsetting. Work with the patient to encourage adherence to the prescribed treatment. When the patient feels that a change should be made in a treatment plan, encourage discussion with the physician.

Written record. Enlist the patient's aid in developing and maintaining a written record of monitoring parameters (such as urine or blood glucose, insulin dosage, pertinent stress factors, exercise level, illnesses, or major changes in diet or other routine) for discussion with the physician (see Figure 16-1). Patients should be encouraged to take this record on follow-up visits.

Fostering compliance. Throughout the hospitalization, discuss medication information and how it will benefit the course of treatment. Seek cooperation and understanding of the following points so that medication compliance may be enhanced:

Patient Education and Monitoring of Therapeutic Outcomes for Patients Receiving Antidiabetic Agents

Medications	Color	To be taken

Name _____

Physician _____

Physician's phone _____

Next appt.* _____

	Parameters	Day of discharge							Comments
Insulin/Oral agent Types: AM PM	Temperature / Weight								
	Site AM / Site PM								
	Units AM / Units PM								
Urine:(use 2nd voided specimen) Sugar/Acetone	Before breakfast								
	Before lunch								
	Before supper								
	Bedtime								
Blood Glucose levels: Insert time (e.g, 1 PM)	Before breakfast: After breakfast:								
	Before Lunch: After lunch:								
	Before Supper: After Supper:								
	Bedtime:								
	Other:								
Diet	Eat all foods allowed								
	Unable to eat								
	Overate or indulged								
Lifestyle	Usual daily activities/exercise								
	Increased amount of exercise								
	Increased stress								
	Normal day-to-day stress								
Injuries or skin integrity	No visible changes in skin of feet								
	Cuts, bruises, open sores								
Hypoglycemia	Sx: Sweating, weak, shaky, hungry								
	Blood Glucose level: Time:								
Hyperglycemia	Sx: Urinating frequently, poor appetite, ↑ thirst, weak, dizzy								
	Blood Glucose level: Time:								

*Please bring this record with you to your next appointment.
Use the back of this sheet for additional information.

Figure 16-1 *Patient education and monitoring of therapeutic outcomes for patients receiving antidiabetic agents.*

1. Name: Be sure that the patient or family member is able to repeat the name of the type of insulin, and the onset, peak, and duration of the insulin or oral hypoglycemic agent prescribed. No change in insulin type, concentration, or brand should be made without medical supervision.
2. Dosage: Instruct the patient about the exact dosage of the prescription, and allow the patient to practice preparation and administration of insulin as ordered.
3. Route and administration times (see Chapters 5, 6, and 7 on administration of medications): Be sure that the patient understands how to administer insulin or oral hypoglycemic agents. If the patient is on a sliding scale of insulin, based on urine or blood glucose values, be certain the patient understands the sliding scale and the amount of *regular* insulin prescribed.
4. Anticipated therapeutic responses: Diabetes is controlled within normal limits of the blood sugar level.
5. Side effects to expect: Fairly constant control of the diabetes with minimal side effects should be expected when the diet and prescription for insulin or oral hypoglycemia agents are followed.
6. Side effects to report: Occasional episodes of hypo- or hyperglycemia may occur if illness, stress, or infection is present, or if there is significant variation in diet or exercise. Frequent episodes should be reported to the physician for adjustment in therapy. (See above for treatment of hypo- or hyperglycemia.)
7. What to do if a dose is missed: A diabetic patient cannot miss a dose of insulin and not develop hyperglycemia. A balanced diet, exercise level, and insulin dosage are crucial to the well-being of the diabetic patient.
8. When, how, or if to refill the medication prescription: Be sure that the patient understands how to refill prescriptions for insulin or oral hypoglycemic agents. When purchasing insulin, have the patient double-check the type and concentration (usually U-100) of insulin and the expiration date. The insulin should be stored in the refrigerator (not the freezer) prior to use. Once it is opened and being used, it can be stored at room temperature.

Difficulty in comprehension. If it is evident that the patient and/or family does not understand all aspects of the continuing therapy being prescribed (such as administration and monitoring of medications, exercises, diets, follow-up appointments) consider the use of social service or visiting nurse agencies.

Associated teaching. Always inform the physician or dentist of any prescription or over-the-counter medication being taken. Over-the-counter medications should not be taken without first discussing them with a physician or pharmacist. Medications such as aspirin and ascorbic acid can interfere with urine testing procedures. When necessary, ask the pharmacist for sugar-free products.

Always report side effects of rash, itching, or hives immediately. Diabetics just starting insulin therapy are more susceptible to allergic reactions at the site of injection. A change in source of insulin may be required.

TAKE ALL OF THE MEDICATION AS PRESCRIBED FOR THE FULL COURSE OF TREATMENT. Do not discontinue use when feeling improved; do not give your medicine to another individual. Sudden discontinuation of certain medications may produce harmful effects.

Keep all medications out of reach of children.

If pregnancy is suspected, consult an obstetrician as soon as possible about continuation of medication therapy and necessary adjustment during pregnancy.

At discharge. Develop a list of specific equipment and supplies the patient will need when discharged. Keep in mind the cost of these supplies. Consider the following:

1. Syringes: Disposable syringes are convenient and presterilized, but are more expensive. (Be sure to tell the patient that disposable syringes are to be used once and then discarded.) Reusable syringes are less expensive, more easily read, and, in some instances, paid for by insurance coverage.
2. Needles: Disposable needles are more convenient, but also more expensive. Stainless steel needles are easily resterilized and reused, but eventually become dull and must be discarded.

   Patients usually use a 26 or 27 gauge, ½ inch needle, but needles should be adjusted to the individual. An obese patient may require a 1 to 1½ inch needle length to properly inject the insulin. Specialty needles with a very fine needle size (28 and 29 gauge) are now available.
3. Specialized equipment: Magni-Guides are available for the visually impaired patient. This aid holds the vial of insulin, acts as a guide in withdrawing insulin, and has a magnifying glass to make reading the syringe scale easier. Special automatic insulin syringes are available for blind patients. A "talking" glucose measuring device is also available for the visually impaired individual to perform self-monitoring of the capillary blood glucose levels.

   Whenever possible, have the family purchase any reusable products the patient will be using. Vary teaching techniques to include the actual equipment the person will use at home.
4. Reusable syringes and needles: Reusable syringes and needles are seldom seen in use today; however when used, teach proper sterilization techniques, including the following: Separate and clean the syringe parts and needles. Place in a strainer in a pan with sufficient water to completely cover all the equipment. Boil for 10 minutes and then remove from the water by lifting the strainer. Once cool, assem-

ble the syringe parts. Store equipment immersed in 91% isopropyl alcohol in a syringe storage container, available at the pharmacy. If stored in this manner, allow to air dry before using with insulin.

If the patient is unable to boil the equipment (such as when traveling), wash all parts thoroughly and then completely immerse them in 91% isopropyl alcohol for 5 to 10 minutes. Allow to air dry thoroughly prior to using for insulin administration.

Items to be sent home with the patient should include the following:

1. Written instructions for use
2. Labels in language and size of print appropriate for the patient
3. If needed, identification cards or bracelets
4. A list of additional supplies to be purchased after discharge (such as syringes, needles, alcohol, cotton balls, insulin, dressings)
5. A schedule for follow-up appointments

Drug Therapy for Diabetes Mellitus

Insulins

OBJECTIVES

1. Explain the role of insulin in the body.
2. Identify the site where insulin is produced.
3. Describe the potential causes of hypoglycemia.
4. State the signs, symptoms, and treatment of an allergic reaction to insulin.
5. Identify the purposes of using a rotation plan for the injection sites for insulin.
6. Describe the onset, peak, and duration of fast-acting, intermediate-acting, and long-acting insulins.
7. Review reading the calibrations on an insulin syringe.
8. Practice preparing two types of insulin in the same syringe.
9. Describe the possible side effects of dehydration on an insulin-dependent diabetic.

KEY WORDS

hyperlipidemia	ketosis
acidosis	desensitization
ketoacidosis	lipodystrophy

Insulin is a hormone produced in the beta cells of the pancreas and is a key regulator of metabolism. Insulins from the pancreases of different animals have similar activity and thus may be used in human beings. Insulin is required for the entry of glucose into skeletal and heart muscle and fat. It also plays a significant role in protein and lipid metabolism. It is not required for glucose transport into the brain or liver tissue.

Insulin deficiency reduces the rate of transport of glucose into cells, producing hyperglycemia. Other metabolic reactions are also inhibited by the lack of insulin, resulting in the conversion of protein to glucose, hyperlipidemia, ketosis, and acidosis.

Insulin was discovered by Sir Frederick Banting, Charles Best, and John Macleod of Toronto, Canada, and was first made available to the public in 1922. Several preparations of insulin isolated from beef and pork pancreas and a biosynthetic form similar to human insulin are now commercially available.

Side effects. Insulin overdose or decreased carbohydrate intake may result in hypoglycemia. If untreated, irreversible brain damage may occur. Hypoglycemia occurs most frequently when the administered insulin reaches its peak action (see Table 16-2). Hypoglycemia must be treated immediately. The following conditions may predispose a diabetic patient to a hypoglycemic (insulin) reaction: improper measurement of insulin dosage, excessive exercise, insufficient food intake, concurrent ingestion of hypoglycemic drugs and discontinuation of drugs (see Drug Interactions), or conditions (such as infection or stress) causing hyperglycemia.

Allergic reactions, manifested by itching, redness, and swelling at the site of injection are common occurrences in patients beginning insulin therapy. These reactions may be caused by modifying proteins in NPH insulin, the insulin itself, the alcohol used to cleanse the injection site or sterilize the syringe, the patient's injection technique, or the intermittent use of insulin. Spontaneous desensitization frequently occurs within a few weeks. Local irritation may be reduced by changing to insulin without protein modifiers (the Lente series) or to insulins derived from another source; using unscented alcohol swabs or disposable syringes and needles; and checking the patient's injection technique. Acute rashes covering the whole body and anaphylactic symptoms are quite rare, but must be treated with antihistamines, epinephrine, and steroids.

Rotation of injection sites is important. Atrophy or hypertrophy of subcutaneous fat tissue may occur at the site of frequent insulin injections. The hypertrophic areas tend to be used more frequently by diabetic patients because the fat pad becomes anesthetized. In addition to the adverse cosmetic effects, the absorption rate of insulin from these sites becomes significantly prolonged and erratic. Loss of diabetic control may result, particularly in unstable, Type I diabetes.

Insulin resistance is an infrequent complication in the control of diabetic symptoms. Acute resistance may develop if the patient acquires an infection or experiences serious trauma, surgery, or emotional disturbances. This type of resistance subsides when the acute episode passes. Chronic insulin resistance may occur with the reinstitution of insulin therapy after a period of discontinuance. Resistance may be reduced by changing the animal sources of the insulin, using "purified" insulins, changing the use of glucocorticoids, or

Table 16-2 Commercially Available Forms of Insulin

TYPE OF INSULIN	MANUFACTURER	STRENGTH (UNITS/ML)	SOURCE	IMPURITIES (PPM)	ONSET (HR)	PEAK (HR)	DURATION* (HR)	GLYCOSURIA†	HYPOGLYCEMIA†
Fast-acting insulin injection									
Humulin R (human)	Lilly	100	Semisynthetic	—	0.5-4	2.5-5	5-16	Early AM(1)	Before lunch(3)
Novolin R (human)	Novo Nordisk	100	Semisynthetic	—	0.5-4	2.5-5	5-16	Early AM	Before lunch
Regular (purified pork) insulin	Novo Nordisk	100	Pork	<10	0.5	2.5-5	8	Early AM	Before lunch
Regular insulin	Novo Nordisk	100	Pork	<25	0.5-1	3-6	6-8	Early AM	Before lunch
Regular Iletin I	Lilly	100	Beef and pork	<25	0.5-1	3-6	6-8	Early AM	Before lunch
Regular Iletin II (Beef)	Lilly	100	Beef	<10	0.5-1	3-6	6-8	Early AM	Before lunch
Regular Iletin II (Pork)	Lilly	100, 500	Pork	<10	0.5-1	3-6	6-8	Early AM	Before lunch
Velosulin	Novo Nordisk	100	Pork	<10	0.5	1-3	8	Early AM	Before lunch
Velosulin (human)	Novo Nordisk	100	Semisynthetic	—	0.5	1-3	8	Early AM	Before lunch
Prompt insulin zinc suspension									
Semilente Iletin I ("new")	Lilly	100	Beef and pork	<25	0.5-1	4-6	12-16	Early AM	Before lunch
Semilente insulin	Novo Nordisk	100	Beef	<25	0.5-1	4-6	12-16	Early AM	Before lunch
Intermediate-acting isophane insulin suspension (NPH)									
Humulin N (NPH)	Lilly	100	Semisynthetic	—	1-4	4-12	16-28	Before lunch(2)	3 PM to supper(3)
Insulatard (NPH)	Novo Nordisk	100	Pork	<10	1.5	4-12	24	Before lunch	3 PM to supper
Insulatard (NPH) human	Novo Nordisk	100	Semisynthetic	—	1.5	4-12	24	Before lunch	3 PM to supper
Novolin N (human)	Novo Nordisk	100	Semisynthetic	—	1-4	4-12	16-28	Before lunch	3 PM to supper
NPH Insulin	Novo Nordisk	100	Beef	<10	1-1.5	8-12	24	Before lunch	3 PM to supper
NPH Iletin I	Lilly	100	Beef and pork	<25	1-1.5	8-12	24	Before lunch	3 PM to supper
NPH Iletin II	Lilly	100	Beef or pork	<10	1-1.5	8-12	24	Before lunch	3 PM to supper
NPH (purified pork) insulin	Novo Nordisk	100	Pork	<10	1.5	4-12	24	Before lunch	3 PM to supper
Isophane insulin suspension and insulin injection									
Humulin 70/30	Lilly	100	Semisynthetic	—	0.5	4-12	24	Before lunch	3 PM to supper
Mixtard	Novo Nordisk	100	Pork	<10	0.5	4-8	24	Before lunch	3 PM to supper
Novolin 70/30 (human)	Novo Nordisk	100	Semisynthetic	—	0.5	4-12	24	Before lunch	3 PM to supper
Insulin zinc suspension									
Humulin L	Lilly	100	Semisynthetic	—	1-4	7-15	16-28	Before lunch	3 PM to supper
Lente Iletin I	Lilly	100	Beef and pork	<25	1-1.5	8-12	24	Before lunch	3 PM to supper
Lente Iletin II	Lilly	100	Beef or pork	<10	1-1.5	8-12	24	Before lunch	3 PM to supper
Lente insulin	Novo Nordisk	40, 100	Beef	<10	1-1.5	8-12	24	Before lunch	3 PM to supper
Lente (purified pork) insulin	Novo Nordisk	100	Pork	<10	2.5	7-15	22	Before lunch	3 PM to supper
Novolin L (human)	Novo Nordisk	100	Semisynthetic	—	1-4	7-15	16-28	Before lunch	3 PM to supper
Extended insulin zinc suspension									
Humulin U Ultralente	Lilly	100	Semisynthetic	—	4-8	12-18	24-28	Supper to bedtime	2 AM to breakfast
Ultralente Iletin I	Lilly	100	Beef and pork	<25	4-8	16-18	36†	Supper to bedtime	2 AM to breakfast
Ultralente insulin	Novo Nordisk	100	Beef	<25	4-8	16-18	36†	Supper to bedtime	2 AM to breakfast

*The times listed are averages based on a newly diagnosed diabetic patient. Factors modifying these times include patient variation, site and route of administration, and dosage.
†Most frequently occurs when insulin is administered at (1) bedtime the previous night; (2) before breakfast the previous day; (3) before breakfast the same day.

using specially prepared insulins with a slightly different chemical structure.

Availability. See Table 16-2.

Over the past decade, significant progress has been made in improving the purity of insulin in an attempt to reduce allergenicity. Conventional insulins have always contained varying concentrations, greater than 10,000 parts per million (ppm), of proinsulin, glucagon, somatostatin, and other proteins from the pancreas. The FDA has named the more highly refined products, with less than 10 ppm of proinsulin, as "purified." All conventional insulins are now "cleaner," with less than 25 ppm of proinsulin content (see Table 16-2). Because purified insulins are more expensive and in limited supply, their use should be restricted to patients with specific indications, such as those using insulin for a short period of time (for example, gestational diabetics, Type II diabetics undergoing surgery, nondiabetics receiving insulin as part of hyperalimentation solutions), patients with insulin resistance (using more than 100 to 200 units per day), patients with local cutaneous allergic reactions, patients with significant lipodystrophy, patients with renal transplants, and patients desensitized to pork insulin. The response is highly variable, but patients usually require less insulin.

Biosynthetic human insulin is now available for selected patients. Onset of action may be slightly more rapid than pork insulin and it is expected to have fewer allergic reactions associated with it than beef and pork insulins. The primary long-range advantage of human insulin is that a new source of insulin is now available to help meet a predicted worldwide shortage in the next decade.

All preparations of insulin (except biosynthetic insulin) are extracted from animal pancreas. The predominant sources are beef and pork, but sheep and fish may also be used. The extract is bioassayed, and the potencies are adjusted to provide concentrations of 100 units/ml (U-100) or 500 units/ml (U-500). Insulin can be modified by adding protein or protamine or by precipitating it in varying concentrations of zinc chloride. Depending on the amount of protamine used, and the type of crystals, insulin can be adjusted to have a short, intermediate, or long duration of action. See Table 16-2 for a comparison of commercially available forms of insulin.

Types of insulin

- *Regular insulin* is used for its immediate onset of activity and short duration of action. It is the only form of insulin that is a clear solution (not a cloudy suspension). Also, it is the *only* dosage form of insulin that may be injected by *intravenous* as well as *subcutaneous* routes of administration. See Table 16-2 for the activity of the regular insulins and Table 16-3 for mixing compatibility with other insulins.
- *Lente insulins* are derived from a manufacturing pro-

Table 16-3 *Compatibility of Insulin Combinations*

COMBINATION	RATIO	MIX BEFORE ADMINISTRATION
Regular + NPH	Any combination	2 to 3 months
Regular + Lente	Any combination	Immediately*
Regular + PZI+	1:1 = action like PZI alone	Immediately
	2:1 = action like NPH	Immediately
	3:1 = action like NPH + regular	Immediately
Lentes	Any combination	Stable indefinitely

*Must be used immediately to retain properties of regular insulin.
+PZI contains excess protamine that binds with regular insulin, prolonging the activity of regular insulin. Regular and PZI should not be mixed but administered at separate sites at approximately the same time.

cess that produces two physical forms, one crystalline and the other noncrystalline. The long-acting, crystalline form is marketed as *Ultralente;* the noncrystalline, fast acting compound is available as *Semilente.* The intermediate-acting *Lente* insulin is a mixture containing approximately 30% noncrystalline Semilente and 70% crystalline Ultralente insulins.
- *Neutral protamine hagedorn (NPH) insulin* is an intermediate-acting insulin containing specific amounts of insulin and protamine. The activity of NPH is similar to that of a mixture of regular insulin and protamine zinc insulin (see Tables 16-2 and 16-3).

Storage of insulin. It is recommended that, whenever possible, insulin be stored under refrigerated conditions. A vial of insulin at room temperature for 1 month can lose about 1.5% of its potency. At temperatures above 86° F, insulins lose potency much more rapidly.

Dosage and administration

Maintenance therapy for newly diagnosed diabetic patients. After ketoacidosis and hyperglycemia have been controlled and the patient can tolerate oral feedings, determine the total amount of regular insulin needed in 24 hours. The usual initial dose is 10 to 20 units of regular insulin, SC. Subsequent doses, administered one-half hour before meals and at bedtime, are based on blood glucose and urine glucose levels. After control is established, the patient is converted to intermediate acting insulin, administered in doses that are 65% to 75% of the total dose of regular insulin required in 24 hours. Regular insulin is used as a supplement based on blood or urine glucose levels. Adjustments in the intermediate-acting insulin doses will be necessary. Divided doses (two-thirds in the morning, one-third in the evening) or combination therapy, using a mixture of insulins (see Table 16-3), may be required to maintain control, especially after the patient leaves the hospital and has changes in exercise and diet.

Maintenance therapy for known diabetic patients. Once ketoacidosis and hyperglycemia have been controlled and the patient can tolerate oral feedings, initiate maintenance therapy of one-half to two-thirds the previous dose of intermediate-acting or combination insulin. Regular insulin is given as a supplement when indicated by blood sugar and urine glucose determinations. Adjust the maintenance dose of insulin until optimal control is achieved for the patient.

NOTE: "Control" of diabetic hyperglycemia is usually easier in the hospital than on an outpatient basis. Adjustments are almost always necessary after discharge due to changes in exercise and diet. Some physicians will allow patients to "spill," or exceed, a ¾% to 1% urine glucose while in the hospital so that after discharge a patient will spill a trace to ¼% as a result of changes in routine. Other physicians will stabilize a patient to a trace to ¼% urine glucose while in the hospital and drop the insulin dosage 5 units on discharge. There is less chance of a hypoglycemic reaction when using the second method, but regardless of the treatment program used, the discharged patient will have to be monitored frequently for medical and emotional adjustment to the new disease.

• **Nursing Interventions: Monitoring insulin therapy**

See also General Nursing Considerations for Patients with Diabetes Mellitus (p. 383).

Three terms (*onset, peak,* and *duration*) are associated with the use of insulin therapy. *Onset* is the time required for the medication to have an initial effect or action; *peak* is when the agent will have the maximum effect; and *duration* is the length of time that the agent remains active in the body. When monitoring insulin therapy, it is quite important to understand these terms and to associate them with the type of insulin being administered to ascertain when a patient is most susceptible to hyperglycemia or hypoglycemia (see Table 16-2).

Side effects to expect and report

HYPERGLYCEMIA. Diabetic or prediabetic patients need to be monitored for the development of hyperglycemia, particularly during the early weeks of therapy.

Assess regularly for abnormal blood glucose and in certain patients, as requested by the physician, for glycosuria and ketones. If symptoms occur frequently, the physician should be notified and the written records maintained by the patient that reflect the results of self-testing should be supplied to the physician for analysis.

Patients receiving insulin may require an adjustment in dosage.

HYPOGLYCEMIA. Monitor for the following signs of hypoglycemia: headache, nausea, weakness, hunger, lethargy, decreased coordination, general apprehension, sweating, blurred or double vision.

Hypoglycemia must be treated immediately. Mild symptoms may be controlled by the oral administration of a glucose source—for example, lump of sugar, or-

ange juice, carbonated cola beverage (not diet), candy (not chocolate)—or ingestion of a commercially prepared substance such as Glutose. Severe symptoms may be relieved by the administration of intravenous glucose, and parenteral glucagon may be prescribed in some instances. If in doubt about whether the patient is hypoglycemic or hyperglycemic, always treat the individual for hypoglycemia to prevent the possible neurologic complications that can occur from untreated hypoglycemia.

ALLERGIC REACTIONS. See Side Effects above. Notify the physician if allergic signs appear. Also check the patient's injection technique.

LIPODYSTROPHIES. Rotation of injection sites is important. Atrophy or hypertrophy of subcutaneous fat tissue may occur at the site of frequent insulin injections. The hypertrophic areas tend to be used more frequently by diabetic patients because the fat pad becomes anesthetized. In addition to the adverse cosmetic effects, the absorption rate of insulin from these sites becomes significantly prolonged and erratic. Loss of diabetic control may result, particularly in unstable Type I patients.

Implementation

MIXING INSULINS. See Chapter 6.

ADMINISTRATION TECHNIQUES. See Chapter 7.

Drug interactions

HYPERGLYCEMIA. The following drugs may cause hyperglycemia (especially in prediabetic and diabetic patients); insulin dosages may require adjustment: acetazolamide, ethanol, corticosteroids, glucagon, dextrothyroxine, lithium, diuretics (thiazides, furosemide, bumetanide), oral contraceptives, diazoxide, phenothiazines, dobutamine, phenytoin, epinephrine, salicylates.

Diabetic or prediabetic patients need to be monitored for the development of hyperglycemia, particularly during the early weeks of therapy.

Assess regularly for glycosuria and report if it occurs with any frequency.

HYPOGLYCEMIA. The following drugs may cause hypoglycemia, thereby decreasing insulin requirements, in diabetic patients: acetaminophen, anabolic steroids (Dianabol, Durabolin), guanethidine, monoamine-oxidase inhibitors, propranolol, salicylates.

Monitor for the following signs of hypoglycemia: headache, nausea, weakness, hunger, lethargy, decreased coordination, general apprehension, sweating, blurred or double vision.

Notify the physician if any of the above symptoms appear.

BETA ADRENERGIC BLOCKING AGENTS. Beta adrenergic blocking agents (propranolol, timolol, nadolol, pindolol, others) may induce hypoglycemia, but may also mask many of the symptoms of hypoglycemia. Notify the physician if you suspect that any of the above symptoms appear intermittently.

Oral hypoglycemic agents
OBJECTIVES

1. Compare the actions of insulin and oral hypoglycemic agents.
2. Explain why insulin cannot be taken orally.
3. Describe criteria for administration of oral hypoglycemic agents rather than insulin by injection.
4. Identify the onset, peak, and duration of the oral hypoglycemic agents.
5. Discuss the possible effect of ingesting alcohol while taking oral sulfonylureas.

All of the oral hypoglycemic agents currently available are sulfonylureas. Sulfonylureas produce hypoglycemia by stimulating the release of insulin from the beta cells of the pancreas. They are of no value in the Type I diabetic, but are effective in Type II diabetic patients where the pancreas still has the capacity to secrete insulin. Sulfonylureas may be effective in the treatment of Type II diabetes mellitus that cannot be controlled by diet alone if the patient is not susceptible to developing ketosis, acidosis, or infections. Patients most likely to benefit from oral hypoglycemic treatment are those who develop signs of diabetes after age 40 and who require less than 40 units of insulin per day.

Side effects. Patients receiving oral hypoglycemic therapy are as susceptible to hypoglycemia as diabetic patients on insulin therapy. Consequently, blood sugar levels and urine sugar levels must be monitored closely, especially in the early stages of therapy.

Side effects of sulfonylureas are infrequent and generally mild. The more common adverse reactions include allergic skin reactions and gastrointestinal symptoms of nausea, vomiting, anorexia, heartburn, and abdominal cramps. Blood dyscrasias, hepatotoxicity, and hypersensitivity reactions have rarely been reported. Sulfonylureas generally should not be administered to patients allergic to sulfonamides. They may also be allergic to sulfonylureas.

Availability. See Table 16-4.

Dosage and administration. See Table 16-4.

Individual dosage adjustment is essential for the suc-cessful use of oral hypoglycemic agents. A patient should be given a 1-month trial on maximum doses of the sulfonylurea being used before the patient can be considered a primary failure. If a patient represents a secondary failure (a patient initially controlled on oral agents), changing to an alternative sulfonylurea is occasionally successful in controlling blood sugar.

• Nursing Interventions: Monitoring sulfonylurea therapy

See also General Nursing Considerations for Patients with Diabetes Mellitus (p. 383).

Side effects to expect

NAUSEA, VOMITING, ANOREXIA, ABDOMINAL CRAMPS. These side effects are usually mild and tend to resolve with continued therapy. Encourage the patient not to discontinue therapy without first consulting the physician.

Side effects to report

HYPOGLYCEMIA. Monitor for the following signs of hypoglycemia: headache, nausea, weakness, hunger, lethargy, decreased coordination, general apprehension, sweating, blurred or double vision.

Hypoglycemia must be treated immediately. Mild symptoms may be controlled by the oral administration of a glucose source—for example, lump of sugar, orange juice, carbonated cola beverage (not diet), candy (not chocolate)—or ingestion of a commercially prepared substance such as Glutose.® Severe symptoms may be relieved by the administration of intravenous glucose, and parenteral glucagon may be prescribed in some instances. If in doubt about whether the patient is hypoglycemic or hyperglycemic, always treat the individual for hypoglycemia to prevent the possible neurologic complications that can occur from untreated hypoglycemia.

Notify the physician immediately if any of the above symptoms appear. The dosage of oral hypoglycemic agents may also have to be reduced.

HEPATOTOXICITY. The symptoms of hepatotoxicity are: anorexia, nausea, vomiting, jaundice, hepatomegaly, splenomegaly, and abnormal liver function tests (ele-

Table 16-4 *Oral Hypoglycemic Agents*

GENERIC NAME	BRAND NAME	AVAILABILITY	INITIAL DOSAGE	DOSAGE RANGE	DURATION* (HOURS)
First generation					
Acetohexamide	Dymelor, ♣Dimelor	Tablets: 250, 500 mg	0.5 g daily	0.25-1.5 g daily	12-18
Chlorpropamide	Diabinese	Tablets: 100, 250 mg	100 mg daily	100-750 mg daily	24-72
Tolazamide	Tolinase	Tablets: 100, 250, 500 mg	100 mg daily	0.1-1 g daily	12-16
Tolbutamide	Orinase, Oramide	Tablets: 250, 500 mg	1 g 2 times daily	0.25-3 g daily	6-12
Second generation					
Glipizide	Glucotrol	Tablets: 5, 10 mg	2.5-5 mg daily	15-40 mg daily	10-24
Glyburide	DiaBeta, Micronase	Tablets: 1.5, 2.5, 5 mg	2.5-5 mg daily	1.25-20 mg daily	24

*The times listed are averages based on a newly diagnosed diabetic patient. Factors modifying these times include patient variation and dosage.
♣Available in Canada only.

vated bilirubin, AST, ALT, GGT, alkaline phosphatase, prothrombin time).

BLOOD DYSCRASIAS. Routine laboratory studies (RBC, WBC, and differential counts) should be scheduled. Stress the need to return for this laboratory work.

Monitor for the development of a sore throat, fever, purpura, jaundice, or excessive and progressively increasing weakness.

DERMATOLOGIC REACTIONS. Report a rash or pruritus immediately. Withhold additional doses pending approval by the physician.

Implementation

PO. Adjust the dosage based on blood and urine sugar levels.

Drug interactions

HYPOGLYCEMIA. The following drugs may enhance the hypoglycemic effects of the sulfonylureas: ethanol, methandrostenolone, chloramphenicol, warfarin, propranolol, salicylates, sulfisoxazole, guanethidine, oxytetracycline, monoamine-oxidase inhibitors, and phenylbutazone.

Monitor for the following signs of hypoglycemia: headache, nausea, weakness, hunger, lethargy, decreased coordination, general apprehension, sweating, blurred or double vision.

Notify the physician if any of the above symptoms appear.

HYPERGLYCEMIA. The following drugs when used concurrently with the sulfonylureas may decrease the therapeutic effects of the sulfonylureas: corticosteroids, phenothiazines, diuretics, oral contraceptives, thyroid replacement hormones, phenytoin, diazoxide, and lithium carbonate.

Diabetic or prediabetic patients need to be monitored for the development of hyperglycemia, particularly during the early weeks of therapy.

Assess regularly for glycosuria and report if it occurs with any frequency.

Patients receiving insulin may require an adjustment in dosage.

BETA ADRENERGIC BLOCKING AGENTS. Beta adrenergic blocking agents (propranolol, timolol, nadolol, pindolol, others) may induce hypoglycemia, but may also mask many of the symptoms of hypoglycemia. Notify the physician if you suspect that any of the above symptoms appear intermittently.

ALCOHOL. Ingestion of alcoholic beverages during sulfonylurea therapy may infrequently result in an Antabuse-like reaction, manifested by facial flushing, pounding headache, feeling of breathlessness, and nausea.

In patients who develop an Antabuse-like reaction to alcohol, the use of alcohol and preparations containing alcohol (such as over-the-counter cough medications and mouthwashes) should be avoided during therapy and up to 5 days after discontinuation of sulfonylurea therapy.

THYROID DISEASE
OBJECTIVES

1. Identify the two classes of drugs used to treat thyroid disease.
2. Describe the signs, symptoms, treatment, and nursing interventions associated with hypothyroidism and hyperthyroidism.
3. State the drug of choice for hypothyroidism.
4. Explain the effects of hyperthyroidism on dosages of warfarin and digitalis glycosides and on persons taking oral hypoglycemic agents.
5. Cite the actions of antithyroid medications on the formation and/or release of the hormones produced by the thyroid gland.
6. State the three types of treatment for hyperthyroidism.
7. Explain the nutritional requirements and activity restrictions needed for an individual with hyperthyroidism.
8. Identify the types of conditions that respond favorably to the use of radioactive Iodine-131.
9. Cite the action of propylthiouracil on the production or synthesis of T_3 and T_4.
10. Identify the correct method for administering Lugol's solution.

KEY WORDS

hypothyroidism	hyperthyroidism
myxedema	cretinism
thyrotoxicosis	Graves' disease
exophthalmic goiter	

Thyroid gland

The thyroid gland is a large, reddish, ductless gland in front of and on either side of the trachea, or windpipe. It consists of two lateral lobes and a connecting isthmus and is roughly butterfly-shaped. It is enclosed in a covering of areolar tissue. The thyroid is made up of numerous closed follicles containing colloid matter and is surrounded by a vascular network. This gland is one of the most richly vascularized tissues in the body.

As with other endocrine glands, thyroid gland function is regulated by the hypothalamus and the anterior pituitary gland. The hypothalamus secretes *thyrotropin releasing hormone* (TRH), which stimulates the anterior pituitary gland to release *thyroid stimulating hormone* (TSH). TSH stimulates the thyroid gland to release its hormones triiodothyronine (T_3) and thyroxine (T_4).

The thyroid hormones regulate general body metabolism. Imbalance in thyroid hormone production may also interfere with the following body functions: growth and maturation; carbohydrate, protein, and lipid metabolism, thermal regulation; cardiovascular function; lactation; and reproduction.

Two general classes of drugs used to treat thyroid disorders are (1) those used to replace thyroid hormones in patients whose thyroid glandular function is inadequate to meet metabolic requirements (hypothyroidism), and (2) antithyroid agents used to suppress synthesis of thyroid hormones (hyperthyroidism). Thyroid hormone replacements available are levothyroxine (T_4), liothyronine (T_3), liotrix, thyroglobulin, and thyroid, USP. Antithyroid agents to be discussed include iodides, prophylthiouracil, and methimazole.

General Nursing Considerations for Patients with Thyroid Disease

Patient Concerns:
Nursing Intervention/Rationale

Hypothyroidism

Hypothyroidism is the result of inadequate thyroid hormone production. It may be caused by excessive use of antithyroid drugs used to treat hyperthyroidism, radiation exposure, surgery, acute viral thyroiditis, or chronic thyroiditis.

Myxedema. *Myxedema* is hypothyroidism that occurs during adult life. The onset of symptoms is usually quite mild and vague. Patients develop a sense of slowness in motion, speech, and mental processes. They often develop more lethargic, sedentary habits; have decreased appetites; are constipated; cannot tolerate cold; gain weight; become weak; and fatigue easily. The body temperature may be subnormal; the skin becomes dry, coarse and thickened; and the face appears puffy. Patients often have decreased blood pressure and heart rate and develop anemia and high cholesterol levels. These patients have an increased susceptibility to infection and are very sensitive to small doses of sedative-hypnotics, anesthetics, and narcotics.

Cretinism. Congenital hypothyroidism occurs when a child is born without a thyroid gland or one that is hypoactive. The historical name of this disease is *cretinism.* Fortunately, this disorder is becoming rare because most states require diagnostic testing of the newborn for hypothyroidism.

In breast-fed infants symptoms are usually not recognized until the child is weaned. Over the next several weeks, the infant develops muscular hypotonia, dyspnea, decreased appetite, retarded growth, and skin and hair changes. The bottle-fed infant becomes a poor feeder, sleeps excessively, and develops bradycardia, subnormal temperature, lethargy, inactivity, and constipation. If the hypothyroidism lasts for several months, permanent mental retardation may result.

Parents of infants who are diagnosed promptly need reassurance that the disease is treatable, but must also understand the need for lifelong treatment.

Parents of infants who were not diagnosed promptly require psychological support as well as direction in providing for additional needs of the infant. The nurse must demonstrate acceptance of the impaired child by caring for the infant in an accepting, caring manner. Emphasize to the parents the normal characteristics the child possesses and teach them how to maximize the learning potential of the infant.

Above all, LISTEN to the parents' concerns. Allow the parents to express their feelings, and respond in a nonjudgmental manner.

Diagnosis. Although the symptoms of hypothyroidism are fairly classical, the final diagnosis is usually not made until diagnostic tests have been completed. These tests include drawing serum levels of circulating T_3 and T_4 hormones. If the levels are low, the patient is considered to be hypothyroid. Further diagnostic testing is required to determine the cause of thyroid hypofunction.

Treatment of hypothyroidism. Hypothyroidism can be treated quite successfully by replacement of thyroid hormones (see individual agents). After therapy is initiated, the dosage of thyroid hormone is adjusted until serum levels of the thyroid hormones are within the normal range.

Hyperthyroidism

Hyperthyroidism is caused by excess production of thyroid hormones. Disorders that may cause hyperactivity of the thyroid gland are Graves' disease, nodular goiter, thyroiditis, thyroid carcinoma, overdoses of thyroid hormones, and tumors of the pituitary gland.

The clinical manifestations of hyperthyroidism are rapid, bounding pulse (even during sleep), cardiac enlargement; palpitations; and arrhythmias. Patients are nervous and easily agitated. They develop tremors, a low-grade fever, and weight loss, despite an increased appetite. Hyperactive reflexes and insomnia are also usually present. Patients are intolerant of heat; the skin is warm, flushed, and moist, with increased sweating; edema of the tissues around the eyeballs produces characteristic eye changes, including exophthalmos. Patients develop amenorrhea, dyspnea with minor exertion, hoarse, rapid speech, and have an increased susceptibility to infection.

Diagnosis. Elevated circulating thyroid hormone tests easily diagnose the hyperthyroidism. Further diagnostic studies are required to determine the cause of hyperthyroidism.

Treatment. Three types of treatment can be used to alter the hyperthyroid state: subtotal thyroidectomy, radioactive iodine, and/or antithyroid medications. Until treatment is under way, the patient requires nutritional and psychological support.

Nutritional status. A high-calorie diet (4,000 to 5,000 calories daily) with balanced nutrients may be required. Minimize stimulants such as tea, coffee, colas, and tobacco.

If the patient has diarrhea, avoid foods with a laxative effect (bran products, raw fruits and vegetables) if not tolerated.

Perform daily weights at the same time, in the same type of clothing on the same scale.

Activity and exercise. Promote rest and limit the extent of ambulation in order to prevent exhaustion. If an activity produces fatigue, discourage the patient from further exposures until the disease process responds to therapy.

Psychological aspects. The hyperactivity caused by the disease requires the nurse to approach the patient calmly. Provide the family with an explanation of the patient's behavior.

Support the patient in working with the change in self-image. Assist with grooming and offer reassurance that treatment will allow a return to the preillness state.

Environment. Providing adequate rest is a nursing challenge because of the hyperactivity associated with the disease. Try to provide a cool room in a quiet area, and encourage the use of frequent back rubs, warm milk, and constructive methods to release nervous tension without overexerting the patient.

Patient Education Associated with Thyroid Disease

Communication and responsibility. Encourage open communication concerning frustrations and anger as the patient attempts to adjust to the diagnosis and the need for prolonged treatment. The patient must be guided to insight into the disorder in order to assume responsibility for the continuation of the treatment. Keep emphasizing the factors the patient can control to alter progression of the disease, including the following:

Nutritional status. A high-protein diet, low in calories and cholesterol, is usually prescribed for patients with hypothyroidism. A weight reduction plan may also be required to reduce obesity.

Constipation. As constipation is quite common among hypothyroid patients, encourage them to eat foods that supply roughage in the form of fresh fruits and vegetables, whole grains, and cereals.

People with constipation frequently drink too little water. Encourage patients to drink 8 to 18 8-ounce glasses of water each day.

Do not encourage elderly patients to use bran or bran products. Due to decreased muscle tone, bran can cause a fecal impaction.

Activity and exercise. Hypothyroid patients are often quite sedentary. With the support of the physician, begin the patient on an exercise plan to develop a pattern of daily activity. As symptoms improve, the patient will start feeling more willing to participate in activities.

Environment. During the severe stages of the disease, control stressors and keep the patient warm. Explain to the family the need to provide a quiet, structured environment because the patient lacks the ability to respond to change and anxiety-producing situations. It is important to inform the patient and family that the patient will return to the pre-illness level of capability when the thyroid levels return to normal.

Expectations of therapy. Discuss the expectations of therapy (such as level of exercise and activity, control of constipation, improved intellectual level, relief of depression, normal blood pressure and pulse, reduced weight, ability to maintain activities of daily living and/or work).

Changes in expectation. Assess changes in expectations as therapy progresses and the patient gains understanding and skill in the management of the diagnosis.

Changes in therapy through cooperative goalsetting. Work with the patient to encourage adherence to the prescribed treatment. (It may be necessary to work initially with family members, because the patient may be experiencing some degree of altered mental status and apathy.) When the patient feels that a change should be made in a treatment plan, encourage discussion first with the physician.

Written record. Enlist the patient's (or family's) aid in developing and maintaining a written record of monitoring parameters. See Figures 16-2 and 16-3 for sample written records.

Prior to discharge, the nurse should start the recording process with the family and patient. Emphasize that the baseline data is a starting point, from which any deviations should be reported. The nurse should explain, in detail, how these data can assist the physician in managing the thyroid disorder. Patients should be encouraged to take this record on follow-up visits.

Fostering compliance. Throughout the hospitalization, discuss medication information and how it will benefit the course of treatment. Seek cooperation and understanding of the following points so that medication compliance may be enhanced:

Thyroid Hormone Replacement:

1. Name
2. Dosage
3. Route and administration times
4. Anticipated therapeutic response: a gradual return to "normal" for the individual; therapeutic response is usually noted after a short time on the medication; reversal of symptoms should be complete within 2 to 3 months
5. Side effects to expect
6. Side effects to report (such as symptoms of hyperthyroidism); notify the physician if the resting pulse rate is 100 or above and do not give the thyroid medication until specific directions are given
7. What to do if a dose is missed
8. When, how, or if to refill the medication

Antithyroid Therapy:

1. Name
2. Dosage
3. Route and administration times

Patient Education and Monitoring of Therapeutic Outcomes for Patients Receiving Thyroid Medications

Medications	Color	To be taken

Name _____

Physician _____

Physician's phone _____

Next appt.* _____

Parameters	Day of discharge							Comments
Pulse								
Temperature								
Weight								
Desire to eat: Eat all the time Normal None 10 5 1								
Use this scale to rate tolerance of Heat Cold Cannot tolerate Moderate toleration Normal 10 5 1								
Fatigue level: Tired all the time Normal Not tired; cannot stop 10 5 1								

Skin condition:
  Dry, leathery
  Oily
  Normal								

How I feel about life: Feel awful Getting better Feel good 10 5 1								
Tolerance for exercise: Difficulty breathing with exercise Normal Endless energy, no problem 10 5 1								

*Please bring this record with you to your next appointment.
Use the back of this sheet for additional information.

Figure 16-2 *Patient education and monitoring of therapeutic outcomes for patients receiving thyroid medications.*

Patient Education and Monitoring of Therapeutic Outcomes for Patients Receiving Antithyroid Medications

Medications	Color	To be taken

Name _____

Physician _____

Physician's phone _____

Next appt.* _____

Parameters	Day of discharge							Comments
Pulse								
Temperature								
Weight								
Desire to eat: Eat all the time / Normal / None 10 — 5 — 1								
Use this scale to rate tolerance of [Heat] [Cold] Cannot tolerate / Moderate toleration / Normal 10 — 5 — 1								
Fatigue level: Tired all the time / Normal / Not tired; cannot stop 10 — 5 — 1								
Skin condition: Dry, leathery Oily Normal								
How I feel about life: Feel awful / Getting better / Feel good 10 — 5 — 1								
Tolerance for exercise: Difficulty breathing with exercise / Normal / Endless energy, no problem 10 — 5 — 1								

*Please bring this record with you to your next appointment.
Use the back of this sheet for additional information.

Figure 16-3 *Patient education and monitoring of therapeutic outcomes for patients receiving anti-thyroid medications.*

4. Anticipated therapeutic response
5. Side effects to report (such as sore throat, fever, general malaise)
6. What to do if a dose is missed
7. When, how, or if to refill the medication

Difficulty in comprehension. If it is evident that the patient and/or family does not understand all aspects of the continuing therapy being prescribed (such as administration and monitoring of medications, exercises, diets, follow-up appointments for laboratory work, and monitoring by the physician), consider the use of social service or visiting nurse agencies.

Associated teaching. Give the patient the following instructions:

Always inform the physician or dentist of any prescription or over-the-counter medications being taken. Over-the-counter medications should not be taken without first discussing them with a physician or pharmacist.

Always report side effects of rash, itching, or hives immediately. Nausea, vomiting, or diarrhea should also be reported for the physician's evaluation if it is a new symptom.

Take all of the medication as prescribed for the full course of treatment. Do not discontinue use when feeling improved; do not save for future use; do not give your medicine to another individual. Sudden discontinuation of certain medications may produce harmful effects.

Keep all medications out of reach of children.

If pregnancy is suspected, consult an obstetrician as soon as possible about continuation of medication therapy.

At discharge. Items to be sent home with the patient should include the following:

1. Written instructions for use
2. Labels in language and size of print appropriate for the patient
3. If needed, identification cards or bracelets
4. A list of additional supplies that may need to be purchased after discharge
5. A schedule for follow-up appointments

Drug Therapy for Thyroid Disease

Thyroid replacement hormones

levothyroxine (le-vo-thy-rok'sen)

> **Synthroid** (sin'throyd), **Letter**

Levothyroxine (T_4) is one of the two primary hormones secreted by the thyroid gland. It is partially metabolized to liothyronine (T_3), so that therapy with levothyroxine provides physiologic replacement of both hormones. It is now considered to be the drug of choice for hormone replacement in hypothyroidism.

Side effects. Adverse effects of thyroid replacement preparations are dose-related and may occur 1 to 3 weeks after changes in therapy have been initiated. Symptoms of adverse effects are tachycardia, anxiety, weight loss, abdominal cramping and diarrhea, cardiac palpitations, arrhythmias, angina pectoris, fever, and intolerance to heat.

Availability

PO—0.0125, 0.025, 0.05, 0.075, 0.1, 0.125, 0.15, 0.175, 0.2, and 0.3 mg tablets.

Injection—100 μg/ml in 6 and 10 ml vials.

Dosage and administration

Adult

PO—Therapy may be initiated in low doses of 0.025 mg daily. Dosages are gradually increased over the next few weeks to an average daily maintenance dose of 0.1 to 0.2 mg.

- **Nursing Interventions: Monitoring levothyroxine therapy**

See also General Nursing Considerations for Patients with Thyroid Disease.

Side effects to expect and report

SIGNS OF HYPERTHYROIDISM. See Side Effects above. These signs are all indications of excessive thyroid replacement. Symptoms may require discontinuation of therapy. Patients may require up to a month without medication for toxic effects to fully dissipate.

Therapy must be restarted at lower dosages after symptoms have stopped.

Implementation

PO. The age of the patient, severity of hypothyroidism, and other concurrent medical conditions will determine the initial dosage and the interval of time necessary before increasing the dosage. Hypothyroid patients are quite sensitive to replacement of thyroid hormones. Monitor patients closely for adverse effects.

Drug interactions

WARFARIN. Patients with hypothyroidism require larger doses of anticoagulants. If thyroid replacement therapy is initiated while the patient is receiving warfarin therapy, the patient should have frequent prothrombin time determinations and should be counseled to observe closely for development of petechiae, ecchymoses, nosebleeds, bleeding gums, dark tarry stools, and bright red or coffee ground emesis.

The dosage of warfarin may have to be reduced by one-third to one-half over the next 1 to 4 weeks.

DIGITALIS GLYCOSIDES. Patients with hypothyroidism require smaller doses of digitalis preparations. If thyroid replacement therapy is started while receiving digitalis glycosides, a gradual increase in the glycoside will be necessary to maintain adequate therapeutic activity.

CHOLESTYRAMINE. To prevent binding of thyroid hormones by cholestyramine, administer at least 4 hours apart.

HYPERGLYCEMIA. Diabetic or prediabetic patients need

to be monitored for the development of hyperglycemia, particularly during the early weeks of therapy.

Assess regularly for glycosuria and report if it occurs with any frequency.

Patients receiving oral hypoglycemic agents or insulin may require an adjustment in dosage.

liothyronine (ly-o-thy'ro-neen)

Cytomel (sy'to-mel)

Liothyronine is a synthetic form of the natural thyroid hormone, triiodothyronine, T_3. Its onset of action is more rapid than levothyroxine's and it is occasionally used as a thyroid hormone replacement when prompt action is necessary. It is not recommended for patients with cardiovascular disease unless a rapid onset of activity is deemed essential.

Side effects. See levothyroxine.

Availability

PO—5, 25, and 50 µg tablets.

Dosage and administration

Adult

PO—The usual starting dose depends on the particular condition but is usually 25 µg daily. The usual maintenance dose is 25 to 75 µg daily.

Nursing interventions. See levothyroxine (p. 400).

liotrix (ly'o-triks)

Euthroid (you'throyd), Thyrolar (thy'ro-lar)

This is a synthetic mixture of levothyroxine and liothyronine in a ratio of 4 to 1, respectively. A few endocrinologists prefer this combination because of the standardized content of the two hormones that results in consistent laboratory test results, more in agreement with the patient's clinical response. The two available commercial preparations of liotrix contain different amounts of each ingredient, so patients should not be changed from one preparation to the other unless differences in potency are considered.

Side effects. See levothyroxine (p. 400).

Availability

PO—Euthroid is available in four combination tablet strengths, and Thyrolar is available in five combination tablet strengths. See the manufacturer's literature for the strengths of each of the combination tablets.

Dosage and administration

Adult

PO—Dosage range is 60 to 180 µg of levothyroxine and 15 to 45 µg of liothyronine, taken as one tablet daily, usually at breakfast.

Nursing interventions. See levothyroxine (p. 400).

thyroglobulin (thy-ro-glob'you-lin)

Proloid (pro'loyd)

Thyroglobulin is a protein obtained from a purified extract of hog thyroid. It contains thyroxine and triiodothyronine. It is effective in the treatment of inadequate thyroid hormone production. The potency of thyroglobulin is equal to that of thyroid, USP, but is twice as costly.

Side effects. See levothyroxine (p. 400).

Availability

PO—32, 65, 100, 130, and 200 mg tablets.

Dosage and administration

Adult

PO—Dosage should be started in small amounts and increased gradually. Maintenance dose is 32 to 200 mg taken once daily, usually in the morning.

Nursing interventions. See levothyroxine (p. 400).

thyroid, USP

Thyroid, USP (desiccated thyroid) is derived from pig, beef, and sheep thyroid glands. Thyroid is the oldest thyroid hormone replacement available and the least expensive. Because of its lack of purity, uniformity, and stability, however, it is generally not the drug of choice for the initiation of thyroid replacement therapy.

Side effects. See levothyroxine (p. 400).

Availability

PO—15, 30, 60, 65, 90, 120, 130, 180, 240, and 300 mg tablets; 60 and 120 mg enteric-coated tablets.

Dosage and administration

Adult

PO—Usual dosage range: 65 to 195 mg daily.

Nursing interventions. See levothyroxine (p. 400).

Antithyroid drugs

The synthesis of thyroid hormones and their maintenance in the bloodstream in sufficient amounts depend on sufficient iodine intake through food and water. Iodine is converted to iodide and stored in the thyroid gland before reaching the circulation.

Excessive formation of thyroid hormones and their escape into the circulatory system causes hyperthyroidism, also known as thyrotoxicosis, exophthalmic goiter, or Graves' disease. Symptoms include increased metabolic rate, increased pulse rate (to perhaps 140 beats per minute), increased body temperature, restlessness, nervousness, anxiety, sweating, muscle weakness and tremors, and a complaint of feeling too warm. This condition is treated with antithyroid drugs or surgical removal of the thyroid gland.

An *antithyroid* drug is a chemical agent that interferes with the formation or release of the hormones produced by the thyroid gland.

radioactive iodine (^{131}I)

Iodine-131 (^{131}I) is a radioactive isotope of iodine. When administered, it is absorbed into the thyroid gland in high concentrations. The liberated radioactivity destroys the hyperactive thyroid tissue, with essentially no damage to other tissues in the body.

Radioactive iodine is most commonly used for treating hyperthyroidism in the following individuals: older patients who are beyond the childbearing years, those with severe complicating diseases, those with recurrent hyperthyroidism after previous thyroid surgery, those who are poor surgical risks, and those who have unusually small thyroid glands.

Side effects. Side effects include radioactive thyroiditis, which causes tenderness over the thyroid area and occurs during the first few days or few weeks after radioactive iodine therapy. Hyperthyroidism seldom recurs after therapy, but it is possible and can be especially dangerous in the patient with severe heart disease. Many patients who receive radioactive iodine develop hypothyroidism, which requires thyroid hormone replacement therapy.

• **Nursing Interventions: Monitoring radioactive iodine therapy**

See also General Nursing Considerations for Patients with Thyroid Disease.

Implementation

ADMINISTRATION OF RADIOACTIVE IODINE. Administration of radioactive iodine preparations seems simple: it is added to water and swallowed like a drink of water. It has no color or taste. The radiation, however, is quite dangerous.

• Minimize exposure as much as possible. Wear rubber gloves whenever administering radioactive iodine or disposing of the patient's excreta.
• If the radioactive iodine or the patient's excreta should spill, follow hospital policy. In general, collect the clothing, bedding, bedpan, urinal, and any other contaminated materials and place them in special containers for radioactive waste disposal.
• AVOID SPILLS! REPORT ANY ACCIDENTAL CONTAMINATION AT ONCE TO YOUR SUPERVISOR, HEAD NURSE, TEAM LEADER, OR INSTRUCTOR AND FOLLOW DIRECTIONS FOR HOSPITAL CONTAMINATION CLEAN-UP TECHNIQUE.
• Fill out an incident report.

propylthiouracil (pro-pil-thy-o-you'rah-sil)

PTU, Propacil, ✦ Propyl-Thyracil

Propylthiouracil is an antithyroid agent that acts by blocking synthesis of T_3 and T_4 in the thyroid gland. Propylthiouracil does not destroy any T_3 or T_4 already produced, so there is usually a latent period of a few days to 2 weeks before symptoms improve once therapy is started. Propylthiouracil may be used for long-term treatment of hyperthyroidism or for short-term treatment prior to subtotal thyroidectomy.

Side effects. The most common reaction (in 5% of all patients) that occurs with PTU is a purpuric, maculopapular skin eruption. Occasionally patients develop headaches, a loss of sense of taste, muscle and joint aches, and enlargement of the salivary glands and lymph nodes in the neck. Rarely, propylthiouracil may cause bone marrow suppression, hepatotoxicity, or nephrotoxicity.

Availability

PO—50 mg tablets.

Dosage and administration

Adult

PO—Initially 100 to 150 mg every 6 to 8 hours. Dosage ranges up to 900 mg daily. The maintenance dose is 50 mg 2 or 3 times daily.

• **Nursing Interventions: Monitoring propylthiouracil therapy**

See also General Nursing Considerations for Patients with Thyroid Disease.

Side effects to expect and report

PURPURIC, MACULOPAPULAR RASH. This skin eruption often occurs during the first 2 weeks of therapy and usually resolves spontaneously, without treatment. If pruritus becomes severe, a change to methimazole may be necessary. Cross-sensitivity is uncommon.

HEADACHES, SALIVARY AND LYMPH NODE ENLARGEMENT, LOSS OF TASTE. These side effects are usually mild and tend to resolve with continued therapy. Encourage the patient not to discontinue therapy without first consulting the physician.

BONE MARROW SUPPRESSION. Routine laboratory studies (RBC, WBC, and differential counts) should be scheduled. Stress returning for this laboratory work.

Monitor the patient for the development of a sore throat, fever, purpura, jaundice, or excessive, progressive weakness.

HEPATOTOXICITY. The symptoms of hepatotoxicity are: anorexia, nausea, vomiting, jaundice, hepatomegaly, splenomegaly, and abnormal liver function tests (elevated bilirubin, AST, ALT, GGT, alkaline phosphatase, prothrombin time).

NEPHROTOXICITY. Monitor urinalyses and kidney function tests for abnormal results. Report increased BUN and creatinine, decreased urine output or decreased specific gravity (despite amount of fluid intake), casts or protein in the urine, frank blood or smoky-colored urine, or RBCs in excess of 0 to 3 on the urinalysis report.

Drug interactions

WARFARIN. Patients with hyperthyroidism require larger doses of anticoagulants. If antithyroid therapy is initiated while the patient is receiving warfarin therapy, the patient should have frequent prothrombin time determinations and should be counseled to observe closely for development of petechiae, ecchymoses, nosebleeds, bleeding gums, dark tarry stools, and bright red or coffeeground emesis.

The dosage of warfarin may have to be reduced over the next 1 to 4 weeks.

DIGITALIS GLYCOSIDES. Patients with hyperthyroidism require larger doses of digitalis preparations. If antithyroid replacement therapy is started while receiving digitalis glycosides, a gradual reduction in the glycoside will be necessary to prevent signs of toxicity. Monitor for the development of arrhythmias, bradycardia, increased fatigue, or nausea and vomiting.

methimazole (meth-im′ah-zoal)

Tapazole (tap′ah-zoal)

Methimazole is another antithyroid agent similar in uses and side effects to propylthiouracil. It is effective for treatment of hyperthyroidism in preparation for subtotal thyroidectomy or radioactive iodine therapy.

Side effects. See propylthiouracil.

Availability

PO—5 and 10 mg tablets.

Dosage and administration

Adult

PO—Initially 5 to 20 mg every 8 hours. Daily maintenance dosage is 5 to 15 mg.

Nursing interventions. See propylthiouracil (p. 402).

CORTICOSTEROIDS

OBJECTIVES

1. Review the functions of the adrenal gland.
2. State the normal actions of mineralocorticoids and glucocorticoids in the body.
3. State the disease states caused by hypersecretion or hyposecretion of the adrenal gland.
4. Identify the baseline assessments needed for a patient receiving corticosteroids.
5. Recall the normal laboratory value for serum electrolytes and the signs and symptoms related to alternations of the major electrolytes.
6. Develop measurable short- and long-term objectives for patient education for persons taking corticosteroids.
7. Prepare a list of the clinical uses of mineralocorticoids and glucocorticoids.
8. Discuss the potential side effects associated with the use of corticosteroids and give examples of specific patient education needed for the patient who will be taking these agents.

KEY WORDS

glucocorticoids   mineralocorticoids
hypopituitarism

Corticosteroids are hormones secreted by the adrenal cortex of the adrenal gland. Corticosteroids are divided into two categories based on structure and biologic activity. The mineralocorticoids (desoxycorticosterone, fludrocortisone aldosterone) are used to maintain fluid and electrolyte balance and to treat adrenal insufficiency caused by hypopituitarism or Addison disease. The glucocorticoids (cortisone, hydrocortisone, prednisone, others) are used to regulate carbohydrate, protein, and fat metabolism. Glucocorticoids have antiinflammatory and antiallergic activity and are prescribed for the relief of symptoms of rheumatoid arthritis, adrenal insufficiency, severe psoriasis, urticaria, chronic eczema, multiple myeloma, Hodgkin's disease, leukemias, and collagen diseases (Table 16-5).

General Nursing Considerations for Patients Receiving Corticosteroids

Minimum assessment data for patients receiving corticosteroids include baseline weights, blood pressure, and electrolyte studies. Monitoring of all aspects of intake, output, diet, electrolyte balance, and state of hydration is important to the long-term success of corticosteroid therapy.

Patient Concerns: Nursing Intervention/Rationale

Baseline assessment and monitoring parameters

Weight. Obtain the patient's weight on admission and use as a baseline in assessing therapy. Patients receiving corticosteroids have a tendency to accumulate fluid and gain weight, so the daily weights are an important tool in assessing ongoing therapy. Always perform daily weights as follows:

1. Using the same scale
2. Using the same approximate weight of clothing
3. At the same time of day

Blood pressure. Take a baseline blood pressure reading in both the supine and sitting positions. Because patients receiving corticosteroids accumulate fluid and gain weight, hypertension may develop. Periodic assessment of the blood pressure will be necessary.

Intake. Accurate I/O records should be kept during every shift and totaled every 24 hours for all patients receiving corticosteroid therapy. Measure and record *accurately* all fluids taken (oral, parenteral, rectal, and via tubes). Ice chips and foods, such as Jell-O, that turn to a liquid state need to be included. Irrigation solutions should be carefully measured, so that the difference between the amount instilled and that returned can be recorded as intake.

Remember to enlist the assistance of the patient, family, or other visitors in this process. Ask them to keep a record of how many glasses of water, glasses of juice, or cups of coffee were consumed. Then convert these to milliliters.

Output. Record all output from the mouth, urethra,

Table 16-5 *Corticosteroid Preparations**

GENERIC NAME	BRAND NAMES	DOSAGE FORMS
Alclometasone	Aclovate	Cream, ointment
Amcinonide	Cyclocort	Cream, ointment, lotion
Betamethasone	Celestone, Valisone, Diprosone, Benisone, Betatrex, others	Tablets, syrup, injection, cream, ointment, lotion, aerosol, gel
Clobetasol	Temovate	Cream, ointment, scalp application
Clocortolone	Cloderm	Cream
Cortisone	Cortisone	Tablets
Desonide	Tridesilon, DesOwen	Cream, ointment
Desoximetasone	Topicort	Cream, ointment, gel
Dexamethasone	Decadron, Dexone, Hexadrol, Decaspray	Cream, aerosol, gel, injection, tablets, inhalant
Diflorasone	Florone, Maxiflor	Cream, ointment
Fludrocortisone	Florinef	Tablets
Fluocinolone	Fluonid, Synalar	Cream, ointment, solution
Fluocinonide	Lidex	Cream, ointment, gel, solution
Flurandrenolide	Cordran, ♣Drenison	Cream, ointment, tape, lotion
Fluticasone	Cutivate	Cream, ointment
Hydrocortisone	Cortef, Solu-Cortef, Hydrocortone, Biosone	Cream, ointment, tablets, enema, gel, lotion, suppositories, injection
Halcinonide	Halog, Halog E	Cream, ointment, solution
Halobetasol	Ultravate	Cream, ointment
Methylprednisolone	Solu-Medrol, Depo-Medrol, Meprolone	Ointment, tablets, enema, injection suspension, gel, lotion
Mometasone	Elocon	Cream, ointment
Paramethasone	Haldrone	Tablets
Prednisolone	Delta-Cortef, ♣Novoprednisolone	Cream, injection, tablets, aerosol, syrup
Prednisone	Deltasone, Orasone, ♣Apo-Prednisone	Tablets, syrup, solution
Triamcinolone	Aristocort, Kenalog, ♣Triamcort	Cream, ointment, lotion, injection, tablets, syrup, aerosol

*Ophthalmic products, Chapter 18; nasal inhalation products, Chapter 12.
♣Available in Canada only.

rectum, wounds, and tubes (such as surgical drains, nasogastric tubes, indwelling catheters).

- Consistency, color, and quantity of liquid stools should be recorded.
- Urine output should include information on quantity, color, pH, odor, and specific gravity.
- All other secretions should be described by color, consistency, volume, and changes from previous collections, if possible.

Daily output is usually 1200 to 1500 cc, or 30 to 50 cc per hour. Always report urine output below this hourly rate. Keep the urinal or bedpan readily available.

Tell the patient and visitors not to "help" by dumping the bedpan or urinal, but rather to use the call light and allow the hospital personnel to empty and record all output.

States of hydration

Dehydration. Assess, report, and record significant signs of dehydration in the patient. Observe for the following signs: poor skin turgor, sticky oral mucous membranes, a shrunken or deeply furrowed tongue, crusted lips, weight loss, deteriorating vital signs, soft or sunken eyeballs, weak pedal pulses, delayed capillary filling, excessive thirst, high urine specific gravity (or no urine output), and possible mental confusion.

Skin turgor. Check skin turgor by gently pinching the skin together over the sternum, forehead, or on the forearm. In the well-hydrated patient elasticity is present and the skin rapidly returns to a flat position. With dehydration, the skin remains pinched or peaked and returns very slowly to the flat, normal position.

Oral mucous membranes. When adequately hydrated, the membranes of the mouth feel smooth and glisten. With dehydration, they are sticky and appear dull.

Laboratory changes. The values of the hematocrit, hemoglobin, BUN, and electrolytes will appear to fluctuate, based on the state of hydration. When a patient is overhydrated, the values appear to drop due to "hemodilution." A dehydrated patient will show higher values due to "hemoconcentration."

Overhydration. Increases in abdominal girth, weight gain, neck vein engorgement, and circumference of the medial malleolus are indications of overhydration.

- Measure the abdominal girth daily at the umbilical level.

- Measure the extremities bilaterally every day, approximately 5 cm above the medial malleolus.
- Weigh the patient daily using the same scale, at the same time, and in similar clothing.

Edema. *Edema* is excess fluid accumulation in the extracellular spaces. Edema is considered to be *pitting* when an indentation remains in the tissue after pressure is exerted against a bony part such as the shin, ankle, or sacrum. The degree is usually recorded at 1+ (slight) to 4+ (deep).

Pale, cool, tight, shiny skin is another sign of edema.

Electrolyte imbalance. Patients taking corticosteroids are particularly susceptible to the development of electrolyte imbalance. Physiologically, corticosteroids cause sodium retention (hypernatremia) and potassium excretion (hypokalemia).

Because the symptoms of most electrolyte imbalances are similar, the nurse should assess changes in the patient's mental status (alertness, orientation, confusion), muscle strength, muscle cramps, tremors, nausea, and general appearance.

Susceptible patients. Patients most likely to develop electrolyte disturbances are those who, in addition to receiving corticosteroids, have a history of renal or cardiac disease, hormonal disorders, massive trauma or burns, or are on diuretic therapy.

Serum electrolytes. Monitor serum electrolyte tests and notify the physician of deviations from normal values.

Hypokalemia. Serum potassium (K^+) levels below 3.5 mEq/liter should be reported.

Hypokalemia is especially likely to occur when a patient receiving corticosteroids develops vomiting, diarrhea, or heavy diuresis. All corticosteroids and diuretics, except the potassium-sparing type, may cause hypokalemia.

Hyperkalemia. Serum potassium (K^+) levels above 5.5 mEq/liter should be reported.

Hyperkalemia occurs most commonly when a patient is given excessive amounts of potassium supplements, either intravenously or orally. It may also occur as an adverse effect of potassium-sparing diuretics.

Hyponatremia. Serum sodium (Na^+) below 135 mEq/liter should be reported.

Hypernatremia. Serum sodium above 145 mEq/liter should be reported.

Remember the phrase "where the sodium goes, water goes." Corticosteroids cause retention of sodium by the kidneys, thus causing fluid retention. Hypernatremia can be aggravated when intravenous fluid intake exceeds output.

Behavioral change. Patients receiving higher doses of corticosteroids are susceptible to psychotic behavioral changes. The most susceptible patients are those with a previous history of mental dysfunction. Perform a baseline assessment of the patient's ability to respond rationally to the environment and the diagnosis of the underlying disease. Make regularly scheduled mental status evaluations and compare the findings. Report the development of alterations.

Hyperglycemia. Corticosteroid therapy may induce hyperglycemia, particularly in prediabetic or diabetic patients. All patients need to be monitored for the development of hyperglycemia, particularly during the early weeks of therapy.

Assess regularly for glycosuria and/or blood glucose and report any frequent occurrences.

History of ulcers. Patients receiving corticosteroid therapy develop a higher incidence of ulcer disease. Ask the patient about any previous treatment for an ulcer, heartburn, or stomach pain. Periodic testing of stools for occult blood may be ordered.

Patient Education Associated with Corticosteroid Therapy

Communication and responsibility. Encourage open communication concerning frustrations and anger as the patient attempts to adjust to the diagnosis and the need for prolonged treatment. The patient must be guided to insight into the disorder in order to assume responsibility for the continuation of the treatment. Keep emphasizing the factors the patient can control to alter progression of the disease including maintenance of general health, nutritional needs, adequate rest and appropriate exercise, continuation of the prescribed medication therapy, and management of the underlying disease process for which the corticosteroids are being prescribed.

Avoid infections. Advise the patient to avoid crowds or people known to have infections. Report even minor signs of an infection (such as general malaise, sore throat, or low-grade fever) to the physician.

Nutritional status. Assist the patient to develop a specific schedule for spacing daily fluid intake and planning sodium restrictions, as prescribed by the physician.

If a high-potassium diet is prescribed, help the patient become familiar with foods that should be consumed.

If weight gain is a specific problem (not related to fluid accumulation), plan for calorie restrictions and spacing of daily intake.

Further dietary needs may include increases in vitamin D and calcium.

Stress. Patients receiving high doses of corticosteroids do not tolerate stress very well. Patients should be instructed to notify the physician prior to exposure to additional stress, such as dental procedures. If a patient sustains an accidental injury or sudden emotional stress, the attending physician should be notified that the patient is receiving steroid therapy. An additional dose may be needed to support the patient through a stressful situation.

Exercise and activity. Encourage the patient to maintain the usual activities of daily living. Help the patient plan for appropriate alterations depending on the disease process and degree of impairment.

Encourage weight-bearing to prevent calcium loss. Active and passive range of motion exercises maintain mobility and joint and muscle integrity.

Expectations of therapy. Discuss the expectations of therapy with the patient. These drugs usually provide improvement of the symptoms for which the medication was prescribed. It must be remembered that the underlying disease process is not being cured through the use of these agents. Thus, for use with rheumatoid arthritis, the anticipated response would be improved mobility as a result of decreased joint pain and edema; for lesions of the skin, a reduction in inflammation; for adrenal insufficiency, gradual improvement of the presenting symptoms.

Changes in expectations. Assess changes in expectations as therapy progresses and the patient gains understanding and skill in the management of the diagnosis. Even after corticosteroid therapy ends, the patient may require reinstitution of therapy during periods of stress, infection, surgery, or accidental injury.

Corticosteroids are usually reserved for treatment when all other therapies have been eliminated. Patients may have difficulty living with the side effects of corticosteroid therapy, but the alternative of the predrug symptoms offers little choice. It may be even more difficult for a patient to understand the need to decrease the dosage and allow incomplete symptom control because of adverse effects experienced.

Changes in therapy through cooperative goal setting. Work with the patient to encourage adherence to the prescribed treatment. When the patient feels that a change should be made in a treatment plan, encourage discussion first with the physician.

Written record. Enlist the patient's aid in developing and maintaining a written record of monitoring parameters (such as blood pressure, pulse, daily weight, degree of pain relief, exercise tolerance) and response to prescribed therapies for discussion with the physician (see Figure 16-4). Patients should be encouraged to take this record on follow-up visits.

Fostering compliance. Throughout the hospitalization, discuss medication information and how it will benefit the course of treatment. Stress the need for regular and long-term treatment, if appropriate to the patient's disease. Seek the patient's cooperation and understanding of the following points so that medication compliance may be enhanced:

1. Name.
2. Dosage: The smallest possible dose is used to control the presenting symptoms for long-term therapy.

NEVER stop taking the medication abruptly. A gradual withdrawal from the drug is required to prevent serious complications. The dosage must be regulated by the physician.
3. Route and administration times: Oral administration is usually done between 6 AM and 9 AM to minimize the suppressive activity on normal adrenal function. To minimize gastric irritation, administer with or after meals.

   Alternate-day therapy is sometimes used for long-term treatment.
4. Anticipated therapeutic response: Improvement in the presenting symptoms for which therapy has been prescribed.
5. Side effects to expect: See the discussion of glucocorticoids.
6. Side effects to report: Hyperglycemia, behavioral changes, signs of infection, exposure to stressful situations, or significant weight gain over a short period of time.
7. What to do if a dose is missed: If one dose is missed, take it when remembered. If more than one is missed, consult your physician.
8. When, how, or if to refill the medication.

Difficulty in comprehension. If it is evident that the patient and/or family does not understand all aspects of the continuing therapy being prescribed (such as administration and monitoring of medications, exercises, diets, follow-up appointments), consider the use of social service or visiting nurse agencies.

Associated teaching. Give patients the following instructions:

Always inform the physician or dentist of any prescription or over-the-counter medication being taken. Over-the-counter medications should not be taken without first discussing them with a physician or pharmacist.

Always report side effects of rash, itching, or hives immediately. Nausea, vomiting, or diarrhea should also be reported for the physician's evaluation if it is a new symptom.

Take all of the medication as prescribed for the full course of treatment. Do not discontinue use when feeling improved; do not save for future use; do not give your medicine to another individual. Sudden discontinuation of certain medications may produce harmful effects.

Keep all medications out of reach of children.

If pregnancy is suspected, consult an obstetrician as soon as possible about continuation of medication therapy.

At discharge. Items to be sent home with the patient should include the following:

1. Written instructions for use
2. Labels in language and size of print appropriate for the patient

Patient Education and Monitoring of Therapeutic Outcomes for Patients Receiving Corticosteroids

Medications	Color	To be taken

Name _____

Physician _____

Physician's phone _____

Next appt.* _____

Parameters		Day of discharge							Comments
Weight									
Blood pressure									
Pulse rate									
Notify doctor of sudden stress in life	Surgery, injury, trauma, death in family or of friend, events such as fights in family								
Pain relief? No relief 10 — Improved 5 — No pain 1									
Assessment of how I feel? Good 10 — Improved 5 — Bad 1									
Breast tenderness	None								
	Occasionally uncomfortable								
	Increasing								
Hair distribution	No changes seen								
	Hair growth increased: site ____								
Edema	Swelling noted (where)? ____								
	Time of day swelling occurs?								

*Please bring this record with you to your next appointment.
Use the back of this sheet for additional information.

Figure 16-4 *Patient education and monitoring of therapeutic outcomes for patients receiving corticosteroids.*

3. Identification cards or bracelets that state the name of the doctor to contact in an emergency, as well as the drug name, dosage, and frequency of use
4. A list of additional supplies to be purchased after discharge
5. A schedule for follow-up appointments

Drug Therapy with Corticosteroids

Mineralocorticoids

desoxycorticosterone (DOCA)
(dez-ok'see-kort-ih-ko-stere-own)

Percorten (per-kort'en)

Desoxycorticosterone is a mineralocorticoid secreted by the adrenal glands. It affects fluid and electrolyte balance by acting on the distal renal tubules causing sodium and water retention, and potassium and hydrogen excretion. Desoxycorticosterone is used in combination with glucocorticoids to replace mineralocorticoid activity in patients who suffer from hypopituitarism or adrenocortical insufficiency (Addison disease), and for the treatment of salt losing adrenogenital syndrome.

Side effects. Because desoxycorticosterone is a natural hormone, side effects are an extension of excessive use of desoxycorticosterone. Most side effects are associated with sodium accumulation and potassium depletion.

Availability
Injection—(Pivalate) 25 mg/ml suspension in 4 ml vials.

Implant—(acetate pellets) 125 mg.

Dosage and administration

Adult

IM—Acetate (short-acting form) 2 to 5 mg daily. Inject into the upper outer quadrant of the gluteal region. Injection into the deltoid muscle should be avoided because of a high incidence of subcutaneous atrophy.

IM—Pivalate (long-acting form) 25 to 100 mg every 4 weeks.

Implant—Pellets are surgically implanted into the subcutaneous tissue every 8 to 12 months.

Drug interactions. See Glucocorticoids.

- **Nursing Interventions: Monitoring desoxycorticosterone therapy**

See General Nursing Considerations for Patients Receiving Corticosteroids (p. 403).

Glucocorticoids

The major glucocorticoid of the adrenal cortex is cortisol. The hypothalamic pituitary axis regulates the secretion of cortisol by increasing or decreasing the output of *corticotropin releasing factor* (CRF) from the hypothalamus. CRF stimulates the release of *adrenocorticotropic hormone* (ACTH) from the pituitary gland. ACTH then stimulates the adrenal cortex to secrete cortisol. As serum levels of cortisol increase, the amount of CRF secreted by the hypothalamus is decreased, resulting in diminished secretion of cortisol from the adrenal cortex.

Glucocorticoids are most frequently prescribed for their antiinflammatory and antiallergic properties. They do not cure any disease, but rather relieve the symptoms of tissue inflammation. When used for the control of rheumatoid arthritis, relief of symptoms is noted within a few days. Joint and muscle stiffness, muscle tenderness and weakness, joint swelling, and soreness are all significantly reduced. When used for this purpose, it is important to assess the patient's predrug activity level. Relief of pain may lead to overuse of the diseased joints. Appetite, weight, and energy are increased, fever is reduced, and sedimentation rates are reduced or return to normal. Anatomic changes and joint deformities that are already present remain unchanged. Symptoms usually return a short time after withdrawal of the glucocorticoids.

Glucocorticoids are also quite effective for relief of allergic manifestations, such as serum sickness, severe hay fever, status asthmaticus, and exfoliative dermatitis. In addition, they may be used for the treatment of shock and for *collagen* diseases, such as lupus erythematosus, dermatomyositis, and acute rheumatic fever.

Side effects. Glucocorticoids are potent agents that produce many undesirable side effects as well as therapeutic benefits. Unless immediate, life-threatening conditions exist, other therapeutic methods should be exhausted before corticosteroid therapy is initiated. Many of the side effects of the steroids are related to dosage and duration of therapy.

Possible side effects of the glucocorticoids include hyperglycemia, glycosuria, aggravation of diabetes mellitus symptoms, negative nitrogen balance, increase in white cell count, reduced resistance to infections, delay in wound healing, peptic ulcer formation, cataract formation, tendency for thrombosis and embolism, a rounded contour of the face, hirsutism, purplish or reddish striae of the skin, potassium depletion, retention of salt and water, and weight gain. Behavioral disturbances, ranging from nervousness and insomnia to manic-depressive (or schizophrenic) psychoses and suicidal tendencies, may develop, particularly with prolonged administration.

These drugs must be used with caution in patients with diabetes mellitus, congestive heart failure, hypertension, peptic ulcer, mental disturbance, and suspected infections.

Availability. See Table 16-5.

Dosage and administration. When therapeutic dosages are administered for a week or longer, one must assume that the internal production of corticosteroids is suppressed. Abrupt discontinuation of the glucocorticoids may result in adrenal insufficiency. Therapy should be withdrawn gradually. The time required to decrease glucocorticoids depends on the duration of treatment, the dosage amount, the mode of administration, and the glucocorticoid being used.

• Nursing Interventions: Monitoring corticosteroid therapy

See also General Nursing Considerations for Patients Receiving Corticosteroids (p. 403).

Side effects to expect and report

ELECTROLYTE IMBALANCE, FLUID ACCUMULATION. The electrolytes most commonly altered are potassium (K^+), sodium (Na^+), and chloride (Cl^-). Of these, *hypokalemia* is most likely to occur.

Many symptoms associated with altered fluid and electrolyte balance are subtle and interspersed with general symptoms of drug toxicity or the disease process itself.

Gather data relative to *changes* in the patient's mental status (alertness, orientation, confusion), muscle strength, muscle cramps, tremors, nausea, and general appearance (drowsy, anxious, lethargic).

Always check the electrolyte reports for early indications of electrolyte imbalance.

Keep accurate records of intake and output, daily weights, and vital signs.

SUSCEPTIBILITY TO INFECTION. Always question the patient, *prior* to initiation of therapy, about any signs and symptoms that would indicate the presence of an infection. Corticosteroid therapy often masks symptoms of infection.

Monitor the patient closely for signs of infection such as sore throat, fever, malaise, nausea, or vomiting.

Encourage the patient to avoid exposure to infections.

BEHAVIORAL CHANGES. Psychotic behaviors are more likely to occur in patients with a previous history of mental instability.

Perform a baseline assessment of the patient's degree of alertness, orientation to name, place, and time, and rationality of responses *prior* to initiating therapy. Make regularly scheduled mental status evaluations and compare the findings. Report the development of alterations.

HYPERGLYCEMIA. Diabetic or prediabetic patients need to be monitored for the development of hyperglycemia, particularly during the early weeks of therapy.

Assess regularly for glycosuria and/or blood glucose and report any frequent occurrences.

Patients receiving oral hypoglycemic agents or insulin may require an adjustment in dosage.

PEPTIC ULCER FORMATION. Before initiating therapy, ask the patient about any previous treatment for an ulcer, heartburn, or stomach pain.

Periodic testing of stools for occult blood may be ordered. Antacids may also be recommended by the physician to minimize gastric symptoms.

DELAYED WOUND HEALING. People who have recently had surgery require close monitoring of surgical sites for signs of dehiscence.

Teach surgical patients to splint the wounds while coughing and breathing deeply.

Inspect surgical sites and report statements such as, "When I coughed, I felt something pop."

VISUAL DISTURBANCES. Visual disturbances noted by patients receiving long-term therapy need to be reported. Glucocorticoid therapy may produce cataracts.

Implementation

ABRUPT DISCONTINUATION. Patients who have received corticosteroids for at least 1 week must not abruptly discontinue therapy.

Symptoms of abrupt discontinuation include fever, malaise, fatigue, weakness, anorexia, nausea, orthostatic dizziness, hypotension, fainting, dyspnea, hypoglycemia, muscle and joint pain, and possible exacerbation of the disease process being treated.

APPLICATION. Topical corticosteroids are applied as directed by the manufacturer. Specific instructions regarding use of an occlusive dressing should be clarified.

ALTERNATE DAY THERAPY. Alternate day therapy may be used to treat chronic conditions. Administration of corticosteroids is usually done between 6 AM and 9 AM to minimize suppression of normal adrenal function. Administer with meals to minimize gastric irritation.

PEDIATRIC PATIENTS. The correct dosage for a child is usually based on the disease being treated, rather than the weight of the patient. (Children may require monitoring of skeletal growth if prolonged therapy is required.)

Drug interactions

DIURETICS (FUROSEMIDE, THIAZIDES, BUMETANIDE, OTHERS). Corticosteroids may enhance the loss of potassium. Check potassium levels and monitor the patient more closely for hypokalemia when these two agents are used concurrently.

Many symptoms associated with altered fluid and electrolyte balance are subtle and interspersed with general symptoms of drug toxicity or the disease process itself.

Gather data relative to *changes* in the patient's mental status (alertness, orientation, confusion), muscle strength, muscle cramps, tremors, nausea, and general appearance (drowsy, anxious, lethargic).

Always check the electrolyte reports for early indications of electrolyte imbalance.

Keep accurate records of intake and output, daily weights, and vital signs.

WARFARIN. This medication may enhance or decrease the anticoagulant effects of warfarin. Observe for the development of petechiae, ecchymoses, nosebleeds, bleeding gums, dark tarry stools, and bright red or coffee ground emesis. Monitor the prothrombin time and adjust the dosage of warfarin if necessary.

The ulcerogenic potential of steroids requires close observation of patients taking anticoagulants to reduce the possibility of hemorrhage.

HYPERGLYCEMIA. Diabetic or prediabetic patients need to be monitored for the development of hyperglycemia, particularly during the early weeks of therapy.

Assess regularly for glycosuria and/or blood glucose and report any frequent occurrences.

Patients receiving oral hypoglycemic agents or insulin may require an adjustment in dosage.

GONADAL HORMONES
OBJECTIVES

1. Describe the body changes that can be anticipated with the administration of androgens, estrogens, or progesterone.
2. Compare the side effects seen with the use of estrogen hormones with those seen with a combination of estrogen and progesterone.
3. Differentiate between the side effects to expect and those requiring consultation with the physician with the administration of estrogen or progesterone.
4. State the uses of estrogens and progestins.
5. State the actions of androgens.
6. Identify the rationale for administering androgens to females who have certain types of breast cancer.
7. Describe the signs and symptoms of hypercalcemia.

KEY WORDS

testosterone   androgens
eunuchism   hypogonadism

The Gonads

The *gonads* are the reproductive glands: the *testes* of the male and the *ovaries* of the female. In addition to producing sperm, the testes produce testosterone, the male sex hormone. Testosterone controls the development of the male sex organs and influences characteristics such as voice, hair distribution, and male body form. *Androgens* are other steroid hormones that produce masculinizing effects.

The *ovaries* produce estrogen and progesterone. These are hormones that stimulate maturation of the female sex organs. They influence breast development, voice quality, and the broader pelvis of the female body form. Menstruation is established because of the hormone production of the ovaries. *Estrogen* is responsible for most of these changes. *Progesterone* is thought to be concerned mainly with body changes that favor the im-

plantation of the fertilized ovum, continuation of pregnancy, and preparation of the breasts for lactation.

General Nursing Considerations for Patients Receiving Gonadal Hormones

A complete physical examination is usually done as a part of the preliminary work-up prior to treatment of any disorders using gonadal hormones.

Patient Concerns:
Nursing Intervention/Rationale

Assessment

Purpose. Ask the patient to describe the current problems that initiated this visit. How long have the symptoms been present? Is this a recurrent problem? If so, how was it treated in the past?

Reproductive history. Have the patient describe the following, as appropriate:

- Age of menarche
- Usual pattern of menses: duration, number of pads used, last menstrual period
- Number of pregnancies, live births, miscarriages, abortions
- Vaginal discharges, itching, infections, and how treated
- Breast self-exam routine (if not being performed regularly, explain the correct procedure)
- Male patients should be asked whether testicular exams are performed (if not being performed regularly, explain the correct procedure)

History of prior illnesses. Any indication of hypertension, heart or liver disease, thromboembolic disorders, or cancers of the reproductive organs is of particular concern.

Medications, smoking. Does the patient currently smoke, or is the patient taking any over-the-counter or prescription medication? Oral contraceptives?

Physical examination. Record basic patient data: height, weight, and vital signs. Blood pressure readings are of particular concern so that recordings on future visits can be evaluated for any change.

Collect urine for urinalysis, and blood samples for hemoglobin, hematocrit, and other laboratory studies deemed appropriate by the physician. Generally, people with a family history of diabetes mellitus should be tested for hyperglycemia prior to starting gonadal hormone therapy.

The physical exam should include a breast examination and a pelvic examination including a Papanicolaou test. Observe the distribution of body hair and the presence of scars. Stress the need for periodic physical examinations while receiving gonadal hormones.

Patient Education Associated with Gonadal Hormone Therapy

Communication and responsibility. Encourage open communication concerning frustrations and anger as the patient attempts to adjust to the diagnosis and the need for prolonged treatment. The patient must be guided to insight into the disorder and to assume responsibility for the continuation of the treatment. Keep emphasizing the factors the patient can control to alter progression of the disease including maintenance of general health, nutritional needs, adequate rest and appropriate exercise, and continuation of the prescribed medication therapy.

Smoking. Explain the risks of continuing to smoke, especially when receiving estrogen or progestin therapy. (The incidence of fatal heart attacks is increased for women over 35 years of age.)

Physical examination. Stress the need for regular periodic medical examinations and laboratory studies.

Expectations of therapy. Discuss the expectations of therapy with the patient (such as degree of pain relief, frequency of use of therapy, relief of menopausal symptoms, sexual maturation, regulation of menstrual cycle, sexual activity, maintenance of mobility and activities of daily living and/or work).

Changes in expectations. Assess changes in expectations as therapy progresses and the patient gains understanding and skill in the management of the diagnosis.

Because there are a number of possible adverse effects, it is necessary to evaluate the effectiveness of the treatment prescribed in relation to the condition being treated and the severity of adverse effects being experienced.

Changes in therapy through cooperative goalsetting. Work with the patient to encourage adherence to the prescribed treatment. When the patient feels that a change should be made in a treatment plan, encourage discussion first with the physician.

Written record. Enlist the patient's aid in developing and maintaining a written record of monitoring parameters (such as blood pressure, pulse, daily weight, degree of pain relief, menstrual cycle information, breakthrough bleeding, nausea, vomiting, cramps, breast tenderness, hirsutism, gynecomastia, masculinization, hoarseness, headaches, sexual stimulation) and responses to prescribed therapies for discussion with the physician. Patients should be encouraged to take this record on follow-up visits.

Fostering compliance. Throughout the hospitalization, discuss medication information and how it will benefit the course of treatment. Seek the patient's cooperation and understanding of the following points so that medication compliance may be enhanced:

1. Name.

2. Dosage: The dosage will depend on the disease being treated and the agent being used.
3. Route and administration: Be certain the patient understands the route of administration and the times of administration in relation to the menstrual cycle.
4. Anticipated therapeutic response: See individual agents.
5. Side effects to expect: See individual agents.
6. Side effects to report: See individual agents.
7. What to do if a dosage is missed.
8. When, how, or if to refill the medication.

Difficulty in comprehension. If it is evident that the patient and/or family does not understand all aspects of the continuing therapy being prescribed (such as administration and monitoring of medications, exercises, diets, follow-up appointments), consider use of social service or visiting nurse agencies.

Associated teaching. Give the patient the following instructions:

Always inform the physician or dentist of any prescription or over-the-counter medication being taken. Over-the-counter medications should not be taken without first discussing them with a physician or pharmacist.

Always report side effects of rash, itching, or hives immediately. Nausea, vomiting, or diarrhea should also be reported for the physician's evaluation if it is a new symptom.

Take all of the medication as prescribed for the full course of treatment. Do not discontinue use when feeling improved; do not save for future use; do not give your medicine to another individual. Sudden discontinuation of certain medications may produce harmful effects.

Keep all medications out of reach of children.

If pregnancy is suspected, consult an obstetrician as soon as possible about continuation of medication therapy.

At discharge. Items to be sent home with the patient should include the following:

1. Written instructions for use
2. Labels in language and size of print appropriate for the patient
3. If needed, identification cards or bracelets
4. A list of additional supplies to be purchased after discharge (such as syringes or dressings)
5. A schedule of follow-up appointments

Drug Therapy with Gonadal Hormones

Estrogens

The natural estrogenic hormone released from the ovaries is comprised of several closely related chemical compounds: *estradiol, estrone,* and *estriol.* The most potent is estradiol. It is metabolized to estrone, which is half as potent. Estrone is further metabolized to estriol, which is considerably less potent. Estrogens are responsible for the development of the sex organs during growth in the uterus and for maturation at puberty. They are also responsible for characteristics such as growth of hair, texture of skin, and distribution of body fat. Estrogens also affect the release of pituitary gonadotropins; cause capillary dilatation, fluid retention, and protein metabolism; and inhibit ovulation and postpartum breast engorgement.

Estrogen products are used for relieving the hot flash symptoms of menopause; for contraception; for hormone replacement therapy after an oophorectomy; for postpartum breast engorgement; in conjunction with appropriate diet, calcium, and physical therapy in the treatment of osteoporosis; and to slow the disease progress (and minimize discomfort) in patients with advanced prostatic cancer and certain types of breast cancer.

Side effects. Estrogen-containing products all have somewhat similar adverse effects with similar dosages. Because estrogens affect so many body functions, many potential adverse effects are associated with therapy. Each patient responds somewhat differently to various estrogenic products and dosages, based on the individual's body chemistry and the duration of the therapy. Adverse effects associated with estrogen therapy, categorized by body system, are as follows:

- Genitourinary: Breakthrough bleeding, changes in menstrual flow, dysmenorrhea, amenorrhea, infertility, and uterine growth changes.
- Gastrointestinal: Nausea, vomiting, abdominal cramps, bloating, jaundice, and colitis. There is a two- to threefold increase in risk of gallbladder disease in women receiving postmenopausal estrogens.
- Breast: Tenderness, enlargement, and secretion.
- Cardiovascular: Hypertension, thrombophlebitis, pulmonary embolism, stroke, and myocardial infarction.
- Skin: Chloasma (pigmentary skin discoloration, usually yellowish brown patches or spots), loss of scalp hair, hirsutism, urticaria, localized dermatitis, erythema multiforme, and hemorrhagic eruption.
- Eyes: Intolerance to contact lenses.
- CNS: Headaches, migraine, dizziness, mental depression.
- Other: Changes in weight, hyperglycemia, edema, changes in libido, aggravation of porphyria.

The use of estrogens for long-term treatment of menopausal symptoms has been associated with a greater risk of endometrial cancer. The risk of endometrial cancer in estrogen users was 4.5 to 13.9 times greater than in nonusers and appears to depend on both duration of treatment and dose. When estrogens are used for the treatment of menopausal symptoms, the lowest dose that will control symptoms should be used, and medication should be discontinued as soon as possible. When prolonged treatment is required, the patient should be examined at least on a semiannual basis to determine the need for continued therapy. Cyclic administration of low doses of estrogen may carry less risk than continuous administration. There is no evidence that "natural" estrogens are more or less hazardous than synthetic estrogens in equivalent doses.

The use of estrogens during early pregnancy is contraindicated. Serious birth defects have been reported, and it has been found that the female offspring have an increased risk of developing vaginal or cervical cancer later in life.

Availability. See Table 16-6.

Dosage and administration. See Table 16-6.

• Nursing Interventions: Monitoring estrogen therapy

See also General Nursing Considerations for Patients Receiving Gonadal Hormones (p. 410).

Side effects to expect

WEIGHT GAIN, EDEMA, BREAST TENDERNESS, NAUSEA. These symptoms tend to be mild and resolve with continued therapy. If they do not resolve, or become particularly bothersome, the patient should consult a physician.

Side effects to report

HYPERTENSION, HYPERGLYCEMIA, THROMBOPHLEBITIS, BREAKTHROUGH BLEEDING, ANY OTHER SYMPTOMS THE PATIENT RECOGNIZED AS BEING OF CONCERN. These are all complications associated with estrogen therapy. It is extremely important that the patient is evaluated by the physician to consider alternative therapy.

Drug interactions

WARFARIN. This medication may diminish the anticoagulant effects of warfarin. Monitor the prothrombin time and increase the dosage of warfarin if necessary.

PHENYTOIN. Estrogens may inhibit the metabolism of phenytoin, resulting in phenytoin toxicity.

Monitor patients with concurrent therapy for signs of phenytoin toxicity, nystagmus, sedation, lethargy. Serum levels may be ordered, and a reduced dosage of phenytoin may be required.

THYROID HORMONES. Patients who have no thyroid function and who start on estrogen therapy may require an increase in thyroid hormone because estrogens reduce the level of circulating thyroid hormones. Do not adjust the thyroid dosage until the patient shows clinical signs of hypothyroidism.

Progestins

Progesterone, and its derivatives (the progestins), inhibit the secretion of pituitary gonadotropins preventing maturation of ovarian follicles, and thus inhibit ovulation. Progestins are used primarily to treat second-

Table 16-6 *Estrogens*

GENERIC NAME	BRAND NAME	AVAILABILITY	USES	DOSES
Chlorotrianisene	Tace	Capsules: 12, 25, 72 mg	Postpartum breast engorgement	PO: 12 mg 4 times daily for 7 days; or 50 mg every 6 hours for 6 doses; or 72 mg every 12 hours for 2 days Administer first dose within 8 hours after delivery
			Prostatic carcinoma	PO: 12-25 mg daily
			Menopause	PO: 12-25 mg daily cyclically*
			Atrophic vaginitis	PO: 12-25 mg daily cyclically*
			Female hypogonadism	PO: 12-25 mg daily for 21 days, followed by 5 days of progestin
Conjugated estrogens	Premarin, Estrocon	Tablets: 0.3, 0.625, 0.9 1.25, 2.5 mg IV: 25 mg/5 ml vial	Menopause	PO: 1.25 mg daily cyclically*
			Atrophic vaginitis	PO: 0.3-1.25 mg daily cyclically*
	✚C.E.S.	Cream: 0.625 mg/g	Female hypogonadism	PO: 2.5-7 mg daily for 20 days, followed by 10 days off
			Ovarian failure or post-oophorectomy	PO: 1.25 mg daily cyclically*
			Osteoporosis	PO: 1.25 mg daily cyclically*
			Breast carcinoma	PO: 10 mg 3 times daily
			Prostatic carcinoma	PO: 1.25-2.5 mg 3 times daily
			Postpartum breast engorgement	PO: 3.75 mg every 4 hours for 5 doses; or 1.25 mg every 4 hours for 5 days
Diethylstilbestrol (DES)	Diethylstilbestrol, ✚Honvol	Tablets: 1, 2.5, 5 mg	Menopause, atrophic vaginitis	PO: 0.2-0.5 mg daily cyclically* Dosage range: up to 2 mg daily
			Female hypogonadism, post-oophorectomy, ovarian failure	PO: 0.2-0.5 mg daily cyclically
			Prostatic carcinoma	PO: 1-3 mg daily
			Breast carcinoma	PO: 15 mg daily
			Postcoital contraception	PO: 25 mg 2 times daily for 5 days. Start within 24 hours, for emergency use only. Do not use routinely.
Esterified estrogens	Estratab, Menest	Tablets: 0.3, 0.625, 1.25, 2.5 mg	Menopause, atrophic vaginitis	PO: 0.3-1.25 mg daily cyclically*
			Female hypogonadism, post-oophorectomy, ovarian failure	PO: 2.5-7.5 mg daily cyclically
			Breast carcinoma	PO: 10 mg 3 times daily
			Prostatic carcinoma	PO: 1.25-2.5 mg 3 times daily

*Cyclically = 3 weeks of daily estrogen followed by 1 week off.
✚Available in Canada only.

Continued.

Table 16-6 *Estrogens—cont'd*

GENERIC NAME	BRAND NAME	AVAILABILITY	USES	DOSES
Estradiol	Estrace	Tablets: 1, 2 mg Injections: Cypionate in oil: 1, 5 mg/ml Valerate in oil: 10, 20, 40 mg/ml	Menopause, atrophic vaginitis, hypogonadism, postoophorectomy, ovarian failure	PO: 1-2 mg daily cyclically* IM: Cypionate: 1-5 mg every 3-4 weeks Valerate: 10-20 mg every 4 weeks
			Postpartum breast engorgement	IM: Valerate: 10-25 mg at end of first stage of labor
			Prostatic carcinoma	PO: 1-2 mg 3 times daily IM: Valerate: 30 mg every 1-2 weeks
	Estraderm	Transdermal patch: 0.05, 0.1 mg	Breast carcinoma Menopause Female hypogonadism Primary ovarian failure Atrophic vaginitis Postoophorectomy	PO: 10 mg 3 times daily Transdermal System: A 0.05 or 0.1 mg patch should be placed on a clean, dry area of the skin on the trunk (usually abdomen) twice weekly on a cyclic schedule (3 weeks of therapy followed by 1 week without). Rotate application site; interval of 1 week between uses of same site.
Estrone	Ogen, Kestrone, ♣Femogen	Tablets: 0.625, 1.25, 2.5, 5 mg Injection: in water: 2, 5 mg/ml	Menopause, atrophic vaginitis	PO: 0.625-5 mg daily cyclically* IM: 0.1-0.5 mg 2-3 times weekly
			Female hypogonadism, postoophorectomy, ovarian failure	PO: 1.25-7.5 mg daily cyclically IM: 0.1-1 mg weekly Dosage range: 0.5-2 mg
			Prostatic carcinoma	IM: 2-4 mg 2 or 3 times weekly
Ethinyl estradiol	Estinyl, Feminone	Tablets: 0.02, 0.05, 0.5 mg	Menopause	PO: 0.02-0.05 mg daily cyclically*
			Female hypogonadism	PO: 0.05 1-3 times daily for 2 weeks followed by 2 weeks of progesterone
			Breast carcinoma Prostatic carcinoma	PO: 1 mg 3 times daily PO: 0.15-2 mg daily
Quinestrol	Estrovis	Tablets: 100 mcg	Menopause, hypogonadism, atrophic vaginitis, postoophorectomy, ovarian failure	PO: Initially, 100 μg daily for 7 days; followed by 100 μg weekly starting 2 weeks after treatment starts

*Cyclically = 3 weeks of daily estrogen followed by 1 week off.
♣ Available in Canada only.

ary amenorrhea, breakthrough uterine bleeding, and endometriosis, but may also be used in combination with estrogens as contraceptives (see Oral Contraceptives in Chapter 20).

Side effects. Side effects associated with administration of progestins are rare, but can include nausea, vomiting, diarrhea, breakthrough bleeding, oily scalp, acne, weight gain, edema, spotting, amenorrhea, headache, cholestatic jaundice, mental depression, and hirsutism.

The use of progestins in early pregnancy has been associated with birth defects. If pregnancy is suspected, the physician should be consulted immediately.

Availability. See Table 16-7.

• Nursing Interventions: Monitoring progestin therapy

See also General Nursing Considerations for Patients Receiving Gonadal Hormones (p. 410).

Table 16-7 *Progestins*

GENERIC NAME	BRAND NAME	AVAILABILITY	USES	DOSES
Hydroxyprogesterone	Delalutin, Pro-Depo, Hylutin	Injection: 125, 250 mg/ml	Amenorrhea; abnormal uterine bleeding	IM: 375 mg
			Uterine carcinoma	IM: 1-7 g weekly
Medroxyprogesterone	Provera, Amen, Curretab	Tablets: 2.5, 5, 10 mg	Secondary amenorrhea	PO: 5-10 mg daily for 5-10 days
			Abnormal uterine bleeding	PO: 5-10 mg daily for 5-10 days, beginning on the 16th or 21st day of the menstrual cycle
Norethindrone	Norlutin	Tablets: 5 mg	Amenorrhea, abnormal uterine bleeding	PO: 5-20 mg starting with the 5th and ending on the 25th day of the menstrual cycle
			Endometriosis	PO: 10 mg for 2 weeks; increase in increments of 5 mg/day every 2 weeks until 30 mg/day is reached
Norethindrone acetate	Norlutate, Aygestin	Tablets: 5 mg	Amenorrhea, abnormal uterine bleeding	PO: 2.5-10 mg starting with the 5th and ending on the 25th day of the menstrual cycle
			Endometriosis	PO: 5 mg for 2 weeks; increase in increments of 2.5 mg/day every 2 weeks until 15 mg/day is reached
Norgestrel	Ovrette	Tablets: 0.075 mg	Oral contraceptive	PO: 1 tablet daily
Progesterone	Progesterone, ♣Gesterol	Injection: 50 mg/ml	Amenorrhea, functional uterine bleeding	IM: 5-10 mg for 6-8 consecutive days

♣Available in Canada only.

Side effects to expect

WEIGHT GAIN, EDEMA, NAUSEA, VOMITING, DIARRHEA, TIREDNESS, OILY SCALP, ACNE. These symptoms tend to the mild and resolve with continued therapy. If they do not resolve, or become particularly bothersome, have the patient consult the physician.

Side effects to report

BREAKTHROUGH BLEEDING, AMENORRHEA, CONTINUING HEADACHE, CHOLESTATIC JAUNDICE, MENTAL DEPRESSION. These are all complications associated with progestin therapy. It is extremely important that the patient is evaluated by the physician to consider alternatives in therapy.

PREGNANCY. Due to the possibility of birth defects, a physician should be consulted immediately.

Drug interactions

RIFAMPIN. Rifampin may enhance the metabolism of progestins. The dosage of progestins may have to be increased to provide therapeutic benefit.

Androgens

The dominant male sex hormone is *testosterone*. It is the primary natural androgen produced by the testicles. Androgens are responsible for the normal growth and development of male sex organs and for maintenance of secondary sex characteristics. These effects include the growth and maturation of the prostate, seminal vesicles, penis, and scrotum; the development of male hair distribution; laryngeal enlargement (Adam's apple); vocal chord thickening; alterations in body musculature, and fat distribution. Androgens are used to treat hypogonadism, eunuchism, androgen deficiency, prevention of postpartum pain, breast engorgement, and palliation of breast cancer in certain postmenopausal women.

Side effects. Women receiving high doses of androgens may develop signs of masculinization manifested by a deepening of the voice, hirsutism, clitoral enlargement, acne, and menstrual irregularities.

In immobilized patients and patients with breast cancer, androgen therapy may cause hypercalcemia.

Androgens cause retention of sodium, potassium, and water. They may also cause gynecomastia and hepatotoxicity.

Androgens should generally not be used in prepubertal children because the drug may cause premature closure of the epiphyses, stopping bone growth.

Availability. See Table 16-8.

• Nursing Interventions: Monitoring androgen therapy

See also General Nursing Considerations for Patients Receiving Gonadal Hormones (p. 410).

Table 16-8 *Androgens*

GENERIC NAME	BRAND NAME	AVAILABILITY	USES	DOSES
Short-acting				
Testosterone in water	Testosterone aqueous, Testaqua, Andro 100	IM: 25, 50, 100 mg/ml	Eunuchism, postpubertal cryptorchidism, impotence due to androgen deficiency	IM: 25–50 mg 2–3 times daily
			Postpartum breast engorgement	IM: 25-50 mg daily for 3-4 days
			Breast carcinoma	IM: 50-100 mg 3 times weekly
Testosterone in oil	Testosterone propionate, Testex	IM: 25, 50, 100 mg/ml	As above	As above
Long-acting				
Testosterone enanthate	Everone, Andryl-200, Delatestryl	IM: 100, 200 mg/ml	Eunuchism, androgen deficiency	IM: 200-400 mg every 4 weeks
			Oligospermia	IM: 100-200 mg every 4-6 weeks
Testosterone Cypionate	Andro-cyp 100, Depotest, Duratest, Testa-C, ♣Depo-testosterone	IM: 50, 100, 200 mg/ml	As for testosterone enanthate	As for testosterone enanthate
Oral products				
Methyltestosterone	Oreton Methyl, Testred, Virilon, ♣Metandren	Tablets: 10, 25 mg Capsules: 10 mg Buccal tablets: 5, 10 mg	Eunuchism	PO: 10-40 mg daily
			Cryptorchidism	PO: 30 mg daily
			Postpartum breast engorgement	PO: 80 mg daily for 3-5 days
			Breast carcinoma	PO: 200 mg daily
Fluoxymesterone	Halotestin, Ora-Testryl, Android-F	Tablets: 2, 5, 10 mg	Male hypogonadism Female:	PO 2-10 mg daily
			breast carcinoma	PO: 10-40 mg daily
			postpartum breast engorgement	PO: 2.5 mg at onset of active labor; then 5-10 mg daily for 4-5 days

♣ Available in Canada only.

Side effects to expect

GASTRIC IRRITATION. If gastric irritation occurs, administer with food or milk. If symptoms persist or increase in severity, report for physician evaluation.

Side effects to report

ELECTROLYTE IMBALANCE, EDEMA. The most commonly altered electrolytes are potassium (K^+), sodium (Na^+), and chloride (Cl^-). Of these, *hyperkalemia* is most likely to occur.

Many symptoms associated with altered fluid and electrolyte balance are subtle and interspersed with general symptoms of drug toxicity or the disease process itself.

Gather data relative to changes in the patient's mental status (alertness, orientation, confusion), muscle strength, muscle cramps, tremors, nausea, and general appearance (drowsy, anxious, lethargic).

Always check the electrolyte reports for early indications of electrolyte imbalance.

Keep accurate records of intake and output, daily weights, and vital signs.

Patients should report weight gains of more than 2 pounds per week. Diuretic therapy, with or without dietary reduction of salt, may be prescribed if edema is significant.

MASCULINIZATION. Females should be monitored for signs of masculinization (deepening of the voice, hoarseness, growth of facial hair, clitoral enlargement, and menstrual irregularities) during androgen therapy. The drug should usually be discontinued when mild masculinization is evident, since some adverse androgenic effects (such as voice changes) may not reverse with discontinuation of therapy. In consultation with her physician, the woman may decide that some masculinization is acceptable during treatment for carcinoma of the breast. Assist patients to adjust to a possible change in self-image or self-esteem due to the effects of masculinization.

Males should be carefully monitored for the development of gynecomastia, priapism, or excessive sexual stimulation. These are indications of androgen overdose.

HYPERCALCEMIA. Monitor patients for nausea, vomiting, constipation, poor muscle tone, and lethargy. These are indications of hypercalcemia, and are indications for discontinuation of androgen therapy.

Force fluids to minimize the possibility of renal calculi. Encourage the patient to drink 8 to 12 8-ounce glasses of water daily.

Perform weightbearing and active and passive exercises to the degree tolerated by the patient to minimize loss of calcium from bones.

HEPATOTOXICITY. The symptoms of hepatotoxicity are: anorexia, nausea, vomiting, jaundice, hepatomegaly, splenomegaly, and abnormal liver function tests (elevated bilirubin, AST, ACT, GGT, alkaline phosphatase, prothrombin time).

Drug interactions

WARFARIN. Androgens may enhance the anticoagulant effects of warfarin. Observe for the development of petechiae, ecchymoses, nosebleeds, bleeding gums, dark tarry stools, and bright red or coffee ground emesis. Monitor the prothrombin time and reduce the dosage of warfarin if necessary.

ORAL HYPOGLYCEMIC AGENTS, INSULIN. Monitor for hypoglycemia: headache, weakness, decreased coordination, general apprehension, diaphoresis, hunger, blurred or double vision.

The dosage of the hypoglycemic agent or insulin may need to be reduced. Notify the physician if any of the above symptoms appear.

CORTICOSTEROIDS. Concurrent use may increase the possibility of electrolyte imbalance and fluid retention. See above for monitoring parameters.

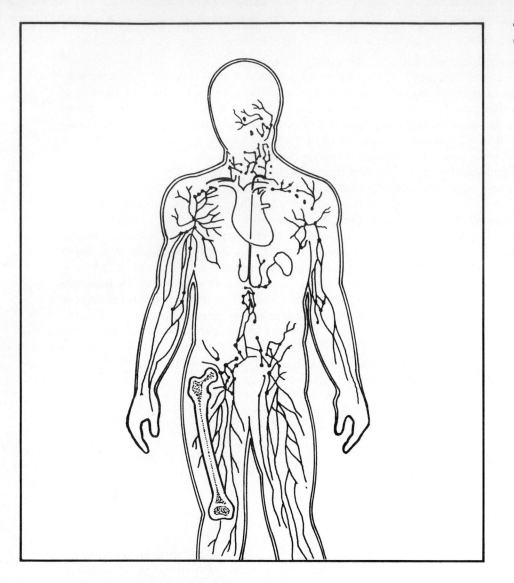

CHAPTER GOALS

After completing this chapter, the student should be able to do the following:

1. Explain the major action and effects of drugs used to provide immunity.
2. Identify baseline data the nurse should collect on a continuous basis for comparison and evaluation of drug effectiveness.
3. Identify important nursing assessments and interventions associated with the drug therapy used to provide immunity.
4. Identify essential components involved in planning patient education for a successful treatment regimen.

NURSING CONSIDERATIONS
AND DRUG THERAPY FOR:

Drug therapy to:
  Induce immunity
    Immune serums (p. 424)

Toxoids   (p. 424)
Vaccines   (p. 427)
Antitoxins   (p. 429)

Induce immunosuppression
  Immunosuppressant   (p. 429)

IMMUNITY

OBJECTIVES

1. Analyze Tables 17-1, 17-2, and 17-3 to determine different recommended immunizations based on the age of the recipient.
2. State the nursing assessments needed to monitor therapeutic response and/or the development of side effects to expect or report from immunizations.
3. Develop measurable objectives for patient education for patients receiving immunizations.
4. Identify locations of immunization clinics in your community.

KEY WORDS

active and passive immunity	antigen
antibodies	toxin
immunization	MMR
DPT	Td

Immunity is a state of resistance to disease. There are two kinds of immunity: natural and acquired (see Figure 17-1). *Natural immunity* is endowed at birth and is retained for life. Microorganisms that live within a host organism such as a human being are harmless to that organism because it has natural defense mechanisms to ward off infection from the microorganism.

Acquired immunity may be *active* or *passive*. Active acquired immunity results when the host organism develops antibodies against the invading antigens, or microorganisms. Active immunity may be induced by artificial means, such as by injection of antigens. Examples of antigens include a suspension of living, inactivated organisms, such as the measles virus in measles vaccine, or a suspension of dead microorganisms, such as in typhoid vaccine. The antigen may be a toxin produced by a bacteria, such as the diphtheria toxin, or it may be an extract from the microorganism, such as the

cell capsules of the influenza viruses used to make influenza vaccine.

Passive acquired immunity can be obtained in two ways: (1) an individual may be given the serum of an animal that has been actively immunized by injections with the specific microorganism that causes a particular disease, or (2) an individual may be given an injection of the serum of an immune person. This serum is rich in antibodies developed to protect the host against the specific disease antigen. *Passive* is used to describe this type of acquired immunity because the recipient's body plays no active part in the preparation of antibodies. The body does not produce antibodies to resist infection as it does in active immunity. As the blood is renewed, the acquired antibodies are lost, so the individual must be reimmunized periodically to maintain protection against that specific microorganism.

General Nursing Considerations for Patients Receiving Immunological Agents

Nurses need to remain current in their knowledge of the recommendations for administration of immunizations. Educating the public about the need for immunizations is a particular challenge because most young people who are now parents have not personally seen the crippling effects of the diseases that immunizations protect against.

In order to comply with immunization recommendations and to foster public health, several states have passed laws that require children to have certain immunizations before entering school. Exceptions are granted for medical reasons if approved by a physician. See Tables 17-1, 17-2, and 17-3 for immunization schedules.

Many people wrongly believe that exposure to someone who has had the disease causes them to be immune to it, too. It should be stressed that exposure does *not* ensure immunity.

A written record of all immunizations should be maintained. At the time of immunization, give the patient (or parents) (1) a record of the *exact* name, dosage, route of administration, and site of injection received (as appropriate to the medication type); (2) discharge instructions for the treatment of symptoms that may develop; and (3) a schedule of additional immunizations that are needed. Suggest recording this information in the child's baby book or the family Bible.

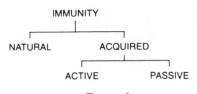

Figure 17-1 *Types of immunity.*

Table 17-1 *Recommended Schedule for Active Immunization of Normal Infants and Children*

RECOMMENDED AGE†	VACCINE(S)§	COMMENTS
2 months	DTP-1¶ + OPV-1** +[HbOC-1¶¶ or PRP-OMP-1§§§]	Can be given earlier in areas of high endemicity
4 months	DTP-2 + OPV-2 + [HbOC-2 or PRP-OMP-2]	6-week to 2-month interval desired between OPV doses to avoid interference
6 months	DTP-3 + HbOC-3	An additional dose of OPV at this time is optional for use in areas with a high risk of polio exposure
12 months	PRP-OMP booster	Completion of primary series of DTP and OPV
15 months††	MMR§§ + DTP-4 + OPV-3 + HbOC booster	Can be given at 18-23 months for children in groups who are thought to be at increased risk of disease, such as day-care–center attendees
4-6 years***	DTP-5, OPV-4	Preferably at or before school entry
14-16 years	Td†††	Repeat every 10 years throughout life

From Centers for Disease Control: *Morbid Mortal Week Rep* 40:1-28, Aug. 8, 1991 and 40:RR-1, Jan. 11, 1991.
†These recommended ages should not be construed as absolute; 2 months can be 6-10 weeks, etc.
§For all products used, consult manufacturer's package enclosure for instructions for storage, handling, and administration. Immunobiologics prepared by different manufacturers may vary, and those of the same manufacturer may change from time to time. The package insert should be followed for a specific product.
¶DTP—Diphtheria and Tetanus Toxoids and Pertussis Vaccine Adsorbed.
**OPV—Poliovirus Vaccine Live Oral; contains poliovirus strains types 1, 2, and 3.
††Provided at least 6 months have elapsed since DTP-3 or, if fewer than three DTPs have been received, at least 6 weeks since last previous dose of DTP or OPV. MMR vaccine should not be delayed just to allow simultaneous administration with DTP and OPV. Administering MMR at 15 months and DTP-4 and OPV-3 at 18 months continues to be an acceptable alternative.
§§MMR—Measles, Mumps, and Rubella Virus Vaccine, Live.
¶¶HbOC—*Haemophilus b* Oligosaccharide Conjugate (diphtheria CRM-197 protein conjugate) Vaccine (HibTITER).
***Up to the seventh birthday.
†††Td—Tetanus and Diphtheria Toxoids Adsorbed (for adult use). Contains the same dose of tetanus toxoid as DTP or DT and a reduced dose of diphtheria toxoid.
§§§PRP-OMP—*Haemophilus b* Polysaccharide Conjugate (meningococcal protein conjugate) Vaccine (Pedvax HIB).

Table 17-2 *Recommended Immunization Schedule for Infants and Children Up to Seventh Birthday Not Immunized at the Recommended Time in Early Infancy**

TIMING	VACCINE	COMMENTS
First visit	DTP-1,† OPV-1,‡ (If child is ≥15 months of age, MMR§ and HbV**)	DTP, OPV, and MMR can be administered simultaneously to children ≥15 months of age
2 months after first DTP, OPV	DTP-2, OPV-2	
2 months after second DTP	DTP-3	An additional dose of OPV at this time is optional for use in areas with a high risk of polio exposure
6-12 months after third DTP	DTP-4, OPV-3	
Preschool‖ (4-6 years)	DTP-5, OPV-4	Preferably at or before school entry
14-16 years	Td¶	Repeat every 10 years throughout life

From Centers for Disease Control: *Morbid Mortal Week Rep* 40:1-28, Aug. 8, 1991 and 40:RR-1, Jan. 11, 1991.
*If initiated in the first year of life, give DTP-1, 2, and 3, OPV-1 and 2 according to this schedule and give MMR when the child becomes 15 months old.
†DTP—Diphtheria and tetanus toxoids with pertussis vaccine. DTP may be used up to the seventh birthday.
‡OPV—Oral, attenuated poliovirus vaccine contains poliovirus types 1, 2, and 3.
§MMR—Live measles, mumps, and rubella viruses in a combined vaccine.
‖The preschool dose is not necessary if the fourth dose of DTP and third dose of OPV are administered after the fourth birthday.
¶Td—Adult tetanus toxoid and diphtheria toxoid in combination, which contains the same dose of tetanus toxoid as DTP or DT and a reduced dose of diphtheria toxoid.
**HbV- *Haemophilus b* Polysaccharide or Conjugate Vaccine.

Table 17-3 *Recommended Immunization Schedule for Persons 7 Years of Age or Older*

TIMING	VACCINE	COMMENTS
First visit	Td-1,* OPV-1,† and MMR‡	OPV not routinely administered to those ≥ 18 years of age
2 months after first Td, OPV	Td-2, OPV-2	
6-12 months after second Td, OPV	Td-3, OPV-3	OPV-3 may be given as soon as 6 weeks after OPV-2
10 years after Td-3	Td	Repeat every 10 years throughout life

From Centers for Disease Control: *Morbid Mortal Week Rep* 40:RR-10, Aug. 8, 1991.
*Td—Tetanus and diphtheria toxoids (adult type) are used after the seventh birthday. The DTP doses given to children under 7 who remain incompletely immunized at age 7 or older should be counted as prior exposure to tetanus and diphtheria toxoids (for example, a child who previously received 2 doses of DTP needs only 1 dose of Td to complete a primary series).
†OPV—Oral, attenuated poliovirus vaccine contains poliovirus types 1, 2, and 3. When polio vaccine is to be given to individuals 18 years or older, IPV is preferred.
‡MMR—Live measles, mumps, and rubella viruses in a combined vaccine. Persons born before 1957 can generally be considered immune to measles and mumps and need not be immunized. Rubella vaccine may be given to persons of any age, particularly to women of childbearing age. MMR may be used, since administration of vaccine to persons already immune is not deleterious.

Patient Concerns: Nursing Intervention/Rationale

Screening before administration of immunologic agents

History of immunizations. Ask patients if they have ever received any previous immunizations, and, if so, if they experienced any symptoms after the immunizations.

History of allergy. Take a thorough medication history BEFORE administering medications. People with a history of allergies, asthma, and chronic rhinitis are particularly susceptible to drug reactions.

Ask specifically about allergies. People with a history of allergy to eggs, feathers, aminoglycoside antibiotics, or horses may require intradermal skin testing before administration of the immunologic agent.

Infections. People with a current infection are generally not given immunizations because it is then difficult to determine whether the symptoms of the patient are due to the infection or are a reaction to the immunization.

Check the policy of your facility concerning the presence of "cold" symptoms; some institutions do give immunizations if symptoms are mild, while others postpone them entirely.

Immunosuppression. Do not administer live, attenuated virus vaccines to those with impaired immune systems. These patients are susceptible to infection from the virus.

People in direct contact with immunosuppressed patients should not receive oral polio vaccine. The live, attenuated virus is excreted from the immunized person's body and may infect the immunosuppressed patient.

Pregnancy. Always ask women of childbearing age if they are pregnant or likely to become pregnant within 3 months after immunization. Depending upon the immunologic agent, there is a risk of birth defects to the fetus.

Nursing actions

Do not administer the medication if the person reports possible allergy, infection, pregnancy, or immunosuppression. Share all information obtained with the physician, who will decide whether to administer the medication.

When a definite drug allergy is identified, the patient's chart, unit Kardex, and identification bracelet should be carefully marked to alert all personnel to the specific agents the patient should *not* receive.

Responding to allergic reactions

Observations. All patients should be watched closely for possible allergy for at least 20 to 30 minutes following the administration of an immunologic agent.

Emergency cart. Know the location of the hospital emergency cart and the procedure for summoning it. In the event of suspected anaphylaxis, summon the physician and the emergency cart immediately.

Sites of reactions. Although a serious reaction may occur with the first administration of a drug, repeated exposures to a previously sensitized substance can be fatal. Respond immediately to any signs of reaction, including the following:

- Swelling, redness, or pain at the site of injection
- Hives, nasal congestion and discharge, wheezing progressing to increasing dyspnea, pulmonary edema, tachycardia, hypotension, stridor, and sternal retractions

Follow-up. Following any reaction, the patient and family should be alerted to inform anyone treating them in the future that they are allergic to a specific drug.

Prevention of disease transmission

Needles and syringes. Always use a separate needle and syringe, regardless of the expense, when administering injections of any type. The recommendations of the Centers for Disease Control (CDC) should be followed precisely to prevent HIV transmission in health-care settings. The "universal blood and body fluid precautions" should be implemented in all health-care settings. The precautions are needed to prevent accidental "needle-sticks" of the health care worker during needle use, cleaning procedures, or disposal of used needles. DO NOT RECAP NEEDLES, DO NOT BEND OR BREAK NEEDLES, and DO NOT REMOVE NEEDLES from the syringe. Place used syringes and needles in a puncture-resistant container located in the immediate vicinity of use. Follow policies that are consistent with the recommendations of the CDC for disposal of used needles and syringes.

Hygiene. Thoroughly wash your hands between patients to prevent possible spread of disease. Gloves should be worn whenever the health-care worker may come in contact with blood or other body fluids and when performing a venipuncture or other vascular access procedure. Wash hands immediately after removing the gloves.

Patient Education Associated with Immunological Agents

Communication and responsibility. Encourage open communication concerning frustrations and anger as the patient attempts to adjust to the diagnosis and need for completion of treatment. The patient must be guided to insight into the need for immunity and to assume responsibility for the continuation of treatment. Keep emphasizing those factors the patient can control to alter the disease progression: maintenance of general health, nutritional needs, adequate rest and appropriate exercise, and continuation of prescribed immunizations to achieve immunity to the disease process, thereby preventing not only development of the disease but also complications that may arise from the disease and drug therapy.

Expectations of therapy. Discuss expectations of therapy with the patient: prevention of the development of communicable disease for which immunization is being given. Assess changes in expectations as therapy progresses and the patient gains understanding of the need to complete all immunizations for effective prevention of disease.

Changes in expectations. Assess changes in expectations as therapy progresses and the patient gains understanding of the immunization required.

Changes in therapy through cooperative goal setting. Work with the patient to encourage adherence to the prescribed treatment. When the patient feels that a change should be made in a treatment plan, encourage a discussion first with the physician.

Written record. Enlist the patient's aid in developing and maintaining a written record of monitoring parameters (Figure 17-2) (rash, general malaise, arthralgias) and response to prescribed therapies for discussion with the physician. Patients should be encouraged to take this record with them on follow-up visits or to call the physician if symptoms become intense.

Fostering compliance. Discuss medication information and how it will benefit the course of treatment. Seek cooperation and understanding of the following points so that medication compliance may be enhanced:

1. Name.
2. Dosage.
3. Route and administration times: Nurses must foster maintenance of the administration schedule and the need to comply rigidly with appropriate storage of the immunologic agents.
4. Anticipated therapeutic response.
5. Side effects to expect: Most immunization clinics have routine orders for health teaching that state the usual symptoms to expect, such as pain, swelling, and tenderness at the injection site.

   The person may develop a subclinical case of the disease for which the vaccine was given. The person needs to understand what symptoms may develop and how to treat fever, general malaise, or rash, should they occur. Check your institution's policies regarding routine orders.
6. Side effects to report: Always tells the patient to contact the physician or go to the nearest emergency room if these symptoms develop.
7. What to do if a dose is missed.
8. When, how, or if to return for the next in a series of immunizations to become sufficiently immunized.

Difficulty in comprehension. If it is evident that the patient and/or family do not understand all aspects of continuing therapy being prescribed (such as need for follow-up appointments and completion of all required immunizations), consider the use of social service or visiting nurse agencies.

Associated teaching. Always provide written information to the patient and family about the specific name of the agent that caused any reactions. Tell them always to inform all health workers (physicians, dentists, industrial nurses) of this reaction before receiving any treatment. Provide them with an allergy identification card and bracelet or necklace, if necessary.

Encourage the patient to report side effects of rash, itching, hives, or dyspnea immediately.

Always give the patient (1) a record of the *exact* name, dosage, route of administration and site of injection received (as appropriate to the medication type); (2) the discharge instructions for the treatment of symptoms that may develop; and (3) a schedule of additional immunizations that are needed. Have the patient maintain a current record of all immunizations received.

Patient Education and Monitoring of Therapeutic Outcomes for Patients Receiving Immune Agents (Vaccines or Immunizations)

Medications	Color	To be taken

Name _____

Physician _____

Physician's phone _____

Next appt.* _____

Parameters		Day of injection								Comments
Temperature	8 AM | 12 N / 5 PM | Bed time									
Pulse										
Skin (rash)	Hivelike, fine red; itching present — (Yes or No)									
Joint discomfort	None									
	Aching									
	Painful									
Irritability	None									
	Mild									
	Unconsolable									
	Last ___ hr./ min.									
How I feel Tired ___ Okay 10 5 1										
Dizziness	Faint when in upright position									
	Occasional									
	None									
Site of injection	Hot, swollen, and painful									
	Swollen, some discomfort									
	No problem									

*Please bring this record with you to your next appointment.
Use the back of this sheet for additional information.

Figure 17-2 *Patient education and monitoring of therapeutic outcomes for patients receiving immune agents (vaccines or immunizations).*

If pregnancy is suspected, consult an obstetrician as soon as possible about continuation of medication therapy or series of immunizations.

Drug Therapy to Induce Immunity

Immune serums

OBJECTIVES

1. Identify the source of immune serums.
2. Cite contraindications for the administration of immune serums.
3. Describe specific equipment and supplies that should be readily available when immune serums are administered.
4. State the sites and routes of administration of immune serums.
5. Describe the signs, symptoms, and immediate treatment necessary for an anaphylactic reaction.
6. State the type of immunity conferred by the administration of an immune serum and explain the duration of the immune response.
7. Explain factors affecting the sequencing of a serum and a vaccine.

KEY WORD

antiimmunoglobulin A antibodies

An immune serum is derived from the serum of a human being who has formed antibodies in the bloodstream against a specific disease. The immune serum is injected into the patient, where specific antibodies that act on disease microorganisms provide passive acquired immunity.

Naturally produced human serums are obtained from the serum of patients who have recovered from a disease and still have the immune antibodies in their blood serum.

All of the immune serums listed in Table 17-4 are obtained from human plasma and contain gamma globulin. The plasma is pooled from blood donors from the general population or from donors who have been immunized against a specific disease. All products are now screened to prevent transmission of human immunodeficiency virus (HIV).

Considerations for use. These products are contraindicated in patients who are allergic to gamma globulin or who have produced antiimmunoglobulin A (IgA) antibodies.

Do not administer skin tests with these products. Local irritation from intradermal injection may easily be misinterpreted as a positive allergic response. True allergic reactions to human gamma globulin administered intramuscularly are extremely rare.

After intramuscular injection, patients may have mild, localized tenderness and stiffness, which may persist for several hours after injection.

Although rare, allergic reactions, manifested by urticaria, angioedema, erythema, and low-grade fever, have been reported. Anaphylactic reaction, although even more rare, is more likely to develop in patients receiving intravenous immune globulin products who have received repeated infusions and who are highly allergic individuals. Epinephrine (1:1000) and other appropriate agents should be available to treat allergic reactions.

Availability. See Table 17-4 for available products.
Administration. See Table 17-4.
IM—Administer these agents intramuscularly (except Immune Globulin, Intravenous), preferably in the gluteal or deltoid region.

• Do not mix with any other product.

IV—Except for Immune Globulin, Intravenous (Gamimune), do not administer these products intravenously. A severe hypotensive reaction may result.

• Immune Globulin, Intravenous, may be diluted with dextrose 5% solution.

• Nursing Interventions: Monitoring immune serum therapy

See also General Nursing Considerations for Patients Receiving Immunologic Agents (p. 419).

Side effects to expect

LOCALIZED TENDERNESS. Inform patients that they may experience stiffness at the site of injection for several days.

FEVER, ARTHRALGIAS, GENERALIZED ACHES AND PAINS. Monitor on a regular basis for the development of these symptoms. Be certain patients (or parents) know how to take a temperature.

Follow routine orders of the physician or clinic concerning the use of analgesics (usually acetaminophen; do not use aspirin or other antiinflammatory agents) for patient discomfort.

Side effects to report

URTICARIA, TACHYCARDIA, HYPOTENSION. Allergic reactions need immediate treatment. Monitor patients for 20 to 30 minutes following administration. Have emergency supplies readily available.

Drug interactions

LIVE VIRUS VACCINES. Antibodies in the immune globulin solutions may interfere with the immune response to live virus vaccination. Do not administer live virus vaccines for at least 3 months after the administration of immune globulin products.

Toxoids

OBJECTIVES

1. Identify the specific type of immune response toxoids produce.
2. Explain contraindications to the administration of toxoids.

Table 17-4 *Immune Serums*

GENERIC NAME	BRAND NAME	AVAILABILITY	COMMENTS
Cytomegalovirus immune globulin (CMV-IVIG)	Same	IV: 2.5 g vial	To be used against CMV disease associated with kidney transplantation
Hepatitis B immune globulin	H-BIG, HyperHep, Hep-B-Gammagee	IM: 1 and 5 ml vials	To be used after accidental exposure by "needle stick" or direct mucous membrane contact from blood, plasma, or serum containing hepatitis B antigen
Immune globulin	Gamimune N, Gammar IV, Sandoglobulin, Gammagard	IV: 5% in 50 and 100 ml vials IM: 2 and 10 ml vials	Used for hepatitis A, hepatitis B, rubeola, rubella exposure IV: Provides immediate antibody levels to provide protection for patients with immune deficiencies IM: Requires 2-7 days for adequate antibody levels
Lymphocyte immune globulin, anti-thymocyte globulin (equine)	Atgam	IM: 50 mg/ml in 5 ml ampules	Used in conjunction with other immunosuppressant therapy to prevent rejection of transplants
Rh₀ (D) immune globulin	RhoGAM, HypRho-D, Gamulin Rh, ♣Winn Rho	IM: 1:1000 dilution, single dose vials	Used in patients who are Rh negative who have been exposed to Rh positive blood; prevents the formation of antibodies that may cause hemolysis if exposed to Rh positive blood again
Tetanus immune globulin	Hyper-Tet	IM: 250 unit vials and pre-filled syringes	For patients exposed to tetanus who have not been immunized with tetanus toxoid
Varicella-zoster immune globulin (VZIG)	Same	IM: 125 units in 2.5 ml vials	For use in immunodeficient children exposed to varicella-zoster (chicken pox)

♣ Available in Canada only.

3. State the signs, symptoms, and immediate treatment of an allergic reaction to the administration of a toxoid.
4. Identify the correct route and technique for administration of toxoids.

KEY WORDS

active acquired immunity
detoxification
toxins

A toxoid is a toxin that has been chemically modified to be nontoxic but still antigenic, thus inducing active, acquired immunity. The agent generally used for the detoxification of toxins is formaldehyde. Toxoids are available in the plain fluid form and as adsorbed and precipitated preparations. Aluminum hydroxide and aluminum phosphate are used to provide an adsorption surface for the adsorbed products, and alum is used for the precipitated products. The adsorbed and precipitated products are absorbed more slowly by the circulating and tissue fluids of the body and are excreted more slowly; thus, they provide immunizing levels longer than the plain fluid form of toxoid.

Considerations for use. These products are contraindicated in patients who are allergic to any one of the individual toxoids. For example, if a patient is allergic to tetanus toxoid, do not administer diphtheria and tetanus toxoids and pertussis vaccine (DPT). The patient may be immunized, however, for diphtheria and pertussis by using individual immunologic products.

In general, do not use these products in patients with an acute infection or who are immunosuppressed. It is difficult to differentiate symptoms of disease from symptoms of reaction to the toxoid if the patient is ill. If a patient is immunosuppressed, it is unlikely that an adequate number of antibodies will be produced against the toxoid, thus the patient will be unprotected.

Infants or children with cerebral damage, neurologic disorders, or a history of febrile convulsions should have their routine immunizations postponed until at least 1 year of age or, in the case of tetanus toxoid, administered first as a small dose to test the patient's tolerance to the toxoid.

DO NOT use toxoids as vaccines for treatment against active infection. Antitoxins or, preferably, specific immune globulins must be administered.

Localized reactions at the site of intramuscular injection are not uncommon. This reaction may be manifested by localized edema, itching, erythema, and induration, which will persist for several days. A nodule may be present at the site for several weeks.

Systemic allergic reactions are quite rare but are manifested by chills, fever, urticaria, generalized aches and pains, flushing, tachycardia, and hypotension. Epinephrine (1:1000) and other appropriate agents should be readily available to treat allergic reactions.

It is recommended that routine immunization schedules be postponed if an outbreak of poliomyelitis should occur. Complete the immunization schedule after the poliomyelitis infection is over.

Availability. See Table 17-5.

Administration

IM—Administer into the deltoid or midlateral muscles of the thigh. Do not inject the same muscle site more than once during the course of the routine immunization schedule.

Table 17-5 *Toxoids*

GENERIC NAME	BRAND NAME	AVAILABILITY	COMMENTS
Tetanus toxoid	Tetanus Toxoid, Fluid; Tetanus Toxoid, Adsorbed	SC: Fluid—0.5 ml syringes and vials, 7.5 ml vials IM: Adsorbed—0.5 ml syringes and vials, 5 ml vials	Tetanus Toxoid, Adsorbed, is recommended for all routine immunization and booster doses Use is recommended for military personnel, farm and utility workers, firemen, and all other persons whose occupation may place them at risk for lacerations and abrasions Do not administer if previous doses resulted in hypersensitivity or neurologic reactions
Diphtheria toxoid	Diphtheria Toxoid Adsorbed (Pediatric)	IM: 5 ml vials	Recommended for use if a patient should not receive either Tetanus Toxoid or Pertussis Vaccine Postpone immunization until age 2 if the infant has a history of seizure activity Do not administer to children over 6 years of age
Diphtheria and tetanus toxoids	Diphtheria and Tetanus Toxoids, Adsorbed, Pediatric and Adult Strengths	IM: 0.5 ml prefilled syringes, 5 ml vials	Administer the pediatric strength (Td) up to age 6 Administer the adult strength (Td) after age 6 Booster injections should be administered every 10 years See comments above
Diphtheria and tetanus toxoids, pertussis vaccine	Diphtheria, Tetanus, Pertussis Vaccine, Adsorbed-Connaught; Tri-Immunol; Ultrafined Triple Antigen	IM: 7.5 vials, 0.5 ml prefilled syringe	Recommended for routine immunizations in children between 2 months and 6 years of age Children beyond the age of 7 years should not be immunized with pertussis vaccine See comments above

SC, IV—DO NOT administer subcutaneously or intravenously.

• **Nursing Interventions: Monitoring toxoid therapy**

See also General Nursing Considerations for Patients Receiving Immunologic Agents (p. 419).

Side effects to expect

FEVER, ARTHRALGIAS, GENERALIZED ACHES AND PAINS. Monitor on a regular basis for the development of these symptoms. Be certain patients (or parents) know how to take a temperature.

Follow routine orders of the physician or clinic concerning the use of analgesics (usually acetaminophen, do not use aspirin or other antiinflammatory agents) for patient discomfort.

Side effects to report

URTICARIA, TACHYCARDIA, HYPOTENSION. Allergic reactions need immediate treatment. Monitor patients for 20 to 30 minutes following administration. Have emergency supplies readily available.

Implementation

IM. Administer intramuscularly using the correct length needle to ensure that the medication is being deposited into the muscle.

Since toxoids may be irritating to the tissues, 0.1 to 0.2 cc of air may be used to flush irritating medications from the needle into the muscle when being injected. (Check your institution's policy before administration.)

Drug interactions

CHLORAMPHENICOL, IMMUNOSUPPRESSANTS. Chloramphenicol, corticosteroids, antimetabolites, and alkylating agents may inhibit production of antibodies against the toxoid. Discontinue chloramphenicol and immunosuppressant therapy before immunization.

Vaccines
OBJECTIVES

1. Identify the specific type of immune response produced by vaccines.
2. Cite contraindications to the use of vaccines.
3. Differentiate among the uses of vaccines, toxoids, and antitoxins.
4. Identify the proper storage method for vaccines.
5. Develop specific questions to be used to screen for allergies prior to the administration of vaccines.

KEY WORDS

attenuated bacteria antigens
antibodies passive immunity
active immunity

Vaccines are suspensions of either live, attenuated or killed bacteria or viruses. They are administered as antigens to stimulate the production of antibodies by the host against the specific bacteria or virus. In contrast to short-term, passive immunity provided by immune se-

rums and antitoxins, vaccines provide long-term, active immunity. Since vaccines must stimulate the production of antibodies, immunity is acquired over several days to weeks. Vaccines are administered prophylactically to prevent infection from specific organisms, whereas antitoxins and immune serums are administered after exposure to a specific organism for immediate protection. See Table 17-6.

Considerations for use. Vaccines are contraindicated in patients who are allergic to the culture media (such as chick embryos), preservatives (such as thimerosal), or antibodies (such as neomycin) used in the manufacturing process.

Live, attenuated viruses should not be administered to patients with immune deficiencies or to those who are immunosuppressed. Replication of the virus may be enhanced in these patients.

Patients should not be immunized during a severe, febrile illness. It is difficult to differentiate symptoms of disease from symptoms of reaction to the vaccine if the patient is ill.

Live, attenuated virus vaccines should not be administered during pregnancy or to women who may become pregnant in the next 3 months. They have potential teratogenic effects on the developing fetus.

DO NOT use vaccines or toxoids for treatment against active infection. Antitoxins, or preferably, specific immune globulins must be administered.

Vaccinations are associated with a low risk of adverse effects, but reactions have been reported for all vaccines. These effects range from mild, local reactions to the very rare, severe systemic illness, such as anaphylaxis or paralysis. See Table 17-4 for precautions on individual vaccines.

Availability. See Table 17-6.

Administration

SC, IM—See individual manufacturer's recommendations.

DO NOT ADMINISTER INTRAVENOUSLY.

Storage at the correct temperature is imperative. DO NOT keep in the refrigerator door, since this temperature is highly variable due to frequent opening. Place on the center shelf in the refrigerator, and periodically monitor the refrigerator temperature.

• **Nursing Interventions: Monitoring vaccine therapy**

See also General Nursing Considerations for Patients Receiving Immunologic Agents (p. 419).

Side effects to expect

FEVER, ARTHRALGIAS, GENERALIZED ACHES AND PAINS. Monitor on a regular basis for the development of these symptoms. Be certain patients (or parents) know how to take a temperature.

Follow routine orders of the physician or clinic concerning the use of analgesics (usually acetaminophen; do not use aspirin or other antiinflammatory agents) for patient discomfort.

Table 17-6 *Vaccines*

GENERIC NAME	BRAND NAME	AVAILABILITY	COMMENTS
Cholera vaccine	Cholera Vaccine	SC, IM: 1, 1.5, 20 ml vials	Killed virus; used primarily for immunity prior to traveling to an area of the world where cholera is still active. Only about 60% of patients injected gain immunity against cholera.
Haemophilus b vaccine	HibTITER	IM: 1, 5, 10 dose vials	*Haemophilus b* oligosaccharide conjugated with diphtheria protein (HbOC). Recommended doses are at 2, 4, and 6 months with a booster at 15 months.
	Pedvax HIB	IM: 0.5 ml powder	*Haemophilus b* polysaccharide conjugated with meningococcal protein (PRP-OMP). Recommended doses are at 2 and 4 months with a booster at 12 months.
	ProHIBiT	IM: 1, 5, 10 dose vials	*Haemophilus b* polysaccharide conjugated with diphtheria protein (PRP-D). A single dose is recommended for unimmunized children 15 months to 5 years of age.
Hepatitis B vaccine	Heptavax-B, Recombivax HB, Engerix-B	IM: 0.5, 1 ml vials	Derived from hepatitis B surface antigen. Vaccination strongly encouraged for all health care workers and patients at high risk for infection with hepatitis B virus. The deltoid muscle is the preferred site in adults.
Influenza vaccine	Fluogen, Fluzone	IM: 0.5, 5, 25 ml vials	Inactivated antigens of virus expected to be prevalent for the next year. Do not administer to patients allergic to eggs, chickens, and chick feathers. Recommended for patients over age 65 due to greater susceptibility and mortality from viral infections.
Measles (rubeola) vaccine	Attenuvax	SC: Single dose vials	Live, attenuated virus; administered to produce a mild measles infection. The mild infection then produces antibodies to prevent future, more serious measles infections.
Rubella vaccine	Meruvax II	SC: Single dose vials	Live, attenuated virus; administered to produce protection against german measles. Absolutely must not be administered to a female who might possibly become pregnant in the next 3 months. Vaccine contains Neomycin. Do not administer to patients allergic to aminoglycosides.
Measles, mumps, rubella vaccine	MMR II	SC: Single dose vials	Live, attenuated viruses. Infants must be at least 15-months of age. Use with caution in children with a history of febrile convulsions, or cerebral injury. Defer vaccination for at least 3 months after blood transfusion. See also measles and mumps vaccines.
Mumps vaccine	Mumpsvax	SC: Single dose vials	Live, attenuated virus. Used for adult and pediatric immunizations against mumps. Mild fevers may occur within 30 days of immunization. Do not administer to patients allergic to aminoglycosides, eggs, chickens, or chick feathers. Discard reconstituted vial after 8 hours.
Pneumococcal vaccine, polyvalent	Pneumovax 23, Pnu-Immune 23	SC, IM: 1 and 5 dose vials	Cell capsules of 23 very prevalent or invasive pneumococcal bacteria that account for 85-90% of pneumococcal bacterial infections. Used in patients who have chronic illnesses who may be at greater risk for viral infections.
Poliovirus vaccine live, oral, trivalent (TOPV)	Orimune	PO: 0.5 ml doses	Live, attenuated viruses; stimulates natural infection without producing symptoms of the disease. Do not administer to immunosuppressed patients. Do not administer during febrile illness. Absolutely do not administer parenterally.

Table 17-6 *Vaccines—cont'd*

GENERIC NAME	BRAND NAME	AVAILABILITY	COMMENTS
Rabies vaccine	Imovax	IM: Single dose vials	Freeze-dried suspension of inactivated rabies virus. Administered for patients who may be exposed to rabies, and for those who may have been exposed. If used post-exposure, an IM dose of rabies immune globulin (human) is also recommended. Soreness and swelling frequently occur and mild febrile responses have been reported. Corticosteroids may interfere with immunity against rabies. Do not administer with rabies vaccine.

Side effects to report

URTICARIA, TACHYCARDIA, HYPOTENSION. Allergic reactions need immediate treatment. Monitor patients for 20 to 30 minutes following administration. Have emergency supplies readily available.

Drug interactions

IMMUNOSUPPRESSANTS. Corticosteroids, antimetabolites, and alkylating agents may inhibit production of antibodies against the vaccine. Discontinue immunosuppressant therapy before immunization.

Do not administer oral poliovirus vaccine to immunosuppressed children or to people who will come in contact with these children. The excreted virus can be transmitted to the immunosuppressed child.

IMMUNE SERUM GLOBULINS. Antibodies in the immune globulin solutions may interfere with the immune response to live virus vaccines up to 3 months after administration of the globulin. It may be necessary to revaccinate persons who received immune globulins shortly after live virus vaccination.

Antitoxins
OBJECTIVES

1. Identify the specific use of an antitoxin.
2. Describe the procedure for performing intradermal skin testing prior to the administration of an antitoxin.
3. Identify characteristics of the reaction to the skin test that would preclude administration of the antitoxin.

KEY WORDS

toxins   antigens
passive immunity   antibodies

Antitoxic serums are formed in the bodies of horses that have been injected with either diphtheria or tetanus toxin. The toxin acts as an antigen, stimulating the formation of antibodies against the toxin. Antitoxins are similar to immune serums in that they produce passive immunity.

Antitoxins are administered to treat a patient who has been exposed to either diphtheria or tetanus. The disadvantage of antitoxins is that there is a high incidence of hypersensitivity to horse blood, even though the products are highly purified. Tetanus immune globulin is recommended for the prevention and treatment of tetanus. The antitoxin should be used only if the immune globulin is not available. There is no immune globulin available for diphtheria.

Tests for sensitivity to horse serum should be made on patients before injection of antitoxins to prevent possibilities of hypersensitivity and anaphylactic shock. The antitoxin should be withheld if a reaction characterized by a red, swollen area develops around the site of the intradermal test injection.

Immunosuppressant
OBJECTIVES

1. Review principles associated with an immune response.
2. Identify monitoring parameters needed to detect renal, hepatic, cardiovascular, neurological and/or hematologic side effects of immunosuppressant agents.
3. Describe specific precautions needed to prevent the immunosuppressed patient from contracting an infection.
4. Review the actions and side effects of corticosteroid therapy.
5. Cite specific assessments needed during the intravenous administration of cyclosporine.
6. Describe the dosing schedule for cyclosporine prior to and following transplantation procedures.
7. State the principles of oral administration of cyclosporine.
8. Identify the proper storage conditions of cyclosporine.
9. Develop measurable short- and long-term objectives for patient education for persons taking cyclosporine.

KEY WORDS

hirsutism	leukopenia
anemia	thrombocytopenia
gingival hyperplasia	lymphocyte proliferation

cyclosporine (syklo-spohr'in)

Sandimmune (sand-im'uhn)

Cyclosporine is a naturally occurring polypeptide antibiotic produced by fungi. It acts as an immunosuppressive agent by selectively inhibiting lymphocyte proliferation and activity that normally would have been associated with cell-mediated immune response that is partially responsible for tissue graft rejection. Unlike azathioprine, cyclosporine does not prevent tissue graft rejection by suppression of the bone marrow. Cyclosporine is used as an immunosuppressant for the prevention of rejection of tissue in transplants of organs such as the liver, kidney, bone marrow, and heart.

Side effects

Renal: The most frequent adverse effect of cyclosporine is nephrotoxicity.

Hepatic: Hepatotoxicity occurs in up to 7% of patients, usually during the first month of therapy when higher doses of cyclosporine are used.

Infection: All immunosuppressed patients are at higher risk for viral, bacterial, and fungal infections.

Cardiovascular: Hypertension has occurred in 25% to 40% of patients receiving cyclosporine therapy. Other rare cardiovascular effects include chest pain, edema, and muscle cramps.

Dermatologic: Hirsutism, sometimes severe, may develop in up to 50% of patients receiving cyclosporine. Gingival hyperplasia may occur in up to 30% of patients. Acne and brittle and abnormal fingernails have also been reported to develop during cyclosporine therapy.

Neurologic: Adverse neurologic complications develop in up to 50% of patients receiving cyclosporine. A fine hand tremor is most common, but headache, paresthesias of the hands and/or feet, flushing, and confusion have also been reported. Seizures have rarely occurred.

Gastrointestinal: Nausea, vomiting, anorexia, abdominal discomfort, hiccups, constipation, difficulty in swallowing, and diarrhea have all been reported with cyclosporine therapy.

Hematologic: Leukopenia, anemia, and thrombocytopenia have been reported to occur during cyclosporine therapy. The frequency has been much lower than that associated with combined azathioprine and corticosteroid therapy.

Availability

PO—100 mg/ml in 50 ml bottles.

Injection—50 mg/ml in 5 ml ampules.

Dosage and administration. NOTE: The manufacturer recommends that corticosteroid therapy be used in conjunction with cyclosporine therapy.

Adult and pediatric

PO—15 mg/kg/day as a single dose 4 to 12 hours before transplantation. This daily single dose is continued postoperatively for 1 to 2 weeks and then tapered gradually to a maintenance level of 5 to 10 mg/kg/day, depending on the patient's renal tolerance of the drug and the systemic cyclosporine concentration.

IV—NOTE: Sensitivity reactions, including anaphylaxis, have occurred in fewer than 2% of patients receiving IV cyclosporine. The allergic reaction may actually be due to solvents within the IV solution that are necessary for stability and solubility. Patients should be under continuous observation for at least the first 30 minutes following the start of the infusion and at frequent intervals thereafter. If anaphylaxis occurs, the infusion should be stopped. An aqueous solution of epinephrine 1:1000 should be available at the bedside as well as a source of oxygen.

Dosage—5 to 6 mg/kg/day as a single dose 4 to 12 hours before transplantation. This single daily dose is continued postoperatively until the patient is able to take oral cyclosporine solution. The usual oral dose is three (3) times the oral dose.

• Nursing Interventions: Monitoring cyclosporine therapy

See also General Nursing Considerations for Patients with Cancer (p. 528) and Patients with Infectious Diseases (p. 457).

Side effects to report

RENAL TOXICITY. Approximately 75% of patients experience at least one episode of renal dysfunction within 2 to 3 months after transplantation, manifested by a rise in serum creatinine and BUN, often without a concomitant fall in urine output. Most cases are reversible with reduction in cyclosporine dosage. Periodic assessment of renal function (BUN, creatinine) and cyclosporine blood level monitoring is essential to minimize this toxicity.

HEPATOTOXICITY. Laboratory signs indicative of hepatotoxicity include increased levels of AST, ALT, GGT, and bilirubin. Reduction of cyclosporine dosage usually reverses the hepatotoxic effects of the drug.

INFECTION. All immunosuppressed patients are at higher risk for viral, bacterial, and fungal infections. Promptly report signs of infection such as sore throat, fever, oral thrush, cough, malaise, anal pruritis, or vaginal discharge.

Teach the importance of meticulous oral and perineal personal hygiene measures.

HYPERTENSION. This effect generally responds to cyclosporine dosage reduction and the use of antihypertensive medication.

GASTROINTESTINAL. Administering the drug with milk, chocolate milk, or orange juice may make it more palatable. Patients with persistent diarrhea of more than 24 to 36 hours' duration should be told to notify their physician, as the dosage of cyclosporine may need to be increased in order to maintain adequate blood concentrations. Malabsorption syndromes are occasionally noted in patients after liver transplantation. Bile salts may be necessary for adequate absorption of cyclosporine in these patients.

Implementation

PO. Using the pipette provided, measure the prescribed dose and transfer to a glass container containing milk, chocolate milk, or orange juice, preferably at room temperature but not hot. After administration, rinse the glass a second time with milk, chocolate milk, or orange juice and administer to be sure that the full therapeutic dose is received. (Do not use styrofoam cups because they are porous and may absorb the drug.) Wipe the pipette with a clean, dry towel before replacing in the container. Do not rinse with water, alcohol, or other solvents, because this may result in clouding of the cyclosporine solution.

COUNSELING. Patient counseling is quite important in the long-term success of immunosuppressant therapy. Patients must understand that they will need to take cyclosporine daily for as long as they have a functioning transplant and that they should take their dose at the same time every day. Since dosage is critical and weight-dependent, daily weighing is recommended. Other critical signs to record include body temperature, 24-hour urine output and blood pressure. Patients must also understand that they must return for periodic laboratory tests to monitor body cyclosporine levels and renal and hepatic function.

STORAGE. Cyclosporine should be stored at temperatures below 85° F (30° C), but not refrigerated. Refrigeration tends to coalesce and separate the product. Once opened, the product must be used within 2 months.

IV. Dilute each 1 ml of cyclosporine IV in 20 to 100 ml of 0.9% sodium chloride injection or 5% dextrose injection and administer in a slow intravenous infusion over 2 to 6 hours.

Drug interactions

AMPHOTERICIN B, AMINOGLYCOSIDES, MELPHALAN, ACYCLOVIR. The nephrotoxic effects of cyclosporine may be potentiated by the concomitant use of these other nephrotoxic agents.

KETOCONAZOLE, CIMETIDINE, CARBAMAZEPINE, ERYTHROMYCIN. These agents increase blood concentrations of cyclosporine by inhibiting hepatic metabolism. Trough serum concentrations of cyclosporine should be monitored, and reduction of cyclosporine dosage or transfer to other immunosuppressant therapy should be considered.

PHENYTOIN, RIFAMPIN, ISONIAZID, PHENOBARBITAL, AND A COMBINATION OF IV SULFAMETHAZINE AND IV TRIMETHOPRIM. These agents decrease blood concentrations of cyclosporine, probably by stimulating hepatic enzymes to enhance metabolism. Monitoring blood cyclosporine concentrations and appropriate dosage adjustment are necessary when any of these drugs is used concomitantly with cyclosporine.

AZATHIOPRINE. The manufacturer recommends that cyclosporine should not be used with other immunosuppressive agents (such as azathioprine) other than corticosteroids, as the risk of lymphoma and other lymphoproliferative disorders and infection is significantly increased with excessive immunosuppression.

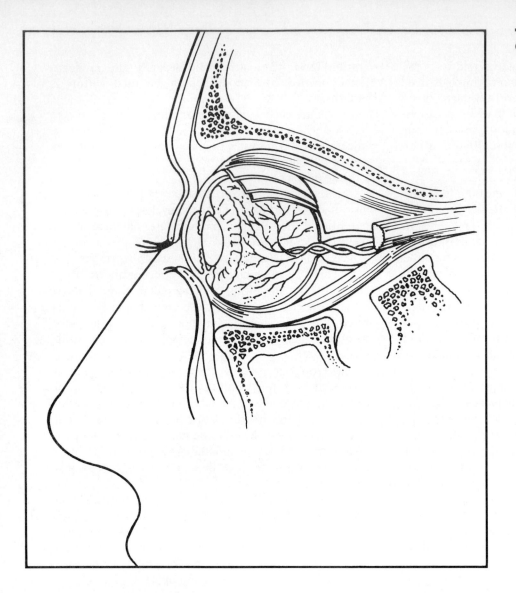

18

Drugs Affecting the Eye

CHAPTER GOALS

After completing this chapter, the student should be able to do the following:

1. Explain the major action and effects of drugs used to treat disorders of the eye.

2. Identify baseline data the nurse should collect on a continuous basis for comparison and evaluation of drug effectiveness.

3. Identify important nursing assessments and interventions associated with the drug therapy and treatment of diseases associated with the eye.

4. Identify essential components involved in planning patient education that will enhance compliance with the treatment regimen.

Disorders of the eye
    Osmotic agents (p. 438)
    Carbonic anhydrase inhibitors
      (p. 439)
    Anticholinergic agents
      (p. 440)
    Antiseptics (p. 441)
      Silver nitrate
    Anesthetics (p. 442)
    Antibacterial agents (p. 442)

Antifungal agents (p. 442)
    Natamycin
Antiviral agents (p. 443)
    Idoxuridine
    Trifluridine
    Vidarabine
Corticosteroids (p. 444)
Other ophthalmic agents (p. 444)
    Fluorescein sodium

Artificial tear solutions
Ophthalmic irrigants
Antiinflammatory agents
Antiallergic agent
Glaucoma
    Cholinergic agents (p. 448)
    Cholinesterase inhibitors (p.
      449)
    Adrenergic agents (p. 450)
    Beta-adrenergic blocking agents
      (p. 451)

DISORDERS OF THE EYE

Objectives

1. Review the anatomical structure of the eye.
2. Describe the physiology of miosis and mydriasis.
3. Describe the normal drainage system of the eye.
4. Explain information that should be obtained when performing a baseline assessment of the eyes.
5. Describe the anticholinergic actions of agents used for refraction.
6. Formulate nursing interventions needed to provide for the safety of a patient with visual impairment.
7. Review the procedure for instilling eye drops or eye ointments.
8. Develop measurable short- and long-term objectives for patient education for persons using cholinergic agents, anticholinergic agents, cholinesterase inhibitors, adrenergic agents, adrenergic blocking agents, osmotic agents, and antifungal or antiviral agents.

KEY WORDS

cornea	aqueous humor
pupil	mydriasis
miosis	accommodation
cycloplegia	Canal of Schlemm
lacrimal canaliculi	exophthalmos
nystagmus	refraction
tonometer	

The Eye

The eyeball has three coats or layers: the protective external, or corneoscleral, coat; the nutritive middle vascular layer, called the choroid; and the light-sensitive inner layer, or retina (Figure 18-1).

The *cornea*, or outermost sheath of the anterior eyeball, is transparent to allow light to enter the eye. The cornea has no blood vessels but receives its nutrition from the aqueous humor and its oxygen supply by diffusion from the air and surrounding vascular structures. There is a thin layer of epithelial cells on the external surface of the cornea that is quite resistant to infection.

An abraded cornea, however, is most susceptible to infection. The cornea has sensory fibers, and any damage to the corneal epithelium will cause pain. Seriously injured corneal tissue is replaced by scar tissue that is usually not transparent. The *sclera*, continuous with the cornea, is nontransparent and is the eye's white portion.

The *iris* is a diaphragm that surrounds the pupil and gives the eye its blue, green, hazel, brown, or gray color. The *sphincter muscle* within the iris encircles the pupil and is innervated by the parasympathetic nervous system. Contraction of the iris sphincter muscle causes the pupil to narrow; this is called *miosis*. The *dilator muscle*, which runs radially from the pupillary margin to

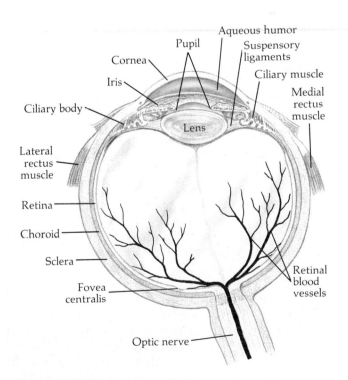

Figure 18-1 *Cross section of the eye. (From Thompson MJ: Mosby's manual of clinical nursing, ed 2, St Louis, Mosby—Year Book, 1989.)*

433

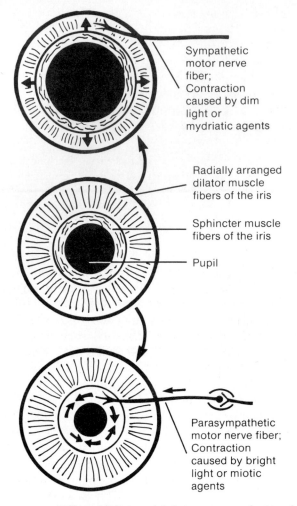

Sympathetic motor nerve fiber; Contraction caused by dim light or mydriatic agents

Radially arranged dilator muscle fibers of the iris

Sphincter muscle fibers of the iris

Pupil

Parasympathetic motor nerve fiber; Contraction caused by bright light or miotic agents

Figure 18-2 *Effect of light or ophthalmic agents on the iris of the eye.*

the iris periphery, is sympathetically innervated. Contraction of the dilator muscle and relaxation of the sphincter muscle cause the pupil to dilate; this is called *mydriasis*. See Figure 18-2.

Drugs that produce miosis (miotics) act similarly to acetylcholine (cholinergic agents) at receptor sites in the sphincter muscle or interfere with cholinesterase activity (cholinesterase inhibitors), prolonging the activity of acetylcholine. Drugs that produce mydriasis (mydriatics) stimulate adrenergic receptors or inhibit the action of acetylcholine. Constriction of the pupil normally occurs with light or when the eye is focusing on nearby objects. Dilation of the pupil normally occurs in dim light or when the eye is focusing on distant objects.

The *lens* is a transparent, gelatinous mass of fibers encased in an elastic capsule situated behind the iris. Its function is to ensure that the image on the retina is in sharp focus. It does this by changing shape (accommodation). This occurs readily in youth, but with age the lens becomes more rigid and the ability to focus close objects is lost. The *near point*, or the closest point that can be seen clearly, recedes. With age, the lens

may lose its transparency and become opaque, forming a cataract. Blindness can occur unless the cataract can be treated or surgically removed.

The lens has ligaments around its edge called *zonular fibers* that connect with the ciliary body. Tension on the zonular fibers helps to change the shape of the lens. In the unaccommodated eye, the ciliary muscle is relaxed and the zonular fibers are taut. For near vision, the ciliary muscle fibers contract, relaxing the pull on the ligaments and allowing the lens to increase in thickness. Accommodation depends on two factors: the ability of the lens to assume a more biconvex shape when tension on the ligaments is relaxed and ciliary muscle contraction. Paralysis of the ciliary muscle is termed *cycloplegia*. The ciliary muscle is innervated by parasympathetic nerve fibers.

The ciliary body secretes aqueous humor, which bathes and feeds the lens, posterior surface of the cornea, and iris. After it is formed, the fluid flows forward between the lens and the iris into the anterior chamber. It drains out of the eye through drainage channels located near the junction of the cornea and sclera into a meshwork that leads into the canal of Schlemm and into the venous system of the eye.

Eyelids, eyelashes, tears, and blinking all protect the eye. There are about 200 eyelashes for each eye. The eyelashes cause a blink reflex whenever a foreign body touches them, closing the lids for a fraction of a second to prevent the foreign body from entering the eye. Blinking, which is bilateral, occurs every few seconds during waking hours. It keeps the corneal surface free of mucus and spreads the lacrimal fluid evenly over the cornea. Tears are secreted by lacrimal glands and contain lysozyme, a mucolytic lubrication for lid movements. They wash away foreign agents and form a thin film over the cornea, providing it with a good optical surface. Tear fluid is lost by drainage into two small ducts (the lacrimal canaliculi) at the inner corners of the eyelids and by evaporation.

General Nursing Considerations for Patients with Disorders of the Eye

The nurse has the important role of educating the public and promoting safety measures to protect the eyes from potential sources of injury. Health professionals can participate in this role during their daily contacts with people at work and in the community. The use of safety glasses in potentially hazardous situations, prevention of chemical burns from common household cleaning items or other agents at home or work, proper cleaning and wearing of contact lenses or glasses, and the selection of safe toys and play activities for children are examples of areas about which the nurse can teach the public. These safety measures could significantly reduce the number of injuries that occur annually.

Nurses also play an important role in detection and

implementation of the treatment process. The information the nurse assesses relative to eye disorders can be used as a baseline for subsequent response to the treatment plan. One of the greatest nursing challenges in the care of chronic eye disorders is to convince the patient of the need for long-term treatment and compliance with the therapeutic regimen.

Patient Concerns: Nursing Intervention/Rationale

Indications of disorders of the eye

Objective data

Eyelids. Observe for complete closure of the eyelid. This is essential for protection of the cornea. All people with corneal anesthesia, fifth cranial nerve surgery, or who are unconscious must be protected from corneal damage.

Eye irrigations, the use of "artificial tears" such as methylcellulose, and closure of the eyes during anesthesia are practices used to insure protection.

Lid edema may be an indication of a systemic disease process or a tumor; report for further evaluation.

Exophthalmus (protusion of the eyeballs) should be evaluated and measures to protect the cornea instituted as part of the treatment plan.

Pupils. Assess pupils for equality of size, roundness, and response to light. Always report irregular contour, unequal size, or decreased or unequal response to light.

Eyelashes. Inspect the eyes to be certain the eyelashes are not turned inward.

Redness, drainage. Persistent redness or discharge from the eyes should be evaluated. Emphasize to the patient that self-treatment with over-the-counter medications or eyewashes, or using another patient's eye medications, can be disastrous. The use of cosmetics near the eyes can also be a source of eye irritation and infection.

Crossed eyes. Eyes that have recently shown signs of deviation from central gaze must be evaluated promptly.

Nystagmus. Report nystagmus that always occurs in the same direction in response to eye movement in either direction.

Hemorrhage or drainage. Drainage observed on the dressing should be reported immediately. Never remove the dressing to inspect the eyes unless given a specific order by the ophthalmologist.

Subjective data

Pain. Pain in the eye is not normal and should always be reported for immediate evaluation. Following ocular surgery, moderate discomfort may be expected; however, increasing pain is always a cause for immediate action. Notify the physician.

Visual alterations. Complaints of "double vision," "halos" around lights, or the sudden occurrence of floating "spots" require physician evaluation.

Blurred vision, unrelated to eye medications, is not normal. All complaints of this should be followed up by examination.

Diagnostic procedures. A *Snellen Visual Chart* can be used to evaluate distance vision. A *Jaeger Card* can be used to evaluate near vision. Visual fields are evaluated using a confrontational test. Color vision is evaluated using an *Ishihara Chart.*

Refraction. Refraction is the part of an eye examination that determines whether a patient will benefit from wearing glasses. Anticholinergic agents are used to obtain the correct degree of dilation and paralysis of the ciliary muscles to allow examination of the interior of the eye.

Tonometry. Pressure within the eye, known as *intraocular pressure,* is measured either directly or indirectly. Direct measurement is made by an instrument known as a *Schiotz tonometer* that is placed directly on the eyeball after the eye has been anesthetized. Indirect measurement comes from a noncontact tonometer. With this methodology a puff of air is directed at the eye and the quantity of force needed to flatten the cornea is determined. No anesthetic is required when this technique is used.

Normal tonometer readings range between 10 and 21 mm Hg. Persons over the age of 40, or individuals with a family history of glaucoma, should have intraocular pressure measurements on a regular basis, usually one or two times per year.

Increased intraocular pressure is treated medically through the use of drugs to control the rising pressure. If medications are ineffective, surgery may be required.

Dyes. Dyes may be used to examine the cornea for abrasions or to identify viral infections. Since these solutions may become contaminated with use, it is imperative that new, sterile solutions be used. Fluorescein angiography is a method of recording the ocular circulation after administration of dye. This is useful in diseases affecting circulation to the retina.

Cultures and smears. Conjunctival or corneal swab and/or scrapings can be taken to identify the etiology of an inflammatory process or exudate found in the eye. This should be done prior to initiation of antibiotic therapy.

Echography. High frequency pulses of ultrasound are produced from a small probe placed on the eye. Lesions of the eye can be detected using this methodology.

Nursing interventions

Visual acuity. Patients with eye disorders should be carefully assessed for the degree of visual impairment. Provide for patient safety through the following measures.

- Orient the patient to new surroundings and leave furnishings in original place
- Place the call light and other needed objects close to the patient

- Assist with ambulation
- Fix the food tray, cut up meat (if necessary), and pour liquids
- Restrict the operation of tools or power equipment as appropriate to the degree of alteration present
- Plan with the patient to call for assistance if needed for daily activities
- If one eye is covered, place the patient in a room where the covered eye is away from the door so the patient can see who enters the room

Disorientation. The blind or those with both eyes patched may suffer from sensory deprivation that may result in disorientation. Employ the following measures:

- Always speak prior to touching a person with impaired vision
- Check on the patient at frequent intervals; hold conversations and regularly orient him or her to date, time, and place
- Try to arrange for a semiprivate room and a roommate who is alert, to provide stimulation
- If the patient is agitated, contact the physician; it may be necessary to obtain an order to remove one eye patch

Injury. Provide for patient safety and prevent personal injury. Following surgery, caution the patient not to rub the eyes or try to touch under the dressings. Following injury it is frequently desirable to place the injured eye at rest. To accomplish this an eye patch is applied. Since both eyes move simultaneously, the unaffected eye may also have to be patched for maximum benefit to occur.

Infection. Always wash your hands before performing any procedure on the eye.

Use only sterile eye medications or dressings on the eyes.

Practice the following personal hygiene measures to prevent the introduction of an infection:

- Do not touch the eyes or rub them
- Wipe one eye from the inner canthus outward; discard the tissue or cotton ball used; wash hands *before* proceeding to the second eye
- When an infection is present, prevent cross-contamination; always use a separate source of medication and droppers for each eye
- Never touch the eyeball or face with the tip of the dropper or opening of the ointment container
- When irrigating the eye, do not allow the solution to flow from one eye to the other
- When inserting or removing contact lenses, wash your hands first, then follow the manufacturer's specific instructions regarding the cleansing and care of the lenses
- Report any persistent redness or drainage from the eyes

Emotional support. Always let the patient know what limitations are being placed on him or her and the *reason* for the restrictions.

Give psychological support to the patient with an eye disorder. Fear of blindness may escalate anxiety and result in further tissue damage. Deal calmly with the patient's concerns. Let him or her vent anxieties.

Administration of medications. See Administration of Eye Drops and Eye Ointments.

Patient Education Associated with Medications Used in the Eye

Communication and responsibility. Encourage open communication concerning frustrations and anger as the patient attempts to adjust to the diagnosis and need for prolonged treatment. The patient must be guided to insight into the condition in order to assume responsibility for the continuation of treatment. Keep emphasizing those factors the patient can control to alter progression of the disease process, including maintenance of general health, nutritional needs, adequate rest and appropriate exercise, and continuation of prescribed medication therapy.

Expectations of therapy. Discuss expectations of therapy with the patient (such as level of exercise, degree of pain relief, frequency of use of medications, relief of visual impairment, ability to maintain activities of daily living and work).

Changes in expectations. Assess changes in expectations as therapy progresses and the patient gains understanding and skill in the management of the diagnosis.

Changes in therapy through cooperative goal setting. Work with the patient to encourage adherence to the prescribed treatment. When the patient feels that a change should be made in a treatment plan, encourage discussion first with the physician.

Written record. Enlist the patient's aid in developing and maintaining a written record of the monitoring parameters (such as blood pressure and pulse with adrenergic agents, degree of visual disturbance, and progression of impairment) and response to prescribed therapies for discussion with the physician (see Figure 18-3). Patients should be encouraged to take this record with them on follow-up visits.

Fostering compliance. Throughout the hospitalization, discuss medication information and how it will benefit the course of treatment. Seek cooperation and understanding of the following points so that medication compliance may be enhanced:

1. Name
2. Dosage
3. Route and administration times: stress the need for maintaining the schedule
4. Anticipated therapeutic response, particularly with

Patient Education and Monitoring of Therapeutic Outcomes for Patients Receiving Eye Medications

Medications	Color	To be taken

Name _____

Physician _____

Physician's phone _____

Next appt.* _____

Parameters		Day of exam							Comments
Blood pressure									
Pain in eye (Right or Left)									
No pain in eyes									
Vision (clarity)	Blurred all the time								
	Occasionally hazy								
	Clear								
Side vision	Must turn head to see								
	Can see without turning head								
Vision since starting eye medication: No improvement 10 Better 5 Much better 1									
Headache	None								
	If yes, location								
	What were you doing when it started?								
Eye Color Redness	Is redness improved by medication?								
Burning	Is burning improved by medication?								
Itching, rash	None								
	Sometimes associated with medication								
	Always occurs with medication								

*Please bring this record with you to your next appointment.
Use the back of this sheet for additional information.

Figure 18-3 *Patient education and monitoring of therapeutic outcomes for patients receiving eye medications.*

glaucoma, control of intraocular pressure, and prevention of blindness

5. Side effects to expect
6. Side effects to report: see individual agents
7. What to do if a dosage is missed
8. When, how, or if to refill the medication prescription; always keep an extra bottle of eye medication on hand; when refilling the prescriptions, always check the label on the new bottle to be sure the new supply is the same as the former bottle

Difficulty in comprehension. If it is evident that the patient and/or family do not understand all aspects of continuing therapy being prescribed (such as administration and monitoring of medications, exercises, diets, follow-up appointments), consider the use of social service or visiting nurse agencies.

Associated teaching. Give patients the following instructions:

Always inform the physician or dentist of any prescription or over-the-counter medication being taken. Over-the-counter medications should not be taken without first discussing them with your physician or pharmacist. This includes the use of eye washes.

Always report side effects of rash, itching, or hives immediately. Nausea, vomiting, or diarrhea should also be reported for the physician's evaluation if it is a new symptom.

Take all of the medication as prescribed for the full course of treatment. Do not discontinue use when feeling improved; do not save for future use; do not give your medicine to another individual. Sudden discontinuation of certain medications may produce harmful effects.

Keep all medications out of reach of children.

If pregnancy is suspected, consult an obstetrician as soon as possible about continuation of medication therapy.

At discharge. Items to be sent home with the patient should include the following:

1. Written instructions for use
2. Labels in a level of language and size of print appropriate for the patient
3. If needed, identification cards or bracelets
4. A list of additional supplies to be purchased after discharge (such as eye dressings, tissues, cotton balls, patches)
5. A schedule of follow-up appointments

Drug Therapy for Disorders of the Eye

Osmotic agents

OBJECTIVES

1. Identify the mechanism of action of osmotic agents that affect intraocular pressure.
2. Explain the reason for using osmotic agents with caution in persons with cardiac or renal disease, or with a patient who has diabetes.
3. Describe patient assessments needed to detect fluid overload or congestive heart failure.
4. Review dosage and administration procedures used with osmotic agents.

KEY WORDS

extravascular space   iridectomy

Osmotic agents are administered intravenously, orally, or topically to reduce intraocular pressure. These agents elevate the osmotic pressure of the plasma, causing fluid from the extravascular spaces to be drawn into the blood. The effect on the eye is reduction of volume of intraocular fluid, producing a decrease in intraocular pressure.

The osmotic agents are used to reduce intraocular pressure in patients with acute narrow-angle glaucoma; prior to iridectomy; preoperatively and postoperatively in conditions such as congenital glaucoma, retinal detachment, cataract extraction, and keratoplasty; and in some secondary glaucomas.

Side effects. Side effects include headache, nausea, vomiting, diarrhea, and thirst.

These agents should be used with caution in patients with cardiac, hepatic, or renal disease; the shift in body water may cause congestive heart failure or pulmonary edema.

In diabetic patients, the metabolism of the glycerin may cause hyperglycemia and glycosuria, so that diabetic patients should be observed for symptoms of acidosis.

Monitor vital signs, fluid and electrolyte balance, and urinary output of all patients.

Availability. See Table 18-1.

Dosage and administration. See individual agents.

- **Nursing Interventions: Monitoring osmotic agent therapy**

See also General Nursing Considerations for Patients with Disorders of the Eye (p. 434).

Side effects to report

THIRST, NAUSEA, DEHYDRATION, ELECTROLYTE IMBALANCE. The electrolytes most commonly altered are potassium (K^+), sodium (Na^+), and chloride (Cl^-).

Many symptoms associated with altered fluid and electrolyte balance are subtle and resemble general symptoms of drug toxicity or the disease process itself.

Gather data relative to *changes* in the patient's mental status (alertness, orientation, confusion), muscle strength, muscle cramps, tremors, nausea, and general appearance (drowsy, anxious, lethargic).

Always check the electrolyte reports for early indicators of electrolyte imbalance.

Keep accurate records of I/O, daily weights, and vital signs.

Table 18-1 *Osmotic Agents*

GENERIC NAME	BRAND NAME	AVAILABILITY	DOSAGE	COMMENTS
Glycerin	Glyrol, Osmoglyn	50, 75% solutions	PO: 1-1.5 g/kg	An oral osmotic agent for reducing intraocular pressure Administer 60-90 minutes prior to surgery Use with caution in diabetic patients; monitor for hyperglycemia
Isosorbide	Ismotic	100 g in 220 ml solution (45%)	PO: 1.5 g/kg (range: 1-3 g/kg) 2-4 times daily	An oral osmotic agent for reducing intraocular pressure Onset of action is 30 minutes, duration is 5-6 hours With repeated doses, monitor fluids and electrolytes The solution will taste better if poured over cracked ice and sipped
Mannitol	Osmitrol	5, 10, 15, 20, 25% solutions for infusions	IV: 1.5-2 g/kg as a 25% solution over 30 minutes	Used intravenously when oral methods are unacceptable When used preoperatively, administer 60-90 minutes prior to surgery Use an in-line filter because mannitol has a tendency to crystallize
Urea	Ureaphil	40 g in 150 ml	IV: 1-5 g/kg	Administer as a 30% solution at an infusion rate not to exceed 4 ml/minute Used when mannitol and oral methods are not available Do not exceed 120 g daily Use extreme caution against extravasation; tissue necrosis may result Do not infuse in veins of lower extremities due to the possibility of thrombus formation

HEADACHE. This is an indication of cerebral dehydration. It can be minimized by keeping the patient lying down.

CIRCULATORY OVERLOAD. These medications act on the blood volume as well by pulling fluid from the tissue spaces into the general circulation (blood). Assess the patient at regularly scheduled intervals for signs and symptoms of fluid overload, pulmonary edema, or congestive heart failure. Perform lung assessments; report the development of rales and increasing dyspnea, frothy sputum, or cough.

Implementation

CATHETER. Be certain the patient has an indwelling catheter if these drugs are used during an operative procedure; check with the physician before scrubbing for the procedure.

IV. Assess the IV site at regular intervals for any signs of infiltration. Tissue necrosis may occur from infiltration into the surrounding tissue. If it occurs, stop the IV, report, then elevate the extremity and follow hospital protocol for extravasation.

Do not use veins in lower extremities for administration of these agents. This will minimize the occurrence of phlebitis and thrombosis.

MANNITOL CRYSTALS. Check the mannitol solution for crystals; DO NOT administer if present. Follow directions in the literature accompanying the medication for a warm bath to dissolve the crystals and then cool the solution prior to administration.

Carbonic anhydrase inhibitors
OBJECTIVES

1. Identify the actions of carbonic anhydrase inhibitors on intraocular pressure.
2. State the adverse effects seen with sulfonamide therapy.
3. Describe the characteristics of electrolyte imbalance and dehydration.

acetazolamide (ah-set-ah-zol′ah-myd)

  Diamox (dy′ah-moks)

dichlorphenamide (dy-klor-fen′ah-myd)

  Daranide (dar′a-neyd)

methazolamide (meth-ah-zol′ah-myd)

  Neptazane (nep′tah-zain)

These three agents are inhibitors of the enzyme carbonic anhydrase. Inhibition of this enzyme results in a decrease in the production of aqueous humor, thus lowering intraocular pressure. These agents are used in conjunction with other treatment modalities to control intraocular pressure in both closed-angle and open-angle glaucoma.

Side effects. Carbonic anhydrase inhibitors are sulfonamide derivatives and thus have the potential to cause adverse effects similar to those associated with sulfonamide antimicrobial therapy. These adverse effects, although rare, include dermatologic, hematologic, and neurologic reactions. For further discussion, see Sulfonamides in Chapter 19.

Patients who are allergic to sulfonamides should not receive carbonic anhydrase inhibitors due to cross-sensitivity.

Side effects associated with carbonic anhydrase inhibitors are usually quite mild. They include gastric irritation, a numbness or tingling of the extremities, diuresis, and, occasionally, drowsiness and confusion.

Although infrequent, treatment with carbonic anhydrase inhibitors may lead to excessive diuresis with water dehydration and electrolyte imbalance.

Availability

Acetazolamide

PO—125, 250 mg tablets, 500 mg capsules.

IV—500 mg per vial.

Dichlorphenamide

PO—50 mg tablets.

Methazolamide

PO—50 mg tablets.

Dosage and administration

Adult

PO—Acetazolamide: 250 mg to 1 g every 24 hours. Dichlorphenamide: 25 to 50 mg 1 to 3 times daily. Methazolamide: 50 to 100 mg, 2 or 3 times daily.

• **Nursing Interventions: Monitoring carbonic anhydrase inhibitor therapy**

See also General Nursing Considerations for Patients with Disorders of the Eye (p. 434).

Side effects to report

ELECTROLYTE IMBALANCE, DEHYDRATION. The electrolytes most commonly altered are potassium (K^+), sodium (Na^+), and chloride (Cl^-). *Hypokalemia* is most likely to occur.

Many symptoms associated with altered fluid and electrolyte balance are subtle and resemble general symptoms of drug toxicity or the disease process itself.

Gather data relative to *changes* in the patient's mental status (alertness, orientation, confusion), muscle strength, muscle cramps, tremors, nausea, and general appearance (drowsy, anxious, lethargic).

Always check the electrolyte reports for early indications of electrolyte imbalance.

Keep accurate records of I/O, daily weight, and vital signs.

DERMATOLOGIC, HEMATOLOGIC, NEUROLOGIC REACTIONS. See Sulfonamides in Chapter 19, "Antimicrobial Agents."

CONFUSION. Perform a baseline assessment of the patient's degree of alertness and orientation to name, place, and time before initiating therapy. Make regularly scheduled subsequent mental status evaluations and compare findings. Report development of alterations.

DROWSINESS. This side effect is usually mild and tends to resolve with continued therapy. Encourage the patient not to discontinue therapy without first consulting the physician.

Persons who are working around machinery, driving a car, pouring and giving medicines, or performing other duties in which they must remain mentally alert should not take these medications while working.

Implementation

SULFONAMIDES. Do not administer to patients allergic to sulfonamide antibiotics without prior physician approval. Observe closely for the development of hypersensitivity.

GASTRIC IRRITATION. If gastric irritation occurs, administer with food or milk. If symptoms persist or increase in severity, report for physician evaluation.

Drug interactions

QUINIDINE. These diuretics may inhibit the excretion of quinidine. If your patient is also receiving quinidine, monitor closely for signs of quinidine toxicity (tinnitus, vertigo, headache, confusion, bradycardia, visual disturbances).

DIGITALIS GLYCOSIDES. Patients receiving these diuretics may excrete excess potassium, which leads to hypokalemia. If your patient is also receiving a digitalis glycoside, monitor closely for digitalis toxicity (anorexia, nausea, fatigue, blurred or colored vision, bradycardia, arrhythmias).

CORTICOSTEROIDS (PREDNISONE, OTHERS). Corticosteroids may enhance the loss of potassium. Check potassium levels and monitor more closely for hypokalemia when these two agents are used concurrently.

Anticholinergic agents

OBJECTIVE

1. Cite the uses of anticholinergic agents for treatment of ophthalmic disorders.

Anticholinergic agents cause the smooth muscle of the ciliary body and iris to relax, producing mydriasis (extreme dilation of the pupil) and cycloplegia (paralysis of the ciliary muscle). Ophthalmologists use these effects to examine the interior of the eye, to measure the proper strength of lenses for eyeglasses (refraction), and to rest the eye in inflammatory conditions of the uveal tract.

Side effects. The pharmacologic effects of anticholinergic agents cause an increase in intraocular pressure. Use these agents with extreme caution in patients with a narrow anterior chamber angle, in infants, children, and the elderly, and in hypertensive, hyperthyroid, and diabetic patients. Discontinue therapy if signs of increased intraocular pressure or systemic effects develop.

Table 18-2 *Anticholinergic Agents*

GENERIC NAME	BRAND NAME	AVAILABILITY	DOSAGE	COMMENTS
Atropine sulfate	Isopto-Atropine, Atropisol	1% ointment; 0.5, 1, 2, 3% solution	Uveitis: 1-2 drops up to 3 times daily	Onset of mydriasis and cycloplegia is 30-40 minutes, duration is 7-12 days Do not use in infants
Cyclopentolate hydrochloride	Cyclogyl, AK Pentolate	0.5, 1, 2% solutions	Refraction: 1 drop followed by another drop in 5-10 minutes	For mydriasis and cycloplegia necessary for diagnostic procedures 1-2 drops of 1-2% pilocarpine allows full recovery within 3-6 hours Central nervous system (CNS) disturbances of hallucinations, loss of orientation, restlessness, and incoherent speech have been reported in children
Homatropine hydrobromide	Isopto-Homatropine, Ak-Homatropine	2 and 5% solutions	Uveitis: 1-2 drops every 3-4 hours	Onset of mydriasis and cycloplegia is 40-60 minutes; duration is 1-3 days
Scopolamine hydrobromide	Isopto-Hyoscine	0.25% solution	Uveitis: 1-2 drops up to 3 times daily	Onset of mydriasis and cycloplegia is 20-30 minutes; duration is 3-7 days
Tropicamide	Mydriacyl	0.5 and 1% solutions	Refraction: 1 or 2 drops, repeated in 5 minutes	Onset of mydriasis and cycloplegia is 20-40 minutes; duration is 6 hours CNS disturbances of hallucinations, loss of orientation, restlessness, and incoherent speech have been reported in children

The only common side effects seen with short-term use are stinging, conjunctival irritation, and sensitivity to bright light.

Prolonged use may result in systemic effects manifested by flushing and dryness of the skin, dry mouth, blurred vision, tachycardia, arrhythmias, urinary hesitancy and retention, vasodilation, and constipation.

Availability. See Table 18-2.

Dosage and administration. See individual agents.

• **Nursing Interventions: Monitoring anticholinergic agent therapy**

See also General Nursing Considerations for Patients with Disorders of the Eye (p. 434).

Side effects to expect

SENSITIVITY TO BRIGHT LIGHTS. The mydriasis produced allows excessive light into the eyes, causing the patient to squint. Use of sunglasses will help reduce the brightness. Caution the patient to temporarily avoid tasks that require visual acuity such as driving or operating power machinery.

CONJUNCTIVAL IRRITATION, LACRIMATION. These side effects are usually mild and tend to resolve with continued therapy. Encourage the patient not to discontinue therapy without first consulting the physician.

Side effects to report

SYSTEMIC SIDE EFFECTS. These are an indication of overdosage or excessive administration. Report to the physician for treatment and dosage adjustment. Children are particularly prone to develop systemic reactions.

Antiseptics
OBJECTIVE

1. Explain the procedure for instillation of silver nitrate in the eyes of a newborn infant.

silver nitrate

Silver nitrate ophthalmic solution is used as an antiseptic agent, primarily as a prophylaxis against gonorrhea infection in the eyes of newborn infants (ophthalmia neonatorum).

Side effects. A mild conjunctivitis manifested by localized erythema is reported in up to 20% of patients.

Availability
Ophthalmic—1% solution in wax ampules.

Dosage and administration
Newborns. Immediately after delivery, instill 2 drops in each eye (see additional instructions below).

• **Nursing Interventions: Monitoring silver nitrate therapy**

See also General Nursing Considerations for Patients with Disorders of the Eye (p. 434).

Side effects to expect

CONJUNCTIVITIS. This side effect is usually mild and tends to resolve within a day.

Implementation

INSTILLATION. Immediately after delivery:

• Wash your hands before and after instillation.
• Using a separate gauze and sterile water for each eye,

wash the unopened lids from the nose outward until free of all blood, mucus, or meconium.

- Separate the eyelids and instill 2 drops of 1% solution into the eye. Separate the lids far enough from the eyeball so that a pool of silver nitrate rests between the lids, on the eye.
- Allow the pool to remain for 30 seconds or longer.
- Do not irrigate the eyes with other solutions after the silver nitrate instillation.
- Take care not to get silver nitrate solution on skin or nails, since they will become discolored.

Anesthetics
OBJECTIVE

1. Name specific ophthalmic anesthetics and describe patient instructions needed when these medications are used.

Local anesthetics (Table 18-3) may be used in such ophthalmic procedures as removal of foreign objects, tonometry, gonioscopy, suture removal, and short corneal and conjunctival procedures. Because the blink reflex is temporarily eliminated, it is wise to protect the eye with a patch after procedures are completed. Caution the patient not to rub the eyes; the patient could damage the eye and yet feel no pain.

Alpha chymotrypsin 1:5000 or 1:10,000 may be used during ocular surgery to dissolve zonular fibers that suspend the cataract in the eye.

Antibacterial agents
OBJECTIVE

1. Cite the rationale for limited use of antimicrobial agents for superficial eye infections.

Antibacterial agents (Table 18-4) are occasionally used in the treatment of superficial eye infections and for prophylaxis against gonorrhea infection in the eyes of newborn infants (ophthalmia neonatorum). Prolonged or frequent intermittent use of topical antibiotics should be avoided because of the possibility of hypersensitivity reactions and the development of resistant organisms, including fungi. If hypersensitivities or new infections appear during use, consult an ophthalmologist immediately. Refer to the Index for a discussion of these antibiotics.

Antifungal agents
OBJECTIVES

1. Cite specific ophthalmic disorders that are treated with antifungal agents.
2. Explain the basis of sensitivity to light associated with the use of antifungal agents.

Table 18-3 *Ophthalmic Anesthetics*

GENERIC NAME	BRAND NAME	AVAILABILITY
Cocaine hydrochloride	Various	1% to 4% solution
Proparacaine hydrochloride	Alcaine, Ophthetic, Ophthaine	0.5% solution
Tetracaine hydrochloride	Pontocaine Eye	0.5% solution, 0.5% ointment

Table 18-4 *Ophthalmic Antibiotics*

ANTIBIOTIC	BRAND NAME	AVAILABILITY
Bacitracin	Bacitracin Ophthalmic	Ointment
Chloramphenicol	Chloromycetin Ophthalmic, Chloroptic, Ophthochlor	Drops, ointment
Chlortetracycline	Aureomycin Ophthalmic	Ointment
Ciprofloxacin	Ciloxan	Drops
Erythromycin	Ilotycin Ophthalmic	Ointment
Gentamicin	Garamycin Ophthalmic	Drops, ointment
Norfloxacin	Chibroxin	Drops
Polymyxin B	Polymyxin B Sulfate	Drops
Sulfacetamide	Sulf-10, Isopto-Cetamide	Drops, ointment
Tetracycline	Achromycin Ophthalmic	Drops
Tobramycin	Tobrex Ophthalmic	Drops, ointment
Combinations		
Trimethoprim/Polymyxin B	Polytrim Ophthalmic	Drops
Neomycin/Polymyxin B	Statrol Ophthalmic	Ointment, drops
Neomycin/Polymyxin B/Bacitracin	Neosporin Ophthalmic, Neotricin	Ointment
Neomycin/Polymyxin B/Gramicidin	Neosporin Ophthalmic	Drops

KEY WORD

fungal keratitis

natamycin (na-tah-my'sin)

Natacyn (na'tah-sin)

Natamycin is an antifungal agent effective against a variety of yeasts, including *Candida*, *Aspergillus*, and *Fusarium*. It is effective in the treatment of fungal blepharitis, conjunctivitis, and keratitis caused by susceptible organisms. If little or no improvement is noted after 7 to 10 days of treatment, resistance to the antifungal agent may have developed. Topical administration does not appear to result in systemic effects.

Side effects. Side effects are quite mild, but include minor blurring of vision and increased sensitivity to light. If eye pain develops, discontinue use and contact an ophthalmologist immediately.

Availability

Ophthalmic—5% suspension.

Dosage and administration. Fungal keratitis: 1 drop in the conjunctival sac at 1 or 2 hour intervals for the first 3 to 4 days. The dosage may then be reduced to 1 drop every 3 to 4 hours. Continue therapy for 14 to 21 days.

• Nursing Interventions: Monitoring natamycin therapy

See also General Nursing Considerations for Patients with Disorders of the Eye (p. 434).

Side effects to expect

SENSITIVITY TO BRIGHT LIGHTS. The slight mydriasis produced allows excessive amount of light into the eyes causing the patient to squint. Use of sunglasses will help reduce the brightness. Caution the patient to temporarily avoid tasks that require visual acuity such as driving or operating power machinery.

BLURRED VISION, LACRIMATION, REDNESS. Provide for patient safety during temporary visual impairment. Instruct the patient not to rub the eyes forcefully while tearing.

These side effects are usually mild and tend to resolve with continued therapy. Encourage the patient not to discontinue therapy without first consulting the physician.

Side effects to report

EYE PAIN. If eye pain develops, discontinue use and consult an ophthalmologist immediately.

THERAPEUTIC EFFECT. If, after several days of therapy the presenting symptoms are not improving or are gradually worsening, consult the physician treating the patient.

Antiviral agents

OBJECTIVES

1. Describe the types of conditions that respond effectively to the treatment with idoxuridine.
2. State the time limit for use of trifluridine.

idoxuridine (i-doks-ur'i-deen)

Dendrid (den'drid), ✦**Stoxil** (stok'sil)

trifluridine (try-flur'i-deen)

Viroptic (vy-rhop'tik)

Idoxuridine and trifluridine are chemically related compounds used to treat herpes simplex keratitis. Idoxuridine is particularly effective against initial infections but is not very effective against deep infections or chronic, recurrent infections. Trifluridine is used to treat recurrent infections in those patients who are intolerant of or resistant to idoxuridine or vidarabine therapy; cross-sensitivity with these other agents has not been reported. Idoxuridine and trifluridine are not effective against bacteria, fungi, and *Chlamydia* infections.

Side effects. Side effects are quite mild, as essentially no systemic absorption takes place. Patients may notice a mild, transient stinging, burning, and redness of the conjunctiva and sclera on instillation.

Other adverse effects that have rarely been reported include stromal edema, hypersensitivity reactions, and increased intraocular pressure.

Use of the ointment form (Stoxil) may cause temporary blurring of vision until the ointment is spread across the eyeball by the eyelid.

Availability

Ophthalmic—Idoxuridine: 0.1% solution and 0.5% ointment.

Trifluridine: 1.0% solution.

Dosage and administration

Idoxuridine. Ophthalmic Solution: Initially 1 drop in each infected eye every hour during the day and every 2 hours after bedtime. After significant improvement, as shown by loss of staining with fluorescein, reduce the dose to 1 drop every 2 hours during the day and every 4 hours at night. Continue therapy for 3 to 5 days after healing appears to be complete to minimize recurrences.

Ophthalmic Ointment: Place a ribbon of ointment in the conjunctival sac of the infected eye 5 times daily, approximately every 4 hours, with the last dose at bedtime. Continue therapy for 3 to 5 days after healing appears to be complete to minimize recurrence.

Trifluridine. Ophthalmic Solution: Place 1 drop onto the cornea of the affected eye every 2 hours. Do not exceed 9 drops daily. Continue for 7 more days to prevent recurrence, using 1 drop every 4 hours (5 drops daily).

NOTE: For both agents, if significant improvement has not occurred in 7 to 14 days, other therapy should be considered. Do not exceed 21 days of continuous therapy due to potential ocular toxicity.

• Nursing Interventions: Monitoring ophthalmic antiviral therapy

See also General Nursing Considerations for Patients with Disorders of the Eye (p. 434).

Side effects to expect

SENSITIVITY TO BRIGHT LIGHTS. The slight mydriasis produced allows excessive amounts of light into the eyes causing the patient to squint. Use of sunglasses will help reduce the brightness. Caution the patient to temporarily avoid tasks that require visual acuity such as driving or operating power machinery.

VISUAL HAZE, LACRIMATION, REDNESS, BURNING. Provide for patient safety during temporary visual impairment. Instruct the patient not to rub the eyes forcefully while tearing.

These side effects are usually mild and tend to resolve with continued therapy. Encourage the patient not to discontinue therapy without first consulting the physician.

Implementation

STORAGE. Idoxuridine and trifluridine should be stored in the refrigerator. (Herplex Liquifilm does not require refrigeration.)

Drug interactions

BORIC ACID SOLUTIONS. Tell the patient not to use boric acid eye washes while using idoxuridine; local irritation may be enhanced.

Vidarabine (vy-dar'a-been)

Vira-A (vy'rah-ay)

Vidarabine is used topically as an ophthalmic ointment to treat keratitis and keratoconjunctivitis caused by herpes simplex virus types 1 and 2. Vidarabine does not show cross-sensitivity to idoxuridine or trifluridine and may be effective in treating recurrent keratitis that is resistant to idoxuridine and trifluridine. Vidarabine is not effective against infections caused by bacteria, fungi, or *Chlamydia*.

Side effects. Minor side effects associated with the use of vidarabine ointment include temporary visual haze, burning, itching, redness, and lacrimation. Photophobia (sensitivity to bright light) occasionally occurs. Allergic reactions have rarely been reported.

Availability

Ophthalmic—3% ointment.

Dosage and administration

Ophthalmic—Place a 1 cm ribbon of ointment inside the lower conjunctival sac of the infected eye 5 times daily at 3 hour intervals. Continue for an additional 5 to 7 days at a dosage of 1 cm twice daily after significant improvement has occurred to prevent recurrence of the infection.

IV—Not for ophthalmic use (see Index).

• Nursing Interventions: Monitoring vidarabine therapy

See also General Nursing Considerations for Patients with Disorders of the Eye (p. 434).

Side effects to expect

VISUAL HAZE, LACRIMATION, REDNESS, BURNING. Provide for patient safety during temporary visual impairment.

Instruct the patient not to rub the eyes forcefully while tearing.

These side effects are usually mild and tend to resolve with continued therapy. Encourage the patient not to discontinue therapy without first consulting the physician.

SENSITIVITY TO BRIGHT LIGHT. The slight mydriasis produced allows excessive light into the eyes, causing the patient to squint. Use of sunglasses will help reduce the brightness. Caution the patient to temporarily avoid tasks that require visual acuity, such as driving or operating power machinery.

Side effects to report

ALLERGIC REACTIONS. Discontinue therapy and consult an ophthalmologist immediately.

Corticosteroids

OBJECTIVE

1. Explain the rationale for the use of corticosteroids for allergic conditions and the contraindications for use with infections.

Corticosteroid therapy is indicated for allergic reactions of the eye and other acute, noninfectious inflammatory conditions of the conjunctiva, sclera, cornea, and anterior uveal tract (Table 18-5). Corticosteroid therapy must not be used in bacterial, fungal, or viral infections of the eye because corticosteroids decrease defense mechanisms and reduce resistance to pathologic organisms. This therapy should be used for a limited time only, and the eye should be checked frequently for an increase in intraocular pressure. Prolonged ocular steroid therapy may cause glaucoma and cataracts.

Other ophthalmic agents

OBJECTIVE

1. Cite the uses of fluorescein solution or strips and the precautions necessary to prevent contamination of the solution.

Fluorescein sodium

Fluorescein sodium is used in fitting hard contact lenses and as a diagnostic aid in identifying foreign bodies in the eye and abraded or ulcerated areas of the cornea. It

Table 18-5 *Corticosteroids*

GENERIC NAME	BRAND NAME	AVAILABILITY
Dexamethasone	Maxidex	Suspension
	AK-Dex	Ointment
Fluorometholone	FML Liquifilm	Suspension
Medrysone	HMS Liquifilm	Suspension
Prednisolone	Econopred Plus, Inflamase,	Solution
	Metreton	Suspension

is also useful for evaluating retinal vasculature for abnormal circulation. When sodium fluorescein is instilled in the eye, it stains the pathologic tissues green if observed under normal light, or bright yellow if viewed under cobalt blue light. Fluorescein sodium is available in 2% topical solution; 0.6, 1, and 9 mg strips for topical application; and 5, 10, and 25% solutions for injection into the aqueous humor. The strips have the advantage of being used once and then discarded. The solution carries the risk of bacterial contamination if used for several different patients. Product names include Fluorescite, Funduscein-25, Ful-Glo, and Fluor-I-Strip.

Artificial tear solutions

Artificial tear solutions are products made to mimic natural secretions of the eye. They provide lubrication for dry eyes. They may also be used as lubricants for artificial eyes. Most products contain variable concentrations of methylcellulose, polyvinyl alcohol, and polyethylene glycol. The dosage is 1 to 3 drops in each eye 3 to 4 times daily, as needed. Product names include Isopto Plain, Lacril, Tears Naturale, Neo-Tears, and Hypotears.

Ophthalmic irrigants

These products are sterile solutions used for soothing and cleansing the eye, removing foreign bodies, in conjunction with hard contact lenses, or with fluorescein. Product names include Eye-Stream, Lavoptik Eye Wash, I-Rinse, Collyrium, and Ocu-Bath Eye Lotion.

Ophthalmic antiinflammatory agents

Flurbiprofen sodium, suprofen, and diclofenac sodium are the first topical nonsteroidal antiinflammatory agents for ophthalmic use. These agents have shown antiinflammatory, antipyretic, and analgesic activity by inhibiting the biosynthesis of prostaglandins that are responsible for an increase in intraocular inflammation and pressure. They also inhibit prostaglandin-mediated constriction of the iris (miosis) that is independent of cholinergic mechanisms. Flurbiprofen and suprofen are used primarily to inhibit miosis during cataract surgery. Diclofenac sodium is used to treat postoperative inflammation following cataract extraction. Flurbiprofen is available as a 0.03% solution (Ocufen) that should be used by instilling 1 drop in the appropriate eye every 30 minutes, beginning 2 hours before surgery (for a total of 4 drops). Suprofen (Profenal) is available as a 1% solution that is instilled (2 drops) into the conjunctival sac at 3, 2, and 1 hour prior to surgery. Diclofenac sodium (Voltaren) is available as a 0.1% solution. One drop is applied to the affected eye 4 times daily beginning 24 hours after surgery and continued for 2 weeks.

Antiallergic agent

Cromolyn sodium is a stabilizing agent that inhibits the release of histamine and SRS-A (slow-reacting substance of anaphylaxis) from mast cells after exposure to specific antigens. It is used to treat allergic ocular disorders such as vernal keratoconjunctivitis, vernal keratitis, and allergic keratoconjunctivitis. It is available as a 4% solution (Opticrom) that is used by applying 1 to 2 drops in each eye 4 to 6 times daily at regular intervals.

Glaucoma
Objectives

1. Differentiate among primary, secondary, and congenital forms of glaucoma.
2. Compare the signs, symptoms, and pharmacological treatment of open-angle and closed-angle glaucoma.
3. Identify specific measures the patient can use to control an increase in intraocular pressure.
4. Describe patient education needed for a person with glaucoma.
5. State specific approaches that can be utilized to insure that a visually impaired patient is using the correct eye medications according to the prescribed directions.

KEY WORD
lacrimation

Glaucoma is an eye disease characterized by abnormally elevated intraocular pressure, which may result from excessive production of the aqueous humor or from diminished ocular fluid outflow. Increased pressure, if persistent and sufficiently elevated, may lead to permanent blindness. There are three major types of glaucoma: primary, secondary, and congenital. *Primary* includes *closed-angle* or *acute congestive* glaucoma and *open-angle*, or *chronic simple* glaucoma. These are diagnosed by the iridocorneal angle of the anterior chamber where aqueous humor reabsorption takes place. *Secondary* glaucoma may result from previous eye disease or may follow a cataract extraction and may require drug therapy for an indefinite period. *Congenital* glaucoma requires surgical treatment.

Open-angle glaucoma develops insidiously over the years as pathologic changes at the iridocorneal angle prevent the outflow of aqueous humor through the trabecular network to the canal of Schlemm and into the veins of the eye. (See Figure 18-4 for the normal pathway of aqueous flow.) Intraocular pressure builds up and, if not treated, will damage the optic disk. Initially, the patient has no symptoms, but over the years there is a gradual loss of peripheral vision. If untreated, total blindness may result. The principle for treatment of open-angle glaucoma is to maintain intraocular pressure at normal levels to prevent further blindness. Mi-

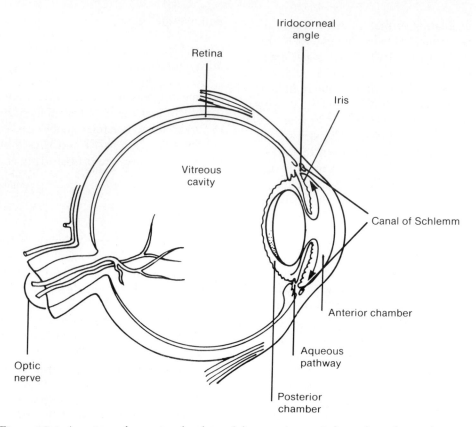

Figure 18-4 *Anterior and posterior chambers of the eye. Arrows indicate the pathway of aqueous flow.*

otic agents are most commonly used to increase outflow of aqueous humor. Other agents that may also be used are the carbonic anhydrase inhibitors (acetazolamide), beta-adrenergic blocking agents (e.g., timolol maleate), and the cholinesterase inhibitors (e.g., echothiophate iodide). The selection of the drug is determined to a great extent by the requirements of the individual patient.

Acute closed-angle glaucoma occurs when there is a sudden increase in intraocular pressure due to a mechanical obstruction of the trabecular network in the iridocorneal angle (Figure 18-5). This occurs in patients who have narrow anterior chamber angles. Symptoms develop gradually and appear intermittently for short periods, especially when the pupil is dilated. (Dilation of the pupil pushes the iris against the trabecular meshwork, causing the obstruction.) Symptoms often reported are blurred vision, halos around white lights, frontal headache, and eye pain. Patients often associate the symptoms with stress or fatigue. An attack can also be precipitated in patients who are administered a mydriatic agent such as atropine or scopolamine for eye examination. Immediate treatment requires the administration of miotic agents to relieve the pressure of the iris against the trabecular network, allowing drainage of the aqueous humor. Mannitol, an osmotic diuretic, may be administered to draw aqueous humor from the eye, and acetazolamide may be administered

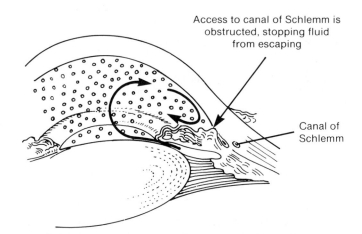

Figure 18-5 *Obstruction to the flow of aqueous fluid, causing closed-angle glaucoma.*

to reduce formation of aqueous humor. Analgesics and antiemetics may be administered if pain and vomiting persist. Surgery is then required to correct the abnormality.

Patient Education Associated with Glaucoma

Communication and responsibility. Encourage open communication concerning frustrations and anger as the patient attempts to adjust to the diagnosis and need for prolonged treatment. The patient must be guided to insight into the condition in order to assume responsibility for the continuation of treatment. Keep emphasizing those factors the patient can control to alter the disease process or progression, including the following:

Prevention. Persons with a family history of glaucoma should receive a yearly eye examination.

Prompt diagnosis. Routine eye examination with tonometry as a part of a yearly physical should be encouraged, particularly in people over 40 years of age.

Patients experiencing alterations in peripheral vision, disturbance in ability to adjust to the dark, eye pain, or a general aching around the eyes should receive diagnostic evaluation as soon as possible.

Nutrition. General dietary intake of a well-balanced variety of nutrients, vitamins, and minerals is essential to good health.

Control. Once diagnosed, *constant control* for the remainder of one's life is essential to prevent blindness.

Medications. Adherence to the *specific* medication regimen prescribed for an individual must be stressed. Do not alter or omit medications; teach specific side effects to expect and how to manage these effects. All medications are directed at decreasing the intraocular pressure through a variety of mechanisms (see individual medications).

Expectations of therapy. Discuss the following expectations of therapy with the patient:

- With simple glaucoma, rigid compliance can control intraocular pressure and prevent further tissue damage. In some cases surgical intervention may be necessary.
- With closed-angle glaucoma, treatment with medications is tried first; surgical intervention is commonly required.

Activities and exercise. To control intraocular pressure, avoid the following:

- Heavy lifting
- Straining with defecation
- Coughing
- Bending and placing the head in a dependent position

Pain relief. With closed-angle glaucoma, the pain may be controlled with potent analgesics.

Nausea, vomiting. Antiemetics to control nausea and vomiting and prevent further increases in intraocular pressure are essential. These symptoms are associated with closed-angle glaucoma.

Improved vision. Degenerated tissue or damage to the optic nerve cannot be reversed. The main goal of therapy is to prevent further damage that may result in blindness.

Personal safety. Provide for personal safety when visual acuity is diminished through the following measures:

- Orient the patient to the surroundings.
- Assist in ambulation as appropriate to the degree of visual impairment.
- Do not allow the operation of equipment that might be dangerous to the visually impaired.

Changes in expectations. Assess changes in expectations as therapy progresses and the patient gains understanding and skill in the management of the diagnosis.

Blurred vision, lacrimation, redness. Many of the medications used cause temporary blurring of vision. With continued therapy this, as well as lacrimation and redness, subsides.

Changes in therapy through cooperative goal setting. Work with the patient to encourage adherence to the prescribed treatment. When the patient feels that a change should be made in a treatment plan, encourage discussion first with the physician.

Written record. Enlist the patient's aid in developing and maintaining a written record of the monitoring parameters: headache, blurred vision, pulse, and blood pressure. (Monitoring should correspond to the medications being taken.) Patients should be encouraged to take this record with them on follow-up visits.

Fostering compliance. Throughout the patient's hospitalization, discuss medication information and how it will benefit the course of treatment. Seek cooperation and understanding of the following points so that medication compliance may be enhanced:

1. Name
2. Dosage
3. Route and time of administration: seek compliance and stress the need for adherence to the schedule to maintain the intraocular pressure at a stable level
4. Anticipated therapeutic response: control of intraocular pressure to prevent blindness
5. Side effects to expect: lacrimation and blurred vision
6. Side effects to report: decreasing vision, pain (see individual agents)
7. What to do if a dose is missed
8. When, how, or if to refill the medication prescription (an extra bottle of medication should be kept on hand in case of contamination of the primary bottle)

   When refilling the prescription, always compare the new bottle with the information on the old prescription: name of drug, concentration or strength, directions, and expiration date.

Difficulty in comprehension. If it is evident that the patient and/or family does not understand all aspects of continuing therapy being prescribed (such as administration and monitoring of medications, restrictions in exercises, need for follow-up appointments), consider the use of social service or visiting nurse agencies. Use of Ocusert may be appropriate depending on the patient's compliance.

Associated teaching. Give patients the following instructions:

Always inform the physician or dentist of any prescription or over-the-counter medication being taken. Over-the-counter medications and eye washes should not be taken without first consulting with the physician or pharmacist.

Always report side effects of rash, itching, or hives immediately. Nausea or vomiting should also be reported for the physician's evaluation if it is a new symptom.

Take all of the medication as prescribed for the full course of treatment. Do not discontinue use when feeling improved; do not save for future use; do not give your medicine to another individual. Sudden discontinuation of certain medications may produce harmful effects.

Keep all medications out of reach of children.

If pregnancy is suspected, consult an obstetrician as soon as possible about continuation of medication therapy.

At discharge. Items to be sent home with the patient should include the following:

1. Written instructions for use
2. Labels in a level of language and size of print appropriate for the patient
3. If needed, identification cards or bracelets
4. A list of additional supplies to be purchased after discharge (such as eye dressings, patches, cotton balls)
5. A schedule of follow-up appointments

Cholinergic agents

OBJECTIVES

1. Explain the action of a cholinergic agent on the pupil shape, the filtration angle, and the intraocular pressure.
2. State the side effects to expect when cholinergic agents are administered for an ophthalmic disorder.
3. Identify the effects of a cholinergic agent on the responsiveness of the eye to light.

KEY WORDS

erythema   myopia

Cholinergic agents produce strong contractions of the iris (miosis) and ciliary body musculature (accommodation). These drugs lower the intraocular pressure in patients with glaucoma by widening the filtration angle, permitting outflow of aqueous humor. They may also be used to counter the effects of mydriatic and cycloplegic agents following surgery or ophthalmoscopic examination.

Advantages of cholinergic agents are that (1) they are effective in many cases of chronic glaucoma, (2) the side effects are less severe and less frequent than those of anticholinesterase agents, and (3) they give better control of intraocular pressure with fewer fluctuations in pressure.

Side effects. A common side effect of cholinergic agents is difficulty in adjusting quickly to changes in light intensity. Reduced visual acuity may be most notable at night by older patients and in those patients developing lens opacities. Other common side effects are headaches in the suborbital or temporal region, conjunctival irritation and erythema, and induced myopia.

Rarely, a patient may develop signs of systemic toxicity, manifested by sweating, salivation, abdominal discomfort, diarrhea, bronchospasm, muscle tremors, hypotension, arrhythmias, and bradycardia. These symptoms are an indication of excessive administration. If accidental overdosage should occur during instillation, flush the affected eye with water or normal saline.

Availability. See Table 18-6.

Dosage and administration. See individual agents.

- **Nursing Interventions: Monitoring cholinergic agent therapy**

See also General Nursing Considerations for Patients with Disorders of the Eye (p. 434).

Side effects to expect

REDUCED VISUAL ACUITY. The miosis induced by the cholinergic agents reduces visual acuity, particularly in areas of poor lighting. Advise patients to use caution while driving at night or performing hazardous tasks in poor light.

Blurred vision occurs particularly during the first 1 to 2 hours after instilling the medication.

Be sure to keep eye medications separate from other solutions.

The ability to read for long periods of time is decreased due to impairment of near-vision accommodation.

Provide for patient safety when visual impairment exists.

- In hospitals, orient to the hospital unit, furniture placement, and call light; place the bed in a low position.
- At home, do not move furniture or the individual's household or personal belongings.

CONJUNCTIVAL IRRITATION, ERYTHEMA, HEADACHE. These side effects are usually mild and tend to resolve with continued therapy. Encourage the patient not to discontinue therapy without first consulting the physician.

PAIN, DISCOMFORT. Because of pupillary constriction, an increase in pain or discomfort may occur, particularly in bright light. Stress the need for compliance and

Table 18-6 *Cholinergic Agents*

GENERIC NAME	BRAND NAME	AVAILABILITY	DOSAGE	COMMENTS
Acetylcholine chloride, intraocular	Miochol Intraocular	1:100 solution	0.5-2 ml instilled into the eye during surgery	Used only during surgery to produce complete miosis within seconds; duration of action is only a few minutes, so pilocarpine may be added to maintain miosis
Carbachol, intraocular	Miostat Intraocular	0.01% solution	0.5 ml	Used only during surgery to produce complete miosis within 2-5 minutes
Carbachol, topical	Isopto-Carbachol	0.75, 1.5, 2.25 and 3% solution	1-2 drops into eye 2-4 times daily	Miotic action lasts 4-8 hours May be particularly useful in patients resistant to pilocarpine
Pilocarpine	Isopto-Carpine, Pilocar, Akarpine, Piloptic, Pilopine HS	0.25, 0.5, 1, 2, 3, 4, 5, 6, 8, 10% solutions; 4% gel	1-2 drops up to 6 times daily; 0.5-4% solutions used most frequently	Safest, most commonly used miotic for glaucoma Also used to reverse mydriasis after eye examination Onset is 15 minutes to 1 hour, and lasts for 2-3 hours

Pilocarpine ocular therapeutic system	Ocusert Pilo-20 Ocusert Pilo-40	—	Inserted weekly, releases either 20 or 40 μg of pilocarpine per hour	A small reservoir containing pilocarpine that is placed in a corner of the eye
				Advantages:
				  Convenience, once-weekly dosing
				  Better continuous control of intraocular pressure
				  Less medication used, lower incidence of toxicity
				Disadvantages:
				  Cost
				  Weekly insertions
				  Conjunctival irritation
				  Variable duration of action
				  May fall out during sleep

assure the patient that this will diminish with continued use.

Side effects to report

SYSTEMIC SIDE EFFECTS. These side effects indicate overdosage or excessive administration. Report to the physician for dosage adjustment. The adverse effects themselves usually do not need to be treated, since they will resolve by withholding cholinergic therapy.

Prevent systemic effects by carefully blocking the inner canthus for 1 to 2 minutes after instilling the medication to prevent absorption via the nasolacrimal duct.

During drug therapy, assess the blood pressure every shift and report significant changes from the baseline data.

Cholinesterase inhibitors
OBJECTIVES

1. Identify the effect of cholinesterase inhibitors on pupil size and intraocular pressure.
2. Explain the underlying problem of cholinesterase inhibitors on the ability of the eyes to adjust to light.
3. Describe the signs, symptoms, and treatment of systemic toxicity from cholinesterase inhibitors.

Cholinesterase is an enzyme that destroys acetylcholine, the cholinergic neurotransmitter. The cholinesterase inhibitors prevent the metabolism of acetylcholine within the eye, causing increased cholinergic activity and resulting in decreased intraocular pressure and miosis. Thus, cholinesterase inhibitors are used in the treatment of glaucoma. Due to higher incidence of side effects, however, they are reserved for patients who do not respond well to cholinergic agents.

Side effects. A common side effect of anticholinesterase inhibitors is difficulty in adjusting quickly to changes in light intensity. Reduce visual acuity may be most notable at night by older patients and in those patients developing lens opacities.

Other common side effects are stinging, burning, headaches, conjunctival irritation and erythema, lid muscle twitching, brow-ache, and induced myopia with blurred vision.

Rarely, a patient may develop signs of systemic toxicity, manifested by sweating, salivation, vomiting, abdominal cramps, urinary incontinence, diarrhea, dyspnea, bronchospasm, muscle tremors, hypotension, arrhythmias, and bradycardia. These symptoms are an indication of excessive administration. If symptoms become severe, parenteral atropine should be administered. If accidental overdosage should occur during instillation, flush the affected eye with water or normal saline.

Availability. See Table 18-7.

Dosage and administration. See individual agents.

Table 18-7 *Cholinesterase Inhibitors*

GENERIC NAME	BRAND NAME	AVAILABILITY	DOSAGE	COMMENTS
Demecarium bromide	Humorsol	0.125, 0.25% solution	1-2 drops 1-2 times daily	Onset is within 1 hour; duration may be several days Due to cumulative doses, use only the minimum dose necessary; wipe excess solution away immediately
Echothiophate iodide	Phospholine Iodide	0.03, 0.06, 0.125, 0.25% solution	1 drop 1-2 times daily	Used most commonly in open-angle glaucoma Onset occurs within 10-45 minutes; duration may be several days After reconstitution, use within 1 month if stored at room temperature, 6 months if refrigerated Tolerance may develop after prolonged use; a rest period will restore response
Isoflurophate	Floropryl	0.025% ointment	¼ inch strip of ointment in conjunctiva every 8-72 hours	When possible, apply at bedtime because of blurred vision Due to cumulative doses, use only the minimum dose necessary
Physostigmine	Eserine, Isopto-Eserine	0.25% ointment 0.25, 0.5% solution	Ointment: small quantity up to 3 times daily Solution: 2 drops up to 4 times daily	May only be needed every other day Do not use if solution turns pink to brown Duration ranges 12-36 hours

• Nursing Interventions: Monitoring cholinesterase inhibitor therapy

See also General Nursing Considerations for Patients with Disorders of the Eye (p. 434).

Side effects to expect

REDUCED VISUAL ACUITY. The miosis induced by the cholinesterase inhibitors reduces visual acuity, particularly in poorly lit areas. Advise patients to use caution while driving at night or performing hazardous tasks in poor light.

CONJUNCTIVAL IRRITATION, ERYTHEMA, HEADACHE, LACRIMATION. These side effects are usually mild and tend to resolve with continued therapy. Encourage the patient not to discontinue therapy without first consulting the physician.

Side effects to report

SYSTEMIC SIDE EFFECTS. These are an indication of overdosage or excessive administration. Report to the physician for treatment and dosage adjustment.

Drug interactions

CARBAMATE AND ORGANOPHOSPHATE INSECTICIDES AND PESTICIDES. Gardeners, farmers, manufacturing employees, and others who are exposed to these pesticides and insecticides and who are receiving cholinesterase inhibitors should be warned of the added risk of systemic symptoms from absorption of these chemicals through the skin and respiratory tract. Respiratory mask and frequent washing and clothing changes are advisable.

Adrenergic agents
OBJECTIVES

1. Review the actions of adrenergic agents.
2. Correlate the systemic effects of adrenergic agents with the alpha, beta-1, and beta-2 actions of this class of medications.

Adrenergic agents have several uses in ophthalmology. Sympathomimetic agents cause pupil dilation, increased outflow of aqueous humor, vasoconstriction, relaxation of the ciliary muscle, and a decrease in the formation of aqueous humor. Adrenergic agents are used to treat open-angle glaucoma, to relieve congestion and hyperemia, and to produce mydriasis for ocular examinations.

Side effects. The only common side effects are stinging, conjunctival irritation, and sensitivity to bright light. Pigmentary deposits in the conjunctiva, cornea, or lids may occur after prolonged use.

Systemic effects from ophthalmic instillation are un-

Table 18-8 *Adrenergic Agents*

GENERIC NAME	BRAND NAME	AVAILABILITY	DOSAGE	COMMENTS
Apraclonidine	Iopidine	1% solution	1 drop 1 hour before surgery	Used to control intraocular pressure after laser surgery
Dipivefrin hydrochloride	Propine	0.1%	1 drop every 12 hours	This drug has no activity itself, but is metabolized to epinephrine; used because it can penetrate the anterior chamber more readily than epinephrine and is less irritating
Epinephrine	Epifrin, Glaucon, Epitrate, Epinal, Eppy/N	0.25, 0.5, 1, 2% solutions	1-2 drops 1-2 times daily	Used to treat open-angle glaucoma, often in combination with cholinergic or beta-blocking agents. Duration of action is about 12 hours
Naphazoline hydrochloride	Vasoclear, Allerest, Naphcon, Albalon Liquifilm	0.012, 0.02, 0.025, 0.03, 0.1% solution	1-2 drops every 3-4 hours	Used as a topical vasoconstrictor
Tetrahydrozoline hydrochloride	Murine Plus, Visine, Optigene	0.05% solution	1-2 drops 2 or 3 times daily	Used as a topical vasoconstrictor

common and minimal. However, systemic absorption may occur via the lacrimal drainage system into the nasal pharyngeal passages. Systemic effects are manifested by palpitations, tachycardia, arrhythmias, hypertension, faintness, trembling, and sweating.

Use with caution in patients with hypertension, diabetes mellitus, hyperthyroidism, heart disease, arteriosclerosis, or long-standing bronchial asthma.

Availability. See Table 18-8.

Dosage and administration. See individual agents.

• **Nursing Interventions: Monitoring adrenergic agent therapy**

See also General Nursing Considerations for Patients with Disorders of the Eye (p. 434).

Side effects to expect

SENSITIVITY TO BRIGHT LIGHTS. The mydriasis produced allows excessive amounts of light into the eyes, which causes the patient to squint. Use of sunglasses will help reduce the brightness. Caution the patient temporarily to avoid tasks that require visual acuity, such as driving or operating power machinery.

CONJUNCTIVAL IRRITATION, LACRIMATION. These side effects are usually mild and tend to resolve with continued therapy. Encourage the patient not to discontinue therapy without first consulting the physician.

Side effects to report

SYSTEMIC SIDE EFFECTS. These are indications of overdosage or excessive administration. Report to the physician for treatment and dosage adjustment.

Prevent systemic effects by carefully blocking the in-

ner canthus for 1 to 2 minutes after instilling the medication to prevent absorption via the nasolacrimal duct.

Monitor the pulse rate and blood pressure and have the patient continue to do this at home; report significant changes from the baseline data.

SWEATING, TREMBLING. Touch the patient and bedding to assess for diaphoresis (sweating), particularly when these agents are used in surgery where the patient is under sterile drapes, anesthetized, and unable to respond to verbal questioning.

Drug interactions

TRICYCLIC ANTIDEPRESSANTS. Tricyclic antidepressants (amitriptyline, imipramine, doxepin, others) may cause additive hypertensive effects.

Monitor carefully for poor blood pressure control or a gradually increasing blood pressure.

Beta-adrenergic blocking agents

OBJECTIVES

1. Compare the actions of adrenergic agents with those of adrenergic blocking agents.
2. Explain monitoring parameters to detect the systemic effects of adrenergic blocking agents.

KEY WORD

aphakic

The beta-adrenergic blocking agents (Table 18-9) are used in ophthalmology to reduce elevated intraocular pressure. The exact mechanism is not known, but these

Table 18-9 *Beta-Adrenergic Blocking Agents*

GENERIC NAME	BRAND NAME	AVAILABILITY	INITIAL DOSAGE	COMMENTS
Betaxolol hydrochloride	Betoptic	5 mg/ml in 5 and 10 ml dropper bottles	1 drop twice daily	A beta-1 selective agent; onset in 30 minutes, duration is 12 hours; several weeks of therapy may be required to determine optimal dosage
Levobunolol hydrochloride	Betagan	0.5% solution in 5 and 10 ml dropper bottles	1 drop once or twice daily	A beta-1,2 agent; onset within 60 minutes, duration is up to 24 hours
Metipranolol	OptiPranolol	0.3% solutions in 5 and 10 ml dropper bottles	1 drop twice daily in affected eye(s)	A beta-1,2 agent; onset within 30 minutes, duration is 12-24 hours
Timolol maleate	Timoptic	0.25, 0.5% solutions in 5, 10, and 15 ml dropper bottles	1 drop of 0.25% solution twice daily	A beta-1,2 agent; onset within 30 minutes, duration is up to 24 hours

agents are thought to act by reducing the production of aqueous humor. Unlike the anticholinergic agents, there is no blurred or dim vision or night blindness, because intraocular pressure is reduced with little or no effect on pupil size or visual acuity. The beta-adrenergic blocking agents are used to reduce intraocular pressure in patients with chronic open-angle glaucoma or ocular hypertension.

Side effects. The only common side effects are stinging and conjunctival irritation upon instillation. Systemic effects are uncommon, but may be manifested by bradycardia, arrhythmias, hypotension, faintness, and bronchospasm. These adverse effects are more frequently observed in patients requiring higher doses of beta-adrenergic blocking agents and in those patients with hypertension, diabetes mellitus, heart disease, arteriosclerosis, or longstanding bronchial asthma.

Availability. See Table 18-9.

Dosage and administration. See Table 18-9.

• **Nursing Interventions: Monitoring beta-adrenergic blocking agent therapy**

See also General Nursing Considerations for Patients with Disorders of the Eye (p. 434).

Side effects to expect

CONJUNCTIVAL IRRITATION, LACRIMATION. These side effects are usually mild and tend to resolve with continued therapy. Encourage the patient not to discontinue therapy without first consulting the physician.

Side effects to report

SYSTEMIC SIDE EFFECTS. These are an indication of overdosage or excessive administration. Report to the physician for treatment and dosage adjustment.

Record the blood pressure and pulse rate at specific intervals.

Drug interactions

BETA-ADRENERGIC BLOCKING AGENTS. Propranolol, atenolol, acebutolol, nadolol, pindolol, labetalol, and metoprolol may enhance the systemic therapeutic and toxic effects of ophthalmic beta-adrenergic blocking agents.

Monitor for an increase in severity of side effects such as fatigue, hypotension, bronchospasm, and bradycardia.

OTHER PHARMACOLOGIC AGENTS

Antimicrobial Agents

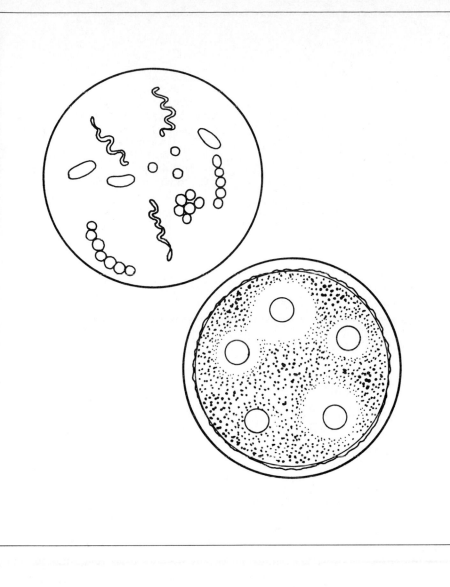

CHAPTER GOALS

After completing this chapter, the student should be able to do the following:

1. Explain the major action and effects of drugs used to treat infectious diseases.

2. Identify baseline data the nurse should collect on a continuous basis for comparison and evaluation of drug effectiveness.

3. Identify important nursing assessments and interventions associated with the drug therapy and treatment of infectious diseases.

4. Identify essential components involved in planning patient education that will enhance compliance with the treatment regimen.

Drug therapy for infectious disease
    Aminoglycosides (p. 461)
    Cephalosporins (p. 462)
    Macrolides (p. 464)
    Penicillins (p. 465)
    Quinolones (p. 467)
    Sulfonamides (p. 469)
    Tetracyclines (p. 471)
    Other antibiotics (p. 472)
        Aztreonam
        Chloramphenicol
        Clindamycin
        Imipenem
        Metronidazole
        Spectinomycin
        Vancomycin
Topical antifungal agents (p. 478)
    Butoconazole

Ciclopirox
Clotrimazole
Econazole
Haloprogin
Ketoconazole
Miconazole
Naftidine
Nystatin
Oxiconazole
Sulconazole
Terconazole
Tioconazole
Tolnaftate
Systemic antifungal agents (p. 480)
    Amphotericin B
    Fluconazole
    Flucytosine

Griseofulvin
Ketoconazole
Miconazole
Drug therapy for tuberculosis
    (p. 487)
    Ethambutol
    Isoniazid
    Rifampin
Drug therapy for viral infections
    (p. 488)
    Acyclovir
    Amantadine
    Idoxuridine
    Ribavirin
    Trifluridine
    Vidarabine
    Zidovudine

Objectives

1. Identify criteria used to select an effective antimicrobial agent.
2. Describe the signs and symptoms of the common side effects associated with antimicrobial agents: (a) an allergic reaction, (b) direct tissue damage, and (c) superinfection.
3. Differentiate between gram-negative and gram-positive microorganisms and between anaerobic and aerobic properties of microorganisms.
4. Describe basic principles of patient care that can be implemented to enhance an individual's therapeutic response during an infection.
5. Review components of a baseline assessment to evaluate the patient's hydration status and assessments needed to detect renal or hepatic toxicity.
6. Identify significant data in a patient history that could alert the medical team that a patient is more likely to experience an allergic reaction.
7. Describe the usual management of nausea, vomiting, and diarrhea when it occurs in conjunction with antimicrobial therapy.
8. State the signs and symptoms of a superinfection and actions that can be encouraged to minimize these effects.
9. Review parenteral administration techniques and the procedure for vaginal insertion of drugs.
10. Develop measurable short- and long-term objectives for patient education for patients receiving aminoglycosides, cephalosporins, penicillins, quinolones, sulfonamides, tetracyclines, antifungal, and antiviral agents.

Key Words

antibiotic   pathogenic organism
gram-negative   gram-positive
bactericidal   bacteriostatic

Antimicrobial agents are chemicals that eliminate living microorganisms pathogenic to the patient. Antimicrobial agents may be of chemical origin, such as the sulfonamides, or may be derived from other living organisms. Those derived from other living microorganisms are called *antibiotics;* for example, penicillin was first derived from the mold *Penicillium notatum.* Most antibiotics used today are harvested from large colonies of microorganisms, purified, and chemically modified into semisynthetic antimicrobial agents. The chemical modification makes the antibiotic more effective against certain specific pathogenic organisms.

The selection of the antimicrobial agent must be based on the sensitivity of the pathogen and the possible toxicity to the patient. If at all possible, the infecting organisms should first be isolated and identified. Culture and sensitivity tests should be completed. The antimicrobial therapy is then started based on the sensitivity results and the clinical judgment of the physician.

Side effects. Side effects common to all antimicrobial agents include: allergy, direct tissue damage, and superinfection.

Allergy. The severity of allergic reaction ranges from a mild rash to fatal anaphylaxis. Allergic reactions may develop within 30 minutes of administration (anaphylaxis, laryngeal edema, shock, dyspnea, or skin reactions) or may occur several days after discontinuance of therapy (skin rashes or fever). All patients must be questioned for previous allergic reactions, and allergy-prone patients must be observed closely. It is important not to label a patient "allergic" to a particular medication without adequate documentation. The medication to which a patient claims an allergy may be a life-saving drug for him or her.

Direct tissue damage. All drugs have at least the potential to damage tissues of certain organs. Examples include kidney damage by the aminoglycosides and penicillins and liver damage by isoniazid. Fortunately, these adverse effects are rare. The physician will order certain laboratory tests during antimicrobial treatment to help monitor the patient's therapy. Patients with preexisting disease, such as renal failure or hepatitis, will require lower doses to prevent toxicity.

Superinfection. Antimicrobial agents may induce overgrowth of resistant bacterial strains or fungal organisms. Superinfections occur most frequently with the use of broad-spectrum antibiotics and with agents that diminish host resistance, such as corticosteroids and antineoplastic agents. Stomatitis, glossitis, itching, and vulvovaginitis are often caused by candidal species of fungi. Viral infections may also develop, especially on the lips (cold sores) and oral mucosa (canker sores).

Common side effects of antimicrobial agents taken orally include nausea, vomiting, and diarrhea. These effects are often dose-related and result from changes in normal bacterial flora in the bowel, from irritation, and from superinfection. Symptoms resolve within a few days and rarely require discontinuation of therapy.

General Nursing Considerations for Patients with Infectious Diseases

Nurses need to consider the entire patient when administering and monitoring antimicrobial therapy. It is essential that the nurse be knowledgeable about the drugs themselves, including physiologic parameters for monitoring expected therapeutic activity, as well as for potential adverse effects.

The following basic principles of patient care should not be overlooked when treating a patient with infections:

1. Adequate rest with as little stress as possible; rest also decreases metabolic needs and enhances the physiologic repair process
2. Nutritional management, including attention to hydration, proteins, fats, carbohydrates, minerals, and vitamins to support the body's needs during an inflammatory response
3. Infection control, as mandated by hospital policy, regarding protective isolation to ensure that the infection is not spread to others
4. Training the patient in personal hygiene measures, such as handwashing techniques, management of their excretions, and wound care
5. Drug therapy specific to the type of microorganism causing the infection

Principles of drug administration need to be followed for all pharmacologic agents administered. (Refer to Chapters 5-7 for a review of specific principles.) The patient may have coexisting medical or surgical diagnoses, be debilitated, or have a suppressed immune system so that an infectious process could be fatal. Routine monitoring of all individuals receiving antimicrobial therapy should include status of hydration, temperature, pulse, respirations, and blood pressure. Monitor at least every 4 hours and more frequently as the patient's clinical status warrants.

Nurses need to perform baseline assessments of their patients for the common side effects associated with each individual agent administered. Further routine assessments should be performed on a scheduled basis to detect and to prevent early indications of allergic reactions, tissue damage (nephrotoxicity, ototoxicity, hepatotoxicity), and superinfections.

The general nursing considerations presented in this section concerning allergic treatment apply to all drug therapy and patient monitoring. However, because antimicrobial therapy is ordered so frequently, it is appropriate to reemphasize them here.

Patient Concerns: Nursing Intervention/Rationale

Allergy

Preventing allergic reactions. Take a thorough nursing history of any prior "allergic" problems that the patient has experienced.

Symptoms. Has the patient taken this medication before? If so, what symptoms (such as nausea, vomiting, diarrhea, rash, itching, or hives) developed when taking it that led him or her to state now that he or she is allergic? Ask the patient to describe the appearance of the rash, where it started, and the course of recovery.

Onset. How soon after starting the medication did the symptoms develop?

Other medications. Was the patient also taking any over-the-counter medications (such as laxatives, antacids, cough or cold preparations, suntanning products, etc.)?

Other allergies. Has the patient previously been allergic to dust, weeds, foods, or other environmental factors?

Asthma. Does the patient have a history of asthma or allergic rhinitis?

Susceptible patients. People with a history of allergies, asthma, rhinitis, taking multiple drug preparations, or kidney or liver dysfunctions are particularly susceptible to drug reactions.

The elderly, because of physiologic changes of aging, need close observations for therapeutic response or for toxicity to drugs administered.

Nursing actions. Do not administer the medication if the person reports possible allergy; share all information obtained with the physician, who will decide whether to administer the drug.

If a definite drug allergy is identified, the patient's chart, unit Kardex, and an identification bracelet should be carefully marked to alert all personnel to the specific drugs the patient should not receive.

Responding to allergic reactions. All patients should be watched carefully for possible allergy for at least 20 to 30 minutes following administration of a medication.

Emergency cart. Know the location of the hospital emergency cart and the procedure for summoning it. In the event of suspected anaphylaxis, summon the physician and the emergency cart immediately.

Sites of reactions. Although a serious reaction may occur with the first administration of a drug, repeated exposures to a previously sensitized substance can be fatal. Respond immediately to any signs of reaction, including the following:

- Swelling, redness, or pain at the site of injection
- Hives, nasal congestion and discharge, wheezing progressing to dyspnea, pulmonary edema, stridor, and sternal retractions

Monitoring. Monitor the patient's vital signs continuously. Report hypotension, increasing pulse, and respirations that become labored and shallow.

Follow-up. Following any reaction, the patient and family should be alerted to inform anyone treating the patient in the future of the allergy to a specific drug.

Preventing and assessing tissue damage

Nephrotoxicity. Monitor urinalysis and kidney function tests for abnormal results. Report an increasing BUN and creatinine, decreasing urine output and/or decreasing specific gravity (despite amount of fluid intake), casts or protein in the urine, frank blood or smoky-colored urine, or RBCs in excess of 0-3 on the urinalysis report.

Many antimicrobial agents are potentially nephrotoxic (aminoglycosides, tetracyclines, cephalosporins). Concomitant therapy with diuretics enhances the likelihood of toxicity, particularly in the elderly or debilitated patient.

When renal function is impaired, most drug dosages must be decreased, or alternate drug therapy employed.

Ototoxicity. Damage to the eighth cranial nerve can occur from drug therapy, particularly from aminoglycosides. This may initially be manifested by dizziness, tinnitus, and progressive hearing loss.

Assess your patient for difficulty in walking unaided and assess the level of hearing daily. Intentionally speak to patients softly; note if they are aware that you said anything. Take particular notice of the patient who repeatedly says, "What did you say?" or who starts talking more loudly or progressively increases the volume on the television or radio.

Hepatotoxicity. Several drugs to be studied in this unit are potentially hepatotoxic (isoniazid, sulfonamides).

The liver is active in the metabolism of many drugs, and drug-induced hepatitis may occur. The actual liver damage may occur shortly after exposure to the pharmacologic agent or may not appear for several weeks after initial exposure. The symptoms of hepatotoxicity are anorexia, nausea, vomiting, jaundice, hepatomegaly, splenomegaly, and abnormal liver function tests (elevated bilirubin, AST, ALT, GGT, alkaline phosphatase, prothrombin time).

Patients with preexisting hepatic disease such as cirrhosis or hepatitis will require lower doses of drugs metabolized by the liver.

Nausea, vomiting, diarrhea. Nausea, vomiting, and diarrhea are the "big three" adverse effects associated with antimicrobial drug therapy. When they occur, gather further data, including the following:

- Does the patient have a history of nausea, vomiting, or diarrhea before starting the drug therapy?
- How soon after starting the medication did the symptoms start?
- Since starting the medication, has the diet or water source changed in any way?
- Was the patient taking other drugs, either by prescription or over-the-counter, before the initiation of antibiotic therapy?
- How much fluid is the patient consuming when taking medications? Sometimes inadequate fluid intake may cause gastritis manifested by nausea. The physician may elect to give the antibiotic with food to decrease irritation even though absorption may be slightly decreased. When reporting any incidence of nausea and vomiting, all significant data should be collected and reported.
- For diarrhea, what was the pattern of elimination before drug therapy? Report diarrhea, and the character and frequency of stools as well as any abdominal pain promptly.

Superinfection

Superinfection may occur in patients receiving broad-spectrum antibiotic therapy, particularly in those who are immunosuppressed. Assess and report white patches in the mouth, cold sores, canker sores, vaginal itching or discharge, diarrhea, and recurrence of any fever. Cultures are taken, and additional antibiotics effective against the new organism are started.

Minimize exposure to people known to have an infection, and practice good personal hygiene measures.

Patient Education Associated with Antimicrobial Therapy

Communication and responsibility. Encourage open communication concerning frustrations and anger as the patient attempts to adjust to the diagnosis and need for prolonged treatment. The patient must be guided to gain insight into the condition in order to assume responsibility for the continuation of treatment. Keep emphasizing those factors the patient can control to alter the progression of the disease: maintenance of general health, nutritional needs, adequate rest and appropriate exercise, and continuation of prescribed medication therapy.

Adequate rest. Rest decreases the metabolic needs of the body and enhances physiologic repair.

Nutrition. Adequate hydration, especially during fever, as well as intake of adequate nutrients to meet the energy needs are paramount so that the body will not break down its proteins and fats to meet energy requirements.

The dietary plan must be individualized to the patient's diagnosis and point of recovery.

Personal hygiene. Teach thorough handwashing techniques to prevent the spread of infection. Protective isolation should be carried out in accordance with the hospital policies and procedures.

Tell the patient who has a wound infection not to touch the infected area.

For those patients with an upper respiratory infection, teaching proper handling and disposal of sputum tissues.

Expectations of therapy. Discuss expectations of therapy with the patient: relief of burning and frequency of urination; relief of cough; end of drainage and healing of a wound; ability to maintain activities of daily living.

Changes in expectations. Assess changes in expectations as therapy progresses and the patient gains understanding and skill in the management of the diagnosis.

Changes in therapy through cooperative goal setting. Work with the patient to encourage adherence to the prescribed treatment. When the patient feels that a change should be made in a treatment plan, encourage the patient to discuss it first with the physician.

Written record. Enlist the patient's aid in developing and maintaining a written record of his/her monitoring parameters (list presenting symptoms: cough with a large amount of phlegm, wound drainage; temperature; exercise tolerance) and response to prescribed therapies for discussion with the physician (Figure 19-1). Patients should be encouraged to take this record on follow-up visits.

Fostering compliance. Throughout the patient's hospitalization, discuss medication information and how it will benefit the course of treatment. Seek cooperation and understanding of the following points, so that medication compliance may be enhanced:

1. Name
2. Dosage
3. Route and administration times
4. Anticipated therapeutic response: decrease in presenting symptoms (such as fever, cough, sore throat, wound drainage)
5. Side effects to expect
6. Side effects to report: failure of presenting symptoms to resolve
7. What to do if a dose is missed
8. When, how, or if to refill the medication prescription

Difficulty in comprehension. If it is evident that the patient and/or family does not understand all aspects of continuing therapy being prescribed (such as administration and monitoring of medications, exercises, diets, follow-up appointments), consider the use of social service or visiting nurse agencies.

Associated teaching. Give patients the following instructions:

Always inform the physician or dentist of any prescription or over-the-counter medication being taken. Over-the-counter medications should not be taken without first discussing them with a physician or pharmacist.

Always report side effects of rash, itching, or hives immediately. Nausea, vomiting, or diarrhea should also be reported for the physician's evaluation if it is a new symptom.

Take all of the medication as prescribed for the full course of treatment. Do not discontinue use when feeling improved; do not save for future use; do not give your medicine to another individual. Sudden discontinuation of certain medications may produce harmful effects.

Keep all medications out of reach of children.

If pregnancy is suspected, consult an obstetrician as

Patient Education and Monitoring of Therapeutic Outcomes for Patients Receiving Antibiotics

Medications	Color	To be taken

Name _____

Physician _____

Physician's phone _____

Next appt.* _____

Parameters		Day of discharge								Comments
Temperature	on arising / 12 noon / 5 PM / 9 PM									
Aspirin	Time; #tabs, e.g 8am 2									
Acetaminophen	Time; #tabs, e.g. 12N 2									
Site of infection Scale + Small ++++ Severe	Redness									
	Pain									
	Drainage									
Cough and sputum Productive:	Color									
	Thickness									
	No cough									
Mouth and throat	Sore throat									
	No problem									
Dizziness	Walk unaided									
	Must use support									
	Walk with help									
Hearing	Had to ↑ volume of radio - TV									
	No difficulty									
Skin	Rash with itching									
	Rash - fine red									
	No itching									
	No rash									
Vaginal itching (Yes or No)										
Rectal itching (Yes or No)										

*Please bring this record with you to your next appointment.
Use the back of this sheet for additional information.

Figure 19-1 *Patient education and monitoring of therapeutic outcomes for patients receiving antibiotics.*

soon as possible about continuation of medication therapy.

At discharge. Items to be sent home with the patient should include the following:

1. Written instructions for use
2. Labels in a level of language and size of print appropriate for the patient
3. If needed, identification cards or bracelets
4. A list of additional supplies to be purchased after discharge (such as syringes or dressings)
5. A schedule for follow-up appointments

Drug Therapy for Infectious Disease

Aminoglycosides

OBJECTIVES

1. Cite the primary uses of the aminoglycosides and the serious side effects that require close monitoring of the patient.
2. Identify precautions needed to prevent incompatibilities between aminoglycosides and other medications.
3. State the method of action of aminoglycosides on the bacterial cell.

KEY WORDS

ototoxicity
nephrotoxicity

The aminoglycoside antibiotics are used primarily against gram-negative microorganisms that cause urinary tract infections, meningitis, wound infections, and life-threatening septicemias. They are a mainstay in the treatment of hospital-acquired gram-negative infections. Kanamycin and neomycin may also be used to re-duce the normal flora content of the intestinal tract prior to surgery. Aminoglycosides act by inhibiting protein synthesis within bacteria.

Side effects. Two serious reactions may occur with the aminoglycosides: ototoxicity, manifested by dizziness, tinnitus, and deafness; and nephrotoxicity, manifested by protein and blood in the urine, particularly in patients receiving high doses, or medications for longer than 10 days. If any of these symptoms should occur, report it immediately. Continue to observe patients for ototoxicity after therapy has been discontinued. These adverse effects may appear several days later.

Availability. See Table 19-1.

• **Nursing Interventions: Monitoring aminoglycoside therapy**

See also General Nursing Considerations for Patients with Infectious Diseases (p. 457).

Side effects to report

OTOTOXICITY. Damage to the eighth cranial nerve can occur from aminoglycoside therapy. This may initially be manifested by dizziness, tinnitus, and progressive hearing loss.

Assess your patients for difficulty in walking unaided and assess their level of hearing daily. Intentionally speak softly; note if he or she is aware that you said anything. Take particular notice of the patient who repeatedly says, "What did you say?" or who starts talking more loudly or progressively increases the volume on the television or radio.

NEPHROTOXICITY. Monitor urinalysis and kidney function tests for abnormal results. Report an increasing BUN and creatinine, decreasing urine output or decreasing specific gravity (despite amount of fluid intake), casts or protein in the urine, frank blood or smoky-colored urine, or RBCs in excess of 0-3 on the urinalysis report.

Table 19-1 *The Aminoglycosides*

GENERIC NAME	BRAND NAME	AVAILABILITY	ADULT DOSAGE RANGE
Amikacin	Amikin	100 mg/2 ml vial 500 mg/2 ml vial 1 g/4 ml vial	IM, IV: 15 mg/kg/24 hr
Gentamicin	Garamycin	2, 10, 40 mg/ml 60 mg/1.5 ml 80 mg/2 ml 100 mg/100 ml	IM, IV: Up to 240 mg/24 hr
Kanamycin	Kantrex, Klebcil	75,500 mg, 1 g vials	IM, IV: Up to 15 mg/kg/24 hr, not to exceed 1.5 gm/24 hr
Neomycin	Mycifradin	500 mg vial	IM: 15 mg/kg/24 hr
Netilmicin	Netromycin	100 mg/ml in 1.5 ml vials	IM, IV: 3-6.5 mg/kg/24 hr
Streptomycin	Streptomycin	400 mg/ml, 1 and 5 g vials	IM: 1-4 g/24 hr
Tobramycin	Nebcin	10 mg/ml in 2 ml vials 40 mg/ml in 1.2 g vials 40 mg/ml in 2 ml vials 60 mg/1.5 ml	IM, IV: Up to 5 mg/kg/24 hr

Implementation

COMPATIBILITIES. DO NOT mix other drugs in the same syringe or infuse together with other drugs. See Drug Interactions for incompatibilities.

LABORATORY. Check with the hospital laboratory regarding timing of aminoglycoside blood level tests.

After levels have been determined, assess whether results are normal or toxic.

RATE OF INFUSION. Consult with a pharmacist or see the individual package literature.

Drug interactions

NEPHROTOXIC POTENTIAL. Cephalosporins and diuretics, when combined with aminoglycosides, may increase the nephrotoxic potential.

Monitor the urinalysis and kidney function tests for abnormal results.

OTOTOXIC POTENTIAL. Aminoglycosides, when combined with ethacrynic acid, bumetanide, and furosemide may increase ototoxicity. Therefore, nursing assessments for tinnitus, dizziness, and decreased hearing should be done regularly every shift.

NEUROMUSCULAR BLOCKADE. Aminoglycoside antibiotics in combination with skeletal muscle relaxants may produce respiratory depression.

Check the anesthesia record in postoperative patients to see if skeletal muscle relaxants such as succinylcholine or pancuronium bromide were administered during surgery.

The nurse should monitor and assess the respiratory rate, depth of respirations, and chest movement, report apnea immediately. As these effects may be seen for up to 48 hours after administration of skeletal muscle relaxants, continue monitoring respirations, pulse, and blood pressure beyond the usual postsurgical vital sign routine.

HEPARIN. Gentamicin and heparin are physically incompatible. DO NOT mix together before infusion.

AMPICILLIN, PIPERACILLIN, TICARCILLIN, MEZLOCILLIN, AZLOCILLIN. These penicillins rapidly inactivate aminoglycoside antibiotics. DO NOT mix together or administer together at the same IV site.

Cephalosporins
OBJECTIVES

1. Compare the action of cephalosporins on gram-negative and gram-positive organisms.
2. State the method of action of cephalosporins on the cell wall.
3. Identify the assessments needed and treatment used for hypoprothrombinemia, thrombophlebitis, and electrolyte imbalances that may occur with the administration of cephalosporins.

KEY WORDS

thrombophlebitis   hypoprothrombinemia

The cephalosporins are chemically related to the penicillins and have a similar mechanism of activity. The cephalosporins may be used with caution as alternatives when patients are allergic to the penicillins, unless they are also allergic to the cephalosporins. The cephalosporins are used for certain pneumonias, urinary tract infections, abdominal infections, septicemias, meningitis, and osteomyelitis.

The cephalosporins act by inhibiting cell wall synthesis in bacteria. The cephalosporins may be divided into groups, or "generations," based primarily on antimicrobial activity. The first-generation cephalosporins have good activity against gram-positive bacteria and relatively moderate activity against gram-negative bacteria. The second-generation cephalosporins have somewhat increased activity against gram-negative bacteria but are much less active than the third-generation agents. Third-generation cephalosporins are generally less active than first-generation agents against gram-positive cocci, although they are much more active against the penicillinase-producing bacteria. Some of the third-generation cephalosporins are also active against Pseudomonas aeruginosa, a very potent gram-negative microorganism.

Side effects. Side effects of the cephalosporins are usually minor. The most common are nausea and diarrhea. Overgrowth of other organisms is manifested by oral thrush, genital and anal pruritus, genital candidiasis, vaginitis, and vaginal discharge.

Transient elevations of liver function tests (AST, ALT, alkaline phosphatase) and renal function tests (BUN, serum creatinine) have been reported. Renal toxicity, as evidenced by proteinuria, hematuria, casts, decreased creatinine clearance, and decreased urine output, has also developed.

Hypoprothrombinemia, with and without bleeding, has been reported. These rare occurrences are most frequent in elderly, debilitated, or otherwise compromised patients with borderline vitamin K deficiency. Treatment with broad-spectrum antibiotics eliminates enough gastrointestinal flora to cause a further reduction in vitamin K synthesis. The hypoprothrombinemia is readily reversed by administration of vitamin K.

A false-positive reaction for glucose in the urine may occur with Clinitest tablets, but not with Tes-Tape or Diastix.

Phlebitis and thrombophlebitis are recurrent problems associated with intravenous administration of cephalosporins. Use small IV needles, large veins, and alternating infusion sites if possible to minimize irritation.

Availability. See Table 19-2.

Table 19-2 *The Cephalosporins*

GENERIC NAME	BRAND NAME	GENERATION	AVAILABILITY	ADULT DOSAGE RANGE
Cefaclor	Ceclor	2	250, 500 mg capsules 125, 187, 250, 375 mg/5 ml suspension	PO: 250-500 every 8 hr; do not exceed 4 g/day
Cefadroxil	Duricef, Ultracef	1	500 mg capsules 1000 mg tablets 125, 250, 500 mg/5 ml suspension	PO: 1-2 g daily in 1-2 doses daily
Cefamandole	Mandol	2	500 mg, 1, 2, 10 g vials	IM, IV: 0.5-1 g every 4-8 hr; do not exceed 12 g/24 hr
Cefazolin	Ancef, Kefzol	1	250, 500 mg, 1, 5, 10, 20 g vials	IM, IV: 250 mg to 1.5 g every 6-8 hr
Cefixime	Suprax	3	200, 400 mg capsules 100 mg/5 ml suspension	PO: 200 mg every 12 hr or 400 mg once daily
Cefmetazole	Zefazone	2	1, 2 g vials	IV: 2 g every 6 to 12 hr
Cefonicid	Monocid	2	500 mg, 1, 10 g vials	IM, IV: 0.5-1 g once daily; do not exceed 2 g daily
Cefoperazone	Cefobid	3	1, 2 g vials	IV: 1-3 g every 6-8 hr
Ceforanide	Precef	2	500 mg, 1 g vials	IM, IV: 0.5-1 g every 12 hr; do not exceed 4 g/day
Cefotaxime	Claforan	3	500 mg, 1, 2, 10 g vials	IV: 1-2 g every 4-8 hr; do not exceed 12 g/day
Cefotetan	Cefotan	3	1, 2, 10 g vials	IM, IV: 1-2 g every 12 hr; do not exceed 6 g/day
Cefoxitin	Mefoxin	2	1, 2, 10 g vials	IM, IV: 1-2 g every 6-8 hr; do not exceed 12 g/day
Ceftazidime	Fortaz, Tazidime, ♣ Magnacef	3	500 mg, 1, 2, 6 gm vials	IM, IV: 1-2 g every 12 hr
Ceftizoxime	Cefizox	3	1, 2, 10 g vials	IV: 1-2 every 8-12 hr
Ceftriaxone	Rocephin	3	250, 500 mg, 1, 2, 10 g vials	IM, IV: 1-2 g once daily; do not exceed 4 g daily
Cefuroxime	Zinacef, Kefurox	2	125, 250, 500 mg tablets; 750 mg, 1.5 g vials	PO: 250-500 mg every 12 hours IV: 750 mg to 1.5 g every 8 hr
Cephalexin	Keflex, ♣ Ceporex	1	250, 500 mg capsules, tablets 1000 mg tablets 100 mg/ml Peds suspension 125, 250 mg/5 ml suspension	PO: 250-1000 mg every 6 hr
Cephalothin	Keflin, ♣ Ceporacin	1	1, 2, 20 g vials	IM, IV: 500 mg to 2 g every 4-6 hr
Cephapirin	Cefadyl	1	500 mg, 1, 2, 4, 20 g vials	IM, IV: 500 mg to 1 g every 4-6 hr
Cephradine	Anspor, Velosef	1	250, 500 mg capsules 125, 250 mg/5 ml suspension 250, 500 mg, 1, 2 g vials	PO: 250-500 mg every 6 hr IM, IV: 500 mg to 1 g every 6 hr; do not exceed 8 g/day
Moxalactam	Moxam	3	1, 2, 10 g vials	IV: 250 mg to 2 g 2-3 times daily; do not exceed 12 g daily

♣ Available in Canada only.

• Nursing Interventions: Monitoring cephalosporin therapy

See also General Nursing Considerations for Patients with Infectious Diseases (p. 457).

Side effects to report

DIARRHEA. Cephalosporins cause diarrhea by altering the bacterial flora of the gastrointestinal tract. The diarrhea is usually not severe enough to warrant discontinuing medication. Encourage the patient not to discontinue therapy without consulting the physician. When diarrhea persists, monitor the patient for signs of dehydration.

SUPERINFECTIONS. With cephalosporins, oral thrush, genital and anal pruritus, vaginitis, and vaginal discharge may occur. Report promptly as these infections are resistant to the original antibiotic used.

Teach the importance of meticulous oral and perineal personal hygiene.

ABNORMAL LIVER AND RENAL FUNCTION TESTS. Monitor returning laboratory data and report abnormal findings to the physician.

HYPOPROTHROMBINEMIA. Assess your patient for ecchymosis following minimal trauma, prolonged bleeding at an infusion site or from a surgical wound, or the development of petechiae, bleeding gums, or nosebleeds. Notify the physician of any of the signs of hypoprothrombinemia. The usual treatment is administration of vitamin K.

THROMBOPHLEBITIS. Carefully assess patients receiving IV cephalosporins for the development of thrombophlebitis.

Inspect the IV area frequently while providing care; inspect during dressing changes and at times the IV is changed to a new site. Always investigate pain at the IV site. Report redness, warmth, tenderness to touch, or edema in the affected part. If in lower extremities, dorsiflexion of the foot may cause pain in the calf area (Homans' sign). Compare findings in the affected limb with the unaffected limb.

ELECTROLYTE IMBALANCE. If a patient develops hyperkalemia or hypernatremia, consider the electrolyte content of the antibiotics. Most of the cephalosporins have a high electrolyte content.

Drug interactions

NEPHROTOXIC POTENTIAL. Patients receiving cephalosporins, aminoglycosides, and diuretics concurrently should be assessed for signs of nephrotoxicity. Monitor urinalysis and kidney function tests for abnormal results. Report an increasing BUN and creatinine, decreasing urine output or decreasing specific gravity (despite amount of fluid intake), casts or protein in the urine, frank blood or smoky-colored urine, or RBCs in excess of 0-3 on the urinalysis report.

PROBENECID. Patients receiving probenecid in combination with cephalosporins are more susceptible to toxicity due to the inhibition of excretion of the cephalosporins by probenecid. Monitor closely for adverse effects.

ALCOHOL. Avoid alcohol consumption during cefamandole, cefoperazone, moxalactam, and possible ceftizoxime therapy. Patients will become flushed, tremulous, dyspneic, tachycardic, and hypotensive. Do not use over-the-counter preparations containing alcohol, such as mouthwash (Cepacol) or cough preparations, because of their alcohol content.

Macrolides
OBJECTIVES

1. Compare the actions of the macrolides and the penicillins on the bacterial cell.
2. Identify the clinical uses of the macrolides.
3. Identify the precautions associated with parenteral erythromycin therapy.
4. Identify the drug interactions associated with macrolide antibiotic therapy.

The macrolide antibiotics (Table 19-3) act by inhibiting protein synthesis in susceptible bacteria. They are bacteriostatic and bacteriocidal, depending on the organism and the concentration of medicine present. Erythromycin is effective against gram-positive microorganisms and gram-negative cocci. Azithromycin is less active against gram-positive organisms than erythromycin, but has greater activity against gram-negative organisms that are resistant to erythromycin. Clarithromycin has a similar spectrum of activity as erythromycin, but has considerably greater potency. Troleandomycin is less effective than erythromycin and offers no advantages over the other macrolide antibiotics. The macrolides are used for respiratory, gastrointestinal tract, skin, and soft tissue infections, and sexually transmitted diseases, especially when penicillins, cephalosporins, and tetracyclines cannot be used.

Side effects. The macrolides are fairly well tolerated with relatively few serious adverse effects. The most common side effects of oral macrolide therapy are diarrhea, nausea and vomiting, and abnormal taste.

Availability. See Table 19-3.

• Nursing Interventions: Monitoring macrolide therapy

See also General Nursing Considerations for Patients with Infectious Diseases (p. 457).

Side effects to expect

GASTRIC IRRITATION. These side effects are usually mild and tend to resolve with continued therapy. Encourage the patient not to discontinue therapy without first consulting the physician.

Side effects to report

THROMBOPHLEBITIS. Carefully assess patients receiving IV erythromycin for the development of thrombophlebitis. Inspect the IV area frequently while providing care; inspect during dressing changes and when the IV is changed to a new site. Always investigate pain at the IV site. Report redness and edema in the affected part. If in lower extremities, dorsiflexion of the foot may cause pain in the calf area (Homans' sign). Compare the affected limb with the unaffected limb.

Table 19-3 *The Macrolides*

GENERIC NAME	BRAND NAME	AVAILABILITY	ADULT DOSAGE RANGE
Azithromycin	Zithromax	PO: 250 mg capsules	PO: 500 mg as a single dose on day 1, followed by 250 mg once daily on days 2-5 for a total dose of 1.5 g
Clarithromycin	Biaxin	PO: 250, 500 mg tablets	PO: 250-500 mg every 12 hr for 7-14 days
Erythromycin	Eryc, Ilosone, E-Mycin, many others	PO: 250, 333, 500 mg enteric-coated tablets; 125, 200, 250, 500 mg chewable tablets; 125, 250, 400, 500 mg film-coated tablets; 125, 250 mg enteric-coated pellets in capsules; 125, 200, 250, 400 mg/5 mg suspension; 100 mg/ml & 100 mg/2.5 ml drops IV: 250, 500, 1000 mg vials for reconstitution	PO: 250 mg 4 times daily for 10-14 days IM: 100 mg every 4-6 hr IV: 15-20 mg/kg/24 hr; up to 4 g/24 hr
Troleandomycin	Tao	PO: 250 mg capsules	PO: 250-500 mg 4 times daily for 10 days

Implementation

PO. Azithromycin and erythromycin should be administered at least 1 hour before or 2 hours after meals. Clarithromycin and troleandomycin may be taken without regard to meals.

IM. Due to pain on injection and the possibility of sterile abscess formation, this route of administration of erythromycin is generally not recommended for multiple-dose therapy.

IV. Dilute the dosage of erythromycin in 100 to 250 ml of saline solution or 5% dextrose and administer over 20 to 60 minutes. Thrombophlebitis after IV infusion is a relatively common side effect.

Drug interactions

TOXICITY CAUSED BY MACROLIDES. Macrolide antibiotics may inhibit the metabolism of several drugs, causing accumulation and potential toxicity. These drugs are: alfentanil, warfarin, bromocriptine, carbamazepine, cyclosporine, disopyramide, and theophyllines. Read individual monographs for monitoring parameters of toxicity from these agents.

Penicillins
OBJECTIVES

1. Compare the actions of the aminoglycosides, cephalosporins, macrolides, and penicillins on the bacterial cell.

2. Identify the clinical uses of the penicillins.
3. Explain the term *penicillin-resistant* in relation to the effectiveness of the penicillin agent prescribed.
4. Cite specific questions that could be asked to screen for a patient with a penicillin allergy prior to administration of the agent.
5. Identify precautions needed to prevent incompatibilities between penicillins and other medications administered via the intramuscular or intravenous routes.

KEY WORD

penicillinase-resistant

The penicillins were the first true antibiotics to be grown and used against pathogenic bacteria in human beings. They remain one of the most widely used classes of antibiotics today.

The penicillins act by interfering with the synthesis of bacterial cell walls. The resulting cell wall is weakened because of defective structure and the bacteria are subsequently destroyed by osmotic lysis. The penicillins are most effective against bacteria that multiply rapidly. They do not hinder growth of human cells, because human cells have protective membranes but no cell wall.

Many bacteria that are initially sensitive to the penicillins develop a protective mechanism and become re-

Table 19-4 *The Penicillins*

GENERIC NAME	BRAND NAME	AVAILABILITY	ADULT DOSAGE RANGE
Amdinocillin	Coactin	500 mg, 1 g vials	IM, IV: 10 mg/kg every 4-6 hr; do not exceed 60 mg/kg/day
Amoxicillin	Amoxil, Trimox, Larotid, Wymox, Polymox	125 and 250 mg chewable tablets 250 and 500 mg capsules 50, 125 and 250 mg/5 ml suspension	PO: 250-500 mg/8 hr
Ampicillin	Amcill, Polycillin, Omnipen, Principen, ♣Apo-Ampi, Totacillin	0.125, 0.25, 0.5, 1, and 2 g vials 250 and 500 mg capsules 125, 250, 500 mg/5 ml suspension	IM, IV: 0.5 to 1 g/4-6 hr PO: 250-500 mg/6 hr
Azlocillin	Azlin	2, 3, 4 g vials	IV: 8-18 g/24 hr in 4-6 divided doses
Carbenicillin	Geopen, Pyopen	1, 2, 5, 10 g vials	IM: Do not exceed 2 g/injection site IV: Up to 40 g/24 hr
Cloxacillin	Tegopen, Cloxapen	250 and 500 mg capsules 125 mg/5 ml suspension	PO: 250-500 mg/6 hr
Dicloxacillin	Dynapen, Pathocil, Veracillin	125, 250, and 500 mg capsules 62.5 mg/5 ml suspension	PO: 125-500 mg/6 hr
Methicillin	Celbenin, Staphcillin	1, 4, 6, 10 g vials	IM, IV: 1 g/4-6 hr
Mezlocillin	Mezlin	1, 2, 3, 4 g vials	IM, IV: Do not exceed 24 g/24 hr
Nafcillin	Nafcil, Unipen	0.5, 1, 2 g vials 250 and 500 mg tablets 250 mg/5 ml suspension	IM, IV: 0.5-1 g/4-6 hr PO: 250-500 mg/4-6 hr
Oxacillin	Bactocill, Prostaphlin	0.5, 1, 2, 4 g vials 250 and 500 mg capsules 250 mg/5 ml suspension	IM, IV: 0.5-1 g/4-6 hr PO: 250-500 mg/4-6 hr
Penicillin G, potassium or sodium	Pfizerpen, Pentids ♣Crystapen	Vials of 0.2, 0.5, 1, 5, and 10 million units Tablets of 1, 2, 2.5, 4, 5, and 800,000 units Suspension of 2, 2.5 and 400,000 units/5 ml	PO: 400,000 to 1.6 million units IM, IV: 600,000 to 30 million units daily
Penicillin V potassium	V-Cillin K, Betapen VK, Pen-Vee-K, Veetids	125, 250, and 500 mg tablets 125 and 250 mg/5 ml suspension	PO: 250-500 mg/6 hr
Piperacillin	Pipracil	2, 3, 4 g vials	IM, IV: 3-4 g every 4-6 hr, not to exceed 24 g/24 hr
Ticarcillin	Ticar	1, 3, and 6 g vials	IM: Do not exceed 2 g/injection site IV: Up to 18 g/24 hr
Combination products			
Amoxicillin and potassium clavulanate	Augmentin, ♣Clavulin	125, 250, and 500 mg tablets 125 and 250 mg/5 ml suspension	PO: 250-500 mg every 8 hr IV: 3.1-3.2 g every 4-6 hr
Ticarcillin and potassium clavulanate	Timentin	3 g ticarcillin/100 mg clavulanate/vial	
Ampicillin and sulbactam sodium	Unasyn	1.5, 3 g bottles and vials	IM, IV: 1.5-3 g every 6 hr

♣Available in Canada only.

sistant to penicillin therapy. These bacteria start producing an enzyme, penicillinase (beta lactamase), which can destroy the antibacterial activity of most bacteria. Penicillinase inactivates the penicillin antibiotics by splitting open the beta-lactam ring of the penicillin molecule. Researchers have developed two mechanisms to prevent this inactivation. The first is to modify the penicillin molecule to "protect" the ring structure while retaining antimicrobial activity. This mechanism culminated in the development of the penicillinase-resistant penicillins (methicillin, nafcillin, oxacillin, cloxacillin, and dicloxacillin). The second method is to add another chemical with similar structure that will more readily bond to the penicillinase enzymes than the penicillin, leaving the free penicillin to inhibit cell wall synthesis. Potassium clavulanate is now added to amoxicillin (Augmentin) and ticarcillin (Timentin) to bond to penicillinases that would normally destroy these antibiotics. Sulbactam has been added to ampicillin (Unasyn) for similar reasons.

The penicillins are used to treat middle ear infections (otitis media), pneumonia, meningitis, urinary tract infections, syphilis, and gonorrhea and as a prophylactic antibiotic prior to surgery or dental procedures for patients with a history of rheumatic fever.

Side effects. The most common side effects of orally administered penicillins are nausea, vomiting, epigastric distress, and diarrhea.

Adverse effects that may develop due to the use of large parenteral doses are: neurologic effects evidenced by hallucinations, hyperreflexia, seizures, and delirium; electrolyte imbalances from sodium or potassium penicillin, ticarcillin, or carbenicillin manifested by cardiac arrhythmias, hyperreflexia, convulsions, and coma; and interstitial nephritis manifested by oliguria, proteinuria, hematuria, casts, azotemia, pyuria, fever and, rarely, a rash. All of these adverse effects are more common in elderly, debilitated patients with impaired renal function.

Availability. See Table 19-4.

• **Nursing Interventions: Monitoring penicillin therapy**

See also General Nursing Considerations for Patients with Infectious Diseases (p. 457).

Side effects to report

DIARRHEA. Penicillins cause diarrhea by altering the bacterial flora of the gastrointestinal tract. The diarrhea is usually not severe enough to warrant discontinuation. Encourage the patient not to discontinue therapy without first consulting the physician. If diarrhea persists, monitor the patient for signs of dehydration.

ABNORMAL LIVER AND RENAL FUNCTION TESTS. Monitor returning laboratory data and report abnormal findings to the physician.

THROMBOPHLEBITIS. Carefully assess patients receiving IV penicillins for the development of thrombophlebitis. Inspect the IV area frequently while providing care; inspect during dressing changes and at times the IV is changed to a new site. Always investigate pain at the IV site. Report redness, warmth, tenderness to touch, and edema in the affected part. If in lower extremities, dorsiflexion of the foot may cause pain in the calf area (Homan's sign). Compare the affected limb with the unaffected limb.

ELECTROLYTE IMBALANCE. The electrolyte content of the antibiotics may cause hyperkalemia or hypernatremia. Most of the penicillins have a high electrolyte content.

Implementation

COMPATIBILITIES. DO NOT mix with other drugs in the same syringe or infuse together with other drugs. See Drug Interactions for incompatibilities.

RATE OF INFUSION. Consult with a pharmacist or see package literature.

Drug interactions

PROBENECID. Patients receiving probenecid in combination with penicillins are more susceptible to toxicity because probenecid inhibits excretion of the penicillins. Monitor closely for adverse effects.

This combination may be used to advantage in the treatment of gonorrhea and other infections where high levels are indicated.

AMPICILLIN AND ALLOPURINOL. When used concurrently, these two agents are associated with a high incidence of rash. Do not label the patient as allergic to penicillins until further skin-testing has verified that there is a true hypersensitivity to penicillins.

ANTACIDS. Excessive use of antacids may diminish the absorption of oral penicillins.

Quinolones
OBJECTIVES

1. Briefly discuss the uses of quinolones and the mechanism of action of these agents.
2. Compare the effectiveness of quinolones with the penicillins, cephalosporins, and aminoglycosides.
3. Describe the effects of antacids on quinolones and the adaptations in scheduling required if both agents are prescribed concurrently.

The quinolone antibiotics are rapidly emerging as an important class of therapeutic agents. This class is not new; the original members—nalidixic acid, oxolinic acid, and cinoxacin—have been available for the treatment of urinary tract infections (see Chapter 15, p. 371) for well over a decade. A new subclass known as the fluoroquinolones is showing great promise as bactericidal agents against a wide range of gram-positive and gram-negative bacteria, including some anaerobes. The fluoroquinolones act by inhibiting the activity of DNA gyrase, an enzyme that is essential for the replication of bacterial DNA. The fluoroquinolones currently available are norfloxacin (Chapter 15, p. 374), ciprofloxacin, and ofloxacin.

ciprofloxacin (sip'roh-floks'ah-sin)

Cipro (sip'roh)

Ciprofloxacin is the first well tolerated, broad-spectrum, oral antibiotic in the quinolone series. It demonstrates rapid bactericidal activity against the bacterial pathogens that cause nosocomial and community-acquired urinary tract infections, most of the strains that cause enteritis, and gonococci, meningococci, *Legionella, Pasturella, Hemophilus influenzae*, methicillin-resistant staphylococci, and some gram-negative bacteria including *Pseudomonas aeruginosa*. The activity of ciprofloxacin against gram-positive and gram-negative cocci is equal to or better than that of the penicillins, cephalosporins, and aminoglycosides, but most anaerobic organisms are resistant.

Side effects. As would be expected with oral administration, the most frequent adverse effects (less than 5%) are nausea, diarrhea, vomiting, and abdominal discomfort. Headache, restlessness, and rash occurred in less than 2% of patients.

Availability

PO—250, 500, 750 mg tablets.
IV—200 and 400 mg vials.

Dosage and administration

Adult

PO—250 to 750 mg every 12 hours.
IV—200 to 400 mg every 12 hours.
Pediatric therapy is not recommended in children due to the potential for causing permanent damage to cartilage.

• Nursing Interventions: Monitoring ciprofloxacin therapy

See also General Nursing Considerations for Patients with Infectious Diseases (p. 457).

Side effects to expect

NAUSEA, VOMITING, DIARRHEA, DISCOMFORT. These side effects are usually mild and tend to resolve with continued therapy. Encourage the patient not to discontinue therapy without first consulting the physician. If the patient should become debilitated, contact the physician.

DIZZINESS, LIGHTHEADEDNESS. Although infrequent, ciprofloxacin may cause these disturbances. They tend to be self-limiting, and therapy should not be discontinued until the patient consults a physician.

Caution the patient against driving or performing hazardous tasks until adjusted to the effects of the medication.

Side effects to report

RASH. Report a rash or pruritis immediately and withhold additional doses pending approval by the physician.

ABNORMAL LABORATORY TESTS. Monitor returning laboratory data and report abnormal findings to the physician.

NEUROLOGIC EFFECTS. Report the development of tinnitus, headache, dizziness, mental depression, drowsiness, or confusion.

Implementation

PO. Ciprofloxacin may be taken with or without meals. The ideal time is 2 hours after a meal. Take with an 8-ounce glass of fluid.

Avoid taking within 2 hours after ingestion of antacids.

IV. Vials must be diluted to 1 to 2 mg/ml prior to administration. Infuse over 60 minutes to minimize pain and venous irritation.

Drug interactions

ANTACIDS. Antacids containing magnesium hydroxide or aluminum hydroxide will decrease the absorption of ciprofloxacin. Administer ciprofloxacin 1 hour before or 2 hours after ingesting antacids.

PROBENECID. Patients receiving probenecid in combination with ciprofloxacin are more susceptible to toxicity because probenecid inhibits excretion of ciprofloxacin. Monitor closely for toxic effects.

The combination may be used to advantage in the treatment of serious or resistant infections where high serum levels of ciprofloxacin are required.

THEOPHYLLINE. Ciprofloxacin, when given with theophylline, may result in theophylline toxicity. Observe for vomiting, dizziness, restlessness, and cardiac arrhythmias. Monitor theophylline serum levels. The dosage of theophylline may have to be reduced.

ofloxacin (oh-floks'ah-sin)

Floxin (floks'sin)

Ofloxacin is a fluoroquinolone antibiotic that has broad spectrum activity against gram-negative, gram-positive, and anaerobic bacteria. It differs from ciprofloxacin by having less activity against *Pseudomonas aeruginosa*, but greater activity against sexually transmitted diseases such as *Neisseria gonorrhoeae, Chlamydia trachomatis*, and genital ureaplasma. Ofloxacin is also less susceptible to drug interactions than other fluoroquinolones. Ofloxacin is used to treat urinary tract infections, prostatitis, skin infections (cellulitis, impetigo), lower respiratory pneumonia, and sexually transmitted diseases other than syphilis.

Side effects. The frequency of adverse effects associated with ofloxacin therapy is 2% to 6%. The most common adverse reactions include gastrointestinal symptoms of nausea, abdominal discomfort, vomiting, and diarrhea. Central nervous system effects are next in frequency and include headache, dizziness, agitation, and sleep disturbance.

Availability

PO—200, 300, and 400 mg tablets.

Dosage and administration

PO—200 to 400 mg every 12 hours. Duration of therapy is dependent upon the type of infection being treated. Acute, uncomplicated gonorrhea can be treated with a single dose, while prostatitis may require 6 weeks of treatment.

Pediatric therapy is not recommended in children due to the potential for causing permanent damage to cartilage.

• Nursing Interventions: Monitoring ofloxacin therapy

See also General Nursing Considerations for Patients with Infectious Diseases (p. 457).

Side effects to expect

NAUSEA, VOMITING, DIARRHEA. These adverse effects are usually mild and tend to resolve with continued therapy. Encourage the patient not to discontinue therapy without first consulting the physician. If the patient should become debilitated, contact the physician.

DIZZINESS. Dizziness tends to be self-limiting, and therapy should not be discontinued until the patient consults a physician. Caution the patient against driving or performing hazardous tasks until adjusted to the effects of the medication.

Side effects to report

RASH. Report a rash or pruritus immediately and withhold additional doses pending approval by the physician.

NEUROLOGIC EFFECTS. Report the development of headache, insomnia, or mental depression.

Implementation

PO. Do not administer ofloxacin with food. Take with an 8-ounce glass of fluid. Maintain adequate hydration.

Avoid taking within 2 hours after ingestion of antacids.

Drug interactions

ANTACIDS. Antacids containing magnesium hydroxide or aluminum hydroxide will decrease the absorption of ofloxacin. Administer ofloxacin 2 hours before or 2 to 4 hours after ingesting antacids.

THEOPHYLLINE. Ofloxacin, when given with theophylline, may result in theophylline toxicity. Observe for vomiting, dizziness, restlessness, and cardiac arrhythmias. Monitor theophylline serum levels. The dosage of theophylline may have to be reduced.

Sulfonamides

OBJECTIVES

1. Cite the method of action of sulfonamides.
2. Identify side effects associated with sulfonamide therapy that require alteration in dosing scheduling and adequate hydration.
3. State the effect of sulfonamide therapy on an individual who is also taking an oral hypoglycemic agent for type II diabetes mellitus.

The sulfonamides are not true antibiotics because they are not synthesized by microorganisms. However, they are highly effective antibacterial agents. Sulfonamides act by inhibiting bacterial biosynthesis of folic acid, which eventually results in bacterial cell death. Human cells do not synthesize folic acid and so are not affected. Sulfonamides are used primarily to treat urinary tract infections and otitis media. They may also be used to prevent streptococcal infection or rheumatic fever in persons who are allergic to penicillin.

Side effects. Due to an increasing frequency of organisms developing a resistance to sulfonamide therapy, and the unreliability of in vitro sulfonamide sensitivity tests, patients should be monitored closely for continued therapeutic response to treatment. This is particularly important in patients being treated for chronic and recurrent urinary tract infections.

Sulfonamides have many side effects, the most common of which are nausea and diarrhea. Rashes may represent more serious underlying disorders and should be reported immediately.

Patients receiving sulfonamides for more than 14 days should have routine red and white cell counts with differential completed periodically.

A false-positive reaction for glucose in the urine may occur with Clinitest tablets, but not with Tes-Tape or Diastix.

Patients should be encouraged to drink water several times daily while receiving sulfonamide therapy. Rarely, crystals form in the urinary tract if the patient becomes too dehydrated.

Availability. See Table 19-5.

• Nursing Interventions: Monitoring sulfonamide therapy

See also General Nursing Considerations for Patients with Infectious Diseases (p. 457).

Side effects to report

NAUSEA, VOMITING, ANOREXIA, DIARRHEA. These side effects are usually mild and tend to resolve with continued therapy. Encourage the patient not to discontinue therapy without first consulting the physician.

If the patient should become debilitated contact the physician.

DERMATOLOGIC REACTIONS. Report a rash of pruritus

Table 19-5 *The Sulfonamides*

GENERIC NAME	BRAND NAME	AVAILABILITY	ADULT DOSAGE RANGE
Sulfacytine	Renoquid	250 mg tablets	PO: Initial dose—500 mg, then 250 mg 4 times daily
Sulfadiazine	Sulfadiazine	500 mg tablets	PO: Initial dose—2-4 g, then 4-8 g/24 hr in divided doses
Sulfamethizole	Thiosulfil Forte	500 mg tablets	PO: 0.5-1 g 3-4 times daily
Sulfamethoxazole	Gantanol, Urobak	500 mg tablets, 500 mg/5 ml suspension	PO: Initial dose—2 g, then 1 g/12 hr
Sulfasalazine	Azulfidine	500 mg tablets, 250 mg/5 ml suspension	PO: Initial therapy—3-4 g daily in divided doses; maintenance dose is 2 g daily
Sulfisoxazole	Gantrisin	500 mg tablets 500 mg/5 ml syrup	PO, IM, IV: Initial dose—2-4 g; maintenance dose is 4-8 g/24 hr divided into 3-6 doses
Triple Sulfas	Triple Sulfa No. 2	Tablets	PO: Initial dose—2-4 g, followed by 2-4 g/24 hr divided into 3-6 hr doses
Co-trimoxazole	Bactrim, Septra	Tablets, suspension, infusion	PO: 2-4 tablets daily, depending on strength, disease being treated IV: 15-20 mg/kg/24 hr (based on trimethoprim) in 3-4 divided doses for up to 14 days
Erythromycin-sulfisoxazole	Pediazole, Eryzole	Suspension	PO: 2.5-10 ml every 6 hr depending on weight of patient

immediately and withhold additional doses pending approval by the physician.

PHOTOSENSITIVITY. The patient should be cautioned to avoid exposure to sunlight and ultraviolet light. Suggest wearing long-sleeved clothing, a hat, and sunglasses when going to be exposed to sunlight. Discourage the use of artificial tanning lamps.

HEMATOLOGIC REACTIONS. Routine laboratory studies (RBC, WBC, and differential counts) are scheduled for patients taking sulfonamides 14 days or longer. Stress returning for this laboratory work.

Monitor for the development of a sore throat, fever, purpura, jaundice or excessive, progressive weakness.

NEUROLOGIC EFFECTS. Report the development of tinnitus, headache, dizziness, mental depression, drowsiness, or confusion.

Implementation

GASTRIC IRRITATION. If gastric irritation occurs, administer with food or milk. If symptoms persist or increase in severity, report for physician's evaluation.

FLUID INTAKE. Adequate intake of 8 to 12 8-ounce glasses of fluid daily is encouraged to prevent crystal formation in the renal tubules. Report the development of hematuria immediately.

Drug interactions

ORAL HYPOGLYCEMIC AGENTS. Sulfonamides may displace sulfonylurea oral hypoglycemic agents (tolbuta-

mide, acetohexamide, tolazamide, chlorpropamide) from protein-binding sites, resulting in hypoglycemia.

Monitor for hypoglycemia, headache, weakness, decreased coordination, general apprehension, diaphoresis, hunger, blurred or double vision.

The dosage of the hypoglycemic agent may need to be reduced. Notify the physician if any of the above symptoms appear.

WARFARIN. This medication may enhance the anticoagulant effects of warfarin. Observe for the development of petechiae, ecchymoses, nosebleeds, bleeding gums, dark tarry stools, and bright red or coffee ground emesis. Monitor the prothrombin time and reduce the dosage of warfarin if necessary.

METHOTREXATE. Sulfonamides may produce methotrexate toxicity when given simultaneously. Monitor patients on concurrent therapy for oral stomatitis and for signs of nephrotoxicity (oliguria, hematuria, proteinuria, casts, etc.).

PHENYTOIN. Sulfisoxazole may displace phenytoin from protein-binding sites, resulting in phenytoin toxicity.

Monitor patients on concurrent therapy for signs of phenytoin toxicity: nystagmus, sedation, lethargy (serum levels may be ordered). A reduced dosage of phenytoin may be required.

Tetracyclines
OBJECTIVES

1. Cite the action of tetracyclines on the bacterial cell.
2. Compare the photosensitivity properties of sulfonamides and tetracyclines.
3. Identify the effect of administering tetracycline during the ages of tooth development and during pregnancy.
4. Describe dosage and administration considerations needed when tetracyclines are prescribed.

The tetracyclines are a class of antibiotics that are effective against both gram-negative and gram-positive bacteria. They act by inhibiting protein synthesis by bacterial cells. The tetracyclines are often used for patients allergic to the penicillins for the treatment of certain venereal diseases, urinary tract infections, upper respiratory tract infections, pneumonia, and meningitis. They are particularly effective against skin (acne), rickettsial, and mycoplasmic infections.

Side effects. The most common side effects of the tetracyclines are gastric upset, loss of appetite, vomiting, and diarrhea. Photosensitivity resulting in an exaggerated sunburn after short exposure has been reported.

Tetracyclines administered during the ages of tooth development (the last half of pregnancy through 8 years of age) may cause enamel hypoplasia and permanent staining of the teeth to a yellow, gray, or brown color. Tetracyclines are secreted in breast milk, so nursing mothers on tetracycline therapy are advised to feed their infants formula or cow's milk, as appropriate.

A false-positive reaction for glucose in the urine may occur between parenteral tetracycline and Clinitest tablets, but not between tetracycline and Tes-Tape or Diastix.

Availability. See Table 19-6.

• Nursing Interventions: Monitoring tetracycline therapy

See also General Nursing Considerations for Patients with Infectious Diseases (p. 457).

Side effects to report

NAUSEA, VOMITING, ANOREXIA, ABDOMINAL CRAMPS, DIARRHEA. These side effects are usually mild and tend to resolve with continued therapy. Encourage the patient not to discontinue therapy without first consulting the physician.

PHOTOSENSITIVITY. The patient should be cautioned to avoid exposure to sunlight and ultraviolet light. Suggest wearing long-sleeved clothing, a hat, and sunglasses when going to be exposed to sunlight. Discourage the use of artificial tanning lamps. Notify the physician for the advisability of discontinuing therapy.

Implementation

PO. Emphasize taking medication 1 hour before or 2 hours after ingesting antacids, milk, or dairy products, or products containing calcium, aluminum, magnesium, or iron (such as vitamins).

Drug interactions

WARFARIN. This medication may enhance the anticoagulant effects of warfarin. Observe for the development of petechiae, ecchymoses, nosebleeds, bleeding gums, dark tarry stools, and bright red or coffee-ground emesis. Monitor the prothrombin time and reduce the dosage of warfarin if necessary.

METHOXYFLURANE. If patients are receiving tetracy-

Table 19-6 *The Tetracyclines*

GENERIC NAME	BRAND NAME	AVAILABILITY	ADULT DOSAGE RANGE
Demeclocycline	Declomycin	150 mg capsules 150 and 300 mg tablets	PO: 150 mg 4 times daily or 300 mg 2 times daily
Doxycycline	Vibramycin, Doxychel	100 and 200 mg vials 50 and 100 mg capsules 25 and 50 mg/5 ml syrup	IV: 100-200 mg 1 or 2 times daily PO: 200 mg on day 1, then 100 mg divided in 2 doses
Methacycline	Rondomycin	150 and 300 mg capsules	PO: 150 mg 4 times daily or 300 mg 2 times daily
Minocycline	Minocin	100 mg vial 50 and 100 mg capsules, tablets 50 mg/5 ml syrup	PO, IV: 200 mg, followed by 100 mg/12 hr
Oxytetracycline	Terramycin, E.P. Mycin, Uri-Tet	50, 125 mg/ml in 2, 10 ml vials 250 mg capsules	IM: 250 mg/24 hr or 100 mg/8 hr IV: 250-500 mg 4 times daily
Tetracycline	Achromycin, Tetralan, Panmycin, Robitet, Sumycin	250, 500 mg vials 100, 250, and 500 mg capsules and tablets 125 mg/5 ml syrup	IM: 250-500 mg/24 hr IV: 250-500 mg/12 hr PO: 250-500 mg 4 times daily

cline and are scheduled for surgery, label the front of the chart "taking tetracycline." Fatal nephrotoxicity has been reported when methoxyflurane is administered to a person taking tetracycline.

IMPAIRED ABSORPTION. Iron, calcium-containing foods (milk and dairy products), calcium, aluminum, or magnesium preparations (antacids), and alkaline products (sodium bicarbonate) will decrease absorption of tetracycline. Administer all tetracycline products 1 hour before or 2 hours after ingesting these foods or products.

Exception: Food or milk does not interfere with the absorption of doxycycline.

PHENYTOIN, CARBAMAZEPINE. These agents reduce the half-life of doxycycline. Monitor patients for lack of clinical improvement from the infection.

TOOTH DEVELOPMENT. Do not administer tetracyclines to pregnant patients or to children under 8 years of age. The infant's or child's tooth enamel may be permanently stained (yellow, gray, or brown).

LACTATION. Nursing mothers need to switch their babies to formula while on tetracyclines, since it is present in the breast milk.

Other antibiotics
OBJECTIVES

1. Cite the effects of aztreonam on pathogens.
2. Describe the current uses of aztreonam.
3. Review the signs and symptoms of phlebitis and nursing actions that can be implemented to prevent it during the administration of intravenous antimicrobial agents.
4. State specific limitations for the use of chloramphenicol.
5. Identify specific nursing assessments needed to detect possible serious hematologic effects from chloramphenicol.
6. Prepare a chart with the following information for each drug in this section: generic name, brand name, mechanism of action, types of microorganisms affected by each agent, side effects to monitor and pertinent information regarding administration, scheduling, and storage of the agents.
7. Describe effective treatment for diarrhea associated with clindamycin therapy.
8. Identify the primary therapeutic use of imipenem/cilastatin.
9. State precautions and specific data that should be sought from the patient before initiating the administration of imipenem/cilastatin.
10. Summarize baseline assessments needed to evaluate a patient's mental status and specific seizure precautions that should be implemented when imipenem/cilastatin therapy is initiated.
11. Identify the specific intravenous recommendations associated with the intravenous infusion of imipenem/cilastatin.
12. State the main uses of metronidazole.
13. Cite specific patient education required to prevent overgrowth of oral and vaginal monilia when metronidazole is prescribed.
14. Identify color alterations in urine that may occur while taking metronidazole.
15. Identify the effectiveness of spectinomycin on gonorrhea and syphilis.
16. Cite specific recommendations for intramuscular administration of spectinomycin.
17. Identify the mechanism of action of vancomycin.
18. State the types of organisms (using gram-staining) that vancomycin may be used to treat.
19. Describe nursing assessments that may be used to detect ototoxicity.
20. Describe the *red man syndrome*.

aztreonam (aze'tree-on-am)

Azactam (aze'ak-tam)

Aztreonam represents the first of a new class of synthetic, bactericidal antibiotics named the monobactams. The monobactams have a high degree of activity against beta-lactamase-producing aerobic gram-negative bacteria, including *Pseudomonas aeruginosa.* Aztreonam has essentially no activity against anaerobes or gram-positive microorganisms. Aztreonam is used to treat urinary tract, lower respiratory tract, skin, intraabdominal, gynecologic, and septicemic infections caused by *Pseudomonas aeruginosa, Neisseria gonorrhoeae* or *meningitidis, Salmonella, Shigella,* and ampicillin-resistant *H. influenzae.* It is recommended that aztreonam be combined with a broad-spectrum antibiotic in the initial treatment of an infection of unknown cause to treat susceptible anaerobes or gram-positive organisms.

Side effects. Adverse effects caused by aztreonam are fairly infrequent. Gastrointestinal disturbances of nausea, vomiting, and diarrhea occur in about 1% of patients. Thrombophlebitis (1.9%) following IV administration and swelling and discomfort (2.4%) following IM administration were reported. Superinfections were reported in 2% to 6% of patients. Patients who are allergic to penicillins or cephalosporins may also be allergic to aztreonam.

Availability

Injection—500 mg, 1 and 2 gm powders in 15 ml and 100 ml bottles for reconstitution.

Dosage and administration

Adult

IM or IV—Urinary tract infections: 0.5 to 1 g every 8 to 12 hours. Moderately severe systemic infections: 1 to 2 g every 8 to 12 hours.

Life-threatening infections: 2 g every 6 to 8 hours.

Dosage adjustment is required in patients with renal impairment.

• **Nursing Interventions: Monitoring aztreonam therapy**

See also General Nursing Considerations for Patients with Infectious Diseases (p. 457).

Side effects to expect

NAUSEA, VOMITING, DIARRHEA. These side effects are usually mild and tend to resolve with continued therapy.

Side effects to report

PHLEBITIS. Avoid IV infusion in the lower extremities or in areas with varicosities. Use proper technique in starting the intravenous solution.

Carefully assess at regularly scheduled intervals for signs of developing phlebitis. Inspect for redness, warmth, tenderness to touch, edema, or pain.

Always assess complaints of pain at the infusion site. If signs of inflammation accompany complaints, discontinue and restart elsewhere.

SUPERINFECTIONS. Oral thrush, genital and anal pruritis, vaginitis, and vaginal discharge may occur. Report promptly, as these infections are resistant to the original antibiotic used. Teach the importance of meticulous oral and perineal personal hygiene measures.

Implementation

IM. Reconstitute a 15 ml vial with at least 3 ml of diluent per gram of aztreonam. After adding diluent to container, shake immediately and vigorously. Inject deeply into the large muscle mass of the gluteus maximus. Discard unused portion of vial.

IV BOLUS. Reconstitute a 15 ml vial with 6 to 10 ml of diluent. Shake immediately and vigorously. Inject directly into a vein or into the tubing of a suitable IV set over 3 to 5 minutes. Discard any unused portion of the vial.

IV INFUSION. Reconstitute the 100 ml bottle with at least 50 ml of diluent. Shake immediately and vigorously. Infuse over the next 30 to 60 minutes.

Drug interactions

CEFOXITIN, IMIPENEM. These antibiotics induce beta-lactamase production in some gram-negative organisms resulting in possible antagonism with a beta-lactam antibiotic such as aztreonam. It is recommended that beta-lactamase antibiotics not be used concurrently with aztreonam.

chloramphenicol (klo-ram-fen′i-kol)

Chloromycetin (klo-ro-my-se′tin)

Chloramphenicol is an antibiotic that acts by inhibiting bacterial protein synthesis of a variety of gram-positive and gram-negative organisms. It is particularly effective in treating rickettsial infections, meningitis, and typhoid fever.

It must not be used in the treatment of trivial infections or when it is not indicated, such as in colds, influenza, throat infections, or as a prophylactic agent to prevent bacterial infection.

Side effects. Serious and possibly fatal bone marrow suppression may occur after therapy is initiated with chloramphenicol. Early signs include sore throat, a feeling of fatigue, elevated temperature, and small petechial hemorrhages and bruises on the skin. If patients describe any of these symptoms, report them to your supervisor immediately.

Chloramphenicol may cause a false-positive urinary glucose reaction when Clinitest is used. Tes-Tape or Diastix may be used instead to test for the presence of glucose.

Gastrointestinal side effects include nausea, vomiting, diarrhea, glossitis, stomatitis, and an unpleasant taste in the mouth.

Availability

PO—250 mg capsules; 150 mg/5 ml suspension.
IV—100 mg/ml in 1 g vials.

Dosage and administration

Adult

PO—50 to 100 mg/kg every 6 hours.
IM—Not recommended due to poor absorption and clinical response.
IV—As for PO administration. Reconstitute by adding 11 mg of sterile water for injection or dextrose 5% to 1 g of chloramphenicol to make a solution containing 100 mg/ml. Administer the calculated dose intravenously over a 1 minute period.

Pediatric

PO—Neonates: 25 mg/kg/24 hours in 4 equally divided doses. Infants over 2 weeks of age: 50 mg/kg/24 hours in 4 equally divided doses.
IM—Not recommended.
IV—As for PO dosages. Administer over 1 minute. Use only chloramphenicol sodium succinate intravenously in children.

• **Nursing Interventions: Monitoring chloramphenicol therapy**

See also General Nursing Considerations for Patients with Infectious Diseases (p. 457).

Side effects to report

HEMATOLOGIC. Routine laboratory studies (RBC, WBC, and differential counts) are scheduled for patients taking chloramphenicol 14 days or longer. Stress returning for this laboratory work.

Monitor for the development of a sore throat, fever, purpura, jaundice or excessive, progressive weakness.

SUPERINFECTIONS. Oral thrush, genital and anal pruritus, vaginitis, and vaginal discharge may occur. Report promptly, as these infections are resistant to the original antibiotic used.

Teach the importance of meticulous oral and perineal personal hygiene.

Drug interactions

WARFARIN. This medication may enhance the anticoagulant effects of warfarin. Observe for the development of petechiae, ecchymoses, nosebleeds, bleeding gums, dark tarry stools, and bright red or coffee-ground emesis. Monitor the prothrombin time and reduce the dosage of warfarin if necessary.

ORAL HYPOGLYCEMIC AGENTS. Monitor for hypoglycemia: headache, weakness, decreased coordination, general apprehension, diaphoresis, hunger, blurred or double vision.

The dosage of the hypoglycemic agent may need to be reduced. Notify the physician if any of the above symptoms appear.

PHENYTOIN. Chloramphenicol inhibits the metabolism of phenytoin.

Monitor patients with concurrent therapy for signs of phenytoin toxicity: nystagmus, sedation, lethargy. Serum levels may be ordered, and the dosage of phenytoin reduced.

clindamycin (klin-dah-my'sin)

Cleocin (klee-o'sin), ✦Dalacin C

Clindamycin is an antibiotic that acts by inhibiting protein synthesis. It is useful against infections caused by gram-negative aerobic organisms as well as a variety of gram-positive and gram-negative anaerobes.

Side effects. Severe diarrhea may develop from the use of clindamycin. If diarrhea of more than five stools per day develops, notify the physician. This may be an indication of drug-induced pseudomembranous colitis. The use of Lomotil, loperamide, or paregoric may prolong or worsen the condition. Large doses of Kaopectate may be effective in diminishing the diarrhea.

Patients may complain of a bitter taste as the medication is secreted in saliva.

Availability

PO—75 and 150 mg capsules, 75 mg/5 ml suspension.

IV—150 mg/ml in 2, 4, and 6 ml ampules.

Dosage and administration

Adult

PO—150 to 450 mg every 6 hours. DO NOT refrigerate the suspension. It is stable at room temperature for 14 days.

IM—600 to 2700 mg/24 hours. DO NOT exceed 600 mg per injection. Pain, induration, and sterile abscesses have been reported. Deep IM injection is recommended to help minimize this reaction.

IV—600 to 2700 mg/24 hours. Dilute to less than 6 mg/ml. Administer at a rate less than 30 mg/minute. Administration by IV push is not recommended.

Pediatric

PO—Suspension: 8 to 25 mg/kg/24 hours in 4 divided doses. Capsules: 8 to 20 mg/kg/24 hours in 4 divided doses. Capsules should be taken with a full glass of water to prevent esophageal irritation.

IM—15 to 40 mg/kg/24 hours in 4 divided doses.

IV—As for IM use. Dilute to less than 6 mg/ml and administer at a rate less than 30 mg/minute.

• **Nursing Interventions: Monitoring clindamycin therapy**

See also General Nursing Considerations for Patients with Infectious Diseases (p. 457).

Side effects to report

DIARRHEA. These side effects are usually mild and tend to resolve with continued therapy. Encourage the patient not to discontinue therapy without first consulting the physician.

SEVERE DIARRHEA. Report diarrhea of five or more stools per day to the physician.

Blood or mucus in the stool should also be reported. *Warn patients not to treat diarrhea themselves when taking this drug.*

Implementation

PO. DO NOT refrigerate the suspension. It is stable at room temperature for 14 days.

IM. Deep IM injection is recommended to help minimize pain, indurations, and possible sterile abscess formation.

IV. It is not recommended that this drug be given by IV push. Dilute to less than 6 mg/ml and administer at a rate less than 30 mg/minute.

Drug interactions

IMPAIRED ABSORPTION. Kaolin-pectin (Kaopectate) absorbs clindamycin. It is effective in stopping diarrhea that may occur with the administration of clindamycin.

NEUROMUSCULAR BLOCKADE. Label charts of patients scheduled for surgery who are taking clindamycin. When combined with surgical muscle relaxants and/or aminoglycosides, neuromuscular blockade may result.

These combinations may potentiate respiratory depression. Check the anesthesia record of surgical patients. Monitor postoperative patients for a prolonged period for respiratory depression. This may occur 48 hours or more after the drug administration.

THEOPHYLLINE TOXICITY. Clindamycin, when given with theophylline, may result in theophylline toxicity. Observe for vomiting, dizziness, restlessness, and cardiac arrhythmias. The dosage of theophylline may need to be reduced.

ERYTHROMYCIN. Therapeutic antagonism has been reported between clindamycin and erythromycin. Do not administer concurrently.

imipenem-cilastatin (imee'pen-ehm si'la-stat'in)

Primaxin (pry-max-in)

Imipenem/cilastatin is a combination product containing a thienamycin antibiotic called imipenem and cilastatin, an inhibitor of the renal dipeptidase enzyme dehydropeptidase I. Cilastatin has no antimicrobial activity but does prevent the inactivation of imipenem by the renal enzyme.

Imipenem is an extremely potent, broad-spectrum antibiotic resistant to beta-lactamase enzymes secreted by bacteria. It acts by inhibition of bacterial cell wall synthesis. It is used in the treatment of lower respiratory tract and intraabdominal infections; infections of the urinary tract, bones and joints, and skin; gynecologic infections; endocarditis; and bacterial septicemia caused by gram-negative or gram-positive organisms. A primary therapeutic role of imipenem/cilastatin will be in the treatment of severe infections due to multiresistant organisms and in mixed anaerobic-aerobic infections, primarily those involving intraabdominal and pelvic sepsis where *Bacteroides fragilis* is a common pathogen. It should be used in combination with antipseudomonal agents due to resistance of *Pseudomonas cepacia* and *P. aeruginosa* to imipenem.

Side effects. Imipenem is classified as a thienamycin derivative that contains a beta-lactam nucleus similar to penicillins and cephalosporins. There have been reports of patients with histories of penicillin allergy who have experienced severe hypersensitivity reactions with other beta-lactams. Before initiating therapy with Primaxin, a careful history should be taken concerning hypersensitivity to any other antibiotics and allergens.

The primary systemic side effects associated with therapy are nausea (2%), diarrhea (1.8%), vomiting (1.5%), rash (0.9%), fever (0.5%), hypotension (0.4%), seizures (0.4%), dizziness (0.3%), pruritus (0.3%), pain (0.7%), erythema at the injection site (0.4%), and vein induration (0.2%).

Seizure activity, including myoclonic activity, focal tremors, confusional states, and other seizures, has been reported with Primaxin. These episodes occurred most frequently in patients with a history of seizure activity.

Availability

IV—250 mg/250 mg and 500 mg/500 mg imipenem/cilastatin powder in 13 ml vials or 120 ml infusion bottles for reconstitution.

IM—500 mg/500 mg and 750 mg/750 mg imipenem/cilastatin powder in vials for reconstitution.

Dosage and administration

Adult

IM, IV—250 mg (imipenem) every 6 hours for mild infections up to 1 g every 6 hours for severe, life-threatening infections. Do not exceed 50 mg/kg/day or 4 g/day, whichever is lower.

Dosage reduction is required in patients with a creatinine clearance rate of less than 70 ml/min/1.73 m².

• **Nursing Interventions: Monitoring imipenem therapy**

See also General Nursing Considerations for Patients with Infectious Diseases (p. 457).

Side effects to expect

NAUSEA, VOMITING, DIARRHEA. These side effects are usually mild and tend to resolve with continued therapy.

Side effects to report

DIZZINESS. Provide for patient safety during episodes of dizziness; report for further evaluation.

CONFUSION, SEIZURES. Perform a baseline assessment of the patient's degree of alertness and orientation to name, place, and time *before* initiating therapy. Make regularly scheduled subsequent mental status evaluations and compare findings. Report development of alterations.

Implement seizure precautions. Make sure the patient continues with anticonvulsant therapy. If seizures develop, provide for patient safety and then record the exact time of seizure onset and duration of each phase, a description of the specific body parts involved, and any progression of the affected parts. Describe the automatic responses seen during the clonic phase: altered, jerky respirations or frothy salivation, dilated pupils and any eye movements, cyanosis, diaphoresis, or incontinence.

PHLEBITIS. Carefully assess patients for the development of thrombophlebitis. Inspect the IV area frequently while providing care; inspect visually during dressing changes and at times the IV is changed to a new site. Report redness, warmth, tenderness to touch, edema in the affected part; if in lower extremities, dorsiflexion of the foot may cause pain in the calf area (Homan's sign). Compare the affected limb with the unaffected limb.

Implementation

HYPERSENSITIVITY. Although this antibiotic is a thienamycin, not a penicillin or cephalosporin, they all contain a beta-lactam nucleus. Cross-hypersensitivity may develop between these classes. Complete a history of hypersensitivity prior to starting therapy. If an allergic reaction to Primaxin occurs, discontinue the infusion. Serious reactions may require epinephrine and other emergency measures.

PREPARATION OF SOLUTION. Reconstitute the 120 mg infusion bottle with 100 ml of diluent and shake until dissolved.

Reconstitute the 13 ml vial with 10 ml of diluent and shake until dissolved. Transfer the contents to a 100 ml infusion solution. DO NOT INFUSE THE SUSPENSION. IT MUST BE DILUTED TO AT LEAST 100 ML. A suggested procedure after reconstitution is to transfer the suspension, and then rinse the 13 ml vial with another 10 ml of diluent and transfer again to the infusion solution. The resulting mixture should be agitated until clear.

RATE. Administer each 250 mg or 500 mg dose over 20 to 30 minutes and each 1 g dose over 60 minutes. If nausea develops, slow the infusion rate.

Drug interactions. Primaxin should not be mixed with or physically added to other antibiotics, but it may be administered concomitantly with other antibiotics such as aminoglycosides.

---

metronidazole (me-trow-nyd'a-zol)

Flagyl (fla'jil)

Metronidazole is a somewhat unusual medication in that it has antibacterial, trichamonicidal, and protozoacidal activity. Its mechanism of action is unknown. It is used to treat trichomoniasis, giardiasis, amebic dysentery, amebic liver abscess, and anaerobic bacterial infections.

Side effects. The most common side effects are nausea, headache, anorexia, and occasionally vomiting, diarrhea, and abdominal cramping. An unpleasant metallic taste is also common. Thrombophlebitis occurs in about 6% of patients receiving parenteral therapy.

The most serious reactions are seizures and peripheral neuropathy. Patients receiving high doses, those with a history of seizure activity, and those with significant hepatic impairment may be at greater risk. Peripheral neuropathy, manifested as numbness of the extremities, has been reported after prolonged therapy. It appears to resolve after discontinuation of therapy, but this may take several weeks.

Overgrowth of oral and vaginal monilia may result in furry tongue, glossitis, vaginal itching and burning, and urethral irritation.

Metronidazole may impart a reddish-brown discoloration to the urine, especially when high doses are used.

Availability

PO—250 and 500 mg tablets.

IV—500 mg/vial.

Dosage and administration

Adult

PO—Trichomoniasis:

1. Males and females—250 mg 3 times daily for 7 days. Sexual partners must be treated concurrently to prevent reinfection.
2. Single doses of 2 g, or 2 doses of 1 g each administered the same day appears to provide adequate treatment for trichomoniasis in both sexes.
   Amebic dysentery: 750 mg 3 times daily for 5 to 10 days.
   Amebic liver abscess: 500 to 750 mg 3 times daily for 5 to 10 days.
   Giardiasis: 250 mg 2 to 3 times daily for 5 to 10 days.

Anaerobic bacterial infections:

1. Start with parenteral therapy initially.
2. The usual *oral* dosage is 7.5 mg/kg every 6 hours. Do not exceed 4 g/24 hours. The usual duration is 7 to 10 days; infections of the bone and joint, lower respiratory tract and endocardium may require longer treatment.

IV—Anaerobic bacterial infections:

1. Loading dose: 15 mg/kg infused over 1 hour.
2. Maintenance dose: 7.5 mg/kg infused over 1 hour every 6 hours. Do not exceed 4 g/24 hours. Convert to oral dosages when clinical condition is stable.
3. Dosage reduction is necessary in patients with hepatic impairment but not renal impairment.

Pediatric

PO—Trichomoniasis: 35 to 50 mg/kg/24 hours in 3 divided doses for 7 days.

Amebiasis: 35 to 50 mg/kg/24 hours in 3 divided doses for 10 days.

Giardiasis: 35 to 50 mg/kg/24 hours in 3 divided doses for 7 days.

• **Nursing Interventions: Monitoring metronidazole therapy**

See also General Nursing Considerations for Patients with Infectious Diseases (p. 457).

Side effects to expect

NAUSEA, VOMITING, ANOREXIA, ABDOMINAL CRAMPS. These side effects are usually mild and tend to resolve with continued therapy. Encourage the patient not to discontinue therapy without first consulting the physician.

Side effects to report

SEIZURES, PERIPHERAL NEUROPATHY. Monitor patients for signs of numbness (paresthesia) in the extremities, report the extent and location. Teach safety measures to the patient experiencing neuropathy. Lack of sensation requires care in testing water temperature before immersing extremities and visual inspection for evidence of skin breakdown.

Assess the patient for development of seizures, nystagmus, muscle twitching, and changes in side effects.

SUPERINFECTIONS. With metronidazole, oral thrush, genital and anal pruritus, vaginitis, and vaginal discharge may occur. Report promptly, because these infections are resistant to the original antibiotic used.

Teach the importance of meticulous oral and perineal personal hygiene.

THROMBOPHLEBITIS. Carefully assess patients receiving IV metronidazole for the development of thrombophlebitis.

Inspect the IV area frequently while providing care; inspect during dressing changes, and when the IV is changed to a new site. Always investigate pain at the IV site. Report redness, warmth, tenderness to touch, and edema in the affected part. If in lower extremities, dorsiflexion of the foot may cause pain in the calf (Homans' sign). Compare the affected limb with the unaffected limb.

Drug interactions

ALCOHOL. Use of alcohol and alcohol-containing preparations, such as over-the-counter cough medications, should be avoided during therapy and up to 48 hours after discontinuation of therapy.

WARFARIN. This medication may enhance the anticoagulant effects of warfarin. Observe for the development of petechiae, ecchymoses, nosebleeds, bleeding gums, dark tarry stools, and bright red or coffee ground emesis. Monitor the prothrombin time and reduce the dosage of warfarin if necessary.

DISULFIRAM. Combined use of disulfiram and metronidazole may result in mental confusion and psychoses. Concurrent therapy is not recommended.

spectinomycin (spek-ti-no-my'sin)

Trobicin (tro'bi-sin)

Spectinomycin is used specifically for the treatment of gonorrhea in both males and females. It has a particular advantage: most bacterial strains of gonorrhea respond to one administration of the recommended dosage. It is not effective in the treatment of syphilis. Serology testing for syphilis should be done prior to initiation of therapy and should be repeated 3 months after spectinomycin therapy. This drug will mask the symptoms of syphilis.

Side effects. Pain at the site of injection is a common side effect. Nausea, chills, urticaria, and fever are other side effects of single-dose therapy.

Availability. 400 mg/ml in 2 and 4 g vials.

Dosage and administration

Adult

IM—A 20-gauge needle is recommended. Injections should be made deep into the upper outer quadrant of the gluteal muscle. The usual dose for both males and females is 2 g. In geographic areas where penicillin-resistant gonorrhea is common, a dose of 4 g is recommended (2 g in each gluteal muscle).

• **Nursing Interventions: Monitoring spectinomycin therapy**

See also General Nursing Considerations for Patients with Infectious Diseases (p. 457).

Implementation

IM. Pain at the injection site is common. Give deeply in a large muscle mass. Devise a plan for rotation of injection sites if more than one injection is administered.

vancomycin (van-ko'my'sin)

Vancocin (van-ko'sin)

Vancomycin is an antibiotic that acts by preventing the synthesis of bacterial cell walls. This site of action is different from the sites sensitive to penicillin and other antibiotics interfering with cell wall synthesis. It is effective only against gram-positive bacteria such as streptococci, staphylococci, *Clostridium difficile*, *Listeria monocytogenes*, and *Corynebacterium* that may cause endocarditis, osteomyelitis, meningitis, pneumonia, or septicemia. It may be used orally against staphylococcal enterocolitis and antibiotic-associated pseudomembranous colitis produced by *C. difficile*. Due to potential adverse effects, vancomycin therapy is reserved for patients with potentially life-threatening infections who cannot be treated with less toxic agents such as the penicillins or cephalosporins.

Side effects. The most prominent and severe adverse effects associated with the use of vancomycin are nephrotoxicity and ototoxicity. These occur with greater frequency and severity in the presence of renal impairment or when large doses are administered. Hearing loss may be preceded by tinnitus and high-tone hearing loss and is often permanent. Elderly patients appear to be particularly susceptible to the ototoxic effects.

Rapid intravenous administration may result in a severe hypotensive episode. These patients develop a *redneck syndrome* or *red man syndrome* characteristic of vancomycin. It is manifested by a sudden and profound hypotension with or without a maculopapular rash over the face, neck, upper chest and extremities. The rash generally resolves within a few hours after termination of the infusion. Rare cases may require the administration of fluids, antihistamines or corticosteroids.

Availability

PO—125 and 250 mg capsules; 1 and 10 g powder for oral solution.

IV—50 mg/ml in 10 ml vial.

Dosage and administration

Adult

PO—500 mg every 6 hours or 1 g every 12 hours. Pseudomembranous colitis produced by *C. difficile*—250 mg to 1 g/day in 3 or 4 divided doses for 7 to 10 days.

IM—Not recommended due to poor absorption and clinical response.

IV—500 mg every 6 hours or 1 g every 12 hours. Dosage must be adjusted for patients with impaired renal function.

Pediatric

PO—Neonates: 10 mg/kg/day in divided doses. Children: 40 mg/kg/day in 4 divided doses; do not exceed 2 g/day.

IM—Not recommended due to poor absorption and clinical response.

IV—Neonates: Initial dose of 15 mg/kg, followed by 10 mg/kg every 12 hours until 1 month of age, then every 8 hours thereafter. Children: 40 mg/kg/day in divided doses.

• **Nursing Interventions: Monitoring vancomycin therapy**

See also General Nursing Considerations for Patients with Infectious Diseases (p. 457).

Side effects to report

OTOTOXICITY. This may initially be manifested by dizziness, tinnitus, and progressive hearing loss. Assess your patients for difficulty in walking unaided and assess their level of hearing daily. Intentionally speak to them softly; note if they are aware that you said anything. Take particular notice of the patient who repeatedly says, "What did you say?" or who starts talking more loudly or progressively increases the volume on the television or radio.

NEPHROTOXICITY. Monitor urinalysis and kidney function tests for abnormal results. Report an increasing BUN and creatinine, decreasing urine output and/or decreasing specific gravity (despite amount of fluid intake), casts or protein in the urine, frank blood or smoky-colored urine, or RBC's in excess of 0-3 on the urinalysis report.

SERUM LEVELS. Serum levels of vancomycin should be routinely ordered to minimize these adverse effects. Notify the physician of any abnormal serum levels reported so that dosage adjustments may be made.

SUPERINFECTIONS. Oral thrush, genital and anal pruritus, vaginitis, and vaginal discharge may occur. Report promptly, as these infections are resistant to the original antibiotic used. Teach the importance of meticulous oral and perineal personal hygiene.

Implementation

RED MAN SYNDROME. This reaction is usually stimulated by too rapid IV administration. Administer the solution diluted to less than 5 mg/ml over at least 60 minutes. Monitor blood pressure during infusion.

PO RECONSTITUTION. Add 115 ml of distilled water to the contents of the 10 g container. Each 6 ml of solution provides approximately 500 mg of vancomycin.

Drug interactions

NEPHROTOXICITY, OTOTOXICITY. Concurrent and sequential use of other ototoxic and/or nephrotoxic agents such as neomycin, streptomycin, kanamycin, gentamicin, viomycin, paromomycin, polymyxin B, colistin, tobramycin, amikacin, cisplatin, furosemide, and bumetanide requires careful monitoring.

Fungal Infections

Fungal infections can generally be divided into two types: superficial (topical) and systemic. The fungi that cause superficial infections do not invade living tissue, but survive on the dead tissue structures of the stratum corneum of the skin, the hair, and the nails. They depend on human-to-human or object-to-human transmission. Predisposing factors include pregnancy, the use of medications such as antibiotics, corticosteroids, and hormones (e.g., oral contraceptives), and illnesses such as diabetes mellitus or those with decreased host immunity (e.g., acquired immunodeficiency syndrome or following radiation or chemotherapy for neoplasms).

Topical antifungal agents
OBJECTIVES

1. Cite the primary disorders for which topical antifungal agents are used.
2. Identify the common methods of transmission of fungal infections.
3. Identify the patients most susceptible to fungal infections.
4. Review the procedures used to administer topical medications to the skin.
5. Review the procedures used to administer intravaginal medications.
6. Review the procedures used to administer oral nystatin and clotrimazole.

The common topical fungal infections caused by several different dermatophytes are: tinea pedis (athlete's foot), tinea cruris (jock itch), tinea corporis (ringworm), and tinea versicolor. *Candida albicans* is the most common cause of oral candidiasis (thrush), cutaneous candidiasis (e.g., diaper rash), and vaginal candidiasis (i.e., moniliasis, "yeast infection"). The topical antifungal agents are listed along with their approved uses in Table 19-7.

Side effects. The topical antifungal agents are generally well tolerated. Some patients have experienced vulvar/vaginal burning, vulvar itching, or discharge, soreness, or swelling from the intravaginal products. Patients applying the topical products rarely report a burning sensation, redness, pain, or the development of a contact dermatitis. Patients receiving larger doses of the oral lozenges have rarely developed nausea, vomiting, and diarrhea. Rarely do the adverse effects of any of these agents require discontinuation of therapy.

Availability. See Table 19-7.

Dosage and administration. See Table 19-7.

• Nursing Interventions: Monitoring topical antifungal therapy

See also General Nursing Considerations for Patients with Infectious Diseases (p. 457).

Side effects to expect and report

IRRITATION. This side effect is usually mild and tends to resolve with continued therapy. Encourage the patient not to discontinue therapy without first consulting the physician.

REDNESS, SWELLING, BLISTERING, OOZING. These signs may be an indication of hypersensitivity. Inform the physician.

Implementation

TOPICAL. Wash hands thoroughly before and immediately after application. Cleanse skin with soap and water and dry thoroughly.

For athlete's foot, the powder is most effective in intertriginous areas and in cases when a dry environment may enhance the therapeutic response. If possible, wear cotton socks (avoid nylon) and change 2 to 3 times daily. Treatments may be required for 6 weeks or more with longstanding infections and in areas of thickened skin.

For jock itch or ringworm, wear well-fitting, ventilated clothing.

For all fungal infections, avoid tight-fitting clothing or occlusive dressings unless otherwise instructed by the physician.

EYE CONTACT. Avoid contact with the eye. Wash eyes immediately if contact should occur.

INTRAVAGINAL. Give the patient the following instructions:

1. Wash the applicator in warm soapy water after each use, so that it does not become a vehicle for reinfection.

Table 19-7 *Topical Antifungal Agents*

GENERIC NAME	BRAND NAME	AVAILABILITY	ADULT USE AND DOSAGE
Butoconazole	Femstat	Vaginal cream: 2%	For vaginal candidiasis: Pregnant patients (2nd and 3rd trimesters only): 1 applicatorful intravaginally at bedtime for 6 days. Nonpregnant patients: 1 applicatorful intravaginally at bedtime for 3 days; may be extended to 6 days, if needed.
Ciclopirox	Loprox	Cream: 1% Lotion: 1%	For ringworm, jock itch, athlete's foot, cutaneous candidiasis, and tinea versicolor: Massage cream or lotion into affected skin twice daily for at least 4 weeks.
Clotrimazole	Gyne-Lotrimin	Vaginal tablets: 100, 500 mg	For vaginal candidiasis: Cream: 1 applicatorful at bedtime for 7-14 nights.
	Mycelex G	Vaginal cream: 1%	Tablets: Insert one 100 mg tablet intravaginally at bedtime for 7 nights or two 100 mg tablets at bedtime for 3 nights; or one 500 mg tablet intravaginally, one time only, at bedtime.
	Mycelex	Cream: 1% Solution: 1%	For ringworm, jock itch, athlete's foot: Apply topically to affected skin morning and evening. Gently rub in.
	Mycelex	Oral lozenges: 10 mg (troches)	For oral candidiasis: Allow 1 lozenge to dissolve slowly in mouth 5 times daily for 14 consecutive days.
Econazole	Spectazole	Cream: 1%	For ringworm, jock itch, athlete's foot, tinea versicolor: Cover affected area once daily. For cutaneous candidiasis: Apply twice daily, morning and evening.
Haloprogin	Halotex	Cream: 1% Solution: 1%	For ringworm, jock itch, athlete's foot, cutaneous candidiasis, and tinea versicolor: Cover affected areas twice daily, morning and evening. Treatment may require 2-4 weeks.
Ketoconazole	Nizoral	Cream: 2%	For ringworm, jock itch, athlete's foot, cutaneous candidiasis, and tinea versicolor: Massage in cream to affected and surrounding tissue once daily. May require 2-4 weeks of treatment. For seborrheic dermatitis: Massage in cream to affected area twice daily for 4 weeks.
		Shampoo: 2%	For dandruff: Moisten hair and scalp with water. Apply shampoo and lather gently for 1 min. Rinse and reapply, leaving lather on scalp for 3 min. Rinse thoroughly and dry hair. Apply shampoo twice weekly for 4 weeks with at least 3 days between shampooing.
Miconazole	Monistat 3	Vaginal suppositories: 200 mg	For vaginal candidiasis: Monistat 3: Insert 1 suppository intravaginally at bedtime for 3 days.
	Monistat 7	Vaginal suppositories: 100 mg Vaginal cream: 2%	Monistat 7: Insert 1 applicatorful or 1 suppository at bedtime for 7 days.
	Micatin	Cream: 2% Powder: 2% Spray: 2%	For ringworm, jock itch, athlete's foot, cutaneous candidiasis, and tinea versicolor: Cover affected areas twice daily, morning and evening. Treatment may require 2-4 weeks.

Continued.

Table 19-7 *Topical Antifungal Agents—cont'd*

GENERIC NAME	BRAND NAME	AVAILABILITY	ADULT USE AND DOSAGE

Naftidine	Naftin	Cream: 1%
		Gel: 1%
			For ringworm, jock itch, athlete's foot:
			  Cream: massage into affected area once daily.
			  Gel: massage into affected area twice daily.

Nystatin	Mycostatin	Vaginal tablets: 100,000 U	For vaginal candidiasis: 1 tablet intravaginally daily for 2 weeks.
	Mycostatin, Nilstat, Nystex	Oral suspension: 100,000 U/ml	For oral candidiasis: 4-6 ml 4 times daily; retain in mouth as long as possible before swallowing.
	Mycostatin, Pastilles	Oral lozenges: 200,000 U (troches)	1-2 tablets 4 or 5 times daily. Do not chew or swallow.
	Mycostatin, Nilstat, Nystex	Cream, ointment, powder	For cutaneous candidiasis: Apply to affected area 2 to 3 times daily.
Oxiconazole nitrate	Oxistat	Cream: 1%	For ringworm, jock itch, athlete's foot: Massage into affected areas once daily at bedtime.
Sulconazole	Exelderm	Cream: 1% Solution: 1%	For ringworm, jock itch, athlete's foot: Massage into affected area twice daily.
Terconazole	Terazol 7	Vaginal cream: 0.4%	For vaginal candidiasis: Insert one applicatorful intravaginally daily at bedtime for 7 consecutive days.
Tioconazole	Vagistat	Vaginal ointment: 6.5%	For vaginal candidiasis: Insert one applicatorful intravaginally daily at bedtime.
Tolnaftate	Tinactin	Cream: 1% Solution: 1% Gel: 1%	For ringworm, jock itch, athlete's foot, cutaneous candidiasis, and tinea versicolor: Cover affected areas twice daily, morning and evening. Treatment may require 2-4 weeks.

2. A pad may be used to protect clothing.
3. Use the number of doses prescribed even if symptoms disappear or menstruation begins.
4. Refrain from sexual intercourse during therapy (or the male should wear a condom to avoid reinfection).
5. Contraception other than a diaphragm or condom should be used when the patient is being treated with the vaginal ointment (i.e., Vagistat). Prolonged contact with petrolatum-based products may cause the diaphragm and condom to deteriorate.

Drug interactions. No clinically significant drug interactions have been reported.

Systemic antifungal agents
OBJECTIVES

1. Cite the primary use of amphotericin B.
2. Describe the systemic side effects seen with intravenous administration of amphotericin B.
3. Identify the monitoring parameters to be used to detect the signs and symptoms of nephrotoxicity.
4. Cite specific dosage and administration characteristics associated with the use of amphotericin B.
5. Describe the effect of light on amphotericin B solution.

6. Identify the drug occasionally added to amphotericin B to prevent venous irritation.
7. Describe the uses of flucytosine.
8. Identify the effects of griseofulvin on a fungal infestation.
9. State laboratory tests needed periodically to monitor for potential renal, hepatic, and hematopoietic function.
10. State the mechanism of action and types of fungal infections for which fluconazole, ketoconazole, and miconazole are used.

KEY WORDS

fungus   proteinuria
oliguria   yeast
thrush

amphotericin B (am-fo-tair'ih-sin)

Fungizone (fun-gi'zone)

Amphotericin B is a fungistatic agent that disrupts the cell membrane of fungal cells, resulting in a loss of cellular contents. Amphotericin B is used primarily for the treatment of systemic fungal infections and meningitis. It can also be used topically for candidal infections.

Side effects. Side effects from topical preparations are usually quite minor. The cream may dry the skin. Both the lotion and the ointment may cause slight irritation, manifested by erythema, pruritus, or a burning sensation. Allergic dermatitis is quite rare.

Systemic side effects from intravenous use include headaches, chills, fever, malaise, muscle and joint pain, cramping, nausea, and vomiting. These adverse effects tend to be dose-related and may be minimized by slow infusion, reduction of dosage, and alternate-day administration. Antipyretics, antihistamines, and antiemetics may provide some symptomatic relief from the side effects.

Renal damage is a potential toxic effect of systemic amphotericin B therapy. Nephrotoxicity may be manifested by increases in excretion of uric acid, potassium, and magnesium, oliguria, granular casts in the urine, proteinuria, and increased BUN and serum creatinine levels. Report input and output, as well as a progressive decrease in daily urine volume or changes in visual characteristics.

Availability

Topical—3% cream, lotion, ointment.
IV—50 mg per vial.

Dosage and administration

Adult

Topical—Apply liberally to candidal lesions 2 to 4 times daily. Any staining from cream or lotion preparations may be removed by soap and warm water, and any staining from amphotericin ointment may be removed by standard cleaning fluids.

IV—Initially 250 μg/kg over 6 hours. The daily dose is gradually increased as the patient develops tolerance. Dosage may range between 1 and 1.5 mg/kg on alternate days.

- Venous irritation may be diminished by the addition of 1200 to 1600 units of heparin and/or 10 to 15 mg of hydrocortisone or methylprednisolone to the infusion solution.
- Amphotericin B must be reconstituted with sterile water for injection without bacteriostatic agent.
- DO NOT use an in-line filter during infusion.
- The infusion must be protected from light during administration.
- The recommended infusion concentration is 1 mg/10 ml of dextrose 5% in water.

- **Nursing Interventions: Monitoring amphotericin therapy**

See also General Nursing Considerations for Patients with Infectious Diseases (p. 457).

Side effects to expect

TOPICAL OINTMENTS/LOTIONS. Slight irritation may occur, causing erythema, pruritus, or burning sensations. If symptoms become severe, report for further evaluation by the physician.

Side effects to report

NEPHROTOXICITY. Monitor urinalysis and kidney function tests for abnormal results. Report an increasing

BUN and creatinine, decreasing urine output or decreasing specific gravity (despite amount of fluid intake), casts or protein in the urine, frank blood or smoky-colored urine, or RBCs in excess of 0-3 on the urinalysis report.

ELECTROLYTE IMBALANCE. The electrolytes most commonly altered are potassium (K^+) and magnesium (Mg^{++}). *Hypokalemia* is most likely to occur.

Many symptoms associated with altered fluid and electrolyte balance are subtle and resemble general symptoms of drug toxicity or the disease process itself.

Gather data relative to *changes* in the patient's mental status (alertness, orientation, confusion), muscle strength, muscle cramps, tremors, nausea, and general appearance (drowsy, anxious, lethargic).

Always check the electrolyte reports for early indications of electrolyte imbalance.

Keep accurate records of I/O, daily weights, and vital signs.

MALAISE, FEVER, CHILLS, HEADACHE, NAUSEA, VOMITING. Check p.r.n. and standing orders for drugs (antihistamines, aspirin, antiemetics) that may alleviate these symptoms.

THROMBOPHLEBITIS. Carefully assess patients receiving IV amphotericin B for the development of thrombophlebitis.

Inspect the IV area frequently while providing care; inspect during dressing changes and when the IV is changed to a new site. Always investigate pain at the IV site. Report redness, warmth, tenderness to touch, and edema in the affected part. If in lower extremities, dorsiflexion of the foot may cause pain in the calf (Homan's sign). Compare the affected limb with the unaffected one.

Implementation

STAINING. Staining on clothing caused by creams or lotion may be removed by soap and water; ointment stains require use of standard cleaning fluids.

IV. See above for reconstitution instructions.

FILTERS. DO NOT use an in-line filter during administration.

LIGHT PROTECTION. Cover the solution to protect it from light during administration.

ADDITIVES. Check for specific orders regarding the addition of heparin, hydrocortisone, or methylprednisone to diminish venous irritation.

RATE. Administer over 6 hours unless specifically ordered otherwise. Maintain close observation for thrombophlebitis.

Drug interactions

CORTICOSTEROIDS (PREDNISONE, OTHERS). Corticosteroids may enhance the loss of potassium. Check potassium levels and monitor more closely for hypokalemia when these two agents are used concurrently.

NEPHROTOXIC POTENTIAL. Combining amphotericin B with other nephrotoxic agents such as aminoglycosides or diuretics should be done with extreme caution. Monitor closely for signs of nephrotoxicity.

fluconazole (flu-kon'azol)

Diflucan (dye-flu-can')

Fluconazole is an antifungal agent chemically related to ketoconazole and miconazole. It acts by inhibiting certain metabolic pathways in fungi that interfere with cell wall synthesis. Fluconazole is approved for oral and IV treatment of cryptococcal meningitis and candidiasis. It is the only antifungal agent currently available that is effective against central nervous system fungal infections.

Side effects. Fluconazole is well tolerated by patients. The most frequently reported adverse effects include nausea, headache, rash, vomiting, abdominal pain, and diarrhea. Hepatotoxicity has been reported rarely.

Availability. 50, 100, and 200 mg tablets; 200 and 400 mg vials.

Dosage and administration
PO—100 to 400 mg daily. Dosage must be individualized to type of infection being treated.
IV—As for PO.

- **Nursing Interventions: Monitoring fluconazole therapy**

See also General Nursing Considerations for Patients with Infectious Diseases (p. 457).

Side effects to expect

NAUSEA, VOMITING, DIARRHEA. These side effects are usually mild and tend to resolve with continued therapy. Encourage the patient not to discontinue therapy without first consulting the physician.

Side effects to report

RASH. Report symptoms for further evaluation by the physician. Do not administer any further doses until so ordered by the physician.

HEPATOTOXICITY. The symptoms of hepatotoxicity are anorexia, nausea, vomiting, jaundice, hepatomegaly, splenomegaly, and abnormal liver function tests (elevated bilirubin, AST, ALT, GGT, alkaline phosphatase, prothrombin time).

Drug interactions

CIMETIDINE. Cimetidine inhibits the absorption of fluconazole. Concurrent use is not recommended.

DIURETICS. Diuretics inhibit the excretion of fluconazole. Monitor patients for an increase in frequency of side effects. The dosage of fluconazole may need to be diminished if concurrent therapy with diuretics is required.

TOXICITY INDUCED BY FLUCONAZOLE. Fluconazole can increase serum concentrations of cyclosporine, phenytoin, and oral sulfonylurea hypoglycemic agents (tolbutamide, glipizide, glyburide). Fluconazole can also potentiate the anticoagulant effects of warfarin. Read in-

dividual monographs for monitoring parameters of toxicity from these agents.

flucytosine (flu-sy'toe-seen)

Ancobon (On-ko-bon'), Ancotil (ahn-co'til)

Flucytosine is an antifungal agent. Its mechanism of action is unknown, but it is effective against susceptible candidal septicemia, endocarditis, urinary tract infections, cryptococcal meningitis, and pulmonary infections.

Side effects. Nausea, vomiting, diarrhea, rash, anemia, leukopenia, thrombocytopenia, and elevation of hepatic enzymes, BUN, and creatinine have been reported. Other side effects include hallucinations, confusion, headache, sedation, and vertigo.

Availability
PO—250 and 500 mg capsules.

Dosage and administration

Adult
PO—50 to 150 mg/kg/day divided into doses every 6 hours. Doses up to 250 mg/kg/day may be required in cryptococcal meningitis.

- Nausea may be reduced if the capsules are given a few at a time over 20 to 30 minutes.

- **Nursing Interventions: Monitoring flucytosine therapy**

See also General Nursing Considerations for Patients with Infectious Diseases (p. 457).

Side effects to expect

NAUSEA, VOMITING, DIARRHEA. These side effects are usually mild and tend to resolve with continued therapy. Encourage the patient not to discontinue therapy without first consulting the physician.

Side effects may be reduced by administering a few capsules at a time over 30 minutes.

Side effects to report

HEMATOLOGIC, RASH. Monitor for the development of sore throat, fever, purpura, jaundice, or excessive, progressive weakness.

NEPHROTOXICITY. Monitor urinalysis and kidney function tests for abnormal results. Report an increasing BUN and creatinine, decreasing urine output or decreasing specific gravity (despite amount of fluid intake), casts or protein in the urine, frank blood or smoky-colored urine, or RBCs in excess of 0-3 on the urinalysis report.

HEPATOTOXICITY. The symptoms of hepatotoxicity are anorexia, nausea, vomiting, jaundice, hepatomegaly, splenomegaly, and abnormal liver function tests (elevated bilirubin, AST, ALT, GGT, alkaline phosphatase, prothrombin time).

Drug interactions

AMPHOTERICIN B. Flucytosine and amphotericin B display enhanced activity when used concurrently.

griseofulvin (griz-ee-o-ful'vin)

Fulvicin (ful'vi-sin), Grifulvin (gri-ful'vin)

Griseofulvin is a fungistatic agent used to treat ringworm of the scalp, body, nails, and feet. After griseofulvin is absorbed, it is incorporated into the keratin of the nails, skin, and hair in therapeutic amounts. The infecting fungus is not killed, but its growth into new cells is prevented. Once the cells are shed or removed, they are replaced by new cells free from the infection. Due to the slow growth of nails, treatment often requires several months.

Side effects. Hypersensitivity reactions, manifested as skin rashes and urticaria, are relatively common adverse effects of griseofulvin. Other side effects include photosensitivity, oral thrush, nausea, vomiting, diarrhea, dizziness, and confusion.

During prolonged therapy, periodic laboratory tests should be completed to warn of changes in renal, hepatic, and hematopoietic function.

Availability

PO—125, 165, 250, 330, and 500 mg tablets and capsules; 125 mg/5 ml oral suspension.

Dosage and administration

Adult

PO—Depending on the specific organism and the location of the infection, 500 mg to 4 g in single or divided doses daily.

- Absorption from the gastrointestinal tract may be increased by administering with a meal high in fat content.

- **Nursing Interventions: Monitoring griseofulvin therapy**

See also General Nursing Considerations for Patients with Infectious Diseases (p. 457).

Side effects to expect

NAUSEA, VOMITING, ANOREXIA, ABDOMINAL CRAMPS. These side effects are usually mild and tend to resolve with continued therapy. Encourage the patient not to discontinue therapy without first consulting the physician.

Side effects to report

URTICARIA, RASH, PRURITUS. Report symptoms for further evaluation by the physician.

Pruritus may be relieved by adding baking soda to the bath water.

CONFUSION. Perform a baseline assessment of the patient's degree of alertness and orientation to name, place, and time *before* initiating therapy. Make regularly scheduled subsequent mental status evaluations and compare findings. Report development of alterations.

DIZZINESS. Provide for patient safety during episodes of dizziness; report for further evaluation.

SUPERINFECTIONS. With griseofulvin, oral thrush, genital and anal pruritus, vaginitis, and vaginal discharge may occur. Report promptly as these infections are resistant to the original antibiotic used.

Teach the importance of meticulous oral and perineal personal hygiene.

PHOTOSENSITIVITY. The patient should be cautioned to avoid exposure to sunlight and ultraviolet light. Suggest wearing long-sleeved clothing, hat, and sunglasses when exposed to sunlight. Discourage the use of artificial tanning lamps. Notify the physician for the advisability of discontinuing therapy.

HEMATOLOGIC. Routine laboratory studies (RBC, WBC, and differential counts) are scheduled for patients taking griseofulvin 30 days or longer. Stress the importance of returning for this laboratory work.

Monitor for the development of a sore throat, fever, purpura, jaundice, or excessive, progressive weakness.

NEPHROTOXICITY. Monitor urinalysis and kidney function tests for abnormal results. Report an increasing BUN and creatinine, decreasing urine output or decreasing specific gravity (despite amount of fluid intake), casts or protein in the urine, frank blood or smoky-colored urine, or RBCs in excess of 0-3 on the urinalysis report.

HEPATOTOXICITY. The symptoms of hepatotoxicity are anorexia, nausea, vomiting, jaundice, hepatomegaly, splenomegaly, and abnormal liver function tests (elevated bilirubin, AST, ALT, GTT, alkaline phosphatase, prothrombin time).

Implementation

PO. Administer with meals high in fat content to increase drug absorption. Stress that the drug may need to be given over a prolonged period to control the infection effectively.

Drug interactions

WARFARIN. This medication may diminish the anticoagulant effects of warfarin. Monitor the prothrombin time and increase the dosage of warfarin if necessary.

BARBITURATES. The absorption of griseofulvin is impaired by combining it with barbiturates. If concurrent therapy cannot be avoided, administer the griseofulvin in divided doses 3 times daily.

ketoconazole (key-toe-kon'a-zol)

Nizoral (nis-o-ral')

Ketoconazole is an antifungal agent chemically related to miconazole. Both act by interfering with cell wall synthesis, causing leakage of cellular contents. Ketoconazole is used orally to treat candidiasis, chronic mucocutaneous candidiasis, oral thrush, candiduria, coccidioidomycosis, histoplasmosis, chromomycosis, and paracoccidioidomycosis.

Side effects. Side effects are usually quite mild and resolve during continued therapy. Nausea and vomiting (3%) are usually controlled by administration just before or with a meal. Other side effects are pruritus (1.5%), abdominal pain (1.2%), rash, dizziness, constipation, diarrhea, fever, chills, and headache.

Gynecomastia has been reported in men but tends to resolve during continued therapy.

Ketoconazole therapy has been associated with hepatotoxicity. Liver function tests are recommended before initiating therapy and biweekly to monthly thereafter. Transient minor elevations in liver enzymes may occur during treatment; treatment should be discontinued if these elevations persist.

Availability
PO—200 mg tablets; suspension: 100 mg/5ml.

Dosage and administration
Adults

PO—200 to 400 mg once daily. Absorption is improved when administered with food.

Pediatrics

PO—44 pounds or less: 50 mg once daily. 44 to 88 pounds: 100 mg once daily. More than 88 pounds: 200 mg once daily.

- **Nursing Interventions: Monitoring ketoconazole therapy**

See also General Nursing Considerations for Patients with Infectious Diseases (p. 457).

Side effects to expect

NAUSEA, VOMITING. These side effects are usually mild and tend to resolve with continued therapy. Encourage the patient not to discontinue therapy without first consulting the physician.

Administer with food or milk to reduce irritation.

Side effects to report

HEPATOTOXICITY. Liver function tests are recommended before initiating therapy, with follow-up tests biweekly to monthly.

The symptoms of hepatotoxicity are anorexia, nausea, vomiting, jaundice, hepatomegaly, splenomegaly, and abnormal liver function tests (elevated bilirubin, AST, ALT, GGT, alkaline phosphatase, prothrombin time).

PRURITUS, RASH. Report symptoms for further evaluation by the physician. Pruritus may be relieved by adding baking soda to the bath water.

Implementation

PO. Administer with food to improve absorption.

Administer at least 2 hours before giving drugs that reduce stomach acidity.

Drug interactions

CIMETIDINE, DICYCLOMINE, ANTACIDS. Anticholinergic agents (dicyclomine, Donnatal, propantheline), antacids, and cimetidine diminish stomach acidity and decrease absorption of ketoconazole. Administer ketoconazole at least 2 hours before these medications.

miconazole (my-kon-a-zol')

Monistat (mon-i'stat), Micatin (my-ka'tin)

Miconazole is an antifungal agent chemically related to ketoconazole. Both act by interfering with cell wall synthesis, causing cellular contents to leak. Parenteral miconazole is used to treat candidiasis, chronic mucocutaneous candidiasis, oral thrush, candiduria, coccidioidomycosis, histoplasmosis, chromomycosis, and paracoccidioidomycosis. Bladder irrigations may be used for fungal cystitis, and intrathecal injections may be used to treat fungal meningitis.

Side effects. Adverse effects associated with parenteral therapy include phlebitis (29%), pruritus (21%), nausea (18%), fever and chills (10%), rash (9%), and emesis (7%). Thrombocytopenia and transient drops in hematocrit and serum sodium values have also been reported. The incidence of nausea and vomiting can be reduced with the use of antihistaminic or antiemetic drugs given before infusion; or by reducing the dose, slowing the rate of infusion, and avoiding administration after mealtime.

Availability. IV—10 mg/ml in 20 ml ampules.

Dosage and administration
Adult

IV—Coccidioidomycosis: 1800 to 3600 mg divided into 3 doses daily.
Cryptococcosis: 1200 to 2400 mg divided into 3 doses daily.
Candidiasis: 600 to 1800 mg divided into 3 doses daily.
Paracoccidioidomycosis: 200 to 1200 mg divided into 3 doses daily.

- Dilute all infusion solutions with at least 200 ml of 0.9% sodium chloride or dextrose 5% and administer over a period of 30 to 60 minutes.

Intrathecal—20 mg every 3 to 7 days as an adjunct to intravenous treatment of fungal meningitis. Administer undiluted by alternating lumbar, cervical, and cisternal punctures.
Bladder instillation—Instill 200 mg of miconazole in a diluted solution into the bladder. Frequency of administration is determined by the infecting microorganism.

- **Nursing Interventions: Monitoring miconazole therapy**

See also General Nursing Considerations for Patients with Infectious Diseases (p. 457).

Side effects to report with parenteral therapy

PHLEBITIS. Avoid IV infusion in the lower extremities and areas with varicosities. Use proper technique in starting the IV solution.

Always assess complaints of pain at the infusion site. If signs of inflammation accompany complaints, discontinue and restart elsewhere.

PRURITUS, RASH, FEVER, CHILLS. Report symptoms for further evaluation by the physician.

Pruritus may be relieved by adding baking soda to the bath water.

NAUSEA, VOMITING, EMESIS. Nausea and vomiting can be reduced by:

- Use of antihistamines or antiemetic agents before infusion

- Reducing doses
- Slowing rate
- Avoiding administration after meals

THROMBOCYTOPENIA. Assess for signs of bleeding: petechiae, ecchymoses, nosebleeds, bleeding gums, dark tarry stools, bright red or coffe ground emesis.

Implementation

IV. Dilute all infusion solutions with a minimum of 200 ml of 0.9% sodium chloride or dextrose 5% and administer over a period of 30 to 60 minutes.

Give antihistamines or antiemetics before infusion; slow the rate of miconazale administration should nausea and vomiting develop.

BLADDER INSTILLATION. Using aseptic technique, catheterize and infuse via an indwelling catheter. Clamp catheter for a specified period; open and drain, as ordered.

Drug interactions

WARFARIN. Parenteral miconazole may enhance the anticoagulant effects of warfarin. Observe for the development of petechiae, ecchymoses, nosebleeds, bleeding gums, dark tarry stools, and bright red or coffee ground emesis. Monitor the prothrombin time, and reduce the dosage of warfarin if necessary.

TUBERCULOSIS

OBJECTIVES

1. Identify the causative organism and mode of transmission of tuberculosis.
2. Describe factors that need consideration to enhance a patient's response during tuberculosis therapy.
3. Develop measurable short- and long-term objectives for patient education for persons receiving antitubercular agents.
4. Compare the mechanism of action of ethambutol, isoniazid, and rifampin.
5. Identify the effect of rifampin on body secretions (such as urine, feces, saliva, sputum).

KEY WORDS

tubercle   hepatitis

Tuberculosis is an infectious disease caused by the bacteria *Mycobacterium tuberculosis*. This microorganism thrives in tissues with a relatively high oxygen content, so the infection is most commonly found in the lungs, kidneys, growing ends of bones, and the cerebral cortex. The organism is spread by airborne droplets from the cough or sneeze of a patient with pulmonary tuberculosis. It is not transmitted on objects such as dishes, clothing, or bedding. Family household contacts and those in institutions (hospitals, nursing homes, prisons) sharing an enclosed environment with a source case are at a major risk for infection.

Due to the long-term courses of therapy required to control tuberculosis, affected individuals must be given particular encouragement to adhere to the treatment plan. The biggest nursing challenge in the treatment of tuberculosis is to educate sufficiently the patient to the need for prolonged drug therapy that may last up to 2 years.

General Nursing Considerations for Patients with Tuberculosis

See also General Nursing Considerations for Patients with Infectious Diseases (p. 457).

Patient Concerns: Nursing Intervention/Rationale

Prevention. The nurse needs to instruct the patient diagnosed with tuberculosis to:

1. Cover nose and mouth thoroughly when coughing or sneezing.
2. Wear a mask when exposed to others until the TB bacillus has been effectively eliminated, or the airborne secretions are no longer contagious, as confirmed by sputum culture. Stress that TB is not communicable after approximately 2 to 3 weeks of continuous drug therapy. Drug therapy is usually continued for 6 months and may be necessary for 1 to 2 years before the disease is cured. After this, it is important for the patient to continue to have periodic testing for a recurrence of the disease.
3. Stress frequent handwashing and proper disposal of tissues in contact with sputum.
4. Proper nutrition and adequate rest are important. Pacing of activities until stamina returns will alleviate periods of exhaustion.

Symptoms. Tuberculosis has a slow, insidious onset; therefore, the individual frequently presents with general complaints of chronic fatigue, anorexia, weight loss, and a low-grade fever that may or may not be accompanied by night sweats. A cough persists with mucopurulent secretions that may be blood streaked.

Diagnosis. Tuberculin skin testing and chest x-rays are done to screen for exposure to tuberculosis. Sputum culture(s) are collected to confirm the presence of M. *tuberculosis*.

Treatment. A combination of drugs is prescribed to treat tuberculosis. Multiple drug therapy is used initially to prevent the development of a drug-resistant bacillus.

Patient Education Associated with Antitubercular Therapy

Communication and responsibility. Encourage open communication concerning frustrations and anger as the patient attempts to adjust to the diagnosis and need for prolonged treatment. The patient must be guided to gain insight into the condition in order to assume responsibility for the continuation of treatment. Keep emphasizing those factors the patient can control to alter the disease process, including maintenance of general health, nutritional needs, adequate rest and appropriate exercise, and continuation of prescribed medication therapy.

Personal hygiene. The patient must be taught to prevent the spread of infection to others by thorough handwashing and by covering the nose and mouth when sneezing or coughing.

The patient should also avoid other people with infections, children, and immunosuppressed or debilitated people.

Nutritional status. Tuberculosis frequently occurs in patients with poor nutritional status. These individuals require a complete evaluation of their nutritional status, correction of deficiencies, and education about how to maintain a balanced diet. An increase in protein, iron, and vitamin C is to be encouraged. Since nausea frequently occurs with the administration of some of the antitubercular drugs, it may be necessary to administer the daily dose at bedtime to alleviate nausea.

Stress. Any person is going to be devastated by the news that he or she has an illness that prevents family socialization and employment, potentially for several months.

Encourage the patient to express feelings about this chronic illness. The adjustment to this situation involves working through great personal fears, frustrations, hostilities, and resentments associated with the loss of control within one's life.

Stress-producing factors within the family setting should be discussed and the individual should be allowed time to vent feelings in a nonthreatening, nonjudgmental atmosphere.

Professional psychological support and assistance from a social worker may be particularly appropriate.

Expectations of therapy. Discuss expectations of therapy with the patient (such as the time he or she will be unable to return to work, length of medication regimen, return to activities of daily living).

Changes in expectations. Assess changes in expectations as therapy progresses and the patient gains understanding and skill in the management of the diagnosis.

Changes in therapy through cooperative goal setting. Work with the patient to encourage adherence to the prescribed treatment. When the patient feels that a change should be made in a treatment plan, encourage discussion first with the physician.

Written record. Enlist the patient's aid in developing and maintaining a written record of the monitoring parameters (such as weekly weights, amount and color of sputum, temperature, frequency of coughing, night sweats, tolerance to daily activities) and response to prescribed therapies for discussion with the physician (Figure 19-1). Patients should be encouraged to bring this record on follow-up visits.

Fostering compliance. Throughout the patient's hospitalization, discuss medication information and how it will benefit the course of treatment. Seek cooperation and understanding of the following points, so that medication compliance may be enhanced:

1. Name
2. Dosage
3. Route and administration times: give daily medications in one dose, usually on arising
4. Anticipated therapeutic response
5. Side effects to expect
6. Side effects to report
7. What to do if a dose is missed
8. When, how, or if to refill the medication prescription

Difficulty in comprehension. If it is evident that the patient and/or family does not understand all aspects of continuing therapy being prescribed (such as administration and monitoring of medications, exercises, diets, follow-up appointments), consider the use of social service or visiting nurse agencies. As this disease requires long-term therapy, it is not uncommon for these agencies to assume the responsibility for administering medications to noncompliant patients. If this approach is not successful, and the patient is still considered to be contagious, the person may require institutionalization.

Associated teaching. Give patients the following instructions:

Always inform the physician or dentist of any prescription or over-the-counter medication being taken. Over-the-counter medications should not be taken without first discussing them with a physician or pharmacist.

Always report side effects of rash, itching, or hives immediately. Nausea, vomiting, or diarrhea should also be reported for the physician's evaluation if it is a new symptom.

Take all of the medication as prescribed for the full course of treatment. Do not discontinue use when feeling improved; do not save for future use; do not give your medicine to another individual. Sudden discontinuation of certain medications may produce harmful effects.

Keep all medications out of reach of children.

If pregnancy is suspected, consult an obstetrician as soon as possible about continuation of medication therapy.

At discharge. Items to be sent home with the patient should include the following:

1. Written instructions for use
2. Labels in a level of language and size of print appropriate for the patient
3. If needed, identification cards or bracelets
4. A list of additional supplies to be purchased after discharge (such as syringes)
5. A schedule for follow-up appointments

Drug Therapy for Tuberculosis

ethambutol (e-tham'bu-tol)

Myambutol (my-am'bu-tol)

Ethambutol inhibits tuberculosis bacterial growth by altering cellular RNA synthesis and phosphate metabolism. Ethambutol must be used in combination with other antitubercular agents to prevent the development of resistant organisms.

Side effects. General side effects that may occur with ethambutol therapy include dermatitis, pruritus, anorexia, nausea, vomiting, headache, dizziness, mental confusion, disorientation, and hallucinations.

Some patients receiving ethambutol develop blurred vision and green color blindness. These adverse effects disappear within a few weeks after therapy is discontinued.

Availability

PO—100 and 400 mg tablets.

Dosage and administration

Adults

PO—Initial treatment: 15 mg/kg administered as a single dose every 24 hours.

Retreatment: 25 mg/kg as a single daily dose. After 60 days, reduce the dose to 15 mg/kg, and administer as a single dose every 24 hours.

• Nursing Interventions: Monitoring ethambutol therapy

See also General Nursing Considerations for Patients with Infectious Diseases (p. 457) and Patients with Tuberculosis (p. 485).

Side effects to expect

NAUSEA, VOMITING, ANOREXIA, ABDOMINAL CRAMPS. These side effects are usually mild and tend to resolve with continued therapy. Encourage the patient not to discontinue therapy without first consulting the physician.

Administer daily dose with food to minimize nausea and vomiting.

Side effects to report

CONFUSION, HALLUCINATIONS. Perform a baseline assessment of the patient's degree of alertness and orientation to name, place and time *before* initiating therapy. Make regularly scheduled subsequent mental status evaluations and compare findings. Report development of alterations. Provide for patient safety during episodes of altered behavior or periods of dizziness.

BLURRED VISION, RED-GREEN COLOR CHANGES. Check for any visual alterations using a color vision chart before initiating therapy. Schedule subsequent evaluations on a regular basis. Report the development of visual disturbances for the physician's evaluation.

Implementation

PO. Administer once daily with food or milk to minimize gastric irritation.

The patient should be warned that omission or interrupted intake may result in drug resistance, reversal of clinical improvement, and increased susceptibility of family members and others to tuberculosis.

Drug interactions. No clinically significant interactions have been reported.

isoniazid (i-so-ny'ah-zid)

INH, Hyzyd (hy'zid), **Nydrazid** (ny'dra-zid), ✦**Rimifon** (rhim-ih-fon')

Isoniazid is used for the treatment of tuberculosis, but its mechanism of action is not known. It should be used in combination with other antitubercular agents for therapy of active disease.

Side effects. Tingling and numbness of the hands and feet, nausea, vomiting, dizziness, and ataxia are relatively common side effects of isoniazid and are dose-related. Pyridoxine, 25 to 50 mg daily, is often recommended to reduce the incidence of these side effects.

Isoniazid may produce a false-positive reaction for urinary glucose with Clinitest tablets, but not with Tes-Tape or Diastix.

The incidence of hepatotoxicity increases with age. This reaction usually occurs within the first 3 months of therapy and is thought to be an allergic reaction. Early symptoms include fatigue, weakness, anorexia, and malaise.

Availability

PO—50, 100, and 300 mg tablets; 50 mg/ml syrup.

IM—100 mg/ml in 10 ml vials.

Dosage and administration

Adult

PO—Treatment of active tuberculosis: 5 mg/kg to a maximum of 300 mg daily. Isoniazid should be used in conjunction with other effective antitubercular agents. Prophylactic therapy: 300 mg daily in single or divided doses.

Concurrent administration of pyridoxine: 25 to 50 mg daily, recommended for prevention of peripheral neuropathies.

IM—As for PO administration.

Pediatric

PO—10 to 30 mg/kg/24 hours in single or divided doses. Infants and children tolerate larger doses than adults. Maximum dose is 500 mg daily.

• Nursing Interventions: Monitoring isoniazid therapy

See also General Nursing Considerations for Patients with Infectious Diseases (p. 457) and Patients with Tuberculosis (p. 485).

Side effects to expect and report

TINGLING, NUMBNESS. Concurrent use of pyridoxine will usually prevent the development of these common symptoms associated with this agent.

When paresthesias are present, the patient must be cautioned to inspect the extremities for any possible skin breakdown because of the diminished sensation.

Also caution patients not to immerse feet or hands in water without first testing the temperature.

Monitor patients with paresthesias for adequate nutrition.

DIZZINESS, ATAXIA. Provide for patient safety and assistance in ambulation until either a dose adjustment or addition of pyridoxine provides symptomatic relief.

HEPATOTOXICITY. The incidence of hepatotoxicity increases with age and the consumption of alcohol.

The symptoms of hepatotoxicity are anorexia, nausea, vomiting, jaundice, hepatomegaly, splenomegaly, and abnormal liver function tests (elevated bilirubin, AST, ALT, GGT, alkaline phosphatase, prothrombin time).

Implementation

PO. Administer on an empty stomach for maximum effectiveness. It is usually given as a single daily dose, but may be given in divided doses.

Pyridoxine is frequently given concurrently with isoniazid to diminish peripheral neuropathies, dizziness, and ataxia.

Drug interactions

DISULFIRAM. Patients may experience changes in physical coordination and mental affect and behavior. Provide for patient safety and monitor the patient's mental status before and during therapy. If possible, avoid concomitant therapy.

RIFAMPIN. Concurrent therapy may rarely result in hepatotoxicity. Patients on combined therapy should have liver function tests periodically.

PHENYTOIN. Isoniazid may inhibit the metabolism of phenytoin. Monitor patients receiving concurrent therapy for signs of phenytoin toxicity: nystagmus, sedation, lethargy. Serum levels may be ordered and the dosage of phenytoin reduced.

CLINITEST. This drug may produce false-positive Clinitest results. Use Clinistix or Tes-Tape to measure urine glucose.

rifampin (rif'am-pin)

Rifadin (rif'ah-din)

Rifampin is used in combination with other agents against tuberculosis. It acts against enzymes within the bacterial cell that are required to produce DNA.

Side effects. The more common adverse gastrointestinal effects are heartburn, anorexia, nausea, vomiting, cramps, gas, and diarrhea. Other side effects include headache, dizziness, mental confusion, visual disturbances, and generalized numbness.

Rifampin may tinge the urine, feces, saliva, sputum, sweat, and tears a red-orange color. No pathologic damage is caused by this color change, and it will disappear when the medication is discontinued.

Availability

PO—150 and 300 mg capsules.
IV—600 mg vials.

Dosage and administration

Adult

PO—600 mg once daily.
IV—As for PO.

Pediatric

PO—10 to 20 mg/kg/24 hours with a maximum daily dose of 600 mg.
IV—As for PO.

• Nursing Interventions: Monitoring rifampin therapy

See also General Nursing Considerations for Patients with Infectious Diseases (p. 457) and Patients with Tuberculosis (p. 485).

Side effects to expect

REDDISH-ORANGE SECRETIONS. Urine, feces, saliva, sputum, sweat, and tears may be tinged a reddish-orange color. The effect is harmless and will disappear after discontinuation of therapy.

Side effects to report

NAUSEA, VOMITING, ANOREXIA, ABDOMINAL CRAMPS. These side effects are usually mild and tend to resolve with continued therapy. Encourage the patient not to discontinue therapy without first consulting the physician.

Administer with food or milk to diminish irritation.

Implementation

PO. See note directly above. Patients should be warned that omission or interrupted intake may result in drug resistance, reversal of clinical improvement, and increased susceptibility of family members to tuberculosis.

Drug interactions

WARFARIN. This medication may diminish the anticoagulant effects of warfarin. Monitor the prothrombin time and increase the dosage of warfarin if necessary.

ISONIAZID. Concurrent therapy may rarely result in hepatotoxicity. Patients on combined therapy should have liver function tests monitored periodically.

QUINIDINE, DIAZEPAM. Rifampin stimulates the metabolism of these agents. Long-term combined therapy may require an increase in dosages for therapeutic effect.

PROBENECID. Probenecid may reduce urinary excretion of rifampin. Monitor closely for rifampin toxicity.

BIRTH CONTROL PILLS. Rifampin interferes with the contraceptive activity of birth control pills. Counseling regarding alternative methods of birth control should be planned.

VIRAL INFECTIONS

OBJECTIVES

1. Differentiate between the treatments used for bacterial and viral infections.
2. Identify the mechanism of action of acyclovir and vidarabine.
3. Prepare a summary of the antiviral agents that includes the generic and brand names, mechanisms of action, clinical uses, and special considerations related to monitoring and administration of antiviral agents.

4. Cite the potential effects of acyclovir on renal function.
5. Identify the first antiviral agent that is effective against respiratory viruses.
6. State specific inhalation administration considerations when giving ribavirin.
7. Review the signs and symptoms of respiratory impairment.
8. Cite the clinical limitations of zidovudine in the treatment of HIV (human immunodeficiency virus).
9. Identify the hematologic tests that should be completed periodically during the use of zidovudine.
10. Describe the effect of zidovudine on transmission of HIV to others through sexual contact or blood contamination.
11. Review current Centers for Disease Control recommendations for handling of body secretions and blood for *ALL* patients.

KEY WORDS

HIV   AIDS

Many viral infections are not treated with antiviral agents, but rather are treated symptomatically depending upon the causative virus. The basic assessments to be done by the nurse depend on the site of the infection, but would include monitoring patient hygiene and routine parameters, such as the vital signs. It is most important to assess the presenting symptoms.

Antiviral agents

acyclovir (a-sy'klo-veer)

Zovirax (zo-veer'ax)

Acyclovir is an antiviral agent that acts by inhibiting viral cell replication. It is used topically to treat initial infections of herpes genitalis and non-life-threatening cases of mucocutaneous herpes simplex virus infections in patients with suppressed immune systems. The intravenous form is used to treat initial and recurrent mucosal and cutaneous herpes simplex type 1 and 2 infections in immunosuppressed adults and children, and to treat severe initial clinical episodes of herpes genitalis who are not immunosuppressed.

Side effects. Common adverse effects associated with topical application include pruritus, rash, and transient burning. Symptoms are mild and usually do not cause discontinuation of treatment.

Side effects that develop upon intravenous administration include phlebitis (14%), transient elevation in serum creatinine (4.7%), and rash or hives (4.7%). The adverse effects reported include diaphoresis, hematuria, hypotension, headache, and nausea. About 1% of patients have neurologic effects manifested by lethargy, obtundation, tremors, confusion, hallucinations, agitation, seizures, or coma.

Patients who are poorly hydrated, have reduced renal function, or who receive boluses of acyclovir are susceptible to renal tubular damage. This adverse effect is manifested by a rise in serum creatinine and blood urea nitrogen (BUN), hematuria, and a decrease in renal creatinine clearance.

Availability
Topical—5% ointment.
IV—500, 1000 mg per vial.
PO—200 mg capsules; 800 mg tablets; 200 mg/5 ml suspension.

Dosage and administration
Adult
Topical—Apply to each lesion every 3 hours, 6 times daily for 7 days. A finger cot or rubber gloves should be used to avoid the spread of virus to other tissues and persons.

- DO NOT apply to the eyes. It is not an ophthalmic ointment.

IV—NOTE: Bolus or rapid intravenous infusions may result in renal tubular damage.

- Acyclovir is reconstituted with 10 ml of preservative-free sterile water for injection to provide a solution concentration of 50 mg/ml. The solution is stable for 12 hours. This solution should be further diluted by a glucose and electrolyte intravenous fluid to a concentration of 1 to 7 mg/ml prior to administration (stable for 24 hours). Infuse over at least 1 hour to well-hydrated patients. Observe for phlebitis at the infusion site.
- Dose for patients with normal function: 5 mg/kg every 8 hours for 5 to 7 days.

PO—Initial treatment of genital herpes: 200 mg every 4 hours, while awake, for a total of 1000 mg daily for 10 days.
Chronic suppressive therapy for recurrent disease: 400 mg 2 times daily for up to 12 months. Some patients require 200 mg 5 times daily.
Intermittent therapy: 200 mg every 4 hours, while awake, for a total of 1000 mg for 5 days. Therapy should be initiated at the earliest sign or symptom (prodrome) of recurrence.
Pediatric
Topical—As for adult patients.
IV—Patients over 12 years of age: 250 mg/m^2 every 8 hours for 7 days, at a constant infusion rate over 1 hour.

- **Nursing Interventions: Monitoring acyclovir therapy**

See also General Nursing Considerations for Patients with Infectious Diseases (p. 457).
Side effects to expect
PRURITUS, RASH, BURNING. Report symptoms for further evaluation by the physician.

Pruritus may be relieved by adding baking soda to the bath water.

Side effects to report

INTRAVENOUS THERAPY. Avoid IV infusion in the lower extremities and areas with varicosities. Use proper technique in starting the IV solution.

Carefully assess at regularly scheduled intervals for signs of developing phlebitis. Inspect for redness, warmth, tenderness to touch, edema, or pain.

RASH, HIVES. Assess, describe, and chart the location and extent of these presenting symptoms. Report for further evaluation.

DIAPHORESIS. Diaphoresis can be serious if the patient is not well hydrated. Assess hydration state, monitor electrolytes, and provide for nursing interventions (such as clean, dry linens, adequate fluid intake).

NEPHROTOXICITY. Monitor urinalysis and kidney function tests for abnormal results. Report an increasing BUN and creatinine, decreasing urine output or decreasing specific gravity (despite amount of fluid intake), casts or protein in the urine, frank blood, or smoky-colored urine, or RBCs in excess of 0-3 on the urinalysis report.

HYPOTENSION. Record the blood pressure in both a supine and sitting position before and during the administration of this drug. Caution the patient to rise slowly from a supine and sitting position.

CONFUSION. Perform a baseline assessment of the patient's degree of alertness and orientation to name, place, and time *before* initiating therapy. Make regularly scheduled subsequent mental status evaluations and compare findings. Report development of alterations.

Implementation

TOPICAL. Apply the ointment using a finger cot or latex gloves to avoid spread to other tissues and persons.

Use meticulous handwashing technique before and after applying the ointment. DO NOT apply to the eyes; it is not an ophthalmic ointment.

IV. See above for instructions on reconstitution.

Bolus or rapid infusion may result in renal damage. Infuse over at least 1 hour to a well-hydrated patient.

Drug interactions

PROBENECID. Probenecid may reduce urinary excretion of acyclovir. Monitor closely for signs of toxicity from acyclovir.

amantadine hydrochloride (ah-man'tah-deen)

Symmetrel (sim'eh-trel)

Amantadine is an antiviral agent that has specific activity against the influenza A virus. Its primary use now, however, is as an anti-Parkinson's disease agent. It does not treat the underlying disease, but reduces its clinical manifestations. It is described in greater detail elsewhere (see p. 178).

idoxuridine (eye-doks-yur'ih-deen)

Stoxil (stok-sil')

Idoxuridine is an antiviral agent used to treat viral infections of the eye. It is discussed in greater detail elsewhere (see p. 443).

ribavirin (ribe-ah-vi'rihn)

Virazole (vi-rah'zohl)

Ribavirin is the first antiviral agent available to be used effectively against respiratory viruses. The mechanisms of action are unknown. Ribavirin has been shown to have inhibitory activity against members of the DNA-type viral families of *Adenoviridae*, *Herpesviridae*, and *Poxviridae*. The RNA viruses for which ribavirin exerts inhibitory activity are the influenza, parainfluenza, and respiratory syncytial viruses. Ribavirin has initially been given FDA approval to be used to treat severe lower respiratory tract infections due to respiratory syncytial virus (RSV) by aerosol administration.

Side effects. Patients must be observed closely for deteriorating pulmonary function when ribavirin aerosol therapy is initiated. Patients with chronic obstructive lung disease or asthma are particularly sensitive to this adverse effect. Patients occasionally complain of dyspnea and chest soreness.

A normochromic, normocytic anemia has been reported with oral or intravenous use. Reticulocytosis has been reported with aerosol use.

Rash and conjunctivitis have been associated with the use of ribavirin aerosol.

Ribavirin is contraindicated in women who are or may become pregnant during exposure to the drug.

Availability

Aerosol powder—20 mg/ml in 100 ml vials for reconstitution.

Dosage and administration. NOTE: Ribavirin must be administered through a specific, small-particle aerosol generator.

1. Using aseptic technique, reconstitute the 6 g of drug by adding 50 ml of sterile water for injection to the 100 ml vial.

2. When dissolved, transfer the contents to a clean, sterilized 500 ml widemouth Erlenmeyer flask and further dilute with sterile water for injection to a final volume of 300 ml. The final concentration is 20 mg/ml.

3. Administer ribavirin at an initial concentration of 20 mg/ml through the reservoir of the small-particle aerosol generator. Treatment is carried out for 12 to 18 hours per day for at least 3 and no more than 7 days. The aerosol is delivered from the generator to the patient via an oxygen hood or face mask. It should not be administered concurrently with any other aerosolized medication.

• **Nursing Interventions: Monitoring ribavirin therapy**

See also General Nursing Considerations for Patients with Infectious Diseases (p. 457).

Side effects to expect

RASH, CONJUNCTIVITIS. These adverse effects tend to occur due to local irritation from poorly placed inhalation equipment. Work with the patient for optimal fit. Methylcellulose eye drops may be applied to reduce conjunctival irritation.

Side effects to report

DIMINISHING PULMONARY FUNCTION. Perform baseline pulmonary function tests to assess whether the patient shows deterioration after therapy is initiated. If initiation of treatment appears to produce sudden deterioration of respiratory function, treatment should be discontinued immediately and reinstituted only with extreme caution and continuous monitoring. Report complaints of chest soreness, shortness of breath, or other adverse effects immediately.

ANEMIA. Reticulocytosis and anemia have been reported during therapy. The severity and significance is not known at this time.

Implementation

PREGNANCY. Ribavirin is contraindicated in women who are or may become pregnant during exposure to the drug. Ribavirin has been reported to cause birth defects in several animal species. It is not completely eliminated from human blood for at least 4 weeks after administration.

PATIENTS ON RESPIRATORS. Ribavirin is not recommended for patients requiring assisted ventilation because precipitation of the drug in the respiratory equipment may interfere with safe and effective use of the ventilator by these patients. If it is deemed necessary to treat a patient with ribavirin who is also receiving ventilatory support, prefilters must be placed in the equipment to prevent precipitation in the endotrachial tube or on the valves and tubing.

Drug interactions. No significant drug interactions have been reported.

trifluridine (tri-flur′ih-deen)

Viroptic (vi-rop′tik)

Trifluridine is an antiviral agent used to treat viral infections of the eye. It is discussed in greater detail elsewhere (see p. 443).

vidarabine (vi-dar′a-been)

Vira-A (vi′ra ay)

Vidarabine is an antiviral agent that acts by inhibiting viral cell replication. It is used intravenously in the treatment of encephalitis caused by herpes simplex virus and topically as an ophthalmic ointment to treat keratitis and keratoconjunctivitis caused by herpes simplex virus types 1 and 2. Vidarabine does not show cross-sensitivity to idoxuridine and may be effective in treating recurrent keratitis that is resistant to idoxuridine.

Side effects. Minor side effects associated with the use of vidarabine ointment include temporary visual haze, burning, itching, redness, and tearing. *Photophobia* (sensitivity to bright light) occasionally occurs, but can be minimized by wearing sunglasses. Allergic reactions have rarely been reported.

The most common side effects from intravenous vidarabine are nausea, vomiting, diarrhea, anorexia, and weight loss. These reactions begin on the second or third day of therapy and resolve in another 1 to 4 days. Hallucinations, psychosis, confusion, tremor, and dizziness may be dose-related and are reversed after discontinuation of therapy.

Intravenous vidarabine should be used with caution in patients with impaired liver or kidney function and in patients susceptible to fluid overload or cerebral edema.

Availability

Topical—3% ophthalmic ointment.

IV—200 mg/ml in 5 ml vials.

Dosage and administration

Adult

Ophthalmic—Place a 1 cm ribbon of ointment inside the lower conjunctival sac of the infected eye, 5 times daily at 3 hour intervals. Continue for an additional 5 to 7 days at a dosage of 1 cm twice daily after reepithelialization has occurred to prevent recurrence of the infection.

IV—15 mg/kg daily for 10 days. Administer for 12 to 24 hours using an in-line filter (0.45 micron or smaller). Make sure that vidarabine is completely dissolved. It requires 2.2 ml of fluid to dissolve 1 mg of vidarabine (1 liter dissolves 450 mg at 77° F). Dissolution may be facilitated by prewarming the IV infusion fluid to 95° to 105° F. Dilute just prior to administration and use within 48 hours. DO NOT refrigerate the solution. Administer with any parenteral fluid, except blood, protein, and lipid products (hyperalimentation fluids).

• **Nursing Interventions: Monitoring vidarabine therapy**

See also General Nursing Considerations for Patients with Infectious Diseases (p. 457).

Side effects to expect and report

OPHTHALMIC OINTMENT

Visual haze, tearing, redness, burning. Provide for patient safety during temporary visual impairment. Instruct the patient not to rub the eyes forcefully when tearing.

These side effects are usually mild and tend to resolve with continued therapy. Encourage the patient not to discontinue therapy without first consulting the physician.

Photophobia. Wearing sunglasses minimizes this effect.

INTRAVENOUS THERAPY

Nausea, vomiting, anorexia. These symptoms usually resolve in 1 to 4 days. Perform daily weights; monitor fluid loss carefully.

Confusion. Perform a baseline assessment of the patient's degree of alertness and orientation to name, place, and time *before* initiating therapy. Make regularly scheduled subsequent mental status evaluations and compare findings. Report development of alterations so that dosage adjustments may be made.

Nephrotoxicity. Monitor urinalysis and kidney function tests for abnormal results. Report an increasing BUN and creatinine, decreasing urine output or decreasing specific gravity (despite amount of fluid intake), casts or protein in the urine, frank blood or smoky-colored urine, or RBCs in excess of 0-3 on the urinalysis report.

Hepatotoxicity. The symptoms of hepatotoxicity are anorexia, nausea, vomiting, jaundice, hepatomegaly, splenomegaly, and abnormal liver function tests (elevated bilirubin, AST, ALT, alkaline phosphatase, prothrombin time).

Blood dyscrasias. Monitor the WBC, RBC, and platelet counts. Report decreasing numbers. Monitor for the development of a sore throat, fever, purpura, or excessive progressive weakness.

Implementation

OPHTHALMIC. Use meticulous handwashing before and after application of eye ointment. DO NOT contaminate the tip of the applicator by touching the eye.

IV. See IV reconstitution instructions above. Be certain it is completely dissolved prior to administration.

Administer with any parenteral solution, except blood, protein, and lipid products (hyperalimentation solutions).

Drug interactions

ALLOPURINOL. In question at the time of this writing is the possibility that the metabolism of vidarabine may be inhibited by allopurinol. Monitor for an increased frequency of toxic effects, if the two agents are used concurrently.

zidovudine (zid-ohv-u′deen)

Retrovir (ret-roh-veer′)

Zidovudine is the first of a new series of antiviral agents that has been shown to be effective for certain patients with human immunodeficiency virus (HIV) infections. It acts by inhibiting replication of the virus. In controlled clinical trials, zidovudine was shown to prolong the lives of patients with acquired immune deficiency (AIDS) and AIDS-related complex (ARC), to reduce the risk and severity of opportunistic infections, and to improve immune status. Unfortunately, zidovudine is not a cure for HIV infections, and patients may continue to acquire illnesses associated with acquired immune deficiency. Zidovudine is indicated for patients who have a confirmed history of *Pneumocystis carinii* pneumonia or an absolute CD4 lymphocyte count of less than 200/mm^3 in the peripheral blood before therapy is begun.

Side effects. Patients treated with zidovudine are already seriously ill with underlying disease with a wide variety of baseline symptoms and clinical abnormalities. The most frequent adverse effect attributable to zidovudine is bone marrow suppression resulting in granulocytopenia and anemia. Other adverse effects that occur in at least 5% of patients include severe headache, nausea, insomnia, and myalgia. Many other adverse effects have been reported, but due to the critical nature of the illnesses, researchers are unable to discern whether the symptoms were due to the drug therapy or the underlying disease.

Availability

PO—100 mg capsules; 50 mg/5 ml syrup.

IV—10 mg/ml in 20 ml vial

Dosage and administration

Adult

PO—Asymptomatic HIV infection: 100 mg every 4 hours while awake (500 mg/day).

Symptomatic HIV infection: 200 mg every 4 hours in a 24-hour period. After 1 month, reduce to 100 mg every 4 hours.

IV—1 to 2 mg/kg infused over 1 hour; administer every 4 hours, 6 times daily.

• Nursing Interventions: Monitoring zidovudine therapy

See also General Nursing Considerations for Patients with Infectious Diseases (p. 457).

Side effects to report

ANEMIA, GRANULOCYTOPENIA. Monitor hematologic indices every 2 weeks to detect serious anemia or granulocytopenia. In patients developing bone marrow suppression, reduction in hemoglobin may occur as early as 2 to 4 weeks, and granulocytopenia usually occurs after 6 to 8 weeks.

It is crucial that patients understand the importance of returning periodically for blood counts while receiving therapy.

Implementation

DOSAGE. Patients must understand the importance of taking the medication every 4 hours around the clock, even though it may interrupt normal sleep.

COMPLIANCE. Patients must also understand that the drug is taken orally and must not be shared with other persons, and that they must not exceed the recommended dose. Potentially fatal adverse effects may result.

TRANSMISSION OF HIV. Zidovudine therapy has not been shown to reduce the risk of transmission of HIV to others through sexual contact or blood contamination.

Drug interactions

NEPHROTOXIC, CYTOTOXIC, HEMATOTOXIC AGENTS. Use of drugs such as dapsone, pentamidine, amphotericin B, flucytosine, vincristine, vinblastine, adriamycin, or interferon may increase the risk of toxicity.

PROBENECID, ASPIRIN, ACETAMINOPHEN, INDOMETHACIN. These agents may inhibit the metabolism and excretion of zidovudine, thus enhancing the potential for toxicity.

Patients must be warned not to use these agents while receiving zidovudine therapy.

Drug Therapy for Urinary Tract Infections

The urinary antiinfective agents, including cinoxacin, methenamine mandelate, nalidixic acid, nitrofurantoin, norfloxacin, and phenazopyridine, are mainstays in urinary antimicrobial therapy. They are discussed in greater detail in Chapter 15, "Drugs Affecting the Urinary System" (p. 371).

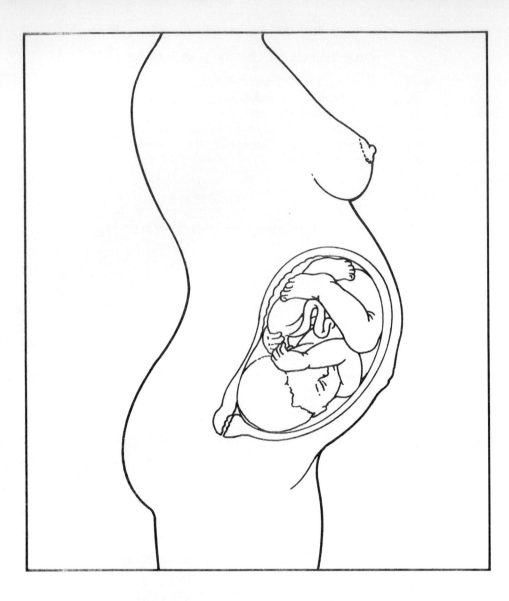

CHAPTER GOALS

After completing this chapter, the student should be able to do the following:

1. Explain the major action and effects of drugs used to treat obstetric and gynecologic disorders.
2. Identify baseline data the nurse should collect on a continuous basis for comparison and evaluation of drug effectiveness.
3. Identify important nursing assessments and interventions associated with the drug therapy and treatment of gynecologic and obstetric disorders.
4. Identify essential components involved in planning patient education that will enhance compliance with the treatment regimen.

OBSTETRICS

OBJECTIVES

1. Identify the factors that must be assessed during the prenatal management of a pregnant woman.
2. Describe nursing assessments and nursing interventions needed for the pregnant patient experiencing bleeding disorders.
3. State the methods and time parameters of each approach to the termination of a pregnancy.
4. Cite the recommended times of administration of Rh$_o$ (D) immune globulin (human) and rubella vaccine in relation to pregnancy.
5. Identify the signs, symptoms, and management of pregnancy-induced hypertension.
6. Describe the nursing assessments and interventions used for pregnancy-induced hypertension.
7. State the purpose of administering glucocorticoids to certain women in preterm labor.
8. Summarize the care needs of the pregnant woman during the normal labor and delivery period.
9. Identify the name, dosage, route of administration, and correct time for administering oxytocic agents and lactation-suppressants.
10. Describe the normal sequence of changes in the appearance of lochia during the postpartum period.
11. Summarize the immediate nursing care needs of the newborn infant following delivery.
12. Cite the rationale for inspection of the placenta and cord following delivery of the newborn.
13. Summarize the Center for Disease Control recommendations for prophylaxis of ophthalmia neonatorum.
14. Identify assessment data that are essential to detect postpartum hemorrhage.
15. State the nursing assessments needed to monitor therapeutic response and/or the development of side effects to expect or report from uterine stimulants, uterine relaxants, lactation suppressants, oral contraceptives, clomiphene citrate, magnesium sulfate, Rh$_o$ (D) immune globulin, erythromycin ophthalmic ointment, and tetracycline ointment and drops.
16. Develop measurable short- and long-term objectives for patient education for patients receiving uterine stimulants, uterine relaxants, lactation suppressants, or oral contraceptives.

KEY WORDS

pregnancy-induced
  hypertension
preeclampsia
placental insufficiency
eclampsia
toxemia of pregnancy
lochia

General Nursing Considerations for Obstetric Patients

See also Drugs Affecting the Endocrine System, Analgesics and Sedatives, and Diuretics.

Patient Concerns:
Nursing Intervention/Rationale

Assessment of the pregnant woman
Prenatal visit
Client history. Obtain basic historical information about the woman and family concerning diseases, surgeries, and deaths.

Menstrual history. Gather data about menstrual pattern (age of initial onset, duration and frequency of monthly periods, date of last full menstrual cycle, any bleeding since the last full menstrual period).

Contraceptive use. Gather data about contraceptive use (use of condoms, foam, diaphragm, sponge, the pill, IUDs).

Obstetrical history. Ask the woman the number of previous live births, stillbirths, miscarriages, or induced abortions. If any of the deliveries were premature, obtain additional information about the infant's age of gestation, survival of the child, any suspected causes, and infections.

Ask if RhoGAM was given for Rh factor incompatibility.

Current information
Medications. Ask the woman if she takes any medications regularly. Include over-the-counter medications.

If she is not currently taking any medications, ask whether any have been taken over the past 6 months. Determine which have been prescribed and for what purpose.

Alcohol or street drugs. Determine use of alcohol or street drugs of any kind, including what, how much, and how frequently.

Health problems. Ask the patient if she has ever been treated for the following:

- Kidney or bladder problems
- High blood pressure, heart disease, or rheumatic fever
- Hypothyroidism or hyperthyroidism
- Diabetes mellitus ("high blood sugar" or "sugar in the urine")
- Allergies to any foods, drugs, or environmental substances
- Sexually transmitted diseases
- Exposure to any communicable diseases since becoming pregnant
- Received blood or blood products

If the woman answers "yes" to any of these questions, gather more information about what physician made the diagnosis, when the disorder occurred, and how it was treated.

Eating and elimination. What are the woman's favorite foods, how often does she eat, and what has she eaten in the last 3 days?

What is the patient's elimination pattern? How often does she have bowel movements; what is the stool consistency and color; is there ever any bleeding; and are laxatives ever needed? If so, how often?

Social history. Capitalize on the individual's strengths.

Determine how the woman feels about this pregnancy (for example, excited; nervous; baby is unwanted).

Who makes up her support group: husband, boyfriend, friends, family?

Ask the woman about her employment status and what type of work she performs.

Determine the woman's level of education and general interest in learning more about effective management of the pregnancy.

Also find out about the woman's economic status. Will referral to social services agencies be necessary?

Physical examination. Assist the individual to undress and prepare for examination.

Urine specimen. Have the individual void and save the specimen. (Give instructions on how to obtain a clean-catch specimen.)

Height and weight. Weigh the woman and measure the current height.

Blood pressure. Try to give the patient time to become more comfortable with the interviewer before taking the initial blood pressure reading. If elevated, recheck in about 10 minutes or when she appears to be more relaxed.

Ask again if any prior treatment has been given for high blood pressure. If so, inquire about the onset, treatment, and degree of control achieved.

Pulse. Count the pulse for 1 full minute. Report irregularities in rate, rhythm, or volume. On subsequent visits, anticipate an increase in rate of approximately 10 beats per minute during the course of the pregnancy.

Respirations. Record the rate of respirations. As the pregnancy progresses, observe for hyperventilation and thoracic breathing.

Temperature. Record the temperature. Tell the client to report any elevations to the physician immediately for further evaluation. If temperature currently is elevated, ask about any signs of infection or exposure to persons with a known infection or communicable disease.

Pelvic exam. Assist the patient to prepare for the pelvic examination. Gather supplies for the physician and assist appropriately. A Papanicolaou (Pap) smear is usually performed as part of the examination. Mark specimens appropriately, noting name, date, age, any hormone therapy, and date of last menstrual period.

Blood studies. Blood samples for CBC, hemoglobin, hematocrit, rubella titer, Rh factor, and, occasionally, a VDRL, may be ordered drawn at this initial visit.

Schedule of follow-up visits. Explain that at each follow-up visit, the following will be done: weighing and necessary dietary teaching; measuring blood pressure, pulse, and respirations; examination of the abdomen with measurement of fundal height and fetal heart sounds. Any problems or concerns will be discussed. Hemoglobin and hematocrit may be periodically rechecked.

The pregnant woman who does not experience complications is usually examined once monthly for the first 6 months, every 2 weeks in the seventh and eighth months, and weekly during the last month of pregnancy. Vaginal exams are usually performed on the initial visit and are not repeated until 2 to 3 weeks prior to the estimated date of confinement (EDC) or "due date," at which time the cervical status, degree of engagement, and fetal presentation are evaluated.

Weight gain. A weight gain of 2 to 4 pounds during the first trimester, 11 pounds during the second trimester, and 11 pounds during the third trimester is usual.

Stress the need to report a weight gain of 2 or more pounds in any 1 week for further evaluation.

Assessment of pregnant patients at risk

Bleeding disorders. Miscarriage and abortion are major causes of bleeding during the first and second trimesters of pregnancy. Bleeding during the third trimester may be due to placenta previa or abruptio placenta.

Bleeding pattern. It is important to take a careful history of the onset and advancement of the bleeding symptoms. Gather specific information about the onset, duration, amount (number of pads used), color, and any clots or tissue seen.

Pain. Ask the patient to describe any pain being experienced. Has she had any backache or pelvic cramping, sharp abdominal pain, faintness, or pain in the shoulder area?

Vital signs. Whenever bleeding is present, the vital signs should be taken and compared to previous baseline data on the patient's records. Continue to monitor the vital signs at regular intervals to detect the development of shock: restlessness, perspiration, pallor, clammy skin, dyspnea, tachycardia, and blood pressure changes. Record the fetal heart rate at regular intervals.

Laboratory studies. When bleeding is present, blood studies for hemoglobin, hematocrit, WBCs, human chorionic gonadotropin (HCG) titer, and type and crossmatch for blood may be ordered.

Other procedures. Other diagnostic procedures such as culdoscopy, sonography, laparoscopy, fetoscopy, and pregnancy tests may be performed.

Activity level. Bedrest and sedation are usually prescribed. Uterine relaxants such as ritodrine may also be required.

Termination of pregnancy. If bleeding occurs near the EDC, the infant may be delivered by cesarean birth.

If it appears that an incomplete abortion (miscarriage) has occurred, the woman may be hospitalized for observation, possible D&C (dilatation and curettage), and fluid replacement.

If a pregnancy is to be terminated (aborted), the following methods may be used:

- Before 12 weeks gestation: Suction curettage or dilatation and evacuation (D&E)
- 12 to 20 weeks gestation: Intraamniotic instillation of hypertonic saline (20% solution) or prostaglandin administered intraamniotically, intramuscularly, or by vaginal suppository
- Intrauterine fetal death after 20 weeks of gestation: Prostaglandin suppositories with or without oxytocin augmentation (see "Uterine Stimulants," p. 504)

RH FACTOR. An Rh-negative mother may receive RhoGAM within 72 hours of the termination of pregnancy (see p. 517).

RUBELLA VACCINE. If the patient's rubella titer is low, an appropriate time for inoculation is immediately after pregnancy.

PATIENT INSTRUCTIONS. Persons having an abortion procedure should be instructed concerning personal care:

- Do not use tampons for 1 to 2 weeks; use pads.
- Do not douche.
- Report bleeding that is heavier than a normal "period" that persists for more than 24 hours.
- Do not engage in sexual intercourse for at least the first week following the abortion.

- Take temperature twice daily (noon and bedtime) for a few days, and report any elevations above 100° F.
- Stress the need for keeping the follow-up visit with the physician.
- Review contraceptive methods if necessary.

PSYCHOLOGIC ASPECTS. Encourage the persons involved in the loss of an infant to talk about their feelings of loss, grief, sadness, or anger. Listen and allow them to vent feelings. Give answers (if known) regarding future pregnancies. Refer for other counseling as appropriate. Anticipate that depression may develop over the next few weeks and may need treatment.

Preeclampsia and eclampsia. Preeclampsia and eclampsia are now called *pregnancy-induced hypertension* (PIH). The term *toxemia of pregnancy* is no longer used because there is no evidence that a "toxin" produces the hypertension, edema, and proteinuria characteristic of the disease. PIH is seen most often in the last 10 weeks of gestation, during labor, and in the first 12 to 48 hours after delivery. The etiology is unknown and the only cure for preeclampsia is termination of the pregnancy. Eclampsia is present when the mother develops seizures and coma in addition to the hypertension, edema, and proteinuria.

PIH occurs in 5 to 7% of all pregnancies. Women predisposed to the disease are those of lower socioeconomic status, teenagers with first pregnancies, and those with a history of chronic hypertension, diabetes mellitus, hydatidiform mole, renal disease, or multiple pregnancy (twins or triplets). Approximately one-third of women who have had PIH will develop it in a subsequent pregnancy.

PIH patients may be treated conservatively at home by limiting daily activity and instruction to eat adequate proteins in the form of lean meat, fish, poultry, and eggs. If the patient develops significant hypertension, edema, weight gain, and proteinuria, she may require hospitalization for more adequate control of the symptoms and to prevent the development of seizures.

History and physical. Carefully assess the patient for a history of predisposing disease or social factors.

Vital signs. Assess vital signs (temperature, blood pressure, pulse, and respirations) and compare to baseline readings. ALWAYS report sudden development of hypertension (an elevation of systolic pressure 30 mm Hg or more above prior readings; or systolic blood pressure of 140 mm Hg or more; or diastolic pressure of 90 mm Hg or more).

Edema. All patients hospitalized for preeclampsia or eclampsia should be monitored for intake and output.

Daily hydration is maintained via oral or intravenous routes. Generally, 1000 ml plus the amount of urine output over the past 24 hours is allowed for intake.

Carefully assess for edema of any body parts (fingers, hands, face, legs, ankles).

Monitor daily weights and instruct the patient to report a weight gain of 2 pounds or more in any 1 week.

Salt intake is generally maintained at a normal level, although heavy use should be discouraged.

Fetal assessment. The status of the fetus may be assessed by fetal movement counts, contraction stress testing, biophysical profile, and ultrasonography for placental placement and measurement of maturity indicators. An amniocentesis may be performed to assess fetal lung maturity.

Laboratory data

URINE. Always use a clean-catch specimen since vaginal discharge or the presence of RBCs may cause a positive test for proteinuria. An indwelling catheter may be necessary in severe cases both to monitor the amount of urine output and to obtain specimens for testing. Test the protein content and specific gravity hourly. Report steadily decreasing hourly output, or output < 30 ml/hr.

ELECTROLYTES. Assess regularly and report abnormal findings.

CLOTTING STUDIES. Assess for possible thrombocytopenia.

BUN. The blood urea nitrogen is usually not elevated unless the patient has renal disease.

URIC ACID. Report increasing serum uric acid levels. There is a fairly good correlation with the severity of the preeclampsia/eclampsia. (Keep in mind that thiazide diuretics cause an increase in uric acid levels.)

HEMATOCRIT. The hematocrit rises as the patient loses water from the intravascular space to the extravascular space or the patient becomes dehydrated due to inadequate hydration.

SERUM ESTRIOLS, L/S RATIO. These laboratory tests give an indication of fetal maturity.

Seizures. Increased drowsiness, hyperreflexia, visual disturbances, and development of severe pain are indications of a worsening condition. Report these symptoms IMMEDIATELY.

If the patient does develop seizures, give supportive care, provide a nonstimulating environment, and have oxygen, suction, and a padded tongue blade available.

Record the respiratory and heart rates, degree of cyanosis, and duration of the seizure.

Continuously monitor fetal heart rate and movements.

Be alert for the start of labor or signs of other complications such as pulmonary edema, disseminated intravascular coagulation, congestive heart failure, abruptio placenta, or cerebral hemorrhage.

Drug treatment

SEDATIVES. A sedative, such as diazepam or phenobarbital, is sometimes given to encourage quiet rest.

ANTIHYPERTENSIVES. The vasodilator hydralazine is generally used to control blood pressure. It may be administered orally or intravenously, depending upon the severity of the condition. If given IV, monitor the maternal and fetal heart rates, and the mother's blood pressure every 2 to 3 minutes after the initial dose, and every 10 to 15 minutes thereafter. The diastolic pressure is usually maintained at 90 to 100 mm Hg.

ANTICONVULSANTS. Magnesium sulfate ($MgSO_4$) is the treatment of choice for seizure activity (see p. 515).

Premature labor. Premature labor is labor that occurs before the end of the 37th week of gestation, resulting in the birth of an infant usually weighing less than 2500 g.

The overall incidence of prematurity in the United States is 9 to 10%; the incidence in blacks is 18 to 19%. Prematurity is responsible for almost two-thirds of infant deaths.

Causes. Among the causes of premature labor are premature rupture of membranes and maternal factors such as diabetes, pregnancy-induced hypertension, uterine anomalies, multiple pregnancies, fetal or uterine infection, and renal and cardiovascular diseases. In approximately two-thirds of cases, no specific cause can be identified.

Fetal assessment. The status of the fetus may be assessed by fetal movement counts, contraction stress testing, biophysical profile, and ultrasonography for placental placement and measurement of maturity indicators. An amniocentesis may be performed to assess fetal lung maturity.

Stopping preterm labor. Early labor may be an indication of obstetrical complications such as infection, fetal death, hemorrhage, or severe pregnancy-induced hypertension. Close assessment by the physician is necessary before it is deemed appropriate to stop labor. (See Figure 20-1.)

NON-DRUG TREATMENT. If it is decided to stop labor, the patient should first be at bedrest, well-hydrated, and possibly sedated to relieve anxiety. These measures alone will stop labor in many patients.

DRUG TREATMENT. If labor does not stop spontaneously, tocolytic agents such as ritodrine, terbutaline, or magnesium sulfate may be used to stop uterine contractions. Isoxsuprine and ethanol have been used in the recent past, but have generally been replaced by more effective agents such as ritodrine (see "Uterine Relaxants," p. 510).

GLUCOCORTICOIDS. Glucocorticoids, usually betamethasone, may be administered IM to the mother to accelerate fetal lung maturation and minimize hyaline membrane disease. It may be used in cases where it is anticipated that premature labor should be stopped for only 36 to 48 hours, such as with premature rupture of the membranes.

Normal labor and delivery

History. Upon admission to the hospital, obtain the following information:

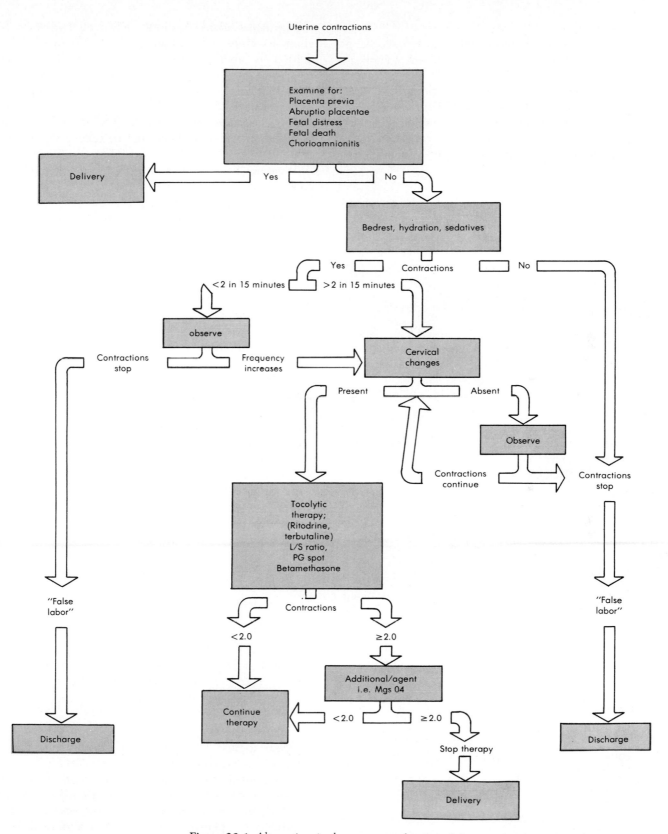

Figure 20-1 *Alternatives in the treatment of preterm labor.*

- Name and age
- Obstetrical history: gravida, para, abortions, fetal deaths, birth weight of previous children, complications during previous deliveries
- Estimated due date, estimated gestational age, and first day of last menstrual period (LMP)
- Prenatal care: type and amount, any significant problems
- Prenatal education: type and extent of childbirth preparation
- Plan for infant feeding
- Status of membranes: intact, ruptured, time ruptured, amount and color of fluid that escaped
- Status of labor: time of onset of contractions, frequency, duration and intensity of contractions, how patient is coping with contractions
- Time of last meal

Physical examination. Assess for the following:

- Height and weight
- Vital signs (temperature, blood pressure, pulse, and respirations)
- Presence of edema
- State of hydration
- Size and contour of abdomen and fundus
- Frequency of contractions
- Fetal heart rate
- Vaginal examination: cervical dilatation and effacement, status of membranes, and presentation and position of fetus

Laboratory tests

Urinalysis. Obtain a clean-catch urine specimen and test for glucose and protein. Send to the lab for microscopic examination.

Blood. Obtain a blood specimen for CBC, hemoglobin, hematocrit, serology tests, and maternal blood type.

Other admission routines

Perineal prep. The physician may order the perineal and pubic area to be shaved, to aid in postpartum repair of the perineum.

Enema. The physician may order this to empty the lower bowel, thus reducing the possibility of contamination during delivery.

Activity and exercise. During the early stages of labor, some women may ambulate. Check the institutional rules.

Basic needs. During labor, provide pain relief, alternate positioning of the mother from side to side (avoid lying flat on the back), back rubs, pelvic rocking, effleurage, and support for the coach and woman when necessary. Encourage rest between contractions throughout labor.

Voiding. Encourage women in labor to void at least every 2 hours. Check for bladder distension.

Nutritional status. Maintain adequate hydration by giving ice chips or clear liquids. Check the status of hydration as labor progresses by observing the mucous membranes, dryness of lips, and skin turgor.

Do not give solid foods unless specifically approved by the physician.

Leg cramps and muscle spasms. Encourage leg extension and dorsiflexion of the foot to relieve spasms and cramping.

Sweating. Keep a sponge available for wiping and cooling the face.

Dry mouth. Provide ice chips, mouthwash, or glycerine swabs, and help the mother brush her teeth if she desires.

Privacy. During the early phases of labor, provide the mother and coach as much privacy as possible. Give correct information when asked, and inform the couple of any procedures to be done.

Ongoing monitoring. As labor progresses, continue to monitor the maternal and fetal vital signs and the frequency, duration, and intensity of uterine contractions.

Report contractions with a duration of 90 seconds or more and those not followed by complete uterine relaxation. Report abnormal patterns on the fetal monitor, such as decreased variability, late decelerations, and variable decelerations.

Continue to assist the coach when necessary.

As vaginal discharge increases, wash the perineum with warm water and dry the area. Change the bedsheets, pad, and gown when necessary.

Monitor patient's temperature every 4 hours while membranes are intact and temperature remains within normal range. Monitor every 2 hours if the patient's temperature is elevated or if the membranes have ruptured.

After delivery. Record the following:

- The time of delivery and position of the infant
- The type of episiotomy and type of suture used in repair, if appropriate
- Any anesthetic or analgesic used during repair
- Time of placental delivery
- Any complications such as additional bleeding or neonatal distress

Medications. Administer and record oxytocic and lactation suppressants, if ordered.

Assessments. The vital signs should be checked every 15 minutes during the first hour or until the woman is stable, then every 30 minutes for the next 2 hours.

Inspect the perineum and note any abnormal swelling or bruising.

Check the fundal height and firmness every 15 minutes for 1 hour, then every 30 minutes for the next 4 hours.

Describe the amount of lochia, the color and the

presence of any clots every 15 minutes for 1 hour; every 30 minutes for 4 hours; hourly for the next 12 hours.

Continue to monitor the state of hydration and elimination.

Support the physiological and psychological needs of the mother and father. Allow them to spend as much time with the infant as possible.

Immediate neonatal care

Before delivery. Before delivery, the maternal history through the current stage of labor should be reviewed to identify potential complications that may arise for the neonate. Although a complete physical examination on the neonate will be performed later, a preliminary assessment and recording of data must be completed at the time of birth.

Immediately after delivery. The following procedures must be completed by the physician or nurse immediately upon delivery:

1. Airway—Ensure that the airway is open and remains so. As soon as the head is delivered, the oral pharynx and nasal passages are suctioned with a small bulb syringe. Immediately after delivery, the newborn baby is held with the head lowered at a 10 to 15 degree angle to help drainage of amniotic fluid, mucus, and blood. Resuction with the bulb syringe as necessary.
2. Clamping of the umbilical cord—When the airway

is opened and the respirations have stabilized, the neonate should be held at the same level as the uterus until pulsations of the cord cease. The cord is then clamped or ligated.

3. Health status—The health status of the neonate is estimated at 1 minute and 5 minutes post delivery using the Apgar rating system (see Table 20-1). Rapid estimation of gestational age is also performed (see Table 20-2).
4. Temperature maintenance—The neonate should be dried immediately and body temperature maintained with the use of prewarmed blankets, a heated bassinet, or an infrared heat lamp. If the neonate is full-term and in stable condition as assessed by the Apgar score, temperature may be maintained by skin-to-skin contact with the mother.
5. Eye prophylaxis—It is a legal requirement that newborn baby's eyes are treated prophylactically for *Neisseria gonorrhoea*. Another rapidly emerging neonatal conjunctival infection is chlamydial ophthalmia neonatorum, which is caused by *Chlamydia trachomatis*. The neonate may have become infected during the birth process if the mother is infected. See box on p. 502 for recommendations for prophylactic treatment for neonatal conjunctivitis caused by *Neisseria gonorrhoea* or *Chlamydia trachomatis*.

Instillation of the ophthalmic agent may be delayed up to 2 hours to facilitate parent-child bonding.

6. Other procedures—While the parents are bonding with the newborn infant, the nurse should prepare an infant identification bracelet and place it on the baby, examine the placenta and cord for anomalies, and verify the presence of one vein and two arteries. Samples of cord blood may be collected for analysis of the Rh factor, blood grouping, and the hematocrit. The baby is then taken to the newborn nursery where it is weighed, measured, and given a complete physical examination. Some physicians also order an intramuscular injection of vitamin K to be administered to the baby as prophylaxis against hemorrhage. Evaluation of the infant's vital signs and color are performed on a continuum. Alterations from baseline are evaluated and reported.

Table 20-1 *The Apgar Scoring System*

SIGN	0	1	2
Heart rate	Absent	Slow (below 100)	Over 100
Respiratory effort	Absent	Slow, irregular	Good, crying
Muscle tone	Flaccid	Some flexion of extremities	Active motion
Reflex irritability	No response	Grimace	Cry
Color	Blue, pale	Body pink, extremities blue	Completely pink

Table 20-2 *Gestational Age*

SITES	36 WEEKS OR LESS	37-38 WEEKS	39 WEEKS OR MORE
Sole creases	Anterior transverse creases only	Occasional creases anterior two thirds	Sole covered with creases
Breast nodule diameter	2 mm	4 mm	7 mm
Scalp hair	Fine, fuzzy	Fine, fuzzy	Coarse and silky
Earlobes	Pliable, no cartilage	Some cartilage	Stiffened by thick cartilage
Testes and scrotum	Testes in lower canal, scrotum small, few rugae	Intermediate	Testes pendulous, scrotum full, extensive rugae

(From Cunningham FG, MacDonald PC, Grant NF: *Williams' obstetrics*, ed 18, Norwalk, Conn., 1989, Appleton & Lange.)

Recommendations for prophylaxis of ophthalmia neonatorum

1. Instillation of a prophylactic agent in the eyes of all newborn infants.
2. Acceptable prophylactic agents that prevent **chlamydial ophthalmia neonatorum** and **gonococcal ophthalmia neonatorum** include the following:
   a. Erythromycin (0.5%) ophthalmic ointment in single-use tubes.
   b. Tetracycline (1%) ophthalmic ointment or drops in single-use tubes or ampules.
3. Prophylactic agents should be given shortly after birth. A delay of up to 1 hour* is probably acceptable and may facilitate initial maternal–infant bonding.
4. The importance of performing the instillation so the agent reaches all parts of the conjunctival surface is stressed. This can be accomplished by careful manipulation of the lids with fingers to ensure spreading of the agent. If medication strikes only the eyelids and lid margins but fails to reach the cornea, the instillation should be repeated. Prophylaxis should be applied as follows:
   a. **Ophthalmic ointment (erythromycin or tetracycline).** Assemble supplies and medication; don gloves:
      (1) Carefully clean eyelids and surrounding skin with sterile cotton, which may be moistened with sterile water.
      (2) Gently open baby's eyelids and place a thin line of ointment, at least 1 to 2 cm (½ in), along the junction of the bulbar and palpebral conjunctiva of the lower lid. Try to cover the whole lower conjunctival area. Carefully manipulate lids to ensure spread of the ointment. *Be careful not to touch the eyelid or eyeball with the tip of the tube.* Repeat in other eye. Use one tube per baby.
      (3) After 1 minute, gently wipe excess ointment from eyelids and surrounding skin with sterile water. *Do not irrigate eyes.*
   b. **Ophthalmic drops (tetracycline).** Assemble supplies and medication; don gloves:
      (1) Carefully clean eyelids and surrounding skin with sterile cotton, which may be moistened with sterile water.
      (2) Gently open baby's eyelids and instill two drops of tetracycline in the conjunctival sac. Allow the ophthalmic drops to run across the whole conjunctival sac. Carefully manipulate lids to ensure spread of the drops. Repeat in the other eye.
      (3) After 1 minute, gently wipe excess tetracycline solution from eyelids and surrounding skin with sterile water. *Do not irrigate eyes.*
5. The eye should not be irrigated after instillation of a prophylactic agent. Irrigation may reduce the efficacy of prophylaxis and probably does not decrease the incidence of chemical conjunctivitis.
6. Infants born to mothers infected with agents that cause ophthalmia neonatorum may require special attention and systemic therapy as well as prophylaxis. A single dose of aqueous crystalline penicillin G, 50,000 units/kg body weight for term and 20,000 units for low-birth-weight infants, should be administered intravenously to infants born to mothers with gonorrhea.
7. The detection and appropriate treatment of infections in pregnant women, which may result in ophthalmia neonatorum, are encouraged.
8. All physicians and hospitals should be required to report cases of ophthalmia neonatorum and etiologic agents to state and local health departments so that incidence data may be obtained to determine the effectiveness of the control measures.

*Center for Disease Control, Atlanta, specifies that up to 2 hours' delay is safe.

Postpartum care

Postpartum is the time between delivery and return of the reproductive organs to prepregnancy status.

Rh factor. An Rh-negative mother may receive RhoGAM within 72 hours of the completion of the pregnancy (see p. 517).

Rubella vaccine. If the mother's rubella titer is low, an appropriate time for inoculation is immediately after pregnancy.

Assessments

Fundus. Continue to assess the fundal height and position until the woman is discharged.

Lochia. The lochia normally progresses from blood red (bright) to darker red with some small clots (1 to 3 days postpartum), to pinkish thin, watery consistency (4 to 10 days), to a yellowish or creamy color (11 to 21 days). The odor should be similar to that of a normal menstrual flow; a foul-smelling odor should be reported. Pads should be changed at frequent regular intervals rather than waiting for them to become heavily laden.

Breastfeeding. On delivery, the breasts secrete a thin yellow fluid called colostrum. Within 3 to 4 days, breast milk becomes available. This may produce some discomfort for the mother as the breasts become congested. She may need to use a breast pump to prevent engorgement.

The quantity of breast milk varies among mothers. The diet, fluid intake, and level of anxiety all effect lactation. Oxytocin nasal spray may be necessary to help encourage milk letdown.

Remind the woman that breastfeeding is not a form of contraception. Alternative methods of contraception should be used if the patient does not desire to become pregnant immediately.

Mothers not desiring to breastfeed can be given lactation suppressants to inhibit milk secretion (see p. 513).

Before discharge. Review methods of contraception if necessary.

Follow-up exam. The mother usually returns for a thorough exam at the physician's office 6 to 8 weeks after delivery.

Patient Education Associated with Pregnancy

Communication and responsibility. Encourage open communication with the expectant family. They must be guided to insight into the pregnancy in order to assume responsibility for the continuation of care. Keep emphasizing those things the family can do to optimize the chances for a healthy baby, including maintenance of general health, nutritional needs, adequate rest and appropriate exercise, and continuation of prescribed medication therapy.

Expectations of therapy. Discuss the expectations of therapy.

Adequate rest, relaxation. Assist the individual to plan for adequate rest periods throughout the day to prevent fatigue, irritability, and overexhaustion.

Talk with the individual about planning rest periods during lunch breaks at work, when preschoolers are napping, or when the husband is home to care for children. A short period of relaxation in a reclining chair or just with her feet up may be beneficial when there is no time for sleep during the day.

Advise the patient to avoid long periods of standing in one place and to perform some daily activities while sitting.

Activity and exercise. Generally, the woman can continue to perform common activities of daily living.

New attempts at strenuous exercise (such as jogging, aerobics) should not be started during pregnancy. Daily walks in the fresh air are encouraged.

Any changes in activity level should be discussed with the physician BEFORE starting.

Encourage good posture and participation in prenatal classes where exercises to strengthen the abdominal muscles and to relax the pelvic floor muscles are taught.

The woman should avoid lifting heavy objects or conditions that might cause physical harm, especially as the pregnancy progresses and her balance may be affected.

Employment. Advice about continued employment should be based on the type of job, working conditions, amount of lifting, standing, or exposure to toxic substances, and the individual's state of health.

General personal hygiene. Encourage maintenance of general hygiene through daily tub baths or showers. Tub baths near the end of pregnancy may be discouraged because of the danger of slipping and falling while getting in and out of the tub. Tub baths should not be taken once the membranes have ruptured.

Encourage the use of plain soap and water to cleanse the genital area and prevent odors. The woman should *not* use deodorant sprays because of possible irritation.

Tell the pregnant woman that an increase in vaginal discharge is common. Discharge that is yellowish or greenish, foul-smelling, or causes irritation and itching should be reported for further evaluation.

Clothing. Encourage the mother to dress in nonconstricting clothing.

As the pregnancy progresses, the mother may be more comfortable with a maternity girdle to support the abdomen. Encourage the mother to wear a well-fitting brassiere to provide proper support for the breasts. She should avoid restrictive circular garters that may impede circulation.

Encourage low-heeled, well-fitting shoes that provide good support. Properly fitting shoes can prevent lower back fatigue as well as tired feet.

Oral hygiene. Encourage the mother-to-be to have a thorough dental exam at the beginning of the pregnancy. She should tell the dentist she is pregnant at the time of the examination.

Encourage thorough daily brushing, flossing, and use of an appropriate mouthwash.

Sexual activity. Refer to an obstetrical text for discussion of alterations in sexuality during pregnancy. The wide range of feelings, needs, and intervention deserve more consideration than can be presented in this text.

Smoking and alcohol. The mother-to-be should be encouraged to abstain from smoking or drinking during pregnancy. A vast amount of data now points out that smoking or drinking is potentially dangerous to the fetus. An increased incidence of neonatal mortality, low birth weight, and prematurity has been reported.

Nutritional needs. Balanced nutrition is always to be encouraged, but is especially important throughout the course of the pregnancy. The Recommended Daily Allowances vary based on the individual's age, weight at the time of pregnancy, and daily activity level. At all times allowances must be made to maintain the nutritional needs of the mother and fetus. Refer to a nutrition text for specific recommendations.

Encourage limiting the caffeine content of the diet during pregnancy. Limit the consumption of coffee, tea, cola beverages, and cocoa. Tell the mother-to-be to check labels for specific caffeine content, as many soft drinks contain a significant quantity of caffeine.

Bowel habits. Assess the individual's usual pattern of elimination and anticipate its continuance until later in pregnancy. Pressure on the lower bowel from the presenting part of the fetus may cause constipation and hemorrhoids. Stool softeners or a mild laxative may be prescribed if problems persist.

Encourage the consumption of fresh fruits, vegetables, whole grain and bran products, along with an adequate intake of six to eight 8-ounce glasses of fluid daily.

Douching. Discourage any type of douching unless specifically prescribed for the individual by the physician.

Be certain when douching is prescribed that the patient is given simple, explicit instructions.

Heartburn. Tell the woman to avoid highly spiced foods and any foods that she knows have caused heartburn in the past. (See Chapter 14.)

Changes in expectations. Assess changes in expectations as pregnancy progresses. Teach the woman how to deal with discomforts such as development of a backache, leg cramps, hemorrhoids, and edema.

Changes in therapy through cooperative goal-setting. Work with the mother-to-be to encourage adherence to the regimen. When she feels that a change should be made in a treatment plan, encourage discussion with the physician.

Written record. Enlist the mother's aid in developing and maintaining a written record of monitoring parameters (blood pressure, pulse, daily weights, presence and relief of discomfort, exercise tolerance, fetal movement) and response to prescribed therapies for discussion with the physician (Figures 20-2 and 20-3). The woman should be encouraged to take this record on follow-up visits.

The woman should always report immediately loss of fluid vaginally, dizziness, double or blurred vision, severe headache, abdominal pain or persistent vomiting, fever, edema of the face, fingers, legs, or feet, and weight gain in excess of 2 pounds per week.

Fostering compliance. Throughout the pregnancy, discuss medication information and how it will benefit the course of treatment. Seek cooperation and understanding of the following points so that medication compliance may be enhanced:

1. Name
2. Dosage
3. Route and administration times
4. Anticipated therapeutic response
5. Side effects to expect
6. Side effects to report
7. What to do if a dose is missed
8. When, how, or if to refill the medication prescription

Difficulty in comprehension. If it is evident that the patient and/or family does not understand all aspects of continuing therapy being prescribed (such as administration and monitoring of medications, exercises, diets, follow-up appointments), consider the use of social service or visiting nurse agencies.

Associated teaching. Give the following instructions:

Always inform the physician or dentist of any prescription or over-the-counter medication being taken. Over-the-counter medications should not be taken without discussing them first with the physician or pharmacist.

Always report side effects of rash, itching, or hives immediately. Nausea, vomiting, or diarrhea should also be reported for the physician's evaluation if it is a new symptom.

Take all of the medication as prescribed for the full course of treatment. Do not discontinue use when feeling improved; do not save for future use; do not give your medicine to another individual. Sudden discontinuation of certain medications may produce harmful effects.

Keep all medications out of reach of children.

At discharge. Items to be sent home with the pregnant woman should include the following:

1. Written instructions for use
2. Labels in a level of language and size of print appropriate for the patient
3. If needed, identification cards or bracelets
4. A list of additional supplies to be purchased after discharge (such as nipple care products, pads, dressings, cord-care supplies)
5. A schedule for follow-up appointments

Drug Therapy with Pregnancy

Uterine stimulants

OBJECTIVES

1. State the primary clinical indications for use of uterine stimulants.
2. Describe specific nursing concerns and appropriate nursing actions when uterine stimulants are administered for induction of labor, augmentation of labor, and postpartum atony and hemorrhage.
3. Explain the limitations of use of oxytocin for the purpose of initiating a therapeutic abortion.
4. Review the procedure for insertion of vaginal suppositories.
5. Differentiate between the uses and actions on the uterus of dinoprostone, ergonovine maleate, methylergonovine maleate, and oxytocin.
6. Identify specific nursing assessments, interventions, and evaluation criteria used during the administration of uterine stimulants.
7. Compare the effects of methylergonovine maleate and ergonovine maleate on lactation.
8. Identify specific actions, dosage and administration, and nursing assessments needed during the use of oxytocin therapy.
9. Describe symptoms of fetal distress.
10. Cite the effect of oxytocin on fluid balance.

KEY WORDS

precipitous labor and delivery
dysfunctional labor
prostaglandins
augmentation

There are four primary clinical indications for the use of uterine stimulants: (1) induction or augmentation of labor, (2) control of postpartum atony and hemorrhage, (3) control of postsurgical hemorrhage (as in cesarean birth), and (4) to induce therapeutic abortion.

Obstetric and Gynecologic Agents

Patient Education and Monitoring of Therapeutic Outcomes for Patients Receiving Prenatal Care

Medications	Color	To be taken

Name _____

Physician _____

Physician's phone _____

Next appt.* _____

Parameters		Day of exam								Comments
Weight										
Blood pressure										
Pulse										
Pain	Cramps?									
	Backache?									
	Abdominal pain?									
Bleeding	With cramps?									
	# pads used per day									
	Describe color (bright or dark red)									
Edema	Morning									
	Evening									
	Other									
	Location: Hands, feet, ankles?									
Fatigue
All day After exercise Normal
10 5 1										
Exercise
Poor toleration Moderate toleration Normal
10 5 1										
Fetal movement	Normal?									
	None?									
Bowel movements
Constipated Normal Diarrhea
10 5 1										

*Please bring this record with you to your next appointment.
Use the back of this sheet for additional information.

Figure 20-2 *Patient education and monitoring of therapeutic outcomes for patients receiving prenatal care.*

Patient Education and Monitoring of Therapeutic Outcomes for Patients Receiving Postpartum Care

Medications	Color	To be taken

Name _____

Physician _____

Physician's phone _____

Next appt.* _____

Parameters		Day of discharge							Comments
Weight									
Blood pressure	AM / PM	/	/	/	/	/	/	/	
Pulse	AM / PM	/	/	/	/	/	/	/	
Lochia	# pads /day ?								
	Color of vaginal discharge								
Cramps Frequent 10 Moderate 5 None 1									
Breast tenderness	↑ discomfort								
	↓ discomfort								
	No problem								
Nipple condition	Sore								
	Cracking								
	No problem								
Sexual activity	Persistently painful								
	Uncomfortable								
	Normal								
Bowel movements	Constipation								
	Normal								

*Please bring this record with you to your next appointment.
Use the back of this sheet for additional information.

Figure 20-3 *Patient education and monitoring of therapeutic outcomes for patients receiving postpartum care.*

Induction of labor. Uterine stimulants, primarily oxytocin, may be prescribed in cases in which, in the physician's judgment, continuation of the pregnancy is considered to be a greater risk to the mother or fetus than the risk associated with drug-induced induction of labor. Such maternal conditions as a history of precipitous labor and delivery, postterm pregnancy, prolonged pregnancy with placental insufficiency, prolonged rupture of the membranes, or pregnancy-induced hypertension may be indications for induction of labor. Vaginal suppositories and gels of prostaglandins are currently being tested as adjunctive therapy to help ripen the cervix.

Augmentation of labor. In general, oxytocin should not be used to hasten labor. The type and force of contraction induced by the oxytocin may be harmful to the mother and fetus. In occasional cases, however, of *dysfunctional labor*, there is a prolonged latent phase of cervical dilatation or arrest of descent through the birth canal. Oxytocin infusions starting with low dosages and continuous fetal monitoring may be beneficial in these cases.

Postpartum atony and hemorrhage. After delivery of the fetus and the placenta, the uterus sometimes remains flaccid and "boggy." Continued intravenous infusions of low-dose oxytocin or intramuscular injections of ergonovine or methylergonovine are frequently used to stimulate firm uterine contractions so as to reduce the risk of postpartum hemorrhage from an atonic uterus. Occasionally, oral dosages of ergonovine or methylergonovine are administered for a few days after delivery to assist in uterine involution.

Therapeutic abortion. Pharmacological agents are usually not effective in evacuating uterine contents until several weeks into the second trimester of pregnancy. Various dosage forms of prostaglandins and hypertonic (20%) sodium chloride may be effective. Uterine smooth muscle is not very responsive to oxytocin stimulation until late in the third trimester, so even large doses of oxytocin are not indicated in therapeutic abortion. Regardless of the stage of pregnancy, stimulants such as ergonovine or methylergonovine may be prescribed after emptying the uterus to control bleeding and maintain uterine muscle tone.

dinoprostone (die'no-prahs-tone)

Prostaglandin E-2, Prostin E-2

Dinoprostone, or prostaglandin E-2, is a uterine and gastrointestinal smooth muscle stimulant. When used during pregnancy, it increases the frequency and strength of uterine contraction and produces cervical softening and dilatation. Dinoprostone is used to expel uterine contents in cases of intrauterine fetal death, benign hydatidiform mole, missed spontaneous miscarriage, and second trimester abortion. Occasionally, oxytocin and dinoprostone are used together to shorten the duration of time required to expel uterine contents.

Side effects. The most frequently observed gastrointestinal side effects are nausea, vomiting, and diarrhea.

Temperature elevations about 38° C (100.6° F) occur within 15 to 45 minutes and continue for up to 6 hours in 50 to 70% of patients.

Headache, chills, and shivering occur in about 10% of patients receiving dinoprostone. Transient hypotension with a drop in diastolic pressure of 20 mm Hg, dizziness, flushing, and arrhythmias have all been reported.

Fragments of uterine contents are frequently left in the uterus after evacuation. Patients should be manually examined to prevent the development of fever, infection, and hemorrhage.

Availability

Vaginal suppository—20 mg.

Dosage and administration

Adult

Intravaginal—Insert 1 suppository high into the posterior vaginal fornix. Patients should remain supine for at least 10 minutes after each insertion. Suppositories should be inserted every 2 to 5 hours, depending on uterine activity and tolerance to side effects.

• Nursing Interventions: Monitoring dinoprostone therapy

See also General Nursing Considerations for Obstetric Patients.

Side effects to expect

NAUSEA, VOMITING, DIARRHEA. Premedication with an antiemetic such as prochlorpromazine and an antidiarrheal agent (loperamide or diphenoxylate) will reduce, but usually not completely eliminate, these adverse effects.

FEVER. Sponge baths with water or alcohol and maintaining fluid intake may provide symptomatic relief.

Aspirin does not inhibit dinoprostone-induced fever.

Patients should be observed for clinical indications of intrauterine infection. Monitor temperature and vital signs every ½ hour.

Side effects to report

ORTHOSTATIC HYPOTENSION. Although this effect is infrequent and generally mild, dinoprostone may cause some degree of orthostatic hypotension manifested by dizziness, flushing, and weakness, particularly when therapy is initiated.

Monitor the blood pressure in both the supine and standing positions.

Anticipate the development of postural hypotension and take measures to prevent its occurrence. For ambulatory patients, teach the patient to rise slowly from a supine or sitting position, and encourage her to sit or lie down if feeling faint. Report rapidly falling blood pressure, as well as bradycardia, paleness, or other alterations in vital signs.

Implementation

WARMING SUPPOSITORY. Prior to removing the tinfoil, allow the suppository to warm to room temperature.

Drug interactions. No clinically significant interactions have been reported.

ergonovine maleate (er-go-no'veen mal-ee-ate)

Ergotrate Maleate (er'go-trayt)

methylergonovine maleate
(meth-il-er-go-no'veen mal-ee-ate)

Methergine (meth'er-jin)

Ergonovine and methylergonovine are structurally similar ergot derivatives that share similar actions. Both drugs directly stimulate contractions of the uterus. Small doses produce uterine contractions with normal resting muscle tone; intermediate doses cause more forceful and prolonged contractions with an elevated resting muscle tone; and large doses cause severe, prolonged contractions. Due to this sudden, intense uterine activity, which is dangerous to the fetus, these agents cannot be used for induction of labor. However, because these agents produce more sustained contractions than oxytocin, small doses of ergonovine and methylergonovine are used in postpartum patients to control bleeding and maintain uterine firmness.

Side effects. The most common side effects are nausea and vomiting, and these are fairly infrequent. Other rare side effects reported include hypertension, dizziness, dyspnea, tinnitus, headache, and palpitations. Patients may also complain of abdominal cramping.

Availability

PO—0.2 mg tablets.

INJ—0.2 mg/ml in 1 ml ampules.

Dosage and administration. NOTE: Use with extreme caution in patients with hypertension, preeclampsia, heart disease, venoatrial shunts, mitral valve stenosis, sepsis, or hepatic or renal impairment.

Adult

PO—0.2 mg every 6 to 8 hours after delivery for a maximum of 1 week.

IM—0.2 mg every 2 to 4 hours, to a maximum of 5 doses.

• **Nursing Interventions: Monitoring ergot therapy**

See also General Nursing Considerations for Obstetric Patients.

Side effects to expect

NAUSEA, VOMITING. These side effects are usually mild and tend to resolve with continued therapy. Encourage the patient not to discontinue therapy without first consulting the physician.

ABDOMINAL CRAMPING. This is normally an indication of therapeutic activity, but, if severe, reduction or discontinuation of dosage may be necessary.

Side effects to report

HYPERTENSION. Certain patients, especially those who are eclamptic or previously hypertensive, may be particularly sensitive to the hypertensive effects of these agents. These patients have a higher incidence of developing generalized headaches, severe arrhythmias, and strokes. Monitor the patient's blood pressure and pulse rate and rhythm. Report immediately if the patient complains of headache or palpitations.

Drug interactions

INHIBITION OF PROLACTIN. Do not use ergonovine in patients who wish to breastfeed. Methylergonovine may be used as an alternative, since it will not inhibit stimulation of milk production by prolactin.

CAUDAL OR SPINAL ANESTHESIA. Hypertension and headaches may develop in patients who have received caudal or spinal anesthesia followed by a dose of either methylergonovine or ergonovine. Monitor the patient's blood pressure and heart rate and rhythm.

oxytocin (ok-se-to'sin)

Pitocin (pih-to'sin)

Oxytocin is a hormone produced in the hypothalamus and stored in the pituitary gland. When released, it stimulates the smooth muscle of the uterus, blood vessels, and the mammary glands. When it is administered during the third trimester of pregnancy, active labor may be initiated.

Oxytocin is the current drug of choice for inducing labor at term and for augmenting uterine contractions during the first and second stages of labor. Oxytocin is routinely administered immediately postpartum to control uterine atony and postpartum hemorrhage. Oxytocin may also be administered intranasally to promote milk letdown and to treat breast engorgement during lactation.

Side effects. Side effects that may occur include nausea, vomiting, hypotension, tachycardia, and arrhythmias.

Oxytocin has some minor antidiuretic activity. When administered in large doses or over prolonged periods with electrolyte-free solutions, water intoxication may occur.

Overdosage of oxytocin may cause hyperstimulation of the uterus, resulting in severe contractions with possible abruptio placentae, cervical lacerations, impaired uterine blood flow, and fetal trauma.

Availability

IV—10 units/ml in 1 and 10 ml vials and 1 ml disposable syringes.

Nasal Spray—40 units/ml in 2 and 5 ml squeeze bottles.

Dosage and administration

Induction of labor. IV—Initial rate: 1 to 2 mU/minute. It is strongly recommended that an infusion pump be used to help control the rate of oxytocin infusion. Most pregnancies close to term will respond well to 2 to 10 mU/minute. Rarely will a patient require more than 20 mU/minute. Those patients at 32 to 36 weeks of gestation often require 20 to 30 mU/min or more to develop a laborlike contraction pattern. Rates of infusion should not be altered more frequently than every 20 to 30 minutes. It is frequently necessary to reduce or discontinue the infusion as spontaneous uterine activity develops and labor progresses.

Augmentation of labor

IV—Occasionally a labor that started spontaneously may not progress satisfactorily. Labor may be augmented by oxytocin infusions at rates of 0.5 to 2 mU/minute.

Postpartum hemorrhage

IM—10 units given after delivery of the placenta.

IV—10 to 40 units may be added to 100 ml of fluid and electrolyte solution and run at a rate necessary to control uterine atony.

Mild letdown

Intranasal spray—1 spray or 3 drops may be instilled into 1 or both nostrils 2 to 3 minutes before nursing or pumping of the breasts.

• Nursing Interventions: Monitoring oxytocin therapy

See also General Nursing Considerations for Obstetric Patients.

Side effects to expect

UTERINE CONTRACTIONS. Oxytocin infusions should be monitored by both a tocometer (measures uterine contractions) and a fetal heart monitor.

Maintain an ongoing record of the frequency, duration, and intensity of uterine contractions. Duration of contractions over 90 seconds requires the flow rate of the oxytocin to be slowed or discontinued.

NAUSEA, VOMITING. Although infrequent, these side effects may occur. Reduction in dosage may control symptoms.

Side effects to report

FETAL DISTRESS. Fetal heart rate should be monitored continuously, but especially closely during uterine contractions. (Normal fetal heart rate = 120 to 160 beats per minute.) Indications of fetal distress may be manifested by tachycardia (>160 bpm) followed by bradycardia (<120 bpm). As the degree of distress progresses, bradycardia occurs more frequently and lasts longer than 15 seconds after contractions.

If the infant develops sudden distress, reduce the oxytocin infusion to the slowest possible rate according to hospital policy, turn the mother to the left lateral position, administer oxygen by nasal cannula or face mask, and call the physician immediately.

HYPERTENSION, HYPOTENSION. Check the mother's blood pressure and pulse rate at least every 30 minutes while infusing oxytocin. Report trends upward or downward, since oxytocin may cause hyper- or hypotension.

WATER INTOXICATION. Oxytocin can alter fluid balance by stimulating antidiuretic hormone, causing the body to accumulate water. This is particularly more likely to occur if oxytocin is administered with electrolyte solutions.

Symptoms of water intoxication include drowsiness, listlessness, headache, confusion, anuria, edema, and, in extreme cases, seizures.

DEHYDRATION. Since mothers are routinely placed NPO during labor, an occasional patient may develop dehydration even though an IV is running. Monitor urine output, dry crusted lips, and requests for water. Report to the physician and request ice chips and additional IV fluids if appropriate.

POSTPARTUM HEMORRHAGE. Early postpartum hemorrhage occurs within the first 24 hours after delivery and is usually defined as a blood loss of 500 ml or greater during this time span.

The hemorrhage may be caused by uterine atony, retained fragments of placenta, or lacerations of the vaginal tract. Less frequent causes include defective blood clotting mechanisms, uterine eversion, and uterine infections.

Oxytocin is routinely administered after delivery of the placenta to cause the uterus to contract and to decrease blood loss. Always check the height of the fundus of the uterus (usually at umbilical level) every 5 minutes following delivery. Report if the uterus is not firm or the height is rising. (This may be an indication of urinary retention or a uterus filling with blood.) When the uterus becomes boggy, uterine massage is necessary until it becomes firm.

Check the vaginal flow rate on each perineal pad at least every ½ hour. With uterine atony or retained placental fragments, the uterus becomes boggy and DARK vaginal bleeding is present; with a laceration of the cervix or vagina, the bleeding is BRIGHT red and the uterus is firm. Regardless of the cause, the woman is observed carefully for signs of hypovolemic shock.

Monitor vital signs as ordered by the physician, or every 15 minutes until stable, every 30 minutes for 2 hours, then every hour until definitely stable. Report an increasing respiratory rate; pulse rate that increases and becomes thready; a pulse deficit; blood pressure that becomes hypotensive; skin that is pale, cold, and clammy; or nail beds, lips, and mucous membranes that are pale or cyanotic. Monitor hourly urine output and report an output of 30 ml/hour or less. Observe for restlessness and complaints of thirst and for any decrease in level of consciousness.

Implementation

STARTING THE INFUSION. Establish records of baseline vital signs, I/O.

Oxytocin administered IV should be added to the solution after the IV is shown to be patent and running.

RATE. Careful monitoring of the prescribed rate of infusion is imperative. Should the IV line suddenly open, the resulting severe contractions could be extremely dangerous to the mother.

INFUSION PUMP. A constant infusion pump is recommended for control of the rate of administration. Keep in mind that a pump can still fail; continue to monitor the number of drops per minute from the drip chamber.

Drug interactions

ANESTHETICS. Monitor the blood pressure and heart rate and rhythm closely. Report significant changes in the blood pressure or pulse.

For those patients receiving a local anesthetic containing epinephrine, report any complaints of sweating, fever, chest pain, palpitations, or severe "throbbing" headache immediately.

Uterine relaxants

OBJECTIVES

1. Compare the effects of uterine stimulants and uterine relaxants on the pregnant uterus.
2. State the effect of hydroxyprogesterone on pituitary hormone secretions.
3. Identify the recommended site of administration for hydroxyprogesterone.
4. Review the effects of adrenergic agents on beta-1 and beta-2 receptors, then identify the relationship of these actions to the side effects to report when adrenergic agents are used to inhibit preterm labor.
5. Cite the effects of adrenergic agents on serum glucose and electrolyte balance.
6. Describe specific assessments needed prior to and during the use of ritodrine or terbutaline.
7. State the baseline laboratory studies needed prior to the initiation of ritodrine or terbutaline therapy.
8. Describe the potential effects of ritodrine or terbutaline on the neonate.

KEY WORD

beta stimulation

Uterine relaxants are used primarily to delay or prevent preterm labor and delivery in selected patients (p. 498).

hydroxyprogesterone (hi-drox'ee-pro-jest'er-own)

Delalutin (del-ah' lew-tin)

Hydroxyprogesterone inhibits the secretion of the pituitary hormones—luteinizing hormone (LH) and follicle-stimulating hormone (FSH)—and inhibits uterine contractions in the pregnant uterus. It is used in obstetrics to prevent habitual miscarriage. It is not effective once premature labor has started, but it may possibly be effective if administered periodically after the 20th week of pregnancy.

Side effects. There are essentially no side effects associated with hydroxyprogesterone therapy. The most common side effect is pain at the injection site. Rarely, hydroxyprogesterone may induce fluid retention. There is a slightly increased incidence of blood clot formation and thrombophlebitis.

Availability

Injection—125 mg/ml in 10 ml vials; 250 mg/ml in 5 ml vials.

Dosage and administration. NOTE: Do not administer during the first 4 months of pregnancy. Teratogenicity may result.

Adult

IM—250 mg once weekly injected deeply into the upper outer quadrant of the gluteal muscle.

• **Nursing Interventions: Monitoring hydroxyprogesterone therapy**

See also General Nursing Considerations for Obstetric Patients.

Side effects to report

FLUID RETENTION. Weigh patients on a regular basis and monitor for an increase in blood pressure or edema.

THROMBOPHLEBITIS. Patients should be encouraged to report any symptoms of pain in the calves or chest, sudden shortness of breath, coughing of blood, severe headache, dizziness, faintness, or changes in vision as soon as possible.

Implementation

IM. Administer by deep injection into the upper, outer quadrant of the gluteal muscle.

Drug interactions. No clinically significant interactions have been reported.

ritodrine hydrochloride (rih'toh-dreen)

Yutopar (u'toh-par)

terbutaline sulfate (ter-bew'tal-een)

Bricanyl (brih-can'il)

Ritodrine and terbutaline are beta adrenergic receptor stimulants, acting predominantly on the beta-2 receptors, but, especially in higher dosages, on the beta-1 receptors as well. Stimulation of the beta-2 receptors produces relaxation of the uterine, bronchial, and vascular smooth muscle. Beta-1 receptor stimulation causes an increased heart rate. Because of selective relaxant properties on the uterus, causing a reduction in the intensity and frequency of uterine contractions, these agents are used in cases of premature labor where it has been determined that there is no underlying pathology that would indicate that pregnancy should not be allowed to progress to completion.

Side effects. Unfortunately, the receptors that are stimulated by beta receptor agents to cause relaxation of the smooth muscle of the uterus are found in other tissues as well as the reproductive system. They are found in the muscles of the heart, blood vessels, bronchopulmonary tree, gastrointestinal, urinary, and central nervous systems. They also help regulate fat and carbohydrate metabolism. For this reason, we can expect to see many side effects from these agents, particularly if used too frequently or in higher doses than recommended.

The most common side effects are dose-related. These include maternal and fetal tachycardia, averaging 130 and 164 beats per minute, respectively; tremor, nervousness, heart palpitations, and dizziness. Maternal systolic blood pressure increases to a range of 96 to 162 mm Hg, while diastolic pressures drop to a range of 0 to 76 mm Hg. Other side effects that may occur less frequently include nausea, vomiting, headache, restlessness, drowsiness, sweating, and tinnitus.

Ritodrine and terbutaline routinely increase serum glucose and insulin levels, though these tend to return to normal within 48 to 72 hours with continued infusion. Diabetic patients should be monitored closely.

Serum potassium levels may drop during IV administration. Urinary losses generally do not increase; much of the losses are actually due to intracellular redistribution, which will return to the blood after discontinuation of therapy.

Patients known to have hypertension, hyperthyroidism, diabetes mellitus, or cardiac disease with arrhythmias may be particularly sensitive to adverse reactions and must be observed closely.

Neonatal adverse effects are infrequent, but hyperglycemia, hypoglycemia, hypocalcemia, hypotension, and paralytic ileus have been reported.

Availability

Ritodrine
PO—10 mg tablets.
Injection—10 mg/ml in 5 ml ampules; 15 mg/ml in 10 ml vials.

Terbutaline
PO—2.5 and 5 mg tablets.
Injection—1 mg/ml in 1 ml ampules.
Dosage and administration. See Tables 20-3 and 20-4 and boxes on p. 512.

• Nursing Interventions: Monitoring ritodrine and terbutaline therapy

See also General Nursing Considerations for Obstetrical Patients

Side effects to report

TACHYCARDIA, PALPITATIONS. Since most symptoms are dose-related, alterations should be reported to the physician. Monitor the mother's and infant's heart rates and rhythms at regular intervals throughout therapy. Report heart rates significantly higher than baseline values.

Always report palpitations and suspected arrhythmias.

TREMORS. Tell the patient to notify the physician if tremors develop after starting any of these medications. A dosage adjustment may be necessary.

NERVOUSNESS, ANXIETY, RESTLESSNESS, HEADACHE. Perform a baseline assessment of the patient's mental status (degree of anxiety, nervousness, alertness); compare at regular intervals to the findings obtained. Report escalation of tension.

NAUSEA, VOMITING. Monitor all aspects of the development of these symptoms.

Table 20-4 *Terbutaline Infusion Rate**

ml/hr	15	20	30	40	50	60	70	80	90
µg/min	5	6.6	10	13	16	20	23	26	30

(From Clayton BD: *Handbook of pharmacology*, ed 4, St. Louis, 1987, Mosby–Year Book.)
*Administer 20 mg/1000 ml or 20 µg/ml.

Table 20-3 *Ritodrine Solution Concentrations and Rates**

5 ml amps/500 ml†		1	2	3	4	5
mg/500 ml		50	100	150	200	250
µg/ml		100	200	300	400	500
µgtts/min	ml/min	µg/min	µg/min	µg/min	µg/min	µg/min
5	0.08	8	16	24	32	40
10	0.16	16	32	48	64	80
15	0.25	25	50	75	100	125
20	0.33	33	66	99	132	165
25	0.41	41	82	123	164	205
30	0.5	50	100	150	200	250
35	0.58	58	116	174	232	290
40	0.66	66	132	198	264	330
45	0.75	75	150	225	300	375
50	0.83	83	166	249	332	415
55	0.91	91	182	273	364	455
60	1.00	100	200	300	400	500

(From Clayton BD: *Handbook of pharmacology*, ed 4, St. Louis, 1987, Mosby–Year Book.)
*Using a microdrip administration set—60 gtts/ml.
†Dilute in 500 ml of 0.9% sodium chloride, dextrose 5%, 10% dextran 40 in 0.9% sodium chloride, 10% fructose, Ringer's solution, or Hartmann's solution.
Usual initial dose is 50 to 100 µ/min. Increase by 50 µg/min every 10 min until desired result is attained. The effective dose usually lies between 150 and 350 µg/min. Frequent monitoring of maternal uterine contractions, heart rate, and blood pressure and of fetal heart rate is mandatory, with dosage individually titrated according to response.

Guidelines for use of ritodrine in premature labor

1. Initiate a control IV of dextrose 5%, Ringer's lactate, or saline solution and administer 400 to 500 ml in 15 to 20 minutes before the initiation of the medication. Then decrease to 100 to 125 ml/hr.
2. Make a ritodrine infusion solution using Table 20-3. The usual concentration is 3 ampules in 500 ml of parenteral solution, but weaker or stronger concentrations may be used depending on the patient's fluid requirements.
3. Have the patient recline in the left lateral position to minimize hypotension.
4. The usual initial dosage is 50 to 100 μg/minute. Increase by 50 μg/minute every 10 minutes until labor is inhibited or side effects prevent further increases in dosage. The effective dose is usually 150 to 350 μg/minute. Frequent monitoring of maternal uterine contractions, heart rate, and blood pressure and fetal heart rate is mandatory, with dosage individually titrated according to response.
5. Fluid input and output, breath sounds, and blood glucose and serum electrolyte levels must be monitored periodically to prevent fluid overload, hyperglycemia, or hypokalemia.
6. The IV infusion is maintained for 8 to 12 hours after cessation of uterine contractions.
7. Start oral ritodrine tablets 30 to 60 minutes before discontinuation of IV therapy. The initial doses are 10 mg every 2 hours for the first 24 hours, then 10 to 20 mg every 4 to 6 hours, depending on uterine activity and side effects.
8. Recurrence of premature labor may be treated starting the guidelines over again. Labor may be arrested on lower IV dosages, depending on the patient's compliance with the oral medication regimen.

Guidelines for use of terbutaline with premature labor*

1. Initiate a control IV of dextrose 5%, Ringer's lactate, or saline solution and administer 400 to 500 ml in 15 to 20 minutes before initiation of the medication. Then decrease to 100 to 125 ml/hr.
2. Add 20 mg of terbutaline to 1000 ml of dextrose 5%.
3. Place the patient in a left lateral, horizontal position with a blood pressure cuff in position.
4. Administer a loading dose of 250 μg IV over 1 to 2 minutes. Monitor very closely for hypotension.
5. Start the infusion at a rate of 10 μg IV (30 ml/hr) using Table 20-4.
6. Increase the infusion rate by 3.5 μg/minute (10 ml/hr) every 10 minutes until labor has stopped or a maximum dose of 26 μg/minute (80 ml/hr) has been attained.
7. Maintain the effective dose for 1 hr or more, then begin decreasing the rate by 2 μg/min (6 ml/hr) every 30 minutes until the lowest effective dose is reached. Maintain the total IV fluid intake at 125 ml/hr.
8. When the lowest effective IV dose is reached, begin PO terbutaline, 2.5 mg every 4 hours.
9. If labor has stopped, discontinue the IV infusion 24 hr after PO administration was initiated if the uterus is not irritable.
10. Continue the PO regimen (2.5 mg every 4 hr or 5 mg every 8 hr) until 36 weeks gestation.
11. If labor begins again, restart the IV infusion as above.

*NOTE: Terbutaline is not approved by the FDA for use in premature labor. It may be used, however, in emergency situations when the physician judges that it is in the best interests of the patient and infant.

When terbutaline is used for premature labor, a sometimes significant drop in blood pressure (due to vasodilatory effects) can be observed at the time of the loading dose and when the infusion is started. Blood pressure and pulse monitoring should be done before and every 5 minutes after the loading dose has been administered and the infusion started, until the patient is stable. Use continuous fetal monitoring. If the maternal pulse exceeds 120 beats/minute and does not decrease with an increase in fluids or when the patient is rolled on her left side, or if there is any evidence of a decrease in uterine perfusion, discontinue the infusion.

Administer the oral medication with food and a full glass of water or milk. Report if the symptoms are not relieved.

DIZZINESS. Provide for patient safety during episodes of dizziness; report for further evaluation.

BASELINE STUDIES. Obtain baseline laboratory data (serum glucose, chloride, sodium, potassium, hematocrit and carbon dioxide) BEFORE initiation of therapy. Monitoring should continue for alterations in baseline data. Report any changes immediately for physician evaluation.

HYPERGLYCEMIA. Diabetic or prediabetic patients need to be monitored for the development of hyperglycemia, particularly during the early days of therapy.

Assess regularly for glycosuria and report if it occurs with frequency.

Insulin requirements may double in these patients during ritodrine or terbutaline therapy.

ELECTROLYTE IMBALANCE. The electrolyte most commonly altered is potassium (K^+). *Hypokalemia* is most likely to occur.

Many symptoms associated with altered fluid and electrolyte balance are subtle.

Gather data relative to *changes* in the patient's mental status (i.e., alertness, orientation, confusion), muscle strength, muscle cramps, tremors, nausea, and general appearance (drowsy, anxious, lethargic).

Always check the electrolyte reports for early indications of electrolyte imbalance.

Keep accurate records of I/O, daily weights, and vital signs.

THE NEONATE. Neonatal adverse effects are infrequent, but hyperglycemia, followed by hypoglycemia, and hypocalcemia, hypotension, and paralytic ileus have been reported. Monitor these newborns closely over the next several hours. Make sure that the infant's sleep after birth is not masking these conditions.

Implementation

IV RATE. Use of an infusion pump is absolutely essential to the safe delivery of these agents.

PO. Administer with food or milk to reduce gastric irritation.

Drug interactions

DRUGS THAT ENHANCE TOXIC EFFECTS. Tricyclic antidepressants (imipramine, amitriptyline, nortriptyline, doxepine, others), monoamine oxidase inhibitors (tranylcypromine, isocarboxazid, pargyline), and other sympathomimetic agents (metaproterenol, isoproterenol, others).

Monitor for increases in severity of drug effects such as nervousness, tachycardia, tremors, and arrhythmias.

DRUGS THAT REDUCE THERAPEUTIC EFFECTS. Beta adrenergic blocking agents (propranolol, timolol, nadolol, pindolol, others).

CORTICOSTEROIDS. Concurrent use may rarely result in pulmonary edema. There is a higher incidence in patients with multiple pregnancy, occult cardiac disease, and fluid overload. Persistent tachycardia may be a sign of impending pulmonary edema. Observe patient closely, monitoring fluid input and output, breath sounds, and heart rate, as well as the patient's anxiety level and state of well-being.

ANTIHYPERTENSIVE AGENTS. Sympathomimetic agents may reduce the therapeutic effects of antihypertensive agents. Monitor blood pressure for an indication of loss of antihypertensive control.

ANESTHETICS. Concurrent use with general anesthetics may result in additional hypotensive effects. Monitor the blood pressure and heart rate and rhythm regularly.

Lactation suppressants
OBJECTIVES

1. State the names of pharmacological agents used to inhibit lactation in the postpartum patient.
2. Compare the dosage and scheduling of administration of bromocriptine, chlorotrianisene, and Deladumone OB.

KEY WORDS
breast engorgement   mastitis

bromocriptine mesylate (bro-mo′krip-teen)

Parlodel (par-lo′del)

Bromocriptine is a nonhormonal, nonestrogenic dopamine receptor stimulant that acts to inhibit secretion of prolactin from the anterior pituitary gland. Administration in postpartum women acts to prevent physiological lactation when therapy is started after delivery and continued for 2 to 3 weeks.

Side effects. Side effects are mild when bromocriptine is used in the relatively low doses needed to suppress lactation. The most frequently occurring adverse reactions are headache (10%), dizziness (8%), nausea (7%), vomiting (3%), fatigue (1%), syncopy (0.7%), and diarrhea and cramps (4%).

Availability

PO—2.5 tablets and 5 mg capsules.

Dosage and administration

Adult

PO—Initially, 2.5 mg twice daily with meals. The dosage must be adjusted according to the patient's response and tolerance. The usual dosage range is 2.5 to 7.5 mg daily. Therapy should be continued for 14 days; however, therapy may be given for up to 21 days if necessary.

• Nursing Interventions: Monitoring bromocriptine therapy

See also General Nursing Considerations for Obstetric Patients.

Side effects to expect

GASTROINTESTINAL EFFECTS. Most of these effects may be minimized by temporary reduction in dosage, administration with food, and use of stool softeners for constipation.

OVULATION. Early resumption of ovulation may occur in women receiving bromocriptine. Women should be informed of the need for contraception.

Side effects to report

NEUROLOGIC. These effects often occur with higher dosages.

Perform a baseline assessment of the patient's degree of alertness and orientation to name, place, and time *prior* to initiating therapy. Make regularly scheduled subsequent mental status evaluations and compare findings. Report development of alterations.

Provide for patient safety; be emotionally supportive.

ORTHOSTATIC HYPOTENSION. Monitor the blood pressure daily in both the supine and standing positions.

Anticipate the development of postural hypotension and take measures to prevent an occurrence. Teach the patient to rise slowly from a supine or sitting position, and encourage her to sit or lie down if feeling faint.

Dosage and administration

TIME OF ADMINISTRATION. Therapy should be started only after the patient's vital signs have stabilized and no sooner than 4 hours after delivery.

PO. Dosage must be adjusted according to the patient's response and tolerance. Side effects can be minimized by administering with food.

Drug interactions

TRICYCLIC ANTIDEPRESSANTS, RESERPINE, HALOPERIDOL, AND PHENOTHIAZINES. These agents increase prolactin levels.

The dosage of bromocriptine may have to be increased for therapeutic activity.

ANTIHYPERTENSIVE AGENTS. Dosage adjustment of the antihypertensive agent is frequently necessary because of excessive orthostatic hypotension.

chlorotrianisene (klo-ro-try-an′e-seen)

Tace (tase)

Chlorotrianisene is a long-acting, synthetic estrogen used in obstetrics to inhibit lactation and reduce the frequency of postpartum breast engorgement in patients who do not wish to breastfeed. It acts by inhibiting the action of prolactin, a pituitary hormone that is necessary for milk production.

Side effects. Side effects associated with short-term estrogen therapy are usually quite minimal. The most common side effect is nausea. There is a slightly increased incidence of blood clot formation and thrombophlebitis. Patients should be encouraged to report any symptoms of pain in the calves or chest, sudden shortness of breath, coughing of blood, severe headache, dizziness, faintness, or changes in vision as soon as possible.

Availability

PO—12, 25, and 72 mg capsules.

Dosage and administration

Adult

PO—Postpartum breast engorgement: 12 mg 4 times daily for 7 days, 50 mg every 6 hours for 6 doses, or 72 mg every 12 hours for 2 days. The first dose must be given within 8 hours after delivery.

• **Nursing Interventions: Monitoring chlorotrianisene therapy**

See also General Nursing Considerations for Obstetric Patients.

Side effects to expect

NAUSEA. Although it is infrequent, a few patients do experience nausea.

Side effects to report

THROMBOPHLEBITIS. Although this is a rare occurrence, patients should report any pain in the calves or chest, sudden shortness of breath, coughing of blood, severe headache, dizziness, faintness, or changes in vision as soon as possible.

Drug interactions

REDUCED THERAPEUTIC RESPONSE. The following agents may counteract the prolactin-inhibiting effects of chlorotrianisene: carbidopa, ethanol, haloperidol, methyldopa, metoclopramide, phenothiazines, reserpine, and thiothixene.

Other agents

OBJECTIVES

1. Describe the method of action of clomiphene citrate.

2. Identify the preliminary screening needed prior to initiation of clomiphene citrate therapy.

3. State the safety precautions needed in the event that visual disturbances occur with the use of clomiphene citrate.

4. Cite the specific time during the menstrual cycle when ovulation can be anticipated with the use of clomiphene citrate.

5. State the action of magnesium sulfate on the central nervous system.

6. State the normal range of blood levels of magnesium sulfate when used as an anticonvulsant.

7. Prepare a list of assessments that must be implemented during the administration of magnesium sulfate to detect toxicity.

8. Explain the rationale for monitoring urine output during magnesium sulfate therapy.

9. Cite methods used to assess deep tendon reflexes and specific findings that would require notification of the physician.

10. Identify treatment used when magnesium sulfate toxicity occurs.

11. Describe specific procedures and precautions needed during the intravenous and intramuscular administration of magnesium sulfate.

12. Identify emergency supplies that should be available in the immediate vicinity during magnesium sulfate therapy.

13. State the action and purpose of administration of Rh$_o$ (D) immune globulin.

14. Identify the specific dosage, administration precautions, and proper timing of the administration of Rh$_o$ (D) immune globulin.

15. State the appropriate treatment of fever, arthralgias, and generalized aches and pains that can be anticipated following Rh$_o$ (D) immune globulin administration.

16. Identify the purpose for the use of erythromycin ophthalmic ointment and tetracycline ointment and drops.

17. Describe the specific procedures used to instill erythromycin ophthalmic ointment and tetracycline ointment and drops.

18. State the causative organisms of ophthalmia neonatorum.

19. Explain the rationale for administering phytonadione to the neonate.

20. Identify the preferred site for intramuscular administration of vitamin K to a neonate.

21. Review the anatomical structures associated with the administration of intramuscular medications in an infant.

22. Describe the side effects to report that are associated with phytonadione therapy.

KEY WORD

biphasic temperature distribution

clomiphene citrate (klom'ih-feen si'trayt)

Clomid (klo'mid)

Clomiphene is a chemical compound that is structurally similar to natural estrogens. When administered, it binds to estrogen-receptor sites, reducing the number of sites available for circulating estrogens. The receptors send back signals to the hypothalamus and pituitary gland, indicating a lack of circulating estrogens. The hypothalamus responds by increasing the secretion of hypothalamic releasing factor. This stimulates the pituitary gland to release luteinizing hormone (LH) and follicle-stimulating hormone (FSH), which in turn stimulate the ovaries to release ova for potential fertilization. Thus, clomiphene is used to induce ovulation in women who were not ovulating due to reduced circulating estrogen levels. Studies indicate that pregnancy occurs in 25 to 30% of patients treated. Ovulation of more than one ovum per cycle with potential of fertilization of multiple ova may occur in 5 to 10% of patients treated.

Side effects. Side effects of clomiphene therapy tend to be quite mild and are generally dose-related. Common side effects include flushing, resembling menopausal hot flashes, and abdominal symptoms, resembling cyclic ovarian pain (mittelschmerz) and premenstrual symptoms. Nausea, vomiting, diarrhea, light-headedness and dizziness, and constipation have been reported less often.

Visual disturbances such as blurred or double vision, irritation from bright lights (photophobia) and "seeing spots before the eyes" may occur, particularly with higher doses.

Availability

PO—50 mg tablets.

Dosage and administration. NOTE: It is mandatory that patients have a complete physical examination to rule out other pathologic causes for lack of ovulation before the initiation of clomiphene therapy.

Patients must be informed of the possibility of multiple fetuses and the importance of timing sexual intercourse at the time of ovulation, usually 6 to 10 days after the last day of treatment.

Clomiphene should not be administered if pregnancy is suspected. Basal temperatures should be followed for the month following therapy. If the body temperature follows a biphasic distribution (peaks twice within a few days), and is not followed by menses, the next course of clomiphene therapy should not be scheduled until pregnancy tests have been completed.

Adult

PO—50 mg daily for 5 days. Start therapy at any time if there has been no recent bleeding. If spontaneous bleeding occurs before therapy, start on or about the fifth day for 5 days.

If ovulation does not occur after the first course, give a second course of 100 mg/day for 5 days. Start this course no earlier than 30 days after the previous course.

A third course may be administered at 100 mg/day for 5 days, but most patients who respond will have done so in the first 2 courses. Reevaluation of the patient is necessary.

- **Nursing Interventions: Monitoring clomiphene therapy**

Side effects to expect

NAUSEA, VOMITING, DIARRHEA, CONSTIPATION, ABDOMINAL CRAMPS. These side effects are usually mild and tend to resolve with continued therapy. Encourage the patient not to discontinue therapy without first consulting the physician.

Side effects to report

SEVERE ABDOMINAL CRAMPS. Patients should be informed to report significant abdominal or pelvic pain and bloating that develop during therapy.

VISUAL DISTURBANCES. Patients developing visual blurring, spots, or double vision should report for an eye examination. The drug is usually discontinued, and visual disturbances pass within a few days to weeks following discontinuation.

Caution the patient to avoid temporarily tasks that require visual acuity, such as driving or operating power machinery.

DIZZINESS. Provide for patient safety during episodes of dizziness; report for further evaluation.

Administration

POSSIBLE PREGNANCY. Clomiphene should not be administered if pregnancy is suspected. Instruct the patient on how to take and record basal temperatures, and how to report a biphasic temperature distribution.

TIMING OF INTERCOURSE. The timing of intercourse is important to the success of therapy. Make sure the patient understands the importance of having intercourse during the time of ovulation, usually 6 to 10 days after the last dose of medication.

Drug interactions. No clinically significant drug interactions have been reported.

magnesium sulfate

Magnesium is an ion normally found in the blood in concentrations of 1.8 to 3 mEq/liter. When administered parenterally in doses sufficient to produce levels above 4 mEq/liter, the drug may depress the central nervous system and block peripheral nerve transmission, producing anticonvulsant effects and smooth muscle relaxation. It is used primarily in obstetrics for the control of seizure activity associated with preeclampsia or eclampsia. It may also be used to inhibit premature labor in patients who cannot tolerate ritodrine. When used as an anticonvulsant or to inhibit labor, blood levels should be maintained at 4 to 8 mEq/liter.

Side effects. Patients maintained at a magnesium serum level between 3 and 5 mEq/liter rarely show any side effects from hypermagnesemia. At levels about 5 to 8 mEq/liter, patients start showing increasing signs of toxicity that correlate fairly well to serum levels. Early signs of maternal toxicity are complaints of "feeling hot all over" and "being thirsty all the time," flushed skin color, and sweating. Patients may then become hypotensive, have depressed patellar, radial, and biceps reflexes, and have flaccid muscles. Later signs of hypermagnesemia are CNS depression shown first by anxiety, then confusion, lethargy, and drowsiness. If serum levels continue to increase, cardiac depression and respiratory paralysis may result. Magnesium sulfate should be administered with extreme caution to patients with impaired renal function and those patients whose urine output is less than 100 ml over the past 4 hours.

Overdosage may be treated with artificial respirations and the administration of calcium gluconate.

Infants born of mothers who receive magnesium sulfate need to be monitored for hypotension, hyporeflexia, and respiratory depression.

Availability
Injection—10, 12.5, 25, and 50% solutions.

Dosage and administration
Anticonvulsant
IM—Loading dose: 10 g of 50% solution (20 ml) is divided into two doses of 5 g each (10 ml) and is injected by deep intramuscular injection into each buttock. (1% lidocaine or procaine may be added to each syringe to reduce the pain on injection.) The IM loading dose is usually administered at the same time as 4 g are administered intravenously (see below). Maintenance dose: 4 to 5 g of 50% solution (10 ml) IM every 4 hours in alternate buttocks.

IV—Loading dose: 4 g of magnesium sulfate is added to 250 ml of 5% dextrose in water and infused slowly at a rate of 10 ml/minute. (The IV loading dose is usually administered at the same time as a 10 g IM loading dose.) Maintenance dose: 1 to 2 g/hr by continuous infusion.

Preterm labor
IV—Loading dose: 4 g of magnesium sulfate intravenously over 15 to 20 minutes. Maintenance dose: 1 to 3 g/hr by continuous infusion.

NOTE: Deep tendon reflexes, intake and output, vital signs, and orientation to the environment must be monitored on a regular, ongoing basis.

• Nursing Interventions: Monitoring magnesium sulfate therapy
Side effects to report
DEEP TENDON REFLEXES. The presence or absence of patellar reflex (knee jerk reflex), biceps reflex, or radial reflex are primary monitoring parameters for magnesium sulfate therapy.

The patellar reflex should be monitored hourly if the patient is receiving a continuous IV infusion, or before every dose if being administered intermittently IM or

IV. If the reflex is absent, further dosages should be withheld until it returns. If the patellar reflex cannot be used due to epidural anesthesia, the biceps or radial reflex may be used.

INTAKE AND OUTPUT. Magnesium toxicity is more likely to occur in patients with reduced renal output. Report urine outputs of less than 30 ml/hr or less than 100 ml over a 4 hour period. Observe the color and measure the specific gravity.

Note any other fluid and electrolyte loss such as vaginal bleeding, diarrhea, or vomiting.

VITAL SIGNS. Vital signs (blood pressure and heart rate and rhythm) should be measured every 15 to 30 minutes when a patient is receiving a continuous IV infusion. Take vital signs before and after each administration for those patients receiving intermittent therapy.

The respiratory rate should be at least 16 breaths per minute before the administration of further doses of magnesium sulfate.

Do not administer additional doses if there is a reduced respiratory rate, drop in blood pressure, fetal heart rate or other signs of fetal distress.

CONFUSION. Perform a baseline assessment of the patient's degree of alertness and orientation to name, place, and time BEFORE initiating therapy. Make regularly scheduled mental status evaluations to assure that the patient is oriented.

OVERDOSE. The antidote for magnesium intoxication (shown by respiratory depression and heart block) is calcium gluconate. A 10% solution of calcium gluconate should be kept at the patient's bedside ready for use. The dosage is 5 to 10 mEq (10 to 20 ml) IV over a 3 minute period.

Administer CPR until the patient responds appropriately.

Administration
IM. Intramuscular injection is very painful. Avoid if possible, or administer in conjunction with a local anesthetic.

IV. It is absolutely essential that an infusion pump be used to help control the infusion of the loading dose and continuous drip.

Drug interactions
CNS DEPRESSANTS. CNS depressants, including barbiturates, analgesics, general anesthetics, tranquilizers, and alcohol will potentiate the CNS depressant effects of magnesium sulfate.

Periodically check the patient's orientation to make sure the patient is not suffering from magnesium toxicity.

NEUROMUSCULAR BLOCKADE. Concurrent use of neuromuscular blocking agents and magnesium sulfate will further depress muscular activity. Monitor the patient closely for depressed reflexes and respiration.

Rh₀ (D) immune globulin (human)

RhoGAM, Hyp-Rho-D, Gamulin Rh, MICRhoGAM, Mini-Gamulin Rh

Rh₀ (D) immune globulin (human) is used to prevent Rh immunization of the Rh-negative patient exposed to Rh-positive blood as the result of a transfusion accident, during termination of a pregnancy, or as the result of a delivery of an Rh-positive infant.

Rh hemolytic disease of the newborn can be prevented in subsequent pregnancies by administering Rh₀ (D) immune globulin (Rh₀ [D] antibody) to the Rh-negative mother shortly after delivery of an Rh-positive child. Rh₀ (D) immune globulin suppresses the stimulation of active immunity by Rh-positive foreign red blood cells that enter the maternal circulation either at the time of delivery, at the termination of a pregnancy, or during a transfusion of inadequately typed blood.

Side effects. Adverse effects are infrequent, but an occasional patient may respond with a slight elevation in temperature. Patients who receive several vials as the result of a mismatched transfusion may report fever, myalgia, and lethargy with mild jaundice.

Availability. Rh₀ (D) immune globulin microdose (MICRhoGAM, Mini-Gamulin Rh): single-dose vial. Rh₀ (D) immune globulin (Gamulin Rh, Hyp-Rho-D, RhoGAM): single-dose vial or prefilled syringe.

Dosage and administration

Pregnancy

POSTPARTUM PROPHYLAXIS— 1 standard dose vial IM. Additional vials may be necessary if there was unusually large fetal-maternal hemorrhage.

ANTEPARTUM PROPHYLAXIS— 1 standard dose vial IM at about 28 weeks gestational age. This must be followed by another vial administered within 72 hours of delivery. Following amniocentesis, miscarriage, abortion, or ectopic pregnancy—<13 weeks of gestation: 1 microdose vial IM within 72 hours. = >13 weeks of gestation: 1 standard dose vial IM within 72 hours.

Transfusion. Rh negative, premenopausal women who receive Rh-positive red cells by transfusion: 1 standard dose vial IM for each 15 ml of transfused packed red cells.

• Nursing Interventions: Monitoring Rh₀ immune globulin therapy

See also General Nursing Considerations for Patients Receiving Immunologic Agents.

Side effects to expect

LOCALIZED TENDERNESS. Inform patients that they may experience stiffness at the site of injection for a few days.

FEVER, ARTHRALGIAS, GENERALIZED ACHES, PAINS. Monitor on a regular basis for the development of these symptoms. Follow routine orders of the physician or hospital concerning the use of analgesics (usually acet-aminophen; do not use aspirin or other antiinflammatory agents) for patient discomfort.

Side effects to report

URTICARIA, TACHYCARDIA, HYPOTENSION. Allergic reactions need immediate treatment. Monitor patients for 20 to 30 minutes following administration. Have emergency supplies readily available.

Implementation

PREVIOUS IMMUNIZATION. Although there is no need to administer Rh₀ (D) immune globulin to a woman who is already sensitized to the Rh factor, there is no more risk than when it is given to a woman who is not sensitized. When in doubt, administer Rh₀ (D) immune globulin.

BEFORE ADMINISTRATION

1. *Never* administer intravenously.
2. *Never* administer to a neonate.
3. *Never* administer to an Rh negative patient who has been previously sensitized to the Rh antigen.
4. *Confirm* that the mother is Rh negative.

erythromycin ophthalmic ointment

Ilotycin

Erythromycin (Ilotycin) is used prophylactically to prevent ophthalmia neonatorum, which is caused by *Neisseria gonorrhea.* It is also effective against *Chlamydia trachomatis.*

Side effects. A mild conjunctival inflammation occurs in the neonate and may interfere with the ability to focus. This side effect generally disappears in 1 to 2 days.

Availability
Ophthalmic ointment— 1, 3.5, and 3.75 g tubes.

Dosage and administration. Instill a ¼-inch narrow ribbon along the lower conjunctival surface of both eyes. Administration should be done within 2 hours of birth.

• Nursing Interventions: Monitoring erythromycin ophthalmic therapy

Side effects to expect

MILD CONJUNCTIVITIS. Assure the family that the redness is only temporary and that it will resolve within 1 to 2 days.

Implementation

OINTMENT TUBE. A new tube should be started for each infant.

WASH HANDS. Wash hands immediately before administration to prevent bacterial contamination. Don gloves.

CLEANSING THE EYES. Using a separate sterile absorbent cotton or gauze pledget for each eye, wash the unopened lids from the nose outward until free of blood, mucus, or meconium.

OPEN THE EYES, INSTILL MEDICATION. Separate the eyelids and instill a narrow ribbon of erythromycin ointment along the lower conjunctival surface.

IRRIGATION. DO NOT irrigate the eyes following instillation.

phytonadione (fy-toe-nah-di'own)

Aquamephyton (ak-wah-mef'i-ton)

Vitamin K is a fat-soluble vitamin necessary for the production of the blood clotting factors prothrombin (factor II), proconvertin (factor VII), plasma thromboplastin component (factor IX), and Stuart factor (factor X) in the liver. Vitamin K is absorbed from the diet and normally is produced by the bacterial flora in the gastrointestinal tract, from which it is absorbed and transported to the liver for clotting factor production. Newborn infants have not yet colonized the colon with bacteria and are often deficient in vitamin K. They also may be deficient in these clotting factors and are thus more susceptible to hemorrhagic disease of the newborn in the first 5 to 8 days after birth. Phytonadione is routinely administered prophylactically to protect against hemorrhagic disease of the newborn.

Side effects. When used as a single recommended dose, no adverse effects other than tenderness and edema at the injection site have been reported.

Availability

Injection—2, 10 mg/ml in 0.5, 1, 2.5, and 5 ml containers.

Dosage and administration

IM—0.5 to 2 mg in the lateral aspect of the thigh.

• **Nursing Interventions: Monitoring phytonadione therapy**

Side effects to report

BRUISING, HEMORRHAGE. Observe for bleeding (usually occurring on the second or third day). Bleeding may be seen as petechiae, generalized ecchymoses, or bleeding from the umbilical stump, circumcision site, nose, or gastrointestinal tract. Assess results of serial prothrombin times.

Implementation

IM. DO NOT administer intravenously! Severe reactions, including hypotension, cardiac arrhythmias, and respiratory arrest, have been reported.

CHOICE OF CONCENTRATION. Although the 2 mg/ml concentration is packaged to be administered to infants (0.5 ml), the 10 mg/ml concentration is often used because the volume to be administered (0.1 ml) intramuscularly is smaller. This is particularly useful in premature or small-for-gestational-age neonates.

Drug Therapy for Oral Contraception

OBJECTIVES

1. Compare the active ingredients in the two types of oral contraceptive agents.

2. Differentiate between the actions and the benefits of the combination pill and the mini-pill.
3. Describe the major adverse effects and contraindications to the use of oral contraceptive agents.
4. Develop specific patient education plans to be used to teach a patient to initiate oral contraceptive therapy using the combination pill and the mini-pill.

KEY WORDS

amenorrhea	libido
chloasma	oligomenorrhea

The oral (hormonal) contraceptives (birth control pills, BCPs) were first available in 1960. They now represent one of the most common forms of artificial birth control in use in the United States. It is estimated that approximately one-third of all women between 18 and 44 years of age use oral contraceptives.

There are two types of oral contraceptives in general use: (1) the combination pill, which is taken for 21 days of the menstrual cycle and contains both an estrogen and a progestin (see Figure 20-4), and (2) the "mini-pill," which is taken every day and contains only a progestin (see Figure 20-5 and Table 20-5). The combination pills are subdivided into fixed combination (monophasic), biphasic, and triphasic products. The monophasic combination pills contain a fixed ratio of estrogen and progestin given daily for 21 days beginning on day 5 of the menstrual cycle. The biphasic product contains a fixed dose of estrogen with a lower

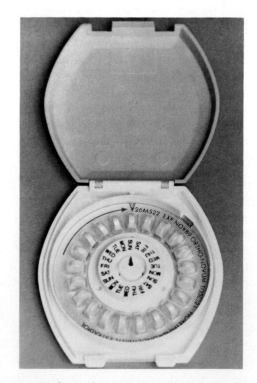

Figure 20-4 *21-day packages. Take oral contraceptive pills for 21 days, wait 1 week, and start a new package on the next Sunday.*

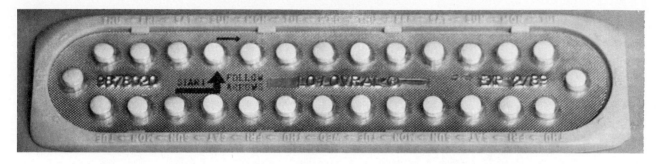

Figure 20-5 *28-day packages. Take 1 pill daily; start a new package on the day after finishing the last package.*

progestin dose on days 1 to 10 than on days 11 to 21 of the menstrual cycle. The triphasic combination pills provide three concentrations of estrogen and progestin. The purpose of the variable concentrations of hormones is to provide contraception with the lowest necessary dose of hormones.

Estrogens and progestins, to some extent, induce contraception by inhibiting ovulation. The estrogens block pituitary release of follicle-stimulating hormone (FSH), preventing the ovary from developing a follicle from which the ovum is released. Progestins inhibit pituitary release of luteinizing hormone (LH), the hormone responsible for release of the ovum from the follicle. Other mechanisms play a contributory role in preventing conception. Estrogens and progestins alter (1) cervical mucus by making it thick and viscous, inhibiting sperm migration, (2) mobility of uterine and oviduct muscle, reducing transport of both sperm and ovum, and (3) the endometrium, impairing implantation of the fertilized ovum.

The mini-pills or progestin-only pills represent a relatively new direction in oral contraceptive therapy. Many of the adverse effects of combination-type contraceptives are due to the estrogen component of the tablet. For those women particularly susceptible to adverse effects of estrogen therapy, the mini-pill provides an alternative. Women who might prefer the mini-pill are those with a history of migraine headaches, hypertension, mental depression, weight gain, and breast tenderness and those who want to breastfeed postpartum. The mini-pill is not without its disadvantages, however. Between 30 and 40% of women on the mini-pill continue to ovulate. Birth control is maintained by progestin activity on cervical mucus, uterine and fallopian transport, and implantation. There is a slightly higher incidence of both uterine and tubal pregnancy. Dysmenorrhea, manifested by irregular periods, infrequent periods, and spotting between periods, is common among women taking the mini-pill.

Side effects. Thirty years of clinical experience with literally millions of women have shown that birth control pills are not as "safe" as indicated by earlier studies. However, use of oral contraceptives must be considered in light of the potential risks and complications stemming from pregnancy. There are minor adverse effects, major adverse effects, and contraindications to use of oral contraceptive therapy.

About 40% of women using oral contraceptives will suffer some side effects. Hormones such as estrogens and progestins have many other actions that affect nearly every organ system within the body. The most common side effects are related to the dose of estrogen and progestin in each product. Nausea, headaches, weight gain, spotting, depression, fatigue, chloasma, yeast infection, vaginal itching or discharge, and changes in libido are common side effects.

Disease states that may be aggravated by continued use of oral contraceptives are hypertension, gallbladder disease, diabetes mellitus, severe varicose veins, seizure disorders, oligomenorrhea or amenorrhea, and rheumatic heart disease.

The list of absolute contraindications to the use of oral contraceptives is somewhat variable depending on the clinician and the particular case history of each woman. However, women with a history of any of the following conditions should strongly consider other forms of contraception: thromboembolic disease, stroke, malignancy of breast or the reproductive system, renal or liver disease, severe mental depression, suspected pregnancy, and repeated contraceptive failure.

Availability. See Table 20-5.

Dosage and administration. The estrogenic component of the combination-type pills is responsible for most of the adverse effects associated with therapy. The FDA has recommended that therapy be initiated with a product containing a low dose of estrogen. Side effects must be reviewed in relation to individual case histories, but many physicians initiate therapy with Norinyl 1 + 50 or Ortho Novum 1/50. Therapy, and therefore products, may be adjusted based on the incidence of side effects.

• **Nursing Interventions: Monitoring oral contraceptive therapy**

Side effects to expect

NAUSEA, WEIGHT GAIN, SPOTTING, CHANGED MENSTRUAL FLOW, MISSED PERIODS, DEPRESSION, MOOD CHANGES, CHLO-

Table 20-5 *Oral Contraceptives*

BRAND NAME	PROGESTIN						ESTROGEN		OTHER INGREDIENTS
	NORETHINDRONE (MG)	NORETHINDRONE ACETATE (MG)	NORGESTREL (MG)	ETHYNODIOL DIACETATE (MG)	NORETHYNODREL (MG)	LEVONORGESTREL (MCG)	ETHINYL ESTRADIOL (MCG)	MESTRANOL (MCG)	
Combination*									
Brevicon (21,28)‡	0.5						35		
Demulen 1/35 (21,28)				1			35		
Demulen 1/50 (21,28)				1			50		
Enovid 5 mg (20)					5			75	
Genora 1/35 (21,28)	1						35		
Genora 1/50 (21,28)	1							50	
Levlen (21,28)						150	30		
Loestrin 1/20 (21)		1					20		
Loestrin Fe 1/20 (28)		1					20		Ferrous Fumarate 75 mg
Loestrin 1.5/3.0 (21)		1.5					30		
Loestrin Fe 1.5/3.0 (28)		1.5					30		Ferrous Fumarate 75 mg
Lo/Ovral (21,28)			0.3				30		
Modicon (21,28)	0.5						35		
Nelova 1/35 E (21,28)	1						35		
Nelova 1/50 E (21,28)	1							50	
Nelova 10/11 (21,28)	10 tabs 0.5 / 11 tabs 1.0						35		
Norcept E 1/35 (21,28)	1						35		
Nordette (21,28)						150	30		
Norethin 1/35 E (21,28)	1						35		
Norethin 1/50 (21,28)	1							50	

Product	Progestin (mg)	Ethinyl Estradiol (µg)	Mestranol (µg)	Other
Norinyl 1 + 35 (21,28)	1	35		
Norinyl 1 + 50 (21,28)	1		50	
Norlestrin 1/50 (21,28)	1	50		
Norlestrin Fe 1/50 (28)	1	50		Ferrous Fumarate 75 mg
Norlestrin 2.5/50 (21)	2.5	50		
Norlestrin Fe 2.5/50 (28)	2.5	50		Ferrous Fumarate 75 mg
Ortho-Novum 1/35 (21,28)	1	35		
Ortho-Novum 1/50 (21,28)	1		50	
Ortho-Novum 10/11 (21,28)	10 tabs-0.5 / 11 tabs-1.0	35		
Ortho-Novum 7/7/7 (21,28)†	7 tabs-0.5 / 7 tabs-0.75 / 7 tabs-1.0	35		
Ovcon-35 (28)	0.4	35		
Ovcon-50 (28)	1	50		
Ovral (21,28)	0.5	50		
Ovulen (21,28)	1		100	
Tri-Levlen (21,28)†	6 tabs-50 / 5 tabs-75 / 10 tabs-125	30 / 40 / 30		
Tri-Norinyl (21,28)†	7 tabs-0.5 / 9 tabs-1.0 / 5 tabs-0.5	35 / 35 / 35		
Triphasil-21 (21,28)†	6 tabs-50 / 5 tabs-75 / 10 tabs-125	30 / 40 / 30		
Progestin only§				
Micronor (28)	0.35			
Nor-QD (42)	0.35			
Ovrette (28)	0.075			

*Products contain 20 or 21 hormone tablets/package
†Triphasic Oral Contraceptives
‡21 hormone tablets/package plus 7 inert tablets
§Products contain all active hormone tablets

ASMA, HEADACHES. These are the most common side effects of hormonal contraceptive therapy. If these symptoms are not resolved after 3 months of therapy, the woman should return to the physician for reevaluation and a possible change in prescription.

Side effects to report

VAGINAL DISCHARGE, BREAKTHROUGH BLEEDING, YEAST INFECTION. These symptoms represent the development of secondary disorders. Examination, a change in oral contraceptive, and possible treatment with other medications may be necessary.

BLURRED VISION, SEVERE HEADACHES, DIZZINESS, LEG PAIN, CHEST PAIN, SHORTNESS OF BREATH, ACUTE ABDOMINAL PAIN. Report as soon as possible. These side effects are usually of minor consequence, but they may be early indications of very serious adverse effects.

Implementation

BEFORE INITIATING THERAPY. The patient should have a complete physical examination that includes blood pressure, pelvic and breast examination, Papanicolaou (Pap) smear, urinalysis, and hemoglobin or hematocrit.

INSTRUCTIONS FOR USING COMBINATION ORAL CONTRACEPTIVES. When to start the pill: Start the first pill on the first Sunday after your period begins. Take one pill daily, at the same time daily, until the pack is gone. If using a 21-day pack, wait 1 week and restart on the next Sunday. If using a 28-day pack, start a new pack the day after finishing the last pack. Use another form of birth control (condoms, foam) during this first month. You may not be fully protected by the pill during the first month.

Missed pills. If you miss 1 pill, take it as soon as you remember it; take the next pill at the regularly scheduled time. If you miss 2 pills, take 2 pills as soon as you remember and 2 the next day. Spotting may occur when 2 pills are missed. Use another form of birth control (condoms, foam) until you finish this pack of pills. If you miss *3 or more,* start using another form of birth control immediately. Start a new pack of pills on the next Sunday even if you are menstruating. Discard your old packs of pills. Use other forms of birth control through the next month after missing 3 or more pills.

Missed pills and skipped periods. Return to your physician for a pregnancy test.

Skipping one period but not missing a pill. It is not uncommon for a woman to occasionally miss a period when on the pill. Start the next pack on the appropriate Sunday.

Spotting for two or more cycles. See your physician.

Periodic examinations. A yearly examination should include tests for blood pressure, pelvic examination, urinalysis, breast examination, and Papanicolaou smear.

Discontinuing the pill for conception. Because of a possibility of birth defects, discontinue the pill 3 months before attempting pregnancy. Use other methods of contraception for these 3 months.

Duration of oral contraceptive therapy. Many physicians prefer to have their patients discontinue the pill for 3 out of every 28 months. This allows the body to return to a normal cycle. Be sure to use other forms of contraception during this time. Long-term use (3 or more years) must be determined on an individual basis.

Side effects to be reported as soon as possible. Severe headaches, dizziness, blurred vision, leg pain, shortness of breath, chest pain, and acute abdominal pain. Although these side effects are usually of minor consequence, absence of serious adverse effects must be confirmed.

NOTE: When being seen by a physician or a dentist for other reasons, be sure to mention that you are currently taking oral contraceptives.

INSTRUCTIONS FOR USING THE MINI-PILL. Starting the mini-pill: start on the first day of menstruation. Take 1 tablet daily, every day, regardless of when your next period is. Tablets should be taken at about the same time every day.

Missed pills. If you miss 1 pill, take it as soon as you remember, and take your next pill at the regularly scheduled time. Use another form of birth control until your next period.

If you miss 2 pills, take 1 of the missed pills immediately and take your regularly scheduled pill that day on time. The next day, take the regularly scheduled pill as well as the other missed pill. Use another method of birth control until your next period.

Missed periods. Some women note changes in the time as well as duration of their periods while using mini-pills. These changes are to be expected. If menses occurs every 28 to 30 days, ovulation may still be occurring. For maximal safety, use alternate forms of contraception on days 10 through 18. If irregular bleeding occurs every 25 to 45 days, ovulation is probably not occurring on a regular basis. You may feel more comfortable if you use other forms of contraception with the mini-pill or discuss switching to an estrogen-containing (combination) contraceptive.

If you have taken all tablets correctly, but do not have a period for over 60 days, speak to your physician concerning a pregnancy test.

NOTE: Report sudden, severe abdominal pain, with or without nausea and vomiting, to your physician immediately. There is a higher incidence of ectopic pregnancy with the mini-pill, since it does not inhibit ovulation in all women.

Side effects to be reported as soon as possible. Severe headaches, dizziness, blurred vision, leg pain, shortness of breath, chest pain, and acute abdominal pain. Although these side effects are usually of minor consequence, absence of serious adverse effects must be confirmed.

Duration of oral contraceptive therapy. Many physicians prefer to have their patients discontinue the pill for 3 out of every 18 months. This allows the body to return to a normal cycle. Be sure to use other forms of contraception during this time. Long-term use (3 or more years) must be determined on an individual basis.

Discontinuing the pill for conception. Because of a possibility of birth defects, discontinue the pill 3 months before attempting pregnancy. Use other methods of contraception for these 3 months.

Drug interactions

WARFARIN. This medication may diminish the anticoagulant effects of warfarin. Monitor the prothrombin time and increase the dosage of warfarin if necessary.

PHENYTOIN. Monitor patients with concurrent therapy for signs of phenytoin toxicity: nystagmus, sedation, lethargy. Serum levels may be ordered, and a reduced dosage of phenytoin may be required.

THYROID HORMONES. Patients who have no thyroid function and who start on estrogen therapy may require an increase in thyroid hormone because the estrogens reduce the level of circulating thyroid hormones. The thyroid dosage is not adjusted until the patient shows clinical signs of hypothyroidism.

PHENOBARBITAL. Phenobarbital may enhance the metabolism of estrogens to the extent that there is inadequate contraceptive protection. Changing to an oral contraceptive with a higher estrogen content or using another form of contraception (foam, condoms) is recommended.

AMPICILLIN, ISONIAZID, RIFAMPIN. The use of another form of contraception (foam, condoms) is recommended.

BENZODIAZEPINES. Oral contraceptives appear to have a variable effect on the metabolism of benzodiazepines. Those that have reduced metabolism with an increase in therapeutic response are alprazolam, chlorazepate, chlordiazepoxide, diazepam, flurazepam, halazepam, and prazepam. Benzodiazepines that have enhanced metabolism and reduced therapeutic activity when taken with oral contraceptives are lorazepam, oxazepam, and temazepam. Adjust the dosage of benzodiazepine accordingly.

PHENYTOIN, PRIMIDONE, CARBAMAZEPINE. The efficacy of the oral contraceptive may be impaired. Breakthrough bleeding may be an indication of this interaction. Adjustment in dosage or oral contraceptive and the use of other methods of contraception (foam, condoms) should be considered.

Drug Therapy for Leukorrhea

OBJECTIVES

1. Identify common organisms known to cause leukorrhea.
2. Cite the generic name and brand names of products used to treat *Candida albicans*, *Trichomonas vaginalis*, and *Gardnerella vaginalis*.
3. Review specific techniques for administering vaginal medications.

4. Develop a plan for teaching self-care to a woman with a sexually transmitted disease. Include personal hygiene measures, medication administration, pain relief, and prevention of spread of infection or reinfection.
5. Discuss specific interviewing techniques that can be used to obtain a sexual history.

KEY WORD
leukorrhea

Secretions from the vagina usually represent a normal physiologic process, but if the discharge becomes excessive, it is known as leukorrhea. Leukorrhea is an abnormal, usually whitish, vaginal discharge that may occur at any age. It affects almost all females at some time in their lives. Leukorrhea is not a disease, but a symptom of an underlying disorder. The most common cause is an infection of the lower reproductive tract, but other physiologic and noninfectious causes of vaginal discharge are well known (see the box on p. 524).

The most common organisms causing the infectious type of leukorrhea are *Candida albicans*, *Trichomonas vaginalis*, and *Gardnerella vaginalis* (Table 20-6). Occasionally, *Candida albicans* infections of the mouth, gastrointestinal tract, or vagina may develop as a secondary infection during the use of the broad-spectrum antibiotics, such as the penicillins, tetracyclines, and cephalosporins.

Pathogens that are frequently transmitted by sexual contact are called sexually transmitted diseases (STDs) (see the box on p. 525). In some cases, such as gonorrhea and genital herpes simplex virus infection, sexual transmission is the primary mode of transmission. In other cases, such as giardiasis, shigellosis, and the hepatitis viruses, other important nonsexual means of transmission exist. Unfortunately, the true incidence of the STDs is not known in the United States because of large numbers of unreported cases.

General Nursing Considerations for Patients with Leukorrhea

See also General Nursing Considerations for Patients with Infectious Disease (p. 457).

Prevention of spread of sexually transmitted diseases

There is a great need for counseling about the current knowledge of the modes of transmission of sexually transmitted diseases (STDs) to all persons who are sexually active. Nurses must be leaders in encouraging persons to report STDs and seek health care as soon as an STD is suspected.

Nurses must also be aware of and practice the recommendations on "Universal Blood and Body Fluid Precautions" by the Center for Disease Control to prevent

Causes of vaginal discharge

Physiologic	Infectious	Noninfectious
Ovulation	Vaginal	Atrophic vaginitis
Coitus	*Candida*	Foreign body
Oral contraceptives	*Trichomonas*	Vaginal adenosis
Pregnancy	*Gardnerella*	Allergic vulvo-vaginitis
Premenstruation	Toxic shock syndrome	Vulvar, vaginal carcinoma
Premenarche	Vulvar	Cervical polyps
Intrauterine device	Herpes	Cervical erosions/ulcers
	Condylomata acuminata	Uterine carcinoma
	Syphilis	Endometrial myoma
	Bartholinitis	Vesicovaginal fistula
	Lymphogranuloma venereum	Enterovaginal fistula
	Chancroid	
	Granuloma inguinale	
	Urethritis	
	Pyoderma	
	Cervical	
	Gonorrhea	
	Chlamydial or bacterial cervicitis	
	Chronic cervicitis	
	Pelvic inflammatory disease	

Reprinted with permission from Reilly BM: *Practical Strategies in Outpatient Medicine.* Philadelphia, 1984, WB Saunders Co.

Table 20-6 *Causative Organisms and Products Used to Treat Genital Infections*

CAUSATIVE ORGANISM	GENERIC NAME	BRAND NAME	DRUG MONOGRAPH, NURSING IMPLICATIONS
Vulvovaginitis			
Candida albicans (fungus)	Butoconazole vaginal cream	Femstat	(p. 479)
	Clotrimazole vaginal cream, vaginal tablets	Gyne-Lotrimin, Mycelex-G	(p. 479)
	Miconazole vaginal cream, suppositories	Monistat	(p. 479)
	Nystatin vaginal tablets, oral tablets	Mycostatin	(p. 480)
	Terconazole vaginal cream	Terazol 7	(p. 480)
	Tioconazole vaginal ointment	Vagistat	(p. 480)
Trichomonas vaginalis (protozoa)	Metronidazole oral tablets	Flagyl	(p. 475)
	Clotrimazole (in pregnancy)	Gyne-Lotrimin, Mycelex-G	
Gardnerella vaginalis (bacteria)	Metronidazole oral tablets	Flagyl	(p. 475)
Gonorrhea			
Neisseria gonorrhea (bacteria)	Ceftriaxone	Rocephin	(p. 463)
	Spectinomycin	Trobicin	(p. 477)
	Amoxicillin + Probenecid		(p. 466)
Syphilis			
Treponema pallidum (spirochete)	Penicillin G, Benzathine	Bicillin C-R	(p. 466)
	Tetracycline	Tetracycline	(p. 471)
	Erythromycin	Erythromycin	(p. 465)
Genital herpes			
Herpes simplex genitalis (virus)	Acyclovir topical ointment	Zovirax	(p. 489)
Chlamydiae			
Chlamydia trachomatis (chlamydia)	Doxycycline	Vibramycin	(p. 471)
	Erythromycin	Erythromycin	(p. 465)
	Sulfisoxazole	Gantrisin	(p. 470)

Sexually transmitted diseases

Bacteria

Neisseria gonorrhea
Gardnerella vaginalis
Treponema pallidum
Hemophilus ducreyi
Shigella species
Campylobacter species
Group B Streptococcus

Chlamydiae

Chlamydia trachomatis

Ectoparasites

Sarcoptes scabei
Phthirus pubis

Fungi

Candida albicans

Mycoplasma

Ureaplasma urealyticum
Mycoplasma hominis

Protozoa

Trichomonas vaginalis
Entomoeba histolytica
Giardia lamblia

Viruses

Herpes simplex virus
Hepatitis A virus
Hepatitis B virus
Cytomegalovirus
Genital wart virus
Molluscum contagiosum virus

---

the spread of disease through inappropriate contact with contaminated fluids.

Anxiety

Sexually transmitted diseases cause a high degree of anxiety. The intimate nature of the questioning required to obtain a sexual history may be embarrassing. Vaginal and/or urethral discharge may also be alarming to the patient seeking health care. Approaching the patient in a nonjudgmental manner, offering emotional support, and openness to listen, and use of good communication techniques can provide reassurance to the patient. It is ethically imperative that the nurse adhere to the policies of confidentiality.

Patient Education Associated with Leukorrhea

Communication and responsibility. The nurse needs to impart current information and recommendations concerning the modes of transmission and prevention of STD. Current information can be obtained by calling the VD National Institute Hotline (1-800-227-8922).

Expectations of therapy. Discuss the expectations of therapy and the degree of relief from symptoms that can be anticipated.

Fostering compliance. Discuss the medication information and how it will benefit the patient's course of treatment. Seek cooperation and understanding of the following points, so that medication compliance may be enhanced and the possibility of a relapse of infection minimized.

1. Name
2. Dosage
3. Route and administration times
4. Anticipated therapeutic response
5. Side effects to expect
6. Side effects to report
7. What to do if a dose is missed
8. When, how, or if to refill the medication prescription

Associated teaching. Encourage the patient to complete the full course of medicine. Do not discontinue use when the symptoms have resolved. Early discontinuation may result in a relapse of infection. If pregnancy is suspected, consult an obstetrician as soon as possible about continuation of therapy.

1. Teach the patient how to correctly administer the medication.
2. The applicator should be washed in warm soapy water after *each* use.
3. Review personal hygiene measures, such as wiping from the front to the back after voiding or defecating.
4. Tell the patient not to douche and to abstain from sexual intercourse after inserting the medication.
5. With most types of infection, both the male and female partners require treatment. To prevent reinfections, partners should abstain from sexual intercourse until both partners are cured.

CHAPTER 21

Antineoplastic Agents

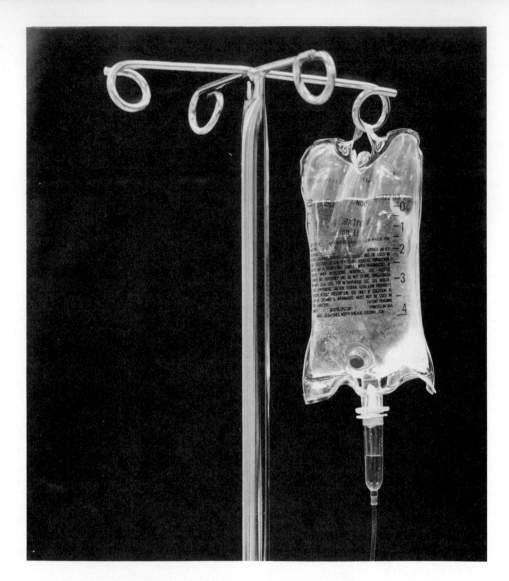

CHAPTER GOALS

After completing this chapter, the student should be able to do the following:

1. Identify baseline data the nurse should collect on a continuous basis for comparison and evaluation of drug effectiveness.

2. Identify important nursing assessments and interventions for drug therapy and treatment of diseases associated with the treatment of cancer.

3. Identify essential components involved in planning patient education that will enhance compliance with the treatment regimen.

Nursing Considerations
and Drug Therapy for:

Drug therapy for cancer: Antimetabolites (p. 527)   Antibiotics (p. 527)
  Alkylating agents (p. 527)   Natural products (p. 527)   Hormones (p. 528)

CANCER AND THE USE OF ANTINEOPLASTIC AGENTS

Cancer is a disorder of cellular growth. It is a collection of abnormal cells that generally proliferate more rapidly than do normal cells, lose the ability to perform specialized functions, invade surrounding tissues, and develop growths in other tissues (metastases).

Cancer is a leading cause of death in the United States. Unfortunately, the number of persons dying from malignant disease increases each year. Early diagnosis and treatment is still one of the most important factors in providing a more optimistic prognosis for those patients stricken with the many forms of neoplastic disease.

Treatment of cancer often requires a combination of surgery, radiation, and chemotherapy. Recent advancements in carcinogenesis, cellular and molecular biology, and tumor immunology have enhanced the role that antineoplastic agents may play in therapy. It is beyond the scope of this chapter to delve into the interrelationships of chemotherapy and neoplastic disease; however, a short discussion of the concepts of cancer chemotherapy will be presented. As a result of rapidly changing approaches to the treatment of specific malignancies and the changing nature of chemotherapeutic regimens, specific agents and dosages have not been discussed.

All cells, whether normal or malignant, pass through a similar series of phases during their lifetime, although duration of time spent in each phase differs with type of cell.

Mitosis (M) is that phase of cellular proliferation when the cell divides into two equal daughter cells. Phase G_1 follows mitosis and is considered a resting phase before the S phase, the stage of active DNA synthesis. G_2 is a postsynthetic phase wherein the cell contains a double complement of DNA. After a period of apparently minimal cellular activity in phase G_2, the M phase again divides the cell into two G_1 daughter cells. G_1 cells may advance again to the S phase or pass into a nonproliferative stage known as G_0. The time required to complete one cycle is called the "generation time."

Many antineoplastic agents are "cell-cycle specific"; that is, the drug is selectively toxic when the cell is in a specific phase of growth. Thus those malignancies most amenable to chemotherapy proliferate rapidly. "Cell-cycle nonspecific" drugs are active throughout the cell cycle and may be more effective against slowly proliferating neoplastic tissue. One implication of cell-cycle specificity is the importance of correlating the dosage schedule of anticancer therapy with the known cellular kinetics of that type of neoplasm. Drugs are usually administered when the cell is most susceptible to the cytotoxic effects of the agent. Table 21-1 lists the more common commercially available drugs, their dosage range, major toxicities, and major indications.

Pharmacology

Chemotherapeutic agents currently used are classified as (1) alkylating agents, (2) antimetabolites, (3) natural products, and (4) hormones. The mechanisms by which these agents cause cell death have not yet been fully determined.

Alkylating agents

The alkylating agents are highly reactive chemical compounds that unite with DNA molecules, causing cross-linking of DNA strands. The interstrand binding prevents the separation of the double-coiled DNA molecule that is necessary for cellular division. Alkylating agents are cell-cycle nonspecific, being capable of combining with cellular components at any phase of the cell cycle. Generally speaking, the development of resistance to one alkylating agent imparts cross-resistance to other alkylators.

Antimetabolites

The antimetabolites (subclassified as folic acid, purine, and pyrimidine antagonists) inhibit key enzymes in the biosynthetic pathways of DNA and RNA synthesis. Many of the antagonists are cell-cycle specific, killing cells during the S phase of cell maturation.

Natural products

Vinca alkaloids. Vincristine and vinblastine are natural derivatives of the periwinkle plant. They are cell-cycle specific agents that block the formation of the mitotic spindle during mitosis, thus inhibiting cell division. Even though there is close structural similarity, cross-resistance does not usually develop between the two agents.

Antibiotics. Through various mechanisms, the antibiotics bind with cellular DNA, preventing its replication as well as RNA synthesis, which is required for subsequent protein synthesis.

Hormones

Adrenocorticosteroids (usually prednisone) may be beneficial in treating lymphomas and acute leukemia because of their lympholytic effects and their ability to suppress mitosis in lymphocytes. Steroids are also used to help reduce edema secondary to radiation therapy and as palliative therapy in temporarily suppressing fever, sweats, and pain, and in restoring, to some degree, appetite, lost weight, strength, and a sense of well-being in critically ill patients. With symptomatic relief, it is hoped that the patient's general physical condition may be improved sufficiently to permit further definitive therapy.

Estrogens and androgens are used in malignancies of sexual organs based on the assumption that these malignancies have hormonal requirements similar to those of nonmalignant sexual organs. Estrogens (usually diethylstilbestrol) are frequently used in prostatic carcinoma. There are regressions in the primary tumor and in soft tissue metastases, with significant symptomatic relief from the point of view of the patient. Androgens may be used in the treatment of metastatic breast cancer of any age group, and estrogens may be used in postmenopausal women with metastatic breast cancer.

Patients often may not complete a course of therapy because of the toxic effects of chemotherapeutic agents on normal as well as malignant cells. Malignant cells that were once susceptible may also develop a resistance to antineoplastic drugs. Several mechanisms may be involved, depending on the sites of action of the drug within the biochemical pathways of the cell. Theories about these mechanisms include a repair mechanism to damaged DNA molecules, altered permeability of the cell to the drug, and increased intracellular concentrations of protective chemicals.

General Nursing Considerations for Patients with Cancer

OBJECTIVES

1. Describe the grieving process of patients and family members in response to the diagnosis of cancer.
2. Analyze role changes and alterations in communication patterns seen in a family unit during cancer therapy.
3. State specific approaches the nurse can use to give the patient a sense of personal control in life management while receiving cancer treatment.
4. State baseline assessments needed during initiation of cancer therapy.
5. Cite the goals of chemotherapy and specific factors affecting the patient dosage, drug identification, drug preparation, and drug administration.
6. Study the nursing interventions needed for persons experiencing adverse effects from chemotherapy.
7. Develop measurable short- and long-term objectives for patient education for persons receiving chemotherapy.

KEY WORDS

alopecia	thrombocytopenia
bone marrow depression	stomatitis

Adaptation to the diagnosis

No other disease seems to evoke fear and anxiety equal to the effect that the diagnosis of cancer has on the patient and family. When the diagnostic workup is completed and revealed to the patient and family, a period of adjustment is needed. The initial response is often one of shock and disbelief. Each member of the patient's support group, as well as the patient himself, has to learn to deal with the diagnosis and establish a personal perspective of its meaning. In addition, some patients must also adjust to an altered body image—for example, due to the loss of a breast or the creation of a colostomy—while simultaneously experiencing a sense of loss of control of their life, their future, and their family unit.

As the days pass, the patient starts to focus on the details of the disease and the prognosis. The patient ultimately views the future in light of the extent of disease involvement that has already occurred. Many patients search for the meaning of their illness and intellectualize the process. Other patients sink into self-blame with thoughts such as "Why didn't I do a breast exam every month?" Some individuals may become passive and withdrawn, while others make a commitment to control the disease.

The family unit

Members of the family unit require careful assessment for the nurse to plan their involvement in the patient's care. Within any family group there are a number of rules, often unspoken, that form the basis of the family's values. During an illness such as cancer, the roles that specific individuals play in the family may be changed. The person with cancer may be so emotionally overwhelmed or incapacitated by the diagnosis that another member of the family may have to assume his role temporarily or permanently. In some families, the adjustment to different persons in new roles may be quite difficult and require time for transition. During this transition, the patient often develops feelings of guilt and frustration in forcing these changes upon the family.

Various patterns of bonding within a family or support group often occur during an illness. Some of the involved parties may experience closeness while others become "outsiders" waiting for acceptance and a chance to be involved. The nurse must be aware of these relationships and make provisions for the needs of all persons affected. Because relationships are ever-changing processes, the nurse must plan for periodic reevaluation of the family unit and shifts within it during the course of the patient's treatment.

When working with the patient's support group, it is important to remember that not all units function effectively, although they may have been operating for some time. Working within the boundaries that exist, rather than trying to change these relationships, may be essential to maintaining communication with the group. Occasionally the nurse will identify a member of the support group who subconsciously wants the patient to remain dependent, and who therefore does not encourage compliance with the treatment plan or help the patient function at an optimal level.

Remember that not everyone is capable of becoming actively involved in the patient's care. Some members want to be active participants, while others are not emotionally capable of tolerating it. The inability to participate may produce guilt, which should not be overlooked when planning and intervening in the care. Incorporation of the family unit should be carefully evaluated so that the degree of participation is individualized to the needs of all parties concerned. Many times the family needs as much support as the patient does, or more.

Trust and positivism

The health team must foster a trusting relationship with the patient. Develop a genuine concern for the patient; take time to be an active *listener,* not a talker. Work with the patient's needs and concerns, then try tactfully to find out what threats the patient perceives from this illness. Answer questions and concerns; take action on even trivial matters so that the patient believes in you and responds with trust. The trust the patient has in the nurse, the physician, and others managing care can have a very significant influence on the response to therapy. Provide the patient with multiple opportunities to verbalize concerns. Frequently the patient is referred to specialists for care and the family physician is only minimally involved. When this occurs, the patient and family members sometimes feel uncertain and hesitate to discuss concerns with new health care providers. It is important to explore the issues and concerns they feel are of the greatest importance. Foster hope for the "control" of the disease, for the prolongation of a functional life, and for the effective management of any difficulties that might be encountered.

Provide alternatives

Give the patient appropriate choices that allow involvement in the decisions to be made concerning selection of care. Encourage the patient to maintain the best health possible within the boundaries of the illness. Include the patient in selection of diet, planning activities, scheduling rest periods, and personal care. Stress what the patient *can* do, not what he or she cannot do.

Limit the amount of information given to the facts that are significant at this point in the plan of care and to the degree of symptoms present. Emphasize the prevention of complications through maintenance of nutrition and hydration, commitment to hygiene, avoidance of exposure to persons with infection, and safety measures to prevent accidental personal injury.

The treatment plan

The treatment plan for the patient is recommended by the physician, based on the specific type of cancer cells (malignancy), the location, and the extent of tissue or organ involvement. The amount of information given the patient is generally decided by the physician. Most individuals are given the facts regarding the disease as it is affecting him or her, and then the patient is actively involved in appropriate decision-making regarding treatment modalities. Before initiation of therapy, the nurse should know the primary site, any metastases the patient has, and the symptoms the patient is experiencing.

Carefully assess all current symptoms the patient is exhibiting so that subsequent data may be compared to these findings for analysis of the therapeutic effectiveness of the agents being used or the detection of adverse effects.

Patient Concerns: Nursing Intervention/Rationale

Assessment of the patient

Type of cancer. Read the patient's chart to determine the type of cancer, location, and extent of involvement.

Perform an initial assessment of the patient and of the current symptoms based on the site of the cancer and degree of tissue or organ involvement.

Ascertain the extent of the patient's knowledge and understanding of the diagnosis. Check the physician's progress notes as well.

Emotional status. Patients often exhibit varying degrees of anxiety or depression as a response to this type of diagnosis.

Tactfully obtain information from the individual regarding fears, feelings, and concerns.

The patient's viewpoint. Try to gain a perspective of the illness from the patient's viewpoint, and how the patient perceives that the cancer will affect the family and close friends. Assist the individual in expressing feelings. Spend time with the patient. Sometimes not much will be said; be patient and understanding. Foster positivism by stressing things the individual can do rather than focusing on significant losses in functioning.

Coping mechanisms. Ask the patient how he or she normally copes with very stressful situations (such as by talking it out, yelling, throwing things, ignoring the situation, drinking, etc.).

Who is the patient's confidant? Involve this individual, if possible, in meeting the patient's care needs.

Verbal and nonverbal messages. Identify both the verbal and nonverbal messages conveyed. Take note of the patient's general appearance, tone of voice, inflections, and gestures. Try to pick up on subtle clues and confirm their meaning with the patient.

Evaluate the psychological issues that the patient is perceiving—loss of control, self-esteem, body part; guilt.

Nursing plans. Plan for nursing intervention based on the alterations that are significant to the patient's behavior, mood, and physical needs.

Pain. It is important to maintain an adequate level of pain relief for the patient with cancer. This requires identification of the underlying cause of the current pain being experienced to allow appropriate interventions to be initiated (e.g., bone and soft tissue pain may respond to local radiation, headaches may be relieved by corticosteroids if the basis is increased intracranial pressure).

Cancer patients experience varying degrees of pain. Careful assessment of the severity, location, duration, and any activities that increase or decrease the pain provides the physician with essential data for analysis of the individual's ever-changing needs for pain management. It is imperative that the nurse record the patient's response to the analgesics administered.

Oral medications are frequently used to provide pain relief. Several analgesics are also available as rectal suppositories. When oral and rectal forms of pain management no longer suffice, patients may require hospitalization for stabilization on parenteral forms of narcotic analgesics. Infusion pumps are frequently used, and spinal morphine may be delivered effectively via epidural or intrathecal catheters.

Nutritional status. Elicit data from the patient about normal eating patterns, food likes and dislikes, and elimination pattern. This information will serve as a baseline for future comparisons.

Weight. Has there been a weight loss or gain in the past year? Record the patient's weight and height on admission and at regular intervals throughout treatment. These data are used to calculate chemotherapy doses and to evaluate the individual's overall response to therapy.

Eating pattern. Ask the patient to describe his or her diet over the past 24 hours. Evaluate the data for types of foods from each of the four food groups, the quantity eaten, and the amount of time spent in eating. Ask if the eating pattern has changed over recent months and to what does the patient attribute any changes identified.

Ask whether certain foods cause bloating, indigestion, or diarrhea, and how much seasoning and spices are put on foods.

Fluid intake. Ask the patient to describe fluid intake. How much water, coffee, teas, soft drinks, fruit juice, and alcoholic beverages?

Personal hygiene

Oral hygiene and dental care. What is the status of the patient's teeth? When was a dentist last seen? Is any dental work currently in progress?

If the patient wears dentures, do they fit well or have there been recent problems in use? How does the patient care for the dentures?

Do not use the glycerin and lemon swabs routinely used in hospitals for oral hygiene. (See Patient Teaching for specific recommendations.)

Bowel habits. Ask the patient to describe a pattern of normal elimination (number of stools per day, color, and consistency). Since most narcotic analgesics produce constipation, an order for a stool softener or bulk laxative to be used on a scheduled basis is generally beneficial.

Administration of chemotherapy

Goal of treatment. Controlling the cancer cell growth, to either eradicate the cancer or to prolong the quality of life, is the primary goal of treatment.

Patient dosage. The dosage and frequency of administration is calculated by the physician. Finding the therapeutic dose that is not too toxic to the patient is done by calculation of the patient's body surface area and body weight as well as by monitoring laboratory tests and the patient's symptomatic response.

Accurate drug identification. Read the physician's order and check the drug name exactly. These drugs are extremely potent and the wrong drug or dose could be fatal to the patient.

Accurate identification of administration route. Chemotherapeutic drugs must be administered by specific routes for optimal effect. It is important to use the specified route.

Look for the details of administration (IV drip, bolus, diluted or undiluted, mixed in a specific solution, or added to a preexisting IV) and whether other medications should also be administered at the same time. (Review Chapters 5 through 7 on administration of medications.)

Mixing the medication. Chemotherapeutic agents that require reconstitution prior to use should *always* be mixed under a laminar vertical flow hood to protect yourself and those around you. Chemotherapeutic agents are potentially carcinogenic, mutagenic, and teratogenic.

Personnel preparing these drugs should follow the agency guidelines for the safe handling and disposal of these agents. Principles are aimed at avoiding direct contact of the antineoplastic agent with the skin and preventing inhalation or ingestion of the agents. A nonabsorbent gown that fastens in the back and has tight-fitting cuffs should be worn. The hands should be washed before donning and after removal of gloves. Wear safety glasses. Safety procedures should be followed for the safe disposal of the drug containers, intravenous apparatus, needles, and other items used during the preparation and administration of the agents.

Adhere closely to policies that define how body excreta, blood, and vomitus will be handled by personnel involved in caring for patients receiving antineoplastic therapy.

Preparation of the agent should be done immediately prior to administration. Always follow specific instructions from the manufacturer regarding the amount and type of diluent used and stability prior to administration.

IV administration. See also Chapter 6, on intravenous administration of medications, for details of vein selection and venipuncture and for complications of IV medication administration. In addition to utilizing short-term peripheral intravenous catheters (e.g., intracatheters, over-the-needle catheters) for administration of chemotherapy, implantable vascular access devices (e.g., Port-a-Cath, Medi-port, A-Port, and Groshong central venous catheters) are being placed for longer term therapy. New to the arena of central access devices is the peripherally inserted central (PIC) catheter. (See p. 106 for more information on the management of these devices.)

Before administering antineoplastic agents intravenously, check the venipuncture patency by giving 5 to 10 ml of normal saline through the needle before giving the agent. After administering the agent, again flush with 5 to 10 ml of saline.

Maintain a constant vigil for extravasation. Stop infusing the drug if the patient complains of burning or stinging. Watch for localized swelling and redness at the injection site. Know the hospital protocol for treatment of an infiltration and have equipment and drugs readily available for use.

Oral administration. Give the drug and dosage exactly as prescribed; usually, all the medication is given at one time, but there may be exceptions.

If vomiting occurs shortly after administration, report to the physician for directions.

Maintain accurate records of the drugs on the medication flow sheet. The flow record should also contain pertinent laboratory data such as WBC, RBC, and platelet counts. With this information, the most appropriate dosing schedule can be established.

When the patient is administering the medications, all aspects of the scheduling, dosage, side effects to expect, and side effects to report must be taught carefully.

Adverse effects associated with chemotherapy

Unfortunately, most chemotherapeutic agents are not very specific in the types of cells destroyed. Many normal cells in addition to abnormal cells are destroyed, thus causing many side effects.

Nausea, vomiting. There are three patterns of emesis associated with antineoplastic therapy: acute, delayed, and anticipatory emesis. Acute emesis occurs during the immediate hours after treatment, delayed emesis begins 12 to 24 hours after treatment, and anticipatory emesis occurs before the treatment starts. The last is caused by a conditioned stimulus as a learned response to the impending therapy. Antiemetic therapy is therefore scheduled differently depending on the pattern of emesis being seen.

Certain antineoplastic agents such as cisplatin, dacarbazine, mechlorethamine, cyclophosphamide, carmustine (BCNU), and dactinomycin are known to be highly emetogenic, and antiemetic therapy is administered prior to and in conjunction with these agents. A combination of agents with different sites of action is frequently used: lorazepam and dexamethasone (act on higher cortical centers), metoclopramide (dopamine antagonist), diphenhydramine (blocks vestibular apparatus and limits extrapyramidal effects of metoclopramide), and ondansetron (serotonin antagonist).

Chart the degree of effectiveness achieved when antiemetics are given. Report poor control to the physician. Changing the antiemetic medication ordered or the route of administration may improve control. Patients having nausea and vomiting need to have daily weighings and need to be monitored for electrolyte values and accurate intake and output.

Hydration. Monitor the patient's state of hydration. Check skin turgor, mucous membranes, softness of the eyeballs, etc. Electrolyte reports require vigilant observation; report abnormal findings to the physician. Fluid replacement via intravenous administration or total parenteral nutrition may be appropriate in some circumstances.

Positioning. Hospitalized patients may be sedated. Position the patient on one side to prevent aspiration.

Changes in bowel patterns. Depending on the treatment, the patient may develop diarrhea or constipation.

Diarrhea. Record the color, frequency, and consistency. Include watery stools in the output record. Check for occult blood. Provide for adequate hydration and administer any drugs ordered to relieve the symptoms.

Check the anal area for irritation, provide for hygiene measures and protect from excoriation with products such as A & D Ointment or zinc oxide ointment.

Encourage adequate fluid intake and dietary alterations such as eliminating spicy foods and those high in fat content. It may be necessary to switch to a clear liquid diet followed by a diet low in roughage. Diarrhea may require high protein foods with high caloric value and vitamin and mineral supplements. Patients with diarrhea should be monitored for fluid intake and output, daily weights, and electrolyte values.

Request an order for antidiarrheal drugs such as Kaopectate or Lomotil and administer appropriately.

Total parenteral nutrition may be necessary if symptoms persist.

Constipation. Compare this symptom with the patient's usual pattern of elimination. Many persons do not normally defecate daily.

Perform daily assessment of bowel sounds when the patient is hospitalized.

When a patient is constipated, the physician usually orders stool softeners or laxatives, fluids, and a diet that enhances normal defecation. Observe carefully for signs of an impaction (the urge to defecate without results, or oozing of a highly colored, watery solution from the rectum). Always report any abdominal pain or absence of bowel sounds.

Persons receiving narcotic analgesics may experience constipation from these agents. Laxatives are prescribed concurrently with the analgesics, and it may be necessary for enemas to be given occasionally.

Oral stomatitis. A comprehensive nursing assessment of oral hygiene and the oral cavity should be performed upon admission for treatment with chemotherapy. Collect data regarding the patient's usual hygiene practices. How many times per day is brushing and flossing done? What kind of toothbrush is used? What type of oral products are used (e.g., toothpaste, mouthwash)? If the person wears dentures, how well do they fit and how long each day are they worn? Have there been any changes in taste of foods or alterations in sensation within the mouth such as burning or tingling? Has there been any difficulty chewing or swallowing?

Stomatitis, manifested by erythema, ulcerations, or white patchy membranes, can be very uncomfortable and may interfere with the patient's nutrition. A scale used to standardize evaluation of stomatitis is listed in the box on this page. Inspect the mouth daily for any signs of bleeding gums or infection. White glistening areas, white patches, or yellow areas, which are usually surrounded by a red halo, should be reported immediately for treatment.

Disruption of the oral mucosa from chemotherapy has an onset within 5 to 7 days after antineoplastic therapy is administered; however, oral hygiene regimens should be initiated when chemotherapy is initiated. Oral hygiene measures should include using a soft-bristled brush, Water-pik on a *low* setting, or sponge-tipped applicators (with severe lesions) to remove debris. With advanced lesions, pain and discom-

---

Stomatitis scale

0 = Pink, moist, intact mucosa; absence of pain/burning
+1 = Generalized erythema with or without pain or burning; scalloped/ridging on tongue or buccal mucosal surfaces
+2 = Isolated small ulcerations and/or white plaques
+3 = Confluent ulcerations with or without white plaques > 25% of mucosal surface
+4 = Hemorrhagic ulcerations on > 25% of mucosal surface

From Engelking, C. Managing stomatitis: a nursing process approach. In Supportive care for the patient with cancer, Richmond, Va., 1988, A.H. Robins Company.

---

fort may be severe and other devices such as a gravity flow irrigating system or an oral syringe may be used to irrigate and cleanse the oral cavity.

Commercially prepared mouthwashes are usually not recommended since they contain alcohol, which may produce further drying of the mouth and irritate rather than relieve symptoms of stomatitis. Alternative solutions for oral hygiene are: one tablespoon of salt or hydrogen peroxide in 8 ounces of water, or ½ teaspoon of baking soda in 8 ounces of water as the mouthwash. There are disadvantages to each of these solutions; however, they remain the hallmark of irrigating solutions in use at this time. The frequency of the oral irrigations is important. They should be performed immediately before and after meals and at bedtime if symptoms are mild. With moderate lesions, increase the frequency to every 2 hours. In patients with severe symptoms, the mouth may be rinsed hourly. When fungal infections are present, the cleansing regimen should be performed immediately prior to administering the topical agents (nystatin liquids as a swish or clotrimazole troches). Performing the cleansing routine immediately prior to the medication will improve the contact of the drug with the denuded surface. Caution the patient not to take food or drink for approximately 15 minutes after the medication.

Dryness in the mouth can be relieved by chewing gum and sucking on ice chips or popsicles. Dry lips can be coated with cocoa butter, KY Jelly, petroleum jelly, or lip balm. Artificial saliva is available (Moi-Stir, Oralub, or Salivart).

Pain associated with oral stomatitis can be a major complication contributing to poor nutrition and hydration. For topical applications of medications for pain to be effective, they must come in contact with the tissue. Therefore, it is advisable to schedule these routines immediately after the cleansing of the oral cavity. The following are routine approaches to treating pain in the oral area:

- Xylocaine: Viscous 2% before meals to relieve pain. Care must be taken to make sure the patient is not burned by the food, since the entire mouth and throat are anesthetized.
- Milk of magnesia can be used to rinse the mouth and coat the mucous membranes.
- Kaopectate stirred in water may be used as a mouthwash to coat painful oral lesions.
- Nystatin liquid can be swished in the mouth for 1 minute then swallowed ("swish and swallow" routine), or clotrimazole troches may be chewed or sucked and then swallowed to reduce candidal oral infections.
- Sucralfate suspensions applied topically have been reported to provide effective pain relief.
- Oral or parenteral analgesics may be administered for severe pain.

Alopecia. Depending upon the type of medication required, patchy hair loss may develop in various parts of the body. When administering certain agents, a scalp tourniquet may be applied before treatment and left in place for 10 to 15 minutes to reduce this effect. Check the hospital procedure manual.

Neurotoxicity. Ask the patient about any changes in sensation or the development of tremors or incoordination. Observe the patient's gait, check tendon reflexes, and watch for foot or wrist drop; assess for alterations in mental status, blurred vision, urinary retention, impotence, and severe constipation.

Musculoskeletal complaints. All complaints of pain over a bony area, muscle weakness, and myalgia require follow-up. Check the calcium level in the laboratory reports at regular intervals and report deviations. Check x-ray reports for any indication of bone metastases. Notify the physician of any complaints that would possibly indicate a fracture. Keep the patient in bed until an examination is completed to rule out a fracture.

Bone marrow depression. Monitor laboratory reports for leukopenia (WBC < 1,000/mm^3); for thrombocytopenia (platelet count < 20,000/mm^3) or for erythropenia (reduced RBCs). Some patients will require transfusions of white cells, platelets, or RBCs. A new class of drugs, granulocyte stimulating agents, is being given to patients experiencing severe myelosuppression. Flu-like symptoms sometimes accompany the administration of these drugs; therefore, acetaminophen may be given concurrently.

Infection. Prevent infection by use of measures appropriate to the degree of suppression (reverse isolation, avoidance of persons with known infections). Use meticulous personal hygiene and report the earliest signs of infections. Staff and visitors should wear masks whenever indicated to protect the immunosuppressed patient from infections.

Three body systems are highly susceptible to infection in the immunocompromised patient. Daily assessments should be done to evaluate the status of the patient's skin and mucous membranes, respiratory system, and genitourinary system.

Immunocompromised patients require careful monitoring of the absolute neutrophil count (% neutrophils × total WBC divided by 100). The risk of infection increases as the neutrophil count decreases. A person with a neutrophil count of >1000/mm^3 is at minimal risk, between 500 and 1,000/mm^3 is at moderate risk, and at 500 cells/mm^3 or below is at severe risk of developing an infection.

Nursing assessments and interventions for the neutropenic patient may include: frequent monitoring of vital signs; observing the patient for chills and the development of a low-grade fever or a subnormal temperature; forcing fluids unless concurrent conditions make this inadvisable; assessment of laboratory studies at regular intervals to detect abnormal values especially in BUN, creatinine, CBC and differential, cultures, and sensitivities. Report abnormal values promptly. Check all IV lines for signs and symptoms of infection, maintain intravenous site dressings, and change intravenous tubings at intervals specified by hospital policy. Observe the color and amount of sputum; assess urine color, odor, and dysuria or frequency; and especially watch for mucus or blood in the urine.

Activity and exercise. Adjust the individual's activity level to the degree of impairment, laboratory alterations, and coordination, gait, or level of strength.

Introduce appropriate measures to conserve the patient's energy and need for oxygen to the tissues. Provide frequent rest periods. Assist with ambulating, if necessary.

It may be necessary to limit the number, frequency, and length of visitors' stays.

Maintain active and passive range-of-motion exercises; introduce measures to prevent foot drop or contractures.

Thrombocytopenia. Provide for patient safety and avoid unnecessary trauma through the following measures:

- Use an electric razor; avoid taking repeated blood pressure readings or using the same extremity for measurement.
- Give parenteral medications only when absolutely necessary. Apply direct pressure to the site for an extended period of time and be certain local bleeding is controlled. Use the smallest gauge needle possible.
- Avoid enemas or rectal temperature and prevent constipation because of the danger of damage to the mucosa and bleeding.
- Test all bowel movements for occult blood.
- Inspect the patient's skin daily for petechiae, ecchymoses, or areas of skin breakdown.

- Follow a specific turning schedule and give thorough skin care. Do not overexpose to the sun.
- Provide for oral hygiene, including lubricating the lips to prevent breakdown with cracking and bleeding. With a thrombocyte count of less than 20,000/mm^3 use sponge-tipped applicators to perform oral hygiene.
- Have the patient report any blood in the urine or blurred vision.

Patient Education Associated with Cancer Chemotherapy

Communication and responsibility. Encourage open communication concerning frustrations and anger as the patient attempts to adjust to the diagnosis and need for prolonged treatment. The patient must be guided to insight into the disorder in order to assume responsibility for the continuation of the treatment. Keep emphasizing those factors the patient can control to alter the progression of the disease, including the following:

Stress management. Some of the stressors observed in the patient coming for chemotherapy may be a belief in the effectiveness of treatment or a lack of faith in its outcomes. Trust in the care-givers and the plan of treatment is of immense importance.

The nurse and patient should discuss the patient's perspective on the illness and its effect on the patient, the family, and their ability to maintain the activities of daily living. Encourage the individual to express feelings about this illness and its effect on lifestyle.

CONTROL. Provide the patient with appropriate choices during care and chemotherapy to make sure he or she does not feel totally dominated by the disease or by the care-givers.

The degree of control will vary with each patient's situation. For example, allow choices in the scheduling of the times of chemotherapy and laboratory studies; try to adjust these so that the person can maintain a work schedule.

Take *time* to explain the procedures. Be calm, supportive, genuine, and warm.

Listen to the patient's concerns; take action to try to resolve appropriate problems, no matter how trivial. Let the patient know that personal *needs* are important.

Encourage the patient to maintain as normal a lifestyle as possible. Stress what the patient *can* do, not what he or she cannot do.

LOSS. Let the patient talk about the loss of a body part, loss of the ability to be a provider, or loss of the ability to receive or convey intimacy.

If the person is unable to provide for personal care, this too may be expressed in various ways (such as frustration, anger, yelling, despondency).

INTIMACY. Care-givers often do not consider the individual's ability to give or accept intimacy. Remember tact and diplomacy to avoid invading the person's privacy.

Involve appropriate members of the support group in the care of the patient to the degree the situation warrants.

ANXIETY. Provide the patient with information about the plan of care and treatment. Do not overwhelm patients with too much information too fast, or with information that is not needed.

Teach relaxation techniques and personal comfort measures, such as a warm bath to relieve stress.

Referral for biofeedback or other relaxation techniques, such as visual imagery, may be appropriate.

Stress produced within the family may be significant. Deal with these problems if possible; refer for professional counseling if necessary.

SUPPORT GROUPS. Support groups such as Make Today Count may be quite helpful. These groups provide the patient and family members with role models who are effectively coping with similar problems.

Nutritional status. Patient teaching must be individualized to the presenting problems, to the patient's experience, and to the nutritional history information. The major goal is to maintain the individual's weight and intake of foods to meet nutritional needs.

WEIGHT LOSS, ANOREXIA, ALTERED TASTE. Encourage the patient to eat favorite dishes (when not experiencing nausea and vomiting) and frequent, small servings of high-protein, bland foods if having difficulty with nausea. If nutritional supplements are needed, serve them attractively.

Encourage the patient to try washing the mouth with saline or sodium bicarbonate mouthwash immediately before eating. This will sometimes relieve the "bad taste" the individual is experiencing.

NAUSEA AND VOMITING. Persons experiencing nausea and vomiting from chemotherapy require special efforts to maintain nutritional needs.

Coke syrup, soda crackers, non-citrus juice, tepid tea, popsicles, or iced beverages may relieve nausea. Experiment with food temperatures—sometimes warm fluid such as broth works well.

The time the individual eats may need to be changed to the evening or late at night. Do not try to feed the patient who is experiencing nausea or vomiting episodes.

Administer antiemetics as prescribed by the physician. Report the effectiveness of response to the physician. Because antiemetics produce a sedative effect, provide for patient safety. Suggest having a family member or friend drive the patient home in the case of outpatient therapy. Have the patient report nausea and vomiting that lasts longer than 24 hours.

Some patients experience anticipatory nausea and vomiting before receiving each dose of medication. Relaxation techniques, visual imagery, and desensitizing techniques are being used effectively to manage these responses. Antiemetic therapy is often not effective in this pattern of emesis.

FLUID INTAKE. Unless contraindicated by co-existing

medical conditions, encourage the patient to maintain a fluid intake of 8 to 12 8-ounce glasses of fluid daily to prevent dehydration.

Oral hygiene. Before starting chemotherapy, any needed dental care should be completed. Have the patient discuss the condition with the physician and dentist.

PATIENT EDUCATION. Teach the patient to practice oral hygiene measures: Inspect the mouth daily for signs of bleeding gums or areas of yellow or white patches with red halos. If found, they should be reported to the physician for evaluation and treatment.

EQUIPMENT. Use a soft-bristled toothbrush or water cleanser (on a low setting) to prevent tissue damage. Use sponge-tipped applicators if degree of pain and mucosal damage reflects the need for this.

FREQUENCY. Oral hygiene measures should be performed immediately prior to and after meals and at bedtime. With more severe stomatitis the routine should be done every 2 hours.

MOUTHWASHES. Recommend that the patient not use commercially prepared mouthwashes. These products contain alcohol, which may cause further drying of the mouth and irritate rather than relieve the problem.

Use one tablespoonful of salt or hydrogen peroxide in 8 ounces of water, or ½ teaspoonful of baking soda in 8 ounces of water.

ORAL DRYNESS. Dryness can be relieved by chewing gum and sucking on ice chips or popsicles. Dry lips can be coated with cocoa butter, KY Jelly, petroleum jelly, or lip balm.

Artificial saliva is available (Moi-Stir, Ora-lub, or Salivart).

PAIN IN THE ORAL AREA. For topical applications of medications for pain to be effective, they must come in contact with the tissue. Teach the patient the regimen that is prescribed for the control of pain due to oral stomatitis. Stress the need to perform oral hygiene measures faithfully on schedule and especially to thoroughly cleanse the mouth immediately prior to performing the prescribed treatment for oral pain. See pp. 532 for description of pain interventions. For painful oral lesions, try using the following:

- Xylocaine: Viscous 2% before meals to relieve pain. Care must be taken to make sure the patient is not burned by the food, since the entire mouth and throat are anesthetized.
- Milk of magnesia can be used to rinse the mouth and coat the mucous membranes.
- Kaopectate stirred in water may be used as a mouthwash to coat painful oral lesions.
- Nystatin liquid can be swished in the mouth for one minute then swallowed ("swish and swallow" routine), or clotrimazole troches may be chewed or sucked and then swallowed to reduce candidal oral infections.

- Sucralfate suspensions applied topically have been reported to provide effective pain relief.
- Oral or parenteral analgesics may be administered for severe pain.

FOOD IRRITANTS. Oral irritation and stomatitis may be aggravated by salty foods, raw vegetables, some spices, alcohol, vinegar, tomatoes, and citrus fruits.

POOR DENTURE FIT. Denture fit should be carefully checked and poor fit discussed with the physician and dentist. Remove the dentures at night to reduce irritation to gum tissue.

Diarrhea. Provide adequate hydration during periods of diarrhea.

Dietary alterations to maintain low residue content should be encouraged in small frequent servings: milk, tender meat, fish, fowl, strained meat-based broth or soup, vegetable puree, ripe bananas, fruit juice, gelatin desserts, puddings, or custard.

During severe symptoms, clear liquids, broth, and clear fruit juices may be tolerated.

Prolonged diarrhea may require more vigorous treatment in a hospital setting. Always report increasing numbers of stools or a lack of response to antidiarrheal therapy.

Encourage the patient to report any black or dark, tarry stools or abdominal pain.

PERSONAL HYGIENE. Teach the patient to cleanse the perianal area thoroughly and to apply protective ointment as needed. Stress that the patient must cleanse hands after this procedure.

Constipation. Instruct the patient about appropriate foods to eat and the need for adequate fluid intake. Foods containing bulk, whole-grain breads or cereal, and stewed prunes may be helpful.

Instruct the patient about the use of any laxative or stool softener that has been prescribed.

Expectations of therapy

Activities and exercise. Maintain the individual's activities of daily living at the highest level consistent with symptoms. The level will vary throughout the course of therapy. Most patients are concerned with being able to continue as much of a normal lifestyle as possible.

- When therapy is first initiated, an increase in fatigue may be experienced for the first 2 to 4 weeks.
- Encourage frequent rest periods to avoid becoming unnecessarily overtired.
- Involve family members in planning assistance with activities, based on the degree of impairment present. Provide for patient safety at all times.

Infection control. Tell the patient to avoid crowds or persons with known infections. Report even the slightest sign of an infection so that vigorous treatment may be started immediately. Teach meticulous personal hygiene measures, especially the importance of handwashing.

Be certain the patient and/or support persons understand how to take a temperature. Go over critical observations that should be reported that are indicative of an infection (e.g., signs and symptoms of genitourinary tract, respiratory, or skin and mucous membrane infection). Teach the patient to use strict aseptic technique when changing dressings on wounds and/or invasive lines. Stress the importance of taking prescribed antibiotics as directed to maintain the blood level of the drug. Further emphasize that no medications should be stopped without specific directions from the physician.

Bleeding. Tell the patient to report bleeding gums, dark tarry stools, nosebleeds, bruises, or developing red spots (petechiae). Prevent accidental injury. Suggest the use of a safety or electric razor, not a standard razor.

Tell the patient not to use aspirin or aspirin-containing products.

Have female patients report menstrual flow that is excessive, bright red in color, or that lasts for a prolonged period of time.

Pain. One of the greatest fears of cancer patients is pain. If this concern is expressed, reassure the patient that pain can be effectively controlled. Additional information is available on pain management under the section on analgesics.

Alopecia. Hair loss may be expected with chemotherapy. Suggest the use of scarves, wigs, or turbans and ask the individual for suggestions.

During treatment, do not use hot curling irons or hair dryers. Avoid brushing, and comb gently. Shampoo less frequently and use a protein-based shampoo.

Tell the patient that hair loss may be evident for several weeks after administration of the chemotherapy. Regrowth usually starts within 8 weeks.

Skin disorders. Rashes and itching may occur with chemotherapy. Suggest the use of products such as Alpha Keri or Calamine lotion, or baking soda baths. Avoid overexposure to the sun.

Sexual activity. The patient should resume sexual activities as soon as possible after hospitalization. Patients need to be told to use birth control during and for 1 to 2 years following treatment with chemotherapy or radiation. (Many chemotherapeutic agents cause sterility or possible teratogenicity.)

Changes in expectations. Assess changes in expectations as therapy progresses and the patient gains understanding and skill in the management of the diagnosis.

Deal with the patient's concerns and questions prior to initiating specific teaching regarding medications or other needs. Determine what symptoms the patient is experiencing and how the patient expects they will be altered.

Changes in therapy through cooperative goal setting. Work with the patient to encourage adherence to the prescribed treatment. When the patient feels that a change should be made in a treatment plan, encourage discussion first with the physician.

Written record. Encourage the patient to return for all scheduled appointments with the physician or for laboratory studies ordered to monitor the individual's response to therapy. Enlist the patient's aid in developing and maintaining a written record of monitoring parameters (fatigue level, weight gain or loss, nausea, vomiting, diarrhea, constipation, pain relief) and response to prescribed therapies for discussion with the physician (Figure 21-1). Patients should be encouraged to bring this record on follow-up visits.

This record will need modification throughout the course of treatment. It should be based on the symptoms exhibited by the patient. The ultimate aim should be to evaluate the therapeutic response achieved when a change in therapy is prescribed.

Fostering compliance. Throughout the course of treatment, discuss medication information and how it will benefit the treatment. Seek cooperation and understanding of the following points so that medication compliance may be enhanced:

1. Name.
2. Dosage.
3. Route and administration times: Teaching must be adapted to the approach being recommended.
4. Anticipated therapeutic response: General improvement in the patient's overall symptoms and mental response (such as decreased pain, increased appetite, and ability to maintain activities of daily living).
5. Side effects to expect: Always research the particular drug your patient is receiving and be able to tell the patient what symptoms are expected. Common side effects include nausea and vomiting, diarrhea or constipation, oral stomatitis, increased fatigue, bleeding complications, alopecia, dyspnea, and peripheral neuropathy.

   Laboratory work to assess the degree of liver and kidney function and bone marrow depression is usually done to monitor the ability of the body to metabolize the antineoplastic agents.

   The nurse should explain the need for regular laboratory studies as a part of the method of evaluating the success of the agents administered. Any alterations from the normal values are reported to the physician for evaluation and modification of treatment.
6. Side effects to report: Always report signs of infection, abdominal pain, inability to defecate, bleeding, or increasing pain that is not controlled by the analgesic currently prescribed. Individualize the reporting of symptoms to the patient's disease state and the medications being used in the treatment plan.
7. What to do if a dose is missed.
8. When, how, or if to refill the medication prescription.

Difficulty in comprehension. If it is evident that the patient and/or family does not understand all aspects of

Patient Education and Monitoring of Therapeutic Outcomes for Patients Receiving Antineoplastic Agents

Medications	Color	To be taken

Name _____

Physician _____

Physician's phone _____

Next appt.* _____

Parameters		Day of discharge							Comments
Temperature	AM / PM								
Pain level — Severe 10 Moderate 5 None 1	8 AM / Noon / 6 PM / Night								
Fatigue level — Exausted with minimal activities 10 / Tired with performance of activities of daily living 5 / Normal 1									
Fear and anxiety — Anxious 10 / 5 / Calm 1									
Nausea: Degree of relief — Good 10 / Moderate 5 / Poor 1	Time of day								
Appetite — Good 10 / Normal 5 / Poor 1									
Oral hygiene — Normal 10 / Moderate pain 5 / Severe pain 1									
Bleeding (Yes or No)	Nosebleeds								
	Bruising								
Bowel movements	Color: brown, tarry								
	Diarrhea: Number of stools								
	Normal								

*Please bring this record with you to your next appointment.
Use the back of this sheet for additional information.

Figure 21-1 *Patient education and monitoring of therapeutic outcomes for patients receiving antineoplastic agents.*

continuing therapy being prescribed (such as administration and monitoring of medications, exercises, diets, follow-up appointments), consider the use of social service or visiting nurse agencies.

Associated teaching. Whenever possible, discuss the need for dental work with the physician and the advisability of having it completed prior to the initiation of chemotherapy.

Always inform the physician or dentist of any prescription or over-the-counter medication or chemotherapy being taken.

Over-the-counter medications should not be taken without first discussing them with a physician or pharmacist.

Always report side effects of rash, itching, or hives immediately. Nausea, vomiting, or diarrhea should also be reported for the physician's evaluation if it is a new symptom.

Take all of the medication as prescribed for the full course of treatment. Do not discontinue use when feeling improved; do not save for future use; do not give your medicine to another individual. Sudden discontinuation of certain medications may produce harmful effects.

Keep all medications out of reach of children.

If pregnancy is suspected, consult an obstetrician as soon as possible about continuation of medication therapy.

At discharge. Items to be sent home with the patient should include the following:

1. Written instructions for use
2. Labels in a level of language and size of print appropriate for the patient
3. If needed, identification cards or bracelets
4. A list of additional supplies to be purchased after discharge (such as for oral hygiene measures, soft-bristled toothbrush, mouthwash substitutes)
5. A schedule for follow-up appointments

Drug Therapy for Cancer

Objectives

1. State the four classes of antineoplastic agents.
2. State the types of tissue/cells affected by antineoplastic agents that result in hair loss, alteration in blood cells, and gastrointestinal symptoms.

Chemotherapeutic agents currently used are classified as (1) alkylating agents, (2) antimetabolites, (3) natural products (plant alkaloids, antibiotics, other synthetic agents), and (4) hormones. The mechanisms by which these agents cause cell death have not yet been fully determined. See Table 21-1 for a list of drug names, dosages, uses, and adverse effects associated with therapy.

Table 21-1 *Cancer Chemotherapeutic Agents*

DRUG	USUAL DOSAGE	TOXICITY		MAJOR INDICATIONS
		ACUTE	DELAYED	
Alkylating agents				
Busulfan (Myleran)	2-8 mg/day for 2-3 weeks PO; stop for recovery; then maintenance	None	Bone marrow depression	Chronic granulocytic leukemia
Carboplatin (Paraplatin)	360 mg/m² every four weeks	Nausea, vomiting	Bone marrow suppression, anemia, nephrotoxicity	Ovarian carcinoma
Carmustine (BCNU; ♣BiCNU)	As single agent: 100-200 mg/m² IV; over 1-2 hr infusion every 6-8 weeks In combination: 30-60 mg/m² IV Use gloves, since solution may cause skin discoloration	Nausea and vomiting; pain along vein of infusion	Granulocyte and platelet suppression Hepatic and renal toxicity	Brain, colon, breast, lung, Hodgkin's disease, lymphosarcoma, myeloma, malignant melanoma
Chlorambucil (Leukeran)	Start 0.1-0.2 mg/kg/day PO; adjust for maintenance	None	Bone marrow depression (anemia, leukopenia, and thrombocytopenia) can be severe with excessive dosage	Chronic lymphocytic leukemia, Hodgkin's disease, non-Hodgkin's lymphoma, trophoblastic neoplasms
Cisplatin (Platinol)	20–100 mg/m² IV; frequency highly variable	Nausea, vomiting	Nephrotoxicity, ototoxicity, blurred vision, changes in color perception	Testicular and ovarian cancers; bladder cancer

♣ Available in Canada only.

Table 21-1 *Cancer Chemotherapeutic Agents—cont'd*

DRUG	USUAL DOSAGE	TOXICITY		MAJOR INDICATIONS
		ACUTE	DELAYED	
Alkylating agents—cont'd				
Cyclophosphamide (Cytoxan)	40-50 mg/kg IV in single or in 2-8 daily doses or 2-4 mg/kg/day PO for 10 days; adjust for maintenance	Nausea and vomiting	Bone marrow depression, alopecia, cystitis	Hodgkin's disease and other lymphomas, multiple myeloma, lymphocytic leukemia, many solid cancers
Fludarabine (Fludara)	25 mg/m^2 daily IV over 30 min for 5 days	Nausea, vomiting	Fever, chills, cough, edema, rash	Chronic lymphocytic leukemia; lymphomas, Hodgkin's disease
Ifosfamide (Ifex)	1.2 g/m^2/day for 5 days IV	Nausea, vomiting, diarrhea	Hematuria alopecia	Testicular, lung, breast, ovarian, pancreatic and gastric cancer
Lomustine (CCNU) (CeeNu)	130 mg/m^2 PO once every 6 weeks	Severe nausea and vomiting; anorexia	Thrombocytopenia, leukopenia, alopecia, confusion, lethargy, ataxia	Brain, colon, Hodgkin's disease, lymphosarcoma, malignant melanoma
Mechlorethamine (nitrogen mustard; HN$_2$, Mustargen)	0.4 mg/kg IV in single or divided doses	Nausea and vomiting	Moderate depression of peripheral blood count	Hodgkin's disease and other lymphomas, bronchogenic carcinoma
Melphalan (1-phenylalanine mustard; Alkeran)	0.25 mg/kg/day for 4 days PO; 2-4 mg/day as maintenance or 0.1-0.15 mg/kg/day for 2-3 weeks	None	Bone marrow depression	Multiple myeloma, malignant melanoma, ovarian carcinoma, testicular seminoma
Streptozocin (Zanosar)	As single agent: 1.0-1.5 mg/m^2/week for 6 consecutive weeks with 4 weeks observation In combination: 400-500 mg/m^2 for 4-5 consecutive days with 6 weeks observation	Hypoglycemia, severe nausea and vomiting	Moderate but transient renal and hepatic toxicity, hypoglycemia, mild anemia, leukopenia	Pancreatic islet cell tumors
Thiotepa (triethylenethiophosphoramide)	0.2 mg/kg IV for 5 days	None	Bone marrow depression	Hodgkin's disease, bronchogenic and breast carcinomas
Antimetabolites				
Cytarabine hydrochloride (arabinosyl cytosine; Cytosar)	2-3 mg/kg/day IV until response or toxicity or 1-3 mg/kg IV over 24 hr for up to 10 days	Nausea and vomiting	Bone marrow depression megaloblastosis	Acute leukemia
Fluorouracil (5-FU, FU)	12.5 mg/kg/day IV for 3-5 days or 15 mg/kg/week for 6 weeks	Nausea	Oral and gastrointestinal ulceration, stomatitis and diarrhea, bone marrow depression	Breast, large bowel, and ovarian carcinoma
Mercaptopurine (6-MP, Purinethol)	2.5 mg/kg/day PO	Occasional nausea and vomiting, usually well tolerated	Bone marrow depression, occasional hepatic damage	Acute lymphocytic and granulocytic leukemia, chronic granulocytic leukemia

Continued.

Table 21-1 *Cancer Chemotherapeutic Agents—cont'd*

DRUG	USUAL DOSAGE	TOXICITY		MAJOR INDICATIONS
		ACUTE	DELAYED	
Antimetabolites—cont'd				
Methotrexate (amethopterin; MTX)	2.5-5.0 mg/day PO; 0.4 mg/kg rapid IV daily 4-5 days (not over 25 mg) or 0.4 mg/kg rapid IV twice/week	Occasional diarrhea, hepatic necrosis	Oral and gastrointestinal ulceration, bone marrow depression (anemia, leukopenia, thrombocytopenia), cirrhosis	Acute lymphocytic leukemia, choriocarcinoma, carcinoma of cervix and head and neck area, mycosis fungoides, solid cancers
Thioguanine (6-TG; ✤Lanvis)	2 mg/kg/day PO	Occasional nausea and vomiting, usually well tolerated	Bone marrow depression	Acute leukemia
Natural products				
Etoposide (Vepesid)	50-100 mg/m² daily for 5 days IV; cycles of therapy are given every 3-4 weeks	Nausea (15%), vomiting, stomatitis, diarrhea	Leukopenia, nadir in 10-14 days, recovery in 3 weeks; thrombocytopenia; alopecia	Testicular tumors, small cell carcinoma of the lung, Hodgkin's disease and non-Hodgkin's lymphoma, acute nonlymphocytic leukemia, breast carcinoma, Kaposi's sarcoma
Vinblastine sulfate (Velban; ✤Velbe)	0.1-0.2 mg/kg/week IV or every 2 weeks	Nausea and vomiting, local irritant	Alopecia, stomatitis, bone marrow depression, loss of reflexes	Hodgkin's disease and other lymphomas, solid cancers
Vincristine sulfate (Oncovin)	0.01-0.03 mg/kg/week IV	Local irritant	Areflexia, peripheral neuritis, paralytic ileus, mild bone marrow depression	Acute lymphocytic leukemia, Hodgkin's disease and other lymphomas, solid cancers
Antibiotics				
Bleomycin (Blenoxane)	10-15 mg/m² once or twice a week, IV or IM to total dose 300-400 mg	Nausea and vomiting, fever, very toxic	Edema of hands, pulmonary fibrosis, stomatitis, alopecia	Hodgkin's disease, non-Hodgkin's lymphoma, squamous cell carcinoma of head and neck, testicular carcinoma
Dactinomycin (actinomycin D; Cosmegen)	0.015-0.05 mg/kg/week (1-2.5 mg) for 3-5 weeks IV; wait for marrow recovery (3-4 weeks), then repeat course	Nausea and vomiting, local irritant	Stomatitis, oral ulcers, diarrhea, alopecia, mental depression, bone marrow depression	Testicular carcinoma, Wilms' tumor, rhabdomyosarcoma, Ewing's and osteogenic sarcoma, and other solid tumors
Daunorubicin (Cerubidine)	30-45 mg/m²/day for 2 or 3 days of combination therapy; never give IM or SC	Nausea, vomiting, diarrhea, fever, chills	Bone marrow suppression, reversible alopecia	Acute nonlymphocytic leukemia in adults; acute lymphocytic leukemia in children and adults
Doxorubicin (Adriamycin)	60-90 mg/m² IV, single dose or over 3 days; repeat every 3 weeks up to total dose 500 mg/m²	Nausea, red urine (not hematuria)	Bone marrow depression, cardiotoxicity, alopecia, stomatitis	Soft tissue, osteogenic and miscellaneous sarcomas, Hodgkin's disease, non-Hodgkin's lymphoma, bronchogenic and breast carcinoma, thyroid cancer, leukemias

✤Available in Canada only.

Table 21-1 *Cancer Chemotherapeutic Agents—cont'd*

DRUG	USUAL DOSAGE	TOXICITY ACUTE	TOXICITY DELAYED	MAJOR INDICATIONS
Antibiotics—cont'd				
Idarubicin (Idamycin)	12 mg/m^2/day for 3 days by slow (10-15 min) IV; do not give IM or SC	Nausea, vomiting, diarrhea	Bone marrow suppression, cardiotoxicity, mucositis, hemorrhage	Acute myelocytic leukemia
Mitomycin C (Mutamycin)	0.05 mg/kg/day IV for 5 days	Nausea and vomiting "flulike syndrome"	Bone marrow depression, skin toxicity; pulmonary, renal, CNS effects	Squamous cell carcinoma of head and neck, lungs, and cervix; adenocarcinoma of the stomach, pancreas, colon, rectum; adenocarcinoma and duct cell carcinoma of the breast
Mitoxantrone (Novantrone)	12 mg/m^2/day for 2-3 days by IV infusion	Nausea, vomiting, diarrhea	Congestive heart failure; GI bleeding; cough, dyspnea	Acute nonlymphocytic leukemia, non-Hodgkin's lymphoma, breast cancer
Plicamycin (Mithracin)	0.025-0.050 mg/kg every 2 days for up to 8 doses, IV	Nausea and vomiting, hepatotoxicity	Bone marrow depression (thrombocytopenia), hypocalcemia	Testicular carcinoma, trophoblastic neoplasms
Other synthetic agents				
Altretamine (Hexalen) ♣ (Hexastat)	260 mg/m^2/day for 14 or 21 days in a 28-day cycle; give daily doses as 4 divided oral doses	Nausea, vomiting	Anemia, leukopenia, thrombocytopenia, peripheral neuropathy	Ovarian cancer
Dacarbazine (DTIC-Dome; DIC)	4.5 mg/kg/day IV for 10 days; repeated every 28 days	Nausea and vomiting "flulike syndrome"	Bone marrow depression (rare)	Metastatic malignant melanoma
Hydroxyurea (Hydrea)	80 mg/kg PO single dose every 3 days or 20-30 mg/kg/day PO	Mild nausea and vomiting	Bone marrow depression	Chronic granulocytic leukemia
Interferon Alfa 2a (Roferon-A)	3 million units daily IM or SC	"Flu-like syndrome"	Bone marrow depression	Hairy cell leukemia
Interferon Alfa 2b (Intron A)	2 million μ/m^2 IM or SC 3 times/week	"Flu-like syndrome"	Bone marrow depression	Hairy cell leukemia
Interferon (Alfa-n3)	Highly variable	Fever, muscle aches, headache, nausea	Bone marrow suppression	Condylomata acuminata; carcinoid tumor; non-Hodgkin's lymphoma
Levamisole (Ergamisol)	50 mg PO every 8 hours for 3 days every 2 weeks	Nausea, diarrhea	Dermatitis, alopecia, leukopenia	Colon cancer
Leuprolide acetate (Lupron)	1 mg SC daily	Hot flashes; initial exacerbation of symptoms	Arrhythmias, edema	Prostatic carcinoma, breast carcinoma
Mitotane (Lysodren)	6-15 mg/kg/day PO	Nausea and vomiting	Dermatitis, diarrhea, mental depression	Adrenal cortical carcinoma
Procarbazine hydrochloride (Methyl hydrazine; ibenzmethylzin; Matulane; ♣Natulan)	Start 1-2 mg/kg/day PO; increase over 1 week to 3 mg/kg; maintain for 3 weeks, then reduce to 2 mg/kg/day until toxicity	Nausea and vomiting	Bone marrow depression, CNS depression	Hodgkin's disease, non-Hodgkin's lymphoma, bronchogenic carcinoma

♣Available in Canada only.

Continued.

Table 21-1 *Cancer Chemotherapeutic Agents—cont'd*

DRUG	USUAL DOSAGE	TOXICITY		MAJOR INDICATIONS
		ACUTE	DELAYED	
Other synthetic agents—cont'd				
Tamoxifen (Nolvadex)	20-40 mg daily in two divided doses	Nausea, vomiting, hot flashes	Increased bone and tumor pain, thrombocytopenia, leukopenia, edema, hypercalcemia	Breast cancer (estrogen sensitive)
Hormones				
Diethylstilbestrol (DES)	15 mg/day PO (1 mg in prostate cancer)	None	Fluid retention, hypercalcemia, feminization, uterine bleeding; if during pregnancy, may cause vaginal carcinoma in offspring	Breast and prostate carcinomas
Dromostanolone propionate (Drolban)	100 mg 3 times a week IM	None	Fluid retention, masculinization, hypercalcemia	Breast carcinoma
Ethinyl estradiol	3 mg/day PO	None	Fluid retention, hypercalcemia, feminization, uterine bleeding	Breast and prostate carcinomas
Fluoxymesterone	10-20 mg/day PO	None	Fluid retention, masculinization, cholestatic jaundice	Breast carcinoma
Flutamide (Eulexin) ♣ (Euflex)	2 capsules PO 3 times daily at 8 hr intervals	Nausea, vomiting	Hot flashes, loss of libido, impotence, gynecomastia	Metastatic prostatic carcinoma
Goserelin (Zoladex)	3.6 mg SC every 28 days in upper abdominal wall; local anesthesia may be used	Anorexia, dizziness, pain	Hot flashes, sexual dysfunction	Carcinoma of the prostate
Hydroxyprogesterone caproate	1 g IM twice a week	None	None	Endometrial carcinoma
Medroxyprogesterone acetate	100-200 mg/day PO; 200-600 mg twice a week	None	None	Endometrial carcinoma, renal cell, breast cancer
Prednisone	10-100 mg/day PO	None	Hyperadrenocorticism	Acute and chronic lymphocytic leukemia, Hodgkin's disease, non-Hodgkin's lymphomas
Testolactone (Teslac)	100 mg 3 times a week IM	None	Fluid retention, masculinization	Breast carcinoma
Testosterone enanthate	600-1200 mg/week IM	None	Fluid retention, masculinization	Breast carcinoma
Testosterone propionate	50-100 mg, IM 3 times a week	None	Fluid retention, masculinization	Breast carcinoma

♣ Available in Canada only.

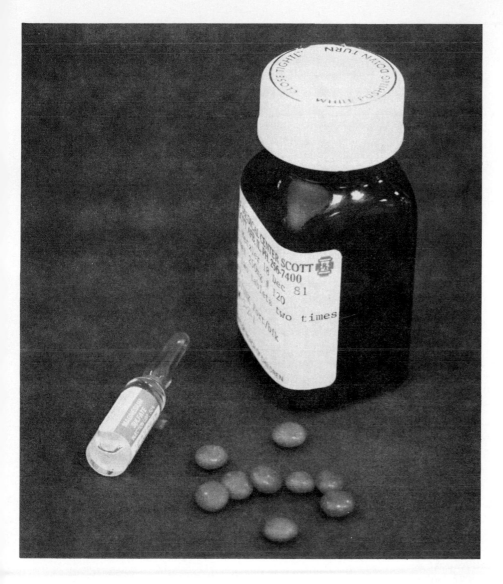

22

Miscellaneous Agents

CHAPTER GOALS

After completing this chapter, the student should be able to do the following:

1. Identify baseline data the nurse should collect on a continuous basis for comparison and evaluation of drug effectiveness.

2. Identify important nursing assessments and interventions associated with the drug therapy.

3. Identify essential components involved in planning patient education that will enhance compliance with the treatment regimen.

General Nursing Considerations for Patients Receiving Medications

Patient Education Associated with Medication Therapy

Communication and responsibility. Encourage open communication concerning frustrations and anger as the patient attempts to adjust to the diagnosis and need for prolonged treatment. The patient must be guided to gain insight into the condition in order to assume the responsibility for the continuation of treatment. Keep emphasizing those factors the patient can control to alter the progression of the disease, including maintenance of general health, nutritional needs, adequate rest and appropriate exercise, and continuation of prescribed medication therapy.

Expectations of therapy. Discuss expectations of therapy with the patient (such as level of exercise, degree of pain relief, frequency of medication use, relief of dyspnea, sexual activity, maintenance of mobility, ability to maintain activities of daily living and/or work).

Changes in expectations. Assess changes in expectations as therapy progresses and the patient gains understanding and skill in the management of the diagnosis.

Changes in therapy through cooperative goal setting. Work with the patient to encourage adherence to the prescribed treatment. When the patient feels that a change should be made in a treatment plan, encourage discussion first with the physician.

Written record. Enlist the patient's aid in developing and maintaining a written record of monitoring parameters (such as blood pressure, pulse, daily weights, degree of pain relief, exercise tolerance) and response to prescribed therapies for discussion with the physician. Patients should be encouraged to bring this record on follow-up visits.

Fostering compliance. Throughout the patient's hospitalization, discuss medication information and how it will benefit the course of treatment. Seek cooperation and understanding of the following points so that medication compliance may be enhanced:

1. Name
2. Dosage
3. Route and administration times
4. Anticipated therapeutic response
5. Side effects to expect
6. Side effects to report
7. What to do if a dose is missed
8. When, how, or if to refill the medication prescription

Difficulty in comprehension. If it is evident that the patient and/or family does not understand all aspects of continuing therapy being prescribed (such as administration and monitoring of medications, exercises, diets, follow-up appointments), consider the use of social service or visiting nurse agencies.

Associated teaching. Give patients the following instructions:

Always inform the physician or dentist of any prescription or over-the-counter medication being taken. Over-the-counter medications should not be taken without first discussing with a physician or pharmacist.

Always report side effects of rash, itching, or hives immediately. Nausea, vomiting, or diarrhea should also be reported for the physician's evaluation if it is a new symptom.

Take all of the medication as prescribed for the full course of treatment. Do not discontinue use when feeling improved; do not save for future use; do not give your medicine to another individual. Sudden discontinuation of certain medications may produce harmful effects.

Keep all medications out of reach of children.

If pregnancy is suspected, consult an obstetrician as soon as possible about continuation of medication therapy.

At discharge. Items to be sent home with the patient should include the following:

1. Written instructions for use
2. Labels in a level of language and size of print appropriate for the patient
3. If needed, identification cards or bracelets
4. A list of additional supplies to be purchased after discharge (such as syringes, dressings)
5. A schedule of follow-up appointments

Drug Therapy

Objectives

1. Compare the effects of allopurinol and colchicine on the formation of urate crystals.
2. State why colchicine is not classified as a uricosuric agent.
3. Identify the assessments and monitoring parameters needed to detect blood dyscrasias caused by allopurinol and colchicine.
4. State the action and uses of disulfiram.

5. Cite the action and uses of lactulose.
6. Describe the usage of nicotine polacrilex (Nicorette) as an aid to cessation of smoking.
7. Identify instructions needed to educate the patient in the proper dosage and use of nicotine polacrilex.

allopurinol (al-o-pu′ri-nol)

Zyloprim (zy′lo-prim)

Allopurinol represents an entirely different approach to the treatment of gout. It blocks the terminal steps in uric acid formation by inhibiting the enzyme xanthine oxidase. This agent can be used for the treatment of primary gout or gout secondary to antineoplastic therapy. It is not effective in treating acute attacks of gouty arthritis.

Allopurinol has an advantage over uricosuric agents in that gouty nephropathy and the formation of urate stones are less likely with allopurinol because the drug reduces the amount of uric acid produced. It may also be used in patients with renal failure, whereas uricosuric agents should not be.

Side effects. The number of gouty attacks may increase during the first 6 to 12 months of treatment. Continue allopurinol therapy without changing doses during these attacks. Treat the acute attack with colchicine or antiinflammatory agents.

General side effects are nausea, vomiting, headache, diarrhea, drowsiness, and a metallic taste in the mouth.

Rarely, allopurinol may produce hepatotoxicity or blood dyscrasias. Periodic laboratory tests, including blood counts and liver function tests, are recommended to avoid complications.

Patients may develop a hypersensitivity to allopurinol manifested by fever, pruritus, and rashes. If these symptoms develop, discontinue therapy.

Availability
PO—100 and 300 mg tablets.
Dosage and administration
Adult
PO—Initially 100 mg daily. Increase the daily dosage by 100 mg/week until the serum urate level falls to 6 mg/100 ml or a maximum dosage of 800 mg daily is achieved.

- The average maintenance dose is 300 mg daily.
- Therapy is better tolerated if the drug is taken with meals.
- Maintain fluid intake at 2 to 3 liters daily.

- **Nursing Interventions: Monitoring allopurinol therapy**

See General Nursing Considerations for Patients with Gout.

Side effects to expect
ACUTE GOUT ATTACKS. Patients should be told that the frequency of gout attacks may increase for the first few months of therapy. The patient should continue therapy without changing the doses during the attacks.

NAUSEA, VOMITING, DIARRHEA, DIZZINESS, HEADACHE. These side effects are usually mild and tend to resolve with continued therapy. Encourage the patient not to discontinue therapy without first consulting the physician.

Side effects to report
HEPATOTOXICITY. The symptoms of hepatotoxicity are anorexia, nausea, vomiting, jaundice, hepatomegaly, splenomegaly, and abnormal liver function tests (elevated bilirubin, AST, ALT, GGT, alkaline phosphatase, prothrombin time).

BLOOD DYSCRASIAS. Routine laboratory studies (RBC, WBC, and differential counts) should be scheduled. Stress returning for this laboratory work.

Monitor for the development of a sore throat, fever, purpura, jaundice, or excessive, progressive weakness.

FEVER, PRURITUS, RASH. Report symptoms for further evaluation by the physician.

Pruritus may be relieved by adding baking soda to the bath water.

Implementation
GASTRIC IRRITATION. If gastric irritation occurs, administer with food or milk. If symptoms persist or increase in severity, report for physician evaluation.

FLUID INTAKE. Maintain fluid intake at 8 to 12 8-ounce glasses daily.

Drug interactions
THEOPHYLLINE DERIVATIVES. Allopurinol, when given with theophylline derivatives, may result in theophylline toxicity. Observe for vomiting, dizziness, restlessness, and cardiac arrhythmias. The dosage of theophylline may need to be reduced.

DICUMAROL (POSSIBLY WARFARIN). This medication may enhance the anticoagulant effects of dicumarol. Observe for the development of petechiae, ecchymoses, nosebleeds, bleeding gums, dark tarry stools, and bright red or coffee ground emesis. Monitor the prothrombin time and reduce the dosage of dicumarol if necessary.

CHLORPROPAMIDE. Allopurinol may reduce the metabolism of chlorpropamide. Monitor for hypoglycemia: headache, weakness, decreased coordination, general apprehension, diaphoresis, hunger, blurred or double vision.

The dosage of the hypoglycemic agent may need to be reduced. Notify the physician if any of the above symptoms appears.

AZATHIOPRINE, MERCAPTOPURINE. When initiating therapy with azathioprine or mercaptopurine, start at one-fourth to one-third of the normal dosage and adjust subsequent dosages to the patient's response.

VIDARABINE. Allopurinol alters the metabolism of vidarabine. Monitor closely for signs of neurotoxicity: pain, itching, tremors of the extremities and facial muscles, and impaired mentation.

Perform a baseline assessment of the patient's degree of alertness and orientation to name, place, and time *before* initiating therapy. Make regularly scheduled subsequent mental status evaluations and compare findings. Report development of alterations.

AMPICILLIN. There is a high incidence of rash when patients are taking both allopurinol and ampicillin. Do not label the patient allergic to either drug until sensitivity tests identify a hypersensitivity reaction.

CYCLOPHOSPHAMIDE. There is a greater frequency of bone marrow depression in patients receiving these agents concurrently. Monitor for the development of a sore throat, fever, purpura, jaundice, or excessive, progressive weakness.

colchicine (kol'chi-sin)

Colchicine is an alkaloid that has been used for hundreds of years to prevent or relieve acute attacks of gout. The exact mechanism of action is not known, but colchicine does interrupt the cycle of urate crystal deposition in the tissues that results in an acute attack of gout. It does not affect the amount of uric acid in the blood or urine, so it is not a uricosuric agent.

Side effects. Nausea, vomiting, and diarrhea are common adverse effects of colchicine therapy. Discontinue therapy when gastrointestinal symptoms develop.

Serious, potentially fatal blood dyscrasias, including anemia, agranulocytosis, and thrombocytopenia, have been associated with colchicine therapy. Although the development of blood dyscrasias is quite rare, periodic differential blood counts are recommended if the patient requires prolonged treatment.

Availability
PO—0.6 mg tablets, 0.5 mg granules.
IV—1 mg/2 ml ampules.

Dosage and administration. NOTE: Use with extreme caution in elderly or debilitated patients and in those patients with impaired renal, cardiac, or gastrointestinal function.

Adult
PO—Acute gout: initially 0.5 to 1.2 mg, followed by 0.6 mg every 1 to 2 hours until pain subsides or nausea, vomiting, and diarrhea develop. A total dosage of 4 to 10 mg may be required. After the acute attack, 0.5 to 0.6 mg should be administered every 6 hours for a few days to prevent relapse. Do not repeat high-dose therapy for at least 3 days. Prophylaxis for recurrent gout: 0.5 to 0.6 mg every 1 to 3 days depending on the frequency of gouty attacks.
IV—Acute gout: initially 2 mg diluted in 20 ml of saline solution. Follow with 0.5 mg every 6 to 12 hours to a maximum of 4 mg in 24 hours. If pain recurs, daily doses of 1 to 2 mg may be administered for several days. Do not repeat high-dosage therapy for at least 3 days. *Avoid extravasation.*
DO NOT ADMINISTER SC OR IM!

• **Nursing Interventions: Monitoring colchicine therapy**

See also General Nursing Considerations for Patients with Gout.

Side effects to expect
NAUSEA, VOMITING, DIARRHEA. Discontinue therapy when gastrointestinal symptoms develop. Always report bright blood or "coffee ground" appearing in vomitus or dark tarry stools.

THERAPEUTIC EFFECTS. Joint pain and swelling begin to subside within 12 hours and are usually gone within 48 to 72 hours following initiation of therapy.

Side effects to report
BLOOD DYSCRASIAS. Routine laboratory studies (RBC, WBC, and differential counts) should be scheduled. Stress returning for this laboratory work.

Monitor for the development of a sore throat, fever, purpura, jaundice, or excessive, progressive weakness. Report immediately.

Implementation
IV. Dilute 2 mg in 20 ml of saline solution and administer slowly over 5 minutes.

EXTRAVASATION. Observe IV site for any change in the color, size, or skin integrity. Pain, swelling, or erythema signify infiltration.

• Clamp, report, and follow hospital protocol for extravasation.
• Elevate the infiltrated area.
• Prepare to assist with administration of drugs to counteract the necrotizing effects.

SC, IM. Do not administer via these routes.

FLUID INTAKE. Monitor intake and output during therapy. Maintain fluid intake at 8 to 12 8-ounce glasses daily.

disulfiram (di-sul'fi-ram)

Antabuse (an'tah-byuse)

Disulfiram is an agent that, when ingested before any form of alcohol, produces a very unpleasant reaction to the alcohol. It is used in alcohol rehabilitation programs for chronic alcoholic patients who want to maintain sobriety. It should be used only in conjunction with other rehabilitative therapy.

The disulfiram-alcohol reaction is manifested by nausea, severe vomiting, sweating, throbbing headache, dizziness, blurred vision, and confusion. The intensity of the reaction is somewhat dependent on the sensitivity of the individual and the amount of alcohol consumed. The duration of the reaction depends on the presence of alcohol in the blood. Mild reactions may last from 30 to 60 minutes, whereas more severe reactions may last for several hours.

Patients must be fully informed of the consequences of drinking alcohol while receiving disulfiram therapy.

As little as 10 to 15 ml of alcohol may produce a reaction. Patients must not drink alcohol in any form, including over-the-counter products such as sleep aids, cough and cold products, after-shave lotions, mouthwashes, and rubbing lotions. Dietary sources, such as sauces and vinegars containing alcohol, are prohibited. A disulfiram-alcohol reaction may occur with the ingestion of any alcohol for 1 to 2 weeks after the discontinuation of disulfiram therapy.

Side effects. Disulfiram generally does not induce many side effects; however, some patients have reported drowsiness, fatigability, impotence, headache, acne, or metallic or garlic taste. These side effects are generally mild and transient. Hypersensitivity reactions manifested by rashes have been reported.

Hepatotoxicity has been reported with disulfiram therapy. Baseline liver function tests are recommended, with follow-up in 10 to 14 days, to detect hepatic dysfunction. Routine liver and kidney function tests, as well as measurement of electrolytes, are recommended every 6 months.

Because of the consequences of a disulfiram-alcohol reaction on other disease states, use disulfiram therapy very cautiously in patients with diabetes mellitus, hypothyroidism, epilepsy, cerebral damage, chronic and acute nephritis, hepatic cirrhosis, or hepatic insufficiency.

Availability

PO—250 and 500 mg tablets.

Dosage and administration. NOTE: Disulfiram must never be administered to patients when they are in a state of intoxication or when they are unaware they are receiving therapy. Family members should also be told of the treatment to help provide motivation and support and to help avoid accidental disulfiram-alcohol reactions.

Do not administer disulfiram until the patient has abstained from alcohol for at least 12 hours.

Adult

PO—Initially a maximum of 500 mg once daily for 1 to 2 weeks. The maintenance dose is usually 250 mg daily (range: 125 to 500 mg). Do not exceed 500 mg daily.

- **Nursing Interventions: Monitoring disulfiram therapy**

Side effects to expect

DROWSINESS, FATIGUE, HEADACHE. These side effects are usually mild and tend to resolve with continued therapy. Encourage the patient not to discontinue therapy without first consulting the physician.

Side effects to report

HEPATOTOXICITY. The symptoms of hepatotoxicity are anorexia, nausea, vomiting, jaundice, hepatomegaly, splenomegaly, and abnormal liver function tests (elevated bilirubin, AST, ALT, GGT, alkaline phosphatase, prothrombin time).

NEPHROTOXICITY. Monitor urinalysis and kidney function tests for abnormal results. Report an increasing BUN and creatinine, decreasing urine output and/or decreasing specific gravity (despite amount of fluid intake), casts or protein in the urine, frank blood or smoky-colored urine, or RBCs in excess of 0-3 on the urinalysis report.

HIVES, PRURITUS, RASH. Report symptoms for further evaluation by the physician.

Pruritus may be relieved by adding baking soda to the bath water.

Implementation

PO. Administer at bedtime to avoid the complications of sedative side effects.

Drug interaction

WARFARIN. This medication may enhance the anticoagulant effects of warfarin. Observe for the development of petechiae, ecchymoses, nosebleeds, bleeding gums, dark tarry stools, and bright red or coffee ground emesis. Monitor the prothrombin time and reduce the dosage or warfarin if necessary.

PHENYTOIN. Disulfiram inhibits the metabolism of phenytoin. Monitor patients with concurrent therapy for signs of phenytoin toxicity: nystagmus, sedation, lethargy. Serum levels may be ordered and the dosage of phenytoin may be reduced.

ISONIAZID. Disulfiram alters the metabolism of isoniazid. Perform a baseline assessment of the patient's degree of alertness (orientation to name, place, and time) and of coordination *before* initiating therapy. Make regularly scheduled subsequent mental status evaluations and compare findings. Report development of alterations.

METRONIDAZOLE. Concurrent administration of disulfiram and metronidazole may result in psychotic episodes and confusional states. Concurrent therapy is not recommended.

lactulose (lak'tu-los)

Cephulac (sef'u-lak), **Duphalac** (du'fah-lak)

Lactulose is a sugar used to treat portal-systemic (hepatic) encephalopathy and hepatic coma by reducing blood ammonia levels. It acts by acidifying the colon, thus preventing the absorption of ammonia, which is implicated as a cause of hepatic encephalopathy and coma. Lactulose may also be used as a laxative.

Side effects. Common adverse effects frequently observed in the early stages of therapy are belching, gaseous distension, flatulence, and cramping. These side effects resolve with continued therapy, but dosage reduction may also be necessary. Diarrhea is a sign of overdosage and responds to dosage reduction.

Use with caution in patients with diabetes mellitus.

Lactulose syrup contains small amounts of free lactose, galactose, and other sugars.

Patients who use lactulose chronically for 6 months or longer should have serum potassium and chloride levels measured periodically.

Availability
PO—10 g of lactulose per 15 ml of syrup.
Dosage and administration
Adult
Laxative:
PO—Initially 15 to 30 ml daily. Increase to 60 ml daily if necessary.
Portal-systemic encephalopathy:
PO—Initially 30 to 45 ml every hour for rapid laxation. Once the laxative effect is achieved, the dosage is reduced to 30 to 45 ml 3 to 4 times daily. Adjust the dose to produce 2 or 3 soft, formed stools daily.
Rectal—Mix 300 ml of syrup with 700 ml of water or normal saline. Instill rectally every 4 to 6 hours with a rectal balloon catheter. Have the patient attempt to retain for 30 to 60 minutes.

- Do not use soap suds or cleansing enemas.

- **Nursing Interventions: Monitoring lactulose therapy**
  Side effects to report
  ELECTROLYTE IMBALANCE, DEHYDRATION. These effects may result from diarrhea. The electrolytes most commonly altered are potassium (K^+) and chloride (Cl^-). *Hypokalemia* is most likely to occur.

  Many symptoms associated with altered fluid and electrolyte balance are subtle and resemble general symptoms of drug toxicity or the disease process itself.

  Gather data relative to changes in the patient's mental status (i.e., alertness, orientation, confusion), muscle strength, muscle cramps, tremors, nausea, and general appearance (drowsy, anxious, lethargic).

  Always check the electrolyte reports for early indications of electrolyte imbalance.

  Keep accurate records of I/O, daily weights, and vital signs.
  Implementation
  PO. Twenty-four to forty-eight hours may be required to produce a normal bowel movement. Administer with fruit juice, water, or milk to make the syrup more palatable.
  RECTAL. See instructions above.
  Drug interactions
  LAXATIVES. Do not administer with other laxatives. Diarrhea makes it difficult to adjust to a proper dosage of lactulose.

  ANTIBIOTICS. Antibiotic therapy may destroy too much of the bacteria in the colon that are necessary for lactulose to work. Monitor patients closely for reduced lactulose activity when concurrent antibiotic therapy is prescribed.

nicotine polacrilex (nik-oh′teen pohl-ah-kry-lex′)
  Nicorette (nik-or′et)
Nicotine polacrilex is used as a temporary aid to the cigarette smoker who wants to quit smoking and who is participating in a behavior modification program under medical supervision. Nicotine polacrilex is a cation-exchange resin that is added to a chewing gum base that has a distinctive, tobacco-like, slightly peppery taste. When chewed, the naturally occurring autonomic stimulant, nicotine, is released and absorbed through the buccal mucosa. Nicotine is a major component of cigarette smoke that is both physiologically and psychologically addicting. The gradual release and absorption provide sufficient nicotine to control withdrawal symptoms but does not produce the "pleasurable effects" often derived from smoking. By reducing or eliminating physical withdrawal symptoms, it permits the smoker to deal more effectively with the social and psychological aspects of smoking. The lack of these effects later helps facilitate gradual withdrawal from the use of the nicotine gum.

Side effects. Common adverse effects of the nicotine gum include burning and soreness of the mouth and throat. Lightheadedness, headache, hiccups, nausea, vomiting, and excess saliva may also occur.

Availability. 2 mg chewing gum squares.

Dosage and administration. NOTE: Behavior modification is an integral component of smoking cessation therapy. Because the gum is used only as an adjunct to the patient's own cessation efforts, the drug should be used only in patients who strongly desire to quit smoking.

The gum should not be swallowed.
Adult
PO—One 2 mg square of gum as needed for cigarette craving.

- **Nursing Interventions: Monitoring nicotine polacrilex therapy**
  Side effects to expect
  BURNING AND SORENESS OF MOUTH. Use cautiously in patients with oral or pharyngeal irritation.

  LIGHTHEADEDNESS, HEADACHE, HICCUPS, EXCESSIVE SALIVATION. These adverse effects can often be minimized by chewing the gum more slowly.
  Implementation
  PO. Emphasize the following points:

1. The patient must stop smoking immediately.
2. The patient should chew one piece of gum whenever there is the urge to smoke.
3. Chew the gum very slowly until the distinctive taste of nicotine or a slight tingling in the mouth is perceived, and then stop chewing (usually about 15 chews).
4. Once this tingling is almost gone (usually within 1 minute), start chewing again, repeating this procedure, for about 30 minutes. This chewing technique

provides constant, slow, buccal absorption of nicotine. Patients should be advised that chewing the gum will not provide the same rapid satisfaction that smoking tobacco provides.

DOSAGE ADJUSTMENT. Patients should titrate their daily use of the gum according to tolerance and response. During the first month of therapy, most patients require approximately 10 pieces of gum daily, 1 piece at a time. The maximum daily usage should not exceed 30 pieces. As the patient's urge to smoke decreases, the number of pieces of gum used each day should be gradually reduced.

DISCONTINUATION OF THERAPY. Patients should be advised not to attempt discontinuing therapy with the resin complex until their craving is satisfied by 1 or 2 pieces of the gum daily. In patients who are successfully abstaining from smoking after 3 months of therapy or when the patient is down to 2 pieces daily, the nicotine polacrilex should gradually be withdrawn.

If the drug is used for longer than 3 months, withdrawal from the gum should be gradual.

Drug interactions

CAFFEINE, THEOPHYLLINE, IMIPRAMINE, PENTAZOCINE, PROPOXYPHENE. Smoking has been shown to increase the metabolism of these agents. Cessation of smoking may result in increased blood concentrations of these drugs. Monitor patients for increased effects of these agents and reduce dosages accordingly.

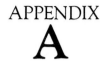
Common Medical Abbreviations

A	Assessment (POMR)	BTL	Bilateral tubal ligation	DSD	Dry sterile dressing
A_2	Aortic second sound	BTFS	Breast tumor frozen section	DT	Delirium tremens
$A_2 > P_2$	Aortic sound larger than second pulmonary sound	BU	Bodansky unit	DTR	Deep tendon reflex
		BUN	Blood urea nitrogen	Dx	Diagnosis
AAL	Anterior axillary line	BVL	Bilateral vas ligation	D_5W	Dextrose 5% in water
Ab	Abortion	BW	Body weight		
Abd	Abdomen, abdominal	Bx	Biopsy		
ABE	Acute bacterial endocarditis			E	Enema
ABG	Arterial blood gases			EBL	Estimated blood loss
ACD	Anterior chest diameter	C	Centigrade, Celsius	ECF	Extracellular fluid
ADH	Antidiuretic hormone	C_2	Second cervical vertebra	ECG	Electrocardiogram
ADT	Alternate-day therapy	CA	Carbonic anhydrase	ECT	Electroconvulsive therapy
AF	Atrial fibrillation; acid fast	Ca	Cancer, calcium	ECW	Extracellular water
AFB	Acid-fast bacteria; acid-fast bacilli	C & A	Clinitest and Acetest	EDC	Expected date of confinement (obstetrics)
A/G	Albumin to globulin ratio	CAD	Coronary artery disease		
AGN	Acute glomerular nephritis	CBC	Complete blood count	EEG	Electroencephalogram
AHF	Antihemophilic factor	CC	Chief complaint	EENT	Eyes, ears, nose, throat
AHFS	American Hospital Formulary Service	CCR	Creatinine clearance	EFA	Essential fatty acids
AHG	Antihemophilic globulin	CCU	Coronary care unit	EH	Enlarged heart
AI	Aortic insufficiency	Ceph floc	Cephalin flocculation	EKG	Electrocardiogram
AJ	Ankle jerk	CF	Complement fixation	EM	Electron microscope
AK	Above knee (amputation)	CHF	Congestive heart failure	EMG	Electromyography
ALD	Alcoholic liver disease	CHO	Carbohydrate	ENT	Ears, nose, and throat
ALL	Acute lymphocytic leukemia	Chol	Cholesterol	ER	Emergency room
ALS	Amyotrophic lateral sclerosis	CI	Color index; contraindication	ESR	Erythroctye sedimentation rate (sed rate)
AMA	Against medical advice	CK	Check		
AMI	Acute myocardial infarction	CLL	Chronic lymphocytic leukemia	EST	Electroshock therapy
ANA	Antinuclear antibodies	CNS	Central nervous system	EUA	Examine under anesthesia
AODM	Adult-onset diabetes mellitus	COAP	Cyclophosphamide, Oncovin, Ara-C, Prednisone		
A & P	Anterior and posterior; auscultation and percussion	C/O	Complains of	F	Fahrenheit
ASAP	As soon as possible	Cong	Congenital	FB	Finger breadths; foreign bodies
AP	Apical pulse, anteroposterior	COP	Cyclophosphamide, Oncovin, Prednisone	FBS	Fasting blood sugar
APB	Atrial premature beats			FEV_1	Forced expiratory volume in one second
AS	Anal sphincter; arteriosclerosis	COPD	Chronic obstructive pulmonary disease		
ASCVD	Arteriosclerotic cardiovascular disease			FF	Filtration fraction
ASHD	Arteriosclerotic heart disease	CPK	Creatine phosphokinase	FFA	Free fatty acids
ASO	Antistreptolysin titer; arteriosclerosis obliterans	C & P	Cystoscopy and pyelography	FH	Family history
		CP	Cerebral palsy; cleft palate	FLK	Funny looking kid
ATN	Acute tubular necrosis	CPR	Cardiopulmonary resuscitation	FP	Family practice; family planning
AV	Arteriovenous; atrioventricular	CR	Cardiorespiratory	FSH	Follicle-stimulating hormone
A & W	Alive and well	CRF	Chronic renal failure	FTA	Fluorescent treponemal antibody
		CRP	C-reactive protein	FUO	Fever of undetermined origin
		CS	Coronary sclerosis	Fx	Fracture; fraction
BAL	British anti-lewisite (dimercaprol)	C & S	Culture and sensitivity		
bands	Banded neutrophils	CSF	Cerebrospinal fluid		
BBB	Bundle branch block; blood-brain barrier	C sect	Cesarean section	G	Gravida
		CT	Circulation time	GA	General appearance
BBT	Basal body temperature	CV	Cardiovascular; costovertebral angle	GB	Gallbladder
BE	Barium enema; base excess	CVA	Cerebrovascular accident	GC	Gonococcus; gonorrhea
BEI	Butanol-extractable iodine	CVP	Central venous pressure	GFR	Glomerular filtration rate
bili	Bilirubin	CX	Cervix, cervical	GI	Gastrointestinal
BJ	Biceps jerk; bone and joint	CXR	Chest X-ray	G6PD	Glucose-6-phosphate dehydrogenase
BK	Below knee (amputation)			G-P-	Gravida-; para-
BLB	A type of oxygen mask			GU	Genitourinary
BLOBS	Bladder observation	DC(D/C)	Discontinue	GYN	Gynecology
BM	Bowel movement; basal metabolism	D & C	Dilatation and curretage		
BMR	Basal metabolic rate	DD	Differential diagnosis		
B & O	Belladonna and opium	DDD	Degenerative disc disease	H	Hypodermic; heroin
BP	Blood pressure; British Pharmacopoeia	DIC	Disseminated intravascular coagulation	HA	Headache
				HAA	Hepatitis-associated antigen
BPH	Benign prostatic hypertrophy	Diff	Differential blood count	HBP	High blood pressure
BRP	Bathroom privileges	DJD	Degenerative joint disease	Hct	Hematocrit
BS	Bowel sounds; breath sounds	DM	Diabetes mellitus	HCVD	Hypertensive cardiovascular disease
BSO	Bilateral salpingo-oophorectomy	DOA	Dead on arrival	HEENT	Head, eyes, ears, nose, throat
BSP	Bromsulphalein	DOE	Dyspnea on exertion	Hgb	Hemoglobin
BT	Breast tumor; brain tumor	DPT	Diphtheria, pertussis, and tetanus	HHD	Hypertensive heart disease

HO	House officer	LVH	Left ventricular hypertrophy	PMI	Point of maximal impulse or maximum intensity
HOB	Head of bed	L & W	Living and well	PMN	Polymorphonuclear neutrophil
HPF	High power field	LWCT	Lee-White clotting time	PMT	Premenstrual tension
HPI	History of present illness	lytes	Electrolytes	PND	Paroxysmal nocturnal dyspnea
HSA	Human serum albumin			PNX	Pneumothorax
HTN	Hypertension	M	Murmur	POMR	Problem-oriented medical record
HTVD	Hypertensive vascular disease	m^2	Square meters of body surface	Postop	After surgery
Hx	History	M_1	First mitral sound	PO	By mouth
		MCH	Mean corpuscular hemoglobin	PP	Postpartum; postprandial
IASD	Intraatrial septal defect	MCHC	Mean corpuscular hemoglobin concentration	PPD	Purified protein derivative
IBC	Iron-binding capacity			PPL	Penicilloyl-polylysine conjugate
IBI	Intermittent bladder irrigation	MCL	Midclavicular line	P & R	Pulse and respiration
ICF	Intracellular fluid volume	MCV	Mean corpuscular volume	Preop	Before surgery
ICM	Intracostal margin	MF	Myocardial fibrosis	PT	Physical therapy; prothrombin time
ICS	Intercostal space	MH	Marital history; menstrual history	PTA	Prior to admission
ICU	Intensive care unit	MI	Myocardial infarction; mitral insufficiency	PUD	Peptic ulcer disease
ICW	Intracellular water			PVC	Premature ventricular contraction
ID	Initial dose; intradermal	MIC	Minimum inhibitory concentration	PZI	Protamine zinc insulin
I & D	Incision and drainage	MJT	Mead Johnson tube		
IDU	Idoxuridine	ML	Midline		
I & O	Intake and Output	MOM	Milk of Magnesia	R	Respiration
IHSS	Idiopathic hypertrophic subaortic stenosis	MS	Morphine sulfate; multiple sclerosis; mitral stenosis	RA	Rheumatoid arthritis; right atrium
				RBC	Red blood cell
IM	Intramuscular	MSL	Midsternal line	RBF	Renal blood flow
Imp	Impression			RCM	Right costal margin
Int	Internal			RF	Rheumatoid factor
IP	Intraperitoneal	N	Normal; Negro	RHD	Rheumatic heart disese; renal hypertensive disease
IPPB	Intermittent positive pressure breathing	NAD	No acute distress; no apparent distress		
				RISA	Radioactive iodine serum albumin
ISW	Interstitial water	NG	Nasogastric	RLL	Right lower lobe
ITh	Intrathecal	NM	Neuromuscular	RLQ	Right lower quadrant
IU	International unit	NPN	Nonprotein nitrogen	RO	Rule out
IUD	Intraterine device (contraceptive)	NPO	Nothing by mouth	ROM	Range of motion
IVP	Intravenous pyelogram	NR	No refill	ROS	Review of systems; review of symptoms
IVPB	Intravenous piggyback	NS	Normal saline		
IVSD	Intraventricular septal defect	NSFTD	Normal spontaneous full-term delivery	RPF	Renal plasma flow; relaxed pelvic floor
		NSR	Normal sinus rhythm	RQ	Respiratory quotient
JRA	Juvenile rheumatoid arthritis	NTG	Nitroglycerin	RR	Recovery room; respiratory rate
JVD	Jugular venous distension	NVD	Nausea, vomiting, diarrhea; neck vein distension	RSR	Regular sinus rhythm
				RTA	Renal tubular acidosis
		NYD	Not yet diagnosed	RTN	Renal tubular necrosis
K^+	Potassium			RUL	Right upper lobe
KO	Keep open			RUQ	Right upper quadrant
17-KS	17-Ketosteroids	O_2	Oxygen	RV	Right ventricle
KUB	Kidney, ureter, and bladder	O	Objective data (POMR)	RVH	Right ventricular hypertrophy
K.W.	Keith Wagner (ophthalmoscopic findings)	OB	Obstetrics; occult blood		
		OOB	Out of bed		
		OOBBRP	Out of bed with bathroom privileges	S	Subjective data (POMR)
		OD	Overdose	S_1	First heart sound
L_2	Second lumbar vertebra	OR	Operating room	S_2	Second heart sound
LA	Left atrium	OT	Occupational therapy	SA	Sinoatrial
Lap	Laparotomy			SBE	Subacute bacterial endocarditis
LATS	Long-acting thyroid stimulator			SC	Subclavian, subcutaneous
LBBB	Left bundle branch block	P	Plan (POMR), pulse	Sed rate	Erythrocyte sedimentation rate
LCM	Left costal margin	P & A	Palpation and auscultation	Segs	Segmented neutrophils
LD	Longitudinal diameter (of heart)	PA	Posteroanterior	SGOT	Serum glutamic oxaloacetic transaminase
LDH	Lactic dehydrogenase	PAT	Paroxysmal atrial tachycardia		
LDL	Low density lipoproteins	PBI	Protein-bound iodine	SGPT	Serum glutamic pyruvic transaminase
LE	Lupus erythematosus	PC	After meals	SH	Social history; serum hepatitis
LFTs	Liver function tests	PCN	Penicillin	SID	Sudden infant death
LHF	Left heart failure	PCV	Packed cell volume (hematocrit)	SL	Sublingual
LKS	Liver, kidneys, and spleen	PE	Physical examination	SLE	Systemic lupus erythematosus
LLE	Left lower extremity	PEEP	Positive end expiratory pressure	SLDH	Serum lactic dehydrogenase
LLL	Left lower lobe	PEG	Pneumoencephalogram	SMA	Serial multiple analysis
LLQ	Left lower quadrant (abdomen)	PERRLA	Pupils equal, round, react to light and accommodation	SOAP	Subjective, objective, assessment plan (POMR)
LMD	Local medical doctor				
LML	Left middle lobe (lung)	PH	Past history	SOB	Shortness of breath
LMP	Last menstrual period	PI	Present illness	S/P	Status post
LOA	Left occipital anterior	PID	Pelvic inflammatory disease	SR	Sedimentation rate (ESR)
LOM	Limitation of motion	PIE	Pulmonary infiltration with eosinophilia	SSE	Saline solution enema; soapsuds enema
LOP	Left occipital posterior				
LP	Lumbar puncture	PKU	Phenylketonuria	SSPE	Subacute sclerosing panencephalitis
lpf	Low power field	PMH	Past medical history	STD	Skin test dose
LUQ	Left upper quadrant				

STS	Serologic test for syphilis	TPN	Total parenteral nutrition	VC	Vena cava
SVC	Superior vena cava	TPR	Temperature, pulse, and respiration	VCU	Voiding cystourethrogram
		TRA	To run at	VDRL	Venereal Disease Research
		T-set	Tracheotomy set		Laboratories (for syphilis)
T	Temperature	TSH	Thyroid-stimulating hormone	VF	Ventricular fibrillation
T_3	Triiodothyronine	TUR	Transurethral resection	VMA	Vanillylmandelic acid
T_4	Thyroxin	TV	*Trichomonas vaginalis*	VP	Venous pressure
T & A	Tonsillectomy and adenoidectomy			VPC	Ventricular premature contraction
TAH	Total abdominal hysterectomy			VS	Vital signs
TAO	Thromboangiitis obliterans	UA(U/	Urinalysis	VSD	Ventricular septal defect
TB	Tuberculosis	A)		VT	Ventricular tachycardia
TBW	Total body water	U & C	Urethral and cervical		
TD	Transverse diameter (of heart)	UCHD	Unusual childhood diseases		
TEDS	Elastic stockings	UGI	Upper gastrointestinal	W	White; widow
TIA	Transient ischemic attack	URI	Upper respiratory infection	WBC	White blood cell; white blood count
TIBC	Total iron-binding capacity	UTI	Urinary tract infection	WDWN-WF	Well-developed, well-nourished, white female
TKO	To keep open				
TLC	Tender loving care			WDWN-WM	Well-developed, well-nourished, white male
TM	Tympanic membrane	V	Vein		
TP	Total protein; thrombophlebitis	Vag hyst	Vaginal hysterectomy	WNL	Within normal limits
TPI	*Treponema pallidum* immobilization	VAH	Veterans' Administration Hospital	Wt	Weight

Prescription Abbreviations

aa, a̅a̅	of each (equal parts)	fl	fluid	q.i.d.	four times daily
a.c.	before meals	gtt	a drop	qod	every other day
ad	to; up to	h.s.	at bedtime	s̄	without
ad lib	as much as desired	o.d.	right eye	sig.	label
b.i.d.	twice daily	o.s.	left eye	ss	one-half
c̄, c	with	o.u.	both eyes	stat	at once
caps	capsules	p.c.	after meals	t.i.d.	three times daily
d	day	p.r.n.	as needed	ung	ointment
et	and	q	every	ut dict.	as directed
ext	an extract	qd	once daily		

Derivatives of Medical Terminology

adeno-	gland	homo-	same	osteo-	bone
adreno-	adrenal gland	hydro-	wet, water	-ostomy	opening
-algia	pain	hystero-	uterus	-otomy	into
angio-	vessel	ileo-	ileum	patho-	disease
arterio-	artery	-itis	inflammation	phago-	eat
arthro-	joint	jejuno-	jejunum	phlebo-	vein
auto-	self	laparo-	loin or flank	-phobia	fear
broncho-	bronchus	laryngo-	larynx	pilo-	hair
brachy-	short	leuko-	white	-plegia	paralysis
brady-	slow	lipo-	fat	pneumo-	lungs; air
carcino-	cancer	litho-	stone	procto-	rectum
cardio-	heart	lympho-	lymph	ptosis	fall
-cele	herniation	macro-	large	pyelo-	pelvis of kidney
-centesis	puncture	masto-	breast	pyo-	pus
chole-	bile	medius	middle	rhino-	nose
chondro-	cartilage	megalo-	huge	-rrhagia	burst forth
costo-	ribs	meningo-	meninges	-rrhaphy	suture
cranio-	head	metra-, metro-	uterus	-rrhea	flow; discharge
cysto-	bladder	micro-	small	sero-	serum
cyto-	cell	myco-	fungus	splanchno-	viscera
derma-	skin	myelo-	bone marrow; spinal cord	spleno-	spleen
diplo-	double	myo-	muscle	-stasis	stop
-ectomy	out	necro-	death	stoma-	mouth
edem-	swell	neo-	new	tachy-	fast; swift
entero-	intestines	nephro-	kidney	thrombo-	clot
erythro-	red	neuro-	nerve	thyro-	thyroid
gastro-	stomach	oculo-	eye	tom-	cut
glomerulo-	glomerulus	oligo-	few	tricho-	hair
glyco-	sweet	-oma	tumor	uretero-	ureter
hem-, hemato-	blood	oophoro-	ovary	urethro-	urethra
hepato-	liver	orchio-, orchido-	testes	uro-	urine
-hesion	join together	os	mouth; bone	vaso-	vessel
hetero-	different	-osis	condition	veno-	vein

Mathematic Conversions

kg = kilograms	ng = nanograms	mEq = milliequivalent
g = grams	m = meter	μm = micron
mg = milligrams	cm = centimeter	L = liter
μg = micrograms	mm = millimeter	ml = milliliter

METRIC SYSTEM

Weight

1 kilogram	=	1000 grams
1 gram	=	1000 milligrams
1 milligram	=	1000 micrograms
1 microgram	=	0.001 milligram
1 milligram	=	0.001 gram
1 gram	=	0.001 kilogram

Volume

1 deciliter	=	100 milliliters
1 liter	=	1000 milliliters
1 milliliter	=	0.001 liter
1 deciliter	=	0.1 liter

Length

1 centimeter	=	10 millimeters
1 decimeter	=	10 centimeters
1 meter	=	10 decimeters
1 kilometer	=	1000 meters
1 millimeter	=	0.1 centimeter
1 centimeter	=	0.1 decimeter
1 decimenter	=	0.1 meter
1 meter	=	0.001 kilometer

COMMON SYSTEM

Apothecary Weight

1 scruple (℈)	=	20 grains (gr)
60 grains	=	1 dram (ʒ)
8 drams	=	1 ounce (℥)
1 ounce	=	480 grains
12 ounces	=	1 pound

Avoirdupois Weight

1 ounce (oz)	=	437.5 grains
1 pound (lb)	=	16 ounces

Apothecary Volume

60 minims (♏︎)	=	1 fluid dram (flʒ)
8 fluidrans	=	1 fluid ounce (fl℥)
1 fluid ounce	=	480 minims
16 fluid ounces	=	1 pint (pt)

Length

12 inches	=	1 foot
36 inches	=	1 yard
3 feet	=	1 yard
5280 feet	=	1 mile
1760 yards	=	1 mile

METRIC AND COMMON SYSTEM EQUIVALENTS

MILLIGRAMS	GRAMS	GRAINS
.1	.0001	1/600
.2	.0002	1/300
.3	.0003	1/200
.4	.0004	1/150
.5	.0005	1/120
.6	.0006	1/100
1.0	.001	1/60
2.0	.002	1/30
10	.01	1/6
15	.015	1/4
30	.03	1/2
45	.045	3/4
60 (65)	.06	1
300 (330)	.3	5
600 (650)	.6	10
1000	1.0	15
2000	2.0	30
3000	3.0	45

1 gram	= 15.4 grains
1 grain	= 64.8 milligrams
1 ounce (℥)	= 31.1 grams
1 ounce (oz)	= 28.3 grams
1 pound (lb)	= 453.6 grams
1 kilogram (kg)	= 2.2 pounds
1 millimeter (ml)	= 16.23 minims
1 minim (♏︎)	= 0.06 ml
1 fluid ounce (fl℥)	= 29.5 ml
1 pint	= 473 ml
1 meter	= 39.3 inches
1 kilometer	= .6 mile
1 mile	= 1.6 mile
1 inch	= 2.54 cm
1 foot	= 30 cm
1 yard	= .9 meter

APPROXIMATE HOUSEHOLD MEASUREMENTS

1 teaspoonful		5 ml
1 dessertspoonful		10 ml
1 tablespoonful	½ fl oz	15 ml
1 jigger	1½ fl oz	45 ml
1 wineglassful	2 fl oz	60 ml
1 teacupful	4 fl oz	120 ml
1 glassful (tumblerful)	8 fl oz	240 ml

Formulas for the Calculation of Infants' and Children's Dosages

CHILDREN'S DOSAGES

Bastedo's rule: Child's approximate dose $= \dfrac{\text{age in years} + 3}{30} \times \text{adult dose}$

Clark's rule: Child's approximate dose $= \dfrac{\text{weight of child (lb)}}{150} \times \text{adult dose}$

Cowling's rule: Child's approximate dose $= \dfrac{\text{age (on next birthday)}}{24} \times \text{adult dose}$

Dilling's rule: Child's approximate dose $= \dfrac{\text{age (in years)}}{20} \times \text{adult dose}$

Young's rule: Child's approximate dose $= \dfrac{\text{age of child (in years)}}{\text{age} + 12} \times \text{adult dose}$

INFANTS' DOSAGES (YOUNGER THAN 1 YEAR OF AGE)

Fried's rule: Infant dose $= \dfrac{\text{age (in months)}}{150} \times \text{adult dose}$

Weight Conversion Table

lb	kg	lb	kg	lb	kg
5	2.3	105	47.7	210	95.5
10	4.5	110	50	220	100
15	6.8	115	52.3	230	104.5
20	9.1	120	54.5	240	109
25	11.4	125	56.8	250	113.6
30	13.6	130	59	260	118.2
35	15.9	135	61.4	270	122.7
40	18.1	140	63.6	280	127.2
45	20.4	145	66	290	131.8
50	22.7	150	68.1	300	136.4
55	25	155	70.5	310	140.9
60	27.3	160	72.7	320	145.5
65	29.5	165	75	330	150
70	31.8	170	77.3	340	154.5
75	34.1	175	79.5	350	159
80	36.4	180	81.8	360	163.6
85	38.6	185	84.1	370	168.2
90	40.9	190	86.4	380	172.7
95	43.2	195	88.6	390	177.2
100	45.4	200	90.9	400	181.8

1 lb = 0.454 kg; 1 kg = 2.2 lb

Temperature Conversion Table

F	C	F	C	F	C
95.0	35.0	98.4	36.9	101.8	38.7
.2	35.1	.6	37.0	102.0	38.8
.4	35.2	.8	37.1	.2	38.9
.6	35.3	99.0	37.2	.4	39.1
.8	35.4	.2	37.3	.6	39.2
96.0	35.5	.4	37.4	.8	39.3
.2	35.6	.6	37.5	103.0	39.4
.4	35.7	.8	37.6	.2	39.5
.6	35.9	100.0	37.7	.4	39.6
.8	36.0	.2	37.8	.6	39.7
97.0	36.1	.4	37.9	.8	39.8
.2	36.2	.6	38.1	104.0	40.0
.4	36.3	.8	38.2	.2	40.1
.6	36.4	101.0	38.3	.4	40.2
.8	36.5	.2	38.4	.6	40.3
98.0	36.6	.4	38.5	.8	40.4
.2	36.7	.6	38.6	105.0	40.5

$C° = \frac{5}{9}(F° - 32°); F° = \frac{9}{5}(C° + 32°)$

Nomogram for Calculating the Body Surface Area of Adults and Children

ADULTS

SA(m²)

Height(H): cm

200
190
180
170
160
150
140
130
120
110
100
90
80
70

2.6
2.5
2.4
2.3
2.2
2.1
2.0
1.9
1.8
1.7
1.6
1.5
1.4
1.3
1.2
1.1
1.0
0.9
0.8
0.7
0.6
0.5

Weight(W): kg

120
110
100
90
80
70
60
50
45
40
35
30
25
20
19
18
17
16
15
14
13
12

CHILDREN

SA(m²)

Height(H): cm

90
85
80
75
70
65
60
55
50
45
40
35
30

0.60
0.55
0.50
0.45
0.40
0.35
0.30
0.25
0.20
0.15
0.10

Weight(W): kg

15
14
13
12
11
10
9
8
7
6
5.5
5
4.5
4
3.5
3
2.5
2
1.5
1

Align a ruler with the height and weight. The point at which the center line is intersected gives the corresponding value for surface area (SA). (From Haycock GB: *J Pediatr* 1978; 93:62-66.)

Commonly Used Laboratory Test and Drug Values

TEST	RANGE	UNITS	CONVERSION FACTOR	SI RANGE	UNITS
Alanine aminotransferase [ALT]	0-35	U/L	0.01667	0-0.58	μkat/L
Albumin, serum	4-6	g/dL	10	40-60	g/L
Alkaline phosphatase	30-120	U/L	0.01667	0.5-2	μkat/L
Aspartate aminotransferase [AST]	0-35	U/L	0.01667	0-0.58	μkat/L
Bilirubin, total (serum)	0.1-1	mg/dL	17.1	2-18	μmol/L
Bilirubin, conjugated	0-0.2	mg/dL	17.1	0-4	μmol/L
Calcium, serum	8.8-10.4	mg/dL	0.2495	2.2-2.58 0-0	mmol/L
Chloride, serum	95-110	mEq/L	1	95-110	mmol/L
Cholesterol					
<29 years	<200	mg/dL	0.02586	<5.2	mmol/L
30-39 years	<225	mg/dL	0.02586	<5.85	mmol/L
40-49 years	<245	mg/dL	0.02586	<6.35	mmol/L
>50 years	<265	mg/dL	0.02586	<6.85	mmol/L
Cortisol, serum					
0800 hours	4-19	μg/dL	27.59	110-520	nmol/L
1600 hours	2-15	μg/dL	27.59	50-410	nmol/L
2400 hours	5	μg/dL	27.59	140	nmol/L
Creatine kinase (CK)					
Isoenzymes	0-130	U/L	0.01667	0-2.167	μkat/L
MB fraction	>5 in myocardial infarction	%	0.01	>0.05	L
Creatinine, serum	0.6-1.2	mg/dL	88.4	50-110	μmol/L
Creatinine clearance	75-125	mL/min	0.01667	1.24-2.08	mL/s
Erythrocyte count					
male	4.3-5.9	$10^6/mm^3$	1	4.3-5.9	$10^{12}/L$
female	3.5-5	$10^6/mm^3$	1	3.5-5	$10^{12}/L$
Erythrocyte sedimentation rate (ESR)					
male	0-20	mm/hr	1	0-20	mm/h
female	0-30	mm/hr	1	0-30	mm/h
Gases, arterial blood					
pO_2	75-105	mm Hg	0.1333	10-14	kPa
pCO_2	33-44	mm Hg	0.1333	4.4-5.9	kPa
Gamma-glutamyltransferase (GGT)	0-30	U/L	0.01667	0-0.5	μkat/L
Glucose, plasma (fasting)	70-110	mg/dL	0.05551	3.9-6.1	mmol/L
Hematocrit					
male	39-49	%	0.01	0.39-0.49	L
female	33-43	%	0.01	0.33-0.43	L
Hemoglobin					
male	14-18	g/dL	10	140-180	g/L
female	11.5-15.5	g/dL	10	115-155	g/L
Iron, serum					
male	80-180	μg/dL	0.1791	14-32	μmol/L
female	60-160	μg/dL	0.1791	11-29	μmol/L
Iron binding capacity	250-460	μg/dL	0.1791	45-82	μmol/L
Lactic dehydrogenase	50-150	U/L	0.01667	0.82-2.66	μkat/L
Leukocyte count differential	3200-9800	mm^3	0.001	3.2-9.8	$10^9/L$
		%	0.01		L

"SI units" is the abbreviation of *système international d'unites*. It is a uniform system of reporting numerical values permitting interchangeability of information among nations and between disciplines.
(From Young DS: Implementation of SI units for clinical laboratory data. *Ann Int Med* 1987; 106:114-129.)

TEST	RANGE	UNITS	CONVERSION FACTOR	SI RANGE	UNITS
Lipoproteins					
low density (LDL)	50-190	mg/dL	0.02586	1.3-4.9	mmol/L
high density (HDL) male	30-70	mg/dL	0.02586	0.8-1.8	mmol/L
female	30-90	mg/dL	0.02586	0.8-2.35	mmol/L
Magnesium, serum	1.8-3	mg/dL	0.4114	0.8-1.2	mmol/L
	1.6-2.4	mEq/L	0.5	0.8-1.2	mmol/L
Mean corpuscular hemoglobin (MCH)	27-33	pg	1	27-33	pg
Mean corpuscular					
hemoglobin concentration (MCHC)	33-37	g/dL	10	330-370	g/L
Mean corpuscular volume (MCV)	76-100	μm^3	1	76-100	fL
Osmolality, plasma	280-300	mOsm/kg	1	280-300	mmol/kg
Osmolality, urine	50-1200	mOsm/kg	1	50-1200	mmol/kg
Phosphate, serum	2.5-5	mg/dL	0.3229	0.8-1.6	mmol/L
Platelet count	130-400	$10^3/mm^3$	1	130-400	10⁹/L
Potassium, serum	3.5-5	mEq/L	1	3.5-5	mmol/L
Reticulocyte count	1-24	#/1000 RBC's	0.001	0.001-0.024	L
Sodium, serum	135-147	mEq/L	1	135-147	mmol/L
Thyroid stimulating hormone (TSH)	2-11	$\mu U/ml$	1	2-11	mU/L
Thyroxine (T4)	4-11	$\mu g/dL$	12.87	51-142	nmol/L
Thyroid binding globulin (TBG)	12-28	$\mu g/dL$	12.87	150-360	nmol/L
Thyroxine, free (serum)	0.8-2.8	ng/dL	12.87	10-36	pmol/L
Triiodothyronine (T_3)	75-220	ng/dL	0.01536	1.2-3.4	nmol/L
T_3 Uptake	25-35	%	0.01	0.25-0.35	L
Transferrin	170-370	mg/dL	0.01	1.7-3.7	g/L
Triglycerides	<160	mg/dL	0.01129	<1.8	mmol/L
Urea nitrogen	8-18	mg/dL	0.357	3-6.5	mmol/L
Zinc, serum	75-120	$\mu g/dL$	0.153	11.5-18.5	$\mu mol/L$

DRUG	RANGE	UNITS	CONVERSION FACTOR	SI RANGE	UNITS
Acetaminophen, toxic	>5	mg/dL	66.16	>330	$\mu mol/L$
Amitriptyline	50-200	ng/mL	3.605	180-720	nmol/L
Carbamazepine	4-10	mg/L	4.233	17-42	$\mu mol/L$
Chlordiazepoxide					
therapeutic	0.5-5	mg/L	3.336	2-17	$\mu mol/L$
toxic	>10	mg/L	3.336	33	$\mu mol/L$
Desipramine	50-200	ng/mL	3.754	170-700	nmol/L
Diazepam					
therapeutic	0.1-0.25	mg/L	3512	350-900	nmol/L
toxic	>1	mg/L	3512	3510	nmol/L
Digoxin					
therapeutic	0.5-2.2	ng/ml	1.281	0.6-2.8	nmol/L
toxic	>2.5	ng/mL	1.281	>3.2	nmol/L
Disopyramide	2-6	mg/L	2.946	6-18	$\mu mol/L$
Doxepin	50-200	ng/mL	3.579	180-720	nmol/L
Imipramine	50-200	ng/mL	3.566	180-710	nmol/L
Isoniazid					
therapeutic	<2	mg/L	7.291	<15	$\mu mol/L$
toxic	>3	mg/L	7.291	>22	$\mu mol/L$
Lidocaine	1-5	mg/L	4.267	4.5-21.5	$\mu mol/L$
Maprotiline	50-200	ng/mL	3.605	180-720	nmol/L
Phenobarbital	2-5	mg/dL	43.06	85-215	$\mu mol/L$
Phenytoin, therapeutic	10-20	mg/L	3.964	40-80	$\mu mol/L$
	>30	mg/L	3.964	>120	$\mu mol/L$
Procainamide					
therapeutic	4-8	mg/L	4.249	17-34	$\mu mol/L$
toxic	>12	mg/L	4.249	>50	$\mu mol/L$
N-acetylprocainamide	4-8	mg/L	3.606	14-29	$\mu mol/L$
Quinidine, therapeutic	1.5-3	mg/L	3.082	4.6-9.2	$\mu mol/L$
	>6	mg/L	3.082	>18.5	$\mu mol/L$
Theophylline	10-20	mg/L	5.55	55-110	$\mu mol/L$
Valproic acid	50-100	mg/L	6.934	350-700	$\mu mol/L$

Sodium, Potassium, and Caloric Content of Selected Foods

FOOD	PORTION	CALORIES	POTASSIUM (MG)	SODIUM (MG)
Fruits				
Apricots, fresh	3	55	301	1
Apricots, large, dried	10 halves	125	470	12
Banana, large	1 large	116	503	1
Breadfruit, raw	3½ oz	103	439	15
Cantaloupe, medium	¼ melon	41	341	17
Casaba, medium	¹⁄₁₀ melon	40	351	17
Dates, dried	10	219	518	1
Elderberries, raw	3½ oz	72	300	—
Figs, dried	7-10	274	640	34
Grapefruit, medium	1 whole	82	270	2
Honeydew, medium	¹⁄₁₀ melon	40	351	17
Lychees, dried	3½ oz	277	1100	—
Orange, 3″ diam. size #72	1 large	87	333	2
Papaya, 1 lb medium	1 whole	119	711	7
Peaches, dried	5	170	618	11
Prunes, cooked dried	½ c	126	347	4
Prunes, pitted uncooked	10	260	708	8
Raisins, dried	½ c	268	553	18
Watermelon, slice	1	108	454	5
Fruit juice				
Apricot nectar	1 c	143	379	trace
Blackberry juice	1 c	74	340	2
Grapefruit juice	1 c	84	324	2
Orange-grapefruit juice	1 c	86	364	2
Orange juice	1 c	112	496	2
Pineapple juice	1 c	138	373	3
Prune juice	1 c	197	602	5
Tangerine juice	1 c	106	440	2
Meat and fish (unsalted)				
Beef meat, cooked	3½ oz	245	370	60
Chicken and turkey (light meat)	3½ oz	182	422	66
Flounder, cooked (baked with margarine)	4 oz	228	664	268
Halibut, cooked	4 oz	192	596	152
Rockfish, steamed	4 oz	120	504	76
Nuts and seeds (unsalted)				
Almonds, whole shelled	½ c	425	549	3
Brazil nuts, whole shelled	½ c	458	500	1
Cashew nuts	½ c	392	325	11
Hazel nuts, whole shelled	½ c	428	475	1
Peanuts, unsalted shelled	⅓ c	332	382	3
Pecans, whole shelled	½ c	371	326	1
Sunflower seeds, hulled	½ c	406	667	22

In general, potassium values for all foods are higher for raw than for cooked, as soaking and/or cooking in water tends to reduce K^+ unless the cooking water is used.

c = cup, T = tablespoon, t = teaspoon

(Adapted from McRae PM: Foods high in potassium. *Hosp Pharm* 1979; 14:730-731.)

FOOD	PORTION	CALORIES	POTASSIUM (MG)	SODIUM (MG)
Milk				
Milk, nonfat	1 c	89	335	127
Vegetables (unsalted)				
Avocado, raw medium	½	188	680	5
Bamboo shoots, raw	1 c	41	806	—
Beans, baby lima cooked	1 c	118	394	129
Beans, lima frozen cooked	½ c	111	426	101
Beans, red cooked	½ c	118	340	3
Beans, soy cooked	1 c	234	972	4
Beans, white cooked	½ c	118	416	7
Chard, Swiss cooked	1 c	26	465	125
Collards	1 c	63	498	—
Cress, garden cooked	1 c	31	477	11
Mustard greens	1 c	32	308	25
Okra, cooked	1 c	70	303	4
Parsnips, cooked	1 c	139	587	12
Peas, black eye, frozen cooked	1 c	210	619	80
Peppers, green raw	1 whole	36	349	21
Potato, baked	1 medium	122	536	4
Potato, baked, with skin	1 medium	145	782	6
Spinach, cooked New Zealand	1 c	23	833	166
Spinach, frozen cooked	1 c	47	683	107
Split peas, cooked	1 c	230	592	26
Squash, butternut, baked, mashed	1 c	139	1248	2
Squash, Hubbard baked	1 c	103	556	2
Tomato juice	1 c	46	552	486
Tomatoes, canned	1 c	51	523	313
Tomatoes, fresh	1	27	300	4
Turnips, frozen, drained	1 c	38	246	28
Turnips, green, canned with liquid	1 c	42	564	548
Miscellaneous				
Molasses, blackstrap	1 T	43	585	19
Salt substitute	¼ t		500	

Template for Developing a Written Record
for Patients to Monitor Their Own Therapy

(Physicians, pharmacists, nurses, and other health practitioners are given permission to make a limited number of copies of this template for direct distribution, without charge, to their patients to aid in monitoring therapy.)

Medications	Color	To be taken

Name _____

Physician _____

Physician's phone _____

Next appt.* _____

Parameters	Day of discharge							Comments

*Please bring this record with you to your next appointment.
Use the back of this sheet for additional information.

Bibliography

Anastasi J, and Rivera JL: AIDS drug update— DDI and DDC, RN 54(11):41–43, 1991.

Beebe A et al: Pain assessment and treatment, JPN 39(11):17–27, 1989.

Billings DM, and Stokes LG: Medical-surgical nursing: Common health problems of adults and children across the life span, ed. 2, St. Louis, 1987, The CV Mosby Co.

Billups NF: American drug index, ed. 35, Philadelphia, 1991, JB Lippincott Co.

Braun AE: Drugs that dissolve clots, RN 54(6):52–57, 1991.

Brodsky PL, and Pelzar EM: Rationale for the revision of oxytocin administration protocols, JOGNN 20(6):440–444, 1991.

Brundage DJ: Renal disorders, St. Louis, 1992, The CV Mosby Co.

Burtis G et al: Applied nutrition and diet therapy, Philadelphia, 1988, WB Saunders Co.

Cahill-Wright C: Managing postoperative pain, Nursing 91 21(12):42–45, 1991.

Cancer manual, Boston, 1990, American Cancer Society.

Cancer update. Pain management: up the ladder, Nursing 90 20(4):61–62, 1990.

Canobbio MM: Cardiovascular disorders, St. Louis, 1991, The CV Mosby Co.

Carlson JH et al: Nursing diagnosis: a case study approach, Philadelphia, 1991, WB Saunders Co.

Carpenito LJ: Nursing Diagnosis, Application to clinical practice, ed. 4, Philadelphia, 1992, JB Lippincott Co.

Centers For Disease Control: Morbid. Mortal. Week. Rep. 40:RR–1, Jan. 11, 1991; 40:1–28, Aug. 8, 1991.

Cerrato P: Hypertension: The role of diet and lifestyle, RN 53(12):46–51, 1990.

Clayton BD: Handbook of pharmacology in nursing, ed. 4, St. Louis, 1987, The CV Mosby Co.

Deglin JH et al: Davis's drug guide for nurses, ed. 2, Philadelphia, 1990, FA Davis Co.

Doane LS et al: How to give peritoneal chemotherapy, AJN 90(4):58–66, 1990.

Doenges ME, and Moorhouse MF: Nurse's pocket guide: nursing diagnosis with interventions, ed. 3, Philadelphia, 1990, FA Davis Co.

Dudjak LA, and Fleck AE: BRM's new drug therapy comes of age, RN 54(10):42–47, 1991.

Ebersole P, and Hess P: Toward healthy aging human needs and nursing responses, ed. 3, St. Louis, 1990, The CV Mosby Co.

Engelking C: Managing stomatitis: a nursing process approach, supportive care for the patient with cancer, Richmond, Va, 1988, AH Robbins Co.

Feury D, and Nash D: Hypertension: the nurse's role, RN 53(11):54–59, 1990.

Fifield MY: Relieving constipation and pain in the terminally ill, AJN 91(7), 1991.

Gilman AG et al, editors: The pharmacological basic of therapeutics, ed. 8, New York, 1990, Permagon Press.

Gordon M: Nursing diagnosis, process and application, ed. 2, New York, 1987, McGraw-Hill Book Co.

Grimes D et al: Infectious diseases, St. Louis, 1991, The CV Mosby Co.

Guyton AC: Textbook of medical physiology, ed. 8, Philadelphia, 1991, WB Saunders Company.

Hahn K: Brush up on your injection technique, Nursing 90 20(9):54–58, 1990.

Hatcher RA et al: Contraceptive technology, 1990-92, ed. 15, New York, 1990, Irvington Publishers.

Hegner BR, and Caldwell E: Geriatrics: a study of maturity, ed. 5, Albany, NY, 1991, Delmar Publishing Inc.

Howard P: Elevated cholesterol: a nurse's guide to drug therapy, RN 54(8):26–30, 1991.

Howard P: Treatment guidelines for hypercholesterolemia, JPN 41(1):15–23, 1991.

Ignataviccius D, and Bayne MV: Medical-surgical nursing: a nursing process approach, Philadelphia, 1991, WB Saunders Co.

Illustrated manual of nursing practice, Springhouse, Pa, 1991, Springhouse Corp.

Koda-Kimble MA, and Young LY, editors: Applied therapeutics, ed. 5, Vancouver, Wash, 1992, Applied Therapeutics Inc.

Kukar PA, and Hill KM: White clot syndrome: when heparin goes haywire, AJN 91(3):59–60, 1991.

Lackner TE: Introduction to transdermal drug delivery systems, JPN 40(1):22–31, 1990.

Lehne R et al: Pharmacological aspects of nursing care, Philadelphia, 1990, WB Saunders Company.

Levine RR: Pharmacology, drug actions, and reactions, Boston, 1973, Little, Brown & Co.

Litwack K: What you need to know about administering preoperative medications, Nursing 91 21(8):44–47, 1991.

Loebb S et al: The nurse's drug handbook, ed. 6, Albany, NY, 1991, Delmar Publishing Inc.

McEvoy G, editor: AHFS drug information, Washington, D.C., 1991, American Society of Hospital Pharmacists Inc.

McGuire L: Administering analgesics: which drugs are right for your patiet, Nursing 90 20(4):34–41, 1990.

McNally JC et al: Guidelines for oncology nursing practice, ed. 2, Philadelphia, 1991, WB Saunders Company.

Madda M: Helping ostomy patients manage medications, Nursing 91 21(3):47–49, 1991.

Medical Letter, New Rochelle, NY, 1991, The Medical Letter Inc.

Medication administration & IV therapy manual process and procedures, Springhouse, PA, 1988, Springhouse Corp.

Melzack R: The McGill pain questionnaire: major properties and scoring methods, Pain 1:277–299, 1975.

Meyer C: New drugs: the class of 1991, AJN 91(12):40–43, 1991.

Moorehouse MF, and Doenges ME: Nurse's clinical pocket manual: nursing diagnoses, care planning and documentation, Albany, NY, 1990, Delmar Publishers.

Nursing 90 drug handbook, Springhouse, Pa, 1990, Springhouse Corp.

Olin BR, and Hebel SK, editors: Facts and comparisons, St. Louis, 1992, Facts and Comparisons, Inc.

Physician's desk reference, Oradell, NJ, 1991, Medical Economics Co.

Porterfield L: Today's antidepressants, Adv Clin Care 5(3), 1990.

Potter P, and Perry AG: Basic nursing theory and practice, ed. 2, St. Louis, 1991, Mosby-Year Book.

Reiss BS, and Evans ME: Pharmacological aspects of nursing care, ed. 3, Albany, NY, 1990, Delmar Publishing Inc.

Rodman MJ: Hypertension: first-line drug therapy, RN 54(1):32–40, 1991.

Rodman MJ: Hypertension: step care management, RN 54(2):24–31, 1991.

Roundtree D: The PIC catheter: a different approach, AJN 91(8):22–28, 1991.

Sause RB, and Mangione RA: Cough and cold treatments with OTC medications, JPN 41(3):15–25, 1991.

Seeley RR et al: Essentials of anatomy and physiology, St. Louis, 1991, The CV Mosby Co.

Spratto GR et al: RN magazine's nurse's drug reference–91, Albany, NY, 1991, Delmar Publishers.

Swearingen PL: Photo atlas of nursing procedures, ed. 2, Redwood City, Calif, 1991, Addison–Wesley Nursing.

Thomason SS: Using a groshong central venous catheter, Nursing 91 21(10):58–60, 1991.

Trissel LA: Handbook on injectable drugs, ed. 5, Bethesda, Md, 1990, American Society of Hospital Pharmacists.

USAN and USP dictionary of drug names, Rockville, Md, 1985, U.S. Pharmacopeial Convention Inc.

U.S. pharmacopeia, ed. 22, Rockville, Md, 1990, U.S. Pharmacopeial Convention Inc.

USP DI–1991, ed. 12, Rockville, Md, 1991, U.S. Pharmacopeial Convention Inc.

Vallerand AH, and Deglin JH: Nurse's guide for IV medications, Philadelphia, 1990, FA Davis Company.

Walker M, and Wong DL: A battle plan for patient's in pain, AJN 21(6), 1991.

Weinstein SM: Intravenous medications, Philadelphia, 1991, JB Lippincott Co.

Wiggins M et al: Guidelines for administering IV drugs, Nursing 90 20(4):145–152, 1990.

Wyngaarden JB, and Smith LH, editors: Cecil's textbook of medicine, ed. 17, Philadelphia, 1985, WB Saunders Co.

Glossary

abruptio placentae Premature separation of the placenta from the uterus.

absorbent Medicine or substance that absorbs liquids or other secretion products; a substance that takes in, or picks up, such as a blotter that absorbs ink.

  pathologic The absorption into the blood of any bodily excretion or morbid product, such as the bile or pus.

acceleration Quickening, as of the pulse rate or respiration.

accommodation Adjustment, especially that of the eye for various distances.

  absolute The accommodation of either eye separately.

  binocular The convergence of the two eyes so as to bring the image of the object seen on each retina.

acetylation Introduction of an acetyl group into an organic molecule.

acetylcholine Acetic acid ester of choline chloride, normally present in many parts of the body and having many important physiologic functions. For example, in the central nervous system it is for the purpose of transmission of nerve impulses. It is used subcutaneously and intravenously to relax peripheral blood vessels.

acetylcholinesterase An esterase in the blood that hydrolyzes any excess of acetylcholine, splitting it into acetic acid and choline.

achlorhydria Absence of hydrochloric acid from the gastric secretions.

acidosis Condition of lessened alkalinity in the body, caused by formation of excess amounts of acid or by lessened amounts of base.

acne Any inflammatory disease of the sebaceous glands, especially acne vulgaris, or common acne. It is chronic and commonly occurs on the chest, back, and face.

acromegaly Enlargement of the bony structure characterized by gigantism and caused by a tumor of the pituitary gland with increased secretion from the gland.

Addison's disease Disease characterized by a bronze-like pigmentation of the skin, severe prostration, progressive anemia, low blood pressure, diarrhea, and digestive disturbances. This condition is caused by lack of function of the adrenal (suprarenal) glands located on top of each kidney and by initial tuberculous infiltration (the last in less than half of the cases today). It is treated with cortisone or hydrocortisone and other hormones and a high-carbohydrate, high-protein diet.

adrenal cortex Outer layer of adrenal gland that manufactures specific hormones.

adrenal gland Gland of internal secretion situated on top of the kidney; also called the suprarenal gland.

adrenalectomy Removal of adrenal bodies.

adrenergic Activated or transmitted by epinephrine (adrenalin); a term applied to that form of autonomic nerves that acts by setting free acetylcholine from their nerve terminations.

adsorbent Substance that acts by gathering up another substance on its surface in a condensed layer.

aerobe A microorganism that can live and grow in the presence of free oxygen.

afferent Carrying, for example, of blood or impulses from the periphery to the center.

aggravate To make worse or to irritate.

aggregation Crowding or clustering together.

agranulocytopenia See *agranulocytosis.*

agranulocytosis Complete or nearly complete absence of the granular leukocytes (granulocytes) from the bone marrow and blood; also called agranulocytopenia.

albumin Protein found in nearly every animal and in many vegetable tissues and characterized by being soluble in water and coagulable by heat. It contains carbon, hydrogen, nitrogen, oxygen, and sulfur.

  albumin A A certain constituent of the blood serum, reduced in amount in cancer patients but increased in cancer cells.

  acetosoluble A form of albumin soluble in acetic acid; sometimes found in urine.

albuminuria The presence of albumin in the urine, indicating either a simple mixture of albuminous matters, such as blood, with the urine or a morbid state of the kidneys that is permitting albumin to pass from the blood.

alkalosis Excessive alkalinity of the body fluids; increased alkali reserve in the blood and other body tissues.

allergy Unusual reaction to a substance that in similar amounts is harmless to most persons.

alopecia Baldness, deficiency of hair, natural or abnormal.

amebiasis State of being infected with amebae.

amenorrhea Absence or abnormal stopping of menstrual flow.

amide Any compound derived from ammonia by substituting an acid radical for hydrogen.

amine Class of compounds derived from ammonia.

amino acids Organic acids in which one or more hydrogen atoms have been replaced by the amino group NH_2. The amino acids are the building blocks of the protein molecule and the end product of protein digestion.

anabolism, anabolic To build up; any constructive process by which simple substances are converted by living cells into more complex compounds; constructive metabolism and assimilation.

anaerobe Any microorganism having the power to live without either air or free oxygen.

analeptic Restorative medicine or agent. Central nervous system stimulants used to antagonize depressant drugs are called analeptics; they restore consciousness and mental alertness.

analgesic Medication to relieve pain, such as aspirin or morphine.

analogue Part or organ having the same function as another, but of a different structure.

analogy Resemblance in structure caused by similarity of function.

anaphylaxis Unusual or exaggerated reaction of an organism or individual to foreign proteins or other substances. These reactions are immediate, shock-like, and frequently fatal within minutes. They include symptoms such as apprehension, burning, prickling

sensations, generalized urticaria or hives, edema, choking sensation, cyanosis, wheezing, cough, incontinence, shock, fever, dilation of pupils, loss of consciousness, and convulsions. Reaction to penicillin is an example. Emergency drugs should always be available whenever injections are administered.

androgen Male sex hormones.

anemia Insufficient blood cells or iron.

anesthetic Drug causing a temporary loss of sensation.

angina pectoris Severe, cramp-like pain of the chest, caused by insufficient circulation and characterized by spasms of the muscles of the coronary arteries surrounding and entering the heart.

angioneurotic edema Giant hives characterized by large wheals or pinkish elevations similar to hives on the skin, with marked itching, nausea, fever, and malaise; generally caused by sensitivity to a food or foods.

anhydrase An enzyme that catalyzes anhydration.

  carbonic An enzyme that catalyzes the release of carbon dioxide from the blood in the tissues and the lungs.

anion Ion carrying a negative charge. They include all the non-metals, the acid radicals, and the hydroxyl ion.

anomalies *(anomaly)* Marked deviations from the normal standard.

anorexia Lack or loss of appetite for food.

anthelmintic Agent to destroy worms.

anthrax Carbuncle or other infection caused by the anthrax bacillus.

  malignant A fatal infectious disease of cattle and sheep caused by the anthrax bacillus and characterized by formation of hard edema or ulcers at the point of inoculation and by collapse symptoms. It may occur in humans.

anti Against.

antibiotic Against life.

antibiotics Medications used to kill living microorganisms that cause infection.

antibodies Substances in the body that react with a specific antigen. They may be present under apparently normal conditions but develop anew in response to the introduction of specific antigen into the tissues or blood. Antibodies include, among others, agglutinins, antienzymes, and antitoxins.

anticoagulant Substance used to prevent blood clotting.

antiemetic Arresting or preventing emesis or vomiting, relieving nausea.

antigen Any substance that will lead to the development of antibodies.

antihistamine Agent given to neutralize histamine produced by the body.

antipyretic Relieving fever; cooling.

antiseptic Drug that tends to prevent or lessen the activity of infection by slowing the growth of microorganisms.

antispasmodic Agent used in relieving muscular contractions, spasms, and convulsions.

antitoxin Serum used to lessen the effects of the toxins or poisons produced by bacteria.

antitussive Relieving or preventing cough.

anuria, anuresis Absolute suppression of urinary secretion.

apical pulse Heartbeat taken with a stethoscope, the bell or disc of the stethoscope being placed over the apex or pointed extremity of the heart.

aplastic anemia Rare condition in which the bone marrow cells cease to produce leukocytes in sufficient amounts to compensate for their destruction.

apnea The transient cessation of breathing that follows forced respiration; asphyxia.

apoplexy Stroke or paralysis caused by rupture of a blood vessel.

apothecary Druggist or pharmacist.

appendicitis Inflammation of the appendix.

appetite Hunger, natural longing, or desire, especially for food.

aqueous humor Fluid filling the anterior and posterior chambers of the eye in front of the lens.

arrhythmia Any variation from the normal rhythm of the heartbeat; irregularities. Some various forms of arrhythmias include sinus arrhythmia, extrasystole, heart block, auricular fibrillation, auricular flutter, and paroxysmal tachycardia.

arteriole Any minute arterial branch.

arteriosclerosis Scarring or hardening of the arteries that results from disease of the arterial walls.

obliterans Proliferation of the intima, or innermost of the three coats of the artery, causing complete obliteration or closing of the lumen of the artery.

arthralgia Neuralgia or pain in a joint.

arthritis Rheumatism characterized by symptoms such as pain, swelling, inflammation, and stiffness of joints.

ascites Accumulation of serous fluid in the peritoneal cavity; dropsy of the abdominal cavity; painless swelling of the abdomen that gives a dull sound on percussion. Causes include local inflammation of the peritoneum and obstruction of the venous circulation by disease of the heart, kidney, or liver.

asphyxia Suffocation or a deficiency of oxygen in the blood.

neonatorum Suffocation in the newborn.

asthma Disease of the bronchi, with difficulty and shortness of breath; often caused by allergies.

asystole Imperfect or incomplete systole; inability of the heart to perform a complete systole.

ataxia Failure of muscular coordination; irregularity of muscle action.

atelectasis Partial collapse of the lung; imperfect expansion of the lung in the newborn.

atherosclerosis Form of arteriosclerosis with marked degenerative changes and fatty degeneration of the connective tissue of the arterial walls.

athetosis A derangement marked by constant recurring series of slow, vermicular movements of the hands and feet, occurring chiefly in children and resulting principally from a brain lesion.

athlete's foot Ringworm of the feet; fungus infection.

atonic Characterized by lack of normal tone, for example, lack of muscle tone.

atrioventricular heart block A blocking at the atrioventricular or auriculoventricular junction (the auricles and ventricles beat independently of each other).

atrium See *auricle*.

atrophy Change or degeneration in a part.

attenuation Act or process of thinning or weakening, especially the weakening of the toxicity of a virus or a microorganism by repeated inoculation and successive culture, adding an agent such as formaldehyde.

auricle Atrium of the heart; chamber at the apex of the heart on either side above the ventricle; divided into right and left auricle or atrium.

autoimmunization Immunization effected by processes within the body.

autonomic Self-governing; independent in function.

azotemia The presence of urea or other nitrogenous bodies in the blood.

chloropenic Condition characterized by deficiency of sodium chloride, fixation of chlorine in the tissues, and azoturia (excess urea and other nitrogenous bodies in the urine).

bactericidal Able to kill bacteria.

bacteriostasis Condition in which bacteria are prevented from growing and spreading. *Bacteriostatic* is more general in its meaning than *antiseptic*.

beriberi An endemic form of polyneuritis prevalent chiefly in Japan, India, China, the Philippines, and the Malay peninsula and often fatal. Characteristic symptoms: spasmodic rigidity of the lower limbs, with muscular atrophy, paralysis, anemia, and neuralgic pains. The disease is thought to result from an almost exclusive diet of overmilled or highly polished rice or other carbohydrate food, which is deficient in the accessory food factor known as antineuritic vitamin.

bilateral Having two sides or pertaining to two sides.

biliary colic Spasm of the gallbladder, hepatic ducts, common bile duct, and cystic duct.

blepharitis Inflammation of the eyelids.

blood pressure Pressure of the blood on the wall of the arteries, dependent on the energy of the heart action, the elasticity of the walls of the arteries, the resistance in the capillaries, and the volume and the viscosity of the blood.

basic That pressure exerted on the blood by the contractile walls independent of the additional pressure caused by the systolic contraction of the heart.

diastolic The lowest arterial pressure at any one time during the cardiac cycle. It results from the recoil of the elastic walls of the aorta and arteries and the pressure this recoil exerts on the blood. It is known as the resting pressure that is being constantly exerted by the aorta and arteries and which the left ventricle must overcome before blood can be ejected into the aorta. This pressure represents the constant minimal load that the arteries must bear at all times.

pulse pressure The difference between systolic and diastolic pressures. Pulse pressure is an important indication of cardiac output and peripheral resistance shown by the width of pulse pressure. A wide pulse pressure is a normal finding if there is bradycardia, and a narrow pulse pressure is normal if there is tachycardia. In hemorrhage, systolic level may fall, but the diastolic level tends to rise. The result is a narrow pulse pressure indicating decreased cardiac output. A pulse pressure as low as 20 mm Hg or as high as 50 mm Hg is pathologic.

systolic The highest arterial pressure at any one time during the cardiac cycle. It is a combination of the ejection of blood from the ventricles during systole and the blood pushing against the elastic walls of the aorta and arteries. It is also known as the active or working pressure. Normal range is about 110 to 140 mm Hg.

blood sugar A simple sugar normally found in the blood.

bolus A rounded mass; a mass of food ready to be swallowed or a mass passing along the intestines. In pharmacy, a rounded mass larger than a pill.

botulism A type of food poisoning caused by a toxin produced by *Clostridium (Bacillus) botulinum* in improperly canned or preserved foods and characterized by vomiting, abdominal pain, disturbances of secretion, motor disturbances, dryness of the mouth and pharynx, dyspepsia, barking cough, mydriasis, paralytic drooping of the eyelid, and prolapse of other parts or organs. It requires immediate medical attention; death can often occur without treatment.

Bowman's capsule Globular dilation that forms the beginning of a uriniferous tubule within the kidney. Each nephron begins as a Bowman's capsule.

bradycardia Abnormal slowness of the heartbeat, as evidenced by slowing of the pulse rate to 60 or less.

broad-spectrum Usually refers to antibiotics and their ability to kill a wide variety of gram-positive and gram-negative bacteria.

bronchial asthma Disease of the bronchi with difficulty and shortness of breath.

bronchiectasis Dilation of the bronchi or of a bronchus, marked by foul breath, paroxysmal coughing, and expectoration of mucopurulent matter.

bronchogenic Originating in a bronchus.

bronchoscopy Examination of the bronchi through a tracheal wound or through an instrument called a bronchoscope.

bronchus Tube-like structure leading to the lung; located between trachea, or windpipe, and lung. There is a left and right bronchus (bronchi).

brucellosis The disease produced by *Brucella*, a bacteria; undulant fever characterized by wavelike changes in fever.

buccal Pertaining to the cheek. In drug administration the mucous-membrane side of the inner cheek.

Buerger's disease Chronic inflammation of the arteries of the extremities with eventual thrombus or clot formation and blocking or occlusion of the blood vessel and gangrene.

buffer Any substance in a fluid that tends to lessen the change in hydrogen ion concentration (reaction), which otherwise would be produced by adding acids or alkalis; any substance that decreases or prevents the reaction that a chemotherapeutic agent would produce if administered alone; the action produced by a buffer.

BUN A laboratory blood: blood urea nitrogen.

Burkitt's lymphoma A rapidly progressive lymphatic tumor that occurs most commonly in the jaw, abdominal cavity, and meninges. Spontaneous regressions have been observed, and many patients are highly responsive to chemotherapy.

bursitis Inflammation of the bursae, or small sacs of tissue, some of which are found in the shoulder and knee.

caduceus Emblem of the medical profession; a wand with wings at the top and two serpents twisted around it.

calcinosis Condition marked by the disposition of calcium salts in nodules under the skin and in the muscles, tendons, nerves, and connective tissue.

Candida, candidal A genus of yeast-like fungi of the family Cryptococcaceae, various species of which have been isolated from pulmonary lesions in man.

Candida albicans A yeast-like fungus that causes an inflammation of the corners of the mouth.

Candida vulva Inflammation of the vulva or external part of the organs of generation in the female, caused by a yeast-like fungus *Candida vulva.*

capillary One of the microscopic blood vessels connecting arteries and veins.

carcinoma Malignant tumor or cancer; new growth made up of epithelial cells that tend to infiltrate and metastasize.

cardiac insufficiency Inability of the heart to perform its function properly.

cardiogenic shock Shock resulting from diminution of cardiac output in heart disease.

cardiospasm Spasm of the cardiac sphincter of the stomach.

carminative Medicine that expels gas from the stomach and intestines.

carotene Yellow pigment found in carrots, sweet potatoes, other vegetables, milk fat, body fat, and egg yolk. It may be converted in the body into vitamin A.

carotenoid Marked by a yellow color resembling that produced by carotene.

catabolism Destructive metabolism; passage of tissue material from a higher to a lower plane of complexity or specialization.

cataract An opacity of the crystalline eye lens or of its capsule.

catecholamines Dopamine, norepinephrine, and epinephrine synthesized, stored, and metabolized in the brain and affecting the central nervous system slightly and the autonomic nervous system to a greater degree.

cation Element or elements of an electrolyte that appears at the negative pole or cathode. Cations include all metals and hydrogen.

cationic See *cation.*

causalgia, causalgic Neuralgia characterized by intense local sensation, as of burning pain.

celiac disease Childhood form of sprue characterized by impaired absorption of fats, perhaps glucose, and with such symptoms as diarrhea (with bulky, pale, frothy, foul-smelling stools), weight loss, vitamin deficiencies, anemia, infantilism, tetany, rickets, and sometimes dwarfism. The disease responds to the elimination of wheat gluten from the diet, administration of oral iron for hypochromic anemia, and vitamin B_{12} for macrocytic anemia. Diet in celiac disease should be high-calorie, high-protein, low-fat, and gluten-free.

cellulitis Inflammation of the cellular tissue, especially purulent inflammation of the loose subcutaneous tissue.

cerebellum That division of the brain behind the cerebrum and above the pons and fourth ventricle; it is concerned with the coordination of movements.

cerebrum Main portion of the brain occupying the upper part of the cranium and consisting of two equal portions called hemispheres, which are united at the bottom by a mass of white matter called the corpus callosum. The cerebrum is the organ of associative memory, reasoning, and judgment.

cervix Lower, neck-like portion of the uterus.

cheilitis Inflammation of the lip.

chemoreceptor Receptor adapted for excitation by chemical substances, such as olfactory and gustatory receptors; a supposed group of atoms in cell protoplasm having the ability to fix chemicals in the same way as bacterial poisons are fixed.

chemotherapeutic agent Agent of chemical nature used in the treatment of disease.

chilblains Inflammation and swelling of the toes, feet, or fingers caused by cold.

cholestatic Resulting from stoppage of bile flow.

cholesterol Fat-like, pearly substance crystallizing in the form of leaflets or plates and found in all animal fats and oils and in bile, blood, brain tissue, milk, egg yolk, kidneys, and suprarenal bodies. It constitutes a larger part of the most frequently occurring gallstones and appears in atheroma of the arteries.

cholinergic Stimulated, activated, or transmitted by choline (acetylcholine); term applied to nerve fibers whose activity is transmitted by acetylcholine; drugs that cause effects in the body similar to those produced by acetylcholine.

cholinesterase Enzyme that hydrolyzes or destroys acetylcholine.

chorea (St. Vitus' dance) Convulsive nervous disease with involuntary and irregular jerking movements and attended with irritability, depression, and mental impairment; it occurs in early age, more commonly in girls than boys, and may be hereditary.

choriocarcinoma Carcinoma (cancer) developed from the epithelium.

chorion The outermost envelope of the growing zygote or fertilized ovum that serves as a protective and nutritive covering.

cicatrice, cicatrix A scar; the mark left by a sore or wound.

ciliary Pertaining to or resembling the eyelashes.

cirrhosis Disease of the liver marked by thickening, atrophy, degeneration, and a granular yellow appearance to the organ caused by coloring from bile pigments.

climacteric Time in life when the body undergoes marked changes and the reproductive organs no longer fully function; menopause.

clitoris A small, elongated, erectile body or organ of the female, situated at the anterior angle of the vulva and homologous with the penis in the male.

clonus Spasm in which there is alternate rigidity and relaxation in rapid succession.

foot A series of convulsive movements of the ankle, induced by suddenly pushing up the foot while the leg is extended.

toe Rhythmic contractions of the great toe, induced by suddenly extending the first phalanx.

wrist Spasmodic contractions of the hand muscles, induced by forcibly bending the hand backward.

Clostridium Genus of Bacillaceae that are anaerobic or microaerophilic and that form clostridial spore forms.

Clostridium oedematiens Strictly anaerobic organism isolated from war wounds in about 40% of the cases. It is gram-positive and forms large subterminal spores.

Clostridium septicum (Clostridium oedematis maligni) Moderately large, motile, gram-positive, rod-shaped organism with rounded ends and oval subterminal spores; infectious for humans only through wounds.

coagulant Agent causing blood or fluid to clot.

coalesce The fusing or blending of parts.

coarctation A straightening or pressing together; a condition of stricture or contraction; for example, of the aorta, with usually severe narrowing of the vessel lumen.

coenzyme A noncolloidal substance that combines with an inactive enzyme to produce activation of the enzyme.

colectomy Excision of a portion of the colon.

colitis Inflammation of the colon.

colloid Glutinous or resembling glue; a state in which the matter is distributed through some form of dispersing medium.

emulsion The dispersing medium is usually water, and the disperse phase consists of highly complex organic substances such as starch or glue, which absorb much water, swell, and become uniformly distributed throughout the dispersion medium.

suspension The disperse or distributing phase consists of particles of any insoluble substance such as metal, and the medium may be gaseous, liquid, or solid.

colostomy The formation of a permanent artificial opening (artificial anus) into the colon.

conduction Transfer of sound waves, heat, nerve influences, or electricity.

conductivity Capacity of a body to conduct a current.

congestive heart failure Result of the inability of the heart to expel sufficient blood for the metabolic demands of the body. Most common causes are hypertension, coronary atherosclerosis, and rheumatic heart disease. Less common causes include chronic pulmonary disease, congenital heart disease, syphilitic aortic insufficiency, calcific aortic stenosis, and bacterial endocarditis.

conjunctiva Mucous membrane lining the inner surface of the eyelids and covering the forepart of the eyeball.

conjunctivitis Inflammation of the mucous membrane conjunctiva. See *conjunctiva.*

constipation Infrequency or difficulty in movements of the bowels.

constriction A constricted part or place, a narrowing.

contract To decrease in size, as muscle tissue.

contractility Capacity for becoming short in response to a suitable stimulus.

cornea Transparent membrane forming the anterior or front part of the outer layer of the eyeball.

coronary occlusion The formation of a clot in a branch of the coronary arteries, which supply blood to the heart muscle, resulting in obstruction of the artery and infarction of the area of the heart supplied by the occluded vessel. Also called cardiac infarction and coronary thrombosis.

cortex Outer part of a gland or structure, such as the rind or bark.

craniotomy Operation on the cranium.

creatine Crystallizable nitrogenous principle, or methyl-guanidine-acetic acid, derived from the juice of muscular tissue; therapeutically, a cardiac, muscular, and digestive tonic.

creatinine Basic substance called creatine anhydride, procurable from creatine and from urine.

cretinism A chronic condition, congenital or developed before puberty, characterized by arrested physical and mental development, with dystrophy of the bones and soft parts. It is regarded as a form of myxedema and is probably caused by deficient thyroid activity.

cryptorchidism Undescended testicle.

crystalluria Formation of crystals in the urine or in the kidneys.

curie Standard unit for measuring the amount of radium emanation. The word curie comes from the discoverer of radium, Marie Sklodowska Curie, a Polish chemist in Paris, who lived 1867-1934.

Cushing's disease Disease caused by overgrowth of the basophil cells of the anterior lobe of the pituitary gland and marked by rapidly developing obesity of the face, neck, and trunk, decreased sexual activity, abnormal growth of hair, abdominal pain, weakness, and sometimes supraclavicular fat pads, striae, and acne.

cutaneous Pertaining to the skin.

cyanosis Blueness of the skin, lips, and often fingernails resulting from cardiac malformations causing insufficient oxygenation of the blood.

cycloplegia Paralysis of the ciliary muscle of the eye.

cystic fibrosis An infant and childhood disease, probably inherited, with pancreatic pathology and digestive and respiratory difficulties. Respiratory failure is most frequently the eventual cause of death. Characteristic symptoms are changes in the activity of the exocrine glands, including sweat (with a salty taste to the skin), salivary, and mucus-producing glands; the newborn manifests meconium ileus, with thick meconium obstructing the lower digestive tract, resulting in the need for emergency surgery. Other infant and childhood symptoms include bulky, offensive stools, protruding abdomen, spindly arms and legs, emaciation of the buttocks, and growth retardation. Foodstuffs, especially proteins and fats, are poorly digested and assimilated; pancreatic digestive enzymes are reduced or absent. Digestive problems improve with additional pancreatic enzymes in the diet. Blocking of the bronchioles, which results from extremely thick and tenacious secretions of the mucus-producing glands of the bronchi, is a serious problem, causing cough, wheezing, respiratory obstruction, emphysema, and frequently infection. The lungs are usually defenseless against microbes. In severe, chronic cases of the disease, patients manifest heart problems, a barrel-like, deformed chest, cyanosis, and clubbing of fingers and toes.

cystitis Inflammation of the bladder.

cystoscopy Examination of the bladder with an instrument called a cystoscope.

cytotoxic Toxin or antibody that has a specific toxic action on cells of special organs.

debilitated, debility Lack or loss of strength.

decrease To lessen or diminish.

defecation The discharge of fecal matter from the bowel.

degradation Reduction of a chemical compound to one less complex, as by splitting off one or more groups.

dehydration Removal of water from a substance or compound; also removal of water from the body; restriction of the water intake.

delirium tremens Condition marked by great excitement with anxiety and mental distress; caused by overuse of alcoholic drinks and characterized by hallucinations.

dementia Insanity characterized by loss or serious impairment of intellect, will, and memory.

demulcent substance Soothing preparation.

deodorant Medicine or substance that covers up, absorbs, or destroys objectionable odors.

depolarization Process or act of neutralizing polarity.

depressor Agent that causes a slowing-up action when applied to nerves and muscles.

derivative Agent that withdraws blood from the seat of a disease; anything that is obtained from another.

dermatitis Inflammation of the skin. Contact dermatitis is caused by contact with an irritating substance followed by an allergic response such as skin reddening, rash, itching, and scaling.

dermatomyositis An inflammatory disease of the voluntary muscles accompanied by characteristic skin lesions. It is attended by violent pains, swellings in the muscles, inflammation of the skin, and edema. Also called multiple myositis.

dermatophyte A plant growth, or species of plant, parasitic on the skin.

dermatoses Skin diseases.

detergent Cleansing agent.

diabetes insipidus Chronic disease, usually of young male adults, characterized by great thirst and the passage of a large amount of urine with no excess of sugar. Huge appetite, loss of strength, and emaciation are often noted. Causes include a deficiency of pitressin secretion from the posterior pituitary gland, impaired function of the supraoptic pathways regulating water metabolism, and, rarely, unresponsiveness of the kidney to pitressin.

diabetes mellitus Metabolic disorder marked by inability of the body to store or utilize carbohydrate.

diaphoresis, diaphoretic Profuse perspiration.

diarrhea Loose, watery bowel movements.

diastolic blood pressure See *blood pressure*.

diffuse Process of becoming widely spread, as through a membrane or fluid.

dilate To enlarge or stretch beyond normal measurements.

diplopia The seeing of single objects as double or two.

disinfectant An agent that destroys disease-producing substances or organisms.

disk (disc) A circular or rounded flat plate or organ.

    choked An inflamed and edematous optic disk, resulting from increased intracranial pressure. Called also papilledema.

    interarticular An interarticular fibrocartilage.

    intervertebral A layer of fibrocartilage between adjacent vertebrae.

distal Remote, farthest from the center, origin, or head; opposed to proximal.

diuresis Increased secretion of urine.

diuretic Drug that increases the flow of urine.

diverticulitis Inflammation of a diverticulum.

diverticulum Sac or pouch protruding from the wall of a tube or hollow organ, for example, from the intestine.

dosage Determination of the amount of medication to be administered to a patient, depending on the patient's weight and age.

ductless Having no excretory duct, as in ductless glands.

duodenum Portion of the small intestine leading from the stomach.

dyscrasias Abnormal composition of the blood.

dysentery Infection of the bowel characterized by inflammation, discharge of liquid and bloody stools, and pain, especially during discharge.

dysmenorrhea Painful menstruation.

dysphoria Disquiet; restlessness; feeling of ill-being; malaise.

dyspnea Difficult or labored breathing.

ecchymosis A discharge or escape of blood; a discoloration of the skin caused by discharge or extravasation of blood.

eclampsia Toxic or poisonous condition usually observed during the last 3 months of pregnancy and characterized by edema or fluid in the tissues, rapid weight gain from the edema, increase in blood pressure, albumin in urine, headache, possible convulsions, and other symptoms.

ectopic Out of the normal place.

edema Increase of tissue fluid in the tissue space; often noticed in the face, hands, fingers, abdomen, ankles, and feet.

efferent Carrying blood or secretion away from a part; carrying impulses away from a nerve center.

effusion Escape of fluid into a part or tissue.

    pleural Presence of fluid in the pleural space or area occupied by the lungs.

electrocardiogram Graphic tracing of the heart action produced by electrocardiography.

electrocardiography Recording of the electric currents in the heart through leads placed on various parts of the body.

electroencephalogram Recording made of the electric currents developed in the cortex by brain activity.

electrolytes Solution that is a conductor of electricity; acids and salts are common electrolytes.

embolism Condition of plugging of an artery or vein by a clot or obstruction that has been brought to its place by the blood current.

embolus Clot or other plug brought by the blood current from a distant vessel and forced into a smaller one, obstructing the circulation.

embryoma A tumor containing embryonic elements or those derived from a rudimentary retained twin parasite.

emetic Substance that causes vomiting, such as mustard and water or the drug apomorphine.

emphysema Presence of air in the alveolar (air sac) tissue of the lungs; distension of the alveoli with air. A few symptoms are exertional dyspnea, prolonged expiratory phase, wheezing, productive cough with difficulty in clearing the bronchi, barrel chest, overuse of accessory muscles of respiration, overaerated lung fields, and flattened diaphragm (only last two indicated in X-rays).

endocarditis Inflammation of the endocardium or epithelial lining membrane of the heart.

bacterial Endocarditis caused by bacterial infection developing as a complication of some infectious diseases.

endometriosis Presence of endometrial tissue in abnormal situations.

internal Occurring in the wall of the uterus or fallopian tube.

external Occurring on the external surface of the uterus, in the ovary, bladder, or intestine, or extraperitoneally.

vesicae Endometriosis involving the bladder.

endometrium Mucous membrane lining of the uterus.

endoscopy Inspection of any cavity of the body, such as the bladder, by means of an endoscope.

endotracheal intubation Insertion of a tube into the larynx through the glottis or into the trachea for the introduction of air; often used during anesthesia to introduce an anesthetic and to keep a proper airway; also used in diphtheria and edema of the glottis to aid breathing.

enhance, enhancing Increasing.

enteric coating Type of coating for tablets and capsules to prevent dissolving until medication reaches intestines, thus preventing stomach juices from destroying certain drugs.

enteritis Inflammation of the intestine, chiefly the small intestine.

enterocolitis Inflammation of the small and the large intestines.

enzymatic Relating to enzyme.

enzyme A chemical ferment formed by living cells. Enzymes are complex organic chemical compounds capable of producing by catalytic action the transformation of some other compound or compounds.

eosinophil Structure, cell, or histologic element readily stained by eosins; particularly an eosinophilic leukocyte or white cell.

eosins Rose-colored stains or dye, the potassium and sodium salts of tetrabromofluorescein. Several other red coal-tar dyes are also called eosins.

epidemic Disease that affects a large group of people in a certain locality at about the same time.

epidermophytosis Fungus infection of the skin.

epigastric Pertaining to the epigastrium.

epigastrium The upper middle portion of the abdomen over or in front of the stomach.

epilepsy Nervous system disease with convulsive seizures.

grand mal Epilepsy in which there are severe convulsions and loss of consciousness, or coma; also called *haut mal.*

Jacksonian A form of epilepsy marked by localized spasm, mainly limited to one side and often to one group of muscles.

petit mal Epilepsy with no decided period of unconsciousness and no obvious spasm or only a slight one.

epistaxis Nosebleed; hemorrhage from the nose.

epithelium Covering of the skin and mucous membranes consisting wholly of cells of varying form and arrangement. The four principal varieties, named according to the shape of the cells, are modified, specialized, columnar, and squamous.

eructate The act of belching; casting up wind from the stomach.

erythema Morbid redness of the skin of many varieties caused by congestion of the capillaries; rose rash.

erythroblastosis fetalis A disease of early infancy showing marked disturbance in the formation of blood.

erythrocytes Red blood corpuscles, circular biconcave disks containing hemoglobin, that carry the oxygen of the blood. Normal red blood cell count (RBC) is 4½ to 5 million/cu ml of blood.

erythrocytosis Increase in the number of red blood corpuscles in the circulation.

eschar A slough produced by burning or by a corrosive application.

esophagitis Inflammation of the esophagus or gullet, which is a musculomembranous canal extending from the pharynx to the stomach.

esterase An enzyme that splits esters.

estrogen Genetic term for many compounds having estrogenic activity; producing effects similar to estrin; a female sex hormone.

eunuch Man or boy deprived of the testes or external genital organs.

eunuchism Condition of a castrated male.

eunuchoidism A defective state of the testicles or of the testicular secretion, with impaired sexual power and eunuch-like symptoms.

euphoria Bodily comfort; well-being; absence of pain or distress.

Ewing's tumor (endothelial myeloma) A form of bone sarcoma that usually involves widening the shaft of long bones by spreading the lamellae apart.

exacerbation Increase in the severity of any symptoms or disease.

excitation Act of irritation or stimulation; a condition of being excited.

excreta Waste matter discharged from the body, particularly fecal matter.

exfoliative dermatitis Inflammation of the skin characterized by a falling off of scales or skin layers and resembling pityriasis rubra, a skin disease.

exophthalmic, exophthalmos Protruding of the eyeballs, sometimes caused by pressure of a goiter on the vessels in the neck leading to the face.

expectorant Medication used to increase secretion and aid in expelling mucus from the respiratory tract or to modify such secretions.

extravasation Discharge or escape, as of blood, from a vessel into the tissues.

fenestration The act of perforating, or the condition of being perforated with openings.

fibrillation Condition in which the groups of muscle fibers of the heart do not contract in unison, causing a rapid and irregular pulse.

fibrin Whitish, insoluble protein formed from fibrigen by the action of thrombin (fibrin ferment), as in the clotting of blood. Fibrin forms the essential portion of the blood clot.

fibrinogen Soluble protein in the blood plasma that is converted into fibrin by the action of thrombin (fibrin ferment), thus producing clotting of the blood.

fibromyositis Inflammation of fibromuscular tissue.

fibrositis Inflammation of muscle fibers.

fimbriae Fringe-like, finger-like tissue projections at the ends of the fallopian tubes of the female reproductive system.

fissure

abnormal Cleft-shaped sore.

normal Groove or cleft, such as one of the fissures of the brain.

flatulence Distension of the stomach or intestines with air or gases.

flexion The act of bending or condition of being bent.

follicle A very small excretory or secretory sac or gland.

graafian Any one of the small spherical vesicular sacs embedded in the cortex of the ovary, each of which contains an egg cell, or ovum. Each follicle contains a liquid supplied with the hormone folliculin, or estrin.

frostbite Condition produced by the freezing of a part, such as fingers, toes, or feet.

fulminant, fulminating Sudden; severe; coming on suddenly with intense severity.

fungus Plant organism characterized chiefly by the absence of chlorophyll.

galactorrhea Excessive or spontaneous secretion of milk.

gallbladder Muscular sac that contains bile; located under the right lobe of the liver.

ganglia Plural of ganglion; any collection or mass of nerve cells that serves as a center of nervous influence.

gangrene Necrosis of tissue combined with invasion by saprophytic organisms.

gastrectomy Removal of the stomach or a portion of it.

gastritis Inflammation of the stomach.

gastroenteritis Inflammation of the stomach and the intestines.

gastrointestinal Pertaining to the stomach and the intestines.

gastroparesis A mild form of paralysis of the stomach. Reversible to some extent.

genetic Congenital or inherited.

geriatrics That branch of medicine that treats the diseases of old age.

gestation Pregnancy; gravidity.

glaucoma A disease of the eye marked by intense intraocular pressure, resulting in hardness of the eye, atrophy of the retina, cupping of the optic disk, and blindness.

globulin Protein substance similar to albumin; examples include cell globulin, fibrinogen, lactoglobulin, and serum globulin.

glomerulonephritis Inflammation of the glomeruli of the kidney.

glomerulus Tuft or cluster; a coil of blood vessels projecting into the expanded end or capsule of each of the uriniferous tubules (channels for the passage of urine).

glossitis Inflammation of the tongue.

gluteus, gluteal Muscles of the buttock commonly used as sites for intramuscular injection of medications.

glycosuria Sugar in the urine.

goiter Enlargement of the thyroid gland, located in the neck.

exophthalmic Enlargement of the thyroid gland, with such symptoms as rapid pulse, sweating, nervousness, muscular tremors, psychic disturbance, emaciation, and increased basal metabolism.

gonads Sex glands; testes in male, ovaries in the female.

gonioscope A kind of ophthalmoscope for examining the angle of the anterior chamber of the eye and for demonstrating ocular motility and rotation.

gonioscopy An examination of the eye with a gonioscope. See *gonioscope.*

gonorrhea Venereal disease of the mucous membrane of the genitalia; can affect the mucous membrane of the eyes.

gout A metabolic disease in which purine substances are deposited in the body, with excess uric acid in the blood, chalky deposits in the cartilages of body joints, and acute arthritis. Characteristic symptoms are acute pain, tenderness, and swelling in body joints, such as in the large toe, ankle, instep, knee, and elbow; elevation of uric acid in the blood; and formation of uric-acid or urate deposits in the cartilage of various parts of the body. These tophi ("chalk stone" or calcareous matter) increase in size and are most often seen along the edge of the ear.

graafian follicle See *follicle, graafian.*

gram-negative Bacteria or tissues that lose the stain or become decolorized by alcohol in Gram's method of staining.

gram-positive Bacteria or tissues that retain the stain in Gram's method of staining.

granulocytes Cells containing granules.

granulocytopenia Abnormal reduction of granulocytes or white blood cells in the blood. See *agranulocytosis.*

Graves' disease See *goiter, exophthalmic.*

gravid Pregnant; with child; containing a fetus.

gripes, gripping Severe and often spasmodic pain in the bowel.

hallucination A sense perception not founded on an objective reality.

hay fever Acute seasonal disease usually caused by an allergy to pollen with characteristic symptoms similar to those of a cold.

heart failure Failure of the heart to work as a pump; characteristic symptoms are fluid in the lungs, ankles, and abdomen.

hemagglutinin Substance that causes agglutination or clumping of red blood corpuscles.

hematocrit Centrifuge for separating corpuscles from plasma or serum of blood.

hematoma Tumor containing effused (spread out, profuse) blood.

hematopoietic Pertaining to or concerned with the formation of blood.

hematuria Discharge of bloody urine.

hemiplegia Loss of function and movement of one side of the body with paralysis.

hemodialysis Installation of an arterial-venal shunt that is connected to the dialyzing machine; the blood is pumped through the dialyzing fluid with a partially porous (semipermeable) plastic membrane to protect the cells. Dialysis is usually performed three times a week for 8 hours each time, but this may vary. It is extremely expensive but lifesaving in chronic renal failure (chronic uremia).

hemoglobin Iron content of the red blood cell.

hemoglobinuria The presence of hemoglobin in the urine resulting from destruction of the blood corpuscles in the vessels or in the urinary passages.

hemolysis Separation of the hemoglobin from the corpuscles and its appearance in the fluid in which the corpuscles are suspended. A few common causes include hemolysins, chemicals, freezing, heating, and placing in distilled water.

hemolytic Causing hemolysis.

hemoperitoneum The presence of extravasated (discharged or escaped) blood into the peritoneal cavity.

hemophilia Congenital condition characterized by delayed clotting of the blood and consequent difficulty in checking hemorrhage; inherited by males through the mother as an x-linked recessive trait.

hemorrhage Massive loss of blood from the body.

hemorrhoids Varicose veins or dilated blood vessels in the anal area.

hemostatic Checking the flow of blood; an agent that arrests the flow of blood.

Henle's loop A U-shaped turn in a uriniferous tubule of the kidney.

hepar Liver.

hepatic Referring to hepar or liver.

hepatitis Infectious inflammation of the liver; a viral infection transmitted by the intestinal-oral route and characterized by symptoms such as anorexia, malaise, nausea, vomiting, fever, enlarged tender liver, jaundice, normal to low white blood cell count, and abnormal hepatocellular liver function tests. The virus is present in the feces and blood during prodromal and acute phases and often in asymptomatic carriers; it may persist for long periods without symptoms after the acute phase. Incubation period is 2 to 6 weeks.

hepatotoxicity Poisoning or toxins destructive to liver cells and originating in the liver.

herpes simplex Skin disease marked by the formation of one or more vesicles on the border of the lip, eye, external nares, or mucous surface of the genitals.

Hg Symbol for mercury; abbreviation for hemoglobin.

hiatus hernia, hiatal hernia Protrusion of any structure through the esophageal hiatus of the diaphragm.

hirsutism Abnormal hairiness, especially in women.

histamine Substance found in the body and in nearly all plant tissues wherever protein is broken down or there is tissue damage.

Hodgkin's disease Characterized by an infectious granulomatous condition (inflammatory enlargement) involving particularly the lymphadenoid tissues of the body. Eosinophils, fibroblasts, giant cells, and frequently *Corynebacterium* organisms, which may be causative agents of the disease, may be found. The glandular enlargement begins at the side of the neck and then extends to the axillary, inguinal, and mediastinal glands and spleen. There is usually a relapsing fever. The disease is called by many names. A few are infectious granuloma, malignant granuloma, malignant lymphoma, lymphadenoma, and lymphosarcoma.

homologous Of similar structure or situation, but not necessarily of similar function.

hormone Chemical product manufactured by some tissue, such as a gland, which is carried by the blood and acts as a messenger to control other tissues, for example, by stimulation or depression, by control of growth sex characteristics, or by effects on the heartbeat.

hydrocholeretics Drugs stimulating the production of bile of a low specific gravity.

hydrogen ion concentration Acidic concentration of hydrogen ions that were formed and given their acid character by acid; has a vital effect on all life processes.

hydrolization, hydrolysis Decomposition resulting from the incorporation of water. The two resulting products divide the water, the hydroxyl group being attached to one and the hydrogen atom to the other.

hydrolyze To subject to hydrolysis.

hydrostatic Pertaining to the pressure exerted by liquids and on liquids; medically, stagnation of fluids.

hydrotropic Chemotropism produced by water; tendency of cells to turn or move in a certain direction under the influence of chemical stimuli.

hyper- A prefix indicating above, beyond, or excessive.

hyperacidity Excessive degree of acidity, often in the stomach.

hyperadrenalism Abnormally increased activity of adrenal gland secretion.

hypercalcemia Abnormally high calcium content in the blood.

hyperchlorhydria Excessive secretion of hydrochloric acid by stomach cells.

hypercholesterolemia Excess of cholesterol in the blood.

hyperflexia, hyperflexion Forcible overflexion or bending of a limb.

hyperglycemia Excess sugar in the blood.

hyperkalemia Abnormally high potassium content in the blood.

hyperoxemia Excessive acidity of the blood.

hyperoxia High oxygen tension in the blood.

hyperplasia Abnormal multiplication or increase in the number of normal cells in normal arrangement in a tissue.

hyperprolactinemia Elevated blood levels of prolactin, the pituitary hormone that causes lactation.

hyperpyrexia A high degree of fever.

hypertension Abnormally high tension, especially high blood pressure.

   benign Essential hypertension that exists for years without producing any symptoms; fluctuating type. Elevation of blood pressure tends to return to normal with rest or sedation.

   essential, primary High blood pressure without previous inflammatory disease of the kidney or urinary tract or any other known cause. A systolic pressure above 150 mm Hg and a diastolic pressure of 100 mm Hg is abnormal at all ages. The upper limit for normal blood pressure, as established by insurance companies, is 140/90 mm Hg.

   malignant Essential hypertension with an acute, stormy onset, development of neuroretinitis, a progressive course, a sustained elevation of blood pressure, and a poor prognosis.

   secondary Elevation of the blood pressure for which the cause is known, such as endocrine, cardiovascular, renal, or neural origin.

hypertensive encephalopathy A complex of cerebral symptoms, including headache, convulsions, and coma, occurring in the course of glomerulonephritis.

hyperthyroid Abnormal condition caused by overactivity of the thyroid gland.

hypertonic Excessive tone, tension, or activity.

hypertrophic, hypertrophy Morbid enlargement or overgrowth of an organ or part.

hypertrophic gastritis Enlargement and inflammation of the stomach.

hyperuricemia Excess of uric acid in the blood.

hyperventilation Abnormally prolonged and deep breathing.

hypnotic Any agent that will produce sleep.

hypo- A prefix denoting a lack or deficiency; also a position under or beneath.

hypocalcemia Reduction of blood calcium below normal.

hypochloremic Pertaining to or characterized by lowered chloride content of the blood.

hypochlorhydria Too small a proportion of hydrochloric acid in the gastric juice.

hypodermic Any method that employs the use of a needle and syringe to place medication under the skin.

hypogenitalism Eunuchoid condition caused by defect of the internal secretion of the testicle or the ovary.

hypoglycemia Deficiency of sugar in the blood.

hypogonadism Decrease of the internal secretion of the gonads; eunuchoidism.

hypokalemia Abnormally low potassium content of blood.

hyponatremia Deficiency of sodium in the blood.

hypoparathyroidism Insufficiency of the parathyroid hormone secretion.

hypopituitarism Condition caused by pathologically diminished activity of the hypophysis or pituitary body and marked by excessive deposits of fat and persistence or acquisition of adolescent characteristics.

hypotassemia Deficiency of potassium in the blood.

hypotension Diminished tension, lowered blood pressure.

hypothalamus The ventral subdivision of the diencephalon or forebrain.

hypothermia Abnormally low temperature.

hypothyroidism Underactivity of the thyroid gland in the neck.

hypoventilation Decrease of the air in the lungs below the normal amount.

hypoxia (hypoxemia) Lack of oxygen and deficient oxygenation of the blood.

idiopathic Morbid state of spontaneous origin; neither sympathetic nor traumatic.

idiosyncrasy Peculiar susceptibility to some drug protein or other substance; exaggerated reaction to drugs.

ileitis Inflammation of the ileus, part of the small intestine.

ileostomy The making of an artificial opening into the ileum.

ileum The distal portion of the small intestine, extending from the jejunum to the cecum.

immunization Method of preventing a first or a second attack of a certain disease.

impacted Driven firmly in, closely lodged.

impermeable Not permitting a passage, as for fluid.

impetigo Low-grade skin infection with small pustules.

incipient Beginning to exist; coming into existence.

increase To enlarge, to grow.

infantilism Condition in which the characters of childhood persist in adult life; marked by mental retardation, underdevelopment of the sexual organs, and often dwarfism.

infarct Area of coagulation necrosis in a tissue caused by local anemia resulting from obstruction of circulation to the area.

inhibits Lessens, decreases.

innervation Distribution or supply of nerves to a part; supply of nervous energy or of nerve stimulus sent to a part.

inoculation Topical or subcutaneous (under the skin) application of bacteria into a human being to produce a mild form of a disease for the purpose of creating an immunity to future attacks.

inotropic To turn or influence; affecting the force or energy of muscular contractions.

   negative Weakening the force of muscular action.

   positive Increasing the strength of muscular contraction.

in situ In the natural or normal place.

insomnia Inability to sleep.

insulin Hormone drug used in the treatment of diabetes mellitus; extract of the islands of Langerhans of the pancreas.

intestines The small and large bowels.

intracranial Within the cranium or skull or brain pan.

intramuscular Into or within the muscle.

intraocular Into or within the eye.

intravenous Into or within the vein.

intrinsic Situated on the inside; situated entirely within or pertaining exclusively to a part.

inulin Polysaccharide found in Inula, Dahlia, and other plants that yield levulose on hydrolysis; also a concentration of resinoid from elecampane root; an aromatic and tonic expectorant.

involution A rolling or turning inward; the return of the uterus to its normal size after childbirth; a retrograde change; the reverse of evolution; involutional, pertaining to, due to, or occurring in involution.

   senile The shriveling of an organ in aged people.

ion Atom or group of atoms having a charge of positive (cation) or negative (anion) electricity.

ionization Dissociation of a substance in solution into its constituent ions.

ionize To separate into ions.

iris Circular pigmented membrane behind the cornea of the eye, perforated by the pupil; made up of circular muscular fibers surrounding the pupil and a band of radiating fibers by which the pupil is dilated.

irradiation Treatment by roentgen rays or other forms of radioactivity.

ischemia Local and temporary deficiency of blood, caused chiefly by contraction of a blood vessel.

isotonic Having a uniform tension. Isotonic solutions are those that have the same osmotic pressure.

isotonic salt solution Solution having the same amount of salt substance as the blood (approximately 0.9% sodium chloride).

isotope Either of two substances chemically identical but with differing atomic weights.

isthmus A narrow strip of tissue or a narrow passage connecting two larger parts; of the thyroid, the band or strip of tissue that connects the lobes of the thyroid gland.

jaundice (icterus) Condition characterized by the presence of bilirubin, a red bile pigment, and deposition of the bile pigment in the skin and mucous membranes, with resulting yellow appearance of the skin and yellow whites of the eyes. It may be caused by obstruction in the biliary system, blockage from a stone that obstructs the passage of bile from the liver to the intestines, or impairment of the liver itself, which produces the bile to aid in the digestion of fats.

juxta- Situated near or in the region of, such as juxtaglomerular—near or in the region of a glomerulus.

keratitis Inflammation of the cornea of the eye.

ketoacidosis A condition of metabolism in which abnormal quantities of acetone bodies are present in the body.

kilogram Unit of weight equal to 1,000 g or 2.2 pounds avoirdupois (the ordinary system of weights in the United States).

labyrinthitis Inflammation of the labyrinth or the intercommunicating cavities or canals of the internal ear: cochlea, vestibule, and canals.

laceration Mangled or torn skin or tissue.

lacrimal canaliculi Tear channels or canals of the eye.

lactation The secretion of milk; the period of the secretion of milk; suckling.

laity The nonprofessional segment of the population.

laryngeal Pertaining to the larynx.

laryngitis Inflammation of the larynx.

larynx Musculocartilaginous, box-like structure, lined with mucous membrane, situated at the top of the trachea and below the root of the tongue and the hyoid bone; located in the midline of the neck. It is the organ of the voice, or voice box.

lateral Pertaining to a side.

laxative Drug having the property of overcoming constipation.

lecithin A monoaminomonophosphatide containing fatty acids and found in animal tissues, especially nerve tissue, semen, yolk of egg, and in smaller amounts in bile and blood. Lecithins are said to have the therapeutic properties of phosphorus and have been given in rickets, dyspepsia, neurasthenia, diabetes, anemia, and tuberculosis; lecithins also are said to be antivenomous.

lens A transparent gelatinous mass of fibers situated behind the iris and pupil of the eye and having the function of giving the image on the retina a sharp focus and of converging or scattering the rays of light.

leprosy Chronic infectious disease caused by a specific microbe (Hansen's bacillus) and marked by a very gradual onset, malaise, headache, formation of nodules, ulcerations, deformities, and loss of sensation in affected parts; often called Hansen's disease.

lethargy Condition of drowsiness of mental origin.

leukemia Often fatal disease with a marked increase in the number of leukocytes in the blood, with enlargement and proliferation of the lymphoid tissue of the spleen, bone marrow, and lymphatic glands. A few characteristic symptoms include progressive anemia, internal hemorrhage, and increasing exhaustion.

leukocyte Any colorless, ameboid cell mass, such as a white blood corpuscle, pus corpuscle, lymph corpuscle, or wandering connective tissue cell, consisting of a colorless granular mass of protoplasm having ameboid movements and varying in size. Normal white blood cell count (WBC) is 5,000 to 10,000/cu ml of blood.

leukocytosis Increase in the number of leukocytes in the blood, generally caused by the presence of infection.

leukopenia Reduction in the number of leukocytes in the blood to 5,000/cu ml of blood or less.

lipids Any one of a group of substances that include the fats and the esters having corresponding properties. The American usage of the term includes fatty acids and soaps, neutral fats, waxes, sterols, and phosphatides. Lipids have a greasy feel.

liver Largest gland of the body, located in the right upper part of the abdomen. It has many functions, including formation and secretion of bile to aid in fat digestion, storage of sugar in the form of glycogen, formation of vitamin A from carotene, and storage of vitamins A and D_2. As a drug it is produced in many forms and has lifesaving properties for many types of anemia.

local Limited to, or pertaining to, one part or spot.

lumen Transverse section of the clear space within a tube; an opening.

lupus erythematosus Chronic, nontuberculous disease of the skin marked by disk-like patches with raised reddish edges and depressed centers and covered with scales or crusts that fall off, leaving off-white scars.

lymphangitis Inflammation of a lymphatic vessel or vessels.

lymphatic system System of vessels carrying lymph (a transparent, slightly yellow liquid, alkaline in reaction) to parts of the body.

lymphocyte Variety of white blood corpuscle with a single nucleus and increased cytoplasm. These corpuscles arise in the reticular tissue of the lymph glands and lymph nodes.

lymphocytic Pertaining to lymphocytes.

lymphoma Any tumor made up of lymphoid tissue.

lymphopenia Decrease in the proportion of lymphocytes in the blood.

lymphosarcoma Malignant neoplasm arising in lymphatic tissue from proliferation of atypical lymphocytes.

lysozyme A mucolytic lubrication for eyelid movements.

macrocytic Condition referring to abnormally large erythrocytes, or red blood corpuscles.

malabsorption Disorder of normal nutritive absorption; disordered anabolism.

malaise Feeling of ill-being; not feeling well.

malignant Virulent; tending to go from bad to worse; progressive.

manic-depressive Insanity in which mania and melancholia alternate.

meconium The fecal matter of the newborn; it consists of a green, sticky substance containing mucus, bile, and epithelial threads.

medulla oblongata Cone of nervous tissue continuous above with the pons of the brain and below with the spinal cord, lying ventral to the cerebellum and forming the floor of the fourth ventricle, with its back; continuation of the spinal cord within the cranium.

megaloblast An erythroblast or primitive red blood corpuscle of large size found in the blood of pernicious anemia.

Ménière's syndrome Disease or inflammatory process and congestion of the semicircular canals in the inner ear with symptoms such as pallor, vertigo, nausea, lack of balance, and several ear and eye disturbances.

meninges The three membranes that envelop the brain and spinal cord, including the dura, the pia, and the arachnoid.

meningitis Inflammation of the meninges of the brain.

menopause Cessation of menstruation; often called "the change of life."

menorrhagia Abnormally profuse menstruation.

menstruation Monthly bloody discharge from the uterus.

mesial Situated in the middle; median; toward the middle line of the body or toward the center line of the dental arch.

metabolism Tissue change; the sum of all the physical and chemical processes by which living organized substance is produced and maintained; the transformation by which energy is made available for the uses of the organism.

metastasis The moving or spreading of infection or cell growth from one area to another.

metorrhagia Profuse bleeding from the uterus at times other than during the menstrual period.

microcurie One-millionth of a curie.

microgram One-millionth part of a gram.

migraine Periodic headache, usually on one side, with such severe symptoms as nausea, vomiting, and light sensitivity.

millicurie One-thousandth of a curie, which is a unit of radiation energy.

milliequivalent One-thousandth of an equivalent combining weight of an atom or ion; an equivalent combining weight, as the weight of an element (in grams) that will combine with 1.008 g of hydrogen.

miosis Excessive contraction of the pupil of the eye.

miotic, myotic Drug that causes the pupil to contract, such as morphine, nicotine, physostigmine, and pilocarpine.

mittelschmerz Intermenstrual pain occurring about halfway through the menstrual cycle, generally during ovulation.

molecule Very small mass of matter; a gathering together or clumping of atoms.

motion sickness Nausea, dizziness, and often vomiting caused by motion of the body when riding in a ship, airplane, automobile, or train.

multipara A woman who has borne several children.

multiple myeloma Tumor composed of cells of the type normally found in the bone marrow; a primary malignant tumor of bone marrow marked by circumscribed or diffuse, tumor-like hyperplasia (abnormal multiplication or increase in number of normal cells in normal arrangement in a tissue) of the bone marrow. It is usually associated with anemia and with Bence Jones protein in the urine. Neuralgic pains and painful swellings on the ribs and skull occur, along with spontaneous fractures.

multiple sclerosis Nervous system disease characterized by scarring of brain and spinal cord that occurs in scattered patches. Patient shows progressive weakness, paralysis, muscle contraction, and muscle cramps. The cause is unknown and the treatment limited.

multisynaptic See *synapse.*

myalgia Pain in a muscle or muscles.

myasthenia gravis Disease characterized by an abnormal weakness of muscles.

mycosis fungoides Fatal fungus skin disease marked by the development of firm, reddish tumors on the scalp, face, and chest that are painful and have a tendency to spread and ulcerate. The disease may last several years.

mydriasis Extreme or morbid dilation of the pupil of the eye.

mydriatic Drug that dilates the pupil of the eye, such as atropine, homatropine, cocaine, phenacaine, hyoscyamine, and ephedrine.

myelin The fat-like substance forming a sheath around the medullated (myelinated) nerve fibers.

myocardium Heart muscle; myocardial infarct; a blockage or clot in the heart muscle.

myoma Any tumor made up of muscular elements; if they are striated, it is a rhabdomyoma, if not, it is a leiomyoma.

myositis Inflammation of muscle.

myxedema Hypothyroid condition causing an edema of tissues, loss of hair, and physical and mental sluggishness in adults.

narcotic Drug that produces sleep or stupor and relieves pain.

nausea Inclination to vomit.

nebulae Very small droplets of water or oil, usually sprayed from an atomizer.

necrosis Death of a circumscribed portion of tissue.

neoplasm Any new and abnormal formation, such as a tumor.

nephritis Inflammation of the kidney.

nephrons Multifunctional units; the renal unit consists of Bowman's capsule, the globular upper end of the tubule, and the tubule, which is concerned with kidney circulation.

nephropathy Disease of the kidneys.

nephrosis Degenerative changes in the kidney without inflammation.

nephrotoxic Toxic or destructive to the kidneys.

neuralgia Nerve pain.

neuritis Inflammation of a nerve, or nerves, with pain.

neuroblastomas Malignant tumors of the nervous system composed chiefly of neuroblasts.

neuroblasts Any embryonic cell that develops into a nerve cell or neuron; an immature nerve cell.

neurogenic Forming nervous tissue, or stimulating nervous energy; originating in the nervous system.

nocturnal Pertaining to, occurring at, or active at night.

node Swelling or protuberance.

    auriculoventricular Remnant of primitive fibers found in all mammalian hearts at the base of the intraauricular septum (separation or partition) and forming the beginning of the bundle of His.

normotensive Characterized by blood pressure within the normal range.

nucleic acid Acid obtained from nuclein, a decomposition product of nucleoprotein.

occlusion Act of closure or state of being closed.

occlusive Effecting a complete occlusion or closure.

occult Obscure, difficult to be observed, hidden.

oculogyric crisis A painful spasm of the eye muscles.

Ocusert A method of administration of eye drops over a continuous, extended period.

oligomenorrhea Scanty or infrequent menstrual flow.

oliguria Deficient secretion of urine.

ophthalmic Pertaining to the eye.

optic Of or pertaining to the eye.

orthopnea Inability to breathe except when sitting up.

orthostatic hypotension Blood pressure lower than normal when the individual is standing or in upright position.

osmosis Passage of pure solvent (liquid used to dissolve) from the lesser to the greater concentration when two solutions are separated by a membrane that selectively prevents the passage of solute (dissolved substance) molecules but that is permeable to the solvent.

osteoarthritis Inflammation of a bony union or joint; it is not as crippling and causes less inflammation than rheumatoid arthritis.

osteomalacia An adult disease marked by increasing softness of the bones so that they become flexible and brittle and attended by rheumatic pains, weakness, and exhaustion, with the patient dying eventually from exhaustion.

osteomyelitis Inflammation of the bone marrow, or bone, or medullary cavity of bone.

osteoporosis Abnormal porousness or loss of density of bone by enlargement of its canals or the formation of abnormal spaces; softening of bone.

otitis media Inflammation of the middle ear.

ototoxicity Poisonous or deleterious to the organs of hearing and balance.

ovary Female sex organ in which ova, or eggs, develop and mature.

palliative Alleviating medicine or treatment offering relief or reducing the severity of pain but not curing the cause.

palpitation Unduly rapid action of the heart felt by the patient.

pancreas Gland of the endocrine system lying behind the stomach and containing the islands of Langerhans, which produce insulin, an internal secretion that reduces the blood and urinary sugar to normal. The pancreas also produces enzymes to aid in the digestion of proteins, carbohydrates, and fats.

pancreatitis Inflammation of the pancreas marked by abdominal pain, pain around the umbilicus or navel, abdominal distension, nausea, and vomiting.

papilla Any small, nipple-shaped elevation.

   optic The optic disk, a round white disk in the fundus oculi medial to the posterior pole of the eyes; corresponds to the entrance of the optic nerve and retinal blood vessels.

papilledema Edema of the optic papilla; a choked disk; optic neuritis caused by intracranial pressure and without inflammatory manifestations.

paralytic ileus Paralysis of the muscular coats of the ileum, a part of the small intestine characterized by possible obstruction of intestinal contents, continuous abdominal pain, distension, vomiting, severe constipation, peritonitis, minimal abdominal tenderness, decreased or absent bowel sounds, history of surgery, and X-ray evidence of gas and fluid in the bowel.

parasympathetic nervous system Part of the autonomic nervous system, including certain nerves whose fibers start from the midbrain, hindbrain, and sacral parts of the spinal cord.

parasympathomimetic drugs Drugs that cause effects in the body similar to those produced by acetylcholine; cholinergic drugs.

parathyroid gland Four small glands, two of which are found on the surface of each lateral lobe of the thyroid. These glands secrete a hormone that regulates calcium-phosphorus metabolism.

parenteral, parenterally Subcutaneous, intramuscular, or intravenous method of administration; treatment by injection.

paresthesia An abnormal sensation, such as burning or prickling.

Parkinson's disease Disease marked by slowing and weakness of voluntary movement, muscular rigidity, and tremor; also known as palsy and paralysis agitans.

paroxysm Sudden recurrence or intensification of symptoms.

patent Wide open.

pathogen Any disease-producing microorganism or material.

pathology The branch of medicine that treats the essential nature of disease, especially the structural and the functional changes caused by disease.

pediculicide Destroying lice; Pediculin is a proprietary remedy for killing lice.

pellagra Endemic skin and spinal disease occurring in southern Europe and southern and central parts of the United States; thought to be caused by deficiency of vitamins B_2 or G, which are found in lean meat, milk, yeast, and other foods. Characteristic symptoms include recurring reddening of the body surface followed by falling off of the skin in layers, along with weakness, debility, digestive disturbances, spinal pain, convulsions, melancholia, and idiocy.

pentagastrin A synthetic peptide that stimulates gastric acid without producing the undesirable side effects of histamine.

peptic ulcer Stomach ulcer.

peptide A compound formed by the union of two or more amino acids. When two amino acids unite, the result is a dipeptide; three form a tripeptide; and more than three form a polypeptide.

perfusion Pouring through or into.

peripheral, periphery Outward part or surface.

   blood vessels Blood vessels near the skin or surface of the body.

   neuropathy Any disease affecting peripheral nerves.

   resistance Ratio of pressure to flow. It is not constant along vessels because of the plastic nature of blood. Resistance is influenced by pressure, viscosity, and vessel lumen size.

peristalsis Worm-like contraction of the muscle tissue of the intestines or certain other organs.

peritoneal cavity Space between the visceral and parietal peritonea.

peritoneum Serous membrane that lines the abdominal walls and invests the contained viscera; holds viscera in place.

   parietal Membrane that lines the abdominal walls, pelvic walls, and undersurface of the diaphragm.

   visceral Membrane reflected at various places over the viscera, forming a complete covering for the stomach, spleen, liver, and many parts of the small and the large intestines.

perlèche Inflammation of the corners of the mouth caused by a yeast-like fungus, *Candida albicans.*

permeability Property or state of being permeable; may be traversed or passed through.

pernicious anemia Chronic disease characterized by a progressive decrease in the number of red corpuscles.

petechiae, petechia Small spots formed by the escape of blood into a part or tissue, as seen in typhus or purpura. See *purpura.*

pH The symbol commonly used in expressing hydrogen ion concentration.

phagocyte Any cell that ingests microorganisms or other cells and substances. The ingested material is often, but not always, digested within the phagocyte. Phagocytes are either fixed, such as endothelial cells, or free, such as leukocytes. The two forms of leukocytes that are phagocytic are the large lymphocyte (macrophage) and the polymorphonuclear leukocyte (microphage). *Polymorphonuclear* means many-shaped nucleus.

pharyngitis Inflammation of the pharynx.

pharynx Tube-shaped passage or musculomembranous sac between the mouth and nares and the esophagus. It is continuous below with the esophagus and above it communicates with the larynx, mouth, nasal passages, and eustachian tubes. It is a passage for both air and food.

pheochromocytoma Tumor of the kidney or adrenal gland consisting of chromaffin cells, which secrete epinephrine.

phlebitis Inflammation of a vein, marked by infiltration of the coats of the vein and the formation of a thrombus of coagulated blood.

phobia Any persistent insane dread or fear.

phosphatide, phosphotidate Phospholipid from which choline or colamine has been split off.

phospholipid Lipin containing phosphorus that yields fatty acids and glycerin on hydrolysis. Lecithin is the best-known example.

photophobia Abnormal sensitivity to or intolerance of light.

pituitary gland (or body) Small, bean-shaped body located in a depression of the sphenoid bone in the skull. It is divided into anterior and posterior lobes, each of which gives off several hormones.

placenta Any cake-like mass; the round, flat organ about 1 inch thick and 7 inches in diameter within the uterus that establishes communication between the mother and child by means of the umbilical cord.

placenta previa A condition in which the placenta is implanted in the lower uterine segment, partially or completely covering the cervical outlet.

platelets Oval disks without hemoglobin found in the blood; they are essential for clotting. Platelets, or thrombocytes, may be manufactured in the red bone marrow. There is wide variance in platelet count, but normal count may be 250,000 to 500,000/cu ml of blood.

pleura The serous membrane that invests the lungs, lines the thorax, and is reflected on the diaphragm. There are two pleurae, right and left, entirely shut off from each other. The pleura is moistened with a serous secretion that eases the movements of the lungs in the chest.

pleural effusion A second-stage inflammation

of the pleura in which exudation of copious amounts of serum occurs. The inflamed surfaces of the pleura may become united by adhesions, which are usually permanent. Symptoms include a "stitch" in the side, and a chill followed by a fever, a dry cough, and pain during breathing. As effusion occurs, there is an onset of dyspnea and a lessening of pain. The patient lies on the affected side.

pleurisy A disease marked by inflammation of the pleura, with exudation into its cavity and on its surface.

polarity Fact or condition of having poles; exhibition of opposite effects at two extremities.

polycythemia vera A disease lasting many years and marked by a persistent increase in the red blood corpuscles (polycythemia), resulting from excessive formation of erythroblasts by the bone marrow and characterized by increased viscosity of the blood, enlargement of the spleen, and cyanotic appearance of the patient.

polymer Any member of a series of substances concerned with, derived from, or pertaining to several pigments.

polymorphonuclear Having nuclei of many forms or shapes, as in certain leukocytes.

polysaccharides Group of carbohydrates that contain more than three molecules of simple carbohydrates combined with each other. They comprise dextrins, starches, glycogens, cellulose, gums, inulin, and pectose.

polyuria Excessive secretion and discharge of urine containing increased amounts of solid constituents.

postpartum Period occurring after delivery or childbirth.

potency Power, strength, as of medicines.

potential Existing and ready for action but not yet active.

precordial Pertaining to the precordium, the region over the heart or stomach; the epigastrium and lower part of the thorax.

precursor Something that precedes or goes before.

priapism Abnormal, painful, and continuous erection of the penis due to disease, usually without sexual desire.

prognosis Forecast as to the probable result of a disease attack; the prospect of recovery from a disease gained through the nature and the symptoms of the case.

proliferation, proliferating Reproduction or multiplication of similar forms, especially of cells and morbid cysts.

prostaglandin A series of chemicals that have pressor, vasodilator, and stimulant effects on the intestinal and uterine muscles.

prostate A gland in the male that surrounds the neck of the bladder and the urethra. It consists of a median lobe and two lateral lobes and is made up of glandular matter, the ducts that empty into the prostatic portion of the urethra, and the muscular fibers that encircle the urethra.

prostatectomy Surgical removal of the prostate or a part of it.

prostatic hypertrophy An enlargement of the prostate gland.

protein Any one of a group of nitrogenized compounds, similar to each other, widely distributed in the animal and vegetable kingdoms, and forming the characteristic constituents of the tissues and fluids of the animal body. They are essentially combinations of α-amino acids and their derivatives.

proteinuria The presence of protein in the urine.

prothrombin Fibrin factor in blood plasma that is supposed to be a precursor of thrombin; also called thrombogen and thrombinogen.

proximal Nearer to or on the side toward the body; opposed to distal.

pruritus Intense itching; a symptom of many skin and other diseases.

psoriasis Chronic inflammatory skin disease marked by the formation of scaly red patches on the surface of the body.

psychomotor Pertaining to or causing voluntary movements.

psychoneurosis Borderline disorder of the mind that is not a true insanity, such as hysteria and neurasthenia.

psychosis Disease or disorder of the mind.

pulmonary embolism Blood clot or foreign material that travels through the circulation and finally lodges in a blood vessel of the lungs.

pulmonary wedge pressure A Swan-Ganz catheter or a special, pliable, multiple-lumen, balloon-tipped catheter is inserted by a highly skilled physician under sterile technique into the subclavian, jugular, or femoral vein and on through the vena cava, the right atrium, and the right ventricle to the pulmonary artery. The large or major lumen of the catheter terminates at the catheter tip and measures pulmonary artery pressure. The small lumen terminates in a latex balloon that can be inflated to surround, but not occlude, the tip of the catheter. When the balloon is inflated and wedged against the pulmonary artery, it continuously measures pulmonary pressure and transmits the measurements to an oscilloscope at the bedside. This procedure is used in congestive heart failure, in myocardial infarction, in measuring left heart pressures and function, and in many other conditions. It is a lifesaving procedure.

pulse pressure See *blood pressure*.

pulvule Proprietary capsule containing a dose of a powdered drug.

pupil Opening in the center of the iris of the eye for the passage of light rays to the retina.

purgative Strong medication administered by mouth to produce bowel evacuation or several movements of the bowels.

purpura Disease characterized by the formation of purple patches on the skin and mucous membranes, caused by the escape of blood into a part or tissue.

purulent Consisting of or containing pus.

pyelitis Inflammation of the pelvis of the kidney; it may be caused by a renal stone, extension of inflammation from the bladder, or stagnation of urine. Symptoms include pain and tenderness in the loins, irritability of the bladder, remittent fever, blood or purulent urine, diarrhea, vomiting, and peculiar pain on flexion of the thigh.

pyelonephritis Inflammation of the kidney and its pelvis.

pyloric spasm Contraction of the pylorus or pyloric sphincter caused by muscle spasm; this will not allow the pylorus to relax and the stomach to empty.

pylorus Gate to the outlet of the stomach; a ring-like band of muscle tissue between the opening of the stomach and the duodenum, or the first part of small intestine.

pyrogen A fever-producing substance.

pyrogenic Inducing fever, also caused by or resulting from fever.

rabies (or hydrophobia, fear of water) Filtrable infectious disease of certain animals, especially dogs, wolves, and squirrels; communicated to man by direct inoculation from the bite of the infected animal—the virus is in the saliva. Incubation period is 1 to 6 months. Symptoms include malaise, depression of spirits, swelling of lymphatics in the region of the wound, choking, spasmodic breathing, and increasing tetanic muscle spasms, especially of respiratory and swallowing muscles, which are increased by attempts to drink water or even by the sight of water. Fever, mental derangement, vomiting, profuse secretion of a sticky saliva, and albuminuria also occur. Disease is almost 100% fatal within 2 to 5 days after onset of symptoms unless rabies vaccine is administered within a short period after the bite occurs.

Raynaud's disease Disease characterized by disturbances in circulation in the blood vessels of the extremities, with the possibility of gangrene and amputation of a limb.

reflux A backward or return flow.

refractory Not readily yielding to treatment.

regurgitation The casting up of undigested food; a backward flowing of the blood through the left atrioventricular opening resulting from imperfect closure of the mitral valve.

remission Period during which symptoms of a disease are abated or lessened in severity.

renal Pertaining to the kidney.

resection Excision of a part of an organ; excision of the ends of bones and other structures forming a joint.

reticulin Albuminoid substance from the connective fibers of reticular tissue; a net-like tissue.

reticulocyte Young red blood cell showing a reticulum or protoplasmic network construction under vital straining.

retin, retinal The innermost tunic (coat, membrane) and perceptive structure of the eye, formed by the expansion of the optic nerve and covering the back part of the eye as far as the ora serrata (the zigzag anterior edge of the retina); often called the nerve of the sense of sight.

retinoblastoma A tumor arising from retinal germ cells.

retinopathy Disease of the retina of the eye.

rhabdomyoma A tumor (myoma) composed of striated muscular fibers.

rhabdomyosarcoma A combined sarcoma and rhabdomyoma.

rheumatic fever Inflammatory joint disease that usually occurs following a streptococcal infection and that is characterized by fever, malaise, joint inflammation and swelling, and transitory pain in the joints. It is usually recurrent and may damage the heart valves.

rheumatic heart disease Chronic disease of the heart valve or valves caused by rheumatic fever.

rheumatoid arthritis Type of arthritis marked by joint pain, swelling of joints, fever, malaise, and crippling of joints.

rhinitis Inflammation of the mucous membrane of the nose; a cold.

rhinorrhea Free discharge of a thin nasal mucus.

rickets Softness of bones in childhood caused by lack of calcium salts, which results in a slowing of the bone-hardening process; lack of vitamin D is a contributing cause.

rickettsiae (Howard Taylor Ricketts' organism) Group of bacteria-like microorganisms that may be transmitted to humans by lice or other parasites. Some diseases caused by rickettsiae include Brill's disease (a form of typhus fever), endemic typhus fever, epidemic typhus fever, and Rocky Mountain spotted fever.

ringworm Parasitic fungus causing a contagious skin disease marked by ring-shaped colored patches; usually on the scalp but can appear on other parts of the body.

roentgen The international unit of roentgen radiation.

roentgen rays Electromagnetic vibrations of waves of very short wavelengths, set in motion when electrons, moving at high velocity, impinge on certain substances, especially the heavy metals. They are able to penetrate most substances, to affect the photographic plate, to bring about chemical reactions, and to produce changes in living matter. They are used in taking photographs of the human body (roentgenograms) or in visualizing portions of the body (fluoroscopy). They reveal foreign bodies in the human body such as calculi (stones) and bullets, as well as fractures of the bone and the functions of such organs as the heart, stomach, and intestines. They are also used in treating various diseases, such as lupus, cancer, and eczema. Also called X-rays.

rubella German measles; an acute eruption rash and febrile disease not unlike measles. After an incubation period of 1 to 3 weeks, the disease begins with slight fever and catarrhal symptoms, sore throat, pains in the limbs, and the eruption of red papules similar to those appearing in measles but lighter in color, not arranged in crescentic masses, and disappearing without peeling or skin flaking within a week.

rubeola A viral disease or measles, characterized by fever, coryza, cough, conjunctivitis, photophobia, and Koplik's spots; the latter usually appear about 2 days before the rash and last 4 days as tiny "table-salt crystals" on the dull red mucous membranes of the inner aspects of the cheeks and often on the inner conjunctival folds and vaginal mucous membranes. Exposure occurs 14 days before the rash. The rash is brick red, irregular, and maculopapular, with onset 4 days after initial symptoms, appearing on the face first, then on the chest, the extremities, and the back. The rash begins fading on the third day in the order that it appeared. Slight desquamation (peeling and flaking of skin) also occurs.

sacroiliac Referring to the sacrum and the ilium bones of the pelvis.

salivation Process of secreting saliva from the salivary glands in the mouth.

salpinx Fallopian or eustachian tube.

saphenous Veins in the legs.

magna The longest vein in the body, extending from the dorsum of the foot to just below the inguinal ligament, where it opens into the femoral vein.

parva Continues the marginal vein from behind the malleolus (ankle joint) and passes up the back of the leg to the knee joint, where it opens into the popliteal vein.

scabies Communicable skin disease caused by the itch mite and attended with intense itching.

schizoid Resembling schizophrenia; reclusive, unsocial, introspective type of personality.

schizophrenia Dementia praecox; adolescent insanity; the term includes a large range of mental disorders that occur early in life and are marked by melancholia; self-absorption; reclusive, unsocial, introspective, withdrawn type of personality; and general mental weakness.

sciatica Inflammation of the sciatic nerve, usually a neuritis. Symptoms include abnormal burning, prickling sensation (paresthesia) of the thigh and leg, tenderness along the course of the nerve, pain that is usually constant, and sometimes a wasting of the calf muscles. It may recur.

sciatic nerve Long nerve with many branches originating in the sacral plexus (a network or tangle of nerves) and distributing through the skin of muscles in thigh, leg, and foot.

sclera The tough, white supporting tunic of the eyeball, covering it entirely except for the segment covered by the cornea; continuous with the cornea; nontransparent; the white portion of the eye.

scurvy Nutritional disease caused by dietetic errors, marked by weakness, anemia, spongy gums, tendency to mucocutaneous hemorrhage, and hardening of the muscles of the calves and legs. Treatment consists of eating fresh potatoes, scurvy grass, onions, lime juice, other citrus fruits such as oranges and lemons, and vitamin C.

sebaceous gland Any gland secreting sebaceous matter (sebum, or a greasy, lubricating substance); chiefly situated in the corium, or true skin.

sedative Quieting or calming type of drug.

serum Watery fluid of the body, especially the fluid left after removal of solid materials of the blood.

SGOT A laboratory blood test: serum glutamicoxaloacetic transaminase.

smallpox Infectious viral disease marked by a rash that passes through several successive stages.

somatic Pertaining to the body tissues, as opposed to reproductive tissues and as distinguished from the psyche.

sperm Mature male cells found in the semen or testicular secretion.

sphincter Ring-like muscle that closes a natural orifice, for example, the pyloric sphincter or the anal sphincter.

spinal cord Cord-like structure contained in the spinal canal and extending from the foramen magnum to the second lumbar vertebra. It is a center for reflex activity and also functions in the transmission of impulses to and from the higher centers in the brain.

splenic flexure syndrome Discomfort originating from the bend of the colon at the junction of the transverse and descending portions.

spondylitis Inflammation of one or more vertebrae.

sprue Chronic disease of disturbed small intestine function characterized by impaired absorption, particularly of fats, and motor abnormalities. Symptoms include bulky, pale, frothy, foul-smelling, greasy stools; weight loss; vitamin deficiencies; impaired intestinal absorption of glucose, vitamins, and fat; large amounts of free fatty acids and soaps in the stool; sore mouth and raw-looking tongue; gastrointestinal catarrh with periodic diarrhea; and change in liver size. The anemia is treated with oral iron for hypochromic anemia and vitamin B_{12} for macrocytic anemia. Therapeutic diet should be high-calorie, high-protein, low-fat, and gluten-free. Sprue occurs mostly in hot countries and is known as tropical sprue. Nontropical sprue is also called intestinal infantilism. See *celiac disease* and *infantilism.*

sputum Substance sent forth from the bronchial tubes and the mouth containing saliva, mucus, and sometimes pus; phlegm.

squamous cell A flat, scale-like epithelial cell.

stasis Stoppage of the flow of blood in any part of the body.

status asthmaticus State or condition of asthma.

status epilepticus A series of rapidly repeated epileptic convulsions with no periods of consciousness.

steatorrhea Presence of excess fat in the stools. *idiopathic* Intestinal infantilism.

stenosis Narrowing or stricture of a duct or canal.

sterol A monohydroxy alcohol of high molecular weight; one of a class of compounds widely distributed in nature, which, because their solubilities are similar to those of fats, have been classified with the lipins. Cholesterol is the best-known member of the group.

stimulant Type of drug that increases activity and hastens action in the body.

stomatitis Inflammation of the mouth.

stratum A layer or set of layers, as in the epidermis, or outermost and nonvascular layer of the skin.

stria (striae atrophicae) Streak or line on the skin. Many of these are often seen on the abdomen of pregnant women or after childbirth, first as reddish streaks, gradually fading to white. They are permanent and caused by atrophy or stretching of the skin.

stricture The abnormal narrowing of a canal, duct, or passage, either from cicatric contraction or the deposit of abnormal tissue.

stye Inflammation of an oil gland of the eyelid.

subaortic Situated below the aorta or the main blood vessel trunk from which the entire systemic arterial system proceeds.

subcapsular cataract Opacity or cloudiness situated beneath the anterior or posterior capsule of the eye lens.

subcutaneous Beneath the skin or in the tissues.

sublingual Beneath the tongue.

substrate A substratum, or lower stratum; the term is applied to the substance on which a ferment or enzyme acts.

supraclavicular Situated above the clavicle, or collar bone.

sympathectomy Surgical removal of a part of a

sympathetic nerve, especially the superior cervical sympathetic ganglion.

sympathetic nervous system Part of the autonomic nervous system; also known as the vegetative or visceral nervous system because the organs controlled by it function unconsciously.

sympathomimetic Resembling the effects produced by disturbance of the sympathetic nervous system. Sympathomimetic drugs relieve the symptoms.

symptom Any disorder of function, appearance, or sensation that the patient experiences.

synapse Anatomic relation of one nerve cell to another; the point of contact between processes of two adjacent neurons, forming the place where a nervous impulse is transmitted from one neuron to another; also called synaptic junction.

syndrome Set of symptoms that occur together.

synovial fluid Fluid secreted by the synovial membrane and contained in joint cavities.

synovitis Inflammation of the synovial membrane, or the covering around joints.

synthesis The artificial building up of a chemical compound by the union of its elements.

syphilis A contagious venereal disease leading to many structural and cutaneous lesions, resulting from a microorganism, the *spirochete pallida*, or *Treponema pallidum*. It is generally propagated by direct venereal contact or by inheritance. Its primary site is a hard or true chancre, whence it extends by means of the lymphatics to the skin, mucosa, and nearly all the tissues of the body, even to the bones and periosteum (the tough, fibrous membrane surrounding bone).

systolic blood pressure See *blood pressure*.

tachycardia Excessive rapidity in the action of the heart, with usually a pulse rate greater than 130 beats per minute.

tachyphylaxis Rapid immunization from the effects of toxic doses of an extract by previous injection of small doses.

tapeworm Flat, tape-like, segmented parasite sometimes found in the intestines of man.

tenacious Holding fast, thick, sticky, adhesive; for example, mucus and sputum.

tenosynovitis Tendon inflammation.

teratogenic Tending to produce fetal monstrosity.

testes Male gonads; organ in reproduction.

tetanus (lockjaw) Acute infectious disease caused by a toxin related by the *Clostridium tetani* (tetanus bacillus) and characterized by more or less persistent tonic spasm of some of the voluntary muscles. Continuous spasm or steady contraction of a muscle without distinct twitching can occur. Spasm can cause locking of the jaw muscles so jaws cannot open, hence its common name.

tetany Nervous affection characterized by muscle twitching, cramps, muscle pains, and convulsions.

thalamus Mass of gray matter at the base of the brain projecting into and bounding the third ventricle.

thrombin The hypothetical fibrin ferment of the blood; the enzyme, present in clotted but not in circulating blood, that converts fibrinogen into fibrin; also called thrombase, fibrin ferment, and fibrinogen.

thromboangiitis obliterans Form of gangrene attributed to a thromboangiitis occurring generally in the larger arteries and veins of the leg, although it may appear in the upper extremity. Also called Buerger's disease and presenile spontaneous gangrene.

thrombocytes Blood platelets.

thrombocytopenia Decrease in the number of blood platelets; same as thrombopenia.

thrombocytopenic purpura Severe form of purpura, with copious hemorrhages from the mucous membranes, marked lessening of the number of blood platelets, marked loss of nuclear substance of blood platelets, and severe constitutional symptoms.

thrombophlebitis Inflammation of a vein or veins resulting from an infection or clot.

thromboplastin substance existing in the tissue that causes clotting of the blood.

thrombosis Formation or development of a thrombus or clot in a blood vessel and remaining at its point of formation.

thyroid gland Gland of internal secretion found in the neck.

thyrotoxicosis Severe condition resulting from abnormal increase of thyroid activity.

tinea corporis Ringworm of the body.

cruris Ringworm of the groin.

pedis Ringworm of the feet, or athlete's foot.

tinnitus Ringing or singing sound heard in the ears; also a clicking sound in the ear heard in chronic catarrhal otitis media or inflammation of the middle ear.

titer Quantity of a substance required to produce a reaction with a given amount of another substance.

agglutination The highest dilution of a serum that causes clumping of bacteria.

colon The smallest amount of a certain substance that indicates the presence of the colon bacillus under standard conditions.

tone In the circulatory system, the factor responsible for a small blood vessel being stiffer or showing more resistance to stretching than a larger vessel, even though the wall material of both small and large vessels possesses exactly the same mechanical properties.

tonometry The measurement of tension, especially intraocular tension.

topical Pertaining to a particular spot; local; medicine for local application, for example, eye drops.

torticollis Wryneck; a contracted state of the cervical or neck muscles producing twisting of the neck and an unnatural position of the head.

trachea Windpipe; the cartilaginous and membranous tube descending from the larynx to the bronchi.

tracheitis Inflammation of the trachea.

tracheostomy Operative formation of an opening into the trachea (windpipe) through the neck and insertion of a trachea tube to aid breathing.

transient Temporary, passing through or over.

trauma Wound or injury.

trifacial neuralgia Pain in the fifth cranial nerve, a nerve of the face. Pain is very severe, shooting, stabbing, searing, or burning in the area of one or more branches of the nerve. Attack frequency varies from many times a day to several times a month or year. Also known as trigeminal neuralgia or tic douloureux.

trigonum vesicae Triangular area of the interior of the bladder between the opening of the ureters and the orifice of the urethra. Called also trigone of bladder and vesical trigone.

trophic Of or pertaining to nutrition.

tuberculosis Infectious disease caused by the tubercle bacillus and marked by presence of tubercles in the affected tissues; most common site is in the lungs.

typhoid fever Contagious disease marked by fever, diarrhea that is sometimes bloody, and malaise. The typhoid bacillus enters the body with food such as milk, watery vegetables such as lettuce, and drinking water.

typhus fever Rickettsial infectious disease characterized by symptoms such as petechial eruptions, high temperature, chills, backache, headache, and great prostration. See *rickettsia*.

urate Any salt or uric acid. Urates, especially that of sodium, are constituents of urine, blood, and tophi or calcerous concretions (a stone or mass containing lime or calcium).

urea White, crystallizable substance, a double amide or compound of carbonic acid, from the urine, blood, and lymph. It is the chief nitrogenous constituent of the urine and is the final product of the decomposition of proteins in the body. It is the form under which the nitrogen of the body is given off. It is thought to be formed in the liver out of amino acids and other compounds of ammonia.

uremia Toxic condition from abnormal urinary constituents in the blood.

ureter The fibromuscular tube that conveys urine from the kidney to the bladder.

ureterosigmoidostomy The operation of implanting the ureter into the sigmoid flexure.

urethra Canal leading from the bladder to the exterior of the body.

uric acid Crystallizable acid, trioxypurine, from the urine of humans and animals, being one of the products of nuclein metabolism. It forms a large portion of certain calculi, or stones, and in the blood causes morbid symptoms, such as those of gout.

uricosuric drugs Drugs administered to relieve pain in gout and increase elimination of uric acid.

urinary retention Retention of urine in the bladder, often caused by a temporary loss of muscle function.

urolithiasis The formation of urinary calculi or stones; also the diseased condition associated with the presence of urinary calculi or stones.

urologic Pertaining to the urine and urinary tract; the term now includes the male and female genitourinary tract.

uropathy Any pathologic change in the urinary tract.

urticaria Hives.

uterus The womb, or organ for containing and nourishing the infant before birth.

vaccination Inoculation with a vaccine as a disease preventive.

vaccine Substance derived from the growth of bacteria and used to confer immunity against certain diseases.

vaccinia Cowpox; a disease of cattle regarded as a form of smallpox. When given to a person via vaccination, it confers a greater or lesser degree of immunity against smallpox.

vagus nerve Tenth cranial nerve, which originates in an area on the floor of the fourth ventricle, extends by small cords from the side of the medulla oblongata, and distributes to larynx, lungs, heart, esophagus, stomach, and most of the abdominal viscera. *Vagus* is a Latin word meaning "wandering." Also called penumogastric nerve.

varicella Chickenpox; an acute contagious disease, principally of young children, marked by slight fever and an eruption of macular vesicles appearing in crops and sometimes followed by scarring.

vascular Pertaining to or full of vessels, often blood vessels.

vasoconstriction Constriction or decrease in size of blood vessels.

vasodilation Dilation or enlargement of the blood vessels.

ventricle Two lower cavities or chambers of the heart; there are right and left ventricles.

venule A minute vein.

vermicular Worm-like in shape or appearance.

vertigo Dizziness, giddiness; disorder of the equilibrating sense marked by a swimming in the head; a sense of instability of apparent rotary movement of the body or of other objects.

Vincent's infection (trench mouth) Inflammation caused by mixed organisms. It was commonly seen among soldiers in the trenches, hence its name. It can involve the throat, stomach, and intestines and is communicable. Also called Vincent's angina.

viscera Internal organs, especially those of the cavities of the chest and abdomen.

viscosity Quality of being sticky or gummy.

vulva The external part of the organs of generation of the female, including the labia majora, labia minora, mons veneris, clitoris, perineum, and vestibulum vaginae.

vulvovaginitis Inflammation of the vulva and vagina, or of the vulvovaginal glands.

wheal A white or pinkish elevation or ridge on the skin, as in urticaria or after the stroke of a whip.

whiplash Inflammation and muscle spasm of the neck and upper back muscles often caused by violent movement during heavy exercise or automobile accidents; often occurs as the result of a sudden backward and forward whipping movement of the neck.

Wilms' tumor A tumor containing embryonic elements; embryoma of the kidney.

Wilson's disease (progressive lenticular disease or hepatolenticular disease) Rare disease characterized by bilateral degeneration of the corpus striatum (a subcortical mass of gray and white matter in front of the thalamus in each cerebral hemisphere) and cirrhosis of the liver with symptoms such as tremor, spastic contractures, increasing weakness and emaciation, and psychic disturbance. Also called dermatitis exfoliativa.

Index

Page numbers followed by T indicate tables.

Nursing process, 142
anticipated therapeutic outcome statements in, 148
applied to pharmacology, 149
assessment in, 142
collaborative problems in, 147
evaluation in, 149
measurable goal statements in, 147
nursing actions in, 149, 150
nursing diagnosis in, 142
nursing implementation in, 149
nursing interventions in, 149
planning in, 147, 151
priority setting in, 147
Nydrazid for tuberculosis, 487
Nyp-Rho-D, obstetric use of, 517
nystatin, 480T, 524T
Nystex, 480T

O

Obstetrical patient, 495; *see also* Pregnant woman
nursing considerations for, 495
Obstetric agents, 504
Obstetrics, 495
Obstructive airway disease, 307
bronchodilators for
anticholinergic, 309
sympathomimetic, 307
xanthine derivative, 310
corticosteroids for, 311
Ocufen, 445
Ocusert Pilo-20 for glaucoma, 449T
Ocusert Pilo-40 for glaucoma, 449T
Official name of drug, 4
Canadian, 5
ofloxacin, 468T
Ogen, 414T
Ointment(s)
administration of, 122
eye, administration of, 131
nitroglycerin, administration of, 126
omeprazole as gastric acid pump inhibitor, 338
Omnipen, 466T
Oncovin for cancer, 540T
ondansetron as antiemetic, 345T
Operative field, sterile, preparing medications for use in, 92
Ophthaine for eye disorders, 442
Ophthalmia neonatorum, prophylaxis for, 502
Ophthalmic irrigants, 445
Ophthetic for eye disorders, 442T
Ophthochlor for eye disorders, 442T
Opiate agonists for pain, 218
Opiate antagonists for pain, 222
Opiate partial agonists for pain, 221
opium
camphorated tincture of, for diarrhea, 352T
with kaolin and pectin for diarrhea, 352T
Opticrom, 445
OptiPranolol, 452T
Optigene for glaucoma, 451
Optimine as antihistaminic decongestant, 315T
Orasone, 404T
Ora-Testryl, 416T
Oral administration of medications
equipment for, 64
liquid-form, 67
solid-form, 66
Oral contraceptives, 518
Oral hygiene, 332
Oral hypoglycemic agents, 349
Oral syringes for drug administration, 65
Oramide for diabetes, 394T
Oretic as diuretic, 365T
Oreticyl-25 as antihypertensive, 281T
Oreton Methyl, 416T
Orflagen, 184T
Orimune, 428T
Orinase for diabetes, 394T
orphenadrine
as centrally acting muscle relaxants, 322T
for Parkinsonism, 184T
Ortho-Novum 1/35, 520T
Ortho-Novum 1/50, 520T
Ortho-Novum 7/7/7, 520T
Ortho-Novum 10/11, 520T

Orudis for pain, 226T
Osmitrol for eye disorders, 439T
Osmoglyn for eye disorders, 439T
Osmotic agents for eye disorders, 438
Otrivin as nasal decongestant, 313T
Ounce, definition of, 33
Ovaries, 410
Ovcon-35, 520T
Ovcon-50, 520T
Over-the-catheter needle, 81
Ovral, 520T
Ovrette, 415T, 520T
Ovulation, induction of, clomiphene citrate for, 515
Ovulen, 520T
oxacillin, 466T
oxazepam for anxiety, 188T
oxiconazole, 480T
Oxistat, 480T
oxtriphylline as bronchodilator, 308T
oxybutynin chloride for urinary system disorders, 368
oxycodone for pain, 219T
oxymetazoline as nasal decongestant, 313T
oxymorphone for pain, 219T
oxyphencyclimine
as anticholinergic agent, 240T
as antispasmodic, 341T
oxytetracycline, 471T
oxytocin as uterine stimulant, 508

P

Pain, 210
acetaminophen for, 228
analgesic therapy for, patient education on, 216
antiinflammatory agents for, 224
drug therapy for, 218
nursing considerations for, 212
nursing interventions for, 212
opiate agonists for, 218
opiate antagonists for, 222
opiate partial agonists for, 221
propoxyphene for, 229
rating scales, 214
Pamelor, 191T
Pamine as antispasmodic, 341T
pancuronium bromide as neuromuscular blocking agent, 325T
Panmycin, 471T
Panwarfin for anticoagulation, 296
papain as digestant, 342T
papaverine for peripheral vascular disease, 277
Paraflex as centrally acting muscle relaxants, 322T
Paral for insomnia, 173T
paraldehyde for insomnia, 173T
paramethasone, 404T
Paraplatin, 538
Parasympatholytic agents, 239
Paregoric for diarrhea, 352T
Parenteral administration of medications, 77
dosage forms for, 83
equipment for, 77
by intradermal route, 94
by intramuscular route, 99
intravenous administration sets for, 82
by intravenous route, 106
needle for, 80
preparation of medication for, 86
by subcutaneous route, 97
syringes for, 77
Parepectolin for diarrhea, 352T
Parkinson's disease
amantadine hydrochloride for, 178
anticholinergic agents for, 183
bromocriptine mesylate for, 179
carbidopa for, 180
characteristics of, 174
drug therapy for, 178
levodopa for, 180
nursing considerations for, 175
patient concerns in, 175
pergolider for, 181
selegiline for, 181
therapy for, patient education on, 176
Parlodel
as lactation suppressant, 513
for Parkinson's disease, 179